PEDIATRIC ANESTHESIA

JAMES (JAMIE) S. FURSTEIN, PhD, DNAP, CRNA, CPNP-AC, FAANA, received his MSN with a concentration in nurse anesthesia from the University of Cincinnati and DNAP and PhD degrees from Virginia Commonwealth University, one of the top-ranked CRNA programs in the United States. He has worked at Cincinnati Children's Hospital Medical Center for over 20 years and is one of the Associate CRNA Directors in the Department of Anesthesia. His efforts are not limited to the clinical arena, however. As Associate Professor and Assistant Program Director for the Nurse Anesthesia Program at the University of Cincinnati College of Nursing, Dr. Furstein was responsible for the curriculum covering pain, pain management, and regional anesthesia, as well as providing hands-on instruction to students in a simulation environment. Dr. Furstein is currently faculty for the Acute Surgical Pain Management Fellowship at the Middle Tennessee School of Anesthesia, where he is responsible for the didactic content pertaining to pediatric pain management and evidence-based practice. To expand his purview beyond the perioperative arena, Dr. Furstein has practiced as a nurse practitioner on the Pain Team and in the pediatric ICU at Cincinnati Children's Hospital Medical Center. He also remains actively involved in research and is currently the primary investigator for several ongoing clinical trials, with his area of focus being pediatric pain.

PEDIATRIC ANESTHESIA

A Comprehensive Approach to Safe and Effective Care

JAMES S. FURSTEIN, PhD, DNAP, CRNA, CPNP-AC, FAANA

EDITOR

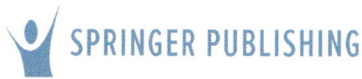
SPRINGER PUBLISHING

Copyright © 2023 Springer Publishing Company, LLC
All rights reserved.

No part of this publication may be reproduced, stored in a retrieval system, or transmitted in any form or by any means, electronic, mechanical, photocopying, recording, or otherwise, without the prior permission of Springer Publishing Company, LLC, or authorization through payment of the appropriate fees to the Copyright Clearance Center, Inc., 222 Rosewood Drive, Danvers, MA 01923, 978-750-8400, fax 978-646-8600, info@copyright.com or on the Web at www.copyright.com.

Springer Publishing Company, LLC
11 West 42nd Street, New York, NY 10036
www.springerpub.com
connect.springerpub.com/

Executive Acquisitions Editor: Joseph Morita
Director, Content Development: Taylor Ball
Compositor: Exeter Premedia Services Private Limited

ISBN: 9780826138743
ebook ISBN: 9780826138750
DOI: 10.1891/9780826138750

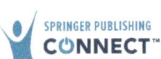 A robust set of instructor resources designed to supplement this text is located at http://connect.springerpub.com/content/book/978-0-8261-3875-0. Qualifying instructors may request access by emailing textbook@springerpub.com.

Instructor's Manual ISBN: 9780826167675
Test Bank ISBN: 9780826167699
PowerPoints ISBN: 9780826167682

22 23 24 25 / 5 4 3 2 1

Medicine is an ever-changing science. Research and clinical experience are continually expanding our knowledge, in particular our understanding of proper treatment and drug therapy. The authors, editors, and publisher have made every effort to ensure that all information in this book is in accordance with the state of knowledge at the time of production of the book. Nevertheless, the authors, editors, and publisher are not responsible for any errors or omissions or for any consequence from application of the information in this book and make no warranty, expressed or implied, with respect to the content of this publication. Every reader should examine carefully the package inserts accompanying each drug and should carefully check whether the dosage schedules therein or the contraindications stated by the manufacturer differ from the statements made in this book. Such examination is particularly important with drugs that are either rarely used or have been newly released on the market.

Library of Congress Cataloging-in-Publication Data

Names: Furstein, James S., editor.
Title: Pediatric anesthesia : a comprehensive approach to safe and
  effective care / edited by James S. Furstein.
Other titles: Pediatric anesthesia (Furstein)
Description: First Springer Publishing edition. | New York, NY : Springer
  Publishing Company, LLC, 2023. | Includes bibliographical references and
  index.
Identifiers: LCCN 2021053876 (print) | LCCN 2021053877 (ebook) | ISBN
  9780826138743 (paperback) | ISBN 9780826138750 (ebook) | ISBN
  9780826167675 (instructor manual) | ISBN 9780826167699 (Test Bank,
  PowerPoints)
Subjects: MESH: Anesthesia--methods | Child | Patient Safety | Infant |
  Nurses Instruction
Classification: LCC RD139 (print) | LCC RD139 (ebook) | NLM WO 440 | DDC
  617.9/6083--dc23/eng/20211124
LC record available at https://lccn.loc.gov/2021053876
LC ebook record available at https://lccn.loc.gov/2021053877

Publisher's Note: **New and used products purchased from third-party sellers are not guaranteed for quality, authenticity, or access to any included digital components.**

Printed in the United States of America by Gasch Printing.

To Dr. Theodore W. "Ted" Striker, a pioneer who was instrumental in defining the field of pediatric anesthesia and who unknowingly influenced generations of pediatric anesthesia providers. Not only was he generous with his vast clinical knowledge, but he also imparted on others the importance of respecting and appreciating all staff. He was genuinely committed to the success of his colleagues and maintained an enduring care for others. As a moral compass and role model to all who knew him, I am forever indebted to Dr. Striker for believing in me and fostering my growth and development as a pediatric anesthesia provider.

CONTENTS

CONTRIBUTORS   XIII
FOREWORD   XXIII
PREFACE   XXV
ACKNOWLEDGMENTS   XXVII
INSTRUCTOR RESOURCES   XXIX

PART I: Foundations of Anesthetic Care

1: Anatomy and Physiology of the Pediatric Patient   2

Nervous System   2
  Mark Blazey

Cardiovascular System   6
  Claire Rizk

Pediatric Airway   11
  Lauren S. Buck, Yann-Fuu Kou, and Matthew M. Smith

Respiratory System   15
  Sarrah L. Schultz and Robert J. Combs

Renal System   21
  Hailey Silverii and Shumyle Alam

Hepatic System   25
  Alison Henry

Thermoregulation   28
  Dawn Elizabeth Bent and Sharifah Wilson

Behavioral and Developmental Milestones   32
  Nicole Garritano

2: Pharmacologic Considerations for the Pediatric Patient   41

Pharmacokinetics and Pharmacodynamics   41
  Chad Watkins and Dennis LaChance

Pharmacologic Agents   49
  Tamara K. Hutson, Andrea Chamberlain, and Trina Devadhar Hemmelgarn

PART II: Perioperative Anesthetic Care

3: Preoperative Evaluation, Testing, and Optimization   76
  Karin J. Detchon and Heather Decker

4: Equipment and Monitoring   82
  Su Chang and Jeanie Skibiski

5: Induction of Anesthesia   95
  Melanie Neal and Carrilee Powell

6: Airway Management   102
  Lauren Irwin, Emily H. Klinefelter, Meaghan O'Meara, and Audrey Rosenblatt

7: Ventilation Management   119
  Saundra L. Smalley

8: Fluids, Electrolytes, and Transfusion Therapy   124
  Christopher A. Allphin, Fernando Franco Cuadrado, and Joseph W. McSoley

9: Temperature Monitoring   133
  Dawn Elizabeth Bent and Sharifah Wilson

10: Postanesthetic Care   140
  Brett J. Morey

PART III: Conditions, Diseases, and Syndromes in Pediatric Patients

SECTION A: Common Conditions and Diseases in Pediatric Patients

11: The Premature Infant   148
  Elise C. Whalen, Jamie Gilley, and Nidhy Paulose Varghese

12: Neurological Conditions   151
  Amanda Ford and Shawn West

13: Ear, Nose, and Throat Conditions   155
  Anita Deshpande, Carol Li, and Charles M. Myer, IV

14: Ophthalmic Conditions   162
  Kathleen Anulao

15: Oral, Maxillofacial, and Dental Conditions   166
  AnnMarie Matusak

16: Endocrine Conditions   172
  James S. Furstein and Aimee Langley

17: Cardiovascular Conditions   180
  Brian J. Gronert, Peace C. Madueme, and Karen S. Bender

18: Gastrointestinal Conditions   204
  Kahleb Graham and Khalil El-Chammas

19: Hematologic Conditions   210
  Marika Highberger, Lindsay Johnson-Bishop, Brandi M. Runnels, and Heather Soni

20: Oncologic-Bone Marrow Transplantation Conditions   217
  Katrina Richardson, Rachael Mohr, and Steffani Maier

21: Genitourinary Conditions 222
   Hailey Silverii and Shumyle Alam

22: Musculoskeletal Conditions 226
   Ramsey S. Sabbagh, Brian M. Grawe, Jagroop M. Parikh, and Shital N. Parikh

SECTION B: Common Syndromes in Pediatric Patients

23: Achondroplasia 229
   Gail Shibata

24: Apert Syndrome 232
   Sarah Milligan

25: Arthrogryposis 233
   Michael Sikora

26: Autism Spectrum Disorder 236
   Amanda Whippey

27: Beckwith–Wiedemann Syndrome 240
   Marianne S. Cosgrove

28: CHARGE Syndrome 243
   Angela Mund

29: Cri du Chat Syndrome 246
   Michael E. Conti

30: Crouzon Syndrome 247
   Kimberly Hunter Olivarez

31: Down Syndrome 250
   Jessica Storey

32: Ehlers–Danlos Syndrome 253
   Michael R. Everhart and Karmella M. Franic-Everhart

33: Epidermolysis Bullosa 255
   Kristen A. Callahan

34: Fetal Alcohol Syndrome 261
   Jennifer McBride Schultz

35: Goldenhar Syndrome 263
   Judy Audas

36: Hurler Syndrome/Hunter Syndrome 266
   Jessica Storey

37: Klippel–Feil Syndrome 269
   Daniel Henz

38: Mitochondrial Myopathy 271
   Leslie Jackson and Matthew McCoy

39: Muscular Dystrophy 273
   Jennifer McBride Schultz

40: Pierre Robin Sequence 275
   Heather J. Rankin, Edgar Soto, and René P. Myers

41: Prader–Willi Syndrome 278
   Aimee Langley

42: Prune Belly Syndrome 280
   Daniel Henz

43: Pulmonary Alveolar Proteinosis 282
   Judy Audas

44: Treacher Collins Syndrome 286
   Marianne S. Cosgrove

45: Tuberous Sclerosis 289
   Brian DeAtley

46: Turner's Syndrome 290
   Judy Audas

47: VACTERL Association 294
   Angela Mund

48: Williams Syndrome 296
   Sean Barclay

PART IV: Common Procedures in Pediatric Anesthetic Care

SECTION A: Neurosurgical Procedures

49: Craniotomy 300
   Jennifer Parks

50: Ventriculoperitoneal Shunt Placement 303
   Amanda Ford

51: Stereotactic Grid Placement 307
   Tiffany Jonasson and Megha Karkera Kanjia

52: Vagal Nerve Stimulator Placement 310
   Kelly Moon

53: Epilepsy Surgery 313
   Jacob Stollard and Whitney Rhoades

54: Dorsal Rhizotomy 320
   Anne M. Que and Meghan Pursley

55: Cranial Vault Reconstruction and Craniosynostosis Repair 322
   Anthony Prickel

56: Myelomeningocele Repair 327
   James S. Furstein and Michael E. Conti

57: Third Ventriculostomy 330
   Anne M. Que

SECTION B: Ear, Nose, and Throat Procedures

58: Myringotomy and Pressure-Equalizing Tubes 333
   Ebone Evans and Andrew Redmann

59: Bone-Anchored Hearing Aid Surgery 335
   Andrew Redmann

60: Tympanoplasty 337
   Andrew Redmann

61: Cochlear Implant Surgery 339
Nicklas Orobello and Andrew Redmann

62: Adenotonsillectomy 342
D. Julie Soelberg

63: Microlaryngoscopy 346
Lauren Freedman

64: Tracheostomy 351
Anita Deshpande and Charles M. Myer, IV

65: Tracheal Resection 354
Carol Li and Charles M. Myer, IV

66: Parotidectomy 358
Michael E. Conti

67: Submandibular Gland Excision 361
Michael E. Conti

68: Septorhinoplasty 362
Alison Henry and Lisa Wahlers

69: Care of Children With Sleep-Disordered Breathing 365
Pornswan Ngamprasertwong and Mario Patino

70: Tongue Base Reduction 369
Hannah Kuhn

71: Drug-Induced Sleep Endoscopy 371
Yann-Fuu Kou, Mohamed A. Mahmoud, and Stacey L. Ishman

SECTION C: Ophthalmic Procedures

72: Ophthalmologic Exam Under Anesthesia 375
Audrey Rosenblatt and Susan P. McMullan

73: Strabismus Repair 376
Priscilla Aguirre and Veronica Y. Amos

74: Nasolacrimal Duct Probing, Irrigation, and Dacryoplasty 379
Audrey Rosenblatt and Susan P. McMullan

75: Retinal Surgery 381
Suzanne M. Wright

76: Ptosis Repair 386
Audrey Rosenblatt and Susan P. McMullan

77: Enucleation 389
Suzanne M. Wright

SECTION D: Oral, Maxillofacial, and Dental Procedures

78: Dental Rehabilitation 393
Corey Southworth and Shannon Zhang

79: Mandibular Distraction 396
Heather J. Rankin, Edgar Soto, and René P. Myers

80: LeFort Osteotomy 401
Terri M. Cahoon and Kris Redden

SECTION E: Plastics Procedures

81: Cleft Lip and Cleft Palate Repair 406
Joshua Lea, Eleanor Mullen, and Julianne Ryan

82: Vascular Malformations 410
Nicole K. Damico and Rajanya S. Petersson

83: Pharyngoplasty 414
D. Julie Soelberg and Tomas Lazo

84: Alveolar Cleft Repair 416
Michele Baker

85: Breast Reduction 418
Nicole K. Damico and Gregory Lynam

86: Microtia Repair 423
Kristen Deveras and Pacifico Tuason

87: Burns 426
Alison Henry and Lisa Wahlers

SECTION F: Endocrine Procedures

88: Thyroidectomy and Parathyroidectomy 432
Tracy Beckham

SECTION G: Cardiovascular Procedures

89: Cardiac Surgery: On-Pump 437
Jamie W. Sinton and Zhe Amy Fang

90: Cardiac Surgery: Off-pump 446
Jamie W. Sinton and Zhe Amy Fang

91: Cardiac Catheterization Laboratory 452
Joanna Rosing Paquin

92: Cardiac Electrophysiology Laboratory Procedures 458
Whitney S. Roberts, M. Leona A. Sayson, and Anne M. Peeke

93: Care of Children With Heart Disease Undergoing Noncardiac Surgery 466
Jamie W. Sinton, Brian J. Gronert, Peace C. Madueme, and Karen S. Bender

SECTION H: General Surgery Procedures

94: Appendectomy 477
Tamra Nicole Kelly

95: Tracheoesophageal Fistula Repair 480
Judith M. Lewis and Ashley J. Austin

96: Hernia Repair 484
Tomas Lazo and Courtney Miller

97: Pectus Excavatum Repair 486
Nicholas Detchon

98: Bowel Resection and Gastrojejunal Tube Placement 491
Caren Bergdahl and Jingjing Sparrow

99: Sleeve Gastrectomy 498
Lisa A. Durako

100: Nissen Fundoplication 502
    Mary J. Scott-Herring and Aileen Mendez

101: Intussusception 504
    Lisa Herbinger and Karen Knight

102: Laparoscopic Surgery 508
    Nathan S. Jones

103: Posterior Sagittal Anorectoplasty 512
    Kimberly Stumpf and Joseph Tobias

104: Pilonidal Cyst 518
    Nathan S. Jones

105: Cholecystectomy 520
    Mary J. Scott-Herring and Aileen Mendez

SECTION I: Gastrointestinal Procedures

106: Endoscopy and Colonoscopy 523
    Ashley J. Austin and Judith M. Lewis

107: Manometry Placement, Esophageal Dilatation, and Botulinum Toxin Injection 526
    Jennifer B. Mills and Jeanie Skibiski

SECTION J: Hematological Procedures

108: Splenectomy 531
    Paula J. Belson

SECTION K: Oncological Procedures

109: Mediastinoscopy and Mediastinal Mass Resection 535
    Barry Swerdlow

110: Lumbar Puncture 539
    Barry Swerdlow

111: Neuroblastoma Resection 543
    Paula J. Belson

SECTION L: Genitourinary Procedures

112: Circumcision 547
    Dawn Elizabeth Bent and Sharifah Wilson

113: Hypospadias Repair 549
    Megan Gdowski, Renee Pederson, and Audrey Rosenblatt

114: Orchidopexy 555
    Heena Pranav and Megha Kanjia

115: Cystoscopy 558
    Dusty C. Pourciau

116: Urolithiasis 560
    Angela Milosh and Sarah Milligan

117: Pyeloplasty 562
    Sarah Milligan and Angela Milosh

118: Lower Urinary Tract Reconstruction 564
    Heather J. Rankin, David B. Joseph, and Ching Man Carmen Tong

SECTION M: Orthopedic Procedures

119: Spinal Fusion 570
    Jason Perry, Abigail Monnig, and Ramsey S. Sabbagh

120: Knee Ligament Reconstruction 578
    Eric Wall and James S. Furstein

121: Mehta Cast Application 581
    Aaron Sundberg

122: Shoulder Surgery 584
    Ramsey S. Sabbagh, James S. Furstein, and Shital N. Parikh

123: Fasciotomy 587
    Carrilee Powell and Ramsey S. Sabbagh

124: Slipped Capital Femoral Epiphysis Surgery 590
    Carrilee Powell

125: Pediatric Amputation 593
    Motaz Awad, Soroush Merchant, Alexandra Szabova, and Kenneth R. Goldschneider

PART V: Special Topics in Pediatric Anesthetic Care

126: Malignant Hyperthermia 598
    Dorothea L. Connolly and Jennifer Raynor

127: Neonatal Emergencies 604
    Carrilee Powell and Vera Winograd-Gomez

128: Trauma 616
    Timothy P. Grannell and Kelly Moon

129: Transplant Surgery 625

   Cardiac Transplantation 625
    Jamie W. Sinton and Zhe Amy Fang

   Liver Transplantation 626
    Lori A. Aronson, Niekoo Abbasian, and Ximena Soler

   Kidney Transplantation 629
    Amanda Ford and Jaclyn Ashline

   Total Pancreatectomy and Islet Autotransplantation 631
    Sean Barclay and Carrilee Powell

130: Fetal Surgery 636

   Minimally Invasive Fetal Surgery 636
    Jagroop Parikh and Mario Patino

   Ex Utero Intrapartum Therapy Procedures 638
    Jagroop Parikh and Mario Patino

131: Pediatric Pain Management 643

   Regional Anesthesia 643
    James S. Furstein, Nancy B. Samol, David L. Moore, and Marc Mecoli

   Patient-Controlled Analgesia Use in Pediatrics 648
    Daniela Herrera

Opioid-Free Anesthesia 650
Tyler A. C. Davis-Sandfoss and Andrew K. Davis-Sandfoss

Anxiety and Anxiolysis 654
David L. Moore

132: Enhanced Recovery After Surgery 658
Marc Mecoli

133: Operative and Anesthetic Care of the Patient With Chronic Pain 662
Soroush Merchant, Motaz Awad, Alexandra Szabova, and Kenneth R. Goldschneider

134: Palliative Care 665
Mark John Meyer and Lori Ann McKenna

135: Procedures in Radiology 668
Christopher A. Allphin and Ali I. Kandil

136: Ultrasound-Guided Vascular Access 675
Nathan Fagan and Manish N. Patel

137: Ethical Considerations in Pediatric Anesthesia 680
Megha Karkera Kanjia and Julie Schackman

138: Quality Improvement and Safety in Pediatric Anesthesia 684
Megha Karkera Kanjia

Appendix A: Common Adjunct Medication Dosing 689

Appendix B: Age-Based Parameters 693

Appendix C: Antibiotic Prophylaxis 695

Appendix D: Case Plan Template 701

INDEX 703

CONTRIBUTORS

Niekoo Abbasian, MD
Assistant Professor of Clinical Anesthesia
Department of Anesthesia
University of Cincinnati College of Medicine
Cincinnati Children's Hospital Medical Center
Cincinnati, Ohio

Priscilla Aguirre, DNP, CRNA
University of Maryland School of Nursing
Nurse Anesthesia Specialty
Baltimore, Maryland

Shumyle Alam, MD
Professor of Urology
College of Medicine
Medical University of South Carolina
Charleston, South Carolina

Christopher A. Allphin, DO
Assistant Professor of Clinical Anesthesia
Department of Anesthesia
University of Cincinnati College of Medicine
Cincinnati Children's Hospital and Medical Center
Cincinnati, Ohio

Veronica Y. Amos, PhD, CRNA, PHCNS-BC
University of Maryland School of Nursing
Nurse Anesthesia Program
Baltimore, Maryland

Kathleen Anulao, BSN, MSN, FNP, APRN, BC, RNFA
Department of Surgery
The Vision Center
Children's Hospital Los Angeles
Los Angeles, California

Lori A. Aronson, MD
Associate Professor of Clinical Anesthesia and Pediatrics
Department of Anesthesia
Director Liver Transplant Anesthesia
University of Cincinnati College of Medicine
Cincinnati Children's Hospital Medical Center
Cincinnati, Ohio

Jaclyn Ashline, MSN, CRNA
Staff CRNA
UPMC Children's Hospital of Pittsburgh
Pittsburgh, Pennsylvania

Judy Audas, DNAP, APRN-CRNA, MSN
Department of Anesthesia
Cincinnati Children's Hospital Medical Center
Cincinnati, Ohio
Program Director, Nurse Anesthesia Program
Northern Kentucky University
Highland Heights, Kentucky

Ashley J. Austin, DNP, APRN, CRNA
Cleveland Clinic Children's Hospital
Case Western Reserve University
Frances Payne Bolton School of Nursing
Cleveland, Ohio

Motaz Awad, MD
Assistant Professor of Anesthesiology
University of Kentucky
Kentucky Children's Hospital
Lexington, Kentucky

Michele Baker, CRNA, MSN
Department of Anesthesia
Norton Children's Hospital
Louisville, Kentucky

Sean Barclay, MSN, CRNA
Department of Anesthesia
Cincinnati Children's Hospital Medical Center
Cincinnati, Ohio

Tracy Beckham, CRNA, DNAP
Assistant Director of School of Anesthesia
Missouri State University
Springfield, Missouri

Paula J. Belson, PhD, MS, CRNA
CRNA Manager, Anesthesiology and Critical Care Medicine
Children's Hospital Los Angeles
Adjunct Clinical Instructor, Anesthesiology
Keck School of Medicine
Los Angeles, California

Karen S. Bender, MD, FAAP
Chief, Division of Cardiac Anesthesiology
Department of Cardiovascular Services
Nemours Children's Hospital
Assistant Professor
University of Central Florida College of Medicine
Orlando, Florida

Dawn Elizabeth Bent, DNP, MSN, CRNA
Program Administrator, Nurse Anesthesia Program
Lecturer N
University of Pennsylvania
Department of Pediatric Anesthesiology
St. Christopher's Hospital for Children
Philadelphia, Pennsylvania

Caren Bergdahl, DNP, CRNA
Instructor, Texas Children's Hospital
Department of Anesthesiology, Perioperative and Pain Medicine
Baylor College of Medicine
Houston, Texas

Mark Blazey, DNP, CRNA
Niagara Frontier Anesthesia
Rochester, New York

Lauren S. Buck, MD
Division of Pediatric Otolaryngology–Head and
   Neck Surgery
Cincinnati Children's Hospital Medical Center
Cincinnati, Ohio

Terri M. Cahoon, DNP, CRNA
Samford University
Birmingham, Alabama

Kristen A. Callahan, MS, CRNA
Department of Anesthesia
Cincinnati Children's Hospital Medical Center
Cincinnati, Ohio

Andrea Chamberlain, PharmD, BCPS, BCPPS
Division of Pharmacy
Cincinnati Children's Hospital Medical Center
Cincinnati, Ohio

Su Chang, DNAP, CRNA
Division of Cardiac Anesthesiology
Department of Cardiovascular Services
Nemours Children's Hospital
Assistant Professor, University of Central Florida College of
   Medicine
Orlando, Florida

Robert J. Combs
Department of Pulmonary Medicine
Cincinnati Children's Hospital Medical Center
Cincinnati, Ohio

Dorothea L. Connolly, MSN, CRNA, APN
Children's Hospital of Philadelphia
Philadelphia, Pennsylvania

Michael E. Conti, PhD, CRNA
Chief Nurse Anesthetist
Johns Hopkins All Children's Hospital
St. Petersburg, Florida

Marianne S. Cosgrove, PhD, DNAP, CRNA, APRN
Program Director
Yale-New Haven Hospital School of Nurse Anesthesia
Staff Affiliate
Yale-New Haven Hospital
New Haven, Connecticut

Fernando Franco Cuadrado, MD
Assistant Professor of Clinical Anesthesia
University of Cincinnati College of Medicine
Department of Anesthesia
Cincinnati Children's Hospital and Medical Center
Cincinnati, Ohio

Nicole K. Damico, PhD., CRNA, FAANA
Herbert T. Watson Endowed Professor
Chair and Associate Professor
Department of Nurse Anesthesia
College of Health Professions
Virginia Commonwealth University
Richmond, Virginia

Andrew K. Davis-Sandfoss, MD
Feinberg School of Medicine
McGaw Medical Center
Northwestern University
Chicago, Illinois

Tyler A.C. Davis-Sandfoss, DNP, CRNA
Ann & Robert H. Lurie Children's Hospital of Chicago
Chicago, Illinois

Brian DeAtley, DNP, CRNA
Department of Anesthesia
Cincinnati Children's Hospital
Cincinnati, Ohio

Heather Decker, DNP, ARNP, PPCNP-BC
Pediatric Nurse Practitioner
Department of Anesthesia
Johns Hopkins All Children's Hospital
St. Petersburg, Florida

Anita Deshpande, MD
Division of Pediatric Otolaryngology-Head and
   Neck Surgery
Cincinnati Children's Hospital Medical Center
Cincinnati, Ohio

Karin J. Detchon, MSN, FNP-BC
Department of Anesthesia
Pre-Anesthesia Consult Clinic
Cincinnati Children's Hospital Medical Center
Cincinnati, Ohio

Nicholas Detchon, MSN, CRNA
Department of Anesthesia
Cincinnati Children's Hospital Medical Center
Cincinnati, Ohio

Kristen Deveras, MSN, DNP, CRNA
Massachusetts General Hospital
Boston, Massachusetts

Lisa A. Durako, MS, CRNA
Department of Anesthesiology and Critical Care
Division of Pediatrics
Saint Louis University
St. Louis, Missouri

Khalil El-Chammas, MD, MS
Associate Professor
Department of Pediatrics
University of Cincinnati
Associate Director, Neurogastroenterology and Motility
   Disorders Center
Division of Gastroenterology, Hepatology, and Nutrition
Cincinnati Children's Hospital
Cincinnati, Ohio

Ebone Evans, MD
Department of Otolaryngology–Head & Neck Surgery
University of Minnesota
Minneapolis, Minnesota

Michael R. Everhart, MS, CRNA
Department of Anesthesia
Cincinnati Children's Hospital Medical Center
Cincinnati, Ohio

CONTRIBUTORS | xv

Karmella M. Franic-Everhart, DNP, CRNA
Department of Anesthesia
Cincinnati Children's Hospital Medical Center
Cincinnati, Ohio

Nathan Fagan, MD
Assistant Professor of Radiology
Cincinnati Children's Hospital Medical Center
Cincinnati, Ohio

Zhe Amy Fang, MD, FRCPC
Department of Anesthesiology and Pain Medicine
Hospital for Sick Children,
Toronto, Canada

Amanda Ford, DNP, CRNA
Staff CRNA, UPMC Children's Hospital of Pittsburgh
Pittsburgh, Pennsylvania

Lauren Freedman, CRNA, MS
Johns Hopkins All Children's Hospital
St. Petersburg, Florida

James S. Furstein, PhD, DNAP, CRNA, CPNP-AC, FAANA
Department of Anesthesia
Cincinnati Children's Hospital Medical Center
Cincinnati, Ohio

Nicole Garritano, DNP, APRN, CPNP-AC
College of Nursing
University of Kentucky
Lexington, Kentucky

Megan Gdowski, MSN, APN, CRNA
Department of Pediatric Anesthesia
Ann & Robert H Lurie Children's Hospital of Chicago
Chicago, Illinois

Jamie Gilley, MSN, APRN, NNP-BC
Instructor
Department of Pediatrics, Neonatology
Baylor College of Medicine
Texas Children's Hospital
Houston, Texas

Kenneth R. Goldschneider, MD
Professor
Clinical Anesthesia and Pediatrics
University of Cincinnati
Pain Management Center
Cincinnati Children's Hospital
Cincinnati, Ohio

Kahleb Graham, MD
Assistant Professor
Department of Pediatrics
University of Cincinnati
Physician, Neurogastroenterology and Motility Disorders Center
Division of Gastroenterology, Hepatology, and Nutrition
Cincinnati Children's Hospital
Cincinnati, Ohio

Timothy P. Grannell, CRNA
Nationwide Children's Hospital
Columbus, Ohio

Brian M. Grawe, MD
Associate Professor of Clinical
Department of Orthopaedics and Sports Medicine
University of Cincinnati
Cincinnati, Ohio

Brian J. Gronert, MD
Division of Cardiac Anesthesiology
Department of Cardiovascular Services
Nemours Children's Hospital
Assistant Professor
University of Central Florida College of Medicine
Orlando, Florida

Trina Devadhar Hemmelgarn, PharmD
Division of Pharmacy
Cincinnati Children's Hospital Medical Center
Cincinnati, Ohio

Alison Henry, MSN, CRNA
Staff CRNA, University of Rochester Medical Center
SRNA Clinical Coordinator
Adjunct Faculty, University of Buffalo School of Nursing
Rochester, New York

Daniel Henz, MS, CRNA
Department of Anesthesia
Cincinnati Children's Hospital
Cincinnati, Ohio

Lisa Herbinger, DNP, CRNA
Samford University
Children's of Alabama
Birmingham, Alabama

Daniela Herrera, RN, MS, CPNP-AC, PPCNP-BC
Division of Anesthesiology, Pain and Perioperative Medicine
Children's National Hospital
Washington, DC

Marika Highberger, MSN, APRN, BMTCN, CPNP
Instructor
Department of Pediatrics
Baylor College of Medicine
Pediatric Nurse Practitioner
Texas Children's Cancer and Hematology Centers
Houston, Texas

Tamara K. Hutson, PharmD
Division of Pharmacy
Cincinnati Children's Hospital Medical Center
Cincinnati, Ohio

Lauren Irwin, MSN, APN, CRNA
Department of Pediatric Anesthesia
Ann & Robert H Lurie Children's Hospital of Chicago
Chicago, Illinois

Stacey L. Ishman, MD, MPH
Department of Otolaryngology–Head and Neck Surgery
University of Cincinnati College of Medicine
Division of Pediatric Otolaryngology-Head and Neck Surgery
Cincinnati Children's Hospital Medical Center
Cincinnati, Ohio

Leslie Jackson, DNP, CRNA
Lead CRNA
Department of Anesthesia and Perioperative Medicine
Nemours A. I. duPont Hospital for Children
Wilmington, Delaware

Lindsay Johnson-Bishop, DNP, APRN, CPNP-AC, CNE
Instructor
Department of Pediatrics
Baylor College of Medicine
Pediatric Nurse Practitioner
Texas Children's Cancer and Hematology Centers
Houston, Texas

Tiffany Jonasson, MD
Department of Anesthesiology
Baylor College of Medicine
Houston, Texas

Nathan S. Jones, MSN, CRNA
Instructor, Texas Children's Hospital
Department of Anesthesiology, Perioperative and Pain Medicine
Baylor College of Medicine
Houston, Texas

David B. Joseph, MD
Department of Urology
University of Alabama at Birmingham
Birmingham, Alabama

Ali I. Kandil, DO, MPH
Associate Professor of Clincial Anesthesia
University of Cincinnati College of Medecine
Department of Anesthesia
Cincinnati Children's Hospital and Medical Center
Cincinnati, Ohio

Megha Kanjia, MD
Assistant Professor
Department of Pediatric Anesthesiology and Perioperative Pain Medicine
Baylor College of Medicine
Texas Children's Hospital
Houston, Texas

Megha Karkera Kanjia, MD
Assistant Professor
Department of Pediatric Anesthesiology and Perioperative Pain Medicine
Baylor College of Medicine
Texas Children's Hospital
Houston, Texas

Tamra Nicole Kelly, DNP, CRNA
Assistant Director, Cardiovascular Division, Nurse Anesthesia
Texas Children's Hospital
Instructor, Baylor College of Medicine
Department of Anesthesia and Perioperative Pain Medicine
Houston, Texas

Emily H. Klinefelter, DNAP, CRNA, APRN
Department of Pediatric Anesthesia
Ann & Robert H Lurie Children's Hospital of Chicago
Chicago, Illinois

Karen Knight, RT(R)
Children's of Alabama
Birmingham, Alabama

Yann-Fuu Kou, MD
Assistant Professor or Otolaryngology
University of Texas Southwestern Medical School
Children's Health Dalls
Dallas, Texas

Hannah Kuhn, MSN, CRNA
Pittsburgh, Pennsylvania

Dennis LaChance, PharmD
Division of Pharmacy
Cincinnati Children's Hospital Medical Center
Cincinnati, Ohio

Aimee Langley, DNP, CRNA, CHSE
Assistant Professor of Anesthesiology and Health Professions
Doctor of Nursing Practice-Nurse Anesthesia Program
Baylor College of Medicine
Houston, Texas

Tomas Lazo, MD
Assistant Professor, Department of Anesthesiology and Perioperative Medicine
Division of Pediatric Anesthesia
Oregon Health & Science University
Portland, Oregon

Joshua Lea, DNP, MBA, CRNA
Boston, Massachusetts

Judith M. Lewis, DNP, APRN, CRNA
Cleveland Clinic Children's Hospital
Case Western Reserve University
Frances Payne Bolton School of Nursing
Cleveland, Ohio

Carol Li, MD
Division of Pediatric Otolaryngology-Head and Neck Surgery
Cincinnati Children's Hospital Medical Center
University of Cincinnati College of Medicine
Cincinnati, Ohio

Gregory Lynam, MD
Richmond Surgical Arts
Richmond, Virginia

Peace C. Madueme, MD, MS, FAAP, FACC, FASE
Medical Director of Non-invasive Cardiac Imaging
Division of Cardiology
Department of Cardiovascular Services
Nemours Children's Hospital
Assistant Professor
University of Central Florida College of Medicine
Orlando, Florida

Mohamed A. Mahmoud, MD
Professor of Clinical Anesthesia
University of Cincinnati College of Medicine
Department of Anesthesia
Cincinnati Children's Hospital and Medical Center
Cincinnati, Ohio

Steffani Maier, MSN, FNP-C, BMTCN
Nurse Practitioner
Bone Marrow Transplant and Immune Deficiency Program
Cancer and Blood Diseases Institute
Cincinnati Children's Hospital
Cincinnati, Ohio

AnnMarie Matusak, DDS, MS
Assistant Professor
Department of Pediatrics
University of Cincinnati
Program Director of Advanced Education in Pediatric Dentistry
Division of Pediatric Dentistry and Orthodontics
Cincinnati Children's Hospital Medical Center
Cincinnati, Ohio

Matthew McCoy, DNP, CRNA
Assistant Director
CCMC Nurse Anesthesia Program
Villanova University
Philadelphia, Pennsylvania

Lori Ann McKenna, MSN, AC/PNP, CHPPN, PMN-BC
Department of Anesthesia
Division of Pain
Cincinnati Children's Hospital Medical Center
Cincinnati, Ohio

Susan P. McMullan, PhD, MSN, CRNA
Associate Professor and Director, Nurse Anesthesia BSN-DNP Pathway
University of Alabama at Birmingham School of Nursing
Staff CRNA, UAB Callahan Eye Hospital
Birmingham, Alabama

Joseph W. McSoley, MS, MD
Assistant Professor of Clinical Anesthesia
University of Cincinnati College of Medicine
Department of Anesthesia
Cincinnati Children's Hospital and Medical Center
Cincinnati, Ohio

Marc Mecoli, MD
Associate Professor of Clinical Anesthesia
University of Cincinnati College of Medicine
Department of Anesthesia
Cincinnati Children's Hospital Medical Center
Cincinnati, Ohio

Aileen Mendez, MS, CRNA
Pediatric CRNA
Division of Anesthesia and Critical Care Medicine
The Johns Hopkins Hospital
Baltimore, Maryland

Soroush Merchant, MD
Fellow
Pain Management Center
Cincinnati Children's Hospital
Cincinnati, Ohio

Mark John Meyer, MD, FAAHPM
Associate Professor
Department of Anesthesia
Director of the Palliative and Comfort Care Team
Cincinnati Children's Hospital Medical Center
Cincinnati, Ohio

Courtney Miller, MD
Resident Physician
Department of Anesthesiology and Perioperative Medicine
Oregon Health & Science University
Portland, Oregon

Sarah Milligan, MSN, CRNA
Cleveland Clinic Foundation
Cleveland, Ohio

Jennifer B. Mills, DNAP, CRNA
Mercy Health Systems
Springfield, Missouri

Angela Milosh, DNP, CRNA
Cleveland Clinic Foundation
Cleveland, Ohio

Rachael Mohr, MSN, RN, CPNP-PC/AC
APRN Clinical Director
Cancer and Blood Diseases Institute and Infectious Diseases
Cincinnati Children's Hospital
Cincinnati, Ohio

Abigail Monnig, MD
Assistant Professor of Clinical Anesthesia
University of Cincinnati College of Medicine
Department of Anesthesia
Cincinnati Children's Hospital Medical Center
Cincinnati, Ohio

Kelly Moon, MSN, CRNA
Nationwide Children's Hospital
Cincinnati, Ohio

David L. Moore, MD
Associate Professor of Clinical Anesthesia
University of Cincinnati College of Medicine
Department of Anesthesia
Cincinnati Children's Hospital Medical Center
Cincinnati, Ohio

Brett J. Morey, DNAP, CRNA, APRN
Lead CRNA, Department of Pediatrics
Yale New-Haven Hospital
New Haven, Connecticut

Eleanor Mullen, MSN, CRNA
Boston, Massachusetts

Angela Mund, DNP, CRNA
Associate Professor
Division Director
Anesthesia for Nurses
Medical University of South Carolina
Charleston, South Carolina

Charles M. Myer, IV, MD
Division of Pediatric Otolaryngology-Head and Neck Surgery
Cincinnati Children's Hospital Medical Center
Department of Otolaryngology-Head and Neck Surgery
University of Cincinnati College of Medicine
Cincinnati, Ohio

René P. Myers, MD
Division of Pediatric Plastic Surgery
University of Alabama School of Medicine
Birmingham, Alabama

Melanie Neal, MSN, CRNA
Department of Anesthesia
Cincinnati Children's Hospital Medical Center
Cincinnati, Ohio

Pornswan Ngamprasertwong, MD, MSc
Associate Professor of Clinical Anesthesia
University of Cincinnati College of Medicine
Department of Anesthesia
Cincinnati Children's Hospital and Medical Center
Cincinnati, Ohio

Meaghan O'Meara, MSN, APN, CRNA
Department of Pediatric Anesthesia
Ann & Robert H Lurie Children's Hospital of Chicago
Chicago, Illinois

Kimberly Hunter Olivarez, MS, CRNA
Department of Anesthesiology, Peri-operative and Pain Medicine
Texas Children's Hospital
Baylor College of Medicine
Houston, Texas

Nicklas Orobello, MD
Department of Otolaryngology–Head & Neck Surgery
University of Minnesota
Minneapolis, Minnesota

Joanna Rosing Paquin, MD
Associate Professor of Clinical Anesthesia
University of Cincinnati College of Medicine
Department of Anesthesia
Cincinnati Children's Hospital Medical Center
Cincinnati, Ohio

Jagroop Parikh, MD
Associate Professor of Clinical Anesthesia
University of Cincinnati College of Medicine
Department of Anesthesia
Cincinnati Children's Hospital and Medical Center
Cincinnati, Ohio

Shital N. Parikh, MD
Professor of Clinical
Department of Orthopaedics and Sports Medicine
Division of Orthopaedic Surgery
Cincinnati Children's Hospital Medical Center
Cincinnati, Ohio

Jennifer Parks, DNP, CRNA
Staff CRNA, Penn State Milton S. Hershey Medical Center
Hershey, Pennsylvania

Manish N. Patel, DO
Assistant Professor of Radiology
Cincinnati Children's Hospital Medical Center
Cincinnati, Ohio

Mario Patino, MD
Associate Professor
Department of Anesthesiology
Cincinnati Children's Hospital and Medical Center
Cincinnati, Ohio

Renee Pederson, DNP, APN, CRNA
Department of Pediatric Anesthesia
Ann & Robert H Lurie Children's Hospital of Chicago
Chicago, Illinois

Anne M. Peeke, MSN, CRNA
Department of Anesthesiology, Critical Care and Pain Medicine
Boston Children's Hospital
Boston, Massachusetts

Jason Perry, CRNA, APRN
Department of Anesthesia
Cincinnati Children's Hospital Medical Center
Cincinnati, Ohio

Rajanya S. Petersson, MD, MS, FACS
Associate Professor
Department of Otolaryngology–Head and Neck Surgery
Virginia Commonwealth University
Section Director, Pediatric Otolaryngology
Children's Hospital of Richmond at VCU
Richmond, Virginia

Dusty C. Pourciau, DNP, CRNA
Los Angeles, California

Carrilee Powell, MSN, CRNA
Instructor
University of Cincinnati College of Nursing
Department of Anesthesia
Cincinnati Children's Hospital Medical Center
Cincinnati, Ohio

Heena Pranav, MD
Assistant Professor
Texas Children's Hospital
Houston, Texas

Anthony Prickel, DNP, CRNA
Cincinnati, Ohio

Meghan Pursley, CRNA
Boston, Massachusetts

Anne M. Que, MS, CRNA
Chief Nurse Anesthetist
Department of Anesthesia,
Critical Care and Pain Medicine
Massachusetts General Hospital
Boston, Massachusetts

Heather J. Rankin, DNP, MBA, CRNA
Nurse Anesthesia Adjunct Faculty
Samford University Ida and Harper School of Nursing
Children's of Alabama
Nurse Anesthesia
Birmingham, Alabama

Jennifer Raynor, DNP, CRNA
Children's Hospital of Philadelphia
Philadelphia, Pennsylvania

Kris Redden, CRNA
Southern Anesthesia Management
Birmingham, Alabama

Andrew Redmann, MD
Department of Otolaryngology–Head & Neck Surgery
University of Minnesota
Ear, Nose, Throat & Facial Plastic Surgery
Children's Minnesota
Minneapolis, Minnesota

Whitney Rhoades, MSN, CRNA
Nationwide Children's Hospital
Columbus, Ohio

Katrina Richardson, MSN, CPNP-AC
Outpatient Oncology Nurse Practitioner
Cancer and Blood Diseases Institute
Cincinnati Children's Hospital
Cincinnati, Ohio

Claire Rizk, MSN, APRN, CPNP-PC/AC
Texas Children's Hospital
Baylor College of Medicine
Houston, Texas

Whitney S. Roberts, MS, CRNA
Department of Anesthesiology, Critical Care and Pain Medicine
Boston Children's Hospital
Boston, Massachusetts

Audrey Rosenblatt, PhD, MSN, CRNA
CRNA Manager
Lurie Children's Hospital
Adjunct Faculty
Rush University College of Nursing
Chicago, Illinois

Brandi M. Runnels, MMS, MS, PA-C
Instructor
Department of Pediatrics
Baylor College of Medicine
Physician Assistant
Texas Children's Cancer and Hematology Centers
Houston, Texas

Julianne Ryan, BSN, RN, SRNA
Boston, Massachusetts

Ramsey S. Sabbagh, MS
Research Fellow
Department of Orthopaedics and Sports Medicine
University of Cincinnati
Cincinnati, Ohio

Nancy B. Samol, MD
Associate Professor
Department of Anesthesia
Cincinnati Children's Hospital Medical Center
Cincinnati, Ohio

M. Leona A. Sayson, MSN, CRNA
Department of Anesthesiology, Critical Care and Pain Medicine
Boston Children's Hospital
Boston, Massachusetts

Julie Schackman, MD
Assistant Professor
Department of Pediatric Anesthesiology and Perioperative Pain Medicine
Baylor College of Medicine
Texas Children's Hospital
Houston, Texas

Jennifer McBride Schultz, MSN, CRNA
Department of Anesthesia
Cincinnati Children's Hospital Medical Center
Cincinnati, Ohio

Sarrah L. Schultz, MSN, APRN, AC-PNP
Pediatric ICU Nurse Practitioner
Cincinnati Children's Hospital Medical Center
Cincinnati, Ohio

Mary J. Scott-Herring, DNP, MS, CRNA
Assistant Professor, Georgetown University
Doctor of Nurse Anesthesia Practice (DNAP) Program
Washington DC

Gail Shibata, MD
Health Science Clinical Professor
UCSF Benioff Children's Hospital
Anesthesia and Perioperative Care at Mission Bay
San Francisco, California

Michael Sikora, MD, MEd
Co-Director, Division of Anesthesia
Associate Professor of Clinical Anesthesia
University of Cincinnati College of Medicine
Department of Anesthesia
Cincinnati Children's Hospital Medical Center
Cincinnati, Ohio

Hailey Silverii, MD
Medical University of South Carolina
Charleston, South Carolina

Jamie W. Sinton, MD
Associate Professor of Clinical Anesthesia
University of Cincinnati College of Medicine
Department of Anesthesia
Cincinnati Children's Hospital Medical Center
Cincinnati, Ohio

Jeanie Skibiski, DNAP, MHA, CRNA
Assistant Professor
School of Anesthesia
Missouri State University
Springfield, Missouri

Saundra L. Smalley, MSN, CRNA
Pediatric Anesthesia Associates
Louisville, Kentucky

Matthew M. Smith, MD
Department of Otolaryngology–Head and Neck Surgery
University of Cincinnati College of Medicine
Division of Pediatric Otolaryngology-Head and Neck Surgery
Cincinnati Children's Hospital Medical Center
Cincinnati, Ohio

D. Julie Soelberg, PhD, MSN, CRNA
Clinical Assistant Professor
Nurse Anesthesia Program
School of Nursing
Clinical Instructor
Department of Anesthesiology and Perioperative Medicine
Division of Pediatric Anesthesia
Oregon Health and Science University
Portland, Oregon

Ximena Soler, MD
Assistant Professor of Clinical Anesthesia
Department of Anesthesia
University of Cincinnati College of Medicine
Cincinnati Children's Hospital Medical Center
Cincinnati, Ohio

Heather Soni, MSN, APRN, CPNP
Instructor
Department of Pediatrics
Baylor College of Medicine
Pediatric Nurse Practitioner
Texas Children's Cancer and Hematology Centers
Houston, Texas

Edgar Soto, BS
University of Alabama School of Medicine
Birmingham, Alabama

Corey Southworth, MSN, CRNA
Massachusetts General/North Shore Center for Outpatient Care
Danvers, Massachusetts

Jingjing Sparrow, DNP, CRNA
Instructor, Texas Children's Hospital
Department of Anesthesiology, Perioperative and Pain Medicine
Baylor College of Medicine
Houston, Texas

Jacob Stollard, MSN, CRNA
Nationwide Children's Hospital
Columbus, Ohio

Jessica Storey, DNP, CRNA
Department of Anesthesia
Cincinnati Children's Hospital Medical Center
Cincinnati, Ohio

Kimberly Stumpf, MSN, CRNA
Department of Anesthesia
Nationwide Children's Hospital
Columbus, Ohio

Aaron Sundberg, MSN, CRNA
Department of Anesthesia
Cincinnati Children's Hospital Medical Center
Cincinnati, Ohio

Barry Swerdlow, MD, FASA
Assistant Professor
Nurse Anesthesia Program
Oregon Health & Science University
Adjunct Clinical Assistant Professor
Department of Anesthesiology, Perioperative and Pain Medicine
Stanford University School of Medicine
Portland, Oregon

Alexandra Szabova, MD
Associate Professor
Clinical Anesthesia and Pediatrics
University of Cincinnati
Pain Management Center
Cincinnati Children's Hospital
Cincinnati, Ohio

Joseph Tobias, MD
Professor of Anesthesiology & Pediatrics
The Ohio State University
Chief, Department of Anesthesiology & Pain Medicine
Nationwide Children's Hospital
Columbus, Ohio

Ching Man Carmen Tong, DO
Department of Urology
University of Alabama at Birmingham
Birmingham, Alabama

Pacifico Tuason, MD
Assistant Professor in Anesthesia
Harvard Medical School
Pediatric Staff Anesthesiologists
Division of Pediatric Anesthesia
Massachusetts General Hospital
Boston, Massachusetts

Nidhy Paulose Varghese, MD
Assistant Professor of Pediatrics
Department of Pediatrics, Pediatric Pulmonology
Baylor College of Medicine
Texas Children's Hospital
Houston, Texas

Lisa Wahlers, DNP, CRNA
Staff CRNA, University of Rochester Medical Center
SRNA Clinical Coordinator
Adjunct Faculty, University of Buffalo School of Nursing
Rochester, New York

Eric Wall, MD
Director, Orthopaedic Sports Medicine
Director, Orthopaedic Fellowship
Professor, UC Department of Surgery
Division of Orthopaedic Surgery
Cincinnati Children's Hospital Medical Center
Cincinnati, Ohio

Chad Watkins, PharmD, MHA
Pharmacy Manager
Cincinnati Children's Hospital
Cincinnati, Ohio

Shawn West, MSN CRNA
Adjunct Faculty, Nurse Anesthesia
University of Pittsburgh
Staff CRNA, Clinical Coordinator
Children's Hospital of Pittsburgh
University of Pittsburgh Medical Center
Pittsburgh, Pennsylvania

Elise C. Whalen, MSN, APRN, FNP-C, CPN
Instructor
Department of Pediatrics, Pediatric Pulmonology
Baylor College of Medicine
Texas Children's Hospital
Houston, Texas

Amanda Whippey, MD, FRCPC
Pediatric Anesthesiologist
McMaster University
Ontario, Canada

Sharifah Wilson, MSN, CRNA
Department of Pediatric Anesthesiology
St. Christopher Hospital for Children
Philadelphia, Pennsylvania

Vera Winograd-Gomez, MD
Cincinnati Children's Hospital Medical Center
Cincinnati, Ohio

Suzanne M. Wright, PhD, CRNA, FAANA
Associate Professor and Chair
School of Nursing
College of Health Sciences
Old Dominion University
Norfolk, Virginia

Shannon Zhang, MD
Anesthesia Site Chief and Medical Director
Massachusetts General/North Shore Center for Outpatient Care
Danvers, Massachusetts

FOREWORD

In the United States, more than 6 million pediatric patients—a quarter of whom are infants—receive anesthesia annually. And yet, pediatric anesthesia as a distinct and separate subspecialty is a relatively recent development. For many years, most anesthetics delivered to pediatric patients were done by anesthesia providers trained in the care of adult patients. Physiologic considerations unique to the pediatric population remained largely unknown and underappreciated. Factors such as temperature regulation and oxygen tension, for example, were ignored. Anesthesia providers were simply charged with using fractional adult quantities to deliver what was thought to be safe, effective care. Fortunately, as the understanding of pediatric-specific physiology and disease processes continues to advance, so do the approaches employed to optimize patient outcomes. Garnering disease and organ-specific insight from pediatric specialists is imperative to discerning and ensuring best practice.

Accounting for nearly half of anesthesia providers in the United States, certified registered nurse anesthetists (CRNAs) are key members of the anesthesia care team, collaborating with surgeons, physician anesthesiologists, dentists, and all health professions to safely administer anesthesia in all practice settings. Notably, CRNAs have evolved to become the primary providers of anesthesia in rural and underserved communities. As such, CRNAs are well equipped with the knowledge and training requisite to administer pediatric anesthesia as a specialized practice.

Pediatric Anesthesia: A Comprehensive Approach to Safe and Effective Care is the first textbook designed to be reflective of the multidisciplinary care teams that offer their expertise to the perioperative care of pediatric patients. Editor James S. Furstein, himself an accomplished educator, has assembled a multidisciplinary set of more than 120 expert perspectives on pediatric anatomy and physiology, pharmacologic considerations for the pediatric patient, and the practice of pediatric anesthesia. An invaluable resource for those in training and practicing anesthesia providers alike, the content in *Pediatric Anesthesia* provides current and evidence-based guidance that is both comprehensive and practical, addressing all aspects of the field. The book effectively provides a strong foundation in pediatric anatomy and physiology, and common syndromes, conditions, and diseases seen in pediatric patients. Through brief and consistently formatted chapters that are organized by body system, *Pediatric Anesthesia* presents state-of-the-art techniques—including indications and contraindications, preoperative evaluation, key assessment points, intraoperative management, complications, and clinical pearls—for safely administering anesthesia in more than 100 of the most common or complex pediatric procedures.

In addition to the breadth of outstanding content in the text itself, instructors who choose to rely on *Pediatric Anesthesia* for teaching will have access to valuable supplements in the form of chapter summaries, additional case studies, multiple-choice questions, and PowerPoint slides to aid lectures and provide study notes. These assets truly set this text apart from others in the field as an effective teaching tool.

I applaud Dr. Furstein's efforts to undertake such a needed project. The result is a set of specialized information that is certain to help ensure those who provide pediatric anesthesia practice collaboratively, safely, and effectively in all settings and in all situations involving the care of our precious our pediatric patients.

Theodore W. Striker, MD*
Professor of Anesthesia
University of Cincinnati
Cincinnati, Ohio

---

* Dr. Striker passed away in October 2021.

PREFACE

Approxiamtely 4 years ago I was approached by a colleague with an idea or, rather, a challenge: to develop a pediatric anesthesia text that offers a new perspective on pediatric anesthesia. Admittedly, this seemed like an insurmountable challenge as we are fortunate to have several revered texts available that have historically guided the practice of pediatric anesthesia. It quickly dawned on me, however, that not all professions who contribute to the perioperative care of pediatric patients have had the opportunity to share their expertise. This text fills that void.

What makes this text unique is the multidisciplinary composition of the authors, with nurse anesthetists, anesthesiologists, nurse practitioners, pharmacists, surgeons, specialty care physicians, and physician assistants all authoring chapters specific to their area of expertise. Ultimately, there is widespread representation from a host of pediatric facilities and academic institutions across the country.

The objective of this text is to provide both the seasoned clinician and the novice provider alike an all-encompassing resource that facilitates the delivery of safe and effective anesthetic care to the pediatric population. The text not only provides a sound foundation in pediatric pharmacology and physiology, but also offers procedure-specific guidance. This includes, but is not limited to, indications, concerns, perioperative algorithms, and a list of common drugs utilized with dosing guidelines. Many sections of the text conclude with case reports to reinforce application of the content presented. Additionally, teaching resources are available to academic institutions to facilitate didactic education related to pediatric anesthesia.

James S. Furstein

ACKNOWLEDGMENTS

It has been said that the ability to acknowledge, absorb, interpret, and implement the wisdom and experience of others facilitates the delivery of optimal patient care. Without question, all the authors who contributed to this text have bolstered the body of knowledge guiding the delivery of safe, effective care to pediatric patients around the world who require anesthesia. I will be forever grateful to them all.

While there is an endless number of colleagues and mentors who have made completion of this text possible, there are a few who deserve special recognition. I would like to thank Rollo Jones, PhD, whose character and unwavering friendship have made him a pillar of strength for decades; Evelyn Overbey, MD, who first challenged me to pursue a career in anesthesia, Theodore W. Striker, MD, whose support was unwavering as I chased my dreams; Wanda Wilson, PhD, CRNA, who inspired me to forever continue my quest to improve clinical practice; Mohamed Mahmoud, MD, who fostered my interests in academic practice and took the time to answer my many questions; Senthilkumar Sadhasivam, MD, MPH, who championed my growth both clinically and academically; Suzanne Wright, PhD, CRNA, who instilled in me a passion for optimizing patient outcomes; Wm. Terry Ray, PhD, CRNA, who offered me my first academic appointment and the trust to play a role in developing burgeoning anesthesia providers; and, finally, the amazing staff at Cincinnati Children's Hospital Medical Center. I consider myself fortunate to learn from and collaborate with so many gifted clinicians who are committed to delivering the best care possible.

Finally, I would like to thank my family. Without their support, the completion of this work would not have been possible. My children, Keala, Matthew, Michael, Elise, and Evelyn, have all made countless sacrifices throughout this journey. My hope is that one day they all will understand my drive to fulfill personal goals and chase their own dreams with equal fervor. Words alone cannot express my gratitude to my amazing wife Sarah who has religiously supported my academic endeavors. Without her support, tolerance, and relentless efforts at home, I would have never reached this point in my life. I look forward to spending the rest of our lives together.

INSTRUCTOR RESOURCES

A robust set of resources designed to supplement this text is located at http://connect.springerpub.com. Qualifying instructors may request access by emailing textbook@springerpub.com.

Available resources include:

- **INSTRUCTOR'S MANUAL:**
  - Case Studies
  - Knowledge Check Discussion Questions and Answers/Rationales

- **TEST BANK:**
  - Multiple-Choice Questions with Answers/Rationales

- **CHAPTER-BASED POWERPOINT PRESENTATIONS**

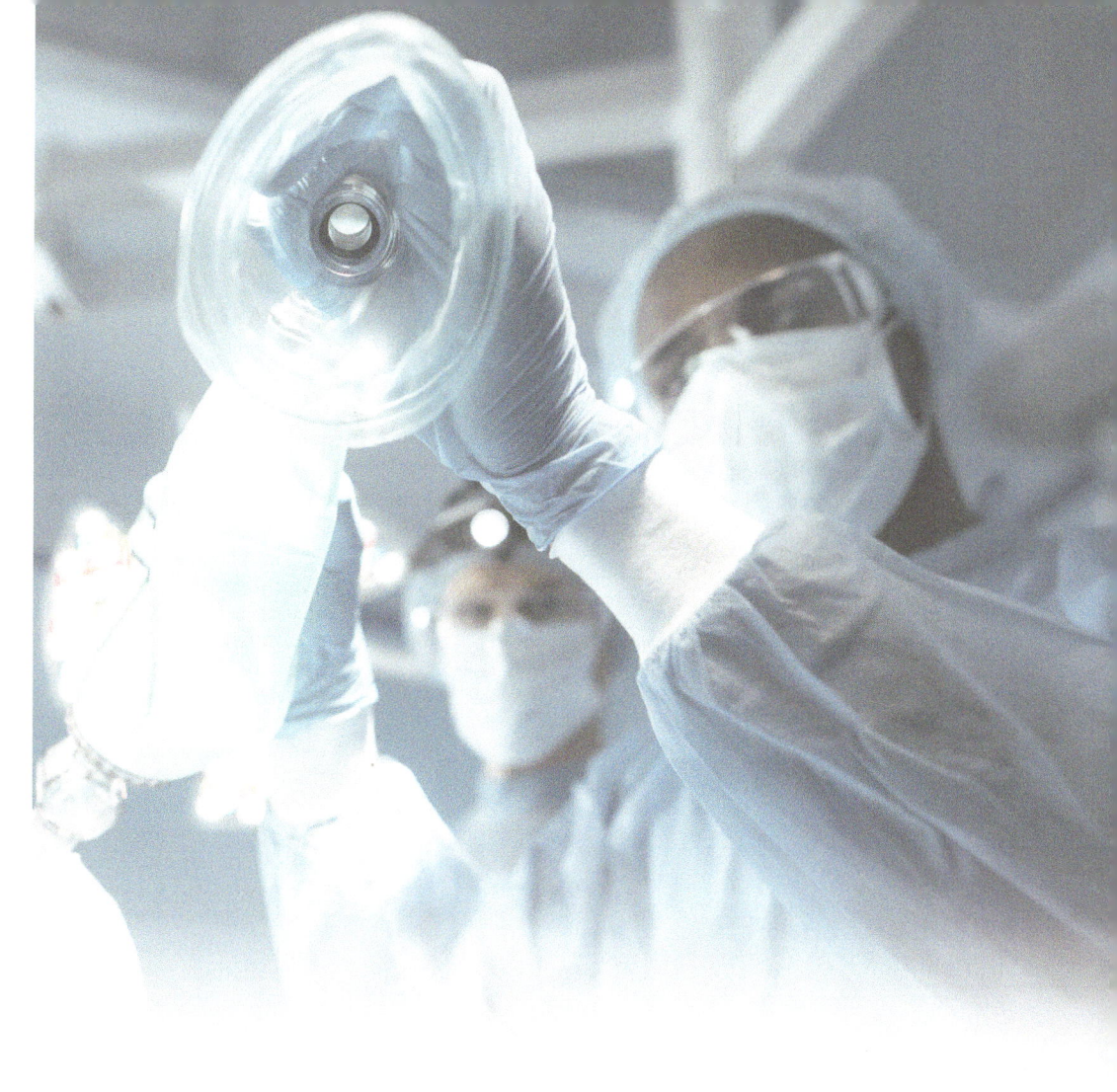

PART I

FOUNDATIONS OF ANESTHETIC CARE

CHAPTER 1

Anatomy and Physiology of the Pediatric Patient

LEARNING OBJECTIVES

- Describe the embryonic development and differentiation of the pediatric nervous system, including the organization of the peripheral and central nervous systems.
- Explain the significance, physiology and pathophysiology, and time frames behind the common newborn reflexes.
- Identify the potential neurocognitive implications of anesthesia on neuroapoptosis in the developing brain.

1.1: NERVOUS SYSTEM

Mark Blazey

INTRODUCTION

Unfortunately, for most of the 20th century, the prevailing thought among the majority of anesthesia providers was that infants did not feel pain or felt it to a much lesser extent than adults. We now know this to be categorically false. This rationale, while flawed, stemmed from the fact that at birth, a newborn possesses only one quarter of the neural cells present in adulthood. It was believed that a newborn's autonomic nervous system was too underdeveloped to be able to transmit painful stimuli to the brain. Certainly, a newborn's inability to articulate needs or recall traumatic experiences did not help dispel this notion. The result, however, was inadequate pain management for the neonatal population as a whole that led to poor surgical, cardiovascular, and developmental outcomes, notwithstanding the obvious ethical issues of inadequately treating surgical pain.

A better understanding of the newborn's neurological development, anatomy, and physiology came about in the 1970s while several research studies reported that newborns demonstrate physiological responses to painful stimuli in the form of hormonal, metabolic, and cardiopulmonary changes to an extent that often exceeded the responses witnessed in adults. Further work in this area was able to correlate physiological changes to meaningful negative outcomes to children who received the standard of care at that time, which consisted of inadequate levels of anesthesia and analgesia. Inadequate anesthesia and analgesia were found to result in an increased incidence of sepsis, disseminated intravascular coagulopathy, cardiac events, such as arrhythmias, and mortality. This section is dedicated to enhancing anesthesia providers' knowledge of the neonatal nervous system. While the overarching goal is to review key aspects of human neurological functions, anatomy, and physiology, we specifically focus on key differences between the pediatric and adult patient rather than a summary of the nervous system as it applies to all human development.

EMBRYONIC DEVELOPMENT

Understanding embryonic development affords anesthesia providers a better appreciation of the key components of the nervous system, as well as the overall function of the human nervous system. Approximately 16 days after an egg is fertilized, the ectoderm (or outer germal layer of the embryo) begins to form the neuroectoderm, which eventually becomes the basic human nervous system. As the cells proliferate and change, the neuroectoderm begins to fold upon itself, forming the neural groove. The two sides of the neural groove ultimately converge to form the neural tube, which lies beneath the ectoderm. At this point, the neural tube is hollow and travels from the anterior end of the embryo to the posterior end. The anterior portion of the neural tube begins to form the brain at 25 days postconception, with the ventricles of the brain arising from the hollow portion of the neural tube. The posterior portion of the neural tube becomes the spinal cord approximately 4 weeks after conception.

With further development, the neural tube separates into three distinct primary vesicles (sacs): the forebrain (prosencephalon), the midbrain (mesencephalon), and the hindbrain (rhombencephalon). In Greek, *cephalon* means "brain," while *pro* represents "beforehand," *mes* denotes "middle," and *rhomben* describes the shape rather than the location. Thus, anatomically, the divisions can be thought of as in the front (anterior), in the middle, and (the rhomboid-shaped sac) in the back (posterior). The brain is a complicated structure, so it should not be a surprise that brain development and differentiation do not stop at three distinct regions and that they further progress into five secondary vesicles: telencephalon, diencephalon, mesencephalon, metencephalon, and myelencephalon. These secondary regions give rise to fully developed anatomical structures present at birth, which anesthesia providers are more commonly familiar with—the cerebellum, cerebrum, and brainstem (**Figure 1.1**).

As the brain develops from the anterior neural tube, the spinal cord rises from the posterior segment. Rather than divide and differentiate as the anterior neural tube, the posterior segment simply elongates, grows, and maintains its long, straight, hollow shape and structure. The side closest to the surface is identified as dorsal, while the deeper side is referred to as ventral aspect. As these neural cells proliferate and differentiate, spinal cord neurogenesis occurs in a ventrodorsal direction beginning with the motor neurons and ending in with the local interneurons in the superficial dorsal horn or substantia gelatinosa. Within the spinal cord, the dorsal tissues develop sensory functions while the ventral tissues develop motor functions. Interestingly, neural development does not fully complete until 12 years of age.

While admittedly nuanced, a basic understanding of embryonic spinal cord development allows a better conceptualization of neural tube disorders, such as spina bifida occulta, meningocele, and myelomeningocele, in which the neural tubes do not close at various levels or degrees.

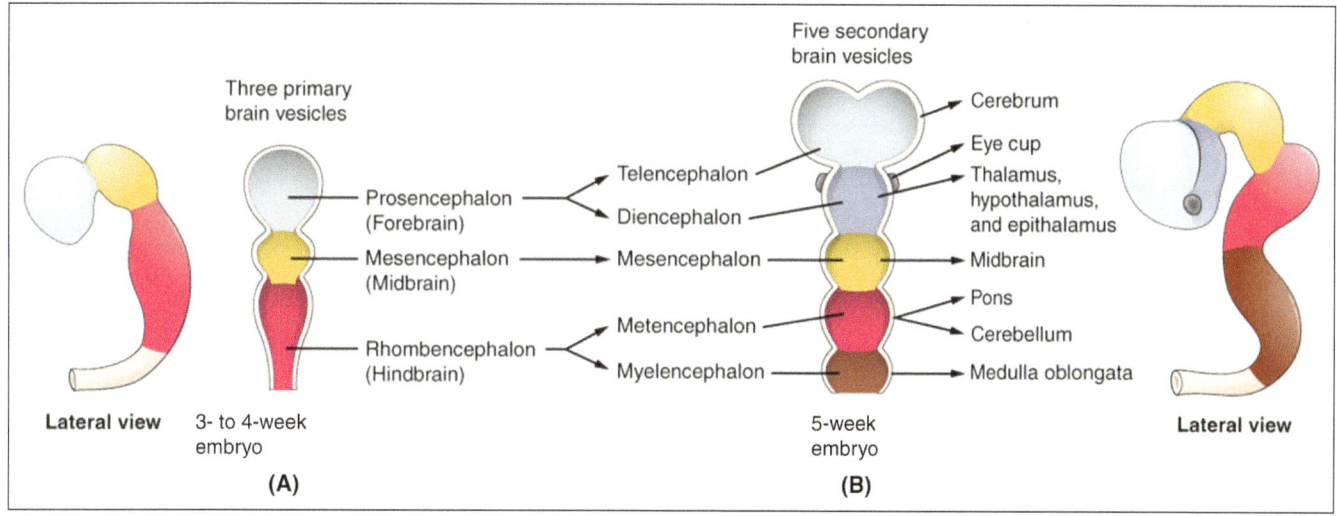

Figure 1.1: (A) Primary and (B) secondary vesicle stages of development.
Source: From https://ecampusontario.pressbooks.pub/neurosciencecdn/chapter/development-of-the-nervous-system-embryologic-perspective.

CENTRAL NERVOUS SYSTEM ANATOMY

By the time of birth, the central nervous system (CNS) is anatomically divided into the brain and the spinal cord. The brain consists of several distinct components, namely, the forebrain, midbrain, and hindbrain. In the cerebral hemisphere, which is a portion of the forebrain, there exist the frontal, temporal, parietal, and occipital lobes. In a rare instance of anatomic convenience, these four lobes share a name with the bone that covers and protects them. A fifth lobe, the insula or Island of Reil, lies deep within the lateral sulcus. The cerebrum interprets impulses, conducts voluntary movements, stores and retrieves information (memory), provides reasoning, is the basis for intellect and personality, and accounts for 75% of all neurons in the nervous system. Other critical structures in the brain include the thalamus, hypothalamus, pons, medulla, cerebellum, and pituitary glands, among others.

The spinal cord begins in the brain at the foramen magnum. At birth, the spinal cord normally ends at the third lumbar vertebrae (L3), which anatomically migrates rostrally to the first or second lumbar vertebrae (L1/L2) by 1 year of age. Likewise, the dural sac shortens from the third sacral vertebrae (S3) to the first sacral vertebrae (S1) by 1 year of age. The spinal cord is essentially a conduit for nerve pathways to and from the brain and brainstem and acts as the center for spinal reflexes. More information about spinal reflexes is provided later in this chapter.

PERIPHERAL NERVOUS SYSTEM ANATOMY

The peripheral nervous system (PNS) is divided into two segments: the somatic nervous system and the autonomic nervous system (ANS). The somatic nervous system connects skin to skeletal muscles with both efferent (motor) and afferent (sensory) nerves, enabling voluntary movement. The somatic nervous system allows us to flex our collective muscles. The PNS contains cranial nerves (CNs) and spinal nerves (SNs), both of which contain somatic fibers and automatic fibers that connect to the viscera. As the name implies, the autonomic fibers are involuntary. Examples include peristalsis in the gut, metabolization of medications, and resting heart rate or blood pressure. The ANS is further divided into the sympathetic nervous system (SNS) and the parasympathetic nervous system (PSNS; Figure 1.2). Both are present at birth, albeit the SNS is underdeveloped while the PSNS is fully developed. The SNS and PSNS have different functions and different target organs. Conceptually, the SNS has been regarded as the "fight or flight" set of reflexes, with the PSNS taking on the role of "resting and digesting." The SNS and PSNS also have complementary roles within each body system.

NEWBORN REFLEXES

Barring several different neurological disorders, all humans have several congenital physiological reflexes. By definition, these are nonpurposeful, automatic, and subconscious movements or responses to some type of stimuli. An example would be the involuntary motor response elicited when the patella tendon or area above the elbow is struck with a rubber. The effects of stimulation are subjectively characterized on a scale 0 to 4, with 0 representing no movement. An exaggerated response (+4) can also be considered abnormal. While these seem innocuous, the lack of reflexes can indicate a neurological change, thus eliciting them is a regular component of many wellness visits and screenings. All reflexes, regardless of age, rely on two neurological tracts that both essentially carry information: the ascending and descending tracts. Simply, the ascending tracts conduct sensory impulses to the brain (e.g., the mallet has hit the patella). The descending tracts conduct motor impulses from the brain to motor neurons, stimulating the target muscles or glands (e.g., the leg or arm extension). This topic is a chapter unto itself, but anesthesia providers should understand that disruption in either tract can result in severe neurological consequences.

Newborns have many more reflexes than older children and adults. These are instinctual survival processes, in every sense of the phrase. They are innate, involuntary, initiated by the CNS, and often key for survival. In fact, a newborn's risk of morbidity and mortality can be estimated by the presence and performance of primitive reflexes, such as the Plantar (Babinski) and Moro (Startle) reflexes. Reflexes can be categorized as being one of two types: primitive (Table 1.1) and postural (Table 1.2). In many cases, reflexes disappear within 4 to 6 months. Others may disappear with myelination,

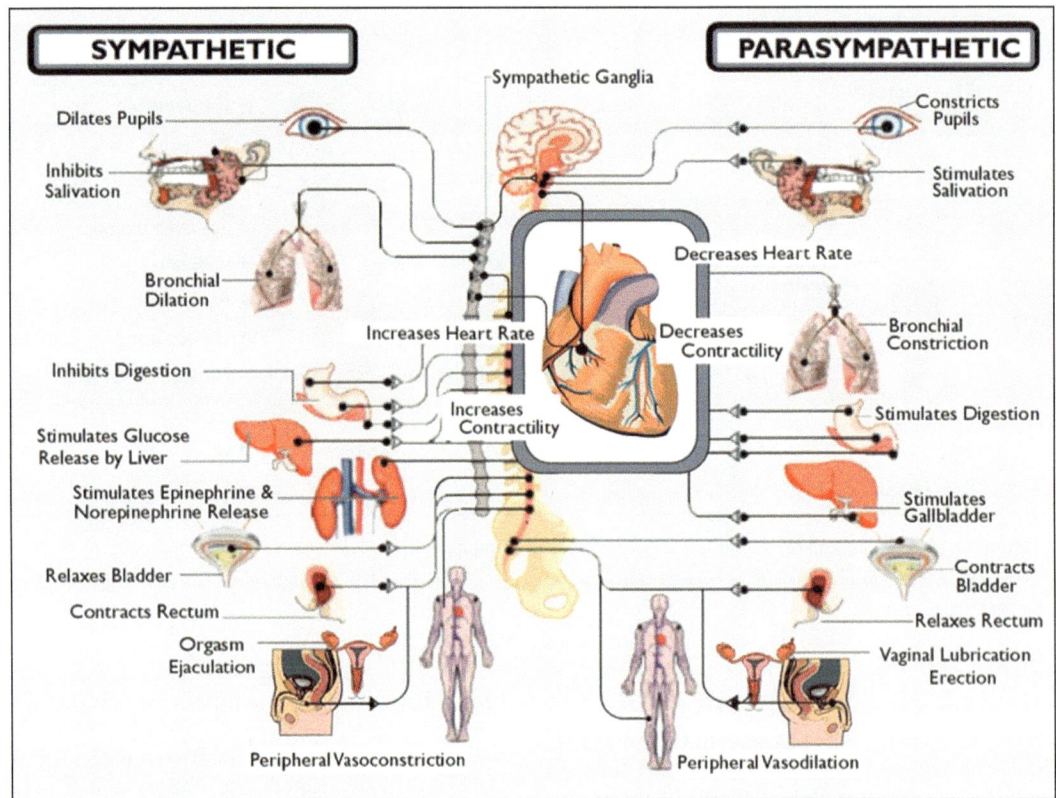

Figure 1.2: Autonomic nervous system: sympathetic and parasympathetic innervation.
Source: From Vinik AI. The conductor of the autonomic orchestra. *Front Endocrinol (Lausanne).* 2012;3:71. doi:10.3389/fendo.2012.00071.

which is generally completed by age 3. Reflexes can remain in certain neurological diseases, such as cerebral palsy from a traumatic birth, or even reemerge in adults as part of a neurological pathophysiological process, such as traumatic lesions, dementia, Parkinson's disease, or stroke.

NEUROCOGNITIVE IMPLICATIONS OF PEDIATRIC ANESTHESIA

Pediatric patients require analgesia and anesthesia for painful stimuli to ensure optimal outcomes and for the ethical reason that they do, in fact, feel and respond to pain. Given the improved, current understanding of the neonatal nervous system, it is important to consider the potential impact anesthetics may have on the developing brain. Early in life, the brain is developing myelin and rapidly forming new neuronal synapses (synaptogenesis) at rates much higher than witnessed in adulthood. Over the past decade, there has been a heighted concern regarding the impact volatile anesthetics (sevoflurane, isoflurane, desflurane, and halothane), hypnotics (propofol, ketamine, and etomidate), benzodiazepines (midazolam and lorazepam), and barbiturates (thiopental) may have on the developing brain.

Given the attention this topic has received, it has become increasingly common for anesthesia providers to be asked if these medications cause neurocognitive delays or deficits later in life. Unfortunately, the answer to this question remains unclear. What is known, however, is that in all tested animal species (rats, cats, mice, monkeys, apes, dogs, sheep, and pigs), the mentioned anesthetic agents cause a dose-, duration-, and timing-related; universal; and histologically similar negative effect on the developing brain. Neuroapoptosis, also known as programmed cell death, is normal when it occurs at a fine balance but accelerates after exposure to all anesthetic agents in the newborn and juvenile stages. The cause of increased neuroapoptosis is multifactorial, but studies clearly demonstrate that the longer the duration of exposure or the higher the dose, the histological changes or apoptosis that ensue are more severe and worse. Likewise, exposure of anesthesia during the peak synaptogenesis in animal models is associated with greater apoptosis. Researchers have linked these changes in brain development to practical or functional applications. The ability and time required to learn new tasks, demonstrate memory, discriminate color, and regulate emotion have all been negatively associated with anesthesia exposure in animal models.

Large longitudinal, epidemiological, population-based studies have demonstrated mixed findings for long-term implications related to anesthesia. Some have found modest decreases in IQ scores and academic performance for those children younger than 5 years old exposed to multiple anesthetics. Others have found an increased risk of having the diagnosis learning disabilities and attention-deficit disorders. By the nature of the type of studies, these must be taken in context to consider countless environmental, social, and genetic factors that may impact these results, as well as the potential to overestimate statistical risk without demonstrating practical or clinical effects.

One of the more frequently cited randomized control trials in humans to date compared children who received a single, brief (less than 1 hour long) anesthetic with vapor to a spinal anesthetic for a hernia repair.[2] Follow-up assessments at 2 and 5 years after the anesthetic supported the hypothesis that a single, brief exposure to anesthesia, even in young children, was not associated with negative neurocognitive outcomes. Furthermore, there was no significant developmental difference between the two cohorts.

Table 1.1	Primitive Newborn Reflexes	
Reflex + Normal Duration	**Cause**	**Effect**
Root: 28 weeks' gestation to 4 months	Touching/stroking corner of mouth	• Turn head and open mouth to follow and "root" in the direction of the stroke • Help find the breast or bottle to begin feeding
Sucking: 32 week's gestation to 4 months	Touching roof of mouth	• Active sucking • Common to all mammals
Moro (Startle): Birth to 4–6 months	Loud sound or movement, including one's own cry	• Extension of head at neck, extension of arms and legs, cry, then pulls the arms and legs back in • Cerebral birth injury if lacking or asymmetric
Asymmetric Tonic Neck (Fencing Posture): Birth to 5–6 months	Head is turned to one side	• Arm toward turned head extends, opposite arm flexes at elbow
Palmar Grasp: Birth to 5–6 months	Stroking the palm of hand	• Closing fingers in a grasp
Tonic Labyrinthine Righting: Birth to 6 months	Body out of orientation/tilting the head back while lying on the back	• Head and body alignment reorientation • Arching back
Plantar (Babinski): Birth to 1–2 years	Firmly stroking sole of foot	• Dorsiflexion (big toe bends back toward the top of the foot and the other toes fan out)
Galant: Birth to 4–6 months	Stroke along the side of back	• Swing toward the side that was stroked
Babkin: Early gestation to 1–2 months	Pressure to both palms	• Combination of head flexion, head rotation, and/or opening of mouth

Table 1.2	Postural Newborn Reflexes	
Reflex + Normal Duration	**Cause**	**Effect**
Stepping (Walking or Dancing): Birth to 5–6 months	Held upright with feet touching a solid surface	• Appears to take steps or dance
Crawling: Birth to 5–6 months	Placed on stomach	• Pulls legs under body and kicks out in crawling motion
Symmetrical Tonic Neck: 6–9 months to 1–3 years	Head flexed forward, extending the back of the neck (or vice versa)	• Upper extremities will contract and the lower extremities will extend
Swimming (Diving): Birth to 4–6 months	Submersion in water	• Waving/kicking of arms like swimming • Rolling over • Open eyes • Bradycardia • Of note the newborn can still aspirate
Head and Body Righting: Birth for lifetime	Rapid loss of balance	• Promotes head control, rolling, sitting, crawling, and standing
Parachuting: 8–9 months to 1 year	Held upright and the body is rotated quickly to face forward (as in falling)	• Extension of arms forward as if to break a fall

The position statement revised in 2017 from the Food and Drug Administration (FDA) currently advises that

> exposure to [anesthetic] medicines for lengthy periods of time or over multiple surgeries or procedures may negatively affect brain development in children younger than 3 years...exposure to general anesthetic and sedation drugs for more than 3 hours can cause widespread loss of nerve cells in the developing brain; and studies in young animals suggested these changes resulted in long-term negative effects on the animals' behavior or learning.

The FDA urges considering combining surgical procedures into one anesthetic, if applicable, and delaying the procedure until after age 3 if not urgent or emergent. This is an ongoing discussion and likely will be for several years. In any event, what is known is that anesthesia, while necessary for surgery, does not positively affect brain development.

KEY TAKEAWAYS

- Newborn patients feel and have a physiological response to pain.
- Neuronal differentiation in embryonic development determines the makeup of the central nervous system, the brain, and spinal cord.
- The brain consists of various lobes, all with different functions, with the cerebrum accounting for 75% of all neurons.
- The peripheral nervous system includes the somatic and autonomic nervous system.
- The somatic nervous system connects skin to skeletal muscles.
- The autonomic nervous system is divided between the parasympathetic and sympathetic nervous system.
- The parasympathetic and sympathetic nervous systems have complimentary roles for each target organ.
- Newborns have innate reflexes critical for processes, such as sucking (feeding) and preventing injury.
- Anesthesia in a duration-, dose-, and timing-related exposure during peak synaptogenesis may promote neuroapoptosis in the developing brain, potentially resulting in impaired cognition, among other issues, later in life.

1.2: CARDIOVASCULAR SYSTEM

Claire Rizk

LEARNING OBJECTIVES

- Conceptualize the anatomic and physiological differences between pediatric and adult heart.
- Understand how fetal embryology and circulation contribute to neonatal hemodynamics.
- Discuss components of cardiac output and cardiopulmonary interactions and their importance for anesthetic care.

INTRODUCTION

The heart continues to grow and develop with the body from the neonatal period through adulthood. Understanding the concepts of cardiac physiology and pathophysiology as they pertain to children is integral to delivering safe, effective care. This section details the important differences in the physiology of pediatric cardiovascular system compared to their adult counterparts. Due to these differences, neonates and young children especially are at higher risk of rapid deterioration and thus developing an appropriate anesthetic plan that considers their fragility reduces morbidity and mortality.

EMBRYOLOGY

The heart is the first organ to form within an embryo and begins functioning during the 4th week of gestation. Formation of the heart begins with the mesoderm of a trilaminar embryo, which differentiates into four cell lines—one being cardiogenic.[1] The cardiogenic mesoderm initially forms a cardiac crescent and then folds to create a linear heart tube. By day 28, the linear tube has looped creating discernible atria and ventricles. The mature heart is developed by day 50 postconception.[2] Disruption to the initial embryogenesis of the heart results in congenital heart defects, which affect approximately 1% of the population.[3]

ANATOMY OF THE HEART
FUNCTIONAL ANATOMY

The fully formed heart consists of four chambers: a right and left atrium in addition to two pumping chambers—the right and left ventricle. The pulmonary artery arises from the right ventricle and carries deoxygenated blood to the lungs, while the aorta arises from the left ventricle and carries oxygen-rich blood to the body. The left ventricle has a thicker myocardium to pump against the systemic vascular resistance of the body, while the right ventricle is thinner walled. In terms of development, as the left ventricle adjusts to increasing systemic blood pressure, it develops more muscle mass.[4] The right atrium is more compliant and thinner walled than the left ventricle.

Contraction of the left ventricle is concentric, whereas the right ventricle is longitudinal. As the ventricles contract to eject blood to their respective circuits, they squeeze against one another creating more force that either ventricle would generate acting alone. Ventricular interactions are an important component of maximizing contraction and thus if one ventricle is underfilled or overdistended, it impedes ejection.[5] The myocardium is supplied with oxygenated blood from the coronary arteries, which arise from the aorta and are filled in diastole. The left ventricle specifically has both a left coronary and circumflex coronary artery, whereas the right ventricle is supplied only by the right coronary artery. Normal cardiac anatomy, pressures, and saturation of each chamber are shown in **Figure 1.3**. The heart size grows with the rest of the body, meaning the heart chambers enlarge and the myocardium continues to thicken until young adulthood.[6]

ELECTRICAL SYSTEM OF THE HEART

The electrical system of the heart is another important component of cardiac anatomy as it carries signals that cause contraction of each chamber in sync with the others and maximize the ejection of the ventricles. Each cardiac cell has the ability to produce an electrical signal. The initial action potential travels from the sinoatrial (SA) node located in the right atrium to cause the atria to contract, sending blood through the atrioventricular (AV) valves to the ventricles. The

then across a patent foramen ovale (PFO) to the left atrium and then left ventricle, where it can be pumped to the fetus's upper body, including brain and myocardium. The other half of the blood is transferred from the umbilical vein to the liver and then to the inferior vena cava (IVC) via the ductus venosus, where it mixes with the deoxygenated blood from the lower part of the body and is then returned to the right atrium and right ventricle, where it is ejected into the pulmonary artery but does not travel to the lungs instead going across the patent ductus arteriosus (PDA) to the descending aorta to supply the lower half of the body. A portion of this blood travels through the umbilical arteries back to the mother's blood supply for reoxygenation. Fetal circulation thus runs in parallel where the brain and myocardium are supplied with well-oxygenated blood via the left side of the heart and the lower body is provided with less oxygenated blood traveling through the right side of the heart (Figure 1.4).[7]

TRANSITIONAL CIRCULATION

Transitional circulation occurs with the birth of the fetus and clamping of the umbilical cord. With the first cry, the baby opens their lungs, which are filled with air, and thus reduces the pulmonary vascular resistance (PVR). Then by clamping the umbilical cord, low-resistance placental circulation ceases, thus raising systemic vascular resistance (SVR). During this time, there is an increase in pulmonary blood flow and thus return of blood to the left atrium, increasing pressure in the chamber relative to pressure in the right atrium, which causes closure of the foramen ovale.[8] Over the next days and weeks, the PDA closes due to rising oxygen levels and decreased circulating

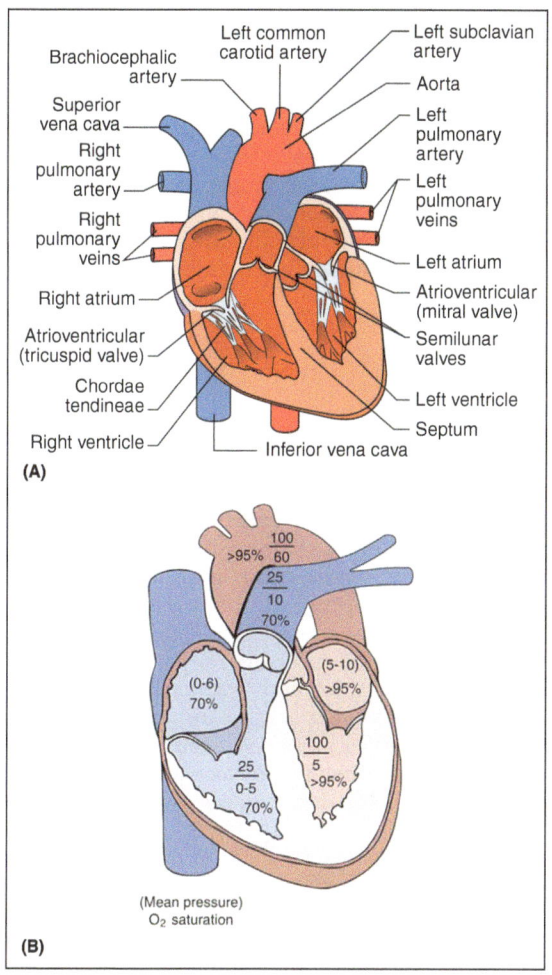

Figure 1.3: (A) Normal cardiac anatomy; (B) normal ventricle pressures.

Source: From Johnson FK, Johnson RA, Rhodes SA. Heart. In: Tkacs NC, Herrmann LL, Johnson RL, eds. *Advanced Physiology and Pathophysiology: Essentials for Clinical Practice.* Springer Publishing. 2020: Fig. 10.39A; Chiang LK, Dunn AE. Cardiology. In: Siberry GK, Iannone R, eds. *The Johns Hopkins Hospital Harriet Lane handbook.* 15th ed. Mosby; 2000:154.

impulse then reaches the AV node, where conduction slows allowing blood to fully empty from the atria. Then the signal travels to the bundle branches where they travel to the apex of the heart. The ventricles contract when the signal travels from the apex through the ventricle walls.[4]

FETAL CIRCULATION

The main job of the heart is to deliver oxygen to the tissue by receiving deoxygenated blood from the body, pumping it to the lungs to become oxygenated and then pumping oxygen-rich blood to the body. However, blood will always travel the path of least resistance, thus optimizing oxygen delivery means taking into account the systemic and pulmonary vascular resistance. In adults, pulmonary vascular resistance is almost always lower than systemic vascular resistance, but in neonates, that is not the case because of fetal circulation and transition to extrauterine life.

During the fetal period, blood flows through placental circulation bypassing the lungs, which are filled with fluid rather than air. Instead, oxygenated blood from the mother passes through an umbilical vein inserted into the placenta. Half of this blood is then sent to the fetus's right atrium and

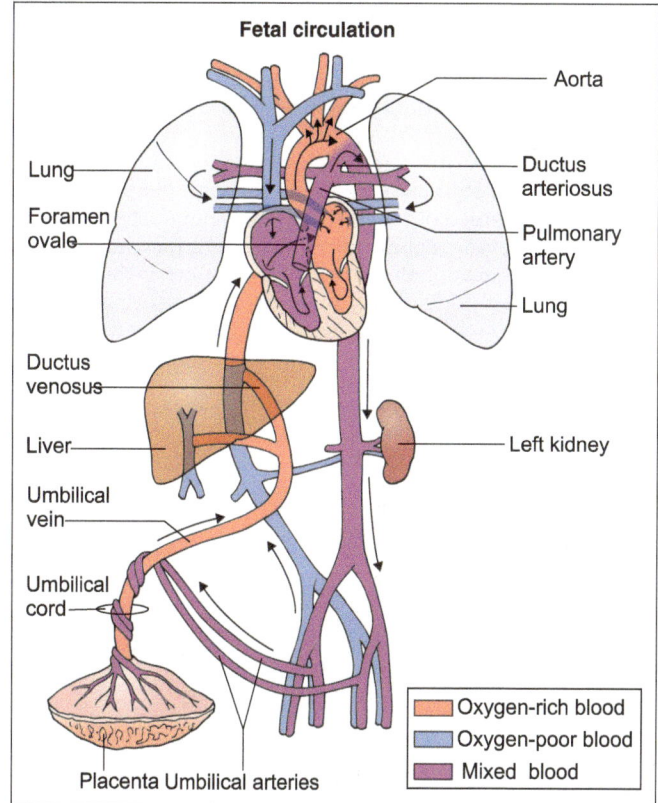

Figure 1.4: Fetal circulation.

Source: From Nantais-Smith L, Herrington C, Kadrofske M. Placental Development and Function. In: Jnah AJ, Trembath AN, eds. *Fetal and Neonatal Physiology for the Advanced Practice Nurse.* Springer Publishing. 2018: Fig. 2.8.

prostaglandin after birth. During periods of stress, such as pain, acidosis, sepsis, and hypothermia, neonates may revert to fetal circulation due to increased PVR, resulting in shunting of blood through the PDA or PFO.[9] The neonate may exhibit differential cyanosis found by measure pre- and postductal saturation (pulse oximetry measured the right limb and lower limb). If there are known right-to-left shunts, more blood is going to the body than the lungs and this should be taken into account when using inhalation of intravenous anesthetic agents.[10]

PHYSIOLOGY

As previously mentioned, the job of the heart is to delivery oxygen to the tissue. However, children, particularly neonates, have higher metabolic demands and less reserve than their adult counterparts, but the job their hearts need to fulfill remains the same. Children's cardiovascular system continues to develop throughout childhood and their physiological differences from adults' place them at higher risk of circulatory compromise, especially during procedures. Thus, understanding and thoughtfulness when developing a care plan are imperative.

CARDIAC OUTPUT

Cardiac output is simply determined by stroke volume multiplied by heart rate. Stroke volume refers to the amount of blood the heart can be ejected per minute and is determined by the preload, contractility, and afterload on the heart. Finally, atrial–ventricular synchrony maximizes ejection volume, and any arrhythmias can reduce cardiac output. Normal heart rate and blood pressure parameters for children by age are described in **Table 1.3**.

Stroke Volume

Preload

Preload is defined as end-diastolic volume in the ventricle after contraction. Volume status, venous return, and ventricular compliance are important components of increasing preload. Based on the Frank–Starling curve (**Figure 1.5**), by increasing preload cardiac output also increases until a plateau is reached because whatever blood is returned through the venous system will be pumped out to the body. As venous return reaches an adequate level, cardiac output no longer increases as evidenced by a plateau in the curve. Venous return is determined by the gradient between mean systemic pressure and right atrial pressure, where mean systemic pressure is influenced by vascular tone and volume. In contrast to arterioles, veins are easily distensible, and two-thirds of the body's volume resides in venous capacitance vessels.[5] Maintaining a low right atrial pressure is key to promoting venous return to maximize preload. In a less compliant ventricle as seen in neonates, increased preload may not result in increased cardiac output.[11] The ventricles in neonates are more fibrous and thus less able to respond to changes in volume.[12] Neonates possess a degree of diastolic dysfunction, meaning their ventricles are unable to relax and fill completely. Essentially, neonates operate along the flat portion of the Frank–Starling curve.[6] Diastolic dysfunction is exacerbated as filling time decreases with increased heart rate.

Contractility

Contractility is the ability of the myocytes to convert electrical signals into the ejection of blood. Cardiac contractility in the neonatal period is operating near full capacity due to high levels of circulating catecholamines and hormones produced during late gestation.[13] However, as mentioned previously, neonatal hearts are composed of fibrous tissue, which is less organized than adult myocardium, limiting the force generated during contraction. Neonatal myocytes rely heavily on calcium as a substrate for contraction due to immature cellular structures and thus optimizing plasma calcium can aid in increasing cardiac output via contractility.[14] Contractility can be modulated with adrenergic agonists like epinephrine and norepinephrine as well as adjunct calcium, but because of already high levels of catecholamines, the neonatal heart may be less responsive to additional agents.[15] The innervation of the heart changes over time, and neonatal hearts are primarily dominated by the parasympathetic system, making them prone to vagal response, including bradycardia. As their nervous system continues to develop, the sympathetic system will become more prominent. Acidosis, hypercarbia, hypoxia, and electrolyte derangements can inhibit myocardial performance.[6] Contractility is negatively affected by anesthetic agents; thus, close monitoring for myocardial depression is essential during induction and throughout procedures.

Afterload

Afterload is described as the pressure the left ventricle pumps against during systole. Neonates are less able to respond to increasing afterload. In terms of modulation,

Table 1.3	Normal Heart Rate and Blood Pressure Parameters for Children		
Age	Heart Rate (beats/min)	Blood Pressure (mm Hg)	Respiratory Rate (breaths/min)
Premature	110–170	SBP 55–75 DBP 35–45	40–70
0–3 months	110–160	SBP 65–85 DBP 45–55	35–55
3–6 months	110–160	SBP 70–90 DBP 50–65	30–45
6–12 months	90–160	SBP 80–100 DBP 55–65	22–38
1–3 years	80–150	SBP 90–105 DBP 55–70	22–30
3–6 years	70–120	SBP 95–110 DBP 60–75	20–24
6–12 years	60–110	SBP 100–120 DBP 60–75	16–22
>12 years	60–100	SBP 110–135 DBP 65–85	12–20

DBP, diastolic blood pressure; SBP, systolic blood pressure.

Source: From Zeno R, Kosla J, Melnyk BM. Evidence-based assessment of children and adolescents. In Gawlik KS, Melnyk BM, Teall AM, eds. Evidence-Based Physical Examination: Best Practices for Health and Well-Being Assessment. Springer Publishing; 2020:57, Table 4.1.

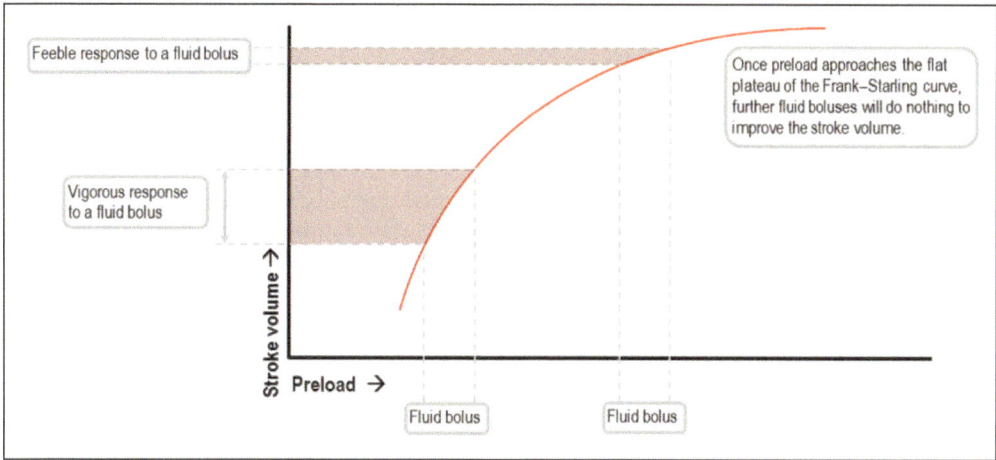

Figure 1.5: Laryngeal cleft extending into through the cricoid cartilage.

afterload can be reduced with medication, whereby preload and contractility can be more challenging to change.[16] Advantageously, neonates and children have less arterial stiffness compared to their adult counterparts (blood pressure increases with age), and thus, afterload tends to be lower. The pressure–volume loops in Figure 1.6 depict how changing the loading conditions of the ventricle can change cardiac output.

Oxygen-Carrying Capacity

In addition to maintaining adequate preload, maximizing oxygen-carrying capacity of the blood flowing through the body can help increase cardiac output. All neonates undergo a period of neonatal anemia related to shorter lifetime of red blood cells compared to adults, shift in the oxygen-dissociation curve from high–oxygen affinity fetal hemoglobin to hemoglobin A, and lower endogenous circulating epopoietin compared to adult.[17]

Heart Rate and Rhythm

Heart rate modulation is a more important component of cardiac output in infants than in older children or adults. Heart rate and rhythm in infants and children can again be significantly affected by hormonal activation, electrolytes, and body temperature. Heart rate in the neonate should be greater than 100 beats per minute (bpm), and some studies show that a heart rate greater than 120 bpm is necessary to ensure adequate cardiac output.[15] Bradycardia may result in inadequate oxygen delivery to the tissue. Ensuring that each heartbeat is synchronous promotes maximal ejection and optimizes cardiac output. In neonates and young children, the ability to increase cardiac output by increasing stroke volume is limited. As infants grow, their heart becomes better able to respond to volume and catecholamines creating increased cardiac reserve.

Variations in Cardiac Output

Signs of low cardiac output include decreased perfusion evidenced by prolonged capillary refill, cool extremity temperature, decreased urine output, evidence of decreased end-organ perfusion (rising blood urea nitrogen/creatinine), low mixed venous saturation measured from the right atrium–superior vena cava junction, and rising lactate.[15] Overall, cognizance of maintaining appropriate cardiac output includes attention to heart rate, AV synchrony, preload, contractility, and afterload to promote good outcomes.

CARDIOPULMONARY INTERACTIONS

Understanding how the lungs and heart work together in the thoracic cavity is integral to maximizing oxygen transport. Both the heart and lungs reside in the thoracic cavity and are composed of elastic structures with both compliance and resistance, which are related to pressure. The transmembrane pressure of a chamber is equivalent to the difference between extracavitary pressure and intracavitary pressures.[5] Using these principles, cardiac output can be augmented to maximize flow through the vessels and promote oxygen delivery. It is important to remember that venous return is governed by mean systemic pressure, which is the blood volume and capacitance of the circulation, and the pressure in the right atrium.

In normal conditions, during inspiration, the pressure in the thoracic cavity is negative, which allows air to rush into the lungs. For the cardiac system, a negative intrathoracic pressure promotes venous return as the right atrium distends because of an increased transmembrane gradient between the chest and right atrium, and the diaphragm distends increasing the pressure of the venous circulation, specifically vessels draining into the IVC. The decreased right atrial pressure and increased pressure of the IVC creates favorable conditions for venous return.[18] However, in patients who are intubated, the ventilator create positive pressure ventilation (PPV) by forcing breaths into the chest and then maintaining end-expiratory pressures (PEEP) that can be supraphysiologic. Positive intrathoracic pressure decreases the transmembrane pressure of the right atrium, which increases its cavitary pressure and decreases the gradient between IVC and right atrial pressure, limiting venous return.[19] In patients with limited compliance of the chambers of the heart, venous return is a key component to cardiac output and thus may need additional volume to maximize preload for adequate cardiac output. Additionally, early removal of PPV may be favorable in some patients with cardiac disease who are preload dependent.[20]

Using the principles discussed earlier by creating positive-intrathoracic pressure through ventilatory strategies, ventricular afterload is reduced because there is reduced transmembrane pressure between the pressure within the ventricle and the pressure of the chest cavity. To eject the ventricle must overcome the transmembrane pressure, and thus negative intrathoracic pressure increases the pressure the ventricle needs

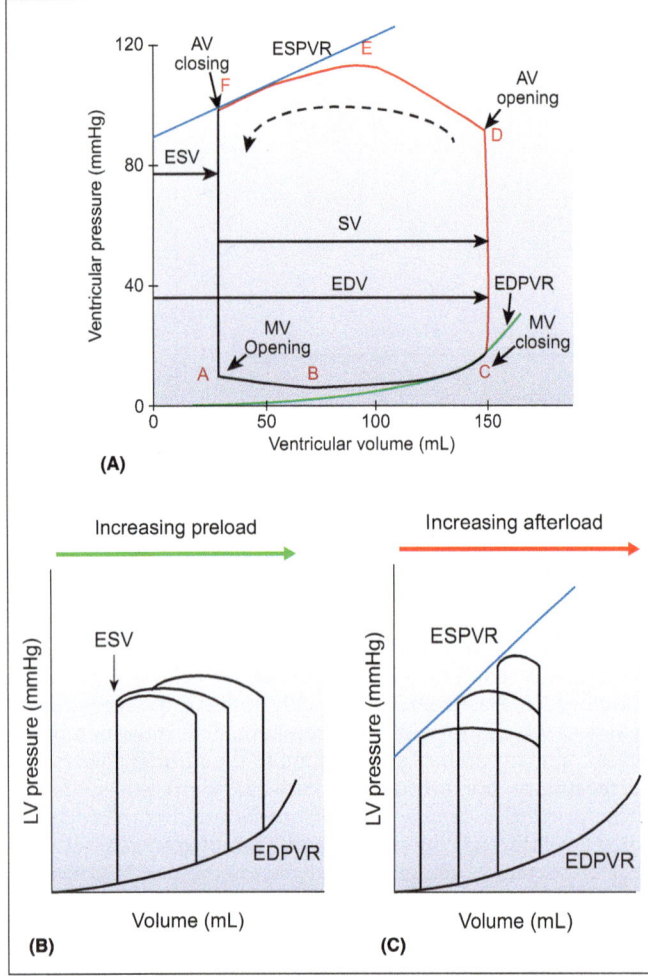

Figure 1.6: Pressure–volume loops (A–C).

(A) Depiction of a left ventricular pressure volume loop in which ventricular volume is on the *x*-axis and pressure is on the *y*-axis. Starting from point A, the mitral valve opens and blood flows into the ventricle, building ventricular volume to point B, where the mitral valve closes. At this point, the ventricle begins to contract, building pressure to point C, where the aortic valve opens, allowing ejection to the body; at this point, volume in the ventricle is decreasing and the aortic valve closes again at point D. From D back to A is a period of isovolumetric relaxation of the ventricle and the cycle begins again. The difference between end-systolic and end-diastolic volume is the "stroke volume" of the ventricle. (B) Effects of preload on stroke volume. As it increases, so does ventricular volume, thus increasing stroke volume. (C) Inverse relationship of afterload on stroke volume. As afterload increases (red loop), isovolumetric contraction phase is prolonged as the ventricle builds enough pressure to overcome LV afterload—this results in less stroke volume and higher LV end-systolic volume. Conversely, the green loop shows that as afterload is decreased so is time for isovolumetric contraction and end-systolic volume thus increasing the stroke volume.

AV, aortic valve; EDPVR, end-diastolic pressure–volume relationship; EDV, end-diastolic volume; ESPVR, end-systolic pressure–volume relationship; ESV, end-systolic volume; LV, left ventricle; MV, mitral valve; SV, stroke volume.

Source: From A–C: A, Johnson FK, Johnson RA, Rhodes SA. Heart. In: Tkacs NC, Herrmann LL, Johnson RL, eds. *Advanced Physiology and Pathophysiology: Essentials for Clinical Practice.* Springer Publishing. 2020: Fig. 10.27, Fig. 10.28, Fig. 10.29 B, B–D, https://www.cvphysiology.com/Cardiac%20Function/CF025.

to generate for ejection.[5] In turn, careful consideration should be given to ventricular function in addition to respiratory mechanics prior to discontinuing PPV.

CONGENITAL HEART DEFECTS

Congenital heart disease (CHD) is the most prevalent congenital anomaly representing eight to nine births per 1,000.[3] Many children born with CHD have associated genetic disorders, such as trisomy 21, Noonan syndrome, and Turner's syndrome.[21] Of the patient diagnosed with CHD, 25% of them will have critical CHD, which will require urgent surgical intervention in the first year of life due to one of three types of lesions: right heart obstructive, left heart obstructive, and mixing lesions.[22]

Right heart obstructive lesions are those that present with hypoxia and are likely related to decrease in pulmonary blood flow. Examples include tetralogy of Fallot, tricuspid atresia, and Ebstein's anomaly. Left heart obstructive lesions present with decreased peripheral pulses, signs of end-organ injury, feeding intolerance, and lethargy. Examples of left heart obstructive lesions include coarctation of the aorta, hypoplastic left heart syndrome, and mitral stenosis. Finally, mixing lesions are consistent with increased work of breathing, tachypnea, and signs of congestive heart failure. Lesions in which mixing occurs include one of the following components: atrial septal defect, ventricular septal defect, or PDA.[23] As patients with congenital heart defects are likely to require anesthesia in the first year of life for surgical or catheter-based interventions, it is imperative that anesthesia providers give careful consideration to the direction of blood flow, resistance of the vascular beds, and expected parameters for oxygen saturation. For additional information regarding the anesthetic management of patients presenting with CHD, please refer to **Chapter 93**, "Care of Children with Heart Disease Undergoing Noncardiac Surgery."

KEY TAKEAWAYS

- The job of the heart is to supply the tissue with oxygen-rich blood to meet metabolic demands.
- Blood will flow the path of least resistance.
- Neonates are at risk of reverting to fetal circulation during periods of stress, which will create shunting from systemic to pulmonary circulation.
- Cardiac Output = Stroke Volume × Heart Rate
  - Stroke volume is preload, contractility, and afterload.
  - Maintaining AV synchrony is imperative
- Infant cardiac output is more heart rate and calcium-dependent than adults.
- Infants have limited ability to augment stroke volume.
- PPV can limit venous return and thus compromise cardiac output.
- PPV, however, can reduce ventricular afterload to promote cardiac output in situations of ventricular dysfunction.
- Congenital heart defects create different physiological conditions than normal hearts that alter the flow of blood and oxygenation to the body.

1.3: PEDIATRIC AIRWAY

Lauren S. Buck, Yann-Fuu Kou, and Matthew M. Smith

> **LEARNING OBJECTIVES**
> - Understand the anatomy of the upper airway, larynx, and trachea.
> - Identify common sites of airway obstruction in the pediatric patient.

INTRODUCTION

Airway management of children during surgical procedures can be difficult. Children can quickly decompensate when the airway is obstructed. It is important for all healthcare providers, especially anesthesia providers who care for children, to be familiar with the entire airway to promptly recognize and intervene for potential airway obstruction. This section provides a brief review of normal airway anatomy and physiology from the nasal cavity down to the trachea. It also briefly identifies common pathologies at each level, which may lead to airway obstruction (Table 1.4).

ANATOMIC SITES OF AIRWAY PATHOLOGY AND OBSTRUCTION

NASAL CAVITY AND NASOPHARYNX

The external nose is composed of superiorly paired nasal bones, upper cartilages supporting the mid-vault, and lower cartilages maintaining patency of the nasal vestibule. Internally, the nasal septum separates the right and left nasal cavity. A septal deviation can cause narrowing and obstruction of the nasal passage and may be present in one-third of children[1]. The lateral wall of the nose has outpouching turbinates, which help humidify the air we breathe. The turbinates separate the nasal cavities into the lower and upper pathway, with the lower pathway between the inferior turbinate and nasal floor and the upper pathway located above the inferior turbinate and below the middle turbinate. The middle turbinate is a vascular structure connected with the cribriform plate; therefore, it is important to stay along the nasal floor when placing any device into the nose, such as a nasopharyngeal airway or endotracheal tube, to avoid excessive bleeding or inadvertent perforation of pyriform fossa (Figure 1.7).

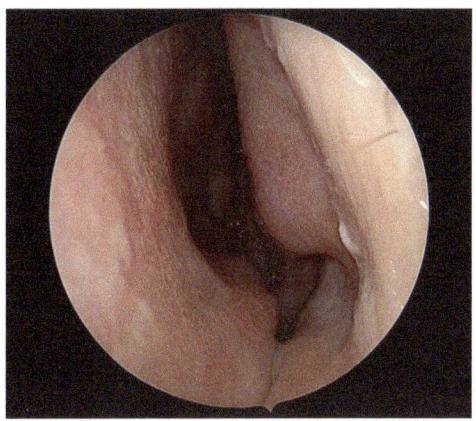

Figure 1.7: Left nasal cavity with left inferior turbinate and prominent septal spur.

Table 1.4	Notable Airway Pathologies by Anatomic Subsite
Anatomic Subsite	**Airway Pathology**
Nasal cavity	Pyriform aperture stenosis Choanal atresia Septal deviation
Nasopharynx	Adenoid hypertrophy
Oral cavity	Macroglossia Micro/retrognathia Temporomandibular joint ankylosis (inability to open mouth)
Oropharynx	Palatine or lingual tonsillar hypertrophy Glossoptosis Vallecular cyst
Larynx	Laryngomalacia Subglottic stenosis Vocal cord paralysis Posterior glottic stenosis
Trachea	Congenital tracheal stenosis (complete tracheal rings) Tracheomalacia Extrinsic compression Acquired tracheal stenosis

The pediatric nose functions similarly to the adult nose, helping to warm and humidify inspired air. Infants, however, are obligate nasal breathers and rely on patent nasal passages to efficiently breathe during the first few months of life. Infants with congenital narrowing or obstruction of the nose will present shortly after birth with significant respiratory distress, especially with feeding.

The posterior nasal cavity opens into the nasopharynx via the choana. In some children, the nasal choanae are narrow/stenotic or never fully opened during development. When there is no opening from the nasal cavity into the nasopharynx, this is known as choanal atresia (Figure 1.8). The superior–posterior wall of the nasopharynx is where the adenoid tissue is attached. Adenoid tissue is lymphatic tissue that is part of Waldeyer's ring, which helps filter environmental antigens. Occasionally, the adenoid tissue can be so enlarged that it completely occludes the nasopharynx and the posterior choanae, leading to nasal obstruction. This adenoid tissue is extremely vascular and can easily bleed when manipulated (Figure 1.9).

ORAL CAVITY AND OROPHARYNX

The oral cavity starts at the vermillion border of the lips and extends to the circumvallate papilla of the tongue. This includes all the maxillary and mandibular dentition. The tongue can be a common site of airway obstruction. Using an oral airway to help bypass the tongue and abate airway obstruction is sometimes needed, especially for children with macroglossia or significant base of tongue collapse. During intubation, the tongue can be swept to the patient's left side with a laryngoscope to view the larynx more easily. Limited mouth opening is important to assess prior to children being

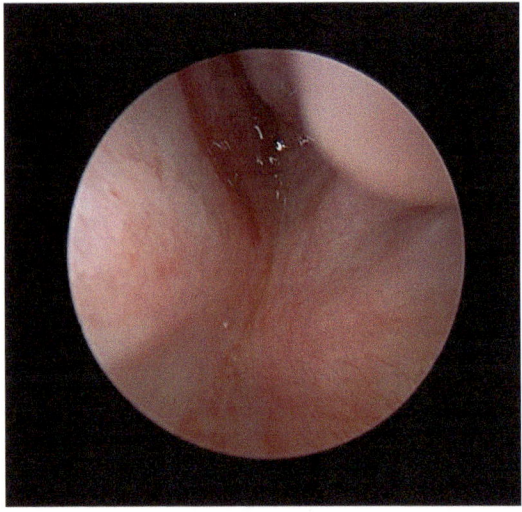

Figure 1.8: Left nasal cavity with choanal atresia.

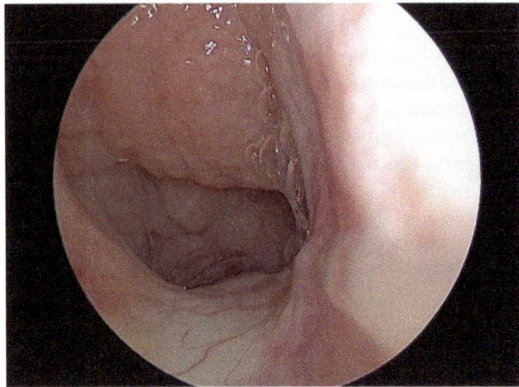

Figure 1.9: View of nasopharyngeal tonsillar tissue, or adenoids, within the nasopharynx from the left nasal cavity.

Table 1.5	Mallampati Classification
Class	Description
I	Easily view the entire soft palate, fauces, uvula, and tonsillar pillars
II	Easily view the soft palate, fauces, and most of the uvula. Cannot view tonsillar pillars easily
III	Easily view the soft palate, base of the uvula. Cannot view the pillars or fauces
IV	Cannot view the soft palate. Only hard palate can be viewed

Source: From Mallampati SR, Gatt SP, Gugino LD, et al. A clinical sign to predict difficult tracheal intubation: a prospective study. *Can Anaesth Soc J.* 1985;32(4):429–434. doi:10.1007/BF03011357.

anesthetized. Microstomia (small mouth opening) can be congenital or secondary due to trauma and can limit the ability to open the mouth, which may make airway manipulation and intubation more challenging. Trismus (inability to open the temporomandibular joint) is also a condition that can limit the opening of the mouth making intubation difficult.

The oropharynx starts at the circumvallate papilla and includes the palatine tonsils, lingual tonsils, tonsillar pillars, soft palate, uvula, and the vallecula. It is important to classify each patient according to the Mallampati classification system in order to understand the amount of oropharyngeal obstruction present[2] (Table 1.5). As mentioned previously, Waldeyer's ring comprises the nasopharyngeal tonsils (adenoids), palatine tonsils ("tonsils"), and the lingual tonsils. The palatine tonsils sit in the lateral oropharynx between the anterior and posterior tonsillar pillars. These are graded by size starting at 0 (absent), 1+ (0%–25% obstruction of the oropharynx), 2+ (26%–50%), 3+ (51%–75%), and 4+ (76%–100%). Lingual tonsils are found on the posterior aspect of the base of tongue. Lingual tonsil hypertrophy can also lead to difficulty with traditional intubation methods.

Pierre–Robin sequence is the association of micrognathia, glossoptosis, and a U-shaped cleft palate. This is nearly always associated with upper airway obstruction. The inciting incident in utero is mandibular hypoplasia leading to glossoptosis, which prevents proper fusion of the soft palate[3]. Children with Pierre–Robin sequence often experience difficulty with anesthesia due to their significant airway obstruction and can be very difficult to expose with direct laryngoscopy. Temporizing measures can include a nasopharyngeal airway and prone positioning.

LARYNX

The larynx is a crucial organ that serves as the branch point between the digestive tract and the airway. As such, it has three major functions: airway patency, airway protection, and phonation. The larynx is divided into three main subsites: the supraglottis (epiglottis, arytenoids, aryepiglottic folds, and false vocal cords), the glottis (true vocal cords), and the subglottis (Figures 1.10 and 1.11). The infant larynx is higher in the neck than the adult larynx, with the cricoid cartilage located roughly at the level of the fourth cervical vertebra. The larynx gradually descends with age to the level of the sixth cervical vertebra.

The rigid framework of the larynx consists of the hyoid bone, thyroid cartilage, and cricoid cartilage. In children, the cricoid cartilage surrounds the subglottic space as the only complete ring of a normal airway, making the subglottis the narrowest portion of the airway in children (Figure 1.12). This makes the subglottis particularly susceptible to airway obstruction due to swelling or scarring. Small changes in the diameter of the airway will cause significant increases in resistance to airflow as explained by Poiseuille's law. Functionally, halving the diameter will increase the resistance to airflow by 16 times.

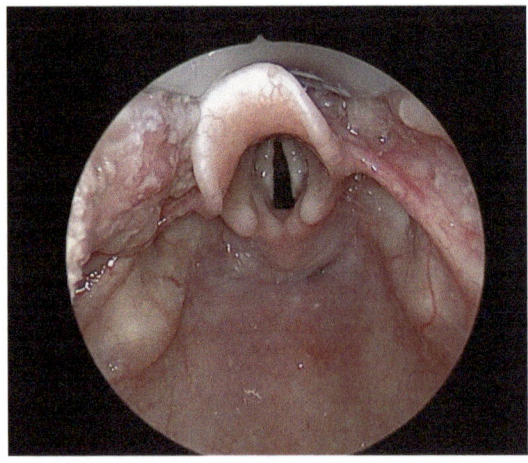

Figure 1.10: Normal larynx.

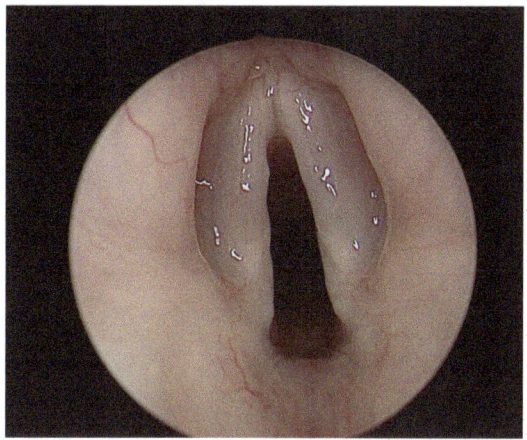

Figure 1.11: Normal vocal cords.

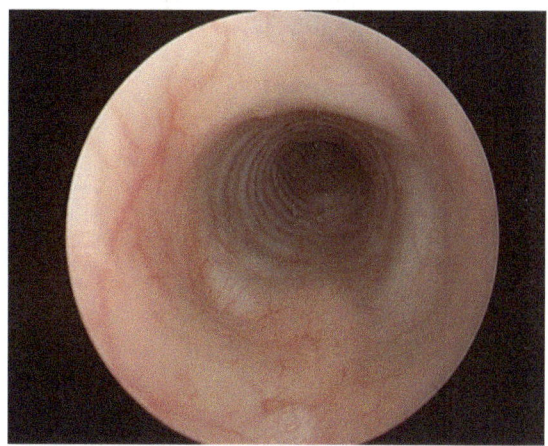

Figure 1.12: Normal subglottis and trachea.

Both motor and sensory innervation of the larynx is from the vagus nerve. The majority of the motor innervation is from the recurrent laryngeal nerve and injury to this nerve can cause vocal cord paralysis. The sensation to the larynx above the glottis is from the internal branch of the superior laryngeal nerve and below the glottis is from the recurrent laryngeal nerve. These nerves facilitate laryngeal reflexes, such as laryngospasm, where the vocal cords remain closed preventing airflow. This event can occur during induction or emergence from anesthesia and warrants prompt recognition and management.

A commonly used descriptor for direct laryngoscopy is the Cormack–Lehane classification system.[4] This system grades the view of the laryngeal anatomy from 1 to 4, with grade 1 being a full view of the glottis and grade 4 being the inability to see any laryngeal structures. A modified version of the scoring system is now commonly used (Table 1.6).[5]

Stenosis can occur at any level of the larynx, but the subglottis is the most common location (Figure 1.13). Subglottic stenosis (SGS) can be congenital but is more commonly acquired. Advances in neonatal care have improved the survival of premature infants but at the cost of prolonged intubation, leading to subglottic stenosis.[6] Previously, rates of subglottic stenosis following prolonged intubation were as high as 8.3%, but recognition of this problem has led to early interventions and changes in practice. Current rates of subglottic stenosis are estimated at 0.63% to 2.0%.[7] The Cotton–Myer system is the most commonly used grading scale for SGS and allows for communication between providers regarding the airway size (Table 1.7).[8]

Scarring at the level of the vocal cords, or glottis, can be congenital or iatrogenic. Iatrogenic webs can be a result of multiple surgeries, such as with recurrent respiratory papillomatosis. Congenital anterior glottic webs are associated with velocardiofacial syndrome.[9] Posterior glottic stenosis (PGS) is often iatrogenic due to prolonged intubation. Long-term immobility of the vocal cords from PGS can eventually lead to cricoarytenoid joint fixation.

A common cause of laryngeal airway obstruction in infants is laryngomalacia (Figure 1.14). Laryngomalacia is the most common cause of stridor in infants. This is often described as immature cartilage or a lack of neuromuscular tone of the larynx, leading to dynamic obstruction. Common findings include an omega-shaped epiglottis that is curled

Table 1.6	Modified Cormack–Lehane Grading System				
	1	2		3	4
Original Cormack and Lehane system	Full view of the glottis	Partial view of the glottis		Only epiglottis visible	Neither glottis nor epiglottis visible
View at laryngoscopy	E / LI	⌣		⌣	⌣
	1	2a	2b	3	4
Modified system	As for original Cormack and Lehane above	Partial view of the glottis	Arytenoids or posterior part of the vocal cords only just visible	As for original Cormack and Lehane above	As for original Cormack and Lehane above

E, epiglottis; LI, laryngeal inlet.

Source: From Yentis SM, Lee DJH. Evaluation of an improved scoring system for the grading of direct laryngoscopy. *Anaesthesia.* 1998;53:1041–1044. doi:10.1046/j.1365-2044.1998.00605.x.

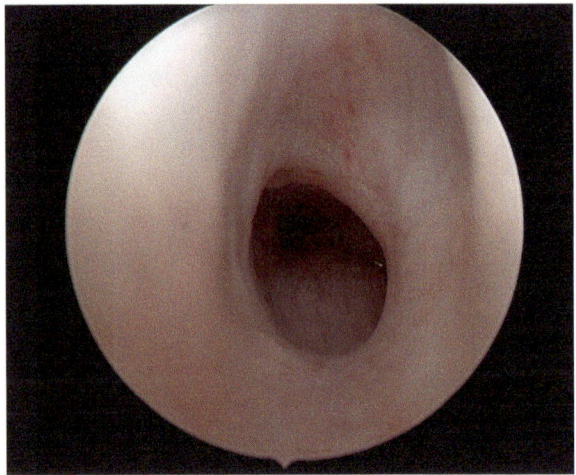

Figure 1.13: Subglottic stenosis.

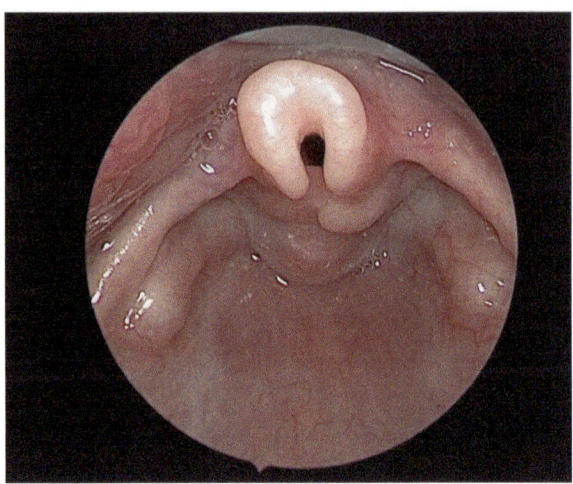

Figure 1.14: Laryngomalacia.

on itself, short aryepiglottic folds, and redundant arytenoid tissue that collapses in with inspiration. Severe cases are associated with failure to thrive, obstructive apneas, and cyanosis.

TRACHEA

The infant trachea when compared to the adult and childhood trachea is highly collapsible. It is composed of incomplete rings of hyaline cartilage with annular ligaments that divide them. The trachealis muscle creates the back wall of the trachea and attaches to the incomplete rings. The distal trachea ends at the carina, which is the branch point of the right and left mainstem bronchi. During development, the trachea and esophagus both originate from the anterior foregut tube. Malformations in this complex process can lead to abnormal connections between the esophagus and trachea, such as tracheoesophageal fistulas and laryngotracheoesophageal clefts (LTECs; Figure 1.15). LTECs vary in length and are classified by the Benjamin–Inglis classification (Figure 1.16). Airway management of these patients is difficult as clefts can be difficult to discern on direct laryngoscopy. Also, during intubation, the endotracheal tube will tend to slip out of the airway, through the cleft, and into the esophagus. Intubation over a rigid or flexible scope to ensure the tube is past the cleft may be ideal, particularly for long clefts, and may require assistance from otolaryngology.

Complete tracheal rings are a rare condition in which the normally incomplete rings are completely closed, thereby narrowing the trachea (Figure 1.17). Symptoms include persistent stridor and worsening respiratory distress over time as

Table 1.7	Cotton–Myer Subglottic Stenosis Grading Scale	
Classification	From	To
Grade I	No obstruction	50% Obstruction
Grade II	51% Obstruction	70% Obstruction
Grade III	71% Obstruction	99% Obstruction
Grade IV	No detectable lumen	

Source: From Cotton RT, Myer CM 3rd, O'Connor DM. Innovations in pediatric laryngotracheal reconstruction. J Pediatr Surg. 1992;27:196–200. doi:10.1016/0022-3468(92)90311-t.

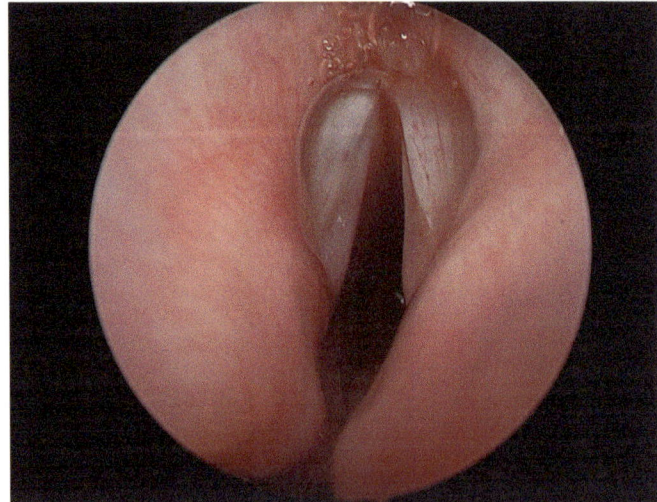

Figure 1.15: Laryngeal cleft extending into through the cricoid cartilage.

CHAPTER 1: ANATOMY AND PHYSIOLOGY OF THE PEDIATRIC PATIENT | 15

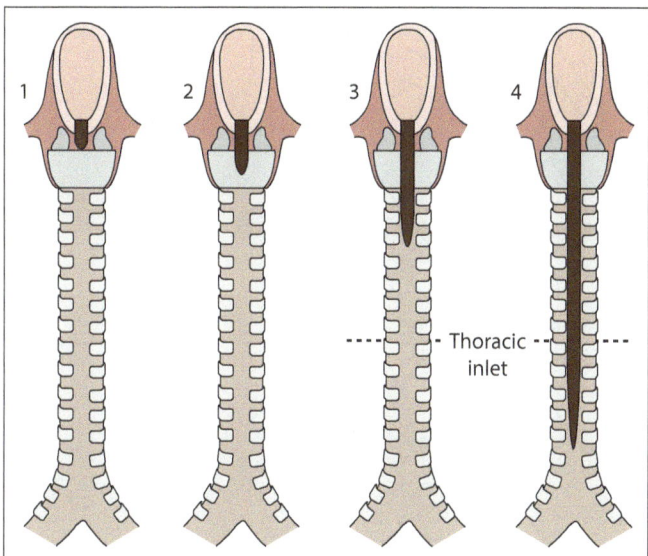

Figure 1.16: Benjamin–Inglis classification of laryngotracheoesophageal clefts. Type 1: to the level of the cricoid cartilage. Type 2: partial cricoid cartilage defect. Type 3: absent posterior cricoid cartilage. Type 4: extends into the trachea.

the airway does not grow in proportion with the child. When treating these children, it is paramount to avoid traumatizing the mucosa in the area of the complete rings as it is more susceptible to airway obstruction due to mucosal edema given the lack of the posterior membranous trachea.

Tracheomalacia is the dynamic collapse of the trachea and can be a significant cause of respiratory distress in infants. External compression of the trachea from aberrant vasculature (pulmonary artery sling and, double aortic arch) can mimic symptoms of tracheomalacia.

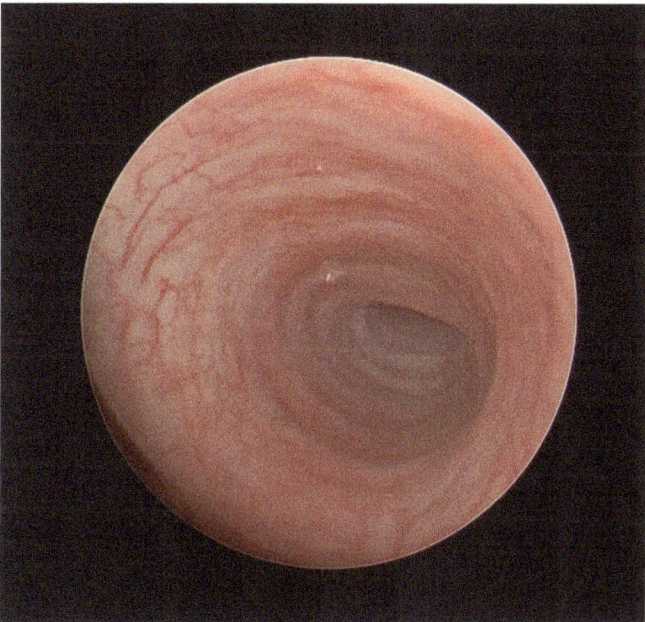

Figure 1.17: Complete tracheal rings.

KEY TAKEAWAYS

- It is essential to understand the anatomy and physiology of the upper airway.
- There are multiple anatomic sites where static or dynamic obstruction can occur in the upper airway.
- Recognition of sites of potential obstruction can help guide management.
- Communication with otolaryngology regarding airway plans and interventions is crucial.

1.4: RESPIRATORY SYSTEM

Sarrah L. Schultz and Robert J. Combs

LEARNING OBJECTIVES

- Adequately describe the anatomy and physiology of the pediatric respiratory system in order to provide safe and effective anesthetic care to pediatric patients.
- Identify which aspects/characteristics of the respiratory system are specific to the pediatric population.
- Understand the mechanics of ventilation in the pediatric patient and the implications for safe delivery of anesthetic care.

INTRODUCTION

To provide safe and effective anesthetic care to pediatric patients, it is vital that anesthesia providers have a fundamental understanding of the anatomy and physiology of the pediatric respiratory system, especially the aspects that are unique to this patient population. The basic functions of the respiratory system are ventilation and perfusion of the alveoli to allow for diffusion of gas into and out of the blood.[1] This statement is universally true regardless of age; however, when caring for pediatric patients, anesthesia providers must take into consideration key developmental factors that make the pediatric respiratory system unique. This section provides an overview of the developmental anatomy and physiology of the pediatric respiratory system, with a particular focus on pulmonary circulation, the developmental mechanics of breathing, and the implications age-related variations have on the delivery of safe and effective anesthetic care to pediatric patients.

LUNG DEVELOPMENT

PRENATAL LUNG DEVELOPMENT

The development of lung tissue begins soon after conception and continues throughout adolescence (Figure 1.18).[2] The embryonic stage of lung development occurs between 3 and 6 weeks' gestation. It is during this time the trachea and two main bronchi form. Following the fourth week of development, the caudal end of the trachea bifurcates to form the left and right primary bronchial buds, with the primary bronchial buds dividing asymmetrically after the fifth week to form the secondary bronchial buds. The new-

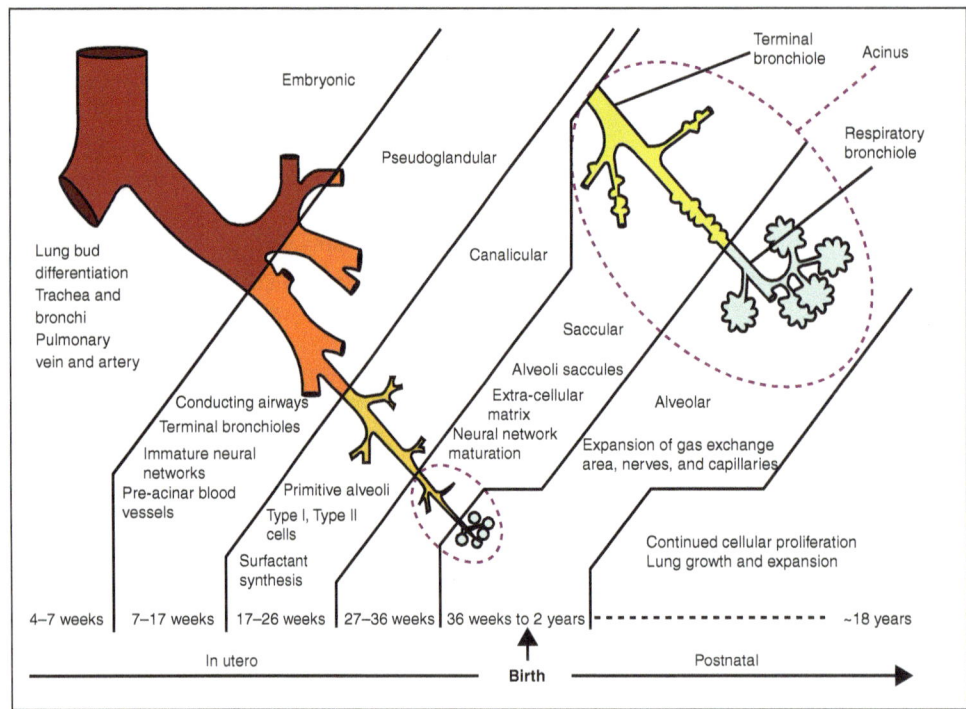

Figure 1.18: Stages of lung development.

Source: From McFadyen JG, Thompson DR, Martin LD. In DS Wheeler, HR Wong, TP Shanley, eds. *Pediatric Critical Care Medicine*. 2nd ed. Springer Publishing; 2014:3–18.

ly formed two bronchial buds on the left and three bronchial buds on the right will ultimately give rise to future lobes of each lung. It is also during this period that the pulmonary vein and artery form. During the pseudoglandular stage (weeks 5–17), the conducting airways are formed as far as the terminal bronchioles and neural networks begin to take shape, and pre-acinar blood vessels are formed. The canalicular phase (weeks 16–25) is most notable for the development of pneumocytes, with Type I cells creating an air–blood barrier where gas exchange will one day occur, and Type II cells responsible for surfactant synthesis. Due to the formation of the gas-exchanging portion of the lungs, some respiration is possible at this stage; therefore, infants born at this stage have the potential to survive if provided with intensive care. During the saccular phase (weeks 24–birth), the extra-cellular matrix develops, neural networks mature, and alveoli saccules form. Pulmonary surfactant production begins in the saccular phase; however, amounts necessary to prevent atelectasis are not produced until 32 weeks. The alveolar phase begins at 36 weeks' gestation and continues for 8 years following birth. This phase is notable for the ongoing expansion of areas of gas exchange with continued alveoli formation as well as pulmonary capillary and nerve networks.

Pulmonary Hypoplasia

Pulmonary hypoplasia is the incomplete development of the lung tissue during the pseudoglandular stage that ultimately limits alveolar development and subsequently impairs gas exchange. The extent of hypoplastic pulmonary tissue depends on the timing of the insult, which can be either primary (idiopathic) in nature or secondary to other congenital anomalies. Clinically, the manifestations range from fatal respiratory insufficiency in neonates (severe form) to chronic lung disease with recurrent respiratory infections (mild form) in adulthood. While the exact incidence is unknown, pulmonary hypoplasia is thought to occur in approximately in 1 out of every 1,000 live births. Incomplete lung development can be classified into three types:[3]

- **Type 1 (agenesis):** the complete absence of pulmonary parenchyma, bronchus, and vessels.
- **Type 2 (aplasia):** the complete absence of pulmonary parenchyma but the presence of a rudimentary bronchus on the affected side.
- **Type 3 (hypoplasia):** the presence of variable amounts of pulmonary parenchyma with a decrease in the number of lung cells, airways, and alveoli.

POSTNATAL LUNG DEVELOPMENT

The lung tissue continues to develop and mature throughout childhood. During the first 2 years of life, enlargement of lungs is a consequence of the increasing number of alveoli; after this point, both the number and size of alveoli increase until the mature lungs form at around 8 years of age. By 8 years of age, the number of alveoli in the lung will reach 300 million, increasing significantly from the 20 million alveolar saccules that are present at birth.[2] This increase in alveoli allows for expansion of surface area from 2.8 m^2 at birth to 75 m^2 by adulthood. Structural changes also occur to facilitate collateral ventilation to distal airways in the event of a proximal obstruction. Pores of Kohn (interalveolar connections) begin to develop during the alveolar stage of lung development, and Lambert's channels (bronchoalveolar connections) begin to develop around 6 years of age. Without these alternative communications, lung tissue is more prone to atelectasis and ventilation and perfusion (V/Q) mismatch, discussed later in this chapter. As such, interbronchiolar connections may develop in diseased lungs to further facilitate collateral ventilation.

VENTILATION

NEUROCHEMICAL CONTROL OF VENTILATION

The neurochemical control system is extremely complex and allows for both involuntary and voluntary breathing.[1] Peripheral chemoreceptors located in the carotid and aortic bodies detect changes in arterial blood oxygenation and relay this information via primary afferent neurons to the medulla oblongata and the pons in the brainstem. In response, respiratory activity is stimulated to maintain normal partial pressure levels of oxygen in the blood. This typically includes increases in both respiratory rate and respiratory volume. In addition, blood flow to the brain and kidneys is increased to prevent deleterious effects secondary to hypoxia. Cardiac output is also increased to maintain blood flood and tissue oxygenation.

Central chemoreceptors located in the medulla oblongata detect changes in arterial partial pressure of carbon dioxide. When changes are detected, impulses are sent to the respiratory center in the brainstem that initiate changes in ventilation aimed at restoring the arterial partial pressure of carbon dioxide to normal. Increase in the arterial partial pressure of carbon dioxide results in an increase in ventilation, which allows more carbon dioxide to be exhaled. Decreases in the arterial partial pressure of carbon dioxide decrease ventilation, thereby increasing the retention of carbon dioxide and allowing the arterial partial pressure of carbon dioxide to return to normal. Central chemoreceptors located near the respiratory center also detect changes in the pH of cerebrospinal fluid (CSF). Small changes in the arterial partial pressure of carbon dioxide lead to alterations in the pH of the CSF, as carbon dioxide freely diffuses across the blood–brain barrier. In an attempt to normalize the pH of the CSF, the respiratory center will stimulate the reparatory center to either decrease or increase ventilation. It is important to note that for approximately the first 3 weeks of life, term neonates have a blunted ventilatory response to hypoxi; however, response to hypercarbia is intact in the term neonate.[4]

A host of airway and pulmonary receptors also contribute to ventilation patterns. Receptors within the lungs also communicate with the respiratory center and provide input to allow for modification of respiratory patterns. Irritant receptors are sensitive to noxious stimulus and trigger the cough reflex, as well as causing increased respiratory rate and bronchoconstriction. Stretch receptors are sensitive to changes in the size or volume of the lungs and signal a decrease in respiratory rate and volume when stimulated. J-receptors (juxtapulmonary capillary receptors) are sensitive to increased pulmonary capillary pressure and result in shallow, rapid breathing, hypotension, and bradycardia when stimulated.

NEONATAL VENTILATION

Ventilation in the neonatal period differs from that of an older child as the newborn is transitioning from intrauterine to extrauterine life. In the neonatal period, hypoxia triggers an increase in minute ventilation, followed by decline in frequency of breathing. This posthypoxic depression is thought to stem from inhibition in the midbrain and other structures rather than a decline in peripheral chemoreceptor firing, although a contribution from the latter cannot be excluded. By the age of 3 weeks, however, hypoxia induces sustained hyperventilation similar to that of older children and adults. Periodic breathing patterns are also a common phenomenon in the neonatal period, with apneic spells lasting typically 5 to 10 seconds. In response to the resulting hypercapnia, newborns will increase ventilation, but to a lesser extent than older children. Should the child be born prematurely, central apnea may be an issue to the immature state of the respiratory center.

LUNG VOLUMES AND CAPACITIES

An understanding of lung volumes and capacities is key to understanding the mechanics of the respiratory systems. Lung volumes are affected by the age and size of a patient, muscle strength, and the static–elastic characteristics of the chest wall and lungs.[2] Tidal volume refers to the amount of gas moved during normal breathing. The tidal volume for both the neonate and adult is approximately 6 mL/kg when at rest. In the neonate, however, the anatomical and physiological dead space is increased, implying an increased portion of the tidal volume is wasted. Residual volume (RV) refers to the amount of gas remaining within the lungs after maximal exhalation. The RV is larger in a neonate than in an adult, primarily due to the increased chest wall compliance, which lacks the ability to maintain a large intrathoracic volume at the end of tidal expiration. The vital capacity is the volume of gas exhaled from the lung following maximal inspiration.[2] Functional residual capacity (FRC) describes the amount of gas remaining in the lung at the end of tidal breath. This serves as an oxygen reservoir during expiration. The FRC of a neonate is similar to that of an adult. The end-expiratory lung volume is usually equal to the FRC; however, it may be higher in pathogenic lungs. Infants end their expiratory phase abruptly when compared to the respiratory pattern of an adult in order to generate positive end-expiratory pressure (PEEP) and avoid derecruitment (**Figure 1.19**). The closing volume, or closing capacity (CC), is the volume of gas that remains in the lung after forced expiration when the small alveoli in the dependent regions of the lungs collapse. In neonates, the CC is increased when compared to that of older children. When CC exceeds FRC, some lung units are closed during tidal breathing, resulting in intrapulmonary shunting.

MECHANICS OF VENTILATION

Neonates and infants have an immature respiratory center, inefficient respiratory muscles, variances in airway and lung anatomy, and altered lung mechanics that, combined with higher basal metabolic requirement of oxygen, yield respiratory physiology that is much different than that of older children and adults. It is imperative that anesthesia providers have a sound understanding of these differences when developing an age-specific anesthetic plan.

ELASTICITY AND RECOIL

Lung tissue is very elastic with a tendency to shrink in size.[2] The chest wall counteracts this tendency with a stiff structure that pulls the lungs open in times of low lung volumes, thereby maintaining adequate expansion and avoiding collapse. Alternately, the chest wall pulls inward at high lung volumes to avoid overexpansion and injury to the lung tissue. Elastin deposition in the lungs begins around 6 years of age and continues throughout the life span, increasing lung recoil with age. Without elastin, lung deflation requires more effort.

Surface Tension and Interdependence

Surface tension is created by the air–fluid interface within the alveoli, enhancing the lung's innate tendency to recoil.[2] Surface tension occurs because of the attractive forces between

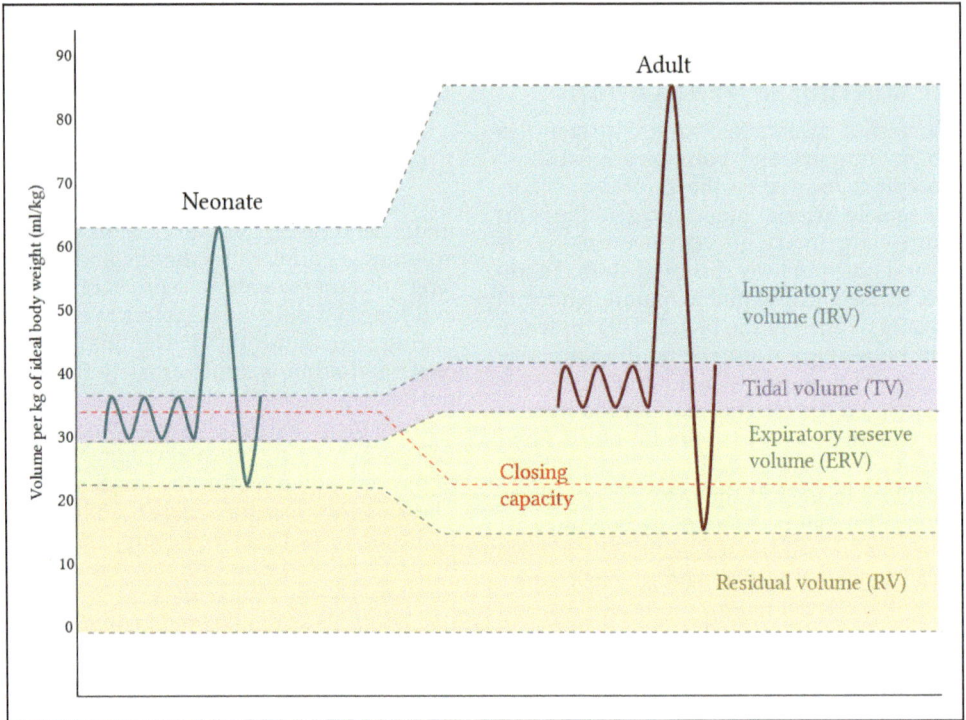

Figure 1.19: Respiratory volumes in neonates and adults.
ERV, expiratory reserve volume; IRV, inspiratory reserve volume; RV, residual volume; TV, tidal volume.
Source: From https://derangedphysiology.com/main/cicm-primary-exam/required-reading/respiratory-system/Chapter%20926/neonatal-respiratory-physiology.

the molecules on the surface layer of the fluid, which leads to collapse of the alveoli. Surfactant is a phospholipid–protein complex that profoundly lowers this surface tension, allowing for adequate lung expansion. The interdependence model of the lung describes the flat, planar walls shared by alveoli, which exert an outward force. Both are key factors contributing to lung stabilization at the alveolar level.

MUSCLE INVOLVEMENT IN VENTILATION

Major Muscles of Inspiration

The diaphragm is a dome-shaped structure that plays a vital part in spontaneous respiration. Contraction of the diaphragm muscle causes the muscle to flatten, thereby increasing the volume within the chest cavity, decreasing the intrathoracic pressure, and allowing air to flow into the airways.[1] In the neonate, the diaphragm is susceptible to fatigue as there are fewer Type I muscle fibers present at birth. Type I muscle fibers are slow endurance muscle fibers that play a role in resistance to fatigue.

The external intercostal muscles are also major muscles of inspiration, although they are not readily utilized during passive inspiration. During periods of increased work of breathing, the external intercostal muscles contract and elevate the anterior portion of the ribs, thereby increasing the anterior–posterior diameter, which in turn increases the volume of the thoracic cavity.

Accessory Muscles of Inspiration

The sternocleidomastoid and scalene muscles are the accessory muscles of inspiration as they increase the volume of the thoracic cavity by increasing the anterior–posterior diameter much like the external intercostal muscles. The accessory muscles of inspiration, however, are much less efficient as their use results in less of an increase in thoracic volume.[1]

Expiration

Expiration is generally a passive process and under normal conditions, there is no need for muscular effort. When active expiration is required, abdominal muscles contract and push the diaphragm up to decrease volume of the thorax. Similarly, interior intercostal muscles will contract, decreasing the anteroposterior diameter, thereby decreasing thoracic volume.

COMPLIANCE

The compliance of the respiratory system is dependent upon the compliance of the lungs and the chest wall. Lung compliance increases by 150% during the first year of life.[2]

Lung Compliance

Lung compliance is described as the change in lung volume per unit of pressure.[2] It is affected by the elasticity of the lung tissue and the lung volume prior to inflation. Lung compliance overall in the neonate is reduced, primarily due to insufficient production of surfactant.

The lungs are found to be least compliant at extremes of inhalation and exhalation. At lower lung volumes, lung compliance is low which correlates with underinflation and atelectasis. As more lung volume is recruited, the compliance increases with a significant change in volume witnessed for a given change in pressure (Figure 1.20). This degree of lung expansion promotes ideal tidal volumes. At higher lung volumes, compliance decreases. The lower airways are also more compliant than older children and adults as well, which gives rise to dynamic collapse during forceful inspiration.

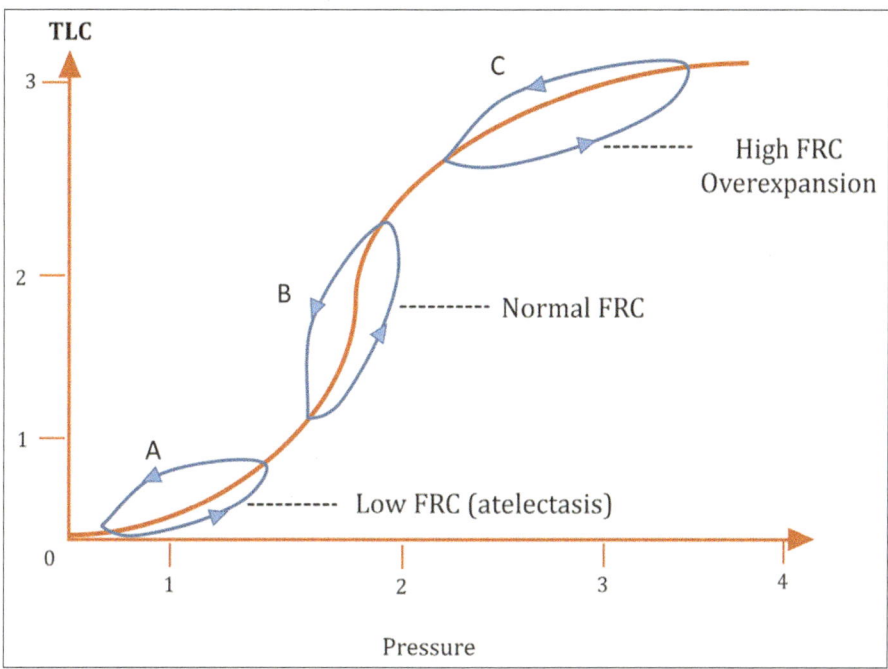

Figure 1.20: Extended compliance or lung expansion curve.
FRC, functional residual capacity.
Source: From Chakkarapani AA, Adappa R, Mohammad Ali SK, et al. Current concepts of mechanical ventilation in neonates - part 1: basics. *Int J Pediatr Adolesc Med.* 2020;7(1):13–18. doi:10.1016/j.ijpam.2020.03.003.

Chest Wall Compliance

An infant's chest wall is highly compliant, which promotes collapse of the lungs. Being three more times compliant than the chest wall of an adult, the elastic recoil of the chest wall is close to zero. In addition, the ribs tend to be more horizontally oriented in infants, limiting the potential for thoracic expansion. Rib cartilage is also less ossified making the chest wall less rigid and allowing the chest wall to retract during episodes of respiratory distress and decrease tidal volume. Thus, the work of inspiration is almost entirely due to diaphragmatic descent, with the diaphragm bearing the majority workload of breathing in neonates and infants.

Inhalation of larger tidal volumes ultimately causes the soft neonatal chest wall to collapse due to the greater negative intrathoracic pressure generated.[2] Hence, there is a greater reliance on respiratory rate to alter minute volume during this period. The lack of chest recoil is also responsible for higher tendency toward lung collapse in the setting of respiratory illness, and results in increased work of breathing requiring use of accessory muscles. The chest wall becomes less compliant with age as the ribs begin to ossify and intercostal muscles tone.

AIRWAY RESISTANCE

There are numerous components of pulmonary resistance to gas flow, including inertia of the respiratory system and friction of the chest wall however, these are considered negligible.[2] Frictional resistance of the lung tissue accounts for about 20%, leaving the frictional resistance of the airways to the flow of air as the largest component of airway resistance. The degree of resistance to flow depends on the type of flow, with smooth, laminar flow causing less resistance than turbulent flow. Turbulent air flow occurs when there is a sudden change in flow rate, a narrowing of the tube, or an acute angle in the tube.

The upper airways are usually thought to be the location of highest resistance to air flow; however, in children under 5 years of age, the resistance to air flow in peripheral lung fields is four times higher than in adult lung tissue.[2] Due to their inherently lower airway diameter, neonates are increasingly vulnerable to further reduction of airway lumen, whether due to inflammation or secretions. At birth, residual fluid in the lung increases respiratory resistance. A reduction in airway diameter results in turbulent flow, which further increases airway resistance. Furthermore, as neonates and young infants are predominantly nose breathers, even a minimal amount of nasal obstruction is already harmful. Additionally, there is a higher incidence of lower airway obstructive diseases in infants and children, which further increases resistance to flow.

Peripheral airway resistance is increased by intraluminal obstruction and extrinsic compression. In addition, the bronchi are smaller in infancy, thereby increasing resistance. Intraluminal sources of obstruction include exogenous material within the peripheral airways, autonomic constriction of bronchial smooth muscle tissue, and low lung volumes. When lungs are adequately inflated, this imparts a radial traction that increases the caliber of the lumen, which in turn decreases resistance to air flow. Extrinsic compression occurs when the airways collapse during forced expiration. This dynamic compression will cause symptoms of airway collapse sooner in patients with malacias or bronchopulmonary dysplasia.

PERFUSION

PULMONARY CIRCULATION

Fetal circulation and neonatal circulation are vastly different. In the womb, gas exchange occurs in the placenta. It is not until birth that the child takes their first breath, driving their lungs to become responsible for oxygenation and ventilation.[5] To fully comprehend pediatric pulmonary circulation, anesthesia providers must have a sound understanding of the transition from fetal to neonatal circulation.

Fetal Pulmonary Circulation

In the womb, fetal circulation relies on two major shunts that direct blood away from lungs: the patent foramen ovale (PFO) and the patent ductus arteriosus (PDA).[5] During development, fetal lung tissue is not capable of accommodating the same degree of blood flow as neonatal lung tissue, largely due to the high pulmonary vascular resistance (PVR). Only about 12% of right ventricular output enters the pulmonary circulation while the remaining 88% crosses the PDA into the aorta. The PFO is located in the right atrium of the heart and shunts blood right to left, while the PDA is located between the aorta and pulmonary artery. Blood flows from the placenta via the umbilical cord, which is made of two arteries and one vein, into the fetus's vasculature. It is shunted away from the lungs through the PDA and PFO, then back to the placenta for gas exchange. The placenta receives deoxygenated blood from the fetus's venous system via the umbilical arteries and returns oxygen-rich blood to the fetus's arterial system via the umbilical vein. The most highly oxygenated blood is first delivered to the myocardium and the brain.

The cause of the high PVR in the fetus is multifactorial. The pulmonary arterioles have high muscle mass and resting tone, the lungs remain collapsed, and resting oxygen tension remains low.[5] The PDA remains patent due to low oxygen tension and the vasodilatory effects of prostaglandins circulating in the blood.

Neonatal Pulmonary Circulation

Once the baby is born and takes their first breath, several physiological changes occur as gas exchange transitions from the placenta to the neonate's alveoli. With this first breath, the lungs expand allowing oxygen, a potent pulmonary vasodilator, to reach the lung tissue, which results in a dramatic fall in PVR.[5] The decrease in PVR promotes blood flow to the pulmonary vasculature as the resistance is less than the systemic vascular resistance (SVR).

Under normal circumstances, a progressive fall in PVR accompanies the immediate rise in SVR that occurs after birth. A transitional circulatory pattern exists for a short period that combines aspects of both the fetal and neonatal circulatory patterns. The decline in the PVR/SVR ratio results in a steady increase in pulmonary blood flow and oxygen uptake in the lung.

Because pressure equalizes between the left and right atria, the PFO is pushed against the atrial septum and closes almost immediately, and the PDA will close usually in 3 to 10 days after birth. The exact mechanism of the PDA closure is not known, but it is thought to be related to an increase in the partial pressure of oxygen and concentration of prostaglandins falling causing ductal constriction. As the shunts close, left ventricular output increases as blood flows through the pulmonary vasculature to the left side of the heart, where the left ventricle pumps oxygenated blood into the systemic circulation.

Persistent Pulmonary Hypertension of the Newborn

Persistent pulmonary hypertension (PPHN) occurs when the pulmonary circulation fails to transition from fetal circulation to normal circulation at birth. PPHN is characterized by elevated PVR that causes labile hypoxemia due to the decreased pulmonary blood flow and right-to-left shunting of blood. The etiology of PPHN can be classified in to one of three groups: (a) abnormally constricted pulmonary vasculature as a result of parenchymal disease; (b) hypoplastic pulmonary vasculature; and (c) normal parenchyma with remodeled pulmonary vasculature.[6]

Two characteristic findings in PPHN are impaired vasorelaxation of pulmonary artery and reduced blood vessel density in the lungs. Treatment of PPHN typically entails general supportive cardiorespiratory care, with the use of vasodilatory agents reserved for severe cases that fail to respond to supportive measures. In those cases, the use of inhaled nitric oxide may be required to reduce the PVR/SVR ratio, or extracorporeal membrane oxygenation may be initiated to provide adequate tissue oxygenation until the PVR decreases.

GAS EXCHANGE

POSTNATAL VENTILATION AND PERFUSION

As the air enters the lungs, gas exchange begins to occur. Oxygen and carbon dioxide exchange takes place between the alveoli and the capillary bed. Ventilation brings oxygen into the lungs and removes carbon dioxide.[7] Perfusion is the blood flow through the pulmonary vasculature down to the pulmonary alveoli. These together are known as V/Q and must be matched appropriately to allow for adequate oxygenation and ventilation.

VENTILATION AND PERFUSION MISMATCH

A V/Q mismatch occurs when areas of the lungs are not well expanded, become atelectatic, and are no longer ventilated, thus precluding gas exchange from occurring at the affected area. This results in low oxygen saturation and possibly increased carbon dioxide levels.[2] When these areas of lung tissue reexpand, anesthesia providers may observe lower oxygen saturation, as blood has been shunted away from these areas that are now being ventilated. As the blood flow returns to these newly recruited areas, there will be improvement in gas exchange and thus an improvement in oxygen saturation.

Perfusion throughout the lungs is very dependent on gravity. This is especially key in respiratory physiology during the neonatal period and early infancy, as the alveoli lack interalveolar communications and remain at risk of collapse and may produce atelectasis in dependent areas of the lung. The lung can be divided into four discrete regions according to the interplay between alveolar pressure, arterial pressure, and venous pressure, known as West's zones (**Figure 1.21**). Zone 1 is where alveolar pressure is higher than arterial or venous pressure. This zone does not exist under normal circumstances and is only present with positive pressure ventilation and profound hypovolemia. Zone 2 is where the alveolar pressure is lower than the arterial but higher than the venous pressure. Zone 3 is where both arterial and venous pressure is higher than alveolar pressure. Zone 4 is where the interstitial pressure is higher than alveolar, arterial, or pulmonary venous pressure.

Alterations in the V/Q ratio are primarily responsible for defects in the exchange of oxygen, with hypercapnia rarely occurring due to the efficiency of the chemoreceptors in keeping the partial pressure of carbon dioxide constant by increasing ventilation (**Figure 1.22**).

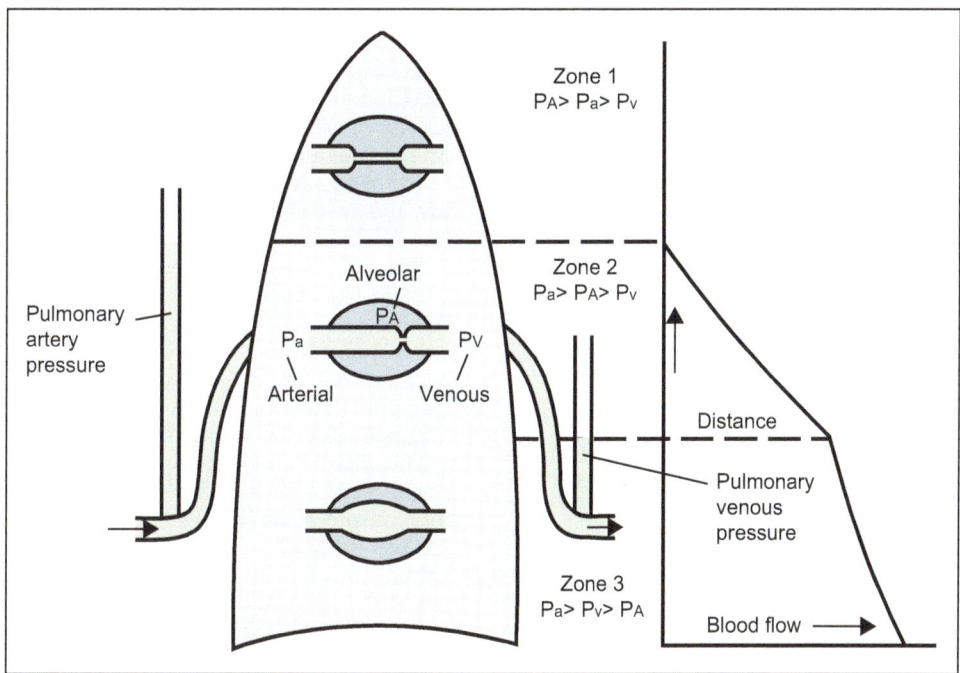

Figure 1.21: West's zones of perfusion and ventilation.

PA, alveolar pressure; Pa, arterial pressure; Pv, venous pressure.

Source: From Sullivan JS, Nkromah TA. Fundamentals of gas exchange and the assessment of oxygenation and ventilation. In: Lucking S, Maffei F, Tamburro R, Thomas N, eds. *Pediatric Critical Care Study Guide.* Springer; 2012. https://doi.org/10.1007/978-0-85729-923-9_1.

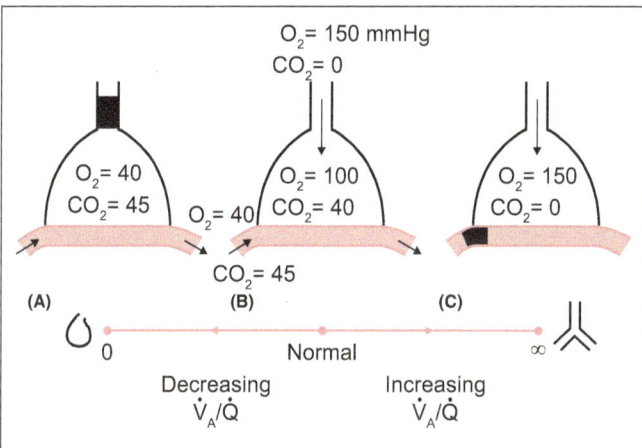

Figure 1.22: Effects of altering the ventilation and perfusion ratio.

Source: From Moretti C, Papoff P. Neonatal pulmonary physiology of term and preterm newborns. In: Buonocore G, Bracci R, Weindling M, eds. *Neonatology.* Springer; 2018. doi:10.1007/978-3-319-29489-6_197.

KEY TAKEAWAYS

- Having a sound understanding of the development of the respiratory system is essential to providing safe and effective anesthesia care to pediatric patients.
- Most cardiac arrests in pediatric patients are respiratory in nature.
- Proper ventilation is essential to maintaining open alveoli following the induction of anesthesia.
- Ventilation and perfusion mismatches can occur following extubation due to hypoventilation.

1.5: RENAL SYSTEM

Hailey Silverii and Shumyle Alam

LEARNING OBJECTIVES

- Review normal development, anatomy, and physiology of the renal system.
- Briefly discuss the pathophysiology of the renal system.

INTRODUCTION

A general understanding of the embryology and development of the genitourinary system allows for an appreciation of the anomalies anesthesia providers may see in a patient secondary to deviation from normal development. This section focuses on congenital anomalies of the kidneys and urinary tract (CAKUT), which are the leading causes of chronic kidney disease (CKD) in the pediatric patient. The CAKUT patient will represent some of the more complex developmental, anatomical, and physiological anomalies of the renal and urinary tracts, highlighting important concepts for the pediatric anesthesia provider to understand prior to providing care for this subset of patients.

CAKUT represents a spectrum of disease ranging from variants of normal to severe. These anomalies occur with deviation from normal renal development and are thought to be due to abnormal signaling and apoptosis during development.[1] Understanding the underlying renal disease in this population will assist in ensuring the delivery of a safe, efficacious anesthetic for this group of patients. In CAKUT patients with CKD, further stressors on the system, such as surgery and anesthesia, may contribute to acute kidney injury (AKI) on CKD, leading to further progression of CKD. The CAKUT spectrum is discussed in detail in subsequent chapters; however, within this section, we review renal physiology key to understanding the potential for renal injury in this group.

EMBRYOLOGY AND DEVELOPMENT

In the developing embryo, there are three separate pairs of renal units, each derived from the intermediate mesoderm. The first of these pairs to form, the pronephros, is a transient, primitive, nonfunctioning kidney that degenerates by the fifth week of gestation. The second pair of kidneys to form, the mesonephros, is also transient; however, it does provide means of excretion for the embryo during the development of the mature renal units called the metanephros. The nephric ducts of the mesonephros form the primitive ureter, which meets the cloaca caudally. Once the mature kidney has formed, by the fourth month, the remaining cranial nephric ducts (wolffian ducts) of the mesonephros form parts of the male reproductive tract: efferent ducts of the testes, epididymis, and vas deferens.[2] In females, the wolffian duct remnants become the nonfunctional structures epoophoron and paroophoron.[3]

The mature kidneys, called the metanephros in the human embryo, start their development around day 28 of gestation. The caudal-remaining mesonephric ducts, in contact with the cloaca, give rise to the ureteric bud, which will become the mature ureter. In the development of the human embryo, the cloaca is the common passageway for feces, urine, and reproduction, at the far end of the hindgut; the structure then divides to form a rectum, a bladder, and genitalia. The metanephros forms when the ureteric bud penetrates the blastema of metanephric mesenchyme at the 28th day of gestation.[4] The metanephric mesenchyme gives rise to the cells that make up the mature nephron and "meat" of the kidney, while the ureteric bud gives rise to the drainage system of the kidney: the collecting ducts, renal calyces, renal pelvis, and ureters. Kidney formation depends on the coordination of complex pathways on a molecular and a cellular level. These pathways are not discussed in detail as it is beyond the scope of this text; however, the takeaway is that these molecular pathways result in cell differentiation, morphogenesis, and regulation of cell number which are crucial to renal development.[3]

The functional unit of the kidney, the nephron, begins development in the fifth week of gestation, which continues through week 36 of gestation in the process of nephrogenesis.[4] Renal growth after the 36th week of gestation consists of maturation of nephrons rather than formation of new nephrons. Despite completion of nephrogenesis by 36 weeks of gestation, the majority of nephron growth and maturation continues through infant life.[5] At birth, a term neonate's glomerular filtration rate (GFR) is approximately 10% of that of an adult; however, GFR doubles at approximately 2 weeks of life.[6] This increase in GFR is a result of drastic changes in renal blood flow and filtration surface area. The infant's ability to concentrate urine continues to improve throughout the first 12 to 24 months of life. GFR maturation is very important during the first 2 years of life. The continued maturation of GFR after birth puts the immature kidneys at risk of fluid and electrolyte loss and may be vulnerable to irreversible injury during times of stress, such as surgery and anesthesia.

PHYSIOLOGY AND HOMEOSTASIS

To minimize risk of renal injury in the vulnerable pediatric patient, an understanding of renal homeostasis is necessary. As described above, the normal yet young kidney is at risk of fluid and electrolyte imbalance due to immature filtration and concentrating mechanisms. A child with an injured kidney or developmentally abnormal kidney is at even higher risk of imbalance and further renal injury if those needs and disease state are not anticipated or planned for during surgery.

The neonatal renal system as described earlier is immature and sees only a small portion of circulating renal blood flow. GFR is dependent upon renal blood flow (RBF), which is determined by renal perfusion pressure (RPP) and renal vascular resistance (RVR).[5] As circulating blood volume and RBF increase with development, GFR increases appropriately (Table 1.8). Of note, premature infants experience delays in reaching mature renal function, typically not achieving this goal until later in childhood.[6] In normal renal units, RBF increases with development until around 2 years of age.[7]

The mature and healthy kidney's autoregulatory ability functions to maintain relatively stable RBF despite changes in blood pressure; however, an immature or abnormal renal unit has difficulty maintaining this RBF and therefore GFR.[5] Animal models demonstrate impairment in autoregulation at the level of the immature glomerulus. The immature nephron sees an incomplete efferent arteriolar vasoconstriction in response to angiotensin II subsequent to a decrease in afferent inflow or afferent vasodilation. This immature nephron response underlines the risk the immature kidney seen with states of decreased circulatory volume or heart failure.[8] Along the same lines, this same immature autoregulatory mechanism is why fetal and neonatal renal function can be drastically impaired by angiotensin-converting enzyme (ACE) inhibitors and nonsteroidal anti-inflammatory drugs (NSAIDs).[9] Therefore, special consideration must be given when considering the use of ketorolac in this patient population. Although widely used in the operating room, it can have significant consequences on the developing renal system.

Table 1.8	Anticipated Glomerular Filtration Rate Based on Age
Age	Range GFR (mL/min/1.73 m²)
*≤30 WGA	<10
*34 WGA	<15
1–3 days	20.8 ± 5.0
3–4 days	39.0 ± 15.1
4–14 days	36.8 ± 7.2
15–19 days	46.9 ± 12.5
1–3 months	85.3 ± 35.1
4–6 months	87.4 ± 22.3
7–12 months	96.2 ± 12.2
1–2 years	105.2 ± 17.3
2.7–11.6 years	127.1 ± 13.5
16.2–34 years	112 ± 13

GFR, glomerular filtration rate; WGA, weeks gestational age.

Source: From Schwartz GJ, Furth SL. Glomerular filtration rate measurement and estimation in chronic kidney disease. *Pediatr Nephrol.* 2007;22(11):1839–1848. doi:10.1007/s00467-006-0358-1; Hunley TE, Kon V, Ichikawa I. Glomerular circulation and function. In: Avner E, Harmon W, Niaudet P, Yoshikawa N, eds. *Pediatric Nephrology.* 6th Ed. Springer; 2009:31–64.

Sodium and water are the biggest factors in maintaining body fluid homeostasis, as sodium concentration largely determines the size of the extracellular space, and therefore intravascular space and perfusion of organs, such as the kidney, are dependent on its balance.[10] Volume sensors throughout the body deliver feedback to the kidneys to influence changes in restoring water and sodium homeostasis. The mechanisms to restore sodium balance largely exist in the kidney, but electrolytes, such as potassium, phosphorus, and calcium, are also regulated in part by the renal system. Neonates tend to have higher potassium levels, which is thought to be due to decreased responsiveness to aldosterone at the level of the tubules, leading to less potassium excretion.[11]

Special consideration must be given to the surgical patient often kept NPO for longer than anticipated from the normal obstacles during a surgical day. Dehydration followed by anesthesia can lead to deleterious effects on the kidney. Given that the system is not physiologically mature, these effects may have downstream consequences. Although children do well after surgery, no one has studied the specific renal effects of anesthesia especially in the vulnerable CAKUT population. An appreciation for the diseased kidney is of utmost importance during anesthesia in determining fluid requirements and drug administration. As one of the main organs for excretion, the kidney is at risk of injury by waste products, (e.g., nephrotoxic medications especially in the setting of an already vulnerable kidney). Renal function also impacts hemodynamic parameters, namely, blood pressure regulation. Decreased GFR, specifically in premature infants, is linked to potential progressive CKD in childhood and is also associated with development of hypertension and heart disease in adulthood.[6]

PATHOPHYSIOLOGY

Decreased nephron endowment and/or renal injury contribute to the development of CKD (Table 1.9), which is defined as a state of irreversible kidney damage that remains stable or progressive over time.[12] Premature babies are born with an incomplete complement of nephrons and are at a distinct disadvantage, as with numerous continued insults in the early neonatal life, nephrogenesis may not ever be completed in these neonates.[8] In the at-risk kidney, AKI is a serious concern for the neonate, especially the neonate with underlying renal injury. Additionally, *AKI* in critically ill children is associated with worse outcomes defined by increased length of stay, length on ventilator, and mortality.[13] Definitions for *AKI* brought forward by Kidney Disease Improving Global Outcomes (KDIGO)[14] have been validated in children[15] and are highlighted in Box 1.1.

There are numerous causes for AKI categorized either by decreased volume status, tubular injury, glomerular injury, vascular injury, infection, or obstruction. These insults may lead to irreversible renal injury especially in an already vulnerable or immature kidney.[11] One of the most at-risk populations for AKI are CAKUT patients. Very few protocols are in place to monitor serum creatinine levels (SCr) in this patient population, especially for outpatient surgery. At times, SCr may be artificially low in neonates and is not considered to be the best marker of renal function in this population. In addition, measures to reduce laboratory draws and testing in the hospital as a cost-saving measure may negatively impact our ability to truly track the outcomes of anesthesia and surgical stress in the population.

MINIMIZING FURTHER RISK OF INJURY

ELECTROLYTES AND ACIDOSIS

Patients with CAKUT and CKD are at risk of increased fluid losses and electrolyte abnormalities specifically hyperkalemia and acidosis for numerous reasons. Acidosis develops in patients with progressive CKD. Patients with CKD without progression can still have significant acidosis with associated hyperkalemia due to renal tubular acidosis (RTA), specifically Type IV. Type IV RTA is due to either an aldosterone deficiency or a lack of response to aldosterone.[16] Acquired resistance to aldosterone is the mechanism of Type IV RTA in CAKUT patients secondary to tubular injury over time from obstruction, reflux, or high pressure. These patients tend to be volume and salt depleted in addition to hyperkalemic and acidotic; therefore, prior to anesthesia, patients should undergo correction of potassium and acidosis in addition to adequate fluid repletion to minimize further risk. Untreated acidosis, irrespective of mechanism, can lead to further renal injury in CKD patients and has been shown as an independent and modifiable risk factor for progression of CKD.[17,18]

FLUID BALANCE

CAKUT patients with CKD will oftentimes have a "fixed urine output," meaning that they have a finite rate of urine production independent of volume status due to tubular damage and glomerular scar over time. These patients can

---

BOX 1.1 DETERMINANTS OF ACUTE KIDNEY INJURY

DEFINITIONS FOR AKI BROUGHT FORWARD BY KDIGO

- Increase in SCr by ≥0.3 mg/dL (≥26.5 µmol/L) within 48 hours

  or

- Increase in SCr to ≥1.5 times baseline, which is known or presumed to have occurred within the prior 7 days

  or

- Urine volume <0.5 mL/kg/hr for 6 hours

KDIGO, Kidney Disease Improving Global Outcomes; SCr, serum creatinine.

Table 1.9	Chronic Kidney Disease Classification by Glomerular Filtration Rate	
Stage	Definition	GFR
1	Normal or decreased GFR with kidney damage	>90
2	Mild decrease in GFR with kidney damage	60–89
3	Moderate decrease in GFR	30–59
4	Severe decrease in GFR	15–29
5	Kidney failure	<5; ESRD

ESRD; end-stage renal disease; GFR, glomerular filtration rate.

quickly become intravascularly deplete, especially in periods of enteral fasting prior to anesthesia. IV fluid hydration prior to induction of anesthesia is recommended for patients with stage III CKD or higher. The risk of dehydration and hypovolemia increases risk of AKI and potential CKD progression in this group; therefore, the goal would be to restore and/or maintain normal circulating blood volume with the administration of hypotonic fluids lost.

BLOOD PRESSURE CONTROL

Poor autoregulation in patients with CKD necessitates close monitoring and tighter parameters for blood pressure during and after anesthesia. In patients with CKD, hypertension is a significant yet modifiable risk factor for CKD progression. The 2004 ESCAPE trial illustrated the importance of maintaining blood pressure control below the 50th age-related percentile in patients with CKD to slow progression of disease in comparison to the previous target of maintaining blood pressure under the 90th percentile.[18] Coinciding with hypertension, proteinuria can identify risk of progression of the disease.

Long-term management of hypertension, proteinuria, and progression of CKD can be accomplished with ACE inhibitors and angiotensin II receptor blockers (ARBs).[19] However, in patients with CKD undergoing anesthesia, it is prudent to hold these agents in order to avoid additional risk of vasoconstriction during surgery. Given the unique pharmacological properties of various ACE inhibitors and ARBs, the appropriate timing for cessation will be different for each medication. Furthermore, questions remain regarding the ideal timing for discontinuing these medications. Therefore, while institutional protocols vary, most recommend holding ACE inhibitors at least 24 hours prior to anesthesia to avert deleterious vasoplegia while under anesthesia. It is important to keep in mind that despite discontinuing longer acting agents prior to surgery, antagonism may still persist into the operative period.

GLOMERULAR FILTRATION RATE ASSESSMENT AND NEPHROTOXIC MEDICATIONS

In patients with CKD, decreases in GFR are due to either decreases in filtration or a decrease in the number of functioning/filtering nephrons; therefore, GFR should be assessed regularly. Various methods to measure GFR exist, though the most accurate measurements are based on clearance of a marker such as inulin.[20] Despite being the gold standard for measuring GFR, inulin clearance has limited use in the clinical setting. Therefore, GFR is often measured using other validated calculations such as the Bedside Schwartz equation (Table 1.10).

Measurement of cystatin C can also be used to guide GFR calculations in CKD. Cystatin C is a protease inhibitor that is filtered at the glomerulus and reabsorbed at the proximal tubule. Its use for measuring GFR in adults has been validated; however, as a standalone value in pediatrics, there are no guidelines recommending its use based on the scarcity of data.[20] However, in support of its use, Bokenkamp et al.[23] identified that as a marker for renal function in children older than 2 years of age, cystatin C is independent of age, gender, height, and body composition in contrast to SCr, which is variable. In patients with CKD, malnutrition is a major problem; therefore, GFR calculations based on creatinine can overestimate GFR due to decreased muscle mass in these patients.

Table 1.10 Formulas to Calculate Glomerular Filtration Rate in the Chronic Kidney Disease Patient

Formula to Calculate GFR	Source	Notes
GFR (mL/min/1.73 m^2) = $0.413 \times$ Ht(cm)/serum creatinine (mg/dL)	Schwartz et al. 2009	"Bedside Schwartz Equation"
GFR (mL/min/1.73 m^2) = $39.8 \times$ (Ht(m)/Scr)$^{0.456}$ (1.8/CystC)$^{0.418}$ (30/BUN)$^{0.079}$ (1.076)^{male} (Ht(m)/1.4)$^{0.179}$	Schwartz et al. 2012	CKiD multivariable equation; Cystatin C and Creatinine
GFR (mL/min/1.73 m^2) = 70.69 (CystC)$^{-0.931}$	Schwartz et al. 2012	Cystatin C only

BUN, blood urea nitrogen; GFR, glomerular filtration rate.

Source: From Schwartz GJ, Muñoz A, Schneider MF, et al. New equations to estimate gfr in children with CKD. *J Am Soc Nephrol.* 2009;20(3):629–637. doi:10.1681/ASN.2008030287; Schwartz GJ, Schneider MF, Maier PS, et al. Improved equations estimating GFR in children with chronic kidney disease using an immunonephelometric determination of cystatin C. *Kidney Int.* 2012;82(4):445–53. doi:10.1038/ki.2012.169.

Finally, CKD and CAKUT alter drug metabolism and excretion of waste products; therefore, all drugs should be dosed according to calculated or expected GFR. In patients with CKD, NSAIDs should be avoided.

END-STAGE RENAL DISEASE AND TRANSPLANTATION

Despite numerous advances in the care of the child with renal disease, there remains approximately 12.9 new end-stage renal disease (ESRD) patients per 1 million children (USRDS, 2019 report). Although many patients progress to renal failure over time, there is not yet a defined plan to minimize the variables that may cause progressive renal injury. Since surgery is often elective and can be planned for in most of these children, it is imperative that anesthesia providers utilize their understanding of the patient's renal physiology based on the disease state to try and minimize harm and the progression to ESRD.

KEY TAKEAWAYS

- Development and physiology of the renal system is complex.
- Anesthesia poses multiple risks of further renal injury in vulnerable pediatric patients with CKD.
- CAKUT is the most common cause of CKD and ESRD in pediatric patients.

RESOURCES

- U.S. Renal Data System 2019 Annual Data Report: Epidemiology of Kidney Disease in the United States

1.6: HEPATIC SYSTEM

Alison Henry

> **LEARNING OBJECTIVES**
>
> - Understand the basic and most critical components of pediatric liver anatomy.
> - Be able to recite the critical physiological functions of the liver.
> - Identify when the liver reaches full maturity.
> - Understand how an immature pediatric liver may affect the anesthesia provider (i.e., drug metabolism, protein synthesis).

Table 1.11	Primary Types of Liver Cells
Cell Type	**Cell Function**
Hepatocyte	Chief parenchymal cells of liver—have several rolls including metabolism, detoxification, and protein synthesis. Compose 80% of total cells in the liver
Endothelial cells	Act as a barrier between blood and hepatocytes
Kupffer cells	Function as macrophages
Stellate cells	Store vitamin A and fat

PEDIATRIC HEPATIC ANATOMY

Liver development in utero is initiated by fetal progenitor cells, which are derived from foregut endoderm and eventually differentiate into mature hepatocytes and cholangiocytes during liver development (Figure 1.23). Despite considerable development during the prenatal period, full maturity can take up to 2 years after birth. Although the liver is not immediately mature, specialized hepatocytes are present at birth and have two distinct functional surfaces. Sinusoidal surfaces receive and absorb oxygenated blood and nutrients from the portal vein, with the canalicular surfaces responsible for the transport of bile and other conjugation and metabolism products, which ultimately end up at the bile ductules.[1]

The liver is composed of four primary cell types: hepatocytes, endothelial, Kupffer, and stellate cells (Table 1.11). In children, the liver is larger than it is in adults when comparing a body-to-weight ratio, with the liver accounting for nearly 4% of a child's body weight compared to only 2% in adults. Despite the differences in body-to-weight ratio, the organ and the vascular anatomy are very similar. The liver has two lobes, right and left, which then further organize into eight segments: the left lobe containing segments 2, 3, and 4 and the right lobe containing 5, 6, 7, and 8. Segment 1 (the caudate lobe) receives its blood supply from both the left and right lobes, which drain into the cava via several short caudate veins. Anatomically, the liver is housed in the right upper quadrant of the abdomen by its attachment to the cava and continuance of assorted ligaments over the surface of the liver and parietal peritoneum as the Glisson's capsule.[2]

The liver has a high energy need, requiring 20% of the body's total oxygen supply. The common hepatic artery, which supplies 25% oxygenated blood to the liver, arises as a branch of the celiac artery, with the portal vein forming from the confluence of the splenic and mesenteric veins. Draining directly into the liver, the portal vein is responsible for approximately 75% of its overall blood flow.[3] The liver drains into the inferior vena cava (IVC) by way of the left middle and right hepatic veins. Substances (e.g., absorbed nutrients or xenobiotics) that enter the body enterally first come into contact with the liver via the portal vein. The hepatic artery is responsible for delivering metabolic products that enter the body through other pathways or portal blood substances not extracted on the first pass.[4]

The hepatic acinus, or functional unit of the liver, has three different zones. Zone 1, bordering the portal tract, helps with hepatocyte regeneration, bile duct proliferation, and gluconeogenesis. Zone 3 borders the central vein and is responsible for aerobic metabolism, glycolysis, and hydrolysis. Zone 2 sits between the two zones and has a mixed set of functions (Figure 1.24).

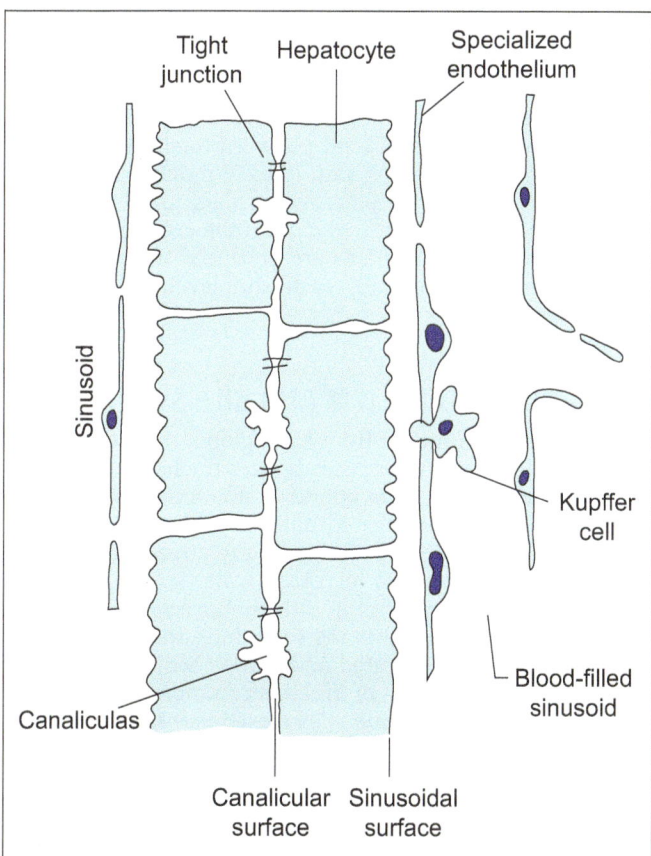

Figure 1.23: Functional surfaces of hepatocytes.

Source: From Beath SV. Hepatic function and physiology in the newborn. In: Seminars in neonatology. 2003;8(5):337–346. doi:10.1016/S1084-2756(03)00066-6.

PEDIATRIC HEPATIC PHYSIOLOGY

As the neonatal liver has only 20% of the hepatocytes that of an adult liver has, its function remains limited during development. The liver performs several critical functions including regulation of glucose, plasma protein synthesis, production of bile, hemoglobin degradation, and biotransformation of substances from the bowel or other organs (such as medications).

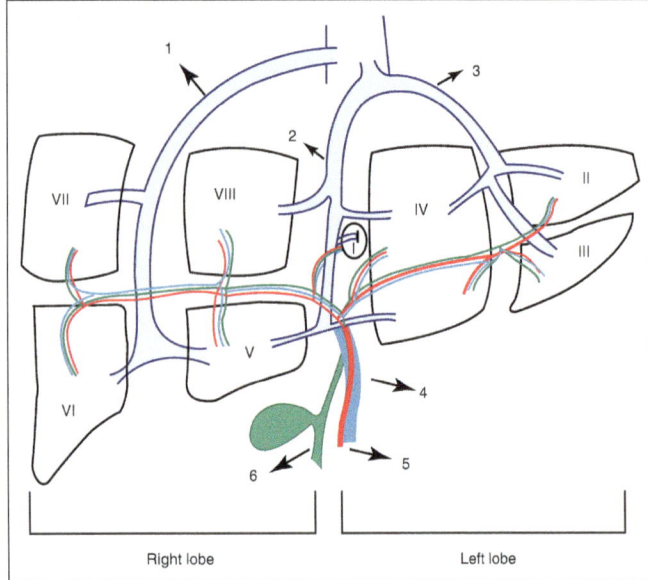

Figure 1.24: Image of the liver's eight segments.

Note: Segments I (caudate lobe), II, III, and IV from the left lobe and V, VI, VII, and VIII from the right lobe. (1) Right hepatic vein, (2) middle hepatic vein, (3) left hepatic vein, (4) portal vein, (5) hepatic vein, and (6) common bile duct.

Source: From Reddy MS. Liver anatomy for pediatric intensivist. *Pediatric Liver Intensive Care.* Springer; 2019:1–5.

GLUCOSE REGULATION

The liver is home to all glucose metabolic pathways (glycogen synthesis, glycogenolysis, gluconeogenesis, and glycolysis). In the liver, glycogen synthesis and degradation are required to maintain blood glucose levels as a whole. Within muscle, these processes are regulated to only meet the needs of the specific muscle itself.[5] Glycogenolysis, which is the breakdown of glycogen into glucose, accounts for approximately one-third of total glucose production during infancy, with gluconeogenesis accounting for most of the remainder of glucose production. The gluconeogenesis pathway produces glucose through noncarbohydrate precursors (e.g., milk—high fat and, low carbohydrate) for further maintenance of glucose levels.[6] Gluconeogenesis is especially important for infants because of their milk-based diet. The glycolysis pathway converts glucose into pyruvate and subsequently Acetyl-CoA, which then enters the Krebs cycle for further energy production (**Figure 1.25**).

LIPID/FATTY ACID METABOLISM

Fatty acid metabolism is another significant source of energy for the neonate. Soon after birth, fat accumulated in the fetal liver is mobilized and oxidized, resulting in increased energy production and ketone formation for peripheral use.[7] Ketones are especially important in the neonatal period as they provide fuel to brain, heart, and skeletal muscle.

In term infants, ketogenesis is considerably increased in the first 3 days of life with it have been suggested that ketones could provide up to 25% of a neonate's basal energy requirement. The ability of the neonate to oxidize fatty acids rapidly also increases in the first few days of life, which again is very important for energy production due to their high-fat, low-carbohydrate diet.

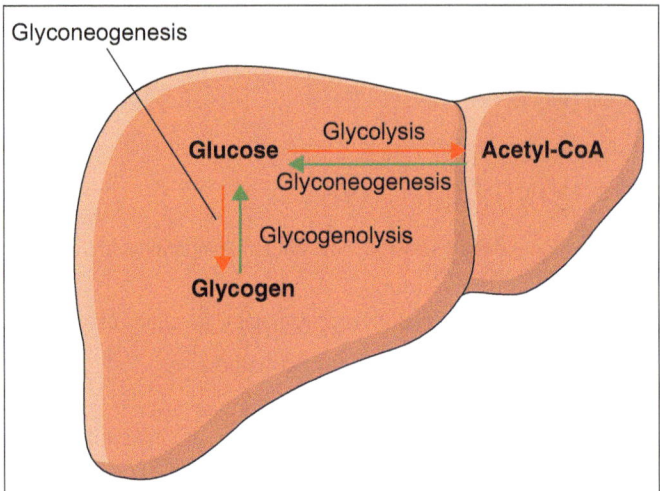

Figure 1.25: Image showing glucose metabolism regulation by glucagon.

Note: The green arrows show glucagon increasing glucose production by stimulating glycogenolysis (breakdown of glycogen to glucose) and glyconeogenesis (formation of glucose from noncarbohydrate sources), while the red arrows show the inhibition of glycolysis (converts glucose into pyruvate) and glycogenesis (formation of glycogen from glucose).

PROTEIN SYNTHESIS

In the fetal liver, alpha-fetoprotein is the primary plasma protein produced, reaching maximal concentration by the end of the first trimester. At approximately the 16th week of gestation, albumin synthesis begins to occur, reaching adult levels by the end of gestation. However, the reduction of circulating plasma proteins (including albumin and alpha-1-acid glycoprotein) increases the bioavailability of highly bound drugs and their active moiety. Total plasma protein levels do not reach normal adult values until 10 to 12 months of age, making it imperative that anesthesia providers adjust a neonate's medication dosing accordingly.[8] With the exception of factor VIII, all coagulation proteins are produced in the liver, and although lower in neonates, reach adult levels within the first several days of life.

BILIRUBIN METABOLISM AND BILE SYNTHESIS

Bilirubin is a by-product from hemoglobin degradation. The reticuloendothelial system metabolizes the heme component into bilirubin, where it is bound to albumin and transported to the liver. Unconjugated bilirubin is lipophilic and hydrophobic making it more difficult to remove from the body. Conjugated bilirubin has increased water solubility making its transportation easier; it is ultimately secreted in the bile where it is then directed to the small intestine to be excreted in the stool or deconjugated and reabsorbed into the blood. During the first 2 weeks of life, it is common to see a rise in unconjugated bilirubin due to increased bilirubin levels without efficient conjugation, as well as increased reabsorption. As the biliary processes mature and the infant develops a normal eating and stooling pattern, the level of unconjugated bilirubin falls.

The primary bile acids, cholate, and chenodeoxycholate increase significantly in the first week of life, with their concentration being much higher than that of an older child or adult. The level of serum bile acids present is multifaceted, with emphasis on hepatic uptake and intestinal absorption, but begins to reach adult levels by 6 months of life. Fetal bile acids have several differences compared to that found in adult patients. Fetal bile acid has an increased ratio of chenodeoxycholic acid to cholic acid, a predominance of taurine conjugation as opposed to the adult glycine-conjugated bile acids, and contains additional hydroxylations at certain carbons of the sterol nucleus. The significance of these findings is not clearly understood, but it has been offered that this possibly serves as increased protection for the immature neonatal liver against hepatoxic substances that it produces.[6]

BIOTRANSFORMATION

The liver plays a critical role in the activation, detoxification, and excretion of both endogenous (ammonium and bilirubin) and exogenous (xenobiotic, poisons, pollutants, etc.) substances. Biotransformation is generally separated into three categories: phase 1 (activation), phase 2 (detoxification), and phase 3 (excretion).

Phase 1 Reactions

Phase 1 involves oxidation, reduction, and hydrolytic reactions, yielding a polar, water-soluble, and often still active metabolite (e.g., morphine's potent metabolite morphine-6 beta glucuronide).

The cytochrome P450 (CYP450) monooxygenases are the main complex involved with phase I reactions. A superfamily composed of CYP450 members causes the oxidative metabolism of a lipophilic substrate. The CYP450 families of 1, 2 and 3 are expressed early in life and have an especially significant role in drug metabolism. Roughly 30% of the CYP450 proteins are present at birth, CYP2E1 and CYP2D6 enzymes rise at the time of birth, with enzymes CYP3A4, 2C9, and 2C19 increasing during the first several weeks of life. Enzyme CYP3A7 has a significant presence at birth and then falls over time, with adult levels being barely measurable. This is contrary to CYP1A2, which is the last enzyme to develop and is not expressed until 1 to 3 months of life. As seen in **Figure 1.26**, none of the CYP450 enzymes develop in a linear fashion, but by 1 to 2 years of age, enzyme activity is similar to that of an adult.[9] However, the overall decrease the CYP450 enzymes are directly proportional to decreased medication half-lives and increased clearance.

Phase 2 Reactions

In phase 2, enzymes conjugate drug molecules to allow for excretion. Phase 2 reactions further increase water solubility of the metabolite by adding endogenous hydrophilic groups to form inactive compounds ready to be excreted. The most common Phase 2 reaction is glucuronidation, but other Phase 2 reactions include methylation, acetylation,

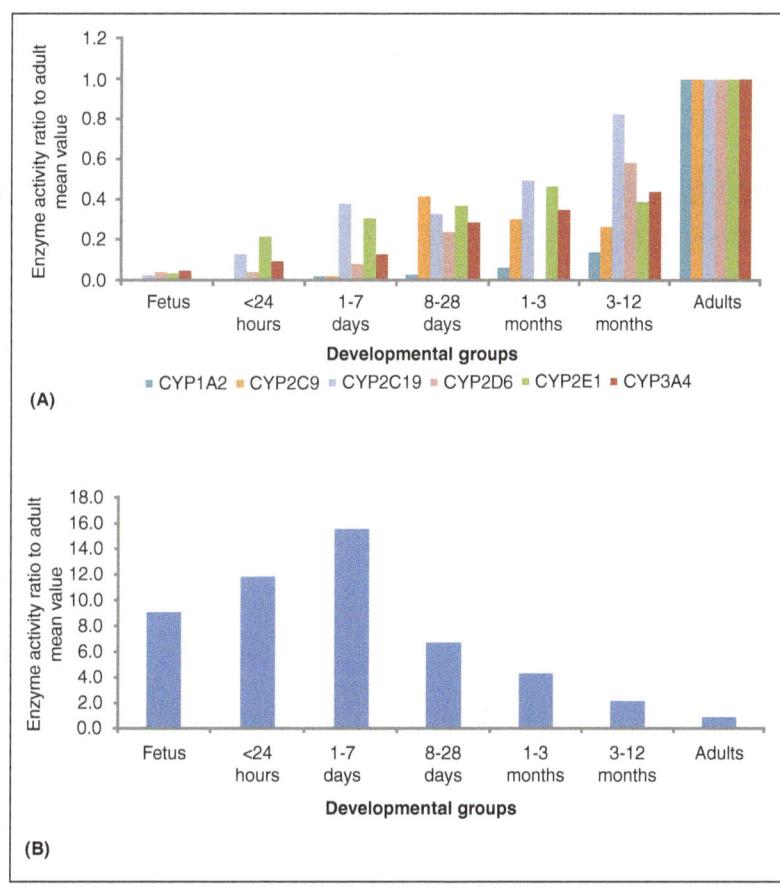

Figure 1.26: (A) The timeline for developmental maturity of six CYP450 enzyme groups. (B) The rise and subsequent fall of the most expressed enzyme at birth, CYP3A7.

CYP450, cytochrome P450.

Source: From Lu H, Rosenbaum S. Developmental pharmacokinetics in pediatric populations. *J Pediatr Pharmacol Ther.* 2014;19(4):262–276. doi:10.5863/1551-6776-19.4.262.

sulfation, glutathione conjugation, and amino acid conjugation (glycine, taurine, glutamic acid).[10] The immaturity and overall low expression of substances needed for Phase 2 reactions to occur further increase plasma half-lives and prolong elimination. For example, neonates express low levels of the uridine 5′-diphospho-glucuronosyltransferase (UDP) glucuronosyltransferase enzyme (UDPGT), only reaching about 30% of adult levels by 3 months of age. UDPGT is present in glucuronidation of many hydrophobic medications, as well as the biotransformation of bilirubin and other endogenous substrates. This reduces the clearance of medications like morphine and acetaminophen that rely on conjugation via glucuronidation pathways.

Phase 3 Reactions

After Phase 2, the now water-soluble product is secreted with bile and ultimately excreted from the body in Phase 3. Excretion is the final process key to the removal of a drug and/or its metabolites from the body. Phase 3 reactions are particularly important for drugs that do not undergo any biotransformation, such as gentamicin. While excretion usually occurs via renal or hepatic routes, it is possible for drugs to leave the body via other routes. The excretion of excipients, which are inactive substances that serve as a vehicle or medium for other active drugs, should also be considered as they have been associated with adverse effects. Hospitalized neonates especially are at risk of being administered large amounts of excipients, with propylene glycol and benzyl alcohol present in many injectable drug formulations, both of which have been associated with serious adverse effects, including death.

KEY TAKEAWAYS

- The liver does not fully mature until approximately 2 years of age.
- The liver contains four primary cell types: hepatocytes, endothelial, Kupffer, and stellate.
- The portal vein is responsible for approximately 75% of blood flow entering the liver, whereas the hepatic artery accounts for only approximately 25%.
- The liver has several critical functions—plasma protein synthesis, production of bile, hemoglobin degradation, regulation of glucose, and biotransformation of substances from the bowel or other organs (such as medications).
- Glycogenolysis accounts for approximately one-third of glucose production.
- Gluconeogenesis is especially important in infancy because of their milk-based diet (high fat, and low carbohydrate).
- Total plasma protein levels do not reach adult levels until 10 to 12 months of age.
- Drug metabolism consists of Phase 1 (activation), Phase 2 (detoxification), and Phase 3 (excretion).
- Approximately 30% of CYP450 enzymes are present at birth, reaching adult levels at about 1 to 2 years of age.

1.7: THERMOREGULATION

Dawn Elizabeth Bent and Sharifah Wilson

LEARNING OBJECTIVES

- Understand the physiological principles of thermoregulation.
- Describe the processes of pediatric heat loss.
- Identify the role of brown adipose tissue.
- Explain mechanisms of thermogenesis.

INTRODUCTION

Thermoregulation is the ability of the body to maintain body temperature in a range that promotes optimal functioning of the body's systems. Humans are endotherms, meaning they use thermoregulation to maintain a consistent internal body temperature even when the external environment changes. If heat loss supersedes that of heat gain, hypothermia ensues. Conversely, should heat gain surpass heat loss, the body becomes hyperthermic. Both hypothermia and hyperthermia have consequential effects on the care and well-being of patients. The balance of heat loss and heat generation must be maintained; otherwise, the human body would cease to function. It is paramount that anesthesia providers have a sound understanding of the physiology driving pediatric thermoregulation in order to provide optimal care for their patients.

PHYSIOLOGY OF THERMOREGULATION

Mammalian thermoregulation relies on transmission of feedback from the periphery to the brain via neural pathways, with negative feedback serving to help maintain the body temperature within narrow limits. Thermoregulation has three mechanisms: afferent thermal sensing, central regulation, and efferent responses. These three processes combine to influence body temperature and its modulation.

AFFERENT THERMAL SENSING

Cold and warm receptors exist in the periphery, with cold receptors being 10 times more prevalent. Cold receptors are generally immediately beneath the dermis, with warm receptors being slightly deeper in the dermis.[1] Afferent nerves transmit temperature impulses from the periphery via A-delta fibers (cold-sensitive receptors) and C fibers (warm-sensitive receptors) to trigeminal and dorsal root ganglia. The signal then travels to the dorsal horn of the spinal cord, ultimately making its way to the preoptic area (POA) of the hypothalamus.[2]

Afferent signaling from the periphery is not the sole source of temperature-related input. Temperature-sensitive cells in the central core tissues also transmit afferent impulses that converge on the hypothalamus.[3] In addition, transient receptor potential (TRP) channels are known to constitute important components of sensory systems, where they participate in the detection or transduction of osmotic, mechanical, thermal, or chemosensory stimuli. These are polymodal cutaneous receptors located in the skin and contribute to thermoregulation. TRPM8, in particular, which is found in the trigeminal and dorsal root ganglia, plays a crucial role in detecting cool to cold temperatures.

CENTRAL REGULATION

The POA receives input from a multitude of tissue throughout the body, with the skin being the largest organ involved. Once afferent signals, both simple and complex, are received by the POA, they are processed and compared to threshold temperatures. Should the temperature remain within threshold limits, or the interthreshold range, no thermoregulatory responses occur (Figure 1.27). The interthreshold range, just as other feedback systems within the body, acts as an autoregulatory response to temperature regulation. Once the temperature exceeds threshold limits, the posterior hypothalamus initiates the efferent response. The mechanism by which the body determines the absolute threshold temperature remains unknown but is thought to be influenced by multiple factors ranging from plasma concentrations of electrolytes and hormones to the influence of circadian rhythms and food intake. Although central regulation is functional in the term neonate, it may not be fully developed in the premature patient.

EFFERENT RESPONSE

The primary autonomic response depends on the afferent information the POA receives from the central core. Once there are temperature deviations outside the interthreshold range, an efferent response will be generated by the posterior hypothalamus, which controls the efferent pathways to the effectors. If internal temperatures grow too cold, the posterior hypothalamus will send signals to the skin, glands, muscles, and organs to increase metabolic heat production and/or decrease environmental heat loss. Likewise, should internal temperatures become too hot, the posterior hypothalamus will send signals triggering sweating, which leads to vasodilatation and ultimately heat loss via evaporation (Table 1.12).

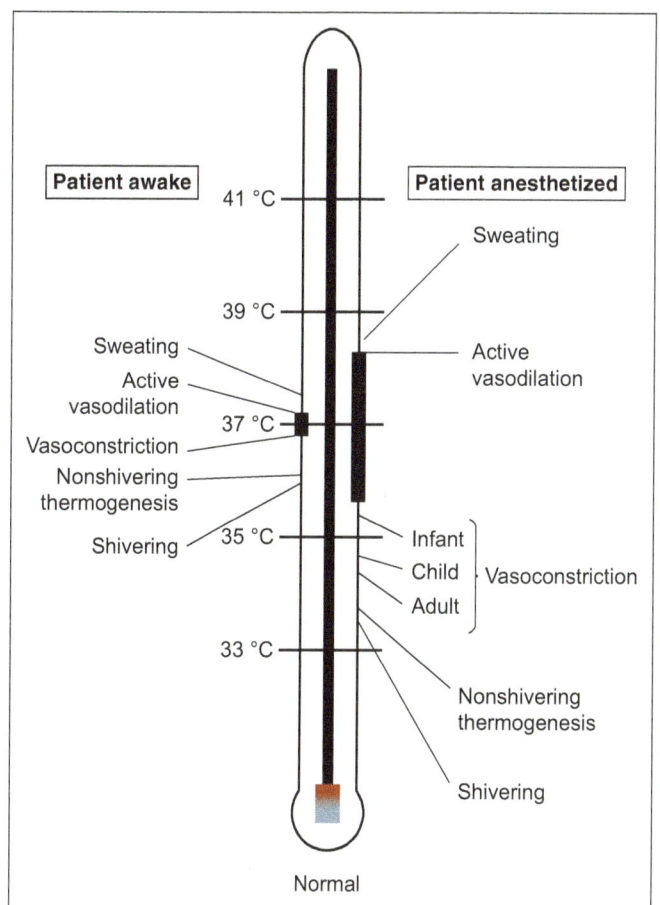

Figure 1.27: Interthreshold range limits.

Table 1.12	Physiological and Behavioral Responses to the Activation of Thermoreceptors			
Body Temperature Stimulus	**Sensors**	**Control Center**	**Effectors**	**Responses**
Increase	Peripheral and central thermoreceptors	Hypothalamus	1. Skin blood vessels 2. Sweat glands 3. Endocrine tissue 4. Behavior	1. Arteriolar and arteriovenous anastomosis vasodilation 2. Sweating 3. Decreased metabolic rate (adrenal and thyroid glands) 4. Reduced activity, stretched body position, and loss of appetite
Decrease	Peripheral and central thermoreceptors	Hypothalamus	1. Skin blood vessels 2. Arrector pili muscles 3. Skeletal muscles 4. Endocrine tissue 5. Behavior 6. Brown adipose tissue	1. Arterior and arteriovenous anastomosis vasoconstriction 2. Piloerection and air trapping 3. Shivering thermogenesis 4. Increased metabolic rate (adrenal and thyroid glands and brown adipose tissue) 5. Increased activity, huddled body position, and increased appetite 6. Nonshivering thermogenesis

Source: From Tansey EA, Johnson CD. Recent advances in thermoregulation. *Adv physiol educ.* 2015;39(3):139–48. doi:10.1152/advan.00126.2014.

MECHANISMS OF HEAT LOSS

Heat loss occurs via two steps. The first step is the controlled dissipation of heat. This requires sufficient intravascular volume and cardiovascular function as the body is attempting to transport rising internal heat to the surface of the skin for release. The rate of heat transfer from the tissue to the blood depends on the rate of energy production within the body, the temperature of the tissue, the temperature of the blood that is moving into the tissue, and the actual blood flow through the tissue.[4] The second step is the transfer of heat from the surface of the skin to the environment (Figure 1.28). The four mechanisms that contribute to heat loss are radiation, convection, evaporation, and conduction. In the pediatric patient, heat loss occurs in the following order: radiation > convection > evaporation > conduction.[5] Table 1.13 defines the four mechanisms of heat loss.

RADIATION

Radiation is the transfer of heat between the surface of the skin and solid objects not directly in contact, but that differ in temperature. Radiative heat loss is based on the Stefan–Boltzmann law of radiation. Heat transfer via radiation does not require direct contact and is not affected by air movement or the distance between the two objects. The emitted radiation transfers energy from the warmer object to the cooler object causing the warmer object to cool. Radiation is the most common mechanism of heat loss after birth.[6]

CONVECTION

Convection is the transfer of heat by the movement of air or liquid across the body. When a body is warm, the density of air molecules in contact with the body is reduced causing the molecules to rise and be subsequently replaced with cooler air. Convection can also occur with a liquid. When the temperature of a liquid in contact with the body is lower than the body's temperature, the body loses heat by warming the water. Overall, the body loses 10% to 15% of its heat through convection.

Table 1.13	Mechanisms of Heat Loss
Mechanism of Heat Loss	**Definition**
Radiation	Heat transfer between objects, no contact
Convection	Heat transfer by air movement
Evaporation	Liquid turning to gas
Conduction	Heat transfer between object, contact

EVAPORATION

While conduction, convection, and radiation can cause both heat loss and heat gain, evaporation is a mechanism of heat loss only. Evaporation is the vaporization of water from the surface of the skin or a mucosal surface. Evaporative heat loss can be attributed to a variety of mechanisms, including sweating, insensible water loss from the skin, respiratory tract, or surgical wound, and the evaporation of liquids applied to the surface of the skin. Evaporation accounts for 10% to 33% of total heat loss, depending on the mechanism of evaporation. The total sweat vaporized from the surface of the skin depends on the following three factors: the surface area exposed to the environment, the temperature and relative humidity of ambient air, and the convective air currents around the body.

Although the sweat mechanism in the pediatric patient is not prominent, full-term neonates have the ability to sweat dependent upon their core body temperature. Once the core rectal temperature surpasses 37.9°C, the full-term neonate may begin to sweat.[7] Anesthesia providers should be aware that some patients do not have the ability to sweat (anhidrosis), predisposing them to physiological stress due to the inability to transfer heat via evaporation.[8]

Greater minute ventilation per kilogram in newborns and infants contributes to greater evaporative heat loss from the respiratory tract. Insensible evaporative losses can be minimized with the use of humidification. A variety of systems are available that help to keep airway gases warm and prevent the drying of gases when ventilating pediatric patients (Figure 1.29).

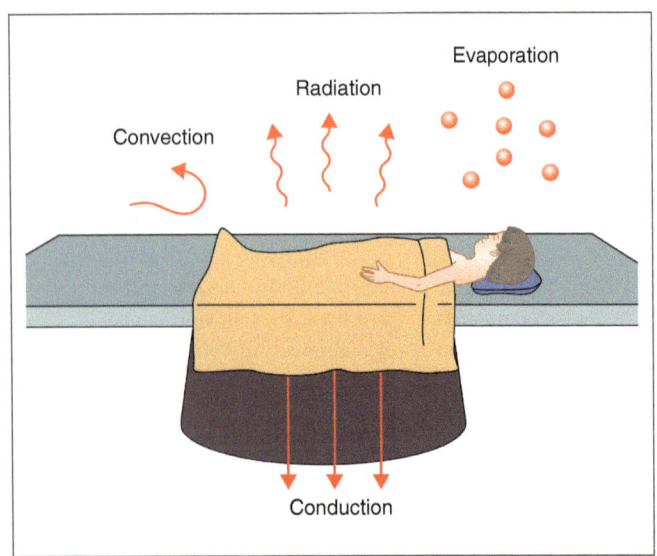

Figure 1.28: Mechanisms of heat loss.

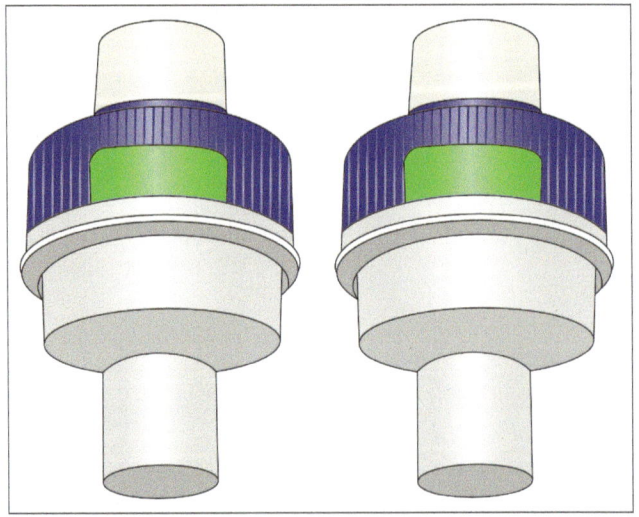

Figure 1.29: Heat and moisture exchanger (HME).

CONDUCTION

Conduction and conductive heat loss require the body to have direct contact with an object. The amount of heat lost is determined by the difference in the temperature between the surface of the skin and the object it is in contact with. Once the temperature of the air near the skin and the temperature of the skin itself are relatively equal, the heat transfer is negligible, and no more heat loss is conducted. Conduction is responsible for approximately 15% of the heat lost by the body.

MECHANISMS OF HEAT GENERATION

The human body has the ability to produce its own heat. Heat creation can be accomplished via four distinct mechanisms: nonshivering thermogenesis, shivering thermogenesis, voluntary muscle activity, and dietary thermogenesis (Figure 1.30).

NONSHIVERING THERMOGENESIS

Newborns lack the muscular structure necessary to produce muscular contractions requisite for heat generation associated with shivering. Nonshivering thermogenesis (NST) is the mechanism of heat production primarily employed by newborns during the first 6 months of life. Although NST is the primary source of thermoregulation in the pediatric patient until the age of 2 years, anesthesia providers should be aware that this method of heat generation is not sustainable, and exogenous sources of heat generation must be utilized in the perioperative period.

As the name indicates, NST does not include voluntary or involuntary muscle activity. Rather, NST utilizes brown adipose tissue (BAT), which is more abundant in newborns than older children or adults. BAT is mainly present in subscapular region, but can also be found in the cervical, perispinal, mediastinal, periaortic, pericardial, and periadrenal areas of the newborn's body (Figure 1.31).[9]

BAT contains adipocytes that act as heat creators or thermogenetic tissue to generate heat. When a newborn receives afferent input signaling cold temperatures beyond the interthreshold range, efferent postganglionic fibers in the sympathetic nervous system release norepinephrine. Norepinephrine then binds to beta 3 (β_3) receptor sites stimulating the transcription of the uncoupling protein 1 (UCP-1) gene, which is located in the inner membrane of the mitochondria of BAT.

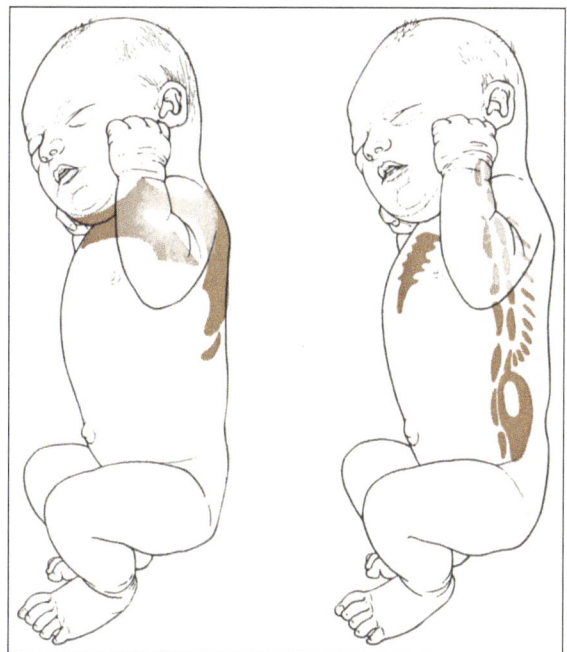

Figure 1.31: Sites of brown adipose tissue.

Source: From Lidell ME. Brown adipose tissue in human infants. In: A Pfeifer, M Klingenspor, S Herzig, eds. *Brown Adipose Tissue*. Handbook of Experimental Pharmacology. Springer; 2018:251.

The activation of UCP-1 initiates the lysis of triglycerides into free fatty acids and increases flow through BAT. The energy derived from the intense catabolic activity is then dissipated as heat in the blood as oxygen and substrates are extracted from the blood at a high rate. BAT has the potential for considerable metabolic activity given the high number of mitochondria and drops of triglycerides present.

Thyroid hormone has also been implicated in having a role in the stimulation of BAT.[9] While there is some indication that glucocorticoids, such as dexamethasone, and mineralocorticoids, such as aldosterone, play a role in triggering NST, there is conflicting literature suggesting glucocorticoids may perhaps inhibit NST.[10]

SHIVERING THERMOGENESIS

Once a pediatric patient is older, typically older than age 2, shivering thermogenesis takes on a larger responsibility in the thermoregulatory process. By definition, shivering thermogenesis is cold-induced involuntary muscle contraction.[11] Typically, contraction of the larger muscles of the trunk is more intense during shivering than that of muscles located in the periphery. Shivering has been noted to increase the metabolic heat production of a patient, as well as increasing oxygen consumption roughly six- to seven fold.[11] The increase in oxygen demand can lead to deleterious effects, including tissue hypoxia.[11]

VOLUNTARY MUSCLE ACTIVITY

Voluntary muscle activity aids in heat production by means of physical activity. When a muscle contraction occurs, hydrolysis of adenosine triphosphate (ATP) occurs and as a result, heat is produced.[4] Muscle activity involving skeletal muscle, being the largest of all muscle fibers in the body, generates the most heat.

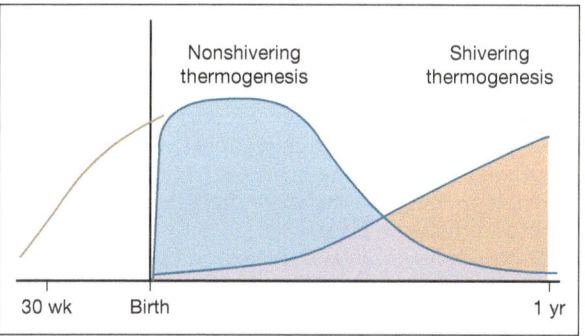

Figure 1.30: Transition from nonshivering thermogenesis to shivering thermogenesis.

Source: From Hull D, Smales ORC: Heat production in the newborn. In: Sinclair JC, ed. *Temperature Regulation and Energy Metabolism in the Newborn*. Grune and Stratton; 1978:129–156.

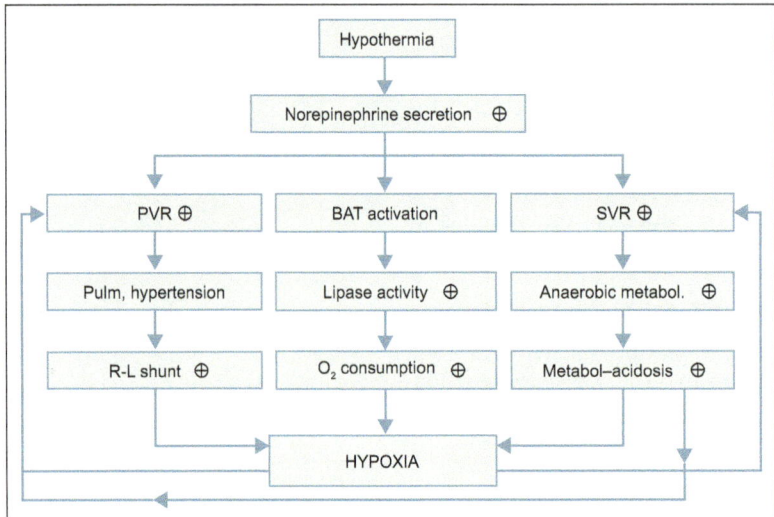

Figure 1.32: Consequences of inadequate thermoregulation in the newborn.

BAT, brown adipose tissue; PVR, pulmonary vascular resistance; SVR, systemic vascular resistance.

Source: From Klaus M, Faranoff A. *Care of the High-Risk Neonate.* Saunders; 1986.

DIETARY THERMOGENESIS

Dietary thermogenesis refers to the heat produced following the ingestion of food. Following consumption of a meal, digestion, absorption, metabolism, and storage of nutrients ensue, leading to increased metabolic activity and ultimately an obligatory increase in heat generation. This heat will contribute to the maintenance of body temperature when the body is exposed to a cold environment.

The generation of heat occurs roughly 1 hour after the ingestion of food and can last up of 7 to 8 hours.[12]

CONSEQUENCES OF INADEQUATE THERMOREGULATION IN THE NEWBORN

Figure 1.32 illustrates consequences of inadequate thermoregulation in the newborn.

1.8: BEHAVIORAL AND DEVELOPMENTAL MILESTONES

Nicole Garritano

LEARNING OBJECTIVES

- Discuss importance of understanding normal pediatric behavioral and developmental milestones.
- Review normal pediatric behavioral and developmental milestones for ages birth through 5 years.
- Understand contributing factors that may impact pediatric behavioral and developmental milestones.

INTRODUCTION

A sound comprehension of anticipated pediatric behavioral and developmental milestones is essential when caring for pediatric patients. It is of particular importance for pediatric anesthesia providers who are charged with caring for patients throughout the entirety of the perioperative period. This includes optimizing patients preoperatively, administration of sedation, monitored anesthesia care, or general anesthesia, and management of key aspects during the postoperative period, such as pain management and respiratory support. Therefore, understanding pediatric behavior and developmental milestones is pivotal in ensuring the delivery of safe, effective anesthetic care in the perioperative environment.

Evaluation of pediatric behavioral and developmental milestones is a fundamental tenet of primary pediatric care. Bright Futures, a national health promotion and prevention initiative led by the American Academy of Pediatrics (AAP) and supported, in part, by the U.S. Department of Health and Human Services, provides theory-based and evidence-driven guidance that healthcare professionals use during all preventive care screenings and well-child visits.[1] It is important to note that the Accreditation Council for Graduate Medical Education requires only 32 half-day education sessions related to pediatric behavior and development for all medical residents, leaving little time to master the content.[2] Therefore, while pediatric specialists rely on the cumulative knowledge that pediatricians document on their patients, it is crucial they also have working knowledge of normal pediatric behavior and development. Not only does this aid in ensuring appropriate age-based care is delivered, but it also facilitates productive interactions between healthcare providers and patients and their caregivers.

Pediatric behavioral and developmental milestones are categorized by age and address the expected growth, physical, language, communication, emotional, and social standards for the patient's age group. Table 1.14 provides an overview of normal parameters for the first 5 years of life as developed by the Centers for Disease Control and Prevention (CDC) and promoted through the AAP's Bright Futures health promotion program.[3] Additional resources for all pediatric age groups provided through the CDC and Bright Futures are provided in the Resources section of this chapter.

Table 1.14	Normal Pediatric Behavioral and Developmental Milestone Guidelines
Age	Milestones
Birth–2 months	Social and emotional • Begins to smile at people • Can briefly calm themselves, bringing hands to mouth • Tries to look at parent Language/Communication • Coos, makes gurgling sounds • Turns head toward sound Cognitive • Pays attention to faces • Begins to follow things with eyes and recognize people at a distance • Begins to act bored (fussy) if activity does not change Movement/Physical development • Can hold head up and begins to push up when lying on tummy • Makes smoother movements with arms and legs
2–4 months	Social and emotional • Smiles spontaneously • Likes to play with people • Copies movements and facial expressions Language/Communication • Begins to babble • Babbles with expression and copies sounds • Cries in different ways for hunger, pain, and tiredness Cognitive • Indicates being happy and sad • Responds to affection • Reaches for toy with one hand • Uses hand and eye together • Follows moving things with eyes • Watches faces closely • Recognizes familiar people and things at a distance Movement/Physical development • Holds head steadily, unsupported • Pushes down on legs when feet are on a hard surface • May roll over from tummy to back • Can hold a toy and shake it and swing at dangling toys • Brings hands to mouth • When lying on stomach, pushes up with elbows
4–6 months	Social and emotional • Knows familiar faces and begins to know if someone is a stranger • Likes to play with others, especially parents • Responds to other people's emotions and often seems happy • Likes to look at self in a mirror Language and communication • Responds to sounds by making sounds • Strings vowels together with babbling • Will take turns when vocalizing • Responds to own name • Makes sounds to show joy and displeasure • Begins to say consonant sounds when jabbering

(continued)

Table 1.14	Normal Pediatric Behavioral and Developmental Milestone Guidelines (*continued*)
Age	Milestones
4–6 months (cont.)	Cognitive • Looks around at nearby objects • Brings things to mouth • Shows curiosity about things and reaches for objects out of reach • Begins to pass objects from one hand to another Movement/Physical development • Rolls over in both directions • Begins to sit without support • When standing, supports weight on legs and may bounce • Rocks back and forth, may crawl backward before forward
6–9 months	Social and emotional • May be afraid of strangers • May be clingy with familiar adults • Has favorite toys Language and communication • Understands "no" • Makes lots of different sounds and strings sounds together • Points at things with finger Cognitive • Watches the path of something falling • Looks for things they sees you hide • Plays peek-a-boo • Puts things in mouth • Moves things smoothly from one hand to another • Picks up things between thumb and index finger Movement/Physical development • Stands, holding on • Can get into a sitting position • Sits without support • Pulls to stand • Crawls
9–12 months	Social and emotional • Is shy or nervous with strangers • Cries when mom or dad leaves • Has favorite things and people • Shows fear in some situations • Hands you a book to hear a story • Repeats sounds and actions for attention • Puts out arm or leg to help with dressing • Plays games such as peek-a-boo or pat-a-cake Language/Communication • Responds to simple spoken requests • Uses simple gestures • Makes sounds with changes in tone • Says *mama* and *dada* • Tries to repeat words

(*continued*)

Table 1.14	Normal Pediatric Behavioral and Developmental Milestone Guidelines (*continued*)
Age	**Milestones**
9–12 months (cont.)	Cognitive • Explores things by shaking, banging, or throwing • Finds hidden things easily • Looks at the correct picture or thing when it is named • Copies gestures • Starts to use things correctly (drink from cup, brush hair) • Puts objects in a container and removes them • Pokes with index finger • Follows simple directions Movement/Physical development • Gets to a sitting position without help • Pulls up to stand, cruises • May take a few steps • May stand alone
12–18 months	Social and emotional • Likes to hand things to others and play • May have temper tantrums • May be afraid of strangers • Shows affection to familiar people • Plays simple pretend • May cling to caregivers in new situations • Points to show others something interesting • Explores alone but with parent close by Language and communication • Says several single words • Says "no" and shakes head • Points to show someone what they want Cognitive • Knows what ordinary things are • Points to get attention • Pretends to feed doll or stuffed animal • Points to one body part • Scribbles on own • Can follow one-step verbal commands without any gestures Movement/Physical development • Walks alone • May walk up steps and run • Pulls toys while walking • Can help undress themselves • Drinks from a cup • Eats with a spoon
18 months–2 years	Social and emotional • Copies others • Gets excited when with other children • Shows more and more independence • Shows defiant behavior • Plays mainly beside other children

(*continued*)

Table 1.14	Normal Pediatric Behavioral and Developmental Milestone Guidelines (*continued*)
Age	Milestones
18 months–2 years (cont.)	Language/Communication • Points to things when they are named • Knows names of familiar people and body parts • Says sentences with two to four words • Follows simple instructions • Repeats words overheard in conversation • Points to things in a book Cognitive • Finds things hidden under two to three covers • Begins to sort shapes and colors • Completes sentences and rhymes in familiar books • Plays simple make-believe games • Builds tower of four or more blocks • Might use one hand more than the other • Follows two-step instructions • Names items in a picture book Movement/Physical development • Stands on tiptoe • Kicks a ball • Begins to run • Climbs onto and down from furniture without help • Walks up and down stairs holding on • Throws ball overhand • Makes or copies straight lines and circles
2–3 years	Social and emotional • Copies adults and friends • Shows affection for friends without prompting • Takes turns in games • Shows concern for crying friend • Understands *mine*, *his*, and *hers* • Shows a wide range of emotions • Separates easily from mom and dad • May get upset with major changes in routine • Dresses and undresses self Language/Communication • Follows 2- to 3-step instructions • Can name most familiar objects • Understands words like in, on, or under • Says first name, age, and sex • Names a friend • Says most first-person pronouns and some plurals • Talks well enough for strangers to understand most of the time • Carries on a conversation using two to three sentences Cognitive • Can work with toys with buttons, levers, and moving parts • Plays make-believe with toys and people • Does puzzles with three to four pieces • Understands what two means • Copies a circle with a pencil or crayon • Turns book pages one at a time • Builds towers of more than six blocks • Screws and unscrews jar lids or turns door handle

(*continued*)

Table 1.14	Normal Pediatric Behavioral and Developmental Milestone Guidelines (*continued*)
Age	Milestones
2–3 years (cont.)	Movement/Physical development • Climbs well • Runs easily • Pedals a tricycle • Walks up and down stairs, one foot on each step
3–4 years	Social and emotional • Enjoys doing new things • Plays "Mom" and "Dad" • Is more creative with make-believe play • Would rather play with other children than alone • Cooperates with other children • Often can't tell what is real and what is make-believe • Talks about what they like or are interested in Language/Communication • Knows some basic rules of grammar • Sings a song or says a poem from memory • Tells stories • Can say first and last name Cognitive • Names some colors and numbers • Understands the idea of counting • Starts to understand time • Remembers parts of a story • Understands the idea of same and different • Draws a person with two to four body parts • Uses scissors • Starts to copy some capital letters • Plays board or card games • Tells you what they think will happen next in a book Movement/Physical development • Hops and stands on one foot up to 2 seconds • Catches a bounced ball most of the time • Pours, cuts with supervision, and mashes own food
4–5 years	Social and emotional • Wants to please friends • Wants to be like friends • More likely to agree with rules • Likes to sing, dance, and act • Is aware of gender • Can tell what's real and what's make-believe • Shows more independence • Is sometimes demanding and sometimes very cooperative Language/Communication • Speaks very clearly • Tells a simple story using full sentences • Uses future tense • Says name and address

(*continued*)

Table 1.14	Normal Pediatric Behavioral and Developmental Milestone Guidelines (*continued*)
Age	**Milestones**
4–5 years (cont.)	Cognitive • Counts 10 or more things • Can draw a person with at least six body parts • Can print some letters and numbers • Copies a triangle and geometric shapes • Knows about things used every day Movement/Physical development • Stands on one foot for 10 seconds or longer • Hops, may be able to skip • Can do a somersault • Uses a fork and spoon and sometimes a table knife • Can use toilet on own • Swings and climbs

Source: From Centers for Disease Control and Prevention (CDC). *CDC's developmental milestones.* 2020. https://www.cdc.gov/ncbddd/actearly/milestones.

FACTORS INFLUENCING NORMAL PEDIATRIC BEHAVIORAL AND DEVELOPMENTAL MILESTONES

Factors that influence pediatric behavior and development can be classified as innate or environmental.[4] The presence and degree of influence of these factors can often be determined by members of the interprofessional team through interactions with the patient and their caregivers. This can include, but is not limited to, nurses, nurse practitioners, physicians, anesthesia providers, social workers, and child life specialists.

Innate factors influencing pediatric behavior and development include genetics, epigenetics, and prenatal and postnatal biological experiences.[4] Influential factors such as this are often readily apparent in patients whose behavior and development fail to align with expected norms for the patient's age.

Anesthesia providers should assess for the presence of environmental factors hampering pediatric behavior and development during the preoperative assessment. Environmental factors that can have a deleterious impact on behavior and development include family birth order, maternal educational level, family dynamics, poverty, child abuse, and strength of religious affiliation.[4] Each of these can have a significant impact on postoperative outcomes, making it imperative that anesthesia providers assess for environmental factors despite achievement of anticipated behavior and development milestones. Early identification of environmental factors affords the healthcare team the opportunity to take corrective measures and provide additional support to allay environmental factors that may preclude optimal patient outcomes. Recognizing when environmental factors may influence the plan of care for a pediatric patient and engaging the support of the interprofessional team when appropriate are key to safeguarding the patient's health and well-being.

KEY TAKEAWAYS

- It is important to assess normal pediatric behavior and development during the preoperative assessment and not rely solely on the documentation of other providers to ensure safe, quality, and patient-centered care.
- Assessing for adverse environmental factors during the preoperative assessment affords the interprofessional team the opportunity to provide additional pre- and postoperative support when appropriate.
- Engaging the interprofessional team to address aberrancies in behavior and development provides a comprehensive approach to patient care that safeguards the patient's health and well-being.

RESOURCES

- CDC Growth Charts
  - https://www.cdc.gov/growthcharts/index.htm
- CDC Pediatric Behavioral and Developmental Milestones
  - https://www.cdc.gov/ncbddd/actearly/milestones/index.html
- Bright Futures
  - https://brightfutures.aap.org/Pages/default.aspx

KEY REFERENCES

Complete references for this chapter are online and available at https://connect.springerpub.com/content/book/978-0-8261-3875-0/part/part01/toc-part/ch001.

1.1: NERVOUS SYSTEM

1. Vinik AI. The conductor of the autonomic orchestra. *Front Endocrinol (Lausanne)*. 2012;3:71. doi:10.3389/fendo.2012.00071
2. Warner DO, Zaccariello MJ, Katusic SK, et al. Neuropsychological and behavioral outcomes after exposure of young children to procedures requiring general anesthesia: The mayo anesthesia safety in kids (MASK) study. *Anesthesiology*. 2018;129(1):89–105. doi:10.1097/ALN.0000000000002232.
3. Anand KJS, Phil D, Hickey PR. Halothane-morphine compared with high-dose sufentanil for anesthesia and postoperative analgesia in neonatal cardiac surgery. *N Engl J Med*. 1992;326(1):1–9. doi:10.1056/NEJM199201023260101
4. Mai JK, Paxinos G, Mai JP. *The Human Nervous System*. Academic Press; 2012.
5. Nguyen L, Rigo JM, Rocher V, et al. Neurotransmitters as early signals for central nervous system development. *Cell Tissue Res*. 2001;305:187–202. doi:10.1007/s004410000343
6. Soriano SG, Eldredge EA, Rockoff MA. Pediatric neuroanesthesia. *Neuroimaging Clin N Am*. 2007;17(2):259–67. doi:10.1016/j.nic.2007.03.010.
7. Soriano S, McClain C, eds. *Essentials of Pediatric Neuroanesthesia*. Cambridge University Press; 2018.
8. U.S. Food and Drug Administration. *FDA approves label changes for use of general anesthetic and sedation drugs in young children*. 2017. https://www.fda.gov/media/104705/download

1.2: CARDIOVASCULAR SYSTEM

1. Kloesel B, DiNardo JA, Body SC. Cardiac embryology and molecular mechanisms of congenital heart disease. *Anesth Analg*. 2016;123(3):551–569. doi:10.1213/ane.0000000000001451
2. Moore KL, Persaud TVN, Torchia M. *The Developing Human: Clinically Oriented Embryology*. Elsevier; 2020.
4. Gordon JB, Young KA, Wise JA, et al. *Anatomy & Physiology*. OpenStax College, Rice University; 2017.
6. Ord H, Griksaitis M. Cardiac output diversity: Are children just small adults? *Physiology News*. 2019;Summer:39–41. doi:10.36866/pn.115.39
9. Singh Y, Tissot C. Echocardiographic evaluation of transitional circulation for the neonatologists. *Front Pediatr*. 2018;6:140. doi:10.3389/fped.2018.00140
13. Vrancken SL, van Heijst AF, de Boode WP. Neonatal hemodynamics: from developmental physiology to comprehensive monitoring. *Front Pediatr*. 2018;6:87. doi:10.3389/fped.2018.00087
15. Saikia D, Mahanta B. Cardiovascular and respiratory physiology in children. *Indian J Anaesth*. 2019;63(9):690–697. doi:10.4103/ija.ija_490_19

1.3: PEDIATRIC AIRWAY

1. Zielnik-Jurkiewicz B, Olszewska-Sosinska O. The nasal septum deformities in children and adolescents from Warsaw, Poland. *Int J Pediatr Otorhinolaryngol*. 2006; 70:731–736. doi:10.1016/j.ijporl.2004.09.014
2. Mallampati SR, Gatt SP, Gugino LD, et al. A clinical sign to predict difficult tracheal intubation: a prospective study. *Can Anaesth Soc J*. 1985;32(4):429–34. doi:10.1007/BF03011357
3. Reddy VS. Evaluation of upper airway obstruction in infants with Pierre Robin sequence and the role of polysomnography – review of current evidence. *Paediatr Respir Rev*. 2016;17:80–87. doi:10.1016/j.prrv.2015.10.001
4. Cormack RS, Lehane J. Difficult tracheal intubation in obstetrics". *Anaesthesia*. 1984;39(11):1105–1111.
5. Yentis SM, Lee DJH. Evaluation of an improved scoring system for the grading of direct laryngoscopy. *Anaesthesia*. 1998;53:1041–1044. doi:10.1046/j.1365-2044.1998.00605.x
6. McDonald IH, Stocks JG. Prolonged nasotracheal intubation. *Br J Anaesth*. 1965;37:161–173. doi:10.1093/bja/37.3.161
7. Walner DL, Loewen MS, Kimura RE. Neonatal subglottic stenosis–incidence and trends. *Laryngoscope* 2001;111:48–51. doi:10.1097/00005537-200101000-00009
8. Cotton RT, Myer CM 3rd, O'Connor DM. Innovations in pediatric laryngotracheal reconstruction. *J Pediatr Surg* 1992;27:196–200. doi:10.1016/0022-3468(92)90311-t
9. Miyamoto RC, Cotton RT, Rope AF, et al. Association of anterior glottic webs with velocardiofacial syndrome (chromosome 22q11.2 deletion). *Otolaryngol Head Neck Surg* 2004;130(4):415–417. doi:10.1016/j.otohns.2003.12.014

1.4: RESPIRATORY SYSTEM

1. Brashers VL. Structure and function of the pulmonary system. In KL McCance, SE Huether, eds. *Pathophysiology: The Biologic Basis for Disease in Adults and Children*. 6th ed. Mosby Elsevier. 2010;1242–1309.
2. McFadyen JG, Thompson DR, Martin LD. In Wheeler DS, Wong HR, Shanley TP, eds. *Pediatric Critical Care Medicine*. 2nd ed. Springer. 2014;3–18.
3. Gott KG, Froh DK. Alterations of pulmonary function in children. In KL McCance, SE Huether, eds. *Pathophysiology: The Biological Basis for Disease in Adults and Children*. 6th ed. Mosby. 2010;1310–1343.
4. Tisekar OR, Ajith Kumar AK. Hypoplastic Lung Disease. In: StatPearls [Internet]. Treasure Island StatPearls Publishing; 2021. https://www.ncbi.nlm.nih.gov/books/NBK562139
5. Murphy P. The fetal circulation. *BJA CEPD*. 2005;5(4):107–112. doi:10.1093/bjaceaccp/mki030
6. Teng RJ, Wu TJ. Persistent pulmonary hypertension of the newborn. *J Formos Med Assoc*. 2013;112(4):177–184. doi:10.1016/j.jfma.2012.11.007
7. Levitzky M. *Pulmonary Physiology*. 9th ed. The McGraw-Hill Companies, Inc. 2018;124–141.
8. Kajekar R. Environmental factors and developmental outcomes in the lung. *Pharmacol Ther*. 2007;114(2):129–145. doi:10.1016/j.pharmthera.2007.01.011
9. West JB, Dollery CT, Naimark A. Distribution of blood flow in isolated lung; relation to vascular and alveolar pressures. *J Appl Physiol*. 1964;19(4):713–724. doi:10.1152/jappl.1964.19.4.713

1.5: RENAL SYSTEM

10. Madden N, Trachtman H. Physiology of the developing kidney: sodium and water homeostasis and its disorder. In: Avner ED, Harmon WE, Niaudet P, eds. *Pediatric Nephrology*. Springer. 2016;181–217.
11. MD MCBMaCJK. Urologic aspects of pediatric nephrology. In: Partin AW, Dmochowski RR, Kavoussi LR, Peters C, eds. *Campbell-Walsh Urology*. 12th ed. Elsevier; 2020.
12. Atkinson MA, Ng DK, Warady BA, et al. The CKiD study: overview and summary of findings related to kidney disease progression. *Pediatr Nephrol*. 2020;36(3):527–538. doi:10.1007/s00467-019-04458-6

16. Quigley R, Wolf MTF. Renal tubular acidosis in children. In: Avner ED, Harmon WE, Niaudet P, eds. *Pediatric Nephrology*. Springer; 2016:1273–1306.
20. VanDeVoorde RG, Wong CS, Warady BA. Management of chronic kidney disease in children. In: Avner ED, Harmon WE, Niaudet P, eds. *Pediatric Nephrology*. Springer; 2016:2207–2266.
24. Rana A, Gruessner A, Agopian VG, et al. Survival benefit of solid-organ transplant in the United States. *JAMA Surg*. 2015;150(3):252–259. doi:10.1001/jamasurg.2014.2038

1.6: HEPATIC SYSTEM

1. Beath SV. Hepatic function and physiology in the newborn. *Semin Neonatol*. 2003;8(5):337–346. doi:10.1016/S1084-2756(03)00066-6
2. Reddy MS. *Liver Anatomy for Pediatric Intensivist*. Pediatric Liver Intensive Care. Springer; 2019:1–5. doi:10.1007/978-981-13-1304-2_1
6. Grijalva J, Vakili K. Neonatal liver physiology. *Semin Pediatr Surg*. 2013;22(4):185–189. doi:10.1053/j.sempedsurg.2013.10.006
7. D'Antiga L, Casotti V. Basic principles of liver physiology. In: D'Antiga L, ed. *Pediatric Hepatology and Liver Transplantation*. Springer; 2019:21–39.
8. Fuhrman BP, Blumer JL. Principles of drug distribution in the critically ill child. In: Fuhrman BP, ed. *Pediatric Critical Care*. 4th ed. Elsevier Saunders; 2011:1538–1552.

1.7: THERMOREGULATION

1. Jänig W. Peripheral thermoreceptors in innocuous temperature detection. *Handb Clin Neurol*. 2018;156:47–56. doi:10.1016/B978-0-444-63912-7.00002-3
2. Tan CL, Knight ZA. Regulation of body temperature by the nervous system. *Neuron*. 2018;98(1):31–48. doi:10.1016/j.neuron.2018.02.022
4. Koop LK, Tadi P. Physiology, heat loss (convection, evaporation, radiation). In: *Stat Pearls*. Stat Pearls Publishing; 2020.
13. Elshazzly M, Anekar AA, Caban O. Physiology, newborn. In: *Stat Pearls*. Stat Pearls Publishing; 2020.
14. Lidell ME. Brown adipose tissue in human infants. *Handb Exp Pharmacol*. 2018;251:107–123. doi:10.1007/164_2018_118
15. Ota W, Nakane Y, Kashio M, et al. Involvement of TRPM2 and TRPM8 in temperature-dependent masking behavior. *Sci Rep*. 2019;9(1):3706. doi:10.1038/s41598-019-40067
21. Miller RD. *Miller's Anesthesia*. Elsevier; 2019
37. Lai L, See M, Rampal S, et al. Significant factors influencing inadvertent hypothermia in pediatric anesthesia. *J Clin Monit Comput*. 2019;33:1105–1112. doi:10.1007/s10877-019-00259-2

1.8: BEHAVIORAL AND DEVELOPMENTAL MILESTONES

1. Sheldrick RC, Schlichting LE, Berger B, et al. Establishing new norms for developmental milestones. *Pediatrics*. 2019;144(6):110. doi:10.1542/peds.2019-0374
2. Voigt RG, Macias MM, Myers SM, Tapia CD. Child development: the basic science of pediatrics. In: Voigt RG, ed. *AAP Developmental and Behavior Pediatrics*. American Academy of Pediatrics; 2018:1–5.
3. Centers for Disease Control and Prevention (CDC). *CDC's developmental milestones*. 2020. https://www.cdc.gov/ncbddd/actearly/milestones
4. Wang P. Nature, nurture, and their interactions in child development and behavior. In Voigt RG, ed. *AAP Developmental and Behavior Pediatrics*. American Academy of Pediatrics; 2018:5–21.
5. Bright Futures. *Bright futures guidelines and pocket guide*. 2020. https://brightfutures.aap.org/materials-and-tools/guidelines-and-pocket-guide/Pages/default.aspx

CHAPTER 2

Pharmacologic Considerations for the Pediatric Patient

LEARNING OBJECTIVES

- Define and apply the principles of pharmacodynamics and pharmacokinetics to the practice of anesthesia.
- Identify important anatomical changes during growth that impact pharmacodynamics and pharmacokinetics.
- Differentiate the concepts of potency versus efficacy.
- Provide a fundamental understanding of dose–response curves modeling.
- Explain physicochemical and physiologic factors that control the absorption, distribution, metabolism, and elimination of pharmacologic agents.
- Describe drug distribution compartment modeling.
- Provide an overview of elimination pharmacokinetic principles that apply to compartment modeling.
- Understand the pharmacology of commonly inhaled and IV anesthetic agents.
- Describe aspects of pharmacology key to pediatric anesthesia.

2.1: Pharmacokinetics and Pharmacodynamics

Chad Watkins and Dennis LaChance

Anatomical maturation has a direct impact on clinical responsiveness to pharmacologic agents. It is inappropriate to extrapolate pharmacodynamic and pharmacokinetic principles from the adult population and apply them to the pediatric population. Physiologic and anatomical variations in pediatric patients have a profound impact on the absorption, distribution, metabolism, and elimination of pharmacologic agents. Further adding to the complexity of pediatric anesthesia is that the pediatric population consists of multiple subgroups, such as neonates, infants, preadolescents, and adolescents. Each subgroup exhibits differing body composition and stages of organ development, which regulate the pharmacologic activity of medications. As a patient progresses through the natural stages of growth and development, their body will respond differently to medications commonly used in anesthesia. This chapter provides a brief overview of the pharmacologic principles necessary to provide safe and effective pediatric anesthesia care.

LIMITATIONS

The approved indications for many pharmacologic agents do not include use among the pediatric population. Over the past several decades, the U.S. Food and Drug Administration (FDA) has placed emphasis on expanding clinical testing among the pediatric population. To garner approval from the FDA for pediatric labeling, there must be clinical data about a pharmacologic agent demonstrating both safe and effective therapy in the pediatric population. The approval process includes an evaluation performed by the Center for Drug Evaluation and Research (CDER). The evaluating team is composed of independent, unbiased physicians, statisticians, chemists, and pharmacologists charged with reviewing clinical data to determine if the proposed labeling supports a therapeutic benefit and outweighs any potential or known risks in a defined patient population. Insufficient or unavailable supporting data ultimately limit the use of many pharmacologic agents, deeming the pediatric population as an off-label indication. Thus, the unknown pharmacodynamics and pharmacokinetics of pharmacologic agents when used in the pediatric population can lead to variances in dosing and outcomes.

GROWTH AND DEVELOPMENT

Therapeutic response to pharmacologic agents has a direct correlation to anatomical growth and development. As an infant progresses through the stages of maturation, developmental changes occur that impact the pharmacokinetic properties of medications. Growth can be defined as a patient's physical increase in size, which over time includes dynamic transformations in body composition. Development involves physiologic changes in function as organs and anatomical systems mature. Both growth and development have a distinct impact on clinical response to pharmacologic agents.

Traditional approaches utilize changes in weight and length to model a patient's growth. Length is an indicator of skeletal growth, while weight directly reflects increase in mass secondary to anatomical development. Weight independently is a nonspecific measurement of growth that represents an overall cumulative change in mass associated with muscle, bone, cartilage, tissue, and fat. The analysis of weight in conjunction with length can be used to predict a patient's overall health and nutritional status. Comparing a patient's values against a standard growth curve will allow the clinician to make assessments of the patient's body composition. Additionally, it is important to understand the anatomical changes in body composition associated with growth. As a patient grows, significant shifts in body composition will directly affect the extent of absorption and distribution of pharmacologic agents. Table 2.1 reflects body composition changes associated with growth and development.[1] The impact of these changes on pharmacokinetics is presented in more detail later in this chapter.

Organ development has a profound impact on a patient's response and tolerance to pharmacologic agents. The immature organ systems of newborns, infants, and children yield significant variations in metabolic and elimination pathways

Table 2.1	Body Composition Changes With Growth and Development						
	Premature Infant (2 kg)	Full-Term Infant (3.5 kg)	1 Year (10 kg)	10 Years (31 kg)	15 Years (60 kg)	Adult (70 kg)	Older Adult (65 kg)
Minerals	2%	3%	3%	4%	4%	6%	4%
Fat	6%	13%	22%	14%	13%	18%	30%
Protein	12%	13%	13%	17%	18%	17%	12%
Water	80%	70%	61%	65%	65%	60%	54%

Source: Puig M. Body composition and growth. In: Walker WA, Watkins JB, eds. *Nutrition in Pediatrics*, 2nd edn. BC Decker; 1996.

when compared with their adult counterparts. It is important that anesthesia providers understand the impact the stages of anatomical development of organ systems have on pharmacokinetic properties. In patients of all ages, metabolic and elimination pathways are regulated by the liver and kidneys. Underdevelopment of these vital organs can result in a reduction of biotransformation processes and decreased renal clearance of pharmacologic agents. These functional differences contribute to prolonged drug half-lives, delayed clearance, and increased reabsorption. These variances increase the relative risk of toxicities associated with increased concentrations. To prevent drug accumulation, when compared with adult dosing, pediatric dosing regimens for many pharmacologic agents will require extended intervals. In particular, premature neonates will require regimens that are carefully adjusted to compensate for underdeveloped organ systems.

Fundamentally, understanding the stages of growth and development will ensure appropriate dosing practices to achieve desirable therapeutic outcomes while preventing toxicities and adverse effects.

Pharmacology studies the relationship between chemical substances and the produced biochemical and physiologic effects on living organisms. Pharmacology can be further subdivided to include the study of pharmacodynamic and pharmacokinetic properties. It is important to recognize the differences between each branch to understand the application to pediatric anesthesia.

PHARMACODYNAMICS

Pharmacodynamics focuses on the chemical effects and functional alterations on biologic systems secondary to the administration of a pharmacologic agent. To abbreviate, pharmacodynamics can be viewed as the effect of the drug on the body. Pharmacodynamics includes understanding the mechanism of action in which a pharmacologic agent produces a therapeutic response. Pharmacologic agents exhibit a variety of mechanisms of action that can either stimulate or inhibit a physiologic response. The primary mechanism of action for most anesthesia-related pharmacologic agents includes activity at the receptor level. Pharmacologic agents that behave as an agonist or antagonist will regulate the response produced from the activation of the target receptor.

POTENCY AND EFFICACY

The pharmacodynamics of a pharmacologic agent is generalized by the potency and efficacy of the drug. This is a concentration-dependent relationship that can greatly differ between the pediatric and the adult population. Potency is the magnitude of the therapeutic response relative to the plasma concentration of the agent. It is important to consider that equivalent weight-based dosing can yield varied plasma concentrations in differing patient populations. Understanding this impact relative to the agent's potency is essential to avoid undesirable effects or potential toxicities in the pediatric patient. Efficacy is the capacity of the pharmacologic agent to produce a therapeutic effect. This can be quantified by determining the maximum response achieved relative to the administered dose. The maximum efficacy (E_{max}) is the threshold at which an increased dose will not yield a greater response. Efficacy and potency between differing agents can be analyzed by plotting the therapeutic effect relative to dose on a dose–response curve.

Graphical analysis between differing pharmacologic agent's dose–response curves will allow anesthesia providers to distinguish between potency and efficacy. In the example illustrated in **Figure 2.1**, both pharmacologic agents have similar activity but yield very different E_{max} values, with Drug A reaching a greater maximum effect than Drug B. It is important to avoid the interpretation that efficacy mirrors superiority. Clinically, the utility of E_{max} may have little influence on achieving appropriate therapeutic outcomes but may offer a greater indication for potential toxicities. For example, for the pharmacologic agents depicted in **Figure 2.1**, consider that an appropriate therapeutic response is achieved at E_{50} for Drug B. Drug A would have an increased potential to result in undesired toxicities with accidental overdoses. Thus, both agents will have adequate clinical efficacy, although Drug A has the potential for an increased effect that may substantiate undesired adverse effects.

Pharmacologic agents with differing potencies are depicted in **Figure 2.2**. The achievable maximum effect for both agents is the same; however, it is accomplished at a much lower dose for Drug A. In this example, it is reasonable to conclude that Drug A has a greater potency when compared with Drug B. Again, it is important to recognize that potency does not reflect superiority. Both agents have equivalent efficacies and when dosed appropriately can achieve optimal therapeutic outcomes.

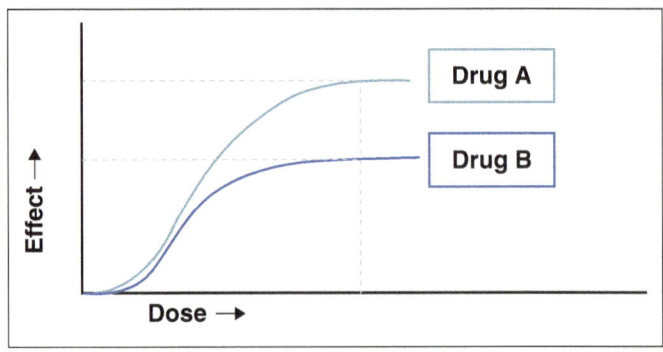

Figure 2.1: Efficacy of pharmacologic agents.

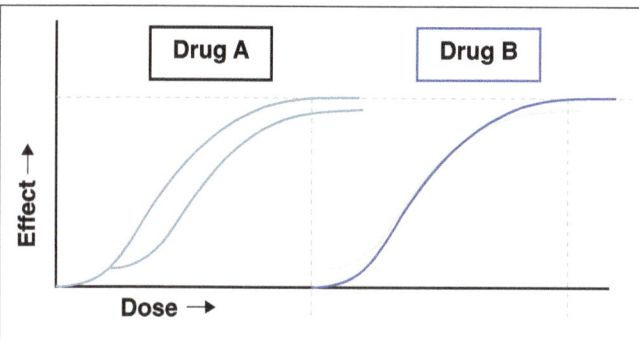

Figure 2.2: Potency of pharmacologic agents.

Dose Response

For the majority of pharmacologic agents, the dose–response curve follows a nonlinear model. A linear effect model would indicate the therapeutic response is directly proportionate to drug concentrations. Thus, this model would assume an infinite therapeutic response defying the principles of efficacy. The linear effect model would be represented by the equation and graph in Figure 2.3.

Maximum Effect Model

The maximum effect model (Figure 2.4) is the fundamental basis of concentration-dependent drug-induced therapeutic responses. The maximum effect model integrates the law of diminishing return by yielding a disproportionate increase of therapeutic effect as concentrations approach E_{max}. This model is represented by a hyperbolic dose–response curve that reaches E_{max} at a threshold concentration. Exceeding the threshold concentration will result in system saturation. This model provides clinical utility in determining a drug concentration that is within a desirable therapeutic range. In practice, EC_{50} is a clinical benchmark utilized in establishing appropriate dosing regimens.

Sigmoidal Maximum Effect Model

The sigmoidal maximum effect model (Figure 2.5) is an extension of the maximum effect model that incorporates the Hill coefficient (n). The Hill coefficient represents the magnitude of substrate binding. Figure 2.5 demonstrates the affinity between the pharmacologic agent and the receptor site on a molecular level. The level of cooperativity has a direct impact on the slope of the response curve. Upon initial substrate binding, a positive cooperative binding effect is represented by a value of n>1 and increased binding affinity to other molecules. Conversely, negative cooperative binding is represented by a value of n<1 and decreased binding affinity to other molecules. Noncooperative binding indicates that substrate binding has no impact on affinity; thus, n = 1, which is represented by the maximum effect model. The sigmoidal maximum effect model is the most accurate representation of a pharmacologic agent that yields an S-shaped dose–response curve.

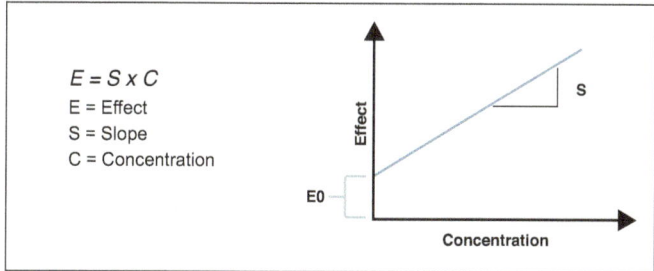

Figure 2.3: Linear effect model.

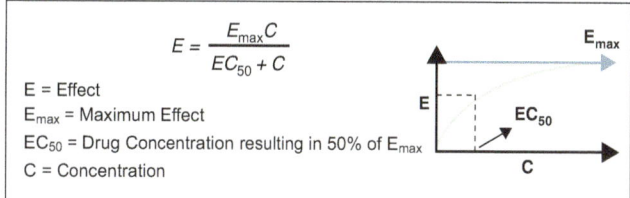

Figure 2.4: Maximum effect model.

PHARMACOKINETICS

The anatomical differences between pediatric and adult patients have a significant impact on the efficacy and therapeutic response to pharmacologic agents. These therapeutic responses are triggered by accumulating drug concentrations, which are determined by the pharmacokinetic properties of the agent. Pharmacokinetics can be summarized as the study of changing drug concentrations in the human body over a defined period. The study of pharmacokinetics can be further dissected to four basic processes: absorption, distribution, metabolism, and elimination. Pharmacokinetics can be mathematically defined by the physiologic processes that regulate the movement of a medication in, through, and out of the body. Crucial pharmacokinetic differences between pediatric and adult patients are summarized in Table 2.2. Understanding the anatomical differences in the pediatric population will allow the clinician to incorporate therapeutic strategies to compensate for the pharmacokinetic differences.

ABSORPTION

The first stage of drug activity is dependent on mechanisms of absorption. The absorption of a pharmacologic agent is predominantly influenced by the route of administration. The process of absorption describes the transit of drug from the site of administration to systemic circulation. Anatomical development and changes in body composition have a profound impact on the extent of systemic absorption. This explains differences in the bioavailability of some medications between pediatric and adult populations.

Bioavailability (F) is the percentage or fraction of the administered pharmacologic agent that reaches the systemic circulation. In anesthesia practice, the majority of medications are administered intravenously. IV pharmacologic agent administered directly into the systemic circulation will exhibit complete absorption (F = 1). However, pharmacologic agents administered via other routes (oral, sublingual, IM, and rectal) must undergo absorption prior to generating a therapeutic response. This process is influenced by two important parameters: rate and extent of absorption. Rate is instrumental in characterizing a pharmacologic agent's onset of action, while the extent of absorption helps identify the effective dose.[2] Drug factors that influence systemic absorption include dosage form disintegration characteristics, drug dissolution properties, drug absorption site stability, and drug substrate affinity for transporters/drug metabolizing enzymes (DMEs).[3] For the majority of non-IV

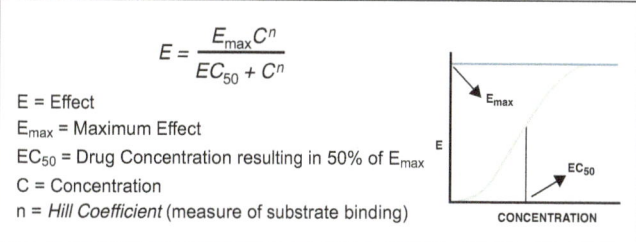

Figure 2.5: Sigmoidal maximum effect model.

Table 2.2 Summary of Pharmacokinetic Differences in Pediatric Versus Adult Patients

Age-Related Difference Compared to Adults	Pharmacokinetic Changes	Examples
Absorption		
Reduced gastrointestinal motility, higher intragastric pH	Higher oral bioavailability for acid-labile drugs Lower oral bioavailability for weak acids Prolonged time to reach maximum concentration after oral administration in general	Penicillin G, ampicillin, phenytoin, phenobarbital
Thinner stratum corneum, greater cutaneous perfusion, greater epidermal hydration	Increased percutaneous absorption, increased systemic exposure	Corticosteroids, lidocaine, povidone iodine
Less muscle mass, weaker muscle contraction, reduced muscle blood flow	Reduced IM bioavailability, erratic IM absorption in general	
Distribution		
Reduced protein binding	Increased unbound plasma concentrations	Phenytoin
Increased water proportion in neonates	Increased volume of distribution of water-soluble drugs Smaller volume of distribution of lipid-soluble drugs	Diazepam
Metabolism		
Reduced metabolizing enzyme activity (phase 1 and 2 metabolism)	Lower clearance	Caffeine, chloramphenicol, morphine
Excretion		
Reduced renal function in neonates	Lower renal clearance	Aminoglycosides, vancomycin, digoxin
Elevated renal clearance per kilogram body weight in children older than 1 year	Higher renal clearance	

pharmacologic agents only a fraction of the administered drug reaches systemic circulation, often yielding a bioavailability less than 100% (F<1). The differing body composition and stages of organ development in the pediatric population directly impact the process of absorption.

In the pediatric population, there are many processes that alter gastrointestinal (GI) absorption of orally administered medications in comparison with adults. Pediatric patients (especially neonates and infants) exhibit extended gastric emptying, decreased intestinal motility, higher gastric acidity, and decreased levels of gastric/intestinal enzymes. Healthy children will reach adult gastric emptying rates by 6 to 8 months of age.[4] In many cases, the reduced GI motility and delayed gastric emptying contribute to an extended absorption period and overall decreased peak concentrations.

Neonates and infants demonstrate a higher gastric pH. The pH decreases to a level of 1 to 3 within 24 to 48 hours of birth, only to return to a neutral value within 8 days. Adult values are not evident until after 2 years of age.[5,6] These higher pH levels may help to preserve the integrity of acid-labile drugs, such as beta-lactams, which increase the overall bioavailability of the pharmacologic agent. Neonatal serum concentrations of penicillin have been observed as five to six times higher than those of older children when administered orally.[7] Conversely, weak acids such as phenytoin, phenobarbital, and acetaminophen may experience decreased absorption due to an increased ionization state.[8,9]

Pediatric anatomical differences also have a significant impact on the absorption of pharmacologic agents administered topically or injected into the tissue. Topical drug absorption is increased secondary to skin that is thin/porous, enhanced epidermal hydration, as well as increased body surface area (BSA) to body weight ratio. Additionally, neonates and infants have higher capillary density in their skin/skeletal muscles, which improves blood flow to the site of administration. Although neonatal skeletal muscle may have enhanced capillary density, decreased skeletal muscle blood flow and drug reservoir capacity may decrease bioavailability following IM administration. This contributes to unpredictable and erratic drug levels, thereby limiting the utility of IM administration in clinical practice.[10,11]

DISTRIBUTION

Upon reaching systemic circulation, the activity of pharmacologic agents becomes dependent on the extent of distribution. The extent of distribution is influenced by both the physiologic characteristics of the host (water mass, circulating plasma/tissue proteins, and tissue transporter expression) and physiochemical properties of the drug (protein binding affinity, acid dissociation constant, partition coefficients). Volume of distribution (Vd) is a proportionality constant that relates a dose to the resulting concentration following administration:

$$\text{Volume of distribution (Vd)} = \frac{\text{Amount of drug}}{\text{Concentration}}$$

Volume of Distribution

In practice, Vd directly impacts the dose required to achieve the desired therapeutic effect. Vd is the overall size/space of all combined compartments and tissues where a dose may disperse after it enters the body. Typically, a low Vd represents a smaller biologic space, such as intravascular volume, extracellular stores, or total body water space (in adults). Small volumes of distribution result in a high-plasma concentration relative to the dose given. Conversely, a large Vd represents extensive dispersal of the drug into the tissues and a coinciding low-plasma concentration per dose administered. Clinically, Vd is an essential variable utilized in calculating loading doses, drug clearance, and a drug's half-life kinetics (discussed later in this chapter; see *First-Order Kinetics*).[12] The Vd of a specific agent is dependent on factors, such as tissue binding, protein binding, and lipid/water solubility.[2]

The most influential developmental difference among age groups is body water composition and its effect on Vd. Total body water content gradually decreases as a neonate progresses through adulthood. Full-term neonates have a total body water content of approximately 70% to 80%, which overtime decreases to approximately 60% by late adolescence.[13] In contrast, body fat increases with age, from 1% to 2% in premature neonates, to 10% to 15% in term neonates, and from 20% to 25% by 1 year of age.[14] Similar constitutional changes are observed with increasing lean muscle mass with age.

Hydrophilic Pharmacologic Agents

Water-soluble pharmacologic agents have a positive correlation with total body water content. In such agents the Vd increases as the total body water content increases. In the neonatal population, higher water content in combination with decreased adipose tissue/lean muscle mass contributes to a greater Vd. For hydrophilic medications, a greater Vd results in more extensive circulation yielding lower concentrations. Under such circumstances, younger patients will require higher dosing regimens to achieve a desired serum concentration or clinical response. Gentamicin is a classic example that illustrates the changes in Vd secondary to body composition changes attributed to growth (**Figure 2.6**). Gentamicin is a hydrophilic agent that widely distributes in extracellular fluid. Neonates with a high total body water content will have greater Vd than an adult patient. Clinically this results in higher weight-based dosing regimens in pediatric patients to achieve therapeutic concentrations.

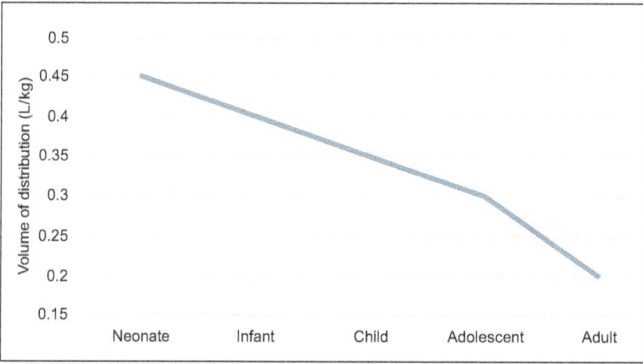

Figure 2.6: Volume of distribution of gentamicin.

Lipophilic Pharmacologic Agents

The opposite is true for pharmacologic agents that exhibit lipophilic characteristics. Lipophilic medications (such as diazepam) saturate adipose tissue, which reduces serum concentrations. Remembering body fat content increases with anatomical growth and development, lipophilic medications will have a decreased Vd resulting in higher serum concentrations in pediatric patients. Thus, younger patients may require lower dosing regimens when relatively compared with adult patients.

Protein Binding

Protein binding has a notable impact on the distribution of many pharmacologic agents utilized in the anesthesia practice. Protein binding restricts the systemic circulation of the free "active" drug. Pharmacologic agents become inactive once bound to a plasma protein such albumin or glycoproteins. In children, moderate to highly protein-bound drugs may have fluctuations in Vd due to a decrease in total protein amount, decreased binding affinity, or the presence of substrates capable of displacing drugs/endogenous substances from protein binding sites. Specifically, many local anesthetics and phenylpiperidine opioids (fentanyl, sufentanil, and alfentanil) bind to alpha-1-acid glycoprotein (AAG). Research indicates infant AAG levels are approximately 25% to 33% of adult levels, with slight increases through 9 to 12 months of age.[15] Excessive free drug concentrations may result in increased hepatic clearance (CLhepatic) of such drugs in infants and increased distribution. AAG is a protein that rapidly increases postoperatively.[16] This increase is observed considerably in infants and to a lesser extent in the adolescent and adult populations. Drugs such as bupivacaine or ropivacaine may experience time-dependent changes in clearance postsurgery.

Impact of Albumin

The albumin level of a patient has a downstream impact on the plasma concentration of the agent. Albumin binds predominately to positively charged acidic drugs. Neonates and infants have lower albumin levels with decreased binding affinity that will produce elevated free drug concentrations with standard dosing regimens of highly protein-bound medications. Thus, desirable therapeutic outcomes could be achieved with decreased dosing. Neonates also have higher concentrations of endogenous substrates (bilirubin, free fatty acids) capable of dislodging substrates from their active sites.[17] Volatile anesthetics are not highly bound to proteins but may displace acidic drugs (such as thiopental sodium) from protein binding sites.[18,19] Although thiopental sodium is highly unbound in neonates, this lower binding seems to be of little importance in the pharmacokinetics of younger patients.[20]

METABOLISM

While several organs (kidney, intestines, lungs, and skin) contain DMEs, the liver is the primary organ responsible for the metabolism of most pharmacologic agents used in anesthesia. The liver encompasses a greater percentage of total body weight (TBW), which leads to greater hepatic clearance in children than in adults when normalized for weight. Due to a relatively larger liver size, hepatic clearance is often converted to BSA in contrast to weight-based dosing in order to consistently predict metabolism through pediatric development.[21] Metabolism may be broken into two distinct phases. Phase 1 metabolism is characterized by reactions that increase renal excretion by decreasing lipophilicity or increasing polarity of a drug. Such Phase 1 reactions include oxidation, reduction, hydrolysis, and methylation. Phase 2 metabolism entails drug molecule manipulations via conjugation of a hydrophilic functional group to enhance water solubility for improved renal excretion. Phase 2 metabolic pathways include glucuronidation, sulfation, and acetylation. Pharmacologic agents requiring metabolism may undergo either one or both phases of metabolism.

Phase 1 Metabolism

Phase 1 metabolism is predominately mediated by the cytochrome 450 (CYPs) enzymes. CYPs are a family of hemeprotein containing oxidases that undergo different levels of expression from neonatal into adult development. The majority of anesthetic drugs are metabolized by CYP3A4.[22] At birth, CYP3A4 levels are very low. Compared with adult values, levels will increase to 30% to 60% within the first week of life and almost 100% by 1 year of age (Figure 2.7). CYP1A2 is a major enzyme in the metabolism of local amide anesthetics. CYP1A2 is the last enzyme to develop, gradually increasing in expression by 1 to 3 months of life and reaching adult levels by 10 years of age. All the enzymes will demonstrate activity similar to adults by 1 to 2 years of age.[23]

Phase 2 Metabolism

Phase 2 metabolism uses binding reactions via glutathione S-transferase (GST), uridine 5′-diphospho-glucuronosyltransferase (UGT), sulfotransferase (SULT), and acetyltransferase to increase water solubility. Most of these Phase 2 enzymes exhibit multiple isoforms with a personalized expression profile. The UGT family of enzymes is critically influential in the practice of pediatric anesthesia. UGTs are responsible for the metabolism of acetaminophen (UGT1A6/1A9) and morphine (UGT2B7) via glucuronidation. Glucuronidation involves the enzymatic addition of glucuronic acid to a drug in order to increase water solubility and improve renal excretion. Each UGT isoform develops along different timelines. UGT1A1 and 2B7 develop very early while UGT1A6 and 1A9 develop slowly through anatomical development. UGT2B7 levels are detectable in the fetus, which increases at birth, only to reach adult levels by 2 to 6 months of age. UGT1A6 is not detected in the fetus, with minimal levels as a neonate. The maturity of Phase 2 enzymes influences dosing requirements, which leads to a balance between therapeutic efficacy and adverse events due to possible limitations in drug metabolism.

In the neonatal population, expression of UGT isoforms plays a significant role in the metabolism of multiple drugs. Morphine is metabolized via UGT2B7 into morphine-6-glucuronide (analgesic substrate) and morphine-3-glucuronide. Due to the minimal activity of UGT2B7 in neonates, the active analgesic metabolite of morphine may experience less renal clearance. This in theory translates to lower dosing requirements for neonates receiving morphine or risk adverse reactions associated with morphine toxicity. In addition, consequences of immature UGT2B7 enzyme activity have been observed in the metabolism of some agents, such as chloramphenicol in neonates. Reduced glucuronidation and clearance of chloramphenicol (a substrate of UGT2B7) have led to "gray-baby" syndrome. Toxic levels of chloramphenicol can result in cyanosis, cardiovascular collapse, and death.[24]

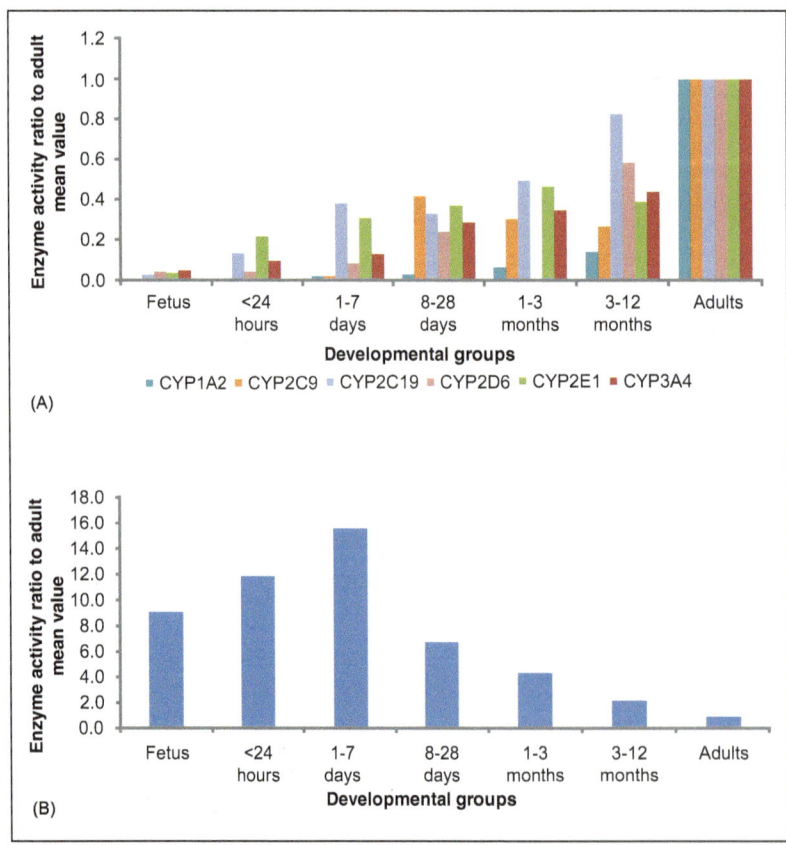

Figure 2.7: CYP enzyme expression by age.

Detoxification Response

The immaturity of Phase 1/2 metabolic pathways in neonates and infants does not always result in increased adverse effects and negative consequences. The detoxification response of the human body is capable of bypassing certain elimination pathways in order to compensate for less developed metabolism mechanisms. This is evident in the metabolism of acetaminophen in neonates and infants. UGT1A6 (glucuronidation) and SULT1A1 (sulfation) are the two primary pathways of acetaminophen metabolism. Sulfation is a process similar to glucuronidation, except substituting sulfonic acid for glucuronic acid. Sulfation is a process well developed at birth, while glucuronidation is decreased in neonates and reaches full capacity by adolescence. Younger patients undergo sulfate conjugation with a transition to glucuronide conjugation by adulthood.[10] Of importance, SULT1A1 metabolism is less efficient than glucuronidation, resulting in a longer overall half-life in infants compared with children and adults. Anesthesia providers should consider the physiochemical properties of the medication, therapeutic index, and alternative metabolic pathways when choosing therapeutic agents.

ELIMINATION

Elimination is the process in which an active drug or metabolite is excreted from the body. The elimination pathway is facilitated by two organs systems: the liver and the kidneys. The liver is dependent on uptake transporters such as organic anion transporting polypeptides (OATPs), organic anion transporters (OATs), and organic cation transporters (OCTs) for the influx of drugs into hepatocytes and excretion via the biliary system. This system is commonly referred to as the Phase 3 hepatic pathway. Few data are available in humans regarding the expression of liver transporters,[25] nor has the clinical significance of developmental differences in transporters across the age spectrum been studied in humans.

Drug elimination via the kidney is divided into three phases: glomerular filtration, tubular excretion/secretion, and tubular absorption/reabsorption. Glomerular filtration entails the passage of free drug from the plasma into the renal tubule, with the glomerular membrane functioning as a filter. Tubule transporters, such as OATs and OCTs, augment renal clearance by facilitating drug influx into the proximal tubule. In addition, other renal transporters efflux drugs into the lumen of the proximal convoluted tubules.

Renal function is less efficient relative to body weight or BSA in preterm/term infants as compared with adults. This inefficiency is due in part to reduced glomerular development/function, low perfusion pressure, reduced renal blood flow, and inadequate osmotic load to produce full countercurrent effects.[26] The maturity of the kidney is directly correlated to postconceptional age. Preterm infants have even further reduced kidney function in comparison with term infants and may necessitate lower dosing or extended interval regimens of renally eliminated agents.[3]

Mathematically, renal clearance (CL_{renal}) equates to the sum of glomerular filtration and tubular secretion, minus the effect of tubular reabsorption. Total clearance considers all elimination pathways:

$$CL_{renal} = CL_{glomerular\ filtration} + CL_{tubular\ secretion} - Tubular\ reabsorption$$
$$CL_{total} = CL_{hepatic} + CL_{renal} + CL_{other}.$$

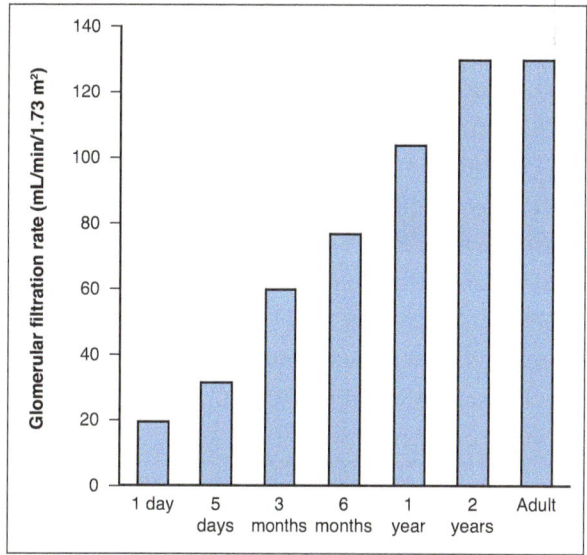

Figure 2.8: Changes in glomerular filtration rate during maturation.

Glomerular filtration rate (GFR) is widely accepted as a reliable marker of renal function. At birth, GFR is only around 10 to 20 mL/min/m² in full-term infants. The GFR doubles within the first weeks of life and reaches adult levels (70 mL/min/m²) by 3 to 5 months, followed by full maturation within 2 years of age (Figure 2.8). Glomerular diameter increases along the stages of anatomical development, which improves renal efficiency. After birth, large-diameter pores have greater abundance than small-diameter pores. Throughout the first year, cardiac output increases almost fourfold. Increased renal perfusion in conjunction with decreased peripheral vascular resistance causes an increase in drug excretion that may even exceed adult levels.[3]

Creatinine is secreted by renal tubules and is freely filtered by the glomerular capillaries. Creatinine-based measurements of GFR are cost-effective and less time-consuming versus endogenous substances, such as the gold standard, inulin.[27] Developed in 1976, the original Schwartz equation has been utilized for estimating GFR to measure creatinine (Table 2.3). New methods with improved accuracy for creatinine calculation have since led to the development of the bedside Schwartz equation and Schwartz cystatin C equation in 2009 and 2012[21] (Box 2.1). However, utility in the neonatal population is limited due to levels still reflecting maternal serum creatinine during the first few days of life.

Table 2.3	Schwartz Equations for Estimating Glomerular Filtration Rate
Age	**K =**
<1 year old, low-birth-weight infant	.33
<1 year old, full-term infant	.45
2–12-year-old child	.55
13–21-year-old female	.55
13–21-year-old male	.7

> **BOX 2.1 CREATININE-BASED MEASUREMENTS OF GLOMERULAR FILTRATION RATE (GFR)**
>
> **Original Schwartz Equation:**
> - GFR (mL/min/1.73m²) = (K × L)/sCr
> - L = length (cm)
> - sCr = serum creatinine (mg/dL)
> - K = see Table 2.3
>
> **Bedside Schwartz Equation (1–18 years):**
> - GFR (mL/min/1.73m²) = .41 × L/sCr
>
> **Schwartz Cystatin C Equation (1–18 years):**
> - GFR (mL/min/1.73m²) = 70.96/(CysC)$^{0.931}$
> - CysC = cystatin C (mg/L)

Tubular secretion is slower to develop than glomerular filtration. The incomplete activity is more pronounced in neonates due to poor blood flow, shorter tubule length, reduced concentrating ability, lower urine pH levels, and decreased energy for minimal transporters. Transporting drugs intracellularly and across the basolateral membrane or brush border (to the lumen) are significant contributors to tubular secretion. OAT activity is low at birth (20%–30% of adult function) and increases independent of kidney maturation until reaching adult capacity at 7 to 8 months of age. Limited data are available regarding OCTs, but animal studies suggest that their development is slower than OATs.[28]

Reaching adult function by 2 years of age, tubular reabsorption is the final phase to fully develop. Although tubular reabsorption is the last to completely mature, certain areas of absorption along the renal tubule develop more rapidly than tubule secretion, such as the proximal tubule. Aminoglycosides have been shown to accumulate due to reabsorption early in life.28 Providers should consider the phases of renal elimination and progression of development when establishing safe dosing regimens.

PHARMACOKINETIC PRINCIPLES

First-Order Single-Compartment Kinetics

Pediatric patients' biologic processes are greatly influenced by age and stage of maturation. Although the dynamic changes that occur throughout development impact the drug's ability to distribute within the human body, the rate of removal predominantly remains consistent following a first-order kinetics or zero-order kinetics model.

Most drugs are removed from the body following a first-order kinetics model. First-order kinetics follow a linear model based on the mathematical formulation that a constant proportion/percentage of drug is removed per unit of time. The amount of drug cleared is proportionately related to the concentration of the drug in the body. IV administration leads to rapid distribution and absorption into body fluids and tissues. The absorption/distribution and metabolism/elimination processes are occurring so quickly and homogenously among the different mediums of the body that the multiple compartments resemble a single compartment model. This is considered first-order single-compartment kinetics. Overall clearance is monoexponential; thus, a constant proportion per unit of time is eliminated from the body. This may be better illustrated using the following equation:

$$C = C_0 e^{-kt}$$

C is the concentration present at any given time, t. C_0 is the initial concentration determined by volume of distribution and dose. The elimination rate constant (k) represents the percentage of the Vd that is cleared over a specified amount of time^{-1}.

$$k = \frac{\text{Clearance}}{\text{Vd}}$$

Taking the natural log (ln) of both sides of a monoexponential equation results in a straight line, where $-k$ is the slope. Graphed on a linear-to-linear axis produces a curvilinear slope, while a semi-logarithmic (log-linear) axis produces a straight line.

The removal of drug is a monoexponential equation (consistent fraction cleared); hence, the log of the differences between two concentrations versus time will create a straight line. This straight line represents the elimination rate constant:

$$k = \frac{\ln(C_1 - C_2)}{(t_2 - t_1)}$$

The elimination rate constant is expressed as a drug's half-life ($t_{1/2}$). The half-life of a drug represents the amount of time required for the total amount of drug in the body to be halved (Table 2.4). The half-life value is applied to calculate the amount of drug that has been removed from the body, and subsequently how much remains. Assuming the serum concentrations are decreased by 50%, then $C_1 = 2 \times C_2$, and $t_2 - t_1 = t_{1/2}$. The half-life may be calculated using the following equation:

$$k = \frac{\ln(2)}{t_{1/2}}$$

$$t_{1/2} = \frac{.693}{k}$$

$$t_{1/2} = \frac{.693 \times \text{Vd}}{\text{Clearance}}$$

A drug is approximately 97% removed from the body after five half-lives following linear kinetics. Additionally, steady state concentrations are achieved after a time period of five half-lives. Steady state is a point of equilibrium between the amount of drug being removed from the body and the amount of drug being administered (peak concentration = trough concentration).[26] The volume of distribution at steady state (V_d^{ss}) accounts for the volume in which this drug is contained. Half-life as an indicator of the fraction of drug remaining in the body is dependent on the process of first-order kinetics. In addition, half-life predominately applies to first-order single-compartment kinetics versus first-order multiple-compartment kinetics.[3]

Table 2.4	Half-Life Elimination Table	
Number of Half-Lives	Remaining Percentage of Drug	Percentage of Drug Removed
1	50%	50%
2	25%	75%
3	12.5%	87.5%
4	6.25%	93.75%
5	3.125%	96.875%
6	1.563%	98.437%

First-Order Multiple-Compartment Kinetics

Most pharmacologic agents used in anesthesia do not follow simple one-compartment model pharmacokinetics, but more commonly a two- or three-compartment model. Drugs following such models are not distributed evenly throughout the body after administration. The rate of distribution is highly dependent on blood flow. The term *compartment* is used to group tissues/organs based on blood flow. In addition, the biochemical properties of a drug determine its ability to cross cellular membranes to exert its effects. Characteristics of drugs with a greater affinity for membrane transfer include low degree of ionization, low molecular weight, high lipid solubility, and high concentration gradient. Applying these principles, a highly lipid-soluble drug with low molecular weight would distribute into numerous body tissues and thus follow a multiple-compartment kinetic model. In contrast, it is probable that a highly ionized drug or hydrophilic agent will be confined to the bloodstream or extracellular fluid. Such agents would indefinitely follow a single-compartment model.

The number of exponential equations used for calculating concentration changes correlates with the type of compartment model. Two-compartment models demonstrate biphasic kinetics, dividing the body into two compartments with differing rates of distribution and elimination. This model includes a central compartment and a peripheral compartment. The central compartment includes plasma and high blood-flow tissues and organs (brain/spinal cord), where the distribution of the drug is almost instantaneous or quickly reaching equilibrium. The peripheral compartment includes tissues in which the distribution and time to reach equilibrium are prolonged. This model is reflected by IV drugs that rapidly partition out of the central compartment and experience rapid hepatic/renal elimination. Two-compartment models use biexponential equations to calculate concentrations. A three-compartment model includes three differing volumes of distribution, composed of a central compartment and two peripheral compartments.

Zero-Order Kinetics

Zero-order kinetics or saturation kinetics is characterized by clearance of a drug that occurs via enzymatic metabolism or transporter-associated elimination. When a drug follows zero-order kinetics, a constant amount of drug is eliminated over a period. Dosing increases may lead to a nonproportional rise in plasma concentrations and area under the plasma concentration curve (AUC) secondary to oversaturation of metabolic enzymes or alternative clearance systems. The Michaelis–Menten pharmacokinetics refers to the rate of drug metabolites formed from enzymatic breakdown. The maximum velocity (V_{max}) is the maximum rate of enzymatic activity in converting active drug to its metabolites. V_{max} is the point when an enzyme is fully saturated and a constant amount of drug is eliminated over a specific time frame. The Michaelis–Menten constant or K_m describes the plasma concentration where the rate of drug metabolism is half. Many drugs are metabolized according to first-order kinetics until reaching K_m. Scenarios such as prolonged infusions, above-standard dosing, enzyme substrate competition, decreases in complementary elimination pathways, and decreased protein binding may contribute to enzyme saturation, resulting in disproportionate concentration increases. Most drugs undergoing enzymatic liver metabolism have therapeutic concentrations lower than K_m values, although exceptions exist phenytoin. It is important anesthesia providers recognize that the reaction rate is independent of concentration. Thus, increases in concentration will not equate to an increased rate of elimination.

2.2: Pharmacologic Agents

Tamara K. Hutson, Andrea Chamberlain, and Trina Devadhar Hemmelgarn

To ensure the delivery of a safe and effective anesthetic, it is imperative anesthesia providers have a sound comprehension of both the foundational tenets of pharmacology and the nuances unique to the pediatric population. This section provides a brief overview of commonly employed inhaled and IV anesthetics, as well as review the pharmacologic agents used to provide muscle relaxation, abate pain, temper nausea and vomiting, and maintain hemodynamic stability.

INHALED ANESTHETICS

The first reports of the use of inhalation anesthetics appear in the mid-1800s, with ether, chloroform, and nitrous oxide among the first agents used. Safety issues, however, led to the development of fluorinated agents that are commonly used today. Halothane and enflurane were two of the earlier compounds used but have given way to safer, more effective, and safer agents in recent years, namely isoflurane, sevoflurane, and desflurane.

Inhalation anesthetics exert their action in a variety of ways. They act on hydrophobic components of the cells (the Meyer–Overton Theory), potentiate the action of gamma-aminobutyric acid (GABA) receptors, inhibit N-methyl-D-aspartate (NMDA) receptors, and interact with potassium and other ion channels to alter the release or response to neurotransmitters. Clinically this leads to reduced arousal, hypnosis, amnesia, and decreased response to pain. In addition to these effects, inhaled anesthetics also produce bronchodilation and skeletal muscle relaxation. The efficacy of these agents depends on their concentrations in the central nervous system (CNS).

Drug solubility is measured in a number of ways, often denoted by partition coefficients that are reflective of the solubility of the inhalation agent in a variety of solvents. Partition coefficients reflect the ratio of the concentration of the solvent in one phase to another. There are several partition coefficients of clinical relevance. The blood–gas partition coefficient indicates the ratio of concentration of a drug in the blood related to the alveoli. A higher blood–gas coefficient, indicative of a higher solubility, results in slower induction and longer recovery from anesthesia. The tissue–blood partition coefficient determines the uptake of the anesthetic gas into the tissues and the time necessary for equilibration between tissues and arterial blood. The oil–gas partition coefficient parallels anesthetic requirements, serving as an index of lipophilicity and has been correlated to anesthetic potency, with a higher coefficient indicating a more potent agent.

Another factor contributing to the efficacy and potency of inhalation anesthetics is the minimum alveolar concentration (MAC). This is the minimum concentration required to suppress movement in 50% of patients in response to surgical incision. Several factors, including age, electrolyte status, and concomitant medications, can affect MAC for inhalation anesthetics and should be taken into consideration when these agents are used.[29,30] In general, MAC is lower in preterm infants and increases with postconceptual age.[31] Thus, infants require lower concentrations than older children. **Table 2.5** summarizes some of the characteristics of inhalation anesthetic agents and the relation of MAC to patient age.

Inhalation anesthetics also have effects on other organ systems that may lead to adverse effects. They all produce

Table 2.5	Characteristics of Inhalation Anesthetics			
	Nitrous Oxide	Isoflurane	Desflurane	Sevoflurane
Blood–gas coefficient	.46	1.4	.4	.65
MAC (% of 1 atmosphere)				
Preterm		1.3		
Term neonate		1.6	9.1	3.3
1–6 months		1.85	9.4	3.2
Children		1.6	8.6	2.5
Adults	104	1.15	6	1.8–2
Percentage metabolized	n/a	0–.2	0–.2	2–5

MAC, minimum alveolar concentration.

Sources: Hudson AE, Herold KF, Hemmings HC. Pharmacology of inhaled anesthetics. In: Hemmings H, Egan TD, eds. *Pharmacology and Physiology for Anesthesia: Foundations and Clinical Application.* 2nd edn. 2019:217–240. https://www.clinicalkey.com/#!/content/book/3-s2.0-B9780323481106000119; Johr M, Berger TM. Paediatric anaesthesia and inhalation agents. *Best Pract Res Clin Anaesthesiol.* 2005;19:501–522. doi:10.1016/j.bpa.2005.01.001; Khan KS, Hayes I, Buggy DJ. Pharmacology of anesthetic agents II: inhalation anesthetic agents. *Crit Care Med.* 2014;14:106–111. doi:10.1093/bjaceaccp/mkt038; McKay RE. Inhaled Anesthetics. In: Pardo M, Miller RD, eds. *Basics of Anesthesia.* 7th edn. 2018:83–103. https://www.clinicalkey.com/service/content/pdf/watermarked/3-s2.0-B9780323401159000074.pdf?locale=en_US&searchIndex=.

dose-related respiratory depression, as well as cardiovascular depression. Isoflurane, desflurane, and sevoflurane also produce decreases in systemic vascular resistance (SVR), which can compound the effect of inhalation anesthetics on blood pressure (see Table 2.6 for a summary of the cardiovascular effects of inhalation anesthetics).

INHALED ANESTHETIC AGENTS

Nitrous oxide is a sweet-smelling gas with low solubility that results in rapid onset and offset of action. It is most commonly used as an adjunct to other inhalation anesthetics for induction of anesthesia (second gas effect), for facilitating IV access, or for decreasing discomfort during moderately painful procedures. In addition, the use of nitrous oxide reduces anesthetic requirements when used in concert with the other more potent inhaled agents. Additionally, it has been suggested that the use of nitrous oxide may reduce the incidence of postoperative pain.[32] While nitrous oxide can be emetogenic, these effects can be tempered with administration of antiemetic agents.

Isoflurane is a pungent agent with slower onset and offset. Because of this it may be less desirable in clinical practice as newer agents with faster offset have become available. Having been used in clinical practice longer than many of the other inhaled agents, isoflurane's MAC values are better known in preterm infants than with other inhaled anesthetic agents.

Desflurane is a completely fluorinated version of isoflurane, which provides very low solubility and potency, which improves onset and offset times compared with isoflurane. It is the most pungent of the inhaled anesthetic agents and often results in laryngospasm, coughing, and bronchospasm, thereby limiting its use with inhalation inductions. It also requires a special vaporizer for administration.

Sevoflurane is the least pungent inhalation anesthetic agent, making it ideal for use during inhalation inductions. It is also completely fluorinated and thus also has low solubility, giving it a relatively rapid onset and offset of action. When compared with isoflurane and halothane, sevoflurane is far less potent. Nonetheless, sevoflurane is a potent respiratory depressant; however, cardiovascular homeostasis is maintained in infants and children at 1 MAC.

Emergence Delirium

Emergence delirium (ED), consisting of delusions, inconsolable crying, confusion, restlessness, and thrashing about, is a common finding and concern in children who receive fluorinated inhalation anesthetic agents. This is generally a self-limiting effect lasting 5 to 30 minutes but can be troublesome to children and their caregivers and may require administration of additional pharmacologic agents to prevent self-injury and maintenance of IV lines, drains, or other medical equipment. Although ED is often associated with the administration of sevoflurane, a study by Locatelli and colleagues revealed a similar incidence of ED in children who received sevoflurane and desflurane.[33]

Table 2.6	Cardiovascular Effects of Inhaled Anesthetics				
	Cardiac Output	Systemic Vascular Resistance	Mean Arterial Pressure	Heart Rate	QTc
Nitrous oxide	↓	↑	↔	↑	↔
Isoflurane	↓	↓	↓/↓↓	↑	↑
Desflurane	↔	↓/↓↓	↓	↑	↑
Sevoflurane	↔/↓	↓	↓	↔	↑

↓, decrease; ↑, increase; ↓↓, marked reduction; ↔, no effect/change.

Sources: Hudson AE, Herold KF, Hemmings HC. Pharmacology of inhaled anesthetics. In: Hemmings H, Egan TD, eds. Pharmacology and Physiology for Anesthesia: Foundations and Clinical Application. 2nd edn., 2019:217–240. https://www.clinicalkey.com/#!/content/book/3-s2.0-B9780323481106000119; Khan KS, Hayes I, Buggy DJ. Pharmacology of anesthetic agents II: inhalation anesthetic agents. *Crit Care Med.* 2014;14:106–111. doi:10.1093/bjaceaccp/mkt038; Inhaled Anesthetics. (2016, July 4). Anesthesia Key. Accessed September 7, 2020. https://aneskey.com/inhaled-anesthetics-4/

Malignant Hyperthermia

Malignant hyperthermia (MH) is one of the most concerning, life-threatening side effects that can occur with use of inhalation anesthetics. The newer anesthetic agents (isoflurane, desflurane, and sevoflurane) appear to have a lower incidence of inducing MH than halothane, although MH can still occur.[29] If signs or symptoms of MH are detected, inhalation anesthetics should be immediately discontinued and IV dantrolene should be administered immediately. The Malignant Hyperthermia Association of the United States (MHAUS) has detailed management recommendations on its website: https://www.mhaus.org/healthcare-professionals/ and also maintains a 24-hour emergency hotline for advice (1-800-644-9737 USA; 001-209-417-3722 outside of USA). For more information regarding MH, please see Chapter 126, "Malignant Hyperthermia."

Neurotoxicity

All commonly used general anesthetics have been shown to cause neurotoxicity in animal models.[34] Accordingly, substantial concerns have been raised regarding the safety of young children undergoing repeated or prolonged general anesthetics. To date, there remains no consensus; however, how the evidence from preclinical and human studies should be interpreted and translated to current pediatric anesthesia practice. This is largely due to the fact that no clear exposure duration threshold below which no structural injury or subsequent cognitive abnormalities occurred has been identified.[35] While some of the biochemical pathways have been identified, the exact molecular mechanisms remain unclear. What is known is that, while scarce, the clinical evidence amounts to associative and not causal relationships.[36] This reinforces the need for high-quality preclinical studies, both basic and translational, to evaluate the mechanisms of toxicity and to inform choice of anesthetic techniques and/or mitigating strategies.[34,36] As no clinical data exist to support alternative anesthetic strategies, there must be a concerted effort moving forward to answer such critically important questions as what is the exact age at which the developing brain is most vulnerable to the effects of anesthetic exposure, whether a particular age exists beyond which anesthetics are devoid of long-term effects on the brain, and whether any specific exposure duration exists that does not lead to deleterious effects.[35]

IV ANESTHETIC AGENTS

There are multiple factors to consider when selecting an IV anesthetic agent for a pediatric patient, such as age-related pharmacokinetics and pharmacodynamics, the length and extent of the surgery or procedure, patient comorbidities, the use of adjunctive medications, and previous exposure to opioids.[37] Table 2.7 reviews many of the pharmacokinetic and pharmacodynamic properties of IV anesthetic agents often used during the delivery of general anesthesia.[38]

BARBITURATES

Thiopental and methohexital are barbiturates that both reach plasma:brain equilibrium rapidly due to their high lipid solubility. These medications may be beneficial for cranial surgeries as cerebral metabolism and oxygen utilization are decreased. When lower doses are used for moderate sedation, anxiolytic and amnestic properties are absent, and delirium and agitation may be observed.

Thiopental is a desirable IV anesthetic agent for patients with cerebral swelling, as its administration is associated with decrease in cerebral blood flow, cerebral metabolic rate, and intracranial pressure. Cerebral perfusion pressure, however, is maintained. Higher doses of thiopental induce burst suppression and may provide protection during profound hypotension, with patients with cerebral emboli and temporary focal ischemia witnessing a reduction in infarct size. However, given the long elimination half-life it is not uncommon to witness prolonged lethargy and residual effects that last for hours after emergence from anesthesia.[39]

Methohexital is an ultra-short-acting barbiturate with dose-dependent effects including depression of the sensory cortex, decreases in motor activity, alterations in cerebral function, and production of dose-dependent sedation and hypnosis. At low doses, methohexital enhances GABA action in the CNS, prolonging the period of chloride channel opening, whereas in higher doses chloride channels open directly, independent of GABA. Methohexital causes an initial increase in the alpha amplitude, followed by progressive decrease in EEG activity, making it useful in neurosurgical procedures involving ablation of seizure foci, as well as in patients undergoing electroconvulsive therapy (ECT). In addition to its antiseizure activity, methohexital has a fast clearance rate with few postoperative effects.

Pentobarbital is a short-acting barbiturate with sedative-hypnotic effects and is often used when analgesia is not required. It can be administered via oral routes, making it useful during diagnostic procedures. Although oral administration requires longer period to produce sedation, it is associated with lower complication rates, especially regarding oxygen saturation.[40,41]

BENZODIAZEPINES

Benzodiazepines are historically the drug of choice for procedural sedation, in addition to being used as anxiolytics preoperatively and adjuvants throughout the perioperative period. Characteristics of the class include a high therapeutic index and a shallow dose response, meaning the dose required to produce desired effects is less than the dose that produces adverse effects or hypnosis.[42] Although there are multiple benzodiazepines available for IV administration, midazolam and diazepam are preferred when IV sedation is desired due to the longer duration of action of lorazepam. Of the two, midazolam is preferred due to its lipid solubility, more rapid onset, slightly shorter duration, and potentially greater amnestic effect.[42] Diazepam and lorazepam are not water-soluble, requiring a nonaqueous vehicle when administered intravenously, which may cause pain and irritation on injection.

Midazolam is the most commonly used benzodiazepine in the perioperative period as it possesses anxiolytic, sedative, amnestic, anticonvulsant, and skeletal muscle relaxant properties, although it should be noted that the amnestic effects of midazolam are more potent than its sedative effects. It has a rapid onset of action in the CNS due to its lipophilic nature at physiologic pH, which aids its transit across the blood–brain barrier. Oral midazolam is the most common oral medication administered preoperatively in children. When given preoperatively midazolam provides reliable sedation and anxiolysis to facilitate parental separation and induction of anesthesia without delaying awakening and discharge postoperatively. As opposed to diazepam and lorazepam, IV midazolam is generally painless since it is not dissolved in propylene glycol and is water-soluble in solution due to the imidazole ring in its structure. Although the solution has a pH of about 3.5 (water-soluble), molecular changes ensue once exposed to physiologic pH resulting in a lipid-soluble compound. The mechanism of action is thought to be facilitation of the effects of GABA.

Table 2.7 Pharmacokinetic and Pharmacodynamic Properties of IV Anesthetic Agents

IV Anesthetic	Mechanism of Action	Protein Binding	Volume of Distribution (L/kg)	Metabolism	Onset of Action	Half-Life	Duration	Route	Notes
Barbiturates									
Thiopental	GABA_AAR agonist; exert different effects on synaptic transmission, mostly those dependent on GABA, and reversibly depress the activity of excitable tissues	72–93%	~.4–3.5 L/kg	Hepatic, metabolized to pentobarbital	30–40 sec	Low doses; first-order elimination: ~5–22 hr Long-term infusion or high doses: ~9–50 hr	20–30 min after a single dose	IV	**Warnings:** Extravasation: Thiopental is an irritant with vesicant-like properties; venospasm, extensive tissue necrosis, and/or sloughing. Ensure proper needle or catheter placement prior to and during infusion.
Methohexital	GABA_AAR agonist; depress the sensory cortex, decrease motor activity, and alter cerebellar function, producing drowsiness, sedation, and hypnosis	Lacks protein binding	2.2 L/kg	Hepatic	IV: immediate IM: 2–10 min Rectal: 5–15 min	1.6–3.9 hr	IM: 1–1.5 hr. IV: time to clinical recovery 5–15 min (psychomotor impairment may continue for up to 8 hr). Rectal: 45–60 min	IM IV Rectal	**Warnings:** More likely to produce cough and hiccups. **Precautions:** Hepatic impairment: Use with caution in patients with hepatic impairment; may prolong or potentiate hypnotic effect. Use with caution in patients with status asthmaticus. **Contraindication:** Porphyria.

| Pentobarbital | GABAnergic inhibition by prolonging the duration of GABAA receptors' opening; reduces excitatory outputs from cortical local circuits | 45 ≥ 70% | .8 L/kg | Hepatic | IM: 10–15 min
IV: almost immediate, within 3–5 min
Oral, rectal: 15–60 min | 26 ± 16 hr | IM: 1–2 hr
IV: 15–45 min
Oral, rectal: 1–4 hr | PO
IV
IM | **Warnings:** Respiratory depression, nausea, and vomiting.
Propylene glycol: Some dosage forms may contain propylene glycol; large amounts are potentially toxic and have been associated with hyperosmolality, lactic acidosis, seizures, and respiratory depression; use with caution. Solution for injection is highly alkaline and extravasation may cause local tissue damage.
Too rapid IV administration may cause respiratory depression, apnea, laryngospasm, or vasodilation with hypotension. |

(continued)

Table 2.7 Pharmacokinetic and Pharmacodynamic Properties of IV Anesthetic Agents (continued)

IV Anesthetic	Mechanism of Action	Protein Binding	Volume of Distribution (L/kg)	Metabolism	Onset of Action	Half-Life	Duration	Route	Notes
Benzodiazepines									
Midazolam	GABA agonist; potentiate GABA-mediated chloride ion influx	~97%	Preterm infants GA: 26–34 wk; PNA: 3–11 d: IV: median: 1.1 L/kg Infants and children 6 months to 16 years: IV: 1.24–2.02 L/kg	Extensively hepatic CYP3A4	Sedation: IM: children: within 5 min IV: 3–5 min Oral: 10–20 min Intranasal (solution, injection): children: 5.55 ± 2.22 min	Preterm infants PNA: 3–11 d: IV: 6.3 hr (range: 2.6–17.7 hr) Neonates: 4–12 hr; seriously ill neonates: 6.5–12 hr Children: IV: 2.9–4.5 hr Syrup: 2.2–6.8 hr	IM: up to 6 hr; mean: 2 hr IV: single dose: <2 hr Intranasal: 23.1 min	Oral IM IN IV Rectal	**Warnings:** Dose-dependent respiratory depression, hypotension, headache, nausea, emesis, cough, and dizziness. Paradoxical reactions (hyperactivity and agitation). **Contraindication:** Acute narrow angle glaucoma, uncontrolled pain, existing CNS depression, and shock.
Diazepam		Intranasal: 95%–98% Oral: Neo-nates: 84%–86%. Adults: 98%. Rectal: 95%–98%	Intranasal: .8–1 L/kg IV: 1.2 L/kg (range: .6–2 L/kg) Oral: 1.1 L/kg (range: .6–1.8 L/kg) Rectal: 1 L/kg	Hepatic CYP3A4 and 2C19	Sedation: Pediatric patients: IV: 4–5 min	IM: Premature neonates (GA: 28–34 wk): 54 hr Infants: ~30 hr Children 3–8 years: 18 hr Intranasal: ~49 hr IV: Parent: 33–45 hr Metabolite: 87 hr Oral: Parent: 44–48 hr Metabolite: 100 hr Rectal: Parent: 45–46 hr Metabolite: 71–99 hr	60–120 min	IV IN Rectal Oral	**Warnings:** Respiratory and cardiovascular depression; ataxia, dizziness, hypotension, bradycardia, blurred vision, and paradoxical agitation.

Lorazepam	~91%	Hepatic	Neonates: .76 ± .37 L/kg (range: .14–1.3 L/kg) Pediatric patients: 5 months to <3 years: 1.62 L/kg (range: .67–3.4 L/kg) 3 to <13 years: 1.5 L/kg (range: .49–3 L/kg) 13 to <18 years: 1.27 L/kg (range: 1–1.54 L/kg)	Hypnosis: IM: 20–30 min Sedation: IV: within 2–3 min	Full-term neonates: IV: 40.2 ± 16.5 hr; range: 18–73 hr Pediatric patients: IV: 5 months to <3 years: 15.8 hr (range: 5.9–28.4 hr) 3 to <13 years: 16.9 hr (range: 7.5–40.6 hr) 13 to <18 years: 17.8 hr (range: 8.2–42 hr)	IM, IV: ~6–8 hr	Oral IV	**Warnings:** Respiratory and cardiovascular depression.
Flumazenil	~50%	BZD antagonist	Hepatic	.5 L/kg	1–2 min; 80% response within 3 min	20–75 min (mean: 40 min)	Range: 19–50 min	IV	**Warnings:** Antagonist only at BZD receptor sites. AE: vomiting, palpitations, ataxia, dizziness, and vertigo. **Precautions:** Hepatic function impairment: moderate: mean total clearance decreased 40%–60%; severe: mean total clearance decreased 75%.

(continued)

Table 2.7 Pharmacokinetic and Pharmacodynamic Properties of IV Anesthetic Agents (continued)

IV Anesthetic	Mechanism of Action	Protein Binding	Volume of Distribution (L/kg)	Metabolism	Onset of Action	Half-Life	Duration	Route	Notes
Other									
Propofol	GABA-A receptor modulator	97–99%	5–10 L/kg	Hepatic	10–50 sec	13–44 hr	3–10 min (dose-dependent)	IV	**Warnings:** AE: PRIS, hypotension (may be more pronounced with hypovolemia), pain with injection, dose-dependent hypoventilation, apnea, and airway obstruction. Antiemetic properties. **Contraindication:** Hypersensitivity to eggs, egg products, soybeans, or soy products.
Etomidate	GABA-A receptor agonist	75%	4.5 L/kg 74.9 L/kg	Hepatic	30–60 sec	2.6 hr	Dose-dependent: 2–3 min (.15 mg/kg dose); 3–5 min (.3 mg/kg dose)	IV PO	Myoclonus (20%–45%), pain on injection, and N/V, adrenocortical suppression. Respiratory depression/oxygen desaturation to <90% or apnea (10%).

| Ketamine | NMDA receptor antagonist | 27% | 2.4 L/kg | Hepatic | IV: anesthetic effect: within 30 sec
IM: anesthetic effect: 3–4 min; analgesia: within 10–15 min
Intranasal: analgesic effect: within 10 min; sedation: children 2–6 years: 5–8 min
Oral: analgesia: 30 min; sedation: children 2–8 years
4 mg/kg/dose: 12.9 ± 1.9 min;
6 mg/kg: 10.4 ± 2.9 min;
8 mg/kg: 9.5 ± 1.9 min | Alpha: 10–15 min; beta: 2.5 hr | IV: anesthetic effect: 5–10 min; recovery: 1–2 hr
IM: anesthetic effect: 12–25 min; analgesia: 15–30 min; recovery: 3–4 hr
Intranasal: analgesic effect: up to 60 min; recovery: children 2–6 years: 34–46 min | IV | **Warnings:** AE: hallucinations, delirium, agitation, and laryngospasm. **Contraindication:** Not to be used in patients with increased ICP or glaucoma; potential for increasing intraocular and intracranial pressures. |
| Fospropofol | GABA-A receptor modulator | 98% | .33 ± .069 L/kg | Hepatic | IV: 4–12 min | .81–.88 hr | 5–18 min | IV | **Warnings:** Paresthesia, perineal discomfort or burning sensation (50%–70%), pruritus (16%–20%), respiratory depression, and hypoxemia (4%). Hypotension, particularly in patients with compromised myocardial function, reduced vascular tone, or reduced intravascular volume. |

5-HT3, 5-hydroxytryptamine; AE, adverse effect; BZD, benzodiazepines; CNS, central nervous system; CYP, cytochrome P450; GABA, gamma-aminobutyric acid; GABA-A, gamma-aminobutyric acid type-A; GABAAR, gamma-aminobutyric acid type-A receptor; ICP, increased intracranial pressure; IM, intramuscular; IV, intravenous; NMDA, N-methyl-D-aspartate; N/V, nausea/vomiting; PRIS, propofol-related infusion syndrome.

Source: Lexicomp Online®, Pediatric & Neonatal Lexi-Drugs®, Cincinnati, Lexi-Comp, Inc.; August 29, 2020; Micromedex Solutions. Truven Health Analytics, Inc. Available at: http://www.micromedexsolutions.com Accessed September 5, 2020.

Diazepam is a highly lipid-soluble benzodiazepine that acts on the limbic system, thalamus, and hypothalamus to produce sedative and anxiolytic actions, although it does so in a variable and unpredictable manner. Generally speaking, it has minimal effects on ventilation and circulation in the absence of other CNS depressant medications. Diazepam has more prolonged duration of action and a long elimination half-life.[43] Although midazolam has largely replaced diazepam for IV sedation, it remains valuable when there is a need for skeletal muscle relaxation. Due to pain associated with injection, it is recommended to be administered by slow rate of infusion through a large vein.[42]

Lorazepam may be the optimal choice for minor procedures in the outpatient setting as it produces more potent sedation and amnesia than midazolam and diazepam, yet the effects on ventilation, cardiovascular status, and skeletal muscle relaxation are similar to that of other benzodiazepines. It should be noted, however, that due to its slow onset of action its use as an IV sedative preoperatively or as an anticonvulsant is limited. In addition, the administration of lorazepam may delay emergence from anesthesia and has the potential to produce amnestic effects for several days following administration.

Benzodiazepine Reversal

Flumazenil is a competitive antagonist used to reverse the somnolence and respiratory depression effects of benzodiazepines. It has high affinity for benzodiazepine receptors, with no affinity for other receptors within the GABA receptor complex.[42] As a selective antagonist flumazenil can be used to reverse only the benzodiazepine component of ventilatory depression that may be witnessed during administration of both an opioid and benzodiazepine. The time for reversal may range from 20 to 60 minutes, with a short duration of action, multiple doses may be needed to prevent recurrence of the undesired effects of longer acting benzodiazepines. Caution should be taken when using this medication in patients with history of chronic panic-anxiety disorders or benzodiazepine-managed convulsive seizures.[42]

SEDATIVE-HYPNOTIC AGENTS

Propofol is a potent hypnotic agent with rapidly increasing levels of sedation resulting in general anesthesia. Favorable properties include rapid onset on induction, predictable effect, and rapid recovery.[44,45] Higher dosing may be needed in pediatric patients due to their higher Vd, shorter elimination half-life, and higher plasma clearance. In addition to being the IV induction drug of choice when inducing general anesthesia, IV propofol can be used when providing monitored anesthesia care, as an adjunct in the treatment of postoperative nausea and vomiting (PONV), as an antipruritic agent, or as an anticonvulsant. Dissolution in surfactant is required to create a state solution for injection due to its lipophilic nature.[44] Administering propofol may decrease cerebral perfusion pressure due to its effect on mean arterial pressure. Propofol-related infusion syndrome (PRIS), a serious side effect with a high mortality rate (up to 33%), may occur with prolonged infusions. Characteristics of PRIS include metabolic acidosis, hyperlipidemia, dysrhythmia (e.g., bradycardia or tachycardia), heart failure, hyperkalemia, and/or rhabdomyolysis or myoglobinuria with subsequent renal failure. In addition, some formulations of propofol use a metabisulfite preservative that may induce bronchoconstriction following administration.

Fospropofol, a recently developed water-soluble sedative-hypnotic agent, is a prodrug that is metabolized by alkaline phosphatases into an active metabolite: propofol. While nonionic and ionic surfactants have been used to formulate propofol microemulsions, fospropofol is more hydrophilic than propofol and hence does not require a surfactant. When compared with propofol, fospropofol has a slower onset of sedation, more sustained levels of bioavailable propofol, and longer duration of action.[46] Because of its chemical composition fospropofol has several potential advantages over propofol, namely less pain on injection and lower risk of bacterial contamination and hypertriglyceridemia.[46] The disadvantages of fospropofol when compared with propofol include prolonged duration of onset and longer duration of recovery.[44]

MISCELLANEOUS AGENTS

Etomidate is a carboxylated imidazole-containing compound that has been used since the early 1970s as a sedative-hypnotic, finally garnering FDA approval in 1983. Chemically, it is unrelated to any other drug used for induction of anesthesia. The onset of action is considered "ultra-fast" (10 seconds), in addition to being short-acting (3–5 minutes) with a short recovery time. Etomidate has limited influence on the cardiovascular and respiratory systems, allowing the maintenance of hemodynamic stability during induction of anesthesia.[41,44] As such, it is ideal for use in patients with cardiac compromise or in hypovolemic patients.[46] In addition, etomidate is a potent direct cerebral vasoconstrictor that decreases cerebral blood flow and oxygen demand, thereby lowering ICP. It does, however, activate seizure foci and result in adrenocortical suppression due to the inhibition of the conversion of cholesterol to cortisol. Etomidate-induced myoclonus can also be witnessed following injection. Therefore, its use is generally limited to single-dose administration for induction of anesthesia, rapid-sequence induction (RSI), and sedation for minor procedures.[45]

Ketamine is a derivative of the hallucinogen, phencyclidine, that achieves sedation with minimal respiratory depression and can be used to induce general anesthesia. The dissociative anesthesia induced by ketamine resembles a cataleptic state, often with a nystagmic gaze. The anesthetic effects of ketamine are due in part to an antagonist effect on excitatory NMDA receptors. Ketamine also acts on norepinephrine, serotonin, and muscarinic cholinergic receptors within the CNS. The administration of ketamine results in increased systemic and pulmonary arterial pressure, heart rate, and cardiac output. Therefore, it should be avoided in patients with glaucoma or elevated intracranial pressure (ICP) due to concerns of enhanced intraocular and ICP.[47] Additionally, critically ill patients with reduced stores of catecholamines may respond to the administration of ketamine with an unexpected decrease in blood pressure and cardiac output. Further undesired side effects associated with ketamine include hallucinations, nausea and vomiting, increased secretion production, and laryngospasm.[47] Ketamine, however, may be beneficial when used in asthmatic patients, as it is a potent bronchial smooth muscle relaxant and affords maintenance of protective airway reflexes.[48]

NEUROMUSCULAR BLOCKING AGENTS

Neuromuscular blocking (NMB) agents are used to facilitate tracheal intubation and can decrease the incidence of postoperative upper airway trauma-related symptoms. The use of NMB agents also decreases the requirements of IV or inhalation anesthetics needed to minimize patient movement intraoperatively and facilitate surgical exposure. As NMB agents do not provide pain control or amnesia, they must be administered in conjunction with other medications with the ability to provide analgesia, sedation, or anesthesia.

Neurotransmission is the process of communication between neurons, with neurotransmitters transferring information from presynaptic cells to postsynaptic cells across a synapse or junction between two neurons. The neuromuscular junction is a synaptic connection between the terminal end of a motor nerve and a muscle. When an action potential reaches the neuromuscular junction, acetylcholine (ACh) is released into the synapse and binds to nicotinic alpha subunits on the ACh receptors on the muscle endplate. This binding causes the influx of sodium and calcium into the postsynaptic neuron and efflux of potassium into the synaptic cleft, resulting in production of an action potential propagation and muscle contraction. Therefore, the nicotinic alpha subunit of ACh receptor is the primary site of action of ACh receptor agonists and antagonists.

The neuromuscular junction develops during fetal development, with maturation of the neuromuscular junction beginning between 24 and 31 weeks' gestational age. This maturation continues through the first 2 months of life. The fetal nicotinic ACh receptor of the muscle is an oligomeric membrane protein composed of five subunits (two alpha and one each of beta, delta, and gamma subunits). The fetal receptor channels depolarize more easily and remain open for a longer period of time, resulting in an increased sensitivity to succinylcholine and risk of hyperkalemia.[31,49] Neonates and infants also have a relatively increased extracellular fluid volume compared with older children and adults, which increases the Vd of the NMB agents. Therefore, response to NMB agents may be different in neonates or young infants than in older children. After birth the adult ACh receptor predominates, in which an epsilon subunit replaces the gamma subunit, and expression of fetal ACh receptors is limited to thymic myoid cells, extraocular muscles, and denervated striated muscle.

The NMB agents can be subdivided into several categories based on their mechanism of action (depolarizing versus nondepolarizing), their primary structure (steroidal versus nonsteroidal), duration of action, and their metabolism/elimination (Table 2.8).

DEPOLARIZING NEUROMUSCULAR BLOCKING AGENT

Succinylcholine is the only depolarizing NMB agent. It is often employed during RSI due to its quick onset and short duration of action. Structurally, succinylcholine is two ACh molecules linked by a methyl group. When bound to the nicotinic ACh receptor, muscle fasciculations ensue, followed by muscle relaxation. Succinylcholine is rapidly hydrolyzed by plasma esterases, resulting in a short duration of action. The duration of action may be prolonged, however, in patients with homozygous atypical plasma cholinesterase and liver disease, as these conditions decrease the overall amount of plasma cholinesterase throughout the body. Some medications, such as oral contraceptives, cyclophosphamide, and monoamine oxidase inhibitors, can also potentiate the duration of action of succinylcholine by antagonizing plasma cholinesterase.

As infants and children have a higher Vd, they often require higher doses of succinylcholine compared with their adult counterparts to achieve the same degree of muscle relaxation and onset of effect. In infants and children, succinylcholine can also induce vagal-mediated bradycardia. Atropine may be administered to infants to mitigate this effect. In the United States, a black-box warning exists, recommending the use of succinylcholine in children be reserved for emergency intubation when immediate airway control is necessary, given reports of acute rhabdomyolysis, hyperkalemia, and cardiac arrest in children with undiagnosed skeletal muscle disorders. Succinylcholine should also be avoided in patients with a personal or family history of MH. Likewise, it should be used with extreme caution in patients with multiple trauma, burns, and renal dysfunction due to the risk of significant hyperkalemia that can occur following the administration of succinylcholine.

NONDEPOLARIZING NEUROMUSCULAR BLOCKING AGENTS

Atracurium is a nondepolarizing NMB agent with a relatively quick onset of action and intermediate duration of effect. It undergoes Hofmann elimination and ester hydrolysis; thus, the duration of action is generally not altered in patients with renal or hepatic dysfunction. One of the by-products produced during the metabolism of atracurium by Hofmann elimination is laudanosine, which is a CNS stimulant and can cause seizures at elevated serum concentrations. Although rare, this should be taken into consideration if prolonged continuous infusions are used. Atracurium can also cause histamine release, which can lead to hypotension, increased bronchial secretions, and wheezing.

Table 2.8 Neuromuscular Blocking Agent Characteristics

Drug	Mechanism of Action	Structure	Onset of Action (Minutes)	Duration of Action (Minutes)	Metabolism/Elimination
Succinylcholine	Depolarizing		1	5–10	Plasma esterases
Atracurium	Nondepolarizing	Benzylisoquinolinium	2–4	30–45	Hofmann elimination and plasma esterases
Cisatracurium	Nondepolarizing	Benzylisoquinolinium	3–5	30–45	Hofmann elimination
Vecuronium	Nondepolarizing	Steroidal	2–4	30–60	Hepatic metabolism and biliary and renal elimination
Rocuronium	Nondepolarizing	Steroidal	1–2	30–60	Biliary and renal elimination
Pancuronium	Nondepolarizing	Steroidal	2–5	60–120	Renal

Sources: Lexicomp Online®, Pediatric & Neonatal Lexi-Drugs®, Cincinnati, Lexi-Comp, Inc.; August 29, 2020; Zuppa AF, Curley MAQ. Sedation analgesia and neuromuscular blockade in pediatric critical care. *Pediatr Clin North Am.* 2017;64:1103–1116. doi:10.1016/j.pcl.2017.06.013; Zafirova Z, Dalton A. Neuromuscular blockers and reversal agents and their impact on anesthesia practice. *Pract Res Clin Anaesthesiol.* 2018;32:203–211. doi:10.1016/j.bpa.2018.06.004; Kaye AD, Fox CJ, Padnos IW, et al. Pharmacologic considerations of anesthetic agents in pediatric patients: a comprehensive review. *Anesthesiol Clin.* 2017;35:e73–e94. doi:10.1016/j.anclin.2017.01.012.

Cisatracurium is the cis-cis isomer of atracurium with a similar duration of effect. Like atracurium, it undergoes Hofmann elimination, and the duration of effect is not impacted significantly by renal or hepatic failure. The incidence of histamine release following cisatracurium is less than atracurium, thus yielding improved cardiovascular stability. Given its greater potency, the onset of action is slightly longer than atracurium. Therefore, a larger dose of cisatracurium is required to achieve a more immediate effect for endotracheal intubation.

Pancuronium is a long-acting steroid-based NMB agent. It is primarily excreted unchanged in the urine with some minor hepatic metabolism. Thus, the duration of action can be prolonged in patients with renal disease or fulminant hepatic failure. As neonates have decreased GFR, pancuronium can have a significantly increased duration of action in this population. Pancuronium also produces tachycardia, increased blood pressure, and increased cardiac output by vagal blockade and release of norepinephrine, which could be an advantage in pediatric patients.

Vecuronium is the 2-desmethyl derivative of pancuronium. It has an intermediate duration of action and lacks hemodynamic side effects as it does not cause release of histamine or catecholamines. It undergoes hepatic metabolism but is primarily cleared through the bile and in the urine. Thus, the duration of action can be prolonged in patients with hepatic failure due to decreased biliary elimination. The 3-desacetyl-vecuronium metabolite has NMB activity about 50% of the parent compound and is felt to contribute to the prolonged duration of action in patients with renal failure. Clearance of vecuronium is similar in children and adults, but the duration of action is longer in infants comparatively. Due to the inherent Vd, infants may require higher initial weight-based doses to achieve desired effects.

Rocuronium is the newest NMB agent and has the advantage of a rapid onset of action, similar to that of succinylcholine. In addition, the lack of histamine promotes hemodynamic stability. The pharmacokinetic/pharmacodynamic profile of rocuronium makes it a favorable choice when selecting an NMB agent to facilitate tracheal intubation. Rocuronium has an intermediate duration of action, although can be increased in some smaller children. It is eliminated primarily through hepatobiliary excretion, which can lead to prolonged effects in patients with hepatic failure.

Reversal of Nondepolarizing Neuromuscular Blocking Agents

Depending on the duration of anesthesia and NMB agent administered, it may be desirable to use a reversal agent at the end of the case to facilitate recovery and help prevent postoperative residual neuromuscular blockade (PRNB). It is reported that PRNB occurs in approximately 20% to 30% of patients following surgery.[50,51] The effects of nondepolarizing NMB agents can be reversed in one of two ways: inhibition of acetylcholinesterase or enhanced elimination of the NMB agent through encapsulation.

Neostigmine is an acetylcholinesterase inhibitor that increases the concentration of ACh at the neuromuscular endplate and competitively overcomes the effect of the NMB agent. Neostigmine is most effective when the concentrations of NMB agent are relatively low and when the patient has a higher train-of-four ratio (TOFR) of .4 to .9. If the TOFR is <.4, administration of reversal agent should be delayed until the ratio is ≥.4 since deeper degrees of neuromuscular blockade may not be fully reversible with neostigmine. The doses of neostigmine administered vary based on the TOFR, with lower doses being given with higher TOFR. With regard to dosing in pediatric patients, it has been found that lower doses are typically needed in children compared with adults.[50] Recovery time from rocuronium-induced blockade is also faster in older children than in younger children and neonates. Pharmacokinetic parameters other than elimination half-life are similar in children and adults.

Because neostigmine increases the amount of ACh at the receptor endplate, it also interacts with muscarinic receptors and can lead to increased parasympathetic effects of bradycardia, prolonged QTc, nausea, vomiting, increased secretions, and bronchospasm. To mitigate these effects, an antimuscarinic agent (glycopyrrolate or atropine) is commonly administered in conjunction with neostigmine. Since neostigmine does not affect NMB agent elimination, it is possible for neuromuscular blockade to recur (recurarization) if the duration of the NMB agent exceeds the time of increased ACh.

Sugammadex is a cyclodextrin compound that forms a complex with rocuronium or vecuronium and encapsulates the drug, thus removing it from the plasma and reducing the circulating concentrations of the drug at the neuromuscular junction. By doing so, it reverses the neuromuscular blockade. One molecule of sugammadex binds one molecule of rocuronium. Sugammadex has 2.5 times higher affinity for rocuronium than vecuronium. A small number of patients who receive sugammadex have PRNB compared with those who receive neostigmine, generally only occurring when the amount of sugammadex is insufficient to bind enough NMB agent. Unlike neostigmine, sugammadex can be used in patients with deeper levels of neuromuscular blockade. Sugammadex also acts more quickly than neostigmine, and time to recovery with rocuronium plus sugammadex was similar to that seen with succinylcholine.[52,53]

Sugammadex does not have FDA approval for use in children; however, several case reports and studies have been published reviewing the use of sugammadex in children and showing it to be efficacious with minimal side effects.[51,54] The pharmacokinetic parameters of sugammadex in pediatric patients are not fully known given the limited formal studies in children. Two pharmacokinetic and pharmacodynamic studies in children have been conducted; however, the results have not been published to date.[55,56] Published parameters in adults are listed in Table 2.9.

The sugammadex:NMB agent complex is excreted in the urine; therefore, sugammadex is not recommended for use used in patients with a creatinine clearance <30 mL/min. Adverse effects seen with sugammadex are generally minor and self-limited and include nausea, vomiting, hypotension, headache, and pain. A mild prolongation of prothrombin and partial thromboplastin times, lasting for 60 minutes, have also been noted when patients receive higher doses of sugammadex, but no clinically significant bleeding has been noted.[51] Bradycardia has been reported in patients receiving sugammadex, which can be severe. Anaphylaxis and hypersensitivity reactions have also been noted and can be treated with an H1 antagonist. Most hypersensitivity reactions have occurred in the first few minutes after administration of sugammadex; therefore, patients should be monitored closely during this time for signs or symptoms of such reactions.

Female patients of childbearing age should be informed that sugammadex interacts with progesterone, as found in progesterone-only and combined oral contraceptive preparations, vaginal rings, implants, and hormonal intrauterine contraceptive devices. Administering sugammadex might temporarily reduce the effectiveness of any hormonal contraceptives and increase the risk of unwanted pregnancy. As such, patients should be advised to use a nonhormonal contraceptive method for the next 7 days.

Table 2.9	Pharmacokinetic and Pharmacodynamic Properties of Nondepolarizing Neuromuscular Reversal Agents						
Drug	Volume of Distribution	Protein Binding	Metabolism	Excretion	Elimination Half-Life (Minutes)	Onset (Minutes)	Duration (Minutes)
Neostigmine	.12–1.4 L/kg	15%–25% albumin	Hepatic	Urine (50% unchanged)	24–113 Infant: 39 Child: 48 Adult: 67	10–30	60–120
Sugammadex	11–14 L	Negligible	n/a	Urine (95% unchanged drug)		<3	120 (longer with renal impairment)

Source: Lexicomp Online®, Pediatric & Neonatal Lexi-Drugs®, Cincinnati, Lexi-Comp, Inc.; August 29, 2020; Lien CA, Eikermann M. Neuromuscular blockers and reversal drugs. In: Hemmings H, Artusio J, eds. *Pharmacology and Physiology for Anesthesia: Foundations and Clinical Application.* 2nd edn. 2019:428–454. https://www.clinicalkey.com/service/content/pdf/watermarked/3-s2.0-B9780323481106000223.pdf?locale=en_US&searchIndex=.

OPIOID ANALGESIC AGENTS

Opioids have a long history of use in medicine and play a crucial role in controlling pain throughout the perioperative period. They have recently fallen under significant scrutiny due to the opioid epidemic, and significant efforts are now placed on incorporating opioid-reducing strategies. Without question, opioids should be used judiciously, especially in the postoperative period and in individuals at risk of addiction.

Opioids produce analgesia by binding to mu-, kappa-, and delta-opioid receptors within the CNS, the highest concentration of which is located in the limbic system, thalamus, striatum, hypothalamus, midbrain, and spinal cord. By binding to the targeted receptor, opioids block the release of a variety of neurotransmitters, including ACh, norepinephrine, and substance P, and alter the release of dopamine. Opioids also bind to peripheral opioid receptors in tissues, leading to many of their side effects. The pharmacology of opioid receptors can be found in Table 2.10.

Certain opioids, including tramadol, oxycodone, fentanyl, methadone, meperidine, codeine, and buprenorphine, have a weak inhibition of serotonin reuptake and have the potential to cause serotonin syndrome when used with other serotonergic agents. Methadone also has activity at the NMDA receptor and antagonizes the effect of glutamate, resulting in the additional relief of neuropathic pain.[57] The pharmacokinetic properties of opioids can be found in Table 2.11.

In recent years, the pharmacogenomic differences in analgesic response to opioid and nonopioid analgesics have been identified. The most well-defined differences in opioid metabolism are due to genetic differences in cytochrome

Table 2.10	Opioid Receptor Agonists and Antagonists		
	Mu (μ)[a]	Delta (δ)[b]	Kappa (κ)[c]
Endogenous Peptides			
Enkephalins	Agonist	Agonist	
B-endorphin	Agonist	Agonist	
Dynorphin A	Agonist		Agonist
Agonists			
Morphine	Agonist		Weak agonist
Codeine	Weak agonist	Weak agonist	
Fentanyl	Agonist		
Meperidine	Agonist	Agonist	
Methadone	Agonist		
Antagonists			
Naloxone	Antagonist	Weak antagonist	Antagonist
Naltrexone	Antagonist	Weak antagonist	Antagonist

[a]Mu 1: analgesia; mu 2: sedation, vomiting, respiratory depression, pruritus, euphoria, anorexia, urinary retention, and physical dependence.
[b]Analgesia and spinal analgesia.
[c]Analgesia, sedation, dyspnea, psychotomimetic effects, miosis, respiratory depression, euphoria, and dysphoria.

Source: Trescot AM, Datta S, Lee M, Hansen H. Opioid pharmacology. *Pain Physician.* 2008;11:S133–S135.

Table 2.11 Pharmacokinetic Properties of Opioid Analgesic Agents

Medication	Absorption	Distribution	Protein Binding	Metabolism	Clearance	Other Information
Opioid Agonists						
Sufentanil	Sublingual: bioavailability 53%	Rapidly and extensively distributes into all tissues. Vd: 1.7–2.9 L/kg	79%–93% (AAG)	Demethylation→active Dealkylation	Urine: 2% unchanged	Onset: 1–3 min Half-life: 164 min
Alfentanil		Vd: .163–.6 L/kg	92% (AAG)	Phase 2 via glucuronidation	Urine: ~1% unchanged	Onset: 1–2 min Half-life: 90–111 min
Remifentanil		Vd: .223–.453 L/kg	70% (AAG)	Esterase metabolism. No active metabolites	Urine	Onset: 1–3 min Half-life: 3–4 min Clearance unaffected by organ dysfunction Very short half-life
Morphine	PO: variable IM	Distributes to skeletal muscle, liver, kidneys, lungs, GI tract, spleen, and brain. Vd: Children: 4.7–7.1 L/kg Adults: 1–6 L/kg	20%–35%	Phase 2 via glucuronidation. Active metabolite	Urine: ~3%–15% unchanged; metabolites Feces: 7%–10%	Onset: 5–10 min Half-life: 3–4 hr Accumulation of active metabolite with renal dysfunction Hypotension due to histamine release
Hydromorphone	PO: rapid (24% bioavailable) IM	Vd: 4 L/kg	8%–19%	Phase 2 via glucuronidation. Active metabolites	Urine: ~7% unchanged; metabolites Feces: 1% unchanged	Onset: 5–10 min Half-life: 2–3 hr Rare neurotoxicity due to metabolite accumulation with renal dysfunction
Codeine	PO: 53% bioavailable	Vd: 3–6 L/kg	7%–25%	CYP2D6→active Phase 2 glucuronidation CYP3A4→inactive	Urine: ~90%; ~10% as unchanged drug Feces	Onset: .5–1 hr Half-life: 3 hr Codeine is contraindicated in patients <12 years of age and in patients <18 years of age following tonsillectomy and/or adenoidectomy (due to CYP2D6 polymorphisms)
Hydrocodone	PO	1300–1400 L	36%	CYP3A4→inactive CYP2D→active	Urine: 26%; ~12% as unchanged drug	Onset: .5–1 hr Half-life: 4 hr Combination product with acetaminophen most commonly used

Oxycodone (immediate release)	PO: 60%–87% bioavailable	2.1–2.6 L/kg	38%–45%	CYP3A4→ active CYP2D6→ active	Urine: >64% as metabolites; ~19% as unchanged drug	Onset: 10–15 min Half-life: 1.8–3.7 hr
Meperidine	PO/IM: erratic and highly variable 50%–60% bioavailable	2.8–8 L/kg	AAG: 52%–85%	Phase 2 hydrolysis, CYP2B6, CYP3A4, and CYP2C19	Urine: as metabolites; ~5% as unchanged drug	Onset: Oral/IM/SubQ: 10–15 min IV: ~5 min Half-life: 2–4 hr (longer in neonates and liver disease) Active metabolite is renally excreted and may cause tremor and seizures; generally avoided due to toxicity
Fentanyl	Bioavailability: Buccal tablet: 65% Lozenge: ~50% Sublingual spray: 76% Sublingual tablet: 54%	Children: 15 L/kg Adults: 4–6 L/kg	79%–87% (AAG and albumin)	CYP3A4→ inactive	Urine: 75%; <7% to 10% as unchanged drug Feces ~9%	Onset: 1–2 min Half-life: 2–4 hr Caution with SSRI and SNRI→ serotonin syndrome possible
Methadone	PO: 36%–100% bioavailable	1–8 L/kg	85%–90% (AAG)	CYP3A4, CYP2B6, CYP2C19, CYP2C9, CYP2D6→ inactive	Urine: <10% as unchanged drug	Onset: .5–1 hr (oral); 10–20 min (IV) Half-life: 8–59 hr Slow release from liver and other tissues may prolong the pharmacologic effect despite low serum concentrations QTc prolongation

(continued)

Table 2.11 Pharmacokinetic Properties of Opioid Analgesic Agents (continued)

Medication	Absorption	Distribution	Protein Binding	Metabolism	Clearance	Other Information
Tramadol (immediate release)	PO: 75% bioavailable	2.6–2.9 L/kg	20%	CYP3A4 → inactive CYP2D6 → active	Urine: 60% as metabolites; 30% as unchanged drug	Onset: within 1 hr Half-life: 6.3 hr Tramadol is contraindicated in patients <12 years and in patients <18 years following tonsillectomy and/or adenoidectomy
Agonist–Antagonists						
Butorphanol	IM/IN: rapid and well absorbed IN bioavailability 60%–70%	305–901 L	~80%	CYP3A4 → active and inactive	Urine: 70%–80%; ~5% as unchanged drug Feces: 15%	Onset: 15 min (IM/IN); 1–3 min (IV) Half-life: 2–9 hr (prolonged in renal and hepatic impairment) Kappa agonist; partial mu agonist
Nalbuphine		3.8 L/kg	~50%	CYP3A4 CYP2C19	Feces Urine: ~7%	Onset: <15 min (IM); 2–3 min (IV) Half-life: 1–5 hr (increases with age) Kappa agonist; mu antagonist

AAG, alpha-1-acid glycoprotein; GI, gastrointestinal; IM, intramuscular; IN, intranasal; IV, intravenous; Vd, volume of distribution.

Sources: Lexicomp Online®, Pediatric & Neonatal Lexi-Drugs®, Cincinnati, Lexi-Comp, Inc.; August 29, 2020; Micromedex Solutions. Truven Health Analytics, Inc. Available at: http://www.micromedexsolutions.com Accessed September 5, 2020; Herndon CM, Ray JB, Kominek C. Pain management. In: DiPiro JT, Yee GC, Posey L, et al. eds. *Pharmacotherapy: A Pathophysiologic Approach, 11e.* McGraw-Hill. Accessed September 09, 2020. https://accesspharmacy-mhmedical-com.proxy.libraries.uc.edu/content.aspx?bookid=2577&sectionid=226724502; Fraser GL, Riker RR. Critical care: pain, agitation, and delirium. In: DiPiro JT, Yee GC, Posey L, et al. eds. *Pharmacotherapy: A Pathophysiologic Approach, 11e.* McGraw-Hill. Accessed September 09, 2020. https://accesspharmacy-mhmedical-com.proxy.libraries.uc.edu/content.aspx?bookid=2577&sectionid=234136370.

P450-2D6 (CPY2D6). Codeine, oxycodone, hydrocodone, and tramadol are all converted either to active or inactive metabolites via CYP2D6. Individuals who possess a variant allele for one or more of these enzymes may have unexpected outcomes, including toxicity or a lack of efficacy at recommended therapeutic doses. Four metabolizer types are recognized currently: poor metabolizers, intermediate metabolizers, extensive metabolizers, and ultra-rapid metabolizers. Poor metabolizers experience a very slow breakdown of certain opioid medications, ultimately yielding little to no analgesic effect. While similar, the effects are not as pronounced with intermediate metabolizers. Extensive metabolizers are considered "normal" with pharmacokinetic and pharmacodynamic profiles as anticipated. Ultra-rapid metabolizers metabolize opioids too quickly, at an unsafe rate. Genotyping may be useful when considering these medications. Table 2.12 shows the most common CYP2D6 phenotype and genotype, as well as recommendations for adjustment for use of codeine in patients based on genetic composition.

REVERSAL OF OPIOID ANALGESIC AGENTS

Naloxone is a competitive antagonist and the most frequently used antagonist in anesthesia. It is a pure opioid antagonist with no agonist activity, completely inhibiting opioid agonists at the mu, delta, and kappa receptor sites. Hence, naloxone is effective in the reversal of opioid-induced cardiovascular and respiratory depression, sedation, hypotension, and biliary tract spasm. It should be administered with caution due to the reversal of analgesia, which may result in increased sympathetic nervous system activity, including tachycardia, cardiac arrhythmias, hypertension, nausea and vomiting, and pulmonary edema. Patients who receive naloxone should be monitored for reoccurrence of undesired opioid-induced effects, as the duration of action of the opioids may exceed that of naloxone.

There are several new opioid antagonists that act peripherally (e.g., naloxegol, methylnaltrexone, naldemedine) to combat opioid-induced constipation without reversing central pain control when used in conjunction with opioids.[58]

ANESTHESIA ADJUNCTS

Acetaminophen and nonsteroidal anti-inflammatory drugs (NSAIDs) are generally preferred as first-line therapies in the treatment of mild to moderate pain. The exact mechanism of acetaminophen is not completely understood but is likely due to an inhibition of central prostaglandin synthesis and elevation of the pain threshold. NSAIDs reversibly inhibit cyclooxygenase-1 and 2 (COX-1 and 2) enzymes, resulting in a decrease in prostaglandins produced in response to noxious stimuli, thereby decreasing pain transmission. Acetaminophen and NSAIDs can result in lower overall opioid requirements when used as part of multimodal analgesic regimen.

Lorazepam binds to stereospecific benzodiazepine receptors on the postsynaptic GABA neurons, enhancing the inhibitory effect of GABA on neuronal excitability and therefore has no analgesic effects. When used as an adjunct for pain management, its action is likely related to its sedative and anxiolytic effects. This may result in less anticipatory anxiety related to painful interventions and add to the sedative effects of other medications being given. Table 2.13 displays the pharmacokinetic parameters of common anesthesia adjunct medications.

ANTIEMETIC AGENTS

A common complication after anesthesia is PONV, which has the potential to result in dehydration, electrolyte disturbances, wound dehiscence, aspiration, and delayed discharge.[59] One of the biggest risk factors for PONV is the sur-

Table 2.12	CYP2D6 Phenotype, Genotype, and Codeine Therapeutic Recommendations			
Phenotype	Genotype	Implications for Codeine Metabolism	Recommendations for Codeine Therapy	Considerations for Alternative Opioids
Ultra-rapid metabolizer	More than two copies of functional alleles	Increased formation of morphine following codeine administration	Avoid codeine use due to potential toxicity	**Alternatives:** Morphine and nonopioid analgesics **Avoid/caution:** Tramadol, oxycodone, and hydrocodone as metabolism is affected by CYP2D6 activity
Extensive metabolizer	Two functional or reduced function alleles, one full and one partial or nonfunctional	Normal morphine formation	Use recommended dosing	
Intermediate metabolizer	One reduced function and one nonfunctional allele	Reduced morphine formation	Use recommended dosing; if no response, consider alternative	Monitor tramadol use for response
Poor metabolizer	No functional alleles	Greatly reduced morphine formation	Avoid codeine use due to lack of efficacy	**Alternatives:** Morphine and nonopioid analgesics **Avoid:** Tramadol, oxycodone, and hydromorphone

CYP2D6, cytochrome P450-2D6.

Table 2.13	Pharmacokinetic Properties of Anesthesia Adjuncts					
Medication	Absorption	Distribution	Protein Binding	Metabolism	Clearance	Pharmacokinetics
Acetaminophen	Enteral: small intestine	~1 L/kg	10%–25%	Hepatic sulfation and glucuronidation; small amount by CYP2E1	Urine (<5% unchanged; 95% as metabolites)	Onset: Enteral: 30 min IV: 15 min $t_{1/2}$: 3–7 hr
Ketorolac	Enteral: 100% absorbed IM: Rapid and complete	.11–.33 L/kg (poor CNS penetration)	99%	Hepatic hydroxylation and glucuronidation	92% urine (~60% as unchanged drug) ~6% feces	Onset: Enteral: ~45 min IM: 30 min $t_{1/2}$: 3–6 hr
Lorazepam	IM: rapid and complete Enteral: readily absorbed	1.27–1.62 L/kg	91%	Hepatic glucuronidation	~88% urine (mostly inactive metabolite) ~7% feces	Onset: IV: 2–3 min IM: 20–30 min Enteral: 1 hr T1/2: 10.5 hr Active metabolites: none

CNS, central nervous system; CYP, cytochrome P450; $t_{1/2}$, half-life.

Source: Lexicomp Online®, Pediatric & Neonatal Lexi-Drugs®, Cincinnati, Lexi-Comp, Inc.; August 29, 2020.

gical procedure as well as the length of the procedure. The medulla houses primary receptor systems involved in the management of nausea and vomiting, in particular the chemoreceptor-triggering zone. This zone has close contact with the cerebrospinal fluid; therefore, irritants can stimulate the area through permeation. Several receptors can activate these pathways, such as cholinergic, dopaminergic, histaminergic, and serotonergic receptors.[59–61] Table 2.14 summarizes the key pharmacokinetic properties, as well as some precautions and side effects, of these medications.

5-HT3 RECEPTOR ANTAGONISTS

5-hydroxytryptamine (5-HT3) receptor antagonists are recommended as the first-line treatment for PONV, as they are effective, nonsedative, and generally well tolerated. Serotonin receptors can be located in the central and peripheral nervous systems, with serotonin activation of the chemoreceptor trigger zone and vagal afferents both triggering the vomiting reflux. Therefore, 5-HT3 receptor antagonists can inhibit stimulation.[60]

Ondansetron is used for both the prevention and treatment of PONV. It is reported to decrease postoperative vomiting when administered prophylactically, without significant side effects.[60] Caution should be used in patients who have prolonged QT interval.

Granisetron is typically used as second line after ondansetron. It is considered more potent, with a longer duration, in comparison with ondansetron. QT prolongation can also occur with granisetron administration.

Dolasetron has 50-fold higher affinity for the 5-HT3 receptor than ondansetron. It is rapidly reduced to its active metabolite hydrodolasetron, which reaches its peak plasma concentration at .5 to .6 hours and has a mean plasma elimination half-life of 4 to 8 hours when given IV, thus having a longer duration of action.[61]

Palonosetron is a second-generation 5-HT3 receptor antagonist, marketed with higher efficacy and sustained prophylactic benefits.[59] In comparison with the other drugs in its class, it has 100-fold greater affinity for the 5-HT3 receptor, and its therapeutic effects last for 72 hours.[60]

DOPAMINE ANTAGONIST

Metoclopramide acts centrally in the chemoreceptor trigger zone and peripherally in the GI tract. It is utilized both as an antiemetic and as an upper GI motility stimulant. Metoclopramide is commonly used for PONV when 5-HT3/droperidol fails. Side effects are rare with small doses when used postoperatively, although it should be used with caution in patients receiving monoamine oxidase inhibitors (MAOIs) inhibitors.[59] Metoclopramide is not recommended in pediatric patients due to the associated increased incidence of extrapyramidal reactions, although it is often used off-label in children for treatment of gastroesophageal reflux (GER), gastroparesis, nausea, and vomiting. It is contraindicated in those with pheochromocytoma, epilepsy, GI hemorrhage, obstruction, or perforation.

H1 ANTAGONIST

Promethazine is a phenothiazine derivative with strong antagonism of the H1 receptor, as well as the muscarinic and postsynaptic mesolimbic dopaminergic receptors in the brain. When bound to the muscarinic receptors, anticholinergic and antiemetic activity ensues. In addition, it has strong alpha-adrenergic blocking effect on hypothalamic and hypophyseal hormone, thus exhibiting antiemetic and sedative properties.[62] Promethazine has been reported to be effective in treating ondansetron failures, although its sedative side effect can delay discharge. Additionally, promethazine may decrease patient opioid consumption in the immediate postoperative period.[63]

Anesthesia providers should be aware that promethazine has a black-box warning from the FDA of severe tissue necrosis following IV administration. Thus, the recommended routes of administration are deep intramuscular (IM), oral (PO), and rectal (PR).[64]

BUTYROPHENONE

Droperidol is a derivative of butyrophenone, which is structurally similar to haloperidol. It interferes with CNS transmission at dopamine, noradrenaline, serotonin, and GABA synaptic sites. Droperidol has been demonstrated to be

CHAPTER 2: PHARMACOLOGIC CONSIDERATIONS FOR THE PEDIATRIC PATIENT | 67

Table 2.14 Pharmacokinetic Properties of Antiemetic Agents

Antiemetic Medication	Route	Protein Binding	Volume of Distribution (L/kg)	Metabolism	Onset of Action	Half-Life	Duration	Timing of Administration	Notes
Serotonin Antagonists (5-HT3 Receptors)									
Ondansetron	IV PO	70%–76%	1–4 months: 3.5 L/kg 5–24 months: 2.3 L/kg 3–12 years: 1.65 L/kg	Hepatic CYP1A2, CYP2D6, and CYP3A4 substrate	~30 min	Infants 1–4 months: 6.7 hr Infants and children 5 months to 12 years: 2.9 hr		End of surgery	AE: headache, constipation
Dolasetron	IV PO	69%–77% (~50% bound to alpha-1-acid glycoprotein)	Children: 5.9–7.4 L/kg	Hepatic	IV: 6 hr Oral: ~1 hr	Oral: Children: 5.5 hr Adolescents: 6.4 hr Adults: 8.1 hr IV: Children: 4.8 hr			AE: headache and dizziness Contraindicated: QT prolongation
Granisetron	IV PO	~65%	2–4 L/kg	Hepatic via CYP1A1 and CYP3A4	IV: 1–3 min	Oral: 6 hr IV: mean range: 5–9 hr SubQ (extended-release): ~24 hr	Oral, IV: generally up to 24 hr SubQ (extended-release): remains detectable in the plasma for 7 days		
Palonosetron	IV	~62%	Mean range: 5.3–6.3 L/kg	Hepatic ~50% metabolized via CYP enzymes	Oral: 5.1 hr	20–30 hr			Use with caution and monitor ECG in patients with other risk factors for QT prolongation Do not give other PRN 5-HT3 antagonists for 72 hr after administration of palonosetron

(continued)

Table 2.14 Pharmacokinetic Properties of Antiemetic Agents (continued)

Antiemetic Medication	Route	Protein Binding	Volume of Distribution (L/kg)	Metabolism	Onset of Action	Half-Life	Duration	Timing of Administration	Notes
Dopamine Antagonist									
Metoclopramide	IV PO IM	85%–90%	~.6 L/kg	Hepatic	3–10 min	~1.7 hr	2–4 hr, may extend to 12 hr	15–30 min prior to end of surgery	Extrapyramidal side effects may be seen with high doses Sedation and hypotension (fast injection) Dose needs to be adjusted in renal dysfunction
H1 Antagonist									
Promethazine	IV Suspension Tablet Suppository	93%	13.4 ± 3.6 L/kg	Hepatic; CYP2D6 CYP2B6 significant first-pass effect	Oral, IM: ~20 min IV: ~5 min	IM: ~10 hr IV: 9–16 hr Supplement syrup: 16–19 hr (range: 4–34 hr)	Usually 4–6 hr (up to 12 hr)		(US boxed warning): Promethazine injection can cause severe tissue injury (including gangrene) regardless of the route of administration Use with caution: bone marrow suppression, CV disease, hepatic impairment, respiratory disease, and seizures

Butyrophenone							
Droperidol	IV	85%–90%	~.6 L/kg	Hepatic	3–10 min	~1.7 hr	2–4 hr	After induction of anesthesia	Psychomimetic, extrapyramidal disturbances, sedation, dizziness, and increased QT interval

Corticosteroids							
Dexamethasone	Oral IV	85%–90%	~.6 L/kg	Hepatic	IV: rapid	ELBW infants with BPD: 9.26 ± 3.34 hr (range: 5.85–16.1 hr) Children 4 months to 16 years: 4.34 ± 4.14 hr (range: 2.33–9.54 hr)	IV: short	After induction of anesthesia	Use with caution in patients at risk of delayed wound healing, hyperglycemia, and risk of infection in patients already at risk. Transient increases in glucose, insomnia and depression, and adrenal suppression

Neurokinin Antagonist							
Aprepitant	Oral	IV: >99% Oral: >95%	IV, oral: ~70 L; crosses the blood-brain barrier	Hepatic via CYP3A4 (major); CYP1A2 and CYP2C19 (minor)	Capsule: ~4 hr Suspension: ~6 hr	~9–13 hr		1–2 hr prior to induction	Headaches, constipation, and fatigue

Atypical Antipsychotics							
Zyprexa	Oral IM	93% bound to albumin	Extensive, 1,000 L	Hepatic CYPP450 and CYP1A2 and CYP2D6 40% removed via first-pass metabolism	1–2 wk	Oral and IM (short-acting): children (10–18 years): 37.2 ± 5.1 hr	IV, oral: ~9–13 hr		Chronic administration, associated with insulin resistance and weight gain, hypercholesterolemia, hyperprolactinemia, QT prolongation, and dystonia and dyskinesia

AE, adverse effect; BPD, bronchopulmonary dysplasia; CV, cardiovascular; CYP, cytochrome P450; ELBW, extremely low birth rate; IM, intramuscular; IV, intravenous.

Source: Lexi-Drugs. Lexicomp. Wolters Kluwer Health, Inc. Accessed September 15, 2020; Available at: http://online.lexi.com.; Micromedex Solutions. Truven Health Analytics, Inc. Available at: http://www.micromedexsolutions.com. Accessed September 5, 2020.

as safe and effective as other antiemetics (e.g., ondansetron), yet more cost-effective. In addition to being an antiemetic, droperidol is a potent anxiolytic, sedative, and hypnotic.[45]

GLUCOCORTICOSTEROID

Dexamethasone is the most commonly used corticosteroid for prevention and treatment of nausea and vomiting. In children a consensus has not been reached on the dose–response relationship in PONV, as various dosing regimens have not shown a difference in PONV rates following procedures. It may be given in combination with a 5-HT3 receptor antagonist to prevent both early and late nausea and vomiting. Although the onset of IV action is rapid, the metabolic side effects can last up to 72 hours. Side effects associated with dexamethasone include tumor lysis syndrome, which has been reported in pediatric patients with hematologic cancers who receive dexamethasone intraoperatively, hyperglycemia, and hypertension.[60,65]

NEUROKININ ANTAGONIST (NK-1 RECEPTOR)

Aprepitant can be used for both prophylaxis and treatment of PONV. It has been shown to prevent both acute and delayed emesis.[45] Although reported to be more effective than ondansetron when used postoperatively, the combination of aprepitant and ondansetron lowers the incidence of emesis and decreases the overall need for rescue antiemetic administration when compared with either drug alone.[45,60]

ATYPICAL ANTIPSYCHOTIC

Olanzapine is an atypical antipsychotic that antagonizes the serotonin 2A receptor (5-HT2A) and has effects on a broad range of receptors. It has been reported to provide effective prophylaxis against chemotherapy-induced nausea and vomiting, which is likely to be due to antagonism of 5-HT3.[58,64]

ANTICHOLINERGIC AGENTS

Anticholinergic agents mainly affect the parasympathetic transmission of impulses at the postganglionic nerve terminals by binding to and blocking ACh binding sites on muscarinic receptors located on smooth muscle, secretory glands, and the CNS. They have little to no effect on sympathetic signal transmission. Anticholinergic agents indirectly reduce salivation by preventing stimulation of ACh receptors. They can be used for a variety of indications, including reduction of secretions, blockade of cardiac inhibitory reflexes during induction of anesthesia and intubation, and abatement of surgically drug- or vagal-induced bradyarrhythmias. In addition, they can limit the muscarinic effects of cholinergic agents (e.g., neostigmine and pyridostigmine) given to reverse the neuromuscular blockade of nondepolarizing NMB agents. Key pharmacokinetic properties of commonly used anticholinergic agents can be found in Table 2.15.

VASOACTIVE AND INOTROPIC AGENTS

During anesthesia, it is crucial to maintain adequate tissue perfusion and blood pressure to decrease the risk of postoperative complications. Perioperative hypotension is associated with increased risk of cardiac events and acute kidney injury.[66,67] Many of the anesthetic agents used during surgery, as well as the use of positive pressure ventilation during anesthesia, result in hypotension that may require corrective intervention. While IV fluid administration is a mainstay in the treatment of hypotension in pediatric patients in the perioperative environment, a multitude of vasoactive agents are routinely employed as well.

Vasoactive agents have an extensive history, with many originally being derived from plants and endocrine glands and working via a host of mechanisms to produce vasoconstriction and inotropy. Some of the more common receptors these medications innervate are listed in Table 2.16. While the mechanism of action of these may vary, most of the clinical effects are mediated through a common endpoint of calcium modulation, leading to cardiac muscle contraction or smooth muscle vasodilation. Refer to Table 2.17 for the different vasoactive medications and their receptor binding and mechanism of action. As with all these medications, the physiologic effects can vary from patient to patient at the same dose, so individual adjustments and dose titration are often necessary to achieve the desired effect.

Dopamine is the most basic catecholamine agent and is the precursor to both norepinephrine and epinephrine.

Table 2.15	Pharmacokinetic Properties of Anticholinergic Agents				
Medication	Absorption	Distribution	Protein Binding	Metabolism	Clearance
Atropine	Rapidly and well absorbed	Widely distributed; crosses blood–brain barrier	14%–44%	Hepatic hydrolysis	Urine: 13%–50% as unchanged drug and metabolites
Glycopyrrolate	Poor oral absorption; variable and erratic Bioavailability 3%	IV: Vd: Children: .7–3.9 L/kg Adults: .42 L/kg Poor CNS penetration	38%–41%	Hepatic oxidation and hydrolysis	Urine (as unchanged drug IM: >80% IV: 85%); bile (as unchanged drug, <5%)
Scopolamine	Poor oral absorption Bioavailability 8%	128 L	~4%	Hepatic conjugation	Urine and feces (varies by route of administration)

CNS, central nervous system; Vd, volume of distribution.

Source: Lexicomp Online®, Pediatric & Neonatal Lexi-Drugs®, Cincinnati, Lexi-Comp, Inc.; August 29, 2020; Micromedex Solutions. Truven Health Analytics, Inc. Available at: http://www.micromedexsolutions.com. Accessed September 5, 2020.

Table 2.16	Adrenergic Receptor Location and Function	
Receptor	Location	Primary Effect of Stimulation or Inhibition
Beta-1	Heart	Stimulation → increased inotropy and chronotropy
Beta-2	Vasculature and lungs	Stimulation → vasodilation and bronchodilation; stimulation of glycogenolysis
Alpha-1	Peripheral vasculature	Stimulation → vasoconstriction
Dopamine (D1)	Renal, coronary, and mesentery vasculature	Stimulation → renal, coronary, mesenteric, and splanchnic vasodilation
Vasopressin (V1 and V2)	V1 → vasculature V2 → renal collecting duct	V1 stimulation → vasoconstriction V2 stimulation → antidiuretic
Phosphodiesterase (PDE3)	Heart and blood vessels	Inhibition → increased inotropy, vasodilation (systemic and pulmonary)

Source: Bauer SR, MacLaren R, Erstad BL. In: DiPiro JT, Yee GC, Posey L, et al. eds. Shock States. Pharmacotherapy: A Pathophysiologic Approach, 11e. McGraw-Hill; 2020. Accessed September 7, 2020. https://accesspharmacy-mhmedical-com.proxy.libraries.uc.edu/content.aspx?bookid=2577&sectionid=223160525.

Dopamine's effects vary in a dose-dependent manner. At low doses, it primarily binds to the dopamine receptor. While binding at the dopamine receptor produces renal, mesentery, and splanchnic vasodilation, using "renal dose dopamine" has not been shown to clinically decrease the rate of renal impairment.[68] Given this information, this practice has largely been abandoned in clinical practice. Until the most recent version, the pediatric surviving sepsis guidelines had recommended dopamine as first line for pediatric septic shock. However, due to increasing reports of worse outcomes in adults receiving dopamine and pediatric studies showing comparable or improved response in patients with septic shock, dopamine has now been replaced by epinephrine.[69-71]

As mentioned previously, epinephrine has replaced dopamine as the drug of choice for pediatric sepsis in recent years.

At lower doses it exerts a primary effect on beta receptors, resulting in an inotropic effect, but at higher doses, its effects are more due to stimulation of alpha receptors. Unlike the other catecholamines, epinephrine is the drug of choice for treatment of anaphylactic reactions as well as for use during cardiac arrest. Outside of the hemodynamic effects of epinephrine it offers several additional advantages, including mast cell stabilization, bronchodilation, and increased glycogenolysis. Epinephrine reduces tissue uptake of glucose and inhibition of release of insulin from the pancreas, resulting in hyperglycemia.

Isoproterenol is the isopropyl derivative of norepinephrine and produces nonselective beta-adrenergic activity. Clinically, isoproterenol is most often used for treatment of refractory bradycardia or for chronotropic support due to its almost

Table 2.17	Receptor Activity of Common Vasoactive and Inotropic Agents					
Drug/Dose	Beta-1	Beta-2	Alpha-1	Dopamine	V1 and V2	PDE 3
Dobutamine	++++	++	0	0	0	0
Dopamine (<3 mcg/kg/min)*	+	0	0	++++	0	0
Dopamine (3–10 mcg/kg/min)*	++++	+	0/+	+++	0	0
Dopamine (>10 mcg/kg/min)*	++++	+	+++	0/+	0	0
Ephedrine	++	++	++	0	0	0
Epinephrine (<.05 mcg/kg/min)*	++++	+++	+	0	0	0
Epinephrine (>.05 mcg/kg/min)*	+++	++	+++	0	0	0
Isoproterenol	++++	++++	0	0	0	0
Milrinone	0	0	0	0	0	++++
Norepinephrine	++	+/++	++++	0	0	0
Phenylephrine	0/+	0	++++	0	0	0
Vasopressin	0	0	0	0	++++	0

Increasing level of activity indicated by +, ++, +++, ++++.
*Effects of dose vary from patient to patient. PDE-3, phosphodiesterase-3.

Sources: Zimmerman J, Lee JP, Cahalan M. Vasopressors and inotropes. In: Hemmings H, Egan TD, eds. Pharmacology and Physiology for Anesthesia: Foundations and Clinical Application. 2nd edn. 2019:520–534. https://www.clinicalkey.com/service/content/pdf/watermarked/3-s2.0-B9780323481106000259.pdf?locale=en_US&searchIndex=; Bauer SR, MacLaren R, Erstad BL. In: DiPiro JT, Yee GC, Posey L, et al. eds. Shock States. Pharmacotherapy: A Pathophysiologic Approach, 11e. McGraw-Hill; 2020. Accessed September 7, 2020. https://accesspharmacy-mhmedical-com.proxy.libraries.uc.edu/content.aspx?bookid=2577&sectionid=223160525.

exclusive action on beta-1 and beta-2 adrenergic receptors. Historically it was used to treat bronchospasm but has been replaced by beta-2 selective agents given the potential for paradoxical bronchoconstriction witnessed with repeated excessive use.

Norepinephrine has both alpha- and beta-receptor affinity; however, it has greater affinity for alpha-1 receptors than beta receptors, thus resulting in primary vasoconstriction at doses used clinically. Because of its lower affinity for beta receptor, norepinephrine has a lower risk of dysrhythmias and myocardial ischemia than norepinephrine or dopamine. It is the drug of choice for adults with septic shock.[72]

Phenylephrine is a noncatecholamine alpha-1 agonist. It is the drug of choice for hypotension during spinal anesthesia, in patients with neurogenic shock, and in patients with increased heart rates. Care must be taken to avoid extravasation as severe tissue necrosis can occur. It can also be used topically to control bleeding or relieve nasal congestion during ear, nose, and throat surgeries.

Ephedrine is given as intermittent bolus doses and for treatment of mild, acute hypotension during anesthesia. However, with repeated doses, tachyphylaxis can occur possibly due to depletion of norepinephrine stores.

Dobutamine is a direct-acting catecholamine that binds to beta-1 and beta-2 receptors, resulting in enhanced contractility and decreased SVR, making it a good choice for short-term treatment of heart failure or inotropic support following cardiac bypass surgery. It has a quick onset and short half-life compared with milrinone, another agent often used for these conditions and so may be preferred in patients with more issues with low blood pressure.

Milrinone, an inodilator, produces increases in cardiac output and decreases in SVR, as well as decreases in pulmonary vascular resistance (PVR). It is used for treatment of pulmonary hypertension and chronic heart failure, or for inotropic support after cardiopulmonary bypass. Hypotension is the most common side effect with milrinone, which is more common following administration of the initial loading dose. It is also renally cleared and will accumulate in patients with renal failure and so dose reductions are necessary in this patient population.

Arginine vasopressin is a hormone released from the pituitary gland. Binding of vasopressin to the V1 receptors produces vasoconstriction, with binding to the V2 receptor producing water retention leading to increased preload. While vasopressin is not first line for treatment of sepsis, it can be used to augment therapy in patients with sepsis or for treatment of patients with diabetes insipidus, although discussion of this is not within the scope of this chapter.

Refer to Table 2.18 for a summary of these clinical effects, as well as common uses and side effects of the medications discussed in this section.

LOCAL ANESTHETICS

Local anesthetics mitigate the physical transmission of pain with less risk of respiratory depression, ileus, and sedation than opioid analgesics. In addition, local anesthetics can help avoid the physiologic disturbances associated with general anesthesia (i.e., respiratory and cardiac depression) when administered as part of a regional anesthetic technique. Local anesthetics reversibly block nerve conduction by decreasing the permeability of sodium ion channels, resulting in an inhibition of depolarization and a blockade of nerve conduction. The threshold for nerve electrical conduction increases, the propagation rate of the action potential decreases, and impulse conduction slows, and eventually, nerve conduction fails. The degree of block by a local anesthetic depends on the degree of nerve stimulation and its resting membrane potential. A resting nerve is less sensitive to local anesthetics than a highly stimulated nerve.[73] See Table 2.19 for details on the pharmacokinetics, common clinical indications, and precautions for use of common local anesthetic agents. Refer to Chapter 131, "Pediatric Pain Management," for additional information regarding the use of local anesthetics with regional anesthesia.

Table 2.18	Physiologic Effects, Common Uses, and Adverse Reactions of Vasoactive and Inotropic Agents						
Drug/Dose	Cardiac Output	Heart Rate	Systemic Vascular Resistance	Mean Arterial Pressure	Post-Void Residual	Common Uses	Adverse Reactions
Dobutamine	↑	0/↑	↓	↓/↑	↓	Heart failure, cardiogenic shock, low cardiac output s/p bypass	Tachycardia, hypotension
Dopamine (<3 mcg/kg/min)*	0	0	0	0	0	Systolic dysfunction, shock	Tachycardia, dysrhythmias, myocardial ischemia, decreased GI motility, immunosuppression
Dopamine (3–10 mcg/kg/min)*	↑	↑	0/↑	↑	0		
Dopamine (>10 mcg/kg/min)*	↑	↑	↑	↑	0		
Ephedrine	↑	↑	↑	↑	0	Hypotension from anesthesia	Hypertension, tachycardia, tremor, tachyphylaxis
Epinephrine (<.05 mcg/kg/min)*	↑	↑	0	↑	0	Septic shock, hypotension, inotropy, cardiac arrest, anaphylaxis	Tachycardia, dysrhythmias, mesenteric hypoperfusion, elevated lactate, hyperglycemia, myocardial ischemia
Epinephrine (>.05 mcg/kg/min)*	↑	↑	↑	↑	0		
Isoproterenol	↑	↑	↓	↓	0	Refractory bradycardia	Myocardial ischemia, tachycardia

(continued)

Table 2.18	Physiologic Effects, Common Uses, and Adverse Reactions of Vasoactive and Inotropic Agents (continued)						
Drug/Dose	Cardiac Output	Heart Rate	Systemic Vascular Resistance	Mean Arterial Pressure	Post-Void Residual	Common Uses	Adverse Reactions
Milrinone	↑	0	↓	↓	↓	Heart failure, post-cardiac bypass, pulmonary hypertension	Hypotension, ventricular arrhythmia, headache
Norepinephrine	0	0	↑	↑	↑	Septic shock	Peripheral ischemia, mesenteric ischemia
Phenylephrine	0	0	↑	↑	↑	Hypotension from anesthesia, neurogenic shock	Peripheral ischemia, bradycardia, pulmonary hypertension
Vasopressin	0	0	↑	↑	0	Shock, post-cardiac bypass	Mesenteric hypoperfusion, peripheral ischemia, hyperbilirubin, increased LFTs

GI, gastrointestinal; LFT, liver function tests; s/p, status post..

*Effects of dose vary from patient to patient.

Sources: Zimmerman J, Lee JP, Cahalan M. Vasopressors and inotropes. In: Hemmings H, Egan TD, eds. *Pharmacology and Physiology for Anesthesia: Foundations and Clinical Application.* 2nd edn. 2019:520–534. https://www.clinicalkey.com/service/content/pdf/watermarked/3-s2.0-B9780323481106000259.pdf?locale=en_US&searchIndex=; Bauer SR, MacLaren R, Erstad BL. In: DiPiro JT, Yee GC, Posey L, et al. eds. *Shock States. Pharmacotherapy: A Pathophysiologic Approach, 11e.* McGraw-Hill; 2020. Accessed September 7, 2020. https://accesspharmacy-mhmedical-com.proxy.libraries.uc.edu/content.aspx?bookid=2577&sectionid=223160525; Lexicomp Online®, Pediatric & Neonatal Lexi-Drugs®, Cincinnati, Lexi-Comp, Inc.; August 29, 2020.

Table 2.19	Pharmacokinetic Properties, Common Uses, and Precautions of Local Anesthetics					
Parenteral Local Anesthetic	Protein Binding	Volume of Distribution (L/kg)	Half-Life	Duration	Main Anesthetic Use/Route	Notes
Bupivacaine	82%–96%	Infants: 3.9 ± 2 Children: 2.7 ± .2	Neonates: 8.1 hr Adults: 2.7 hr	Epidural: 2–7.7 hr Infiltration: 2–8 hr Dental injection: up to 7 hr Spinal: 1.5–2.5 hr	Infiltration Peripheral nerve blockade Epidural Spinal	Infants may be at greater risk of bupivacaine toxicity due to lower AAG concentrations
Lidocaine	60%–80% (AAG)	.7–2.7 (usual 1.5 ± .6)	Biphasic Initial: 7–30 min Terminal: Infants: 3.2 hr Adults: 1.5–2 hr	10–20 min	Infiltration Peripheral nerve blockade Epidural Spinal Topical	Substrate of CYP1A2 (major), 2C9 (minor), 3A4 (major) Half-life prolonged with congestive heart failure, liver disease, shock, and severe renal dysfunction
Ropivacaine	94%	Children: Epidural infusion: 2.1–4.2 Adults: Intravascular infusion: 41 ± 7 L	Children: Epidural: 4.9 hr (3–6.7 hr) Adults: Epidural: 5–7 hr IV: 111 ± 62 min	3–15 hr	Infiltration Peripheral nerve blockade Epidural	Widespread use in regional blocks due to its long duration of action and improved safety profile in terms of cardiac and neurological toxicity Substrate of CYP1A2 (major), 2D6 (minor), 3A4 (minor)
Levobupivacaine	>97%	54–66.9 L	2.06–2.6 hr	4–10.7 hr	Infiltration Peripheral nerve blockade Epidural	

AAG, alpha-1-acid glycoprotein; CYP, cytochrome P450; IV, intravenous.

Sources: Anesthetics-Local:Meditext. In Micromedex (Columbia Basin College Library ed.) [Electronic version]. Greenwood Village, CO:Truven Health Analytics. 2016. Accessed November 22, 2016. http://www.micromedexsolutions.com/; Lexicomp Online®, Pediatric & Neonatal Lexi-Drugs®, Cincinnati, Lexi-Comp, Inc.; August 29, 2020; McCloskey JJ, Haun SE, Deshpande JK. Bupivacaine toxicity secondary to continuous caudal epidural infusion in children. *Anesth Analg.* 1992;75(2):287–290; Dillane D, Finucane BT. Local anesthetic systemic toxicity. *Can J Anaesth.* 2010;57:368–380. doi:10.1007/s12630-010-9275-7; Hansen TG, Ilett KF, Lim SI, et al. Pharmacokinetics and clinical efficacy of long-term epidural ropivacaine infusion in children. *Br J Anaesth.* 2000;85:347–353. doi:10.1093/bja/85.3.347; Berde 2015.

KEY TAKEAWAYS

- The pediatric population introduces a great level of variability that can pose many challenges to anesthesia providers.
- Even within itself, the pediatric population consists of many differing subpopulations all at differing stages of physiologic and anatomical development.
- Although research has guided treatments the past several decades, the medical community is still in need of additional research to enhance treatment regimens to establish safe and precise dosing.
- It is imperative anesthesia providers recognize that dosing regimens utilized in the adult population cannot be linearly extrapolated to pediatrics.
- In order to provide safe and effective dosing regimens, anesthesia providers must recognize the differing physiology of the developing child and the impact on pharmacokinetics.

KEY REFERENCES

Complete references for this chapter are online and available at https://connect.springerpub.com/content/book/978-0-8261-3875-0/part/part01/toc-part/ch002.

2.1: PHARMACODYNAMICS AND PHARMACOKINETICS

2. Lu H, Rosenbaum S. Developmental pharmacokinetics in pediatric populations. *J Pediatr Pharmacol Ther.* 2014;19(4):262–276. doi:10.5863/1551-6776-19.4.262

26. Cote C. Pharmacokinetics and pharmacology of drugs used in children. In: Cote C, Lerman J, Todres ID, eds. *A Practice of Anesthesia for Infants and Children.* 6th ed. Elsevier; 2018:89–146.

28. Ruggiero A, Ariano A, Triarico S, et al. Neonatal pharmacology and clinical implications. *Drugs Context.* 2019;8:212608. doi:10.7573/dic.212608

2.2: PHARMACOLOGIC AGENTS

30. Hudson AE, Herold KF, Hemmings HC. Pharmacology of inhaled anesthetics. In: Hemmings H, Egan TD, eds. *Pharmacology and Physiology for Anesthesia: Foundations and Clinical Application.* 2nd ed., 2019:217–240. https://www.clinicalkey.com/#!/content/book/3-s2.0-B9780323481106000119

42. Becker DE. Pharmacodynamic considerations for moderate and deep sedation. *Anesth Prog.* 2012;59(1):28–42. doi:10.2344/0003-3006-59.1.28

47. Khumari N, Patel P, Kraus M, Trentman T. Pharmacologic considerations for pediatric sedation and anesthesia outside the operating room: a review for anesthesia and non-anesthesia providers. *Pediatr Drugs.* 2017;19(5):435–446. doi:10.1007/s40272-017-0241-5

54. Won YJ, Lim BG, Lee DK, et al. Sugammadex for reversal of rocuronium-induced neuromuscular blockade in pediatric patients: a systematic review and meta-analysis. *Medicine.* 2016;95:e4678. doi:10.1097/MD0000000000004678

59. Cao X, White PF, Ma H. An update on the management of postoperative nausea and vomiting. *J Anesth.* 2017;31(4):617–626. doi:10.1007/s00540-017-2363-x

68. Bauer SR, MacLaren R, Erstad BL. In: DiPiro JT, Yee GC, Posey L, et al. eds. *Shock States. Pharmacotherapy: A Pathophysiologic Approach, 11e.* McGraw Hill; 2020. Accessed September 7, 2020. https://accesspharmacy-mhmedical-com.proxy.libraries.uc.edu/content.aspx?bookid=2577&sectionid=223160525

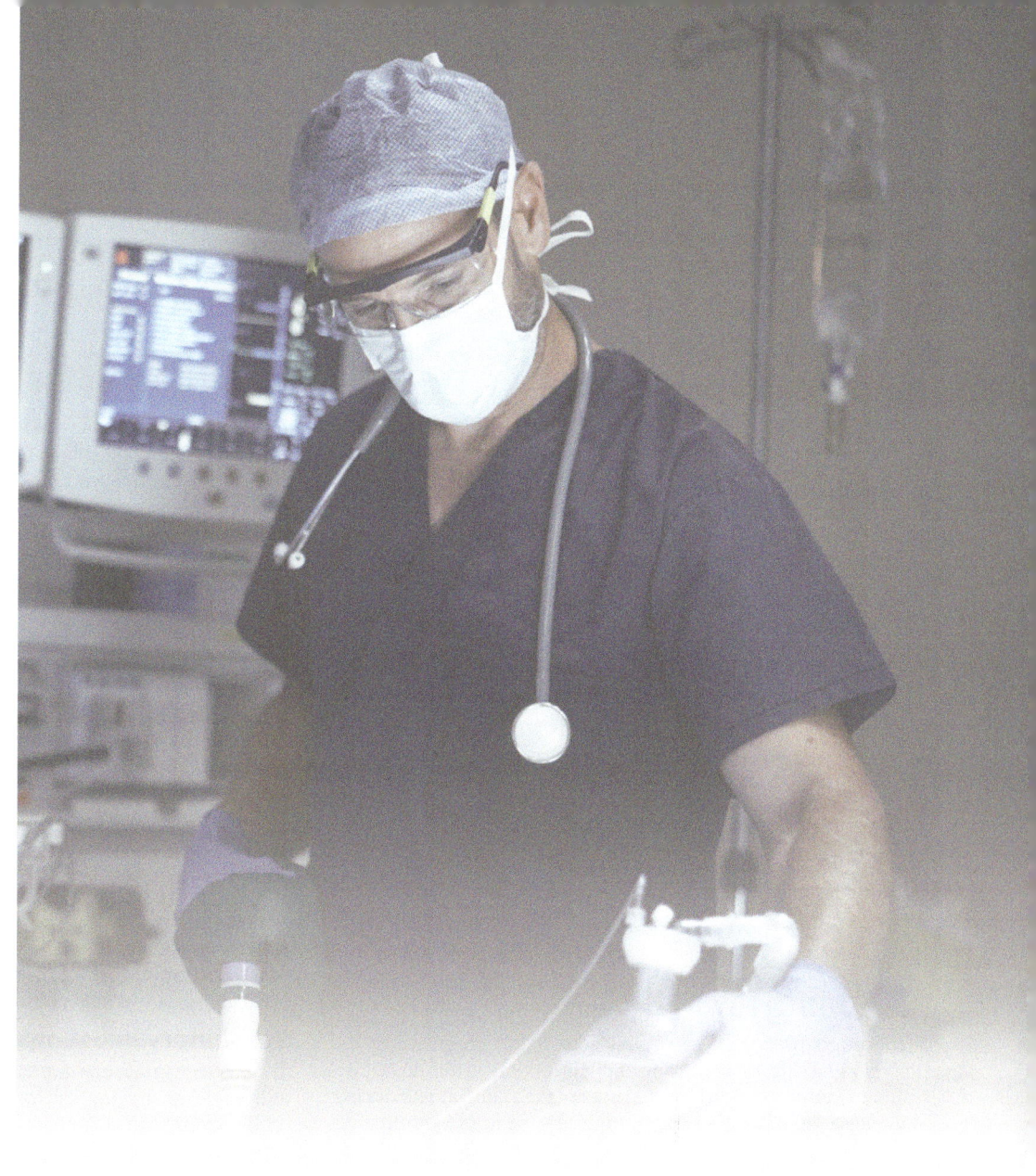

PART II

PERIOPERATIVE ANESTHETIC CARE

CHAPTER 3

Preoperative Evaluation, Testing, and Optimization

Karin J. Detchon and Heather Decker

LEARNING OBJECTIVES

- Understand the importance of the preanesthetic assessment.
- Define key components of the pediatric preanesthetic assessment.
- Review the importance of assessing current or recent respiratory illness.
- Explain the use of the current signs and symptoms, onset of symptoms, presence of lung disease, airway device used during the surgery, and surgery type scoring system.
- Discuss the importance of assessing preanesthesia fasting status.
- List pediatric preoperative fasting guidelines.
- Describe emerging modalities for assessing preoperative fasting status.

INTRODUCTION

A thorough preanesthesia assessment is key to ensuring the delivery of a safe, effective anesthetic. Not only is this an opportunity to identify conditions that may place a child at risk during anesthesia, but also it is a requirement by the Joint Commission for the Accreditation of Healthcare Organizations.[1,2] A complete preoperative evaluation should include a comprehensive physical exam, review of available pertinent laboratory results and imaging studies, and audit of previous anesthesia and medical records, if available. As the preoperative evaluation ultimately guides development of an individualized anesthetic plan, it is the opportune time for anesthesia providers to determine the need for additional testing, optimization, or premedication.

PREOPERATIVE EVALUATION AND TESTING

PREOPERATIVE EVALUATION

The medical history obtained during a preanesthesia assessment is the most important component of a preoperative evaluation. Should a recent history and physical exam be available from the child's primary care provider, it can be used to guide questions regarding the patient's health history or as a prompt to elicit further details as parents are frequently poor historians. This should also cue anesthesia providers that certain aspects of the physical exam warrant close examination or perhaps consultation with a specialist. If it is known that a patient has a complex medical history prior to the day of surgery, it is recommended an anesthesia consult be scheduled before the day of surgery to ensure adequate time for assessment and planning prior to the procedure.

A preanesthetic assessment should include a complete and thorough review of all systems. Other key components to be included are a review of all medications, including the time of the patient's last dose and a review of allergies (including medications, foods, and products) and reactions. It is important that anesthesia providers inquire about the child's birth history to assess for prematurity (less than 37 weeks' gestation) and any associated complications.

It is imperative that anesthesia providers ask about patient or family history of malignant hyperthermia (MH) during each preoperative evaluation, as 52.1% of all MH reactions occur in children.[3] For additional information about MH, please refer to Chapter 126, "Malignant Hyperthermia." If the patient has previous experience with anesthesia, it is important to vet if there were any complications or postoperative concerns. Potential complications, such as pseudocholinesterase deficiency, postoperative nausea and/or vomiting, and bleeding disorders should all be discussed to ensure an appropriate anesthesia plan is developed. Equally important, anesthesia providers should ask the child's parents about known family issues with anesthesia. Once a thorough preanesthesia history and physical exam has been performed, the American Society of Anesthesiologists (ASA) Physical Status Classification System can be used communicate a patient's preanesthesia medical comorbidities to providers.

Respiratory Infections

Respiratory infections are common among pediatric patients, with children having six to eight upper respiratory infections (URIs) each year. Of all children presenting for elective surgery, approximately 30% will present on the day of surgery with an active URIs, making this a frequently encountered issue in the preoperative setting.[4] It is important that anesthesia providers assess for sign and symptoms of a current or recent respiratory illness in all patients scheduled for anesthesia, especially those 2 years of age and younger as recent or active URI can have a negative impact on the child's well-being during an anesthetic. The smaller diameter of the pediatric airway inherently places this population at an increased risk of airway complications during anesthesia even when healthy. The incidence of airway complications increases significantly when a child has a URI, with the potential for devastating outcomes. Common perioperative complications associated with recent or ongoing URIs include laryngospasm, bronchospasm, atelectasis, postextubation croup, and postoperative pneumonia.

There are no formal rules for proceeding with anesthesia or canceling the case in the presence of a current or recent URI, and each case should be managed on an individual basis. Clinical algorithms, however, such as the COLDS (current signs and symptoms, onset of symptoms, presence of lung disease, airway device used during the surgery, and surgery type) scoring system offered by Lee and August,[5] can help determine the risk of perioperative respiratory adverse events when a child presents with a current or recent URI (Figure 3.1). The COLDS scoring system takes into consideration current signs and symptoms, the onset of symptoms, history of lung disease, planned airway instrumentation, and the type of surgery. Each risk factor is given a score based on presence or severity, with the total possible scores ranging from a

	1	2	5
C	None	Mild (parent confirms URI AND/OR congestion, rhinorrhea, sore throat, sneezing, low fever, and dry cough)	Moderate/severe (purulence, wet cough, abnormal lung sounds, lethargy, toxic appearance, or high fever)
O	>4 wk ago	2–4 wk ago	<2 wk ago
L	None	Mild (Hx of RSV, mild interrmittent asthma, BPD if >1 y/o, loud snoring, or passive smoker)	Moderate/severe (moderate persistent asthma, infant with BPD, OSA, or pulmonary hypertension)
D	None or face mask	LMA or Supraglottic Airway	Endotracheal tube
S	Other (including PE tubes)	Minor airway (T/A, nasal lacrimal duct probing, flexible bronchoscopy, and dental extractions)	Major airway (cleft palate, rigid bronchoscopy, and maxillofacial surgery)

Figure 3.1: COLDS scoring tool. C, current signs and symptoms; O, onset of symptoms; L, presence of lung disease; D, airway device used during the surgery; S, surgery type

*Each of these subcomponents of the COLDS score represents known risk factors for perioperative respiratory adverse events.

URI, upper respiratory infection.

Source: From Lee LK, Bernardo M, Grogan TR, et al. Perioperative respiratory adverse event risk assessment in children with upper respiratory tract infection: validation of the COLDS score. *Paediatr Anaesth.* 2018;28(11):1007–1014. doi:10.1111/pan.13491.

minimum score of 5 to a maximum score of 25. The higher the score, the greater the perioperative risk.

The COLDS score has good predictive value and can help quantify the risk of perioperative respiratory adverse events when a patient has had a recent or current respiratory illness. When studied in a clinical setting, the COLDS score had an intraclass correlation coefficient of .99, indicating high interrater reliability. The predictive ability of the COLDS score performed best in younger age groups 0 to <2 years of age (area under the curve [AUC] of 0.70, 95% CI: .61–.79) and 2 to 4 years of age (AUC = .71, 95% CI: .61–0.81), although there was still good predictability in ages 4 to 6 (AUC = .66, 95% CI: .56–.77).[4] Of note, case cancelations occurred at a COLDS score of 19 and higher.[4] While the decision to proceed or cancel a case is up to the anesthesia team caring for the patient, using the COLDS scoring system may help the anesthesia team, the surgery team, and the patient's family make a more informed decision regarding anesthesia risk.[4]

An experienced pediatric anesthesia provider may be comfortable with proceeding if mild rhinorrhea or nasal congestion is the only symptom, depending on the age of the patient, the comorbidities present, and the surgical procedure scheduled. It is especially important to consider the patient's chronic respiratory medical history, such as asthma, recurrent croup, and chronic lung disease when making this decision. It is also common for elective procedures to be canceled in the presence of an active or recent URI if the increased anesthesia-related risks associated with an ongoing or recent URI outweigh the benefit or urgency of the procedure. If canceled, elective procedures should be rescheduled 4 to 6 weeks following resolution of all respiratory symptoms as the airways can remain inflamed and reactive during, recovery thereby heightening the potential for adverse events.[3]

Preoperative Fasting

Preoperative fasting before elective surgery is a universally applied guideline to minimize the risk of pulmonary aspiration of gastric contents, as the administration of anesthetic agents can result in regurgitation and the loss of protective airway reflexes.[6] Noncompliance with preoperative fasting guidelines can result in negative sequelae in the perioperative environment, making it important for anesthesia providers to establish the patient's nothing by mouth (NPO) status early in the preanesthesia assessment. Gathering details about the patient's NPO status early in the preanesthetic assessment will allow the anesthesia team to make a timely decision about proceeding as scheduled, delaying, or canceling an elective surgery.

The 2017 ASA guidelines on preoperative fasting and the use of pharmacological agents to reduce the risk of pulmonary aspiration are the most widely accepted and recommended guidelines regarding preoperative fasting, although implementation of these guidelines may vary slightly from institution to institution. The ASA guidelines on preoperative fasting state that patients should remain NPO for 8 hours following a heavy meal, fried foods, fatty

Table 3.1	Preoperative Fasting Guidelines		
Up to 2 Hr Before Anesthesia	Up to 4 Hr Before Anesthesia	Up to 6 Hr Before Anesthesia	Up to 8 Hr Before Anesthesia
Clear liquids	Breast milk	Infant formula, nonhuman milk, a light meal	A heavy meal, fried foods, fatty foods, meat

foods, and meat; 6 hours following a light meal, infant formula, and nonhuman milk, 4 hours following human milk/breast milk, and 2 hours following the consumption of clear liquids (Table 3.1). Definitions of *light meal* may differ among anesthesia providers, parents, and patients. Therefore, gathering details of what foods were consumed and what amount, along with the time consumption ended, is extremely important in assessing preoperative fasting status and will help the anesthesia provider determine if an 8- or 6-hour preoperative fasting period is warranted.

Approximately 7% of children presenting for ambulatory surgery present with an inadequate preoperative fasting time.[7] Patient compliance and successful preoperative fasting require clear communication when educating a parent or caregiver about expected preoperative fasting times. Your institution should have a process in place to ensure the parent or caregiver understands the preoperative fasting instructions before the day of surgery, including the difference between solid foods, formula, human milk, and clear liquids, as well as their associated fasting times. When providing preoperative fasting instructions, it is important to inform parents/caregivers to keep food and drink out of reach of children during the period that they should be observing preoperative fasting. This is more obvious in their home, but it is important to have them check car seats, cribs, and the like for leftovers or forgotten drinks or food pieces that, when hungry, children will find and consume. Despite clear communication of preoperative fasting expectations, there is inevitably still noncompliance in some patients. Age-appropriate children will usually tell the truth when asked if they have had anything to eat or drink recently, so asking the patient directly can be useful when parents or caregivers are not with the child in the hours before surgery (i.e., school or day care).

Although the ASA preoperative fasting guidelines are revered and widely accepted, it has been offered that revision of the guidelines may have the potential to yield improved patient outcomes and optimize safety. Many times, preoperative fasting far exceeds the minimum preoperative fasting times recommended in the 2017 ASA guidelines, which can be detrimental to pediatric patients. Prolonged preoperative fasting can result in dehydration, ketoacidosis, hypoglycemia, and cardiovascular instability.[6] Given the potential negative impact prolonged preoperative fasting can have, there has been a heightened interest in revisiting fasting guidelines prior to anesthesia for the pediatric populaiton.

Clear Fluids
Although patients are allowed to have clear fluids up to 2 hours before anesthesia, recent literature suggests decreasing the minimum NPO time for clear liquids to 1 hour before general anesthesia for otherwise healthy children presenting for elective surgery.[8] Further research is required before definitive changes in practice can be made, especially for specialty populations, such as neonates, emergency surgery patients, and patients with gastrointestinal disorders.[6] Patients who will likely not be eligible for reductions in the NPO time for clear liquids to 1 hour include those with a history of gastroesophageal reflux, renal failure, enteropathy, esophageal strictures, achalasia, and diabetes mellitus with gastroparesis.[8] Longitudinal studies from institutions that have implemented a 1-hour NPO time for clear liquids will be beneficial in vetting if the formal guideline should be revisited.

Carbohydrate Drinks
Enhanced recovery after surgery (ERAS) protocols have gained popularity in recent years as they have been proven effective in optimizing postoperative outcomes following a plethora of surgeries in the adult population. A common practice among ERAS protocols is to have the patient consume a carbohydrate drink 2 hours before surgery. In a study published in the *British Journal of Anaesthesia*, the gastric volume in pediatric patients was assessed preoperatively using ultrasound after fasting for 8 hours and then again 2 hours after drinking a carbohydrate drink. It was reported that consuming the carbohydrate drink 2 hours before general anesthesia reduced gastric volume and increased parent satisfaction because the carbohydrate drink reduced their child's thirst and irritability.[9] While the science regarding NPO status, and the consumption of carbohydrate drinks preoperatively continues to evolve, anesthesia providers should continue to adhere to the long-standing recommended guidelines.

Gastric Ultrasound
Inappropriate preoperative fasting results in delays, cancellations of elective surgeries, parental dissatisfaction, and inefficient use of health resources.[7] When questions arise regarding NPO fasting times, gastric ultrasound can be used to assess the nature and volume of gastric contents. Gastric ultrasound is a simple tool that has the potential to reduce adverse respiratory events from pulmonary aspiration and may limit the need to delay or cancel surgeries.[7] Furthermore, it is an exam that is easy to learn and perform, in additional to being noninvasive and reproducible. The use of gastric ultrasound can also be helpful in the emergency setting when deciding if a rapid-sequence intubation is warranted or not.[8] While not currently standard practice, the use of gastric ultrasound preoperatively continues to increase when verbal assessment alone is unreliable or inconclusive.

PREMEDICATION AND OPTIMIZATION

PREOPERATIVE ANESTHESIA CLINICS
The perioperative period is often an unfamiliar experience and can be highly stressful for patients and families alike. Setting appropriate expectations can help reduce anxiety of the patient and their parent or caregiver on the day of surgery.[10] It is imperative that anesthesia providers remain cognizant of age-related variances in behavior and cognitive abilities when preparing a child for anesthesia. If possible, an open dialogue should be fostered to better understand the child's specific fears and concerns. The use of preoperative anesthesia clinics

has become increasingly popular, as they can provide patients and families the opportunity to tour the unit and discuss the procedure in an age-appropriate manner. This experience can help prepare the child psychologically for the surgery and may aid the development of a plan for the day of surgery.

PREOPERATIVE MEDICATION

Prior to anesthesia, medication administration in the preoperative area may be required for a host of reasons. The primary indication is often the management of preoperative anxiety. If it is not adequately managed, anxiety can heighten stress in the child and increase parental anxiety. It is associated with emergence delirium and postoperative behavioral changes.[11] For more information regarding anxiety, please see Chapter 131, "Pediatric Pain Management." Preoperative anxiety is not the sole indication for preoperative medications, however. This section discusses medications commonly administered in the preoperative environment. Further information regarding pharmacological agents can be found in Chapter 2, "Pharmacological Considerations for the Pediatric Patient."

Sedatives

Midazolam is the most widely used sedative in pediatric and adult patients and has been found to be more effective in tempering separation anxiety and improving mask acceptance compared to many other sedatives.[12,13] Midazolam is available in oral, nasal, IM, IV, and rectal formulations. When administered orally, midazolam has a bitter taste, which limits it acceptance among children. If agreeable and in compliance with institutional policies, involving parents may improve patient acceptance of oral medications and decrease patient apprehension.

Midazolam is not the sole anxiolytic used in practice. Multiple medications or combinations of medications have been used in the pediatric population, with practice varying by institution and geographical region. Once the drug of choice, chloral hydrate has become less commonly employed as an anxiolytic and is more often used for procedural sedation. Table 3.2 reviews some the more commonly used sedatives in pediatrics.

Melatonin

Melatonin is a hormone synthesized by the pineal gland and released in response to darkness. The release of melatonin does not begin until after sundown, peaks in the middle of the night, and slowly decreases throughout the night following a circadian rhythm that mirrors sleep patterns. Consuming exogenous forms of melatonin prompts drowsiness and sleep as well as assists with regulation of blood pressure and autonomic cardiovascular regulation.[14] Its primary role as a premedication has been to facilitate sleep or sedation. Melatonin has been found to significantly decrease the amount of propofol required for induction and results in faster recovery from anesthesia compared to children who received midazolam.[15] Comparable studies have noted preoperative anxiety and emergence delirium to be decreased with the use of melatonin.[16]

Nonopioid Analgesics

Acetaminophen is an antipyretic and an analgesic that is available in a multitude of formulations. Administering acetaminophen perioperatively can decrease postoperative analgesia and minimize opioid requirements. Anesthesia providers must remain cognizant that hepatotoxicity can occur should excessive or duplicate doses be administered, so safeguards should be in place to present this. Ibuprofen is a nonsteroidal anti-inflammatory medication that is also available in oral (liquid, chewable tablet, or tablet) or IV formulations. Nonsteroidal anti-inflammatory drugs have several known side effects that anesthesia providers should be aware of, including gastric ulcers, impacting clotting time, and decreasing renal blood flow in patients with a history of renal disease.

Antiemetics

Postoperative nausea and vomiting is one of the most common, yet undesirable side effects of anesthesia. Several modifiable and unmodifiable risk factors have been identified. Children have almost a twofold increased risk of developing postoperative nausea and vomiting compared with adults.[17] Pediatric risk factors include (a) age greater than 3 years, (b) surgical time greater than 30 minutes, (c) strabismus surgery, and (d) previous history of postoperative nausea and vomiting or family member with postoperative nausea and vomiting.[18] Determining the need for a single drug versus a multimodal antiemetic approach can be determined based on risk factors (Box 3.1).

5-Hydroxytryptamine Antagonists

Ondansetron is the first-line drug of choice in preventing postoperative nausea and vomiting. Although not commonly used in infants, it can be administered to children as young as 1 month. In combination with dexamethasone, it has been found to the most effective treatment for children. Ondansetron, dolasetron, and granisetron are the most commonly used 5-HT3 antagonists in children, each of which block serotonin peripherally in the gastrointestinal system and centrally in the chemoreceptor trigger areas. Ondansetron has been known to cause prolonged QT intervals; thus, a careful history should be taken prior to administration, and caution should be used in patients with a history of prolonged QT syndrome.

Corticosteroids

The antiemetic mechanism of acting of dexamethasone is not fully understood, although it is thought to be multifactorial. Dexamethasone is not commonly used as a single agent of treatment for postoperative nausea and vomiting; however, it has been a proven agent when used in combination with other antiemetics.

Table 3.2	Frequently Used Oral Preoperative Medications	
Medication	**Oral Dose**	**Onset**
Midazolam	.25–.5 mg/kg/dose, maximum dose 20 mg	5–15 min
Diazepam	.2–.5 mg/kg/dose, maximum dose 10 mg	15–60 min
Chloral hydrate	25–50 mg/kg/dose, maximum dose 1000 mg	30–60 min
Melatonin	.5 mg/kg/dose, maximum dose 20 mg	20–30 min

BOX 3.1	COMBINATION ANTIEMETIC THERAPY REGIMENS FOR CHILDREN
Ondansetron .05 mg/kg + dexamethasone .015 mg/kg	
Ondansetron .1 mg/kg + droperidol .015 mg/kg	
Tropisetron .1 mg/kg + dexamethasone .5 mg/kg	

Table 3.3	Recommended Antibiotic Prophylaxis for Pediatric Infective Endocarditis	
Condition	Medication	Dose Single Dose Given 30 Min Prior to Procedure
Oral	Amoxicillin	50 mg/kg IV or IM
IV or IM	Ampicillin Cefazolin or ceftriaxone	50 mg/kg IV or IM 50 mg/kg IV or IM
Allergic to penicillins, oral administration	Cephalexin Clindamycin Azithromycin or Claromycin	50 mg/kg 20 mg/kg 15 mg/kg
Allergic to penicillins IV or IM	Cefazolin or ceftriaxone Clindamycin	50 mg/kg IV or IM 20 mg/kg IV or IM

Anticholinergic

Transdermal scopolamine is an effective adjunctive medication; however, it not a first-line agent. It can be applied preoperatively the night before surgery or in the preoperative period on the day of surgery and remain in place for up to 72 hours. Its main side effects are dry mouth, drowsiness, dizziness, visual changes, and irritation at the site of the patch, which are all reversed after patch removal.

Subacute Bacterial Endocarditis Prophylaxis

Infective endocarditis is an infection of the endocardium that if left untreated can damage the heart valves. In 2017, the American Heart Association and the American College of Cardiology published an update to their previous guidelines for antibiotic prophylaxis for dental and surgical procedures. Patients requiring antibiotic prophylaxis include those with (a) prosthetic cardiac valves, (b) prosthetic material used in cardiac surgery, and (c) congenital heart disease with subcategories of those that have unrepaired cyanotic defects, repaired congenital heart defects with prosthetic material, repaired congenital heart defects with residual shunts or valvular regurgitation, or cardiac transplant recipients with valvular regurgitation. Patients do not require antibiotic prophylaxis if they are undergoing a gastrointestinal or genitourinary tract procedure. The Committee of Infective Endocarditis: Guidelines from the American Heart Association (2007) established recommended antibiotics for prophylaxis (Table 3.3).

NONPHARMACOLOGICAL APPROACHES TO ANXIOLYSIS

While medications have been found to be very effective in reducing preoperative anxiety in children, the side effects, potential for paradoxical reactions, and perceived impact on postoperative recovery time may limit their use. A number of nonpharmacological distraction methods have been identified to assist reducing postoperative distress for the entire family.

A multidisciplinary approach that employs a family-centered care approach and incorporates a child life therapist in the process is beneficial. Child life specialists are specially trained in psychologically preparing the child in a developmentally appropriate manner and can identify strategies to improve the experience and support the child and family throughout all phases of perioperative care.[19]

The incorporation of child-sized toy cars for transportation to the operating room and music therapy are both beneficial in reducing anxiety for children as well as their parents.[20,21] In school-aged children, relaxation-guided imagery, the use of virtual reality glasses, and web-based clinical games were noted to decrease pain and stress.[22,23] It should be noted that while parents may provide a calming effect for the anxious child, they can also have a negative impact on a child's emotional sense if they themselves are exceptionally anxious.[24] Therefore, parental presence during induction remains a controversial topic with a wide variety of opinions espoused.[25]

KEY TAKEAWAYS

- A thorough preanesthesia assessment is critical, including early assessment of current or recent respiratory illness.
- A COLDS score is a helpful decision-making tool to help quantify the risk of perioperative respiratory adverse events in the setting of a current or recent respiratory illness.
- Assessing preoperative fasting status early on in the preanesthesia assessment is important.
- The generally accepted preoperative fasting guidelines remain the gold standard of care.
- Research is evolving regarding preoperative fasting time frames, and new modalities, such as ultrasound, are being examined as an adjunct to evaluate fasting status and to facilitate safe anesthesia care.

RESOURCE

- Validation of COLDS Scoring System: A Preanesthetic Risk Assessment Tool
    - http://www.asaabstracts.com/strands/asaabstracts/abstract.htm?year=2015&index=16&absnum=3880

KEY REFERENCES

Complete references for this chapter are online and available at https://connect.springerpub.com/content/book/978-0-8261-3875-0/part/part02/toc-part/ch003.

1. Lerman J. Preoperative assessment and premedication in paediatrics. *Eur J Anaesthesiol*. 2013;30(11):645–650. doi:10.1097/EJA.0b013e328360c3e2
3. Basel A, Baji, D. Preoperative evaluation of the pediatric patient. *Anesthesiol Clin*. 2018;36(4):689–700. doi:10.1016/j.anclin.2018.07.016
4. Lee LK, Bernardo M, Grogan TR, et al. Perioperative respiratory adverse event risk assessment in children with upper respiratory tract infection: Validation of the COLDS score. *Paediatr Anaesth*. 2018;8(11):1007–1014. doi:10.1111/pan.13491
6. Frykholm P, Schindler E, Sümpelmann R, et al. Preoperative fasting in children: review of existing guidelines and recent developments. *Br J Anaesth*. 2018;120(3):469–474. doi:10.1016/j.bja.2017.11.080
10. Adler AC, Leung S, Lee B H, et al. Preparing your pediatric patients and their families for the operating room: reducing fear of the unknown. *Pediatr Rev*. 2018;39(1):13–26. doi:10.1542/pir.2017-0011
12. Hanna AH, Ramsingh D, Sullivan-Lewis W, et al. A comparison of midazolam and zolpidem as oral premedication in children, a prospective randomized double-blinded clinical trial. *Paediatr Anaesth*. 2018;28(12):1109–1115. doi:10.1111/pan.13501
13. Agrawal N, Kumari S, Usha G, et al. Comparison of oral clonidine, oral dexmedetomidine, and oral midazolam for premedication in pediatric patients undergoing elective surgery. *Anesth Essays Res*. 2017;11(1):185. doi:10.4103/0259-1162.194586
17. Harvey M, Geary T. Preoperative assessment and preparation for safe paediatric anaesthesia. *Anaesth. Intensive Care Med*. 2018;19(8):401–408. doi:10.1016/j.mpaic.2018.05.004
19. H.R, Thompson P. *The Handbook of Child Life: A Guide for Pediatric Psychosocial Care*. Charles C Thomas Pub Ltd. 2018.
20. Liu PP, Sun Y, Wu C, et al. The effectiveness of transport in a toy car for reducing preoperative anxiety in preschool children: a randomized controlled prospective trial. *Br J Anaesth*. 2018;121(2):438–444. doi:10.1016/j.bja.2018.02.067
22. Vagnoli L, Bettini A, Amore E, et al. Relaxation-guided imagery reduces perioperative anxiety and pain in children: a randomized study. *Eur J Pediatr*. 2019;178(6):913–921. doi:10.5152/TJAR.2019.67503
23. Buffel C, van Aalst J, Bangels AM, et al. A web-based serious game for health to reduce perioperative anxiety and pain in children (clinipup): pilot randomized controlled trial. *JMIR Serious Games*. 2019;7(2):e12431. doi:10.2196/12431
24. Bizzio R, Cianelli R, Villegas N, et al. Exploring non-pharmacological management among anesthesia providers to reduce preoperative distress in children. *J Pediatr Nurs*. 2020;50:105–112. doi:10.1016/j.pedn.2019.11.005
26. Practice Guidelines for Preoperative Fasting and the Use of Pharmacologic Agents to Reduce the Risk of Pulmonary Aspiration: Application to Healthy Patients Undergoing Elective Procedures: An Updated Report by the American Society of Anesthesiologists Task Force on Preoperative Fasting and the Use of Pharmacologic Agents to Reduce the Risk of Pulmonary Aspiration. *Anesthesiology*. 2017;126(3):376–393. doi:10.1097/ALN.0000000000001452
28. Hickman SR, Mathieson KM, Bradford LM, et al. Randomized trial of oral versus intravenous acetaminophen for postoperative pain control. *Am J Health Syst Pharm*. 2018;75(6):367–375. doi:10.2146/ajhp170064
30. Manoj M, Satya Prakash MVS, Swaminathan S, et al. Comparison of ease of administration of intranasal midazolam spray and oral midazolam syrup by parents as premedication to children undergoing elective surgery. *J Anesth*. 2017;31(3):351–357. doi:10.1007/s00540-017-2330-6
31. McHale B, Badenhorst CD, Low C, et al. Do children undergoing bilateral myringotomy with placement of ventilating tubes benefit from pre-operative analgesia? A double-blinded, randomised, placebo-controlled trial. *J Laryngol Otol*. 2018;132(8):685–692. doi:10.1017/S0022215118001111
32. Uritis I, Orhurhu N, Jones MR, et al. Postoperative nausea and vomiting in paediatric anaesthesia. *Turk J Anaesthesiol Reanim*. 2020;48(2):88–95. doi:10.5152/TJAR.2019.67503
33. Viswanath A, Oreadi D, Finkelman M, et al. Does pre-emptive administration of intravenous ibuprofen (caldolor) or intravenous acetaminophen (ofirmev) reduce postoperative pain and subsequent narcotic consumption after third molar surgery? *J Oral Maxillofac Surg*. 2019;7(2):262–270. doi:10.1016/j.joms.2018.09.010
34. Wilson W, Taubert KA, Gewitz M, et al. Prevention of infective endocarditis: a guideline from the American Heart Association: a guideline from the American Heart Association Rheumatic Fever, Endocarditis, and Kawasaki Disease Committee, Council on Cardiovascular Disease in the Young, and the Council on Clinical Cardiology, Council on Cardiovascular Surgery and Anesthesia, and the Quality of Care and Outcomes Research Interdisciplinary Working Group. *Circulation*. 2007;116(15):1736–1754. doi:10.1161/CIRCULATIONAHA.106.183095

CHAPTER 4

Equipment and Monitoring

Su Chang and Jeanie Skibiski

LEARNING OBJECTIVES

- Review equipment commonly used when delivering anesthesia to children.
- Describe indications for invasive pediatric monitoring devices.
- Describe standard monitors used in pediatric anesthesia.
- State the minimum monitoring requirements for pediatric patients undergoing anesthesia.

INTRODUCTION

Patient safety is the primary goal during every anesthetic. Change can rapidly ensue during the course of an anesthetic. Thankfully, advances in monitoring have made anesthesia very safe in the modern era.[1] Nonetheless, it is imperative that anesthesia providers continually monitor the patient's physiologic parameters and intervene accordingly before the patient suffers harm. To do so effectively, anesthesia providers need to be able to interpret information provided by key monitors, as well as have a sound understanding of proper indications, contraindications, and how to trouble potential complications that may arise.[2]

Pediatric monitoring standards are the same as those that govern monitoring of adult patients undergoing anesthesia.[3] Accordingly, the anesthesia workstation is composed of an anesthetic gas delivery system, as well as associated monitoring, alarms, and protection devices. However, due to a lack of evidence, validity, and size constraints, the use of advanced monitoring techniques for children under anesthesia differs at times from that of their adult counterparts.

ANESTHESIA MACHINE

All anesthesia machines have the ability to deliver volatile anesthetic agents into a breathing system and provide mechanical ventilation no matter the size of the patient. Adaptations and safeguards, however, must be implemented when preparing to anesthetize a child or neonate. The U.S. Food and Drug Administration (FDA) recognizes the consensus standards for anesthetic workstations that include standards outlined by the International Organization for Standardization (ISO) standards for medical electrical equipment.[4] ISO standard 4135:2001 specifically addresses anesthesia equipment. Anesthesia machines are typically composed of two systems: the electrical and the pneumatic systems.

ELECTRICAL SYSTEM

A master switch activates both the electrical and pneumatic systems. Turning the machine on and off will reboot the computer, which is necessary for optimal function. Several components of the modern anesthesia machine may be electronic, such as the ventilator and vaporizers for desflurane.[5] In addition, the master switch is responsible for activating the flow of gases into the intermediate pressure circuit of the anesthesia machine. The electrical system is also necessary for the Anesthesia Information Management Systems (AIMS) that records clinical data, as well as housing the computer hardware and software.

PNEUMATIC SYSTEM

The anesthesia machine controls the flow and composition of the delivered fresh gas, as well as that of volatile agents in a controllable concentration. Within the pneumatic system, there are three distinct systems based on the amount of pressure associated within each system: the high-, intermediate-, and low-pressure systems. The high-pressure system includes the gas cylinders on the anesthesia machine, as well as the hanger yoke assembly. The high-pressure system is responsible for receiving gases at variable pressures, which can be up to 1900 psig when coming from oxygen cylinders. Gases pass from the cylinders through the hanger yoke assembly and ultimately through the pressure regulator, which then converts the highly variable gas pressure into a lower, more constant pressure that is suitable for use in the anesthesia machine. Anesthesia machines utilize the medical gas pin index safety system that incorporates specific pin configurations to ensure that the correct medical gas cylinder is hung in the correct yoke and prevent erroneous misconnections of gas supplies.

The intermediate-pressure system of the anesthesia machine includes components that receive gases at reduced pressures, usually in the range of 37 to 55 psi. This includes, but is not limited to, the oxygen failure alarms, flow meter assembly, and oxygen flush valve. The oxygen flush valve activates oxygen within the intermediate-pressure system and allows for oxygen flows at 35 to 75 L/min with a pressure of 45 to 60 psig. Anesthesia providers must be cognizant that there is potential for barotrauma in the pediatric lung with excessive use of the oxygen flush valve. The flow meter assembly controls, measures, and indicates the rate of gas flow in the machine.

The low-pressure system is the part of the machine downstream of the flow meters. This includes the vaporizers, back pressure safety devices, and the common gas outlet. In the low-pressure system, pressure exerted by gases is slightly above atmospheric pressure.

SCAVENGING SYSTEM

To prevent contamination of the operating room with waste anesthetic gases, an active or passive gas disposal system must be in place. Factors contributing to operating room pollution include use of high-flow techniques as often seen with inhalation induction techniques. Components of a scavenging system for gas collection are shown in **Figure 4.1**.[6]

CARBON DIOXIDE ABSORPTION

The ability to absorb carbon dioxide (CO_2) with an absorbent allows for the use of a circle system breathing circuit. CO_2 absorption occurs by employing the general principle of a

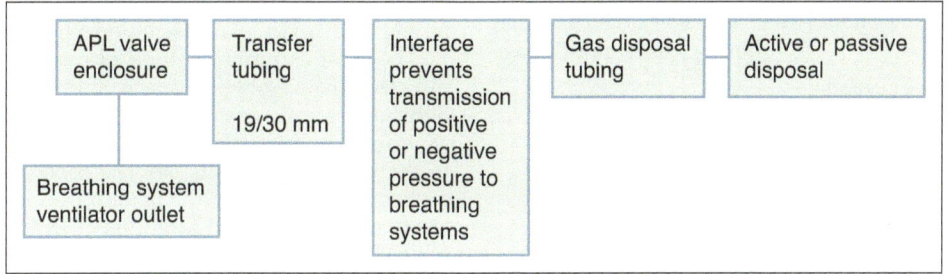

Figure 4.1: Components of a scavenging system.
APL valve, adjustable pressure-limiting valve.

base neutralizing an acid. The acid is carbonic acid from the reaction of CO_2 with water to form carbonic acid. The base is a hydroxide of an alkali (soda lime). The product of the reaction is generation of water and a carbonate.[7]

Should soda lime absorbent become desiccated, adverse reactions between volatile agents, and the absorbent can occur. In the presence of desiccated soda lime, ether anesthetics can degrade to carbon monoxide with the potential for carbon monoxide production greatest from desflurane followed by isoflurane, sevoflurane, and halothane. When combined, sevoflurane and desiccated soda lime may produce compound A, which has been reported to result in renal injury in animal studies. Newer absorbents have been developed that do not contain the strong alkali agents NaOH and KOH and are inert to the ether anesthetics.[8]

HUMIDIFICATION

Inhaled gases are administered at room temperature with little to no humidification. Dry gases must then be humidified and warmed by the upper respiratory tract, which accounts for approximately 15% of the body's total base heat expenditure.[9] Prolonged humidification has the potential to result in negative sequelae, such as atelectasis and ventilation/perfusion mismatch. To avoid such undesired outcomes, anesthesia providers should employ either active passive or active humidification techniques. Humidification and warming of inspired gases are especially important with neonates and infants.

Passive humidification can be achieved with the use of a heat and moisture exchanger (HME). HMEs typically contain hygroscopic material that aids in the retention of heat and moisture. Using small pleated hydrophobic filters is recommended if extra humidity is desired.[10] An HME may also serve as a barrier to droplet transmission and are recommended to prevent transmission of the SARS-CoV-2 virus.[11] Anesthesia providers must be aware that the use of a HME can increase dead space, leading to greater rebreathing of exhaled carbon dioxide, as well as contribute to increased airway resistance and difficulties with ventilation. Accordingly, use of an HME should be avoided with neonates weighing less than 2.5 kg.[10] HME use may also affect capnography measurement, particularly with smaller tidal volumes. Sampling may be done on either the patient or the machine side of the filter, but there may be differences in CO_2 measurement.[10] Using a circle breathing circuit with low gas flows is an alternate approach to providing condensation and water vapor.

Active humidification requires a water supply and external power and are more effective than passive humidification in preserving moisture and heat. A variety of active humidifiers are available, including bubble humidifiers, nebulizers, and heated humidifiers. Bubble humidifiers work by passing the fresh gas through a water reservoir. In doing so, the bubbles absorb water vapor as they pass to the surface of the reservoir. Rather than vaporizing the liquid, nebulizers produce a mist of droplets that suspend in the gas. Heated humidifiers employ a heated chamber of water that evaporates when heated. Gases are then passed through the chamber becoming saturated. Regardless of technique used, a water trap should be used to collect excess condensate as it is a potential locus for colonization of bacteria.

ANESTHESIA MACHINE CHECK

Anesthesia providers should incorporate a validated anesthesia machine checklist, such as the one developed jointly by the American Society of Anesthesiologist, the American Association of Nurse Anesthetists, and the American Society of Anesthesia Technicians, to ensure the delivery of safe, effective care. The 15-item checklist may be part of an automated checkout procedure, but the completion of the checklist will allow for supporting essential life functions (Table 4.1). The checklist should be employed at beginning of the day and prior to the start of each subsequent case performed.[12]

OXYGEN, CARBON DIOXIDE, AND ANESTHETIC AGENT MONITORING

OXYGEN DELIVERY

Documentation of the percentage of inspired oxygen is a requirement according to practice standards put forth by both the American Society of Anesthesiologists and the American Association of Nurse Anesthetists.[3,12] An oxygen analyzer should be placed in the inspiratory limb of the anesthesia circuit to ensure delivery of adequate oxygen concentrations to the patient.

Oxygen delivery must be precisely calibrated for the pediatric patient, especially the premature infant in whom retinopathy of prematurity is a concern.

There are three types of oxygen analyzers that are commonly used in anesthesia machines: polarographic or Clark electrodes, galvanic or fuel cell, and paramagnetic;[14] Polarographic electrodes uses a cathode made of platinum, gold, or palladium; an anode made of silver; an electrolyte gel; and a Teflon membrane to determine the dissolved oxygen concentration in a liquid (usually blood). As oxygen reacts with the electrodes, a current is generated proportional to the dissolved oxygen concentration value. Galvanic or fuel cell analyzers employ two electrodes in a potassium hydroxide bath. Similar to the polarographic electrodes, as oxygen flows through a Teflon membrane, an electric current is generated proportional to the partial pressure of oxygen.[15] Paramagnetic oxygen analyzers rely on the fact that oxygen is a strong parametric gas. Using an electromagnetic field and a pressure transducer, a differential pressure is generated between the reference sample and the anesthetic gas

Table 4.1	Anesthesia Machine Checkout	
Task to Be Done	Daily	Between Cases
Verify auxiliary oxygen cylinder and manual ventilation device (Ambu Bag) are available and functioning	X	
Verify patient suction is adequate to clear the airway	X	X
Turn on anesthesia delivery system and confirm that AC power is available	X	
Verify availability of required monitors, including alarms	X	X
Verify that pressure is adequate on the spare oxygen cylinder mounted on the anesthesia machine	X	
Verify that the piped gas pressures are ≥50 psig	X	
Verify that vaporizers are adequately filled and, if applicable, that the filler ports are tightly closed	X	X
Verify that there are no leaks in the gas supply lines between the flow meters and the common gas outlet	X	
Test scavenging system function	X	
Calibrate, or verify calibration of, the oxygen monitor and check the low oxygen alarm	X	
Verify carbon dioxide absorbent is fresh and not exhausted	X	X
Perform breathing system pressure and leak testing	X	X
Verify that gas flows properly through the breathing circuit during both inspiration and exhalation	X	X
Document completion of checkout procedures	X	X
Confirm ventilator settings and evaluate readiness to deliver anesthesia care anesthesia time out	X	X

sample. This is converted to a direct current voltage proportional to the oxygen concentration. Paramagnetic oxygen analyzers require use of a water trap as they are affected by water vapor.[15]

CAPNOGRAPHY

Capnography is the continuous monitoring of the CO_2 with a graphic display. Monitoring ventilation by observation and confirmation of continuous expired CO_2 during all types of anesthesia is required per the Standards for Nurse Anesthesia Practice and the American Society of Anesthesiologists.[3,13] Qualitative capnography may be used for confirmation of endotracheal intubation, while quantitative capnography may measure adequacy of resuscitation efforts during cardiac arrest.

The most common method of measurement of CO_2 is the infrared (IR) absorption spectrometry method. Using an IR light, the sample gas absorbs light in proportion to the concentration of CO_2 (Beer–Lambert Law), the light then goes to the IR detector to display the concentration.[15] CO_2 shows a strong absorption in the far-infrared light at 4.3 μm. There are two common configurations of IR CO_2 monitors, each of which has a distinct location where CO_2 is monitored. These are known as nondiverting and diverting capnography.

Nondiverting, or mainstream, capnographs measure CO_2 passing through an adaptor within the breathing circuit. Mainstream gas analyzers have several advantages. They do not extract gas from the circuit and hence have faster response times and are less likely to become obstructed with secretions.[16] Unfortunately, mainstream analyzers are heavy and may obstruct a small endotracheal tube (ET), which can be especially problematic in pediatric anesthesia. Diverting, or sidestream, analyzers continuously remove gas from the breathing circuit and are the most common type of CO_2 monitoring. Diverting analyzers may prove helpful for trend monitoring during high frequency ventilation.[16] High aspiration rates coupled with limited dead space sampling typically increase sensitivity and decrease sampling lag time. Diverting sampling lines are prone to becoming obstructed with water or secretions.

As capnography is frequently used to adjust ventilation parameters, anesthesia providers should be aware of the differences that exist between partial pressure of carbon dioxide ($PaCO_2$) and end-tidal carbon dioxide ($ETCO_2$) values. Typical difference is assumed to be .5 kPa, though the potential exists for an overestimation of $ETCO_2$ in children who are mechanically ventilated resulting in unrecognized hypocarbia.

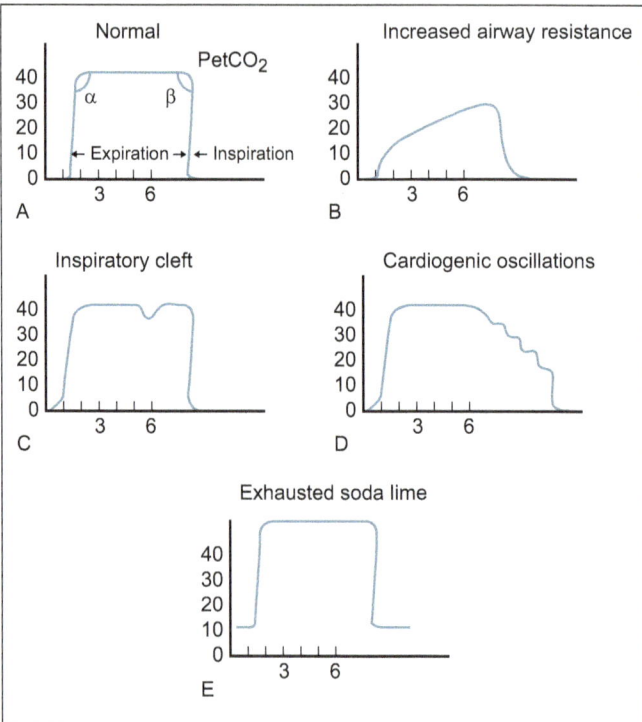

Figure 4.2: Normal and abnormal capnograms. (A) Normal; (B) increased airway resistance; (C) inspiratory cleft; (D) cardiogenic oscillations; and (E) exhausted soda lime.

$PetCO_2$, patient end-tidal carbon dioxide.

Table 4.2	Comparison of Agent Analyzers			
Analyzer Type	**Analysis Method**	**Speed**	**Advantages**	**Disadvantages**
Mass spectrometer	Spreads gases into a spectrum according to mass/charge ratios	Fast response time if using a stand-alone unit Shared units have slower times	Multiple gas Multiple agent Low cost to operate	Measures only the pre-programmed gases and may have calibration errors Long warm-up time May have distorted signal for pediatrics
Rahman spectroscopy (Ohmeda RASCAL II)	Laser light striking gas molecules. Energy is reabsorbed and re-emitted at a wavelength specific for each agent	Slower than mass spectroscopy	Multiple gas Multiple agent Short start-up time if not turned off Calibration every 30 days	May be large and heavy Argon and helium cannot be measured High initial cost Inaccurate with fruit-flavored scents Artifacts with nitric oxide
IR gas analysis	Gases absorb IR energy at wavelengths specific to five inhaled anesthetic gases, CO_2 and N_2O	Fast response time	Multiple gas Portable Short warmup time No interference by argon or nitric oxide	Oxygen and nitrogen not measured by IR spectroscopy Inaccurate with alcohols and propellants Water vapor interference Interference among gases

IR, infrared spectroscopy.

A volume capnogram (Figure 4.2) may be divided into two segments: inspiratory and expiratory. As expiration occurs, there is a sharp upstroke as the dead space gas mixes with CO_2 exhaled from the alveoli followed by a plateau phase. The end of the plateau is the best estimation of $ETCO_2$. The inspiratory segment is seen as a sharp downstroke as fresh gas enters the lungs. There are two angles that can be measured within the capnogram as well. The alpha angle is measured at the beginning of the plateau and is normally 100° to 110°, though may increase with airway obstruction. The beta angle is measured at the end of the plateau phase and the downstroke of inspiration and is normally 90° but increases when rebreathing occurs.[15]

Capnography use in the postanesthesia care unit (PACU) is not considered to be a standard monitor, although capnography use may improve the recognition of hypoventilation and apnea.[17] Mainstream capnography can be achieved in the PACU with specially designed masks or oxygen cannulas, such as the cap-ONE® mask. This design allows for measurement of CO_2 that is less affected by administered oxygen.[18]

AGENT ANALYZERS

Measuring volatile anesthetic gases is not yet a standard of care in the United States. Nonetheless, it is important anesthesia providers monitor the delivery of volatile agents to assess adequate anesthetic delivery, uptake, and distribution.[19] This can also aid in detecting breathing circuit disconnections.

A variety of technologies are available for analysis of inhalational anesthetic agents (Table 4.2). These include Raman spectroscopic analysis, mass spectroscopy, IR photoacoustic spectrometry, IR simple spectrometry, and piezoelectric crystal agent analysis. The most common method being IR spectrometry.[15]

BASIC PHYSIOLOGIC MONITORING

PRECORDIAL STETHOSCOPE

The pretracheal or precordial stethoscope is a simple, inexpensive, and easy-to-use tool for respiratory monitoring (Figure 4.3).

The precordial stethoscope is a weighted bell attached to the patient's precordium or pretracheal area with double-sided adhesive disks depending on the focus of continuous assessment. If monitoring for heart sounds, the precordial stethoscope should be placed over the precordium. If using a precordial stethoscope for respiratory sound monitoring, it should be placed in the pretracheal area. When properly used, a precordial stethoscope can detect airway obstruction before oxygen desaturation occurs. Combining a precordial stethoscope with capnography and pulse oximetry has been shown to be most effective in detecting airway obstruction in children receiving propofol sedation.[20] Monitoring of ventilation by capnography or precordial stethoscope is strongly recommended by the American Academy of Pediatrics in their 2019 Guidelines for Monitoring and Management of Pediatric Patients Before, During, and After Sedation for Diagnostic and Therapeutic Procedures.[21]

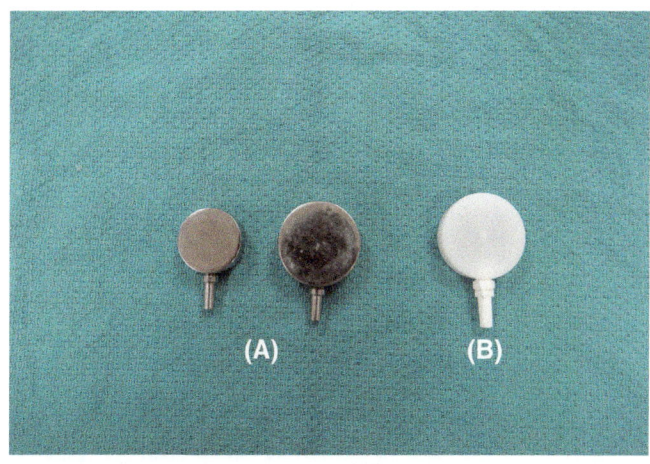

Figure 4.3: Precordial stethoscopes. (A) Precordial stethoscopes in infant and child sizes. Nonferrous stethoscope for MRI use and (B) precordial stethoscope with double-stick disk.

PULSE OXIMETRY

Continuous pulse oximetry can signal impending hypoxemia.[3] Pulse oximetry measures oxygen saturation by illuminating the skin via a distally placed probe (Figure 4.4). Changes in light absorption of oxygenated (oxyhemoglobin) and deoxygenated blood (reduced hemoglobin) is then measured using two light wavelengths: 660 nm (red) and 940 nm (IR). The amount of light absorption at each light frequency depends on the degree of oxygenation of the hemoglobin molecule. This information is then processed, and the ratio of absorbance at these two wavelengths is calculated and calibrated against direct measurements of arterial oxygen saturation (SaO_2) to establish the pulse oximeter's measure of arterial saturation (SpO_2).

For optimal results and functioning, the probe should be placed on an extremity that allows for transillumination, such as finger, toe, or earlobe. The oxygen saturation data are collected over 5 to 20 pulses, depending on the manufacturer. The pulse rate is also calculated from the number of LED cycles between successive pulsatile signals and averaged out over a period.

All pulse oximeter probes are subject to motion artifact. In an actively moving child, pulsatile movement of fluids may occur and lead to falsely low saturation reading. To combat this known issue, many manufacturers utilize additional algorithms to reject motion artifact and reduce false alarms.[23] Reflection pulse oximetry uses reflected rather than transmitted light on a single-sided monitor, allowing these probes to be applied to the forehead, which may limit movement-related artifact.

Multiple wavelength pulse CO-oximetry has been expanded to provide noninvasive measurement of total hemoglobin. This technology has been found to provide accurate trend data in children undergoing major surgical procedures associated with substantial blood loss.[24] In trauma victims, however, multiple wavelength pulse CO-oximetry is not precise enough to provide a transfusion trigger and may be most effective in determining when an invasive test of hemoglobin is needed.[25] Hemoglobinopathies, such as methemoglobin or carboxyhemoglobin, can interfere with the accuracy of the standard pulse oximeter. The accuracy of multiple-wavelength pulse oximetry, however, is not impact by hemoglobinopathies.[23]

ELECTROCARDIOGRAM

Monitoring of a patient receiving anesthesia is a standard when monitoring circulation per both the Standards for Nurse Anesthesia Practice and American Society of Anesthesiologists.[3,12] For pediatric patients, the HR is a critical monitor with bradycardia being an indicator of hypoxia and

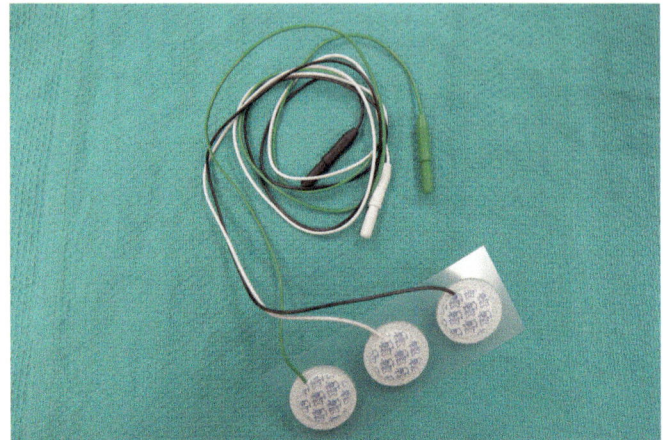

Figure 4.5: Infant ECG electrodes.

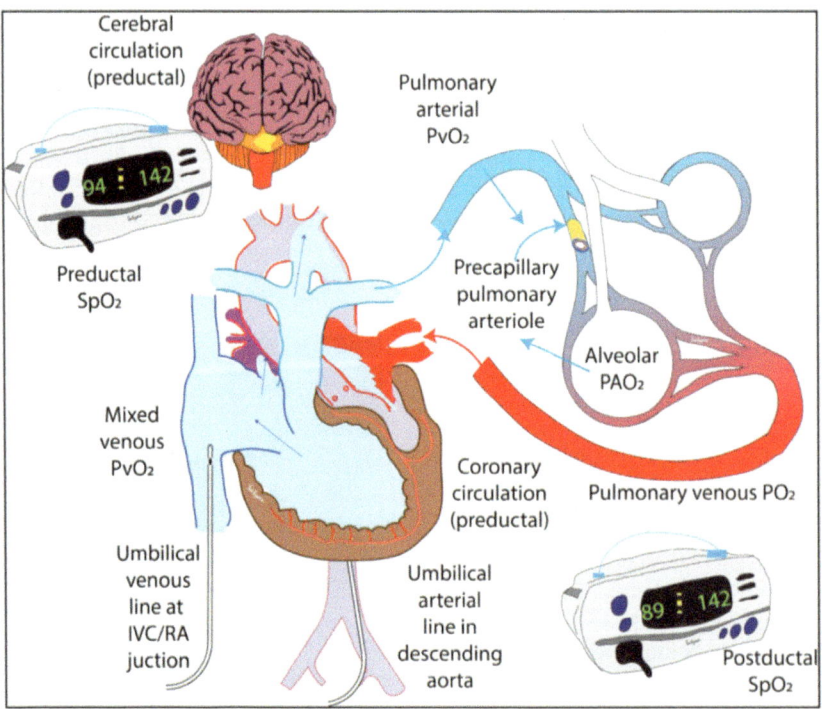

Figure 4.4: Pulse oximetry.

IVC, inferior vena cava; PAO2, partial pressure of oxygen in the alveoli; PO2, partial pressure of oxygen; PvO2, normal mixed venous oxygen tension; RA, right atrium; SpO2, oxygen saturation.

Source: From Chandrasekharan P, Rawat M, Lakshminrusimha S. How do we monitor oxygenation during the management of PPHN? Alveolar, arterial, mixed venous oxygen tension or peripheral saturation? *Children.* 2020;7(10):180. doi:10.3390/children7100180.

tachycardia being an indicator of volume status, infection, or pain. For general pediatric anesthesia, three-lead monitoring is sufficient to detect arrhythmias and the basic HR. Using a five-lead ECG should be considered for pediatric cardiac anesthesia or critically ill patients.[26] Infant-sized electrodes are available when caring for neonates and infants (Figure 4.5). Anesthesia providers must be sure to use nonferrous ECG leads for patients receiving an MRI to avoid potential burn injuries.

NONINVASIVE BLOOD PRESSURE MONITORING

Noninvasive blood pressure (NIBP) measurement is done via oscillometry. During cuff inflation, complete arterial compression occurs to prevent antegrade blood flow, and the cuff is gradually deflated (Figure 4.6). As blood flow resumes, oscillations develop. The point of maximal oscillations defines the mean arterial pressure; the systolic and diastolic blood pressures are then calculated based on algorithms.[27] During measurement, shivering or motion can induce errors leading to erroneous measurements.

Proper measurement of blood pressure in neonates and infants can be technically challenging.

Using the correct size NIBP cuff is necessary for an accurate measurement. A narrow cuff will overestimate the NIBP, while a wide cuff will underestimate. The International Neonatal Consortium recommends that when selecting a NIBP cuff, there should be a cuff width to arm circumference ratio of 0.5. The right upper arm is the recommended location for oscillometric measurements.[28]

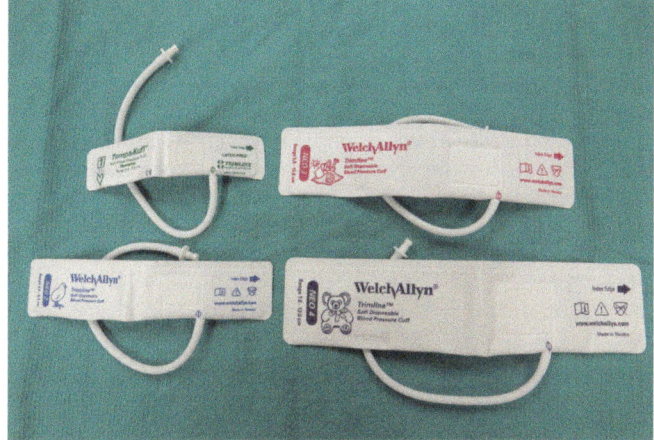

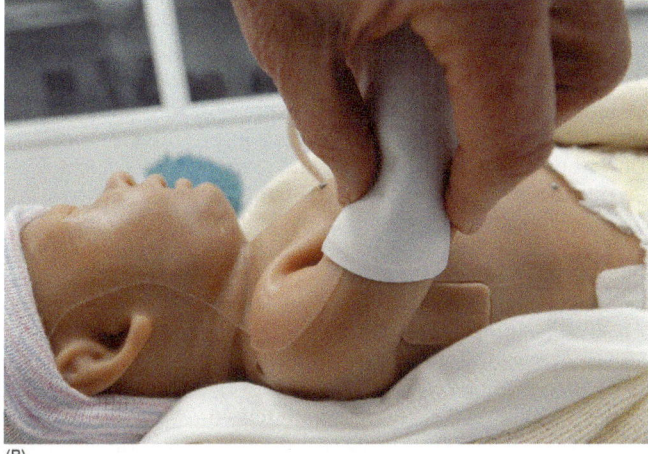

Figure 4.6: Neonatal noninvasive blood pressure cuff. (A) Cuff sizes and (B) demonstration for checking infant blood pressure cuff size.

TEMPERATURE MONITORING

Thermoregulation during general anesthesia occurs in three phases: internal redistribution of heat, heat loss to the environment, and thermoregulatory response. General anesthesia impairs internal redistribution of heat. When providing anesthesia for pediatric patients, heat conservation is critical due to the higher rate of heat loss when compared to adults. Active or passive methods for warming a child are available, with implementation of a standardized temperature management algorithm decreasing the incidence of hypothermia by 53%.[29] For more information on thermoregulation and temperature monitoring, see Chapters 1.7 and 9 in this text.

URINE OUTPUT MONITORING

Intraoperative monitoring of urine output is indicated in the procedures where large shifts in fluid, blood, or hemodynamics are anticipated. Examples include during cardiac surgery and neurosurgery, when caring for patients with significant burns, when the use of hemodilution is planned, or if use of diuretics is planned. In the neonate, urine output is not a sensitive measure of intravascular volume as they lack the ability to concentrate urine until approximately 1 year of age.[30]

Invasive methods include insertion of Foley catheters; size 6 Fr for full-term neonates or smaller feeding tube for premature infants. Urinary bladder catheter should be connected to a urinometer capable of measuring small volumes or to a vented 10- to 20-mL syringe.[23] Noninvasive methods include the use adhesive-backed collection bags or weighing diapers.

ADVANCED MONITORING EQUIPMENT AND TECHNIQUES

Advanced hemodynamic monitoring helps detect hemodynamic alterations, diagnose underlying causes, and optimize oxygen delivery to the tissues. The adequacy of therapeutic interventions, such as volume expansion or vasoactive medications, can be evaluated by advanced hemodynamic monitoring though they are not routinely utilized outside of the critical care setting and even less so in the pediatric noncardiac patients.

ARTERIAL BLOOD PRESSURE MONITORING

In the clinical setting, NIBP monitoring is acceptable in most clinical scenarios unless the need for accurate, reliable, beat-to-beat measurement of blood pressure is necessary (Box 4.1). In this scenario, an arterial catheter may need to be placed for continuous measurement of the arterial blood pressure (ABP).[27] Not only are NIBP and ABP monitoring used in different circumstances, but they often yield different values with NIBP tending to be higher than radial ABP during periods of hypotension and lower than ABP during periods of hypertension. Accordingly, concomitant use of NIBP and ABP is associated with decreased rates of blood transfusion and lees need for vasopressors and antihypertensives when compared with blood pressure monitoring via ABP alone.[27]

Site Selection

The distal radial site is the preferred site and has several advantages, such as collateral blood flow can be readily assessed, the risk of ischemic complications is low, aseptic technique and line management are easy to maintain, and the right radial artery blood gas measurements accurately reflect cerebral

> **BOX 4.1 ARTERIAL BLOOD PRESSURE MONITORING**
>
> **Indications**
>
> - Continuous beat-to-beat monitoring of blood pressure during shock, major surgery, hypertensive emergency, vasopressor therapy, or if the blood pressure is labile.[31]
> - Continuous monitoring of cardiac output and evaluation of respirophasic variations in the arterial pressure waveform to predict fluid responsiveness.[32]
> - Frequent arterial blood gasses and other laboratory draws are necessary.[31]
>
> **Contraindications**[32]
>
> - Avoid sites with overlying skin infection or abscess for indwelling arterial catheters.
> - Distorted anatomy at the puncture site from previous surgical interventions, congenital or acquired malformations, burns, aneurysm, stent, AV fistula, or vascular graft.
> - Disrupted or compromised collateral circulation.
> - Severe peripheral vascular disease of the artery selected.
> - A history of or active Raynaud's syndrome or evidence of poor peripheral perfusion.
> - Supratherapeutic coagulopathy and infusion of thrombolytic agents. Avoid repeated arterial sticks when the INR is >3 and/or the ACT is >100. Therapeutic anticoagulation is not a contraindication for arterial needle puncture, but it is a relative contraindication for an indwelling catheter.
> - Avoid arterial catheter insertion when the platelet count is <50 × 109/L.
>
> INR, international normalized ratio; ACT, activated clotting time

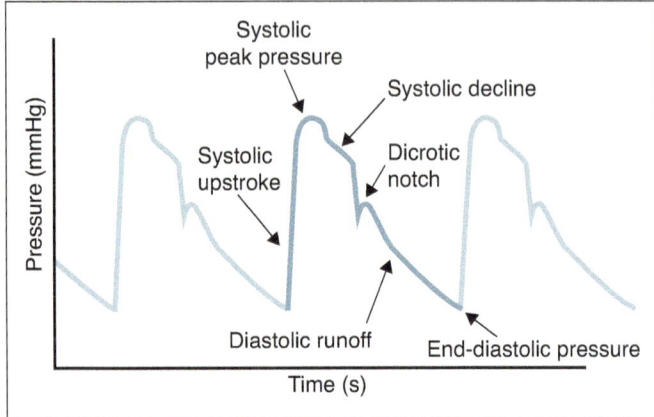

Figure 4.7: Arterial waveform.

oxygenation and perfusion pressure in children with congenital heart disease.[31] The average diameter of the radial artery is 1.2 mm ± .3 mm in pediatric patients younger than 2 years of age, and cannulation can be difficult. First attempt success rate of pediatric radial artery cannulation ranges from 18% to 56% with pulse palpation technique. Ultrasound guidance provides a significant improvement in the success rate of radial artery cannulation from 48% to 83%.[33] For more information regarding the use of ultrasound for vascular access, please refer to Chapter 136, "Ultrasound-Guided Vascular Access."

Locations alternate to the radial artery may also be used for cannulation, with the ulnar artery preferred to the femoral artery in neonates and young infants. It has been offered that the ulnar artery may be the preferable location as it is more palpable than the radial artery, more superficial and better developed than the radial artery, and readily identified under ultrasound guidance.[34] The posterior tibial artery is also preferred to the femoral site in neonates and young infants, as is the dorsalis pedis artery.[31] Prior to cannulizing the dorsalis pedis artery collateral flow should be assessed by occluding the dorsalis pedis artery and confirming a rapid return of color to the great toe when the nail bed is compressed.[31]

The femoral artery is used when arterial access in the wrist or foot is not achievable. Anesthesia providers should be aware that cannulizing the femoral route may lead to thrombosis and distal embolization to the foot therefore the patient must be closely monitored.[31] The brachial artery should be avoided because of limited collateral flow to the distal arm, especially in neonates and young infants.[31] Axillary artery is typically avoided in neonates and young infants but may be used in older children with poor perfusion when cannulation of other sites is unsuccessful.[31]

Arterial Waveform Interpretation

The arterial waveform results from ejection of blood from the left ventricle into the aorta during systole, followed by peripheral runoff during diastole. The normal arterial pressure waveform is shown in the Figure 4.7. Unusual radial arterial pressure waveforms may occur due to pathology in the ascending aorta or aortic valve, or with decreases in systemic blood pressure or systemic vascular resistance (Figure 4.8).[32] Pulse pressure is the difference between systolic and diastolic pressures, which can be used to assess intravascular volume status. Elevated pulse pressure indicates age-associated vascular stiffness, increases in stroke volume (SV) and/or decreases in systemic vascular resistance. A decrease in pulse pressure can be caused by hypovolemia, decreases in SV, and increases in systemic vascular resistance.

Potential Complications Related to Arterial Cannulation

Clinically significant complications of arterial cannulation are uncommon, with the greatest complication rates among neonates and infants. Proper site selection, sterile technique, and ultrasound guidance during cannulation can minimize the incidence of complications. Complications of arterial cannulation in children in descending order of frequency include arterial obstruction, hematoma formation, infection, arterial thrombosis, arterial embolism, and iatrogenic blood loss. Rare complications include air embolism, pseudoaneurysm, and arteriovenous (AV) fistula.[31]

The risk of arterial obstruction is increased with younger patient age and a longer duration of cannulation. Transient arterial obstruction may cause dampening of the arterial waveform, blanching, pain, induration, and rarely skin necrosis.[31] Vasospasm should be suspected if the child reports pain in the extremity, if there is a decrease in ABP, severe damping of the arterial waveform, a loss of the arterial pulse, or a significant decrease in the oximetry plethysmogram signal quality index distal to the arterial cannulation site. Risk factors associated with higher complication rates include female sex, a history of

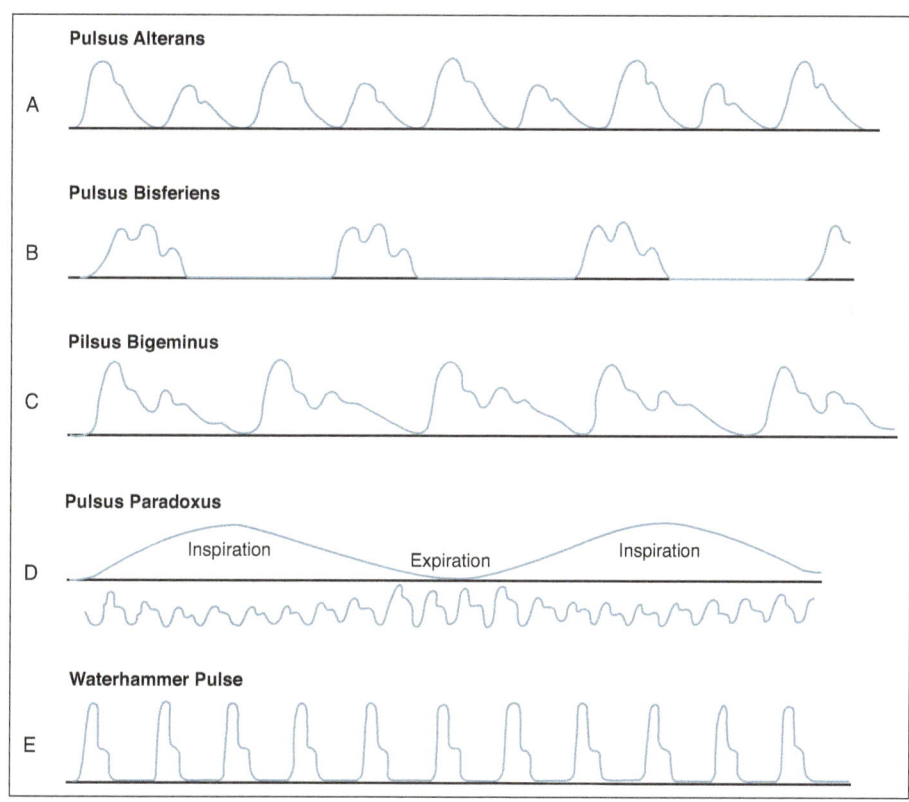

Figure 4.8: Abnormal arterial waveforms and possible causes.
(A) Pulsus alterans, variation in pulse amplitude occurring with alternate beats while the rhythm is regular. Primary cause is left ventricular failure. (B) Pulsus bisferiens, best detected by palpation of the carotid artery, characterized by two systolic peak and a midsystolic dip. Primarily seen in aortic stenosis with significant aortic regurgitation. (C) Pilsus bigeminus, normal pulsation followed by a premature contraction where the amplitude is less than the normal pulsation. Can be seen in alternate premature beats, A. V block, and sinoatrial block with ventricular escape. (D) Pulsus paradoxus, characterized by an exaggerated decrease (>10 mm Hg) in amplitude during inspiration and an increase in amplitude during expiration. Can be seen in superior vena cava obstruction, asthma, emphysema or airway obstruction, pericardial effusion, constrictive pericarditis, and severe congestive heart failure. (E) Waterhammer pulse, which a greater amplitude than expected, a rapid rise to a narrow summit, and a sudden descent. Can be seen in fever, alcohol consumption and pregnancy, and high-output states such as anemia, beriberi or cor pulmonale, cirrhosis, Paget's disease, AV fistula, thyrotoxicosis, cardiac lesions such as aortic regurgitation, PDA, aortopulmonary window, and systolic hypertension.

AV, arteriovenous; PDA, patent ductus arteriosus.

diabetes mellitus, and the ratio of catheter size to radial artery size.[32] Arterial thrombosis should be suspected in patients with decreased distal pulses, dampened or lost arterial waveform, or cyanotic digits. Risk factors for thrombosis include a duration of catheterization greater than 72 hours, the use of a larger catheter, smaller blood vessels, low-flow states such as those seen with low CO, and the presence of peripheral artery disease or vasospastic disorders such as Raynaud's phenomenon.[32]

TRANSCUTANEOUS MONITORING OF THE PARTIAL PRESSURE OF CARBON DIOXIDE

Transcutaneous monitoring of the partial pressure of carbon dioxide ($TcCO_2$) is a noninvasive alternative to arterial blood gas sampling that is frequently used in the neonatal intensive care unit. $TcCO_2$ monitors measure the CO_2 that diffuses through the skin by a sensor that is heated above body temperature (40°C–44°C) to achieve local arterialization. Although substantial variability can exist between $TcCO_2$ and $PaCO_2$, several devices are available that have been shown to be accurate when placed on the earlobe.[35]

CENTRAL VENOUS CATHETERS

Central venous catheters (CVCs) have a wide array of uses care of a critically ill child. Not only are they a reliable means of administering large volumes of fluids, but they can also be used to collect blood samples and as a conduit for advanced hemodynamic monitoring in infants and children, such as central venous pressure or mixed venous oxygen saturation.[36] In addition, CVCs can be used to administer medications that require direct delivery to the central circulation or potentially irritating solutions and can be a viable means of establishing venous access in patients who have proved to be challenging in securing or maintain peripheral venous access. Peripherally inserted central catheter (PICC) lines can also be inserted in patients requiring long-term antibiotics, chemotherapy, or total parental nutrition.[37] Ultimately, the choice of venous access depends on the indication, infusate characteristics, and the anticipated duration of the access. Patient factors, such as obesity, thrombophlebitis, or a history of multiple hospitalizations, may result in using a CVC due to limited peripheral venous access.[38] Common contraindications to CVC placement include inherited or acquired coagulopathy, infection at the insertion site, or surgical manipulation or trauma at the insertion site.[36] Inserting a CVC at noncompressible sites is considered a relative contraindication due to the risk of hemorrhage, especially in patients with coagulopathies.

The internal jugular, subclavian, and femoral veins are the three primary sites for central venous access in infants and children, with the umbilical vein being the preferred site in neonates younger than 10 days of age. The right internal jugular vein is preferred to the left as the catheter is more likely to pass directly from the innominate vein into the superior vena cava, and there is a lower risk of pneumothorax or damage to the thoracic duct.[38] If the left internal jugular vein must be accessed, anesthesia providers must remember that the length of the catheter will be longer than if the right side were to be accessed. Cannulation of the subclavian vein in children has a lower complication rate than cannulation of the internal jugular vein. The femoral vein is not suitable for long-term access in a mobile patient and should not be cannulated in patients who have suspected disruption of the inferior vena cava. For more information regarding the use of ultrasound for vascular access, please refer to Chapter 136, "Ultrasound-Guided Vascular Access."

Central Venous Pressure Monitoring

Central venous pressure (CVP) is a measure of pressure in the vena cava via a CVC. To accurately measure the CVP, the distal tip of a CVC should be inserted in the superior vena cava just proximal to the right atrium. The pressure measured at this location should be equal to that in the right atrium, assuming there is no obstruction to the vena cava. The pressure within the right atrium varies throughout the cardiac cycle, as well as with respiration. CVP is most accurately measured with the patient lying flat, at the end of diastole, and at the end of expiration with the transducer placed at the level of the fourth intercostal space in the midaxillary line, which correlates to the location of the right atrium (**Figure 4.9**). Absolute values for CVP are not commonly used in clinical practice, as monitoring the trend in values generated is often of greater significance.[37]

Central venous lines are essential in anesthesia for major surgical procedures, and the use of CVP targets in pediatric cardiac surgery is still commonplace. That said, various other methods and devices continue to be developed for volume assessment.[39] This is largely due to the poor relationship between CVP and blood volume, as well as the inability of CVP monitoring to predict the hemodynamic response to a fluid challenge.

Cardiac Output Monitoring

Cardiac output (CO) is the product of cardiac SV and heart rate (HR) and can be monitored via a pulmonary artery (PA) catheter inserted through a CVC (**Figure 4.10**). The use of a PA catheter is warranted when there is a need for simultaneous monitoring of PA pressure, cardiac filling, CO, and mixed venous oxygen saturation. Additional indications include severe circulatory shock, right ventricular failure, acute respiratory failure due to pulmonary edema requiring complex fluid management evaluation, diagnosis of pulmonary hypertension, cardiac tamponade or constrictive pericarditis, or assessment of right-sided valvular disease, congenital heart disease, and cardiac shunts, when surgical repair is planned.[40,41]

Modern thermodilution techniques involves placement of a specialized catheter within the PA, the most common example being the Swan–Ganz catheter. PA catheters have a temperature probe at the distal end, as well as a proximal port, which lies in the right atrium. Following injection of a cold solution through the proximal port into the right atrium, temperature changes relative to the dilution within the blood are detected by the temperature probe at the distal end of the catheter allowing accurate measurement of CO.

As the indications for the use of PA catheters in child are few, their use in pediatrics remains limited. In addition, there is a lack of evidence in improving mortality, and the placement of PA catheters can be technically challenging in small children, especially those in a state of low CO. Moreover, the associated risks such as bleeding, cardiac perforation, knotting, inadvertent persistent wedge positioning, thromboembolism, and infection often outweigh the potential benefit.

An alternate means of monitoring continuous hemodynamic status in pediatrics is the use of a pulse index continuous CO (PiCCO) catheter, which combines the tenets of transpulmonary thermodilution and pulse contour analysis (**Table 4.3**). Essentially, a PiCCO catheter is arterial line with a thermistor on the distal end that is able to provide complete hemodynamic monitoring by integrating a wide array of both static

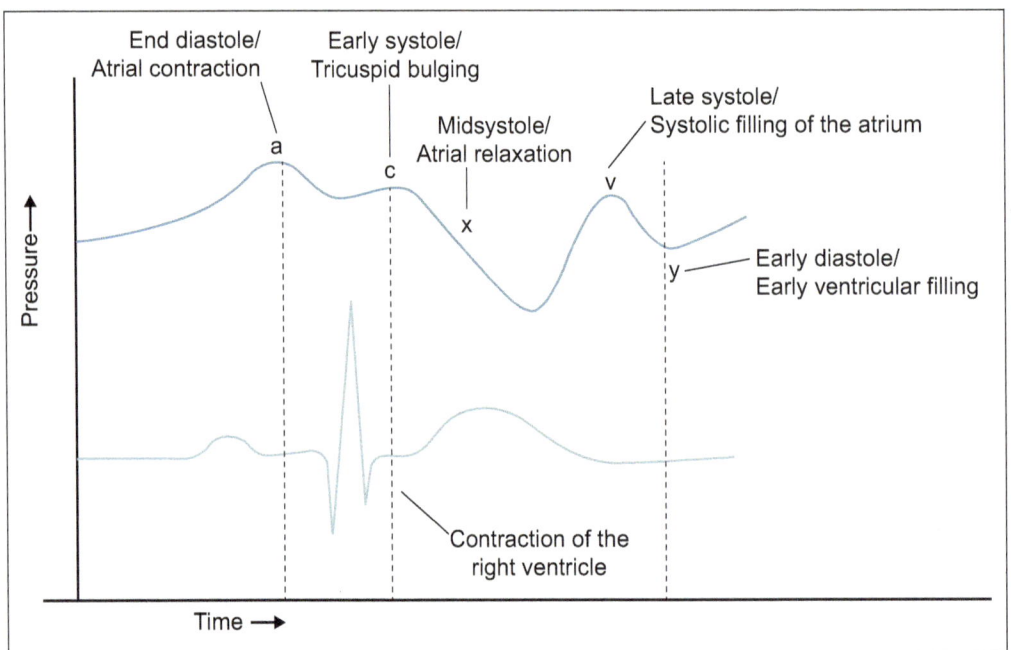

Figure 4.9: Central venous pressure waveform and correlation to the cardiac cycle. *a* wave, end diastole/atrial contraction; *c* wave, early systole/tricuspid bulging; *x* descent, mid-systole/atrial relaxation; *v* wave, late systole/systolic filling of the atrium; *y* descent, early diastole/early ventricular filling.

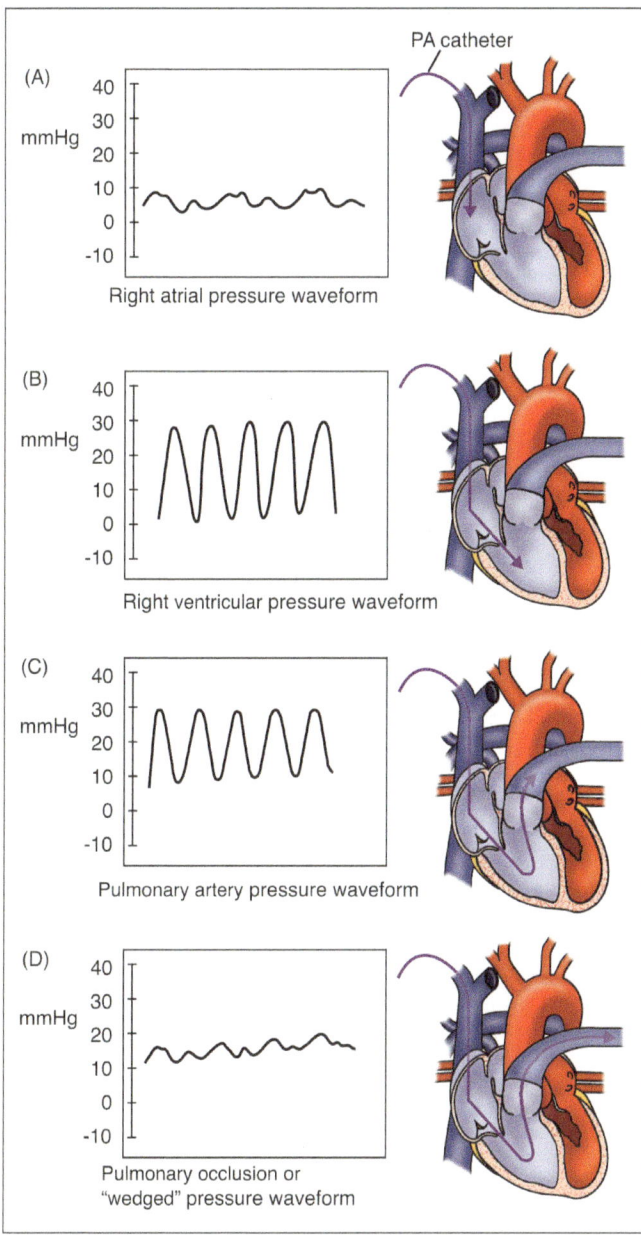

Figure 4.10: Pulmonary artery catheter waveform.

and dynamic data. The use of a PiCCO catheter can be especially useful in presence of complex mixed forms of shock (e.g., septic, cardiogenic), although their performance substantially degrades at extremes of physiology.[42] Furthermore, the lower weight limit of application is generally considered to be 3.5 kg.

Mixed Venous Oxygenation Monitoring

Although CO is one of the main determinants of oxygen delivery, analysis of mixed venous oxygen saturation better allows anesthesia providers to interpret whole-body tissue oxygenation.[1,42-44] Mixed venous oxygen saturation (SvO2) is the percentage of oxygen bound to hemoglobin in blood returning to the right side of the heart. A low mixed venous saturation correlates with high oxygen extraction, indicating there is more demand for oxygen than there is supply.[42] Ideally, blood samples for SvO2 analysis are obtained from the tip of the PA catheter to all the venous blood returning from the head and arms (via superior vena cava), the gut and lower extremities (via the inferior vena cava) and the coronary veins (via the coronary sinus).

Should there not be a PA catheter in place, central venous oxygen saturation (ScvO2) can be used as a surrogate and interpreted in the same manner as a SvO2 sample. Blood for ScvO2 analysis are typically obtained from a CVC placed in the internal jugular or subclavian vein. While this is only reflective of blood returning from the head and the upper extremities, the interpretation is considered to be similar to that of a SvO2 sample.

Potential Complications Related to Central Venous Catheters

The insertion site does not seem to influence the infection rate in infants and children; however, infectious complications are frequent and are related to the duration of indwelling time, younger patient age, the use of extensive guidewire exchange during repositioning or replacement of the central line, and techniques or handling/maintenance of the indwelling catheter. Adherence to strict protocols have reduced the incidence of infections, and antibiotic prophylaxis is not recommended but is often practiced. In addition, subcutaneous tunneling for long-term use of CVCs is recommended.[45] In addition to the complications from placement of a CVC, the complications related to the use of a PA catheter include pulmonary infarction, PA rupture, catheter knotting, and endocardial damage (Table 4.4).[40]

TRANSESOPHAGEAL ECHOCARDIOGRAPHY

With the advent of miniaturized probes, transesophageal echocardiography (TEE) is now possible with pediatric patients. When combined with clinical examination and additional monitoring techniques, echocardiography provides rapid and reliable diagnostic assessment of cardiac anatomy allowing for real-time estimates of intracardiac pressures, pressure gradients across valves or defects, direction of blood flow, and fluid responsiveness.[46] TEE therefore not only has a role in the assessment of cardiac structures, but it can also provide valuable feedback regarding surgical repairs and catheter-based interventions. Perioperative echocardiography also offers accurate assessment of volume status, cardiac function, and presence of structural heart disease. Clinically, echocardiography is superior to catheter-based pressure measurements as the cardiac chamber volume can be directly calculated rather than inferred from a pressure–volume curve. While not commonly used in the perioperative environment, TEE can prove to be a valuable addition to standard monitors when caring for a critically ill child.[47] Echocardiography can also be employed in a variety of settings, including the preassessment clinic, ICU, operating room, and catheterization laboratory.

Certain structures such as the major aorto-pulmonary collateral vessels, distal pulmonary arteries and some parts of the aortic arch are difficult to see with the TEE, and a transthoracic echocardiogram may provide better visualization of such structures. In some instances, some intracardiac shunts may be difficult to identify during a TEE, and a direct pressure measurement or blood gas analysis may need to be employed.[47] Also, anything preventing the acoustic signal reflection, such as air, bone, bandages, or other foreign bodies, will decrease the quality of the images.[46]

An absolute contraindication to placing a TEE probe is significant esophageal pathology, such as previous esophageal surgery for tracheoesophageal fistula. The incidence

Table 4.3 Invasive and Noninvasive Cardiac Output Monitoring Devices

Device Name	Technology Used	Advantage	Disadvantage
Minimally Invasive			
PiCCO	Pulse contour analysis	Continuous CO monitoring, external calibration for precision, well validated	Central access required
LiDCO	Pulse contour analysis	Continuous CO monitoring, external calibration for precision, well validated, no central access	Lithium injection required, contraindicated in pregnancies, can interfere with chronic lithium therapy or NMBA
Flo Trac/Vigileo	Pulse contour analysis	Continuous CO monitoring, easy to use, no calibration required	Least accurate of the three, inconsistent tracking, prone to drift over time
Noninvasive			
ClearSight	Pulse contour analysis	Finger cuff used without need for intra-arterial access	Not well validated
Thoracic electrical bioimpedance	Bioimpedance	Continuous CO monitoring, easy to place	Not well validated, changes in thoracic fluid volume can impede with results
Transthoracic echocardiography	Ultrasound, Doppler	Highly accurate, well-validated, easy to establish diagnosis in experienced hands	Operator dependent, requires training, only intermittent measurement

CO, cardiac output; LiDCO, lithium dilution cardiac output; NMBA, neuromuscular blocking agent; PiCCO, pulse index continuous cardiac output.

Table 4.4 Central Venous Catheter Complications

On Insertion	Postinsertion
Air embolism	Accidental dislodgement
Arrhythmias	Catheter-associated blood stream infections
Arterial puncture	Catheter malfunction
Brachial plexus injury	Catheter migration/displacement
Cardiac tamponade	Device occlusion
Failure	Extravascular infusion
Guidewire knotting/fracturing	Infection at exit site
Hematoma at insertion site	Line fracture ± embolization
Hemorrhage	Right atrial perforation ± cardiac tamponade
Hemothorax	Subcutaneous extravasation
Phrenic nerve injury	Venous perforation
Pneumothorax	Venous stenosis
Thoracic duct trauma ± chylothorax	Venous thrombosis
Vascular damage (e.g., perforation/dissection)	
Tricuspid valve damage	

Table 4.5 Contraindications to Transesophageal Echocardiography

Absolute	Relative
Perforated viscus	History of radiation to neck/mediastinum
Esophageal stricture	History of GI surgery
Esophageal tumor	Recent upper GI bleed
Esophageal perforation, laceration	Barrett's esophagus
Esophageal diverticulum	History of dysphagia
Active upper GI bleed	Restriction of neck mobility
Recent pharyngeal, esophageal, or gastric surgery	Symptomatic hiatal hernia
	Facial or airway trauma
	Esophageal varices
	Coagulopathy, thrombocytopenia
	Active esophagitis
	Active peptic ulcer disease

GI, gastrointestinal.

Source: From Hahn et al, 2013, American Society of Echocardiography and the Society of Cardiovascular Anesthesiologists, O'Rourke MC, Goldstein S, & Mendenhall BR. Transesophageal Echocardiogram. In *StatPearls*. StatPearls Publishing; 2020. https://pubmed.ncbi.nlm.nih.gov/28723055.

Table 4.6	Common EEG Waveforms		
Wave Form	Frequency	Amplitude	Conditions Associated With Wave
Beta	13–30 Hz	30 µV	Awake patient thinking
Alpha	8–13 Hz	30–50 µV	Relaxed patient
Theta	4–7 Hz	50–100 µV	Light sleep
Delta	.5–5 Hz	100–200 µV	Deep sleep and coma

of TEE-related complications is low but may include dislodgement or movement of the endotracheal tube, issues with ventilation, traumatic damage to teeth, tongue, oral mucosa, pharynx, upper gastrointestinal tract, compression of vascular structures, and traumatic or thermal damage to esophagus or stomach during probe insertion or removal (Table 4.5).[47]

NEAR-INFRARED SPECTROSCOPY

Near-infrared spectroscopy (NIRS) is a noninvasive technique to continuously monitor regional tissue oxygenation and assess tissue health. While not yet standard monitoring equipment for noncardiac pediatric patients requiring general anesthesia, cerebral NIRS monitoring has become a standard monitoring tool in many pediatric cardiac neonatal intensive care units.[1]

NIRS works by measuring the transmission of near-IR light and its differential absorption by chromophores (usually oxyhemoglobin and deoxyhemoglobin) across brain tissues. Approximately 75% of the information gathered via NIRS monitoring is from venous blood flow, with the remaining data gathered from by measuring the transmission of near-IR light and its differential absorption across arterial blood flow.[42] The normal range of regional cerebral oxygen saturation is between 55% and 75%, with a significant drop in values suggesting cerebral ischemia.

When used as a trend monitor to evaluate the balance between tissue oxygen delivery and consumption, NIRS can aid in early identification of abnormalities in hemodynamics and cerebral perfusion. It can also be used to assess the impact of interventions intended to increase oxygen delivery such as augmenting CO or transfusing blood or to assess the efficacy of interventions intended to decrease oxygen extraction, such as reducing the work of breathing or treating fever or infection.[48] The information garnered is independent of blood flow as NIRS interrogates arterial, venous, and capillary blood in totality to generate a weighted value.[48] NIRS should not be confused with pulse oximetry as the technology is different.[1]

ELECTROENCEPHALOGRAPHY

Electroencephalography (EEG) is a composite of postsynaptic cortical neuronal potentials, recorded as a mixture of oscillations measured in both amplitude and frequency. EEG signals are detected at the skin surface and can be used as surrogate indicators of level of consciousness. EEG signals can be impacted by a number of factors. Not only can detection of the signals be sensitive to interference, but age-related alterations are also expected with infants younger than 6 months of age having a globally lower amplitude on an EEG.[51]

Dose-dependent changes in EEG amplitude occur with general anesthesia, with some anesthetic drugs having unique effects on EEG waveforms (Table 4.6). At subanesthetic doses hypnotics induce rapid oscillations, primarily of beta waves. Following the administration of anesthetic doses of hypnotics, the amplitude of alpha and beta waves decreases as that of slower theta and delta waves increase. During very deep states of anesthesia, the EEG waveform changes into a burst and suppression pattern, finally becoming flat.[52] Propofol and volatile anesthetics produce similar effects generating low-frequency, large amplitude oscillations. Ketamine and nitrous oxide, however, cause high-frequency, low-amplitude oscillations.[51] Deep levels of sevoflurane-induced anesthesia may produce complex epileptiform EEG activity.[52]

A variety of EEG-derived indices have been developed to assist providers, such as the bispectral index (BIS) manufactured by Covidien, Entropy manufactured by GE, and Narcotrend manufactured by Schiller monitors. All use individual algorithms to produce scores and require at least 15 seconds of monitoring to process a score. The BIS (Covidien, USA) monitor has been on the market the longest of the three devices, and its use has been studied in children. The BIS monitor measures a single frontal EEG signal but may also pick up electromyographic signals from the supraorbital muscles. The BIS index is calculated from input from three sources: the spectral analysis, the bispectral analysis, and the temporal analysis. The XP version of the BIS monitor subtracts the electromyograph contribution.[52] In children younger than 1 year of age, the unprocessed EEG may need to be monitored if there is concern as the BIS algorithm may not be appropriate for this age group.[51]

The Entropy (GE, UK) monitor is based on an analysis of the frontal EEG signal using a public algorithm that employs two frequency intervals to calculate a score: the state entropy calculated on the frequency interval of 0 to 32 Hz and the response entropy calculated on the interval of 0 to 47 Hz. Entropy monitors also calculate a percentage of time with a nearly flat EEG during deep anesthesia. Values produced by the Entropy monitor follow a similar trend to the BIS under anesthesia.[52]

The Narcotrend (Monitor Technik, Germany) monitor is the only EEG monitor that employs a pediatric-specific algorithm. This monitor uses a frontal electrode to differentiate the EEG into six lettered stages (A–F), each of which corresponds to various states of consciousness ranging from awake to burst suppression. The Narcotrend index is derived from these stages, generating a score of 100 (awake) to 0 (burst suppression).[53] Of note, the Narcotrend monitor has been found to correlate accurately with the MAC of Sevoflurane for infants older than 4 months of age.[53]

EQUIPMENT AND MONITORING DURING TRANSPORT

Hypoxemia can quickly occur while transporting a child from the operating room to the PACU and can be a life-threatening adverse event. Quite often a restless child emerging from anesthesia is not cooperative with a close-fitting face mask leading to the use of blow-by oxygen during transport. Anesthesia providers must remember that the face mask must be less the 5 cm from the face with a flow rate greater than 10 L/min to deliver an fraction of inspired oxygen (FiO2) concentration greater than 50%.[54] As such, the Joint Commission has recommended that pulse oximetry should be routinely used during transport of patient from the operating room to the PACU.[55]

Transport of extremely low-birth-weight or premature neonates should be done in an isolette to allow for active warming and temperature monitoring. A standardized bundle of interventions when transporting to and from the neonatal intensive care unit to the operating room has proved to increase the average postoperative temperature from 36.4°C to 36.8°C.[56] Anesthesia providers should consider the use of an active warming device, such as a gel-filled, thermostable, disposable mattress that can provide up to 2 hours of warming, when cold stress is a concern and the child is too large for use of an isolette.[57]

RESOURCES

- **Anesthesia Machine**
  - https://healthprofessions.udmercy.edu/academics/na/agm/01.htm
- **Capnography**
  - https://www.capnography.com/speciality-applications/pediatrics?id=135
- **Monitoring Standards**
  - https://www.aana.com/practice/practice-manual
  - https://www.asahq.org/standards-and-guidelines/standards-for-basic-anesthetic-monitoring
- **Pediatric Anesthesia Safety Resources**
  - http://wakeupsafe.org
  - https://smarttots.org

KEY TAKEAWAYS

- The basic monitoring skills of palpation and auscultation should always be used. Do not make the mistake of relying too heavily on monitoring equipment as our eyes, ears, and hands are the most valuable monitoring tools.
- As guardians of the airway, anesthesia providers should monitor airway patency by using auscultation, observation, and capnography when available. Inadequate ventilation is the most common cause of morbidity and mortality in pediatric anesthesia.
- The monitoring plan will vary depending on the procedure and the patient's anesthetic risk. Anesthesia monitoring primarily focuses on the cardiovascular and pulmonary systems to enable early detection of anesthetic complications; therefore, monitoring multiple variables enables early detection of anesthetic complications.
- Vigilant perioperative monitoring is crucial in assessing the adequate depth of anesthesia and minimize any insult to normal homeostasis that can be caused by anesthetic drugs directly, from underlying disease states, and by direct surgical manipulation.

KEY REFERENCES

Complete references and bibliography for this chapter are online and available at https://connect.springerpub.com/content/book/978-0-8261-3875-0/part/part02/toc-part/ch004.

29. Kim P, Taghon T, Fetzer M, Tobias JD. Perioperative hypothermia in the pediatric population: a quality improvement project. *Am J Med Qual.* 2013;28(5):400–406. doi:10.1177/1062860612473350
32. Theodore A, Manaker S, Finlay G. *Arterial blood gases.* 2020. https://www.uptodate.com/contents/arterial-blood-gases
42. Skowno JJ. Hemodynamic monitoring in children with heart disease: overview of newer technologies. *Paediatr Anaesth.* 2019;29(5):467–474. doi:10.1111/pan.13590
48. Deng Y, Markan S, Navarro JC, Navarro JC. Advances in anesthesia monitoring. *Oral Maxillofac Surg Clin North Am.* 2019;31(4):611–619. doi:10.1016/j.coms.2019.07.005
52. Constant I, Sabourdin N. The EEG signal: a window on the cortical brain activity. *Paediatr Anaesth.* 2012;22(6):539–552. doi:10.1111/j.1460-9592.2012.03883.x

CHAPTER 5

Induction of Anesthesia

Melanie Neal and Carrilee Powell

> **LEARNING OBJECTIVES**
>
> - Review indications and contraindications for inhalation and IV inductions.
> - Describe inhalation induction techniques.
> - Identify various IV induction techniques that can be employed with children.
> - Discuss potential complications that can occur during induction of anesthesia.

INTRODUCTION

Induction of general anesthesia in infants and children can be a challenging and precarious time that mandates anesthesia providers remain ever vigilant and ready to adapt to the changing patient state. In addition to the presenting comorbidities, there are age-specific and developmental influences that may impact airway management, hemodynamic stability, and the pharmacokinetics and pharmacodynamics of various induction agents. While many factors must be considered when determining whether an inhalation or IV induction technique will be used, both inhalation and IV induction techniques have a well-established role when caring for the pediatric patient. Ultimately, anesthesia providers are charged with determining the most appropriate technique on a patient-specific basis and should defer to the technique that is safest for the patient and best minimizes stress, anxiety, and trauma.

PATIENT PREPARATION PRIOR TO INDUCTION

As with any anesthetic, preparation is key as anesthesia providers must be ready to navigate untoward events at a moment's notice. This includes, but is not limited to, warming the operating room, performing an anesthesia machine checkout, having suction on and ready, ensuring appropriate monitors and airway supplies are readily available, and having induction agents and emergency drawn up and within reach. Having supplies and medications prepared can help minimize distractions when the child is being induced. In addition, monitors should be placed on the patient prior to the induction of anesthesia if possible. Other considerations include ensuring the patient is appropriately fasted when possible and assessing the need for a preoperative anxiolytic.

Preoperative anxiety is common among pediatric patients. Fortunately, there is an ever-evolving host of tools and strategies to anesthesia providers can employ to temper a child's anxiety. Child life therapists play an important role in preparing children for anesthesia as they are specifically trained to recognize and allay anxiety and fear in an age-specific fashion. They are well versed at incorporating age-appropriate distraction techniques, such as decorating the anesthesia mask, encouraging role play as an astronaut or scuba diver to improve mask acceptance, and pretending to blow out birthday candles, all of which can assist in easing the child's anxiety.

Gamification, or the use of game design elements in non-game contexts, has become more commonly employed as a distraction technique with the advent of apps and technology that incorporate the anesthesia circuit in an immersive game during an inhalation induction.[1] Tablets or cellular phones can also be used as a distraction tool (Figure 5.1). Allowing a child to view a movie or play a game during the induction process has been shown to increase compliance and decrease anxiety during induction of general anesthesia.[1] Virtual reality has also been harnessed to facilitate mask inductions, therapeutic procedures, and even awake fiberoptic intubations.

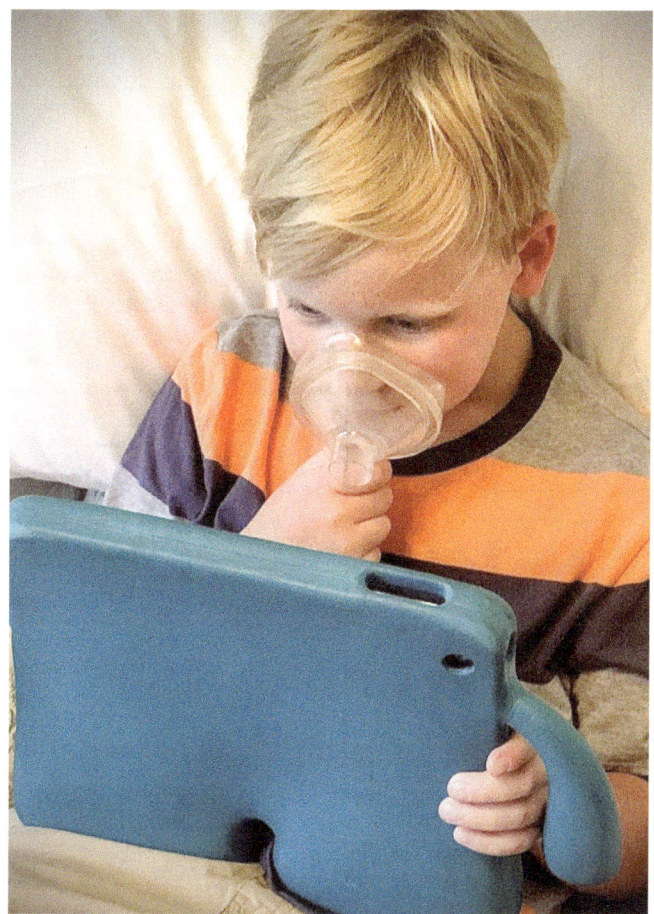

Figure 5.1: Distraction during inhalation induction.

While parental presence during inhalation induction remains controversial, parental presence has been reported to lessen a child's anxiety during induction of anesthesia.[2] If parental presence is allowed and indicated, it is important to prepare a safe and comfortable space for the parents to participate. Anesthesia providers should remember that watching their child being induced can also be stressful for the parents, making it important a chair is available for them to sit if needed. Having a discussion with the parent about what they might see during the induction process prior to the start of induction can help prepare them for the changes they witness as their child transitions through the stages of anesthesia. A thorough explanation of excitation behavior, such as eye rolling, jerky movements, or exaggerated breathing noises, better prepares the parent so they can focus their efforts on reassuring and comforting their child.

INHALATION INDUCTION

The most common technique for inducing anesthesia in infants and children is an inhalation induction. With this technique, a mask is placed on the child's face covering their nose and mouth, allowing the child to inhale a titratable mixture of oxygen, nitrous oxide, and a volatile anesthetic agent. Selecting a mask for the infant or child that fits appropriately is important, as the mask should cover both the nose and mouth to minimize a leak during inhalation induction to expedite the process and minimize exposure of others in the room to volatile anesthetic agents (**Figure 5.2**). Anesthesia providers can place a flavor in the mask to help distract from the strong smell of the volatile agent (lip balm on the mask or flavor sprays are often used).

Most commonly, sevoflurane is the volatile agent of choice for inhalation inductions. Sevoflurane is a potent bronchodilator that is not irritating to the airway and is considered to be far less pungent than other volatile agents. Furthermore, the pharmacokinetics of sevoflurane allow for both a rapid induction and recovery.[3] Desflurane is used for maintenance of anesthesia but is not recommended for induction as it is very pungent and can be irritating to the airway, resulting in coughing, increased secretions, and potentially laryngospasm.

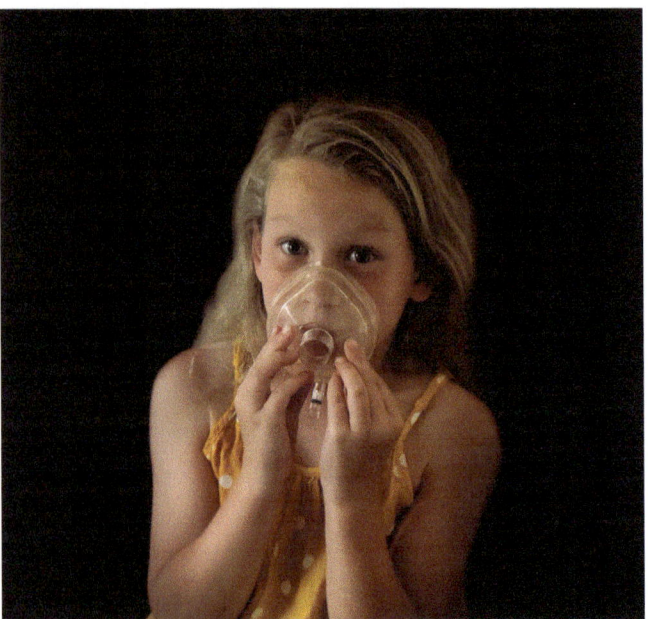

Figure 5.2: Proper mask fitment.

There are several specific inhalation induction techniques that can be employed based on the child's developmental age, level of sedation, and ability to cooperate.

STEAL INDUCTION

If a child is already asleep upon arrival to the induction room or operating room, a steal induction can be performed. In this scenario, the anesthesia provider attempts to keep the child asleep while slowly titrating in a mixture of oxygen, nitrous oxide, and a volatile anesthetic agent to induce anesthesia. Holding the mask near the sleeping child's face with a mixture of oxygen and nitrous oxide for a few minutes first may help further sedate the child, allowing sevoflurane to be introduced and increased incrementally up to 8%. As the child becomes more sedated, the mask can be moved closer to their face and placed on their face without waking them. This technique causes the least amount of trauma by avoiding the child's awareness of separation and avoiding exposure to the strange surroundings.

INHALATION INDUCTION WITH PARENTAL PRESENCE

While a steal induction is ideal, most children do not present to the operating room already asleep. As such, anesthesia providers should employ age-appropriate strategies to foster success. For toddlers, it may be helpful for the patient to sit on a parent's lap, whereas it is more practical to have older children sit on the bed or a stretcher. Also, consider incorporating a security item such as a stuffed animal or a blanket in the induction process. If the child is cooperative, the mask can be placed on the child's face with a mixture of oxygen and nitrous oxide initially, followed by incremental increases of sevoflurane with the pace of induction dictated by the child. In the event that the child is uncooperative, it may be necessary to employ additional strategies, such as allowing the patient to watch a favorite movie or play a game on an electronic device or having a parent hold the patient. If distraction does not work and the child becomes combative, it may also be necessary to gently hold the child's hands and/or feet to prevent them from inadvertently hurting themselves. It is especially important to supporting the child's head and neck should they become combative or uncooperative. In order to keep the mask on the child's face, anesthesia providers may have to hold the mask with one hand and the back of the child's head with the other to ensure the mask stays on their face throughout despite movement.

When patients are extremely fearful of separation from their parents or are extremely fearful of the mask, an anxiolytic can be administered preoperatively if not contraindicated. Anxiety and fear are not always identified or present in the preoperative phase, however. If the patient presents without receiving an anxiolytic and becomes increasingly anxious, it can be extremely difficult to get the mask close to the child's face for an inhalation induction. An alternate approach is to use the circuit without the mask initially, holding the end of the circuit close to the child's face with a cupped hand. This strategy may take longer but may allow the anesthesia provider to sedate the patient enough with a mixture of oxygen and nitrous oxide before applying the mask. It may also be feasible for the anesthesia provider to incorporate gamification techniques, although some creativity may be required to encourage the child to be cooperative.

SINGLE-BREATH INDUCTION

Single-breath inhalation induction, also known as vital capacity induction, is an appropriate technique to use with a cooperative child. With a single-breath induction, the anesthesia circuit is primed with 8% sevoflurane and a high gas flow rate of 100% O_2 by occluding the circuit for at least 30 seconds.[4] Children are asked to completely exhale their residual volume several times in a row, at which point the mask is placed securely on their face as the children take a deep breath in and hold it. After holding their breath for as long as they can, normal breaths can be taken until the children are asleep. Typically, the older the children, the more apt they are to have success with this technique. The biggest advantage to this technique is the rapid onset of anesthesia induction.[5]

STAGES OF ANESTHESIA

Originally developed in 1937, Guedel's classifications of the stages of anesthesia continue to be referenced despite the advent of new anesthetic agents and induction techniques.[4] Stage I is initiated after a premedication is administered in the preoperative setting or when nitrous oxide is used during induction. At this stage, the child's heart rate and breathing are regular and slow, and they are calm. Once unconscious, Stage II begins. Stage II provides the anesthesia provider with the most challenges. Irregular breathing, tachycardia, and involuntary movements are hallmarks of this stage. Airway reflexes are intact and sensitive to manipulation, making the risk of laryngospasm high.

Allowing the patient to enter Stage III before stimulating procedures take place, such as patient repositioning, IV catheter placement, or placement of noninvasive monitors, is recommended. Once children enter Stage III, their heart rate begins to decrease; rapid eye movements cease; and their respiratory pattern becomes more regular. Proceeding with stimulating activities during this stage is generally tolerated.[4]

INTRAVENOUS INDUCTION OF ANESTHESIA

IV induction is becoming more common in pediatric anesthesia (Table 5.1). While historically reserved for the older child who will tolerate IV catheter placement while awake, IV inductions are increasingly being performed in infants and younger children. Although the preferred technique of induction for young children is an inhalation induction, not all children can participate in an inhalation induction.

While contraindications to inhalation induction are rare, they do exist and often are secondary to genetic syndromes or diseases, such as malignant hyperthermia. It has been reported that IV induction of anesthesia is associated with a lower risk of adverse respiratory events, such as coughing and breath holding, when compared to inhalation induction techniques.[6] Ultrasound guidance and the use of child life therapists have greatly helped with placement of IV catheters in awake infants and children. An alternative to awake IV catheter placement is placing an IV catheter while the child is inhaling a mixture of oxygen and nitrous oxide in the operating room. Administering a 50% to 70% mix of oxygen and nitrous oxide through a face mask often provides adequate sedation to facilitate placement of an IV catheter. For additional information regarding specific IV induction agents, please refer to Chapter 2, "Pharmacological Considerations for the Pediatric Patient."

INTRAVENOUS INDUCTION AGENTS

Propofol

Propofol is the most common drug used for IV induction. It has several properties that make its use more advantageous than other anesthetic agents, including a rapid onset of amnesia, rapid elimination, and a low association with emergence delirium and respiratory complications. Following administration, a decreased level of consciousness is obtained by acting on the central inhibitory neurotransmitter gaba-aminobutyric acid. There is plethora of literature describing the use of propofol use in children. Although the Food and Drug Administration has approved its use for children older than 3 years of age, it is widely used in infants and children younger than 3 years of age.[7]

Propofol dosing requirements to induce anesthesia are generally higher in healthy children when compared to their adult counterparts. It is common for children to require 2 to 5 mg/kg to induce anesthesia due to their rapid metabolism, smaller central compartment, and larger volume of distribution. However, the dose required can be dramatically decreased if a benzodiazepine or opioid is administered concurrently. A major disadvantage to propofol is pain at the injection site, particularly if the IV catheter is in a small vein. A variety of techniques can be used in an attempt to lessen the pain associated with injection, such as pretreatment with lidocaine or ondansetron, or administration at a slower rate.[7]

Ketamine

Ketamine is a commonly used drug for induction of anesthesia in pediatric patients with congenital heart disease and cardiovascular compromise, as this patient population generally does not tolerate the vasodilatory effects associated with propofol. An advantage of ketamine is that it produces analgesia without marked respiratory depression, as well as a dissociative effect by acting as an antagonist on the N-methyl-D-aspartate and glutamate receptors. The loss of consciousness is rapidly obtained with an induction dose of 1 to 2 mg/kg IV and generally lasts for 10 minutes.[6] Adverse effects of ketamine administration are potential increases in oral secretions, postoperative nausea and vomiting, and hallucinogenic effects following administration.

Etomidate

Etomidate is indicated for induction of anesthesia for critically ill children presenting with hypovolemia, congenital heart disease, or traumatic brain injury. Etomidate better maintains hemodynamic stability than propofol; however, its use is associated with potential adrenal suppression for up to 24 hours following a single dose and pain on injection. Furthermore, the current recommendation is that is not be administered to patients with ongoing sepsis.[8] The recommended dosage is .2 to .3 mg/kg, although this can be adjusted based on the patient's myocardial instability.

RAPID-SEQUENCE INDUCTION

Patients presenting for emergency surgery often require a rapid-sequence induction (RSI) be performed due to having

Table 5.1	Common Intravenous Induction Agents
Drug	Dose
Propofol	2–5 mg/kg
Ketamine	1–2 mg/kg
Etomidate	.2–.3 mg/kg
Succinylcholine	2 mg/kg
Rocuronium	.6–1.2 mg/kg

a full stomach or comorbidities that could result in aspiration during the induction of anesthesia. Unlike RSI for adults, where having emergency medications and intubation equipment available, suction readily available, using short-acting neuromuscular blocking medications, and performing preoxygenation with cricoid pressure for intubation, it can be far more challenging to adhere to standard RSI algorithms as many of the expectations are not practical for children.

A crying infant or uncooperative child can hinder preoxygenation attempts and actually increase oxygen consumption.[9] Furthermore, short periods of apnea are not well tolerated by infants and children, with hypoxemia rapidly occurring due to the child's increased metabolic rate. Infants especially do not tolerate periods of apnea due to their immature respiratory system and decreased functional residual capacity. Securing IV access can also be difficult to obtain in the uncooperative, awake child.

It has been offered that the technique for applying of cricoid in children differs from that for their adult counterparts. In the young child, the cricoid cartilage is smaller and located more cephalad, making it difficult to identify. In children younger than 8 years of age, the esophagus may lie lateral to the cricoid cartilage.[9] The typical 30 N of pressure required to compress the esophagus during RSI for adults is often too much pressure when used for a small child as it can distort the airway. Therefore, the force applied to the cricoid cartilage should be decreased to 7.7 N, which is adequate to prevent pulmonary aspiration of gastric contents.[9]

As with adults, classic and modified RSI techniques may be employed when caring for children. Classic RSI includes preoxygenation, no ventilation, and cricoid pressure followed by intubation using a rapid-acting neuromuscular blocking agent. The preferred neuromuscular blocking agents to facilitate endotracheal intubation are succinylcholine (2 mg/kg) or rocuronium (1.2 mg/kg).[10] The advent of sugammadex for immediate reversal of rocuronium has greatly assisted in the inability to ventilate or intubate patient scenarios. The modified RSI technique adds gentle face mask ventilation using decreased ventilatory pressures to avoid gastric insufflation along with cricoid pressure.

Advances in technology have greatly decreased complications related to RSI in children. The addition of an ultrasound gastric scan preoperatively to assess for gastric contents is generally well tolerated and reliable. Gastric contents are visualized in the antrum of the stomach with the use of an ultrasound. These findings can assist the anesthesia provider in determining the best route for induction in addition to the patient's medical history and reported last time of oral intake.[10]

Pyloric Stenosis

Infants with pyloric stenosis present with projectile vomiting, dehydration, and electrolyte abnormalities and are at an increased risk of aspiration of gastric contents due to a hypertrophy of the pylorus muscle layers. In an effort to prevent aspiration during induction, a vented suction catheter is placed in the awake infant in the supine position. The infant is then turned to the left lateral and right lateral positions to remove gastric contents prior to induction of anesthesia.[11] These infants may benefit from an ultrasound scan to assess effectiveness of removal of gastric contents with a suction catheter prior to induction of anesthesia. For more information regarding the anesthetic management of pyloric stenosis, please refer to Chapter 127, "Neonatal Emergencies."

Posttonsillectomy Bleeding

Managing posttonsillectomy bleeding is one of the most common pediatric surgeries performed. When a child presents to the operating room with posttonsillectomy bleeding, the anesthesia provider must be prepared as this is considered an emergency with potential serious complications. The volume of blood loss can be difficult to assess due to the unknown amount of swallowed blood. This coupled with a scared and anxious child makes assessment difficult. IV access should be established prior to induction and anesthesia providers should have the difficult airway cart in the room or nearby. It is recommended to have a smaller endotracheal tube than used prior readily available given the likelihood of airway edema. In addition, two suction canisters with Yankauer attachments should be readily available. RSI is most commonly performed due to increased risk of aspiration. The most common adverse events associated with posttonsillectomy bleeding are hypoxemia, bradycardia with induction, hypotension, and difficult intubation.[12]

COMPLICATIONS DURING INDUCTION

Children, especially infants, more commonly experience adverse events during the induction of anesthesia compared to adults.[13] Commonly reported complications during induction include laryngospasm, airway obstruction, hypoxemia, and bradycardia. Differences in infant airway anatomy and physiology may contribute to the occurrence of adverse events during the induction of anesthesia.

LARYNGOSPASM

Laryngospasm occurs when there is partial or complete glottis closure resulting in blockage of airway movement to the trachea and lungs. A lack of recognition or delay in treatment of a laryngospasm can be a life-threatening complication in pediatric patients, potentially resulting in hypoxemia, pulmonary edema, bradycardia, cardiac arrhythmias, and potential death. Closure of the vocal cords occurs with repetitive simulation of either the internal branch of the superior laryngeal nerve or the intrinsic and extrinsic muscles of the larynx. During a complete laryngospasm, the vocal cords will be tightly sealed closed, making ventilation impossible. During a partial laryngospasm, the vocal cords will be adducted, but a small opening will remain, allowing a minimal amount of air movement for ventilation. Depending on the degree of obstruction, the patient may exhibit paradoxical chest movement, intercostal retractions, diminished or absent breath sounds, and hypoxemia. A high-pitched stridor or "crowing" may be heard during a partial laryngospasm.[14,15]

The overall incidence of pediatric laryngospasm is reported to be about 1.7%. Laryngospasm is more common in the pediatric population than the adult population, occurring two times more frequently in older children and three times more frequently in younger children compared to adults. Preexisting risk factors for pediatric laryngospasm include recent upper respiratory tract infection (4–6 weeks after resolution of an upper respiratory tract infection), exposure to cigarette smoke, obese children with sleep-disordered breathing, and younger age. Surgical risk factors for laryngospasm mainly involve the type of procedure the child is undergoing including procedures of the ear, nose, and throat; esophageal endoscopy; plastic surgery; appendectomy; and urological surgery. Anesthetia-related risk factors include an inadequate depth of anesthesia, secretions or blood stimulating the vocal cords, instrumentation of the airway by a nasal or oral airway, laryngoscope, laryngeal mask airway or suction catheter. An inadequate depth of anesthesia most commonly occurs during Stage II of anesthesia, thereby placing the patient at greatest risk of laryngospasm during induction and emergence.[14,15]

Initially treatment of laryngospasm includes removal of stimulus, deepening of anesthetic with the volatile agent or propofol (.5 mg/kg IV), and administration of 100% oxygen with continuous positive airway pressure (CPAP). Administration of propofol will not only deepen the anesthetic but also inhibit airway reflexes. Positive pressure ventilation via face mask can help alleviate the compression of soft tissue of the larynx and supraglottic obstruction as well as open the vocal cords up in a partial laryngospasm. Care should be taken during positive pressure ventilation with a face mask to minimize stomach distention and diaphragm elevation. Pressure on the laryngospasm notch, also known as Larson's maneuver, can also be implemented to try to relieve a laryngospasm. The laryngospasm notch is located cephalad to the earlobe, between the mastoid process and mandibular condyle.[14] The anesthesia provider should apply firm and inward pressure at this notch while also performing a jaw thrust, causing an afferent impulse, causing cord relaxation.

If the preceding measures have failed to relieve the laryngospasm or severe deterioration of patient status occurs the gold standard treatment for laryngospasm is the administration of succinylcholine. If the patient has an established IV catheter, 1 to 2 mg/kg of succinylcholine can be administered. Additionally, .02 mg/kg atropine IV should be administered to negate the succinylcholine side effects of bradycardia and other cardiac arrhythmias. If no IV catheter is present, intramuscular (IM) succinylcholine 3 to 4 mg/kg can be administered via IM injection, typically in the quadriceps. IM atropine administration should follow IM succinylcholine. Full effect of the IM succinylcholine is reported to occur 3 to 4 minutes after administration, but relaxation of airway tissue occurs within 1 minute of administration.[14,15]

AIRWAY OBSTRUCTION

Upper airway obstruction is a frequent complication in anesthetized children that are spontaneously breathing. Smaller airway dimensions; enlarged soft tissue, especially in the tonsil and adenoid area; and administration of medications that reduce pharyngeal muscle tone collectively increase upper airway resistance and reduce airway patency resulting in upper airway obstruction. Various maneuvers, including change in body position, a chin lift, opening the mouth with a jaw thrust, or CPAP, can be implemented to reduce upper airway obstruction and promote patency. Changing a child's positioning from supine to lateral can promote airway patency by minimizing the force of gravity on the epiglottis and soft palate, preventing these structures from moving backward against the pharyngeal wall. In the supine position, placing the child in sniffing position or elevation of the shoulders with a shoulder roll will promote upper airway patency. Frequently, the epiglottis of an anesthetized child will be displaced posteriorly leading to obstruction, which can typically be relieved, with a single-handed jaw thrust. If the jaw thrust alone is not sufficient, the anesthetist can perform a two-handed jaw thrust from the mandibular angles with an upward and anterior manner, which will also allows the mouth to open, relieving the obstruction. A CPAP at 10 cm H_2O pressure can be used to promote airway patency through continuous positive pressure that increases the size of the airway. Care should be taken with CPAP to not inflate the stomach.[16]

Infants are known to have more anterior airways, a reduced functional residual capacity (FRC), and increased oxygen consumption. Due to these challenges, multiple laryngoscopy attempts may be performed to secure an airway in an infant, placing the infant at risk of hypoxemia, bradycardia, and potentially cardiac arrest; in infants, hypoxemia can occur for a variety of reasons including reduced FRC, atelectasis, bronchospasm, laryngospasm, sections, prolonged laryngoscopy, or multiple laryngoscopy attempts. Although hypoxemia may present independently, it has the potential to lead to bradycardia with possible progression to cardiac arrest. Please refer to Chapter 1.3 in this text for additional information regarding the pediatric airway and potential challenges with airway management.

BRADYCARDIA

Bradycardia frequently occurs during induction of children with Down syndrome as inhalation and induction agents are known to depress the cardiovascular system. Up to 57% of patients with Down syndrome may experience bradycardia and hypotension during an inhalation induction, which is significantly higher than those without Down syndrome (12%).[17] Prior to induction of anesthesia, previous anesthetic records should be reviewed for history of bradycardia during induction to determine if preinduction administration of an anticholinergic is warranted. It should be noted, however, that preinduction administration of an anticholinergic medication may not always prevent bradycardia. Patients with Down syndrome may require a slower inhalation induction with lower concentrations of inhalation agent compared to those patients without Down syndrome. For more information about the anesthetic management of patients with Down syndrome, please refer to Chapter 31, "Down Syndrome."

SPECIAL CONSIDERATIONS

Preexisting conditions and comorbidities in infants and children present anesthesia providers with unique challenges during the induction of anesthesia. Therefore, special consideration should be given to several patient populations in an effort to minimize adverse events and complications during the induction of anesthesia.

ASTHMA

The prevalence of asthma is 9.5% of children aged 0 to 17 years old and continues to increase, making it one of the most common chronic diseases in children.[18] Hyperreactivity and inflammation of the airways increase the risk of perioperative complications, including bronchospasm. Prior to the induction of anesthesia, a thorough history and physical evaluation should be performed. Control of asthma symptoms, home medications, room air oxygen saturation, history of hospital visits, and steroid must all be vetted. Also, auscultation of the lungs to assess wheezing and coughing should be performed.

Before induction of anesthesia, an inhaled beta-2 adrenergic agonist, such as albuterol, can be administered 1 to 2 hours prior to surgery to optimize the child's lungs prior to surgery. Theoretically, as administration of oral or IV midazolam will reduce anxiety, thereby decreasing the incidence of bronchospasm. The bronchodilatory effects of sevoflurane make it an excellent choice to use during inhalation induction of anesthesia with patients who have a history of asthmatics.

During an IV induction, lidocaine 1.0 to 1.5 mg/kg can be administered to decrease airway hyperreactivity and IV glycopyrrolate or atropine can be administered to reduce secretions and further enhance bronchodilation. Propofol is the IV induction agent of choice for asthmatic patients because of its potential to decrease bronchospasm and airway resistance. IV ketamine produces smooth muscle relaxation and direct bronchodilation effects and should be considered the IV induction agent of choice for asthmatic patients who are hemodynamically unstable.[18] Laryngeal mask placement is preferred over tracheal intubation to avoid bronchospasm if not contraindicated.

BRONCHOPULMONARY DYSPLASIA

Bronchopulmonary dysplasia (BPD) is one of the most prevalent complications in preterm infants, especially those with low birth weights and low gestational ages.[18] Lung injury occurs from oxygen toxicity and positive pressure ventilation requirements, as well as impaired angiogenesis resulting in ventilation–perfusion mismatch. Consequences of this injury include decreased surface area for alveolar–capillary gas exchange, increased risk of respiratory infections, and potential for pulmonary hypertension.[19] During induction of anesthesia for patients with BPD, care should be taken to avoid excessive positive pressure ventilation while optimizing gas exchange and preventing bronchospasm. Excessive positive pressure can lead to increased lung injury and potential for a tension pneumothorax due to friable lung tissue.[19]

During an inhalation induction, sevoflurane can be slowly titrated to prevent a dose-dependent decrease in cardiac contractility and decrease in systemic vascular resistance (SVR). IV inductions using propofol should also be done with caution, being sure to slowly administer doses in an incremental fashion to avoid sudden decreases in SVR. Should there be sudden decreases in SVR, increases in pulmonary vascular resistance may be potentiated, leading to a pulmonary hypertensive crisis. Swift treatment of decreases in SVR to avoid pulmonary hypertension includes inhaled nitric oxide due to its rapid onset of action. Inotropic medications that do not further decrease SVR, such as epinephrine and dopamine, should also be considered. Neuromuscular blocking agents causing a release in histamine should be avoided.[18]

CONGENITAL HEART DISEASE

Congenital heart disease (CHD) is one of the most common congenital anomalies seen in pediatric anesthesia.[20] Therefore, it is essential anesthesia providers have an extensive knowledge of the effects on the uptake and delivery of anesthetic agents when caring for pediatric patients with CHD. This is especially true for patients with CHD presenting for noncardiac surgeries as they are at an increased risk for perioperative morbidity and mortality,[21] Please refer to Chapter 93 in this text for more information regarding the anesthetic care of children with heart disease undergoing noncardiac surgery.

Sevoflurane can depress myocardial contractility which can cause rapid decompensation in a patient with CHD. A decrease in myocardial contractility in a patient with CHD, especially one with already compensated ventricular function, is generally not well tolerated. Propofol decreases SVR and mean arterial pressure and is typically avoided in patients with CHD and those who have right-to-left shunting.[22] Fentanyl has relatively low cardiovascular side effects and is a stable choice to use during induction, as are etomidate and ketamine.[21,22] Prolonged induction times correlate with the presence of a right-to-left shunt.[20] Dilutional mixing of the inhalational agent in the left ventricle impedes the uptake to the brain due to decreased pulmonary flow secondary to the right-to-left shunt. Care must be taken by anesthesia providers to not overdose the inhalational agent and slowly titrate to effect.

OBESITY

The frequency of obese children between the ages 2 and 17 years presenting to the operating room for general anesthesia continues to increase. The Centers for Disease Control and Prevention defines obesity as having a body mass index greater than the 95th percentile for age and gender.[23] Childhood obesity presents several challenges for anesthesia providers, including difficulties with mask ventilation, positioning concerns, increased preoxygenation requirements, and challenges in determining appropriate medication dosage administration to prevent adverse outcomes during induction.

An appropriate mask fit is essential to effective ventilation. Depending on the age of the child and degree of cooperation, preoxygenation can be challenging. Anesthesia providers should position the patient in the sniffing position to yield more effective ventilation and greater success with intubation. Placing sheets or pillows under their shoulders may be necessary to achieve this position. Medications typically dosed on total body weight can have adverse effects, such as hemodynamic instability and prolonged time to wake from anesthesia for the obese child.[23] For the obese child, a propofol dose of 2.0 mg/kg based on the actual body weight should be administered for induction as the ED95 to induce loss of consciousness during induction of anesthesia is significantly lower in obese children.[23]

KEY TAKEAWAYS

- It is imperative that anesthesia providers adequately prepare patients and their family members in an attempt to decrease anxiety and fear related to anesthesia.
- A variety of induction techniques are available for anesthesia providers to use with the pediatric population.
- Sound knowledge of induction drugs and doses, as well as the potential complications associated with pediatric induction of anesthesia, well prepares the anesthesia provider to deliver safe, effective care.
- When caring for a pediatric patient with coexisting diseases or severe illness, anesthesia providers must possess an in-depth understanding of all physiological processes involved to ensure the patient remains stable during induction.

KEY REFERENCES

Complete references for this chapter are online and available at https://connect.springerpub.com/content/book/978-0-8261-3875-0/part/part02/toc-part/ch005.

1. Ryu JH, Park JW, Nahm FS, et al. The effect of gamification through a virtual reality on preoperative anxiety in pediatric patients undergoing general anesthesia: a prospective, randomized, and controlled trial. *J Clin Med*. 2018;7(9):284. doi:10.3390/jcm7090284

3. Gupta A, Datta PK. Sevoflurane consumption during inhalational induction in children: a randomized comparison of minute ventilation-based techniques with standard fixed fresh gas flow technique. *AANA J.* 2020;88(3):177–182.
4. Ramgolam A, Hall GL, Zhang G, et al. Inhalational versus intravenous induction of anesthesia in children with a high risk of perioperative respiratory adverse events: a randomized controlled trial. *Anesthesiology.* 2018;128(6):1065–1074. doi:10.1097/ALN.0000000000002152
10. Gagey AC, de Queiroz Siqueira M, Monard C, et al. The effect of pre-operative gastric ultrasound examination on the choice of general anaesthetic induction technique for non-elective paediatric surgery. A prospective cohort study. *Anaesthesia.*2018;73(3):304–312. doi:10.1111/anae.14179
14. Collins S, Schedler P, Veasey B, et al. Prevention and treatment of laryngospasm in the pediatric patient: a literature review. *AANA J.* 2019;87(2):145–151
22. Yuki K, Lee S, Staffa SJ, DiNardo JA. Induction techniques for pediatric patients with congenital heart disease undergoing noncardiac procedures are influenced by cardiac functional status and residual lesion burden. *J Clin Anesth.* 2018;50:14–17. doi:10.1016/j.jclinane.2018.06.022

CHAPTER 6

Airway Management

Lauren Irwin, Emily H. Klinefelter, Meaghan O'Meara, and Audrey Rosenblatt

> **LEARNING OBJECTIVES**
>
> - Understand how to perform an age-appropriate pediatric airway assessment.
> - Recognize pediatric-specific difficult airway risk factors.
> - Optimize mask management of a pediatric patient.
> - Identify the role of supraglottic airways in pediatric anesthesia.
> - Utilize properly sized airway equipment across the age spectrum.
> - Discuss methods and strategies utilized to intubate the pediatric patient.
> - Explain a rapid sequence intubation in the pediatric patient.
> - Describe management of the pediatric patient with a tracheostomy.
> - Classify airway management techniques and strategies for pediatric difficult airway.
> - Summarize extubation strategies and criteria for normal and difficult pediatric airways.

INTRODUCTION

Airway management is vital to the administration of any safe anesthetic and is a basic and fundamental skill of anesthesia practice. Pediatric anesthesia providers must have a specialized set of skills to ensure competent management of the pediatric airway. Airway management varies according to patient factors, such as age, weight and size, medical history and comorbidities, airway assessment and anomalies, and surgical considerations, such as airway manipulation and ventilation requirements. The anesthesia provider must be prepared to manage anticipated and unanticipated airway complications. Early recognition of a difficult airway obstruction, or the inability to ventilate and/or intubate, is crucial to avoiding patient deterioration and progression to hypoxemia, cardiac arrest, and potential neurological sequelae. This chapter presents the basic principles of pediatric airway management including strategies for the management of the difficult pediatric airway.

PREOPERATIVE ASSESSMENT

Careful preanesthetic evaluation and clinical assessment are the pillars of airway management, and identification of a potential difficult airway is the first step in preventing a catastrophic outcome. An airway-focused history should include a review of previous anesthesia and medical records as well as a detailed physical examination. Performing an airway examination can be challenging in young patients who are unable or unwilling to cooperate, yet efforts should be made to complete this important component of the preoperative assessment. An airway examination should include an assessment of facial symmetry, degree of mouth opening, presence or absence of oral pathology, upper incisor length and alignment, thyromental distance, length and circumference of the neck, and neck range of motion.[1] It should be noted that the Mallampati score is not useful in infants and younger children; however, it has been shown to correlate with Cormack–Lehane laryngoscopic view in children older than 4 years.[2]

Review of previous airway management and intubation records can provide valuable information about the patient's airway and successful or unsuccessful airway management strategies during previous encounters. For patients who are suspected of having a difficult airway or a history of a difficult airway, the time should be taken to request and receive records from other facilities and anesthesia providers. The ease of mask ventilation, need for airway adjuncts, type of laryngoscope used, number of attempts at laryngoscopy, and laryngoscopic view ultimately achieved should all be noted.[1] It is important to keep in mind that the airway evolves with growth, maturation, and previous surgical intervention.

AIRWAY MANAGEMENT

MASK MANAGEMENT

Inhalation induction is common practice in pediatric anesthesia and necessitates skilled mask management and familiarity with devices that optimize oxygenation and ventilation. Selecting the proper mask size is crucial to obtaining a seal that will allow for comfortable bag mask ventilation. Inflating the soft outer portion of the mask allows for optimal seal. Ideal mask fit will rest on the bridge of the nose and encompass the mandible.[3] Basic hand position involves the anesthesia provider's thumb securing the top portion of the mask, while the first digit wraps around the bottom of the mask (**Figure 6.1**). The fifth digit can assist by subluxing the temporomandibular joint anteriorly, displacing the tongue and soft tissue and creating a more patent airway. Careful attention should be paid so as not to compress the submandibular soft tissue, causing partial obstruction.[4] Adequate ventilation will yield chest rise, condensation within the mask, reservoir bag movement, and end-tidal carbon dioxide production. Ventilation can be assisted by the anesthesia provider with gentle administration of continuous positive airway pressure (CPAP) by means of the adjustable pressure limiting "pop-off" valve.[3] However, it is important to note that gastric distension may result from positive pressure ventilation, which can impair successful ventilation.[4] Pediatric mask management can be a challenging skill to conquer especially when there is a considerable differential between a small face and an adult anesthesia provider's hand. Experienced hands demonstrate mastery of this technique with added finesse, allowing for optimal oxygenation and ventilation.

Oropharyngeal Airways

Oropharyngeal airway devices are designed to overcome upper airway obstruction caused by soft tissue collapse

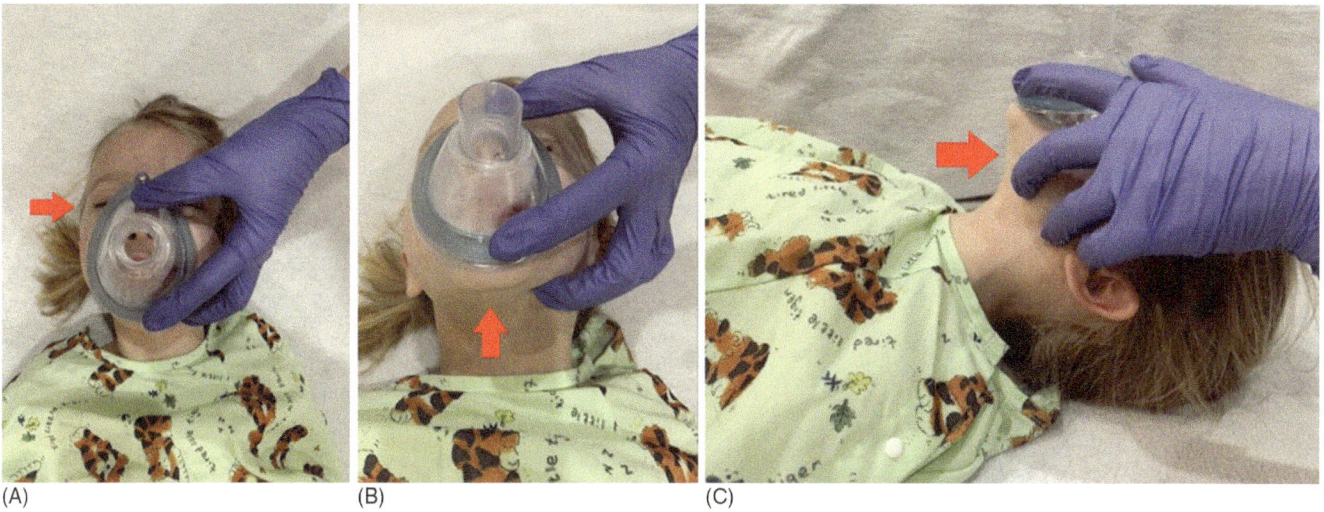

Figure 6.1: Basic hand position for pediatric mask ventilation.
Pediatric mask management requires special attention to avoid patient eyes and submandibular soft tissue.

including posterior tongue displacement, which commonly occurs during deep sedation or general anesthesia.[5] The proportionally large tongue of infants can also create obstruction to mask management. Proper use and sizing of an oral airway will displace the tongue forward from the posterior pharyngeal wall thereby opening the airway and easing mask management efforts. Appropriate oropharyngeal airway size selection is essential for ventilation optimization and is based largely on length (Figure 6.2). Table 6.1 provides an age-based airway sizing guide. Correct sizing can be estimated by placing the oral airway to the patient's cheek. The tip of the oral airway should rest cephalad to the angle of the mandible, while the flange lies near the patient's mouth.[3] Improper sizing can impede airway exchange. An oropharyngeal airway that is too small may cause further obstruction by pushing the tongue posteriorly, whereby an oropharyngeal airway that is too large can displace the epiglottis onto the glottic opening while also causing trauma to the pharyngeal structures (Figure 6.3).[3,5] A tongue depressor can be used to facilitate insertion. Careful attention should be paid to ensure the lip is not pinched between the teeth and oral airway causing trauma to the lip or gums. Oral airways can also be useful to prevent biting of the endotracheal tube (ETT) during emergence of anesthesia and for purposes of suctioning.[3]

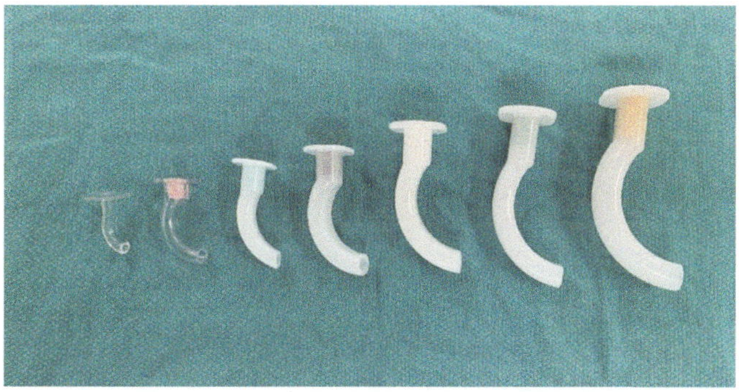

NASOPHARYNGEAL AIRWAYS

Nasopharyngeal airways serve as another way to overcome upper airway obstruction by providing a patent conduit through the nare. The placement of a nasopharyngeal airway can be advantageous anytime upper airway obstruction is suspected; however, oropharyngeal airways are more commonly used in conjunction with mask management due to their ease of placement. The placement of a nasopharyngeal airway can be stimulating, but once in place they are usually well tolerated. Proper sizing is based on length and is selected by measuring from the nare to the angle of the mandible.[3] Sizing ranges from 12 French (smallest) to 34 French (largest) and should be considered prior to insertion (Figure 6.4). When inserting a nasopharyngeal airway, lubricate well with a water-based lubricant and insert into the nose aiming posteriorly with the beveled edge facing medially to prevent damage to the turbinate with the tip of the device. If resistance is met, it is prudent to remove the airway due to the risk of trauma or bleeding and attempt insertion in the opposite nare. Some nasopharyngeal airways have a collar, or flange, which sits at the nare and can be adjusted to decrease the depth. Do not remove this collar as it could slip back into the nose and become irretrievable. Nasopharyngeal airways are also a useful adjunct to place prior to extubation in a patient who is at risk of upper airway obstruction.

ADVANCED MASK VENTILATION TECHNIQUES

While the use of an oropharyngeal or nasopharyngeal airway can facilitate bag-mask ventilation, difficult bag-mask ventilation (DBMV) may persist. When the anesthesia provider encounters difficult ventilation, it is important to rule out bronchospasm or laryngospasm as causes or contributing factors. Inadequate depth of anesthesia can be a contributing cause of DBMV as well.[6] Position manipulations, such as chin lift, jaw thrust, and the placement of a shoulder roll, are initial steps that can be utilized to open the airway. Two-person bag-mask ventilation techniques can also be an effective strategy to enhance air exchange. The anesthesia provider inserts an oropharyngeal airway and raises the mandible with two

Figure 6.2: Oropharyngeal airway sizes 30–90 mm.

Table 6.1 Age-Based Pediatric Airway Guide

Age	Oropharyngeal Airway (mm)	Blade	Cuffed ETT	Insertion Depth (cm)
Preemie (1000–2500 g)	30	Miller 0	2.5–3 uncuffed	7–9
Neonate	30–40	Miller 1 Phillips 1	3.0	9–10
Infant (<6 months)	40–50	Miller 1 Phillips 1	3.0–3.5	10
Infant (6–12 months)	40–50	Miller 1 Phillips 1	3.5	10–11
1 year	50–60	Miller 1 Phillips 1 Wis-Hipple 1.5	4.0	11–12
2 years	60	Wis-Hipple 1.5 Mac 2	4.0–4.5	12–13
3 years	60	Wis-Hipple 1.5 Mac 2	4.0–4.5	13–14
4 years	60–70	Wis-Hipple 1.5 Mac 2	4.5	14
5 years	70	Mac 2	5.0	15

Notes: Sizing are estimates based on average weight and size per age; children off the growth curve need specific assessment.

When using an uncuffed ETT, select one-half size larger.

ETT, endotracheal tube.

Source: From Fiadjoe JE, Litman RS, Server JF, et al. The pediatric airway. In Cote CJ, Lerman J, Anderson B, eds. *A Practice of Anesthesia for Infants and Children, Sixth Edition*. Saunders-Elsevier; 2019:297–339.

hands while another person ventilates by squeezing the reservoir bag.[5] This allows for optimal mask to face seal and opens the upper airway allowing exchange and ventilation. If these strategies are unsuccessful, placing the patient in the lateral position may open the airway facilitating mask ventilation.[6]

In patients with DBMV, gastric distention can become a concern. Using the lowest pressure that allows for adequate ventilation will help limit gastric distention. The anesthesia provider should consider decompressing the stomach if this is exacerbating the ventilation difficulty.

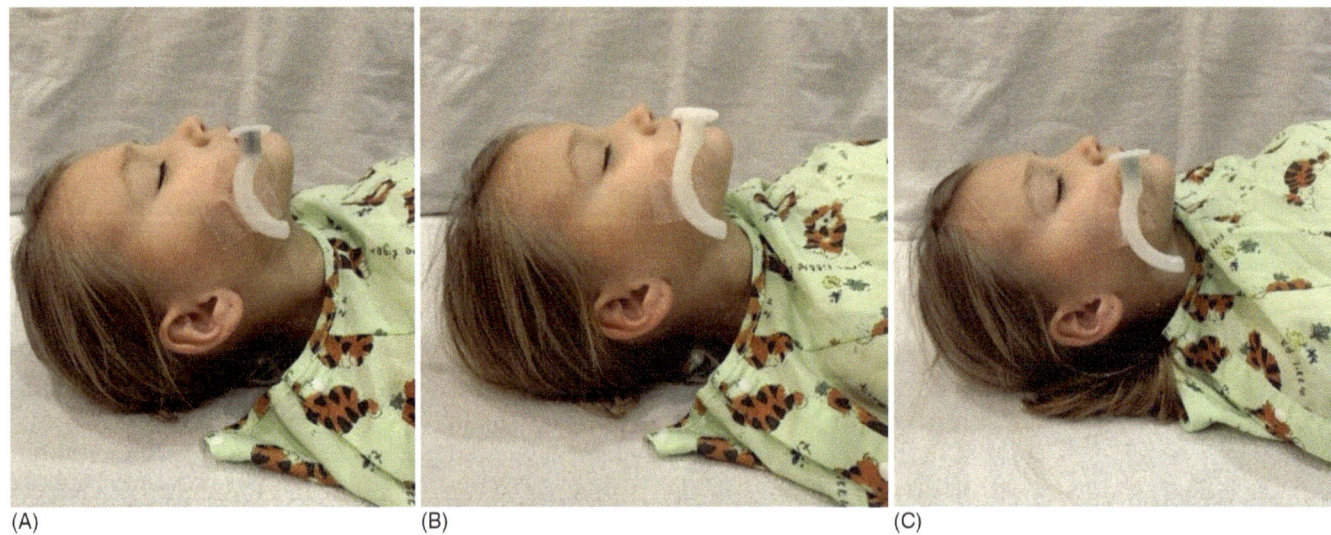

Figure 6.3: Oropharyngeal airway sizing.
(A) 60 mm oropharyngeal airway (OA), which is too small for this child and would likely displace the tongue posteriorly causing further obstruction.
(B) 70 mm OA which is the appropriate size for this child.
(C) 80 mm OA, which is too large for this child and would likely displace the epiglottis and potentially cause obstruction and trauma in this airway.

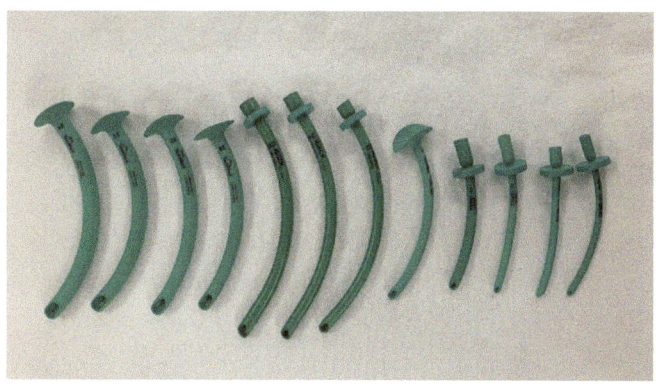

Figure 6.4: Nasopharyngeal airways.

Note: There is variation in the moveable flange to adjust the length of the nasopharyngeal airways.

SUPRAGLOTTIC AIRWAYS

The evolution of supraglottic airways has revolutionized airway management, specifically in the pediatric population. Since the introduction of the laryngeal mask airway (LMA), multiple other supraglottic devices have been developed, which are shown in Figure 6.5. The supraglottic airway (SGA) is a well-established airway management strategy and plays a safe and important role in pediatric anesthesia.[7] The goal of supraglottic device placement is to create a perilaryngeal seal through which ventilation can occur.[7] These devices can be electively used when tracheal intubation is not necessary.[7] SGA use can also serve as a rescue device in cases of unexpected difficult airway (e.g., difficult ventilation and failure to intubate) and emergency airway management.[7] SGA use in the pediatric population yields lower failure rates than in the adult population (0.86% vs 1.1%); therefore, its use is often an acceptable and safe airway option for both manual and assisted ventilation.[8] SGAs are safe and effective and, depending on surgical requirements, may be preferable to intubation, particularly for infants and small children. SGAs in infants may reduce the risk of perioperative respiratory events as compared to ETTs.[9]

There are multiple different types of SGAs, each with unique characteristics, which are outlined in Figure 6.6. Prior to SGA use, comparison of the various features of each can guide selection of the correct device. These devices are classified as first or second generation based on the incorporation of a gastric access channel that serves as a gastric vent and/or allows gastric tube placement.[10] Characteristics of the second-generation SGA design are intended to ease insertion, provide positive pressure ventilation, and assist in tracheal intubation.[10] The LMA Classic, LMA ProSeal, and LMA Unique are all older original model devices and are accepted within pediatric anesthesia. While older SGA models, specifically the LMA Classic and LMA Unique, can be used in children, limitations exist, including possible mask movement, resulting in poor seal, and potential epiglottic displacement, causing obstruction.[6] Newer SGA devices, such as air-Q®, Ambu Aura-i®, and i-gel®, offer easier placement, better seating, and reduced need for troubleshooting efforts.[10] For infants, the LMA ProSeal®, air-Q®, or i-gel® may offer superior stability.[10] The LMA ProSeal® and i-gel® may also provide better means for positive pressure ventilation, while the air-Q® and the Ambu Aura-i® serve as the best conduits for tracheal intubation.[10] While device selection may be limited by the supply chain at a given facility, understanding design features can be useful to daily practice.

Complications with SGA placement are not uncommon; thus, insertion and placement may require troubleshooting efforts. Limitations of SGA placement can include mask displacement, poor seal, gastric insufflation, and reflex activation of the airway.[10] This may necessitate manipulation of the device or utilization of an alternate airway plan. Placement of supraglottic devices can be via a midline or rotational technique.[6] The midline approach requires device insertion over the tongue along the hard palate until seated into the posterior pharynx.[6] The rotational technique involves inverted initial insertion, followed by 180-degree rotation of the device at the level of the soft palate during advancement to the final position in the posterior pharynx.[6] Due to pediatric anatomy and a more acute posterior pharyngeal angle, the rotational approach may allow for easier placement in children.[6]

Innovations in supraglottic devices have allowed for more advanced intubating techniques ultimately providing safer intubating options in pediatric anesthesia. During difficult airway management, the SGA can be useful for ventilation or as a conduit for endotracheal intubation.[6] SGA use and its place in the difficult airway algorithm are discussed later in this chapter.

ENDOTRACHEAL TUBES

ETTs provide a secure and patent airway for positive pressure ventilation, often during the administration of general anesthesia. The choice to intubate is guided by the patient's medical condition, the surgical indications, and the duration

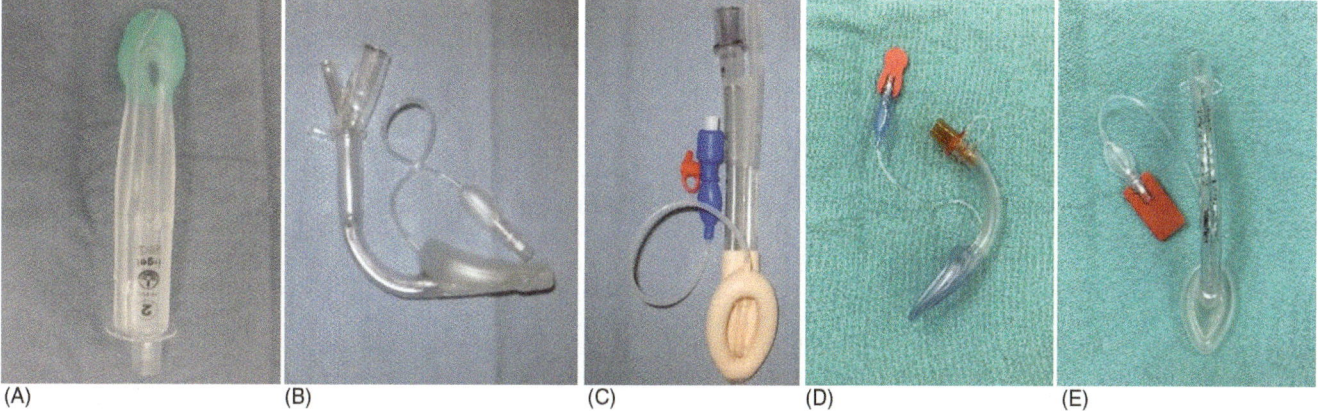

Figure 6.5: Common pediatric supraglottic devices. (A) i-gel®. (B) LMA Supreme®. (C) LMA ProSeal®. (D) air-Q®. (E) LMA Unique®.

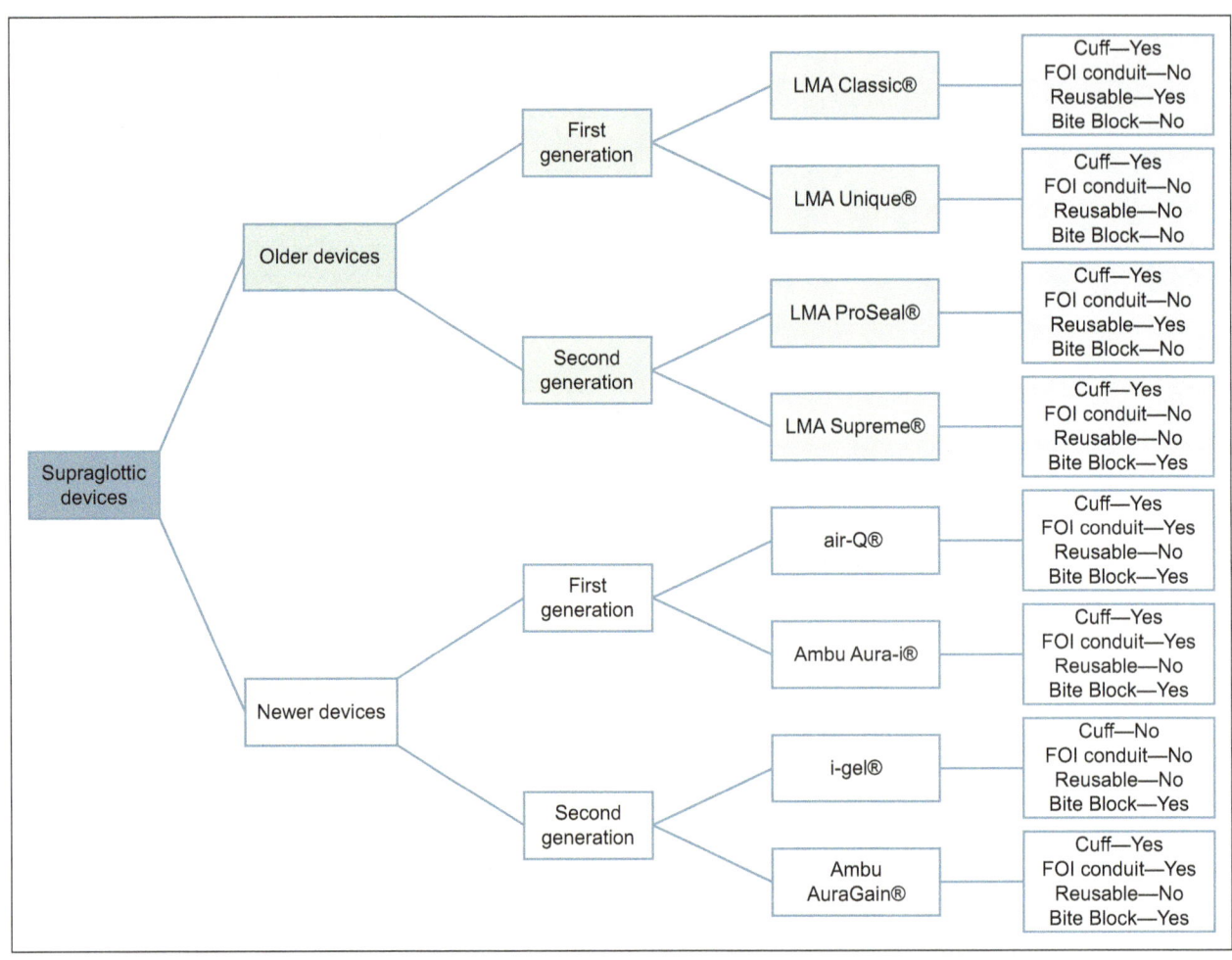

Figure 6.6: Pediatric supraglottic airway characteristics comparison.
First-generation devices have no gastric access, while second-generation devices have gastric access capabilities.
FOI, fiberoptic intubation.

of the procedure. While SGAs are often favored due to ease of placement and reduction of possible postoperative airway complications, their use is not suitable for all patients and surgical procedures. When intubation is indicated, proper selection of an ETT is paramount. Basic management involves selection of an appropriately sized cuffed or uncuffed ETT, as well as strategies to confirm proper size, depth, and acceptable leak pressure.

The selection of a cuffed versus uncuffed ETT is a unique pediatric consideration. In current clinical practice, most pediatric intubations for general anesthetics utilize a cuffed ETT. Considerations for placing an uncuffed ETT are small patient size, young age, and the plan for postoperative intubation and ventilation. Previous models of ETTs have had high-pressure, low-volume cuffs. These ETTs are not ideal for pediatrics due to the risk of postintubation croup and subglottic stenosis related to increased pressure on the trachea from the ETT cuff. The majority of ETTs in current practice are high-volume, low-pressure cuffs, which make these tubes safer in the pediatric airway. Microcuff tubes are a subset of ETTs specifically designed for the pediatric airway. These tubes consist of a rectangular cuff to ensure a more even distribution of pressure on the trachea and the absence of a murphy eye, allowing the cuff to be positioned more distally on the ETT to prevent pressure on the cricoid cartilage.[3] **Table 6.2** outlines in greater detail the pros and cons of the use of uncuffed versus cuffed ETTs in pediatric patients.

A properly sized ETT is important to ensure effective ventilation while minimizing risk of airway complications. Age and weight are the major determining factors when selecting the proper ETT size; however, sizing is unique to each patient.[3] The size of the ETT is based on the internal diameter (ID). It should be noted that the external diameter (OD) varies among manufacturers and can account for some irregularities in appropriate sizing for a patient of equal age and weight.[3] Appropriate ETT sizes based on age can be seen in **Table 6.1** and **Table 6.3**. A variety of formulas can be used to guide selection of the correct size of ETT to prevent airway mucosal injury. Cuffed ETTs should be 0.5 to 1.0 mm smaller than an uncuffed ETT selected for the same patient. In children >2 years, Cole's formula is used to select an uncuffed ETT [ID (mm) = (age/4) + 4.0].[11] For a cuffed ETT, the most commonly used formulas are those offered by Khine [ID (mm) = [age/4] + 3] and Motoyama [ID (mm) = (age/4) + 3.5]. The Khine formula, for example, results in selection of the appropriate cuffed ETT size with 99% accuracy.[12] In newborns to infants <1 year, ID 3.0 mm cuffed ETT and, in children from 1 to 2 years, ID 3.5 mm cuffed ETTs should be used. When using second-generation Microcuff PETs, Salgo proposed a new recommendation, which allows selection of larger ID cuffed tracheal tubes than previously recommended.[13]

Table 6.2	Cuffed Versus Uncuffed Endotracheal Tubes
Cuffed Endotracheal Tubes	**Uncuffed Endotracheal Tubes**

Pros
• Lower incidence of reintubation
• Ability to adjust cuff size can provide patient-specific sizing
• May provide more optimal ventilation conditions due to the ability to make small cuff size adjustments
	Pros
	• Increased internal diameter of ETT
	  ◦ Radius has an exponential effect on flow resistance
	• Poiseuille's law
	  ◦ $\Delta p = (8\mu LQ/\pi R^4)$
	• Decreased focal pressure on the trachea

Cons
• Increased variation in external diameter
• Need to downsize internal diameter of ETT to accommodate for cuff
  ◦ Especially problematic in small infants needing longer term intubation
• Possible increase in incidence of laryngospasm
• Possible increase in postintubation croup (unlikely)
	Cons
	• No ability to adjust the seal around the ETT to improve ventilation
	• Reintubation to upsize or downsize the ETT can result in loss of airway or trauma from repeated laryngoscopies and intubations
	• Sizing is rigid in half size increments
	  ◦ Example: a patient with no leak around a 4.0 uncuffed ETT at 30 cmH$_2$O may have a free leak around a 3.5 uncuffed ETT

ETT, endotracheal tube.

Source: From Fiadjoe JE, Litman RS, Server JF, et al. The pediatric airway. In CJ. Cote, J. Lerman, B. Anderson, eds. *A Practice of Anesthesia for Infants and Children, Sixth Edition.* Saunders-Elsevier. 2019:297–339, and Harless J, Ramaiah R, Bhananker SM. Pediatric airway management. *Int J Crit Illn Inj Sci.* 2014;4(1):65–70. doi:10.4103/2229-5151.128015.

Table 6.3	Recommendations for Age-Based Cuffed ETT Sizing		
Age (Years)	Khine et al.[a]	Motoyama et al.[b]	Salgo et al.[c]
Birth to <0.5	3.0	3.0	3.0
0.5 to <1.0	3.0	3.0	3.5
1.0 to <1.5	3.5	3.5	3.5
1.5 to <2.0	3.5	3.5	4.0
2.0 to <3.0	3.5	4.0	4.0
3.0 to <4.0	4.0	4.0	4.5
4.0 to <5.0	4.0	4.5	4.6

ETT, endotracheal tube.

[a]Motoyama EK. Endotracheal intubation. In: EK Motoyama, PJ Davis, eds. *Smith's Anesthesia for Infants and Children.* 5 ed. C.V. Mosby. 1990;269–275.

[b]Salgo B, Schmitz A, Henze G, et al. Evaluation of a new recommendation for improved cuffed tracheal tube size selection in infants and small children. *Acta Anaesthesiol Scand.* 2006;50:557–61.

[c]Bhardwaj N. Pediatric cuffed endotracheal tubes. *J Anaesthesiol Clin Pharmacol.* 2013;29(1):13–18. doi:10.4103/0970-9185.105786 .

Source: From Khine HH, Corddry DH, Kettrick RG, et al. Comparison of cuffed and uncuffed endotracheal tubes in young children during general anaesthesia. *Anesthesiology* 1997;86:627–31.

Once endotracheal intubation has been verified, the ETT must be secured at the appropriate depth. The goal is to secure the tube at a depth where the tip of the ETT is below the cricoid cartilage and above the carina. The following equation serves as a guide to proper depth after the age of 2 years: age(years)/2 + 12 = depth in centimeters.[3] This equation does not apply to children younger than 2 years old. Another equation frequently used for determining depth is 3 x ETT size in centimeters.[14] This method is useful as there are no age restrictions. While these equations are useful guides, the main determinants of appropriate insertion depth are the presence of bilateral breath sounds and chest expansion. In neonates and infants, minor variations in patient positioning can be the difference between mainstem bronchial intubation, tracheal intubation, and extubation. It is prudent to auscultate breath sounds even after minor changes in positioning in this patient population. Note that even the removal of a shoulder roll or the placement of a head donut may be enough to displace an ETT. A small, but persistent drop in oxygen saturation, can indicate endobronchial intubation and should always be evaluated.[3]

Prior to securing the ETT at the appropriate depth, the anesthesia provider should verify that the ETT is the appropriate size. Smooth insertion during intubation is a rudimentary sign of proper size and may also indicate that the ETT is too small. If the tube is difficult to pass, it may be too large. Even if the tip of the ETT moves past the vocal cords, it must also pass easily through the cricoid cartilage. A leak test should be performed to verify appropriate ETT size. Performing a leak test serves to confirm appropriate sizing and proper cuff inflation by evaluating the airflow, or leak, around the ETT. **Box 6.1** outlines the process of performing a leak test. An air leak at 20 to 25 cmH$_2$O is recommended as risk of tracheal injury and/or ischemia is reduced at these pressures. It should be noted that higher pressures can be tolerated for short-term intubations, but use caution as this does not preclude airway complications.[3] If muscle relaxant is not used for intubation, ensure adequate depth of anesthesia prior to performing a leak test as laryngospasm around the ETT can mimic an ill-fitting ETT.[3]

A variety of specially designed ETTs are available and constructed for varying surgical indications. Many of these

---

BOX 6.1 — PERFORMING A LEAK TEST

- Confirm endotracheal intubation.
  - Presence of end-tidal CO$_2$, auscultation of bilateral breath sounds and presence of bilateral chest expansion
- Place stethoscope on the neck or above the mouth.
- Set the anesthesia machine to manual with the adjustable pressure limiting (APL) valve to 0.
- Turn the APL valve to 20.
- Listen as the pressure rises in the circuit and watch the pressure gauge on the anesthesia machine.
- If no noise is heard and the circuit holds 20 cm H$_2$O, increase the APL valve to 30.
- The presence of an audible leak and a plateau of pressure in the circuit is the place at which a leak occurred.
- Inflate the cuff to adjust the pressure; goal 20–25 cm H$_2$O.

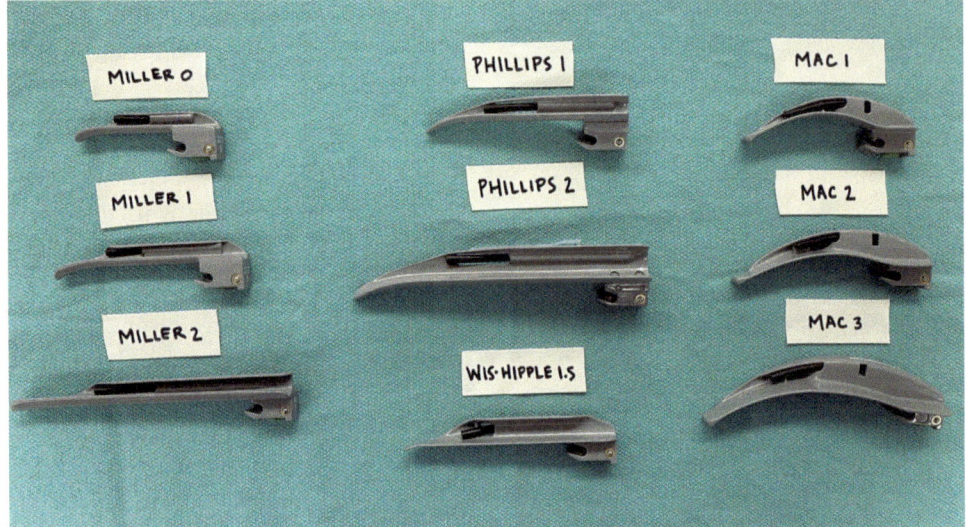

Figure 6.7: Laryngoscope blades of varying sizes and shapes utilized in pediatric anesthesia.

specialized ETTs are utilized for head and neck surgery. Since these tubes are often placed to facilitate surgical exposure, effective communication with surgical colleagues is important. Oral Ring–Adair–Elwyn (RAE) ETTs have a 90-degree angle to help aid in the visualization and exposure for oral surgeries. The angle of the oral RAE ETT lies flat along the chin or in the corner of the mouth to facilitate exposure without kinking. Nasal RAE tubes have a special shape and length to account for nasal anatomy, which similarly prevents kinking. The prefixed bend may not provide the needed length and can be a drawback to nasal and oral RAE ETTs. This is especially true for patients with subglottic stenosis or those who are off the growth curve for height. Reinforced ETTs contain coiled wires to prevent kinking and maintain the shape of the tube when extreme positioning of the neck or head is needed for surgical exposure. A drawback of the reinforced tube is that it can become permanently obstructed if bitten or damaged. A laser ETT, a type of reinforced tube, is impregnated with metal, often aluminum, to reduce the risk of airway fire when surgical lasers are needed in the airway. Due to the high risk of airway fire, saline is typically instilled in the cuff instead of air. A neural integrity monitor electromyogram tracheal tube (NIM-EMG ETT) allows the surgeon to assess the recurrent laryngeal nerve and thus vocal cord function during neck surgeries, such as a neck dissection or thyroidectomy.[15] NIM-EMG ETT is often placed with video laryngoscopy (VL), so that surgical colleagues can verify the placement of the nerve monitoring portion of the NIM-EMG ETT.

Methods and Techniques for Placement of ETT
Direct Laryngoscopy
The most common method for placement of an ETT is direct laryngoscopy (DL). The selection of the proper laryngoscope is based on age and body mass of the child.[3] There are two types of laryngoscope blades: straight and curved. Straight blades, such as a Miller, Phillips, or Wis-Hipple, are the superior choice for intubating infants and small children. Straight blades provide a *direct* view of the glottis by physically lifting the epiglottis and base of the tongue to expose the vocal cords. Due to the large epiglottis and tongue relative to size in infants and small children, the straight blade provides the best exposure of the vocal cords in patients under the age of 4 years old.[16] The curved blade, known as a Macintosh and commonly referred to as Mac, is utilized in older children and adults to achieve an *indirect* view of the glottis. Placing the tip of the blade in the vallecula and lifting causes an indirect elevation of the epiglottis, exposing the vocal cords.[16] Figure 6.7 demonstrates the different laryngoscope blades.

To perform DL successfully, patient positioning is paramount. The goal of proper positioning is to obtain alignment of the oral, pharyngeal, and tracheal axes required for the visualization of the glottis.[16] Depending on the age and body habitus, different positions are optimal. For children of all ages, ensure the neck is in neutral position. If head stabilization is needed, consider the use of a foam or gel donut. In infants, this can unfavorably flex the head forward; the foam donut can be torn to create a halo that holds the head in a neutral position. See Figure 6.8, which demonstrates poor positioning of an infant. Next, ensure that there is slight head extension. When positioning infants and small children, the back of the head is relatively large and more pronounced. The use of a shoulder roll can facilitate proper head and neck alignment for this age group (Figure 6.9).[16] In older children, this can be achieved with the patient lying flat on the operating room table or in some cases with the use of a folded blanket under the head and shoulders. Teenage, adult-sized patients with body mass index greater than 30 may need a ramp of blankets under the upper shoulders or a positioning device to optimize DL.

Once the patient is properly positioned, the mouth can be opened with varying techniques. In children approximately age 3 and older, the scissors technique can be used to manually open the mouth. To perform the scissors technique, place a gloved hand in the right corner of the patient's mouth and use the thumb to push the lower incisors caudad and the index or middle finger to stabilize against the upper incisors. Often, head position is adjusted simultaneously into slight extension to facilitate mouth opening. In school-age children, pressure on loose primary teeth should be avoided. In infants and small children, mouth opening can be achieved by placing the heel of the anesthesia provider's right hand on the forehead of the child, securing the head with gentle downward pressure. Then, using the middle or index finger, open the mouth by applying pressure to right side of the mandible (Figure 6.10). This method keeps the right oral commissure free to allow optimal introduction of the laryngoscope blade.

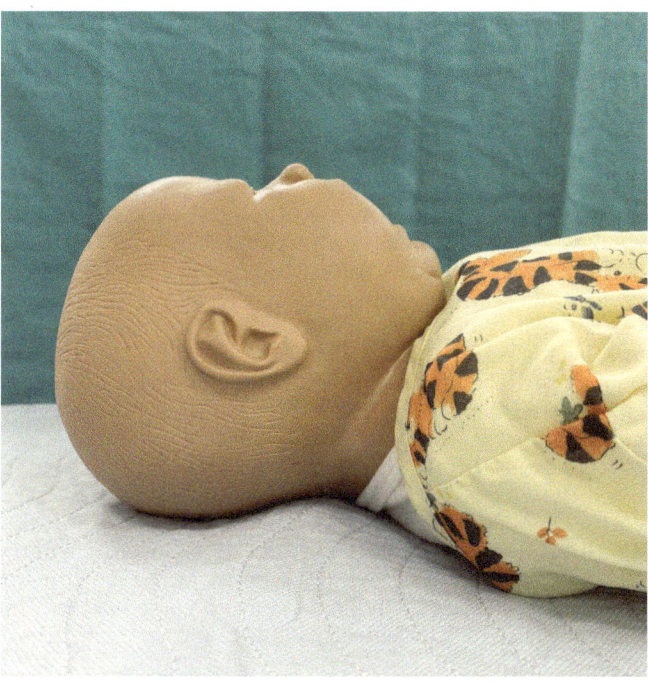

Figure 6.8: Improper infant positioning.
The large occiput creates neck flexion and poor alignment of the oral, pharyngeal, and tracheal axes.

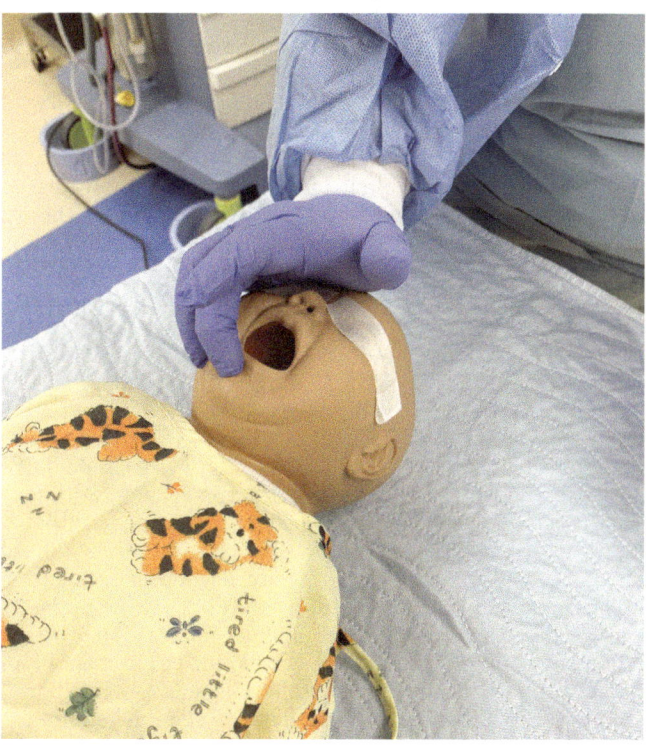

Figure 6.10: Scissors mouth-opening technique.

Occasionally, neck extension alone will allow the mouth to open enough to introduce the blade.

DL technique varies depending on what blade the anesthesia provider is using. When using a curved blade, insert the blade into the right side of the mouth, sweeping the tongue to the left as the blade moves midline. Advance the blade into the vallecula and lift, in a toasting fashion, to indirectly lift the epiglottis, exposing the vocal cords. If your first view is of the epiglottis, advance the blade further into the vallecula before exposing again. When using a straight blade, insert into the mouth just right of midline, sweeping the tongue to the left. Advance the blade under direct visualization past the tongue base toward the epiglottis with the goal of directly lifting the epiglottis to expose the vocal cords. If the epiglottis cannot be directly lifted, it is acceptable to insert the tip of the blade into the vallecula to elevate the epiglottis indirectly. If there is only a partial view of the cords, gentle external laryngeal pressure can be exerted on the neck to bring the vocal cords into better view.[17]

Video Laryngoscopy

Although DL remains the gold standard for placement of an ETT, VL has gained popularity in the last two decades. VL has continued to gain momentum in the management of the pediatric airway as it has proved to be a safe and reliable intubating method. VL has also become less expensive and more accessible, as many brands have made more pediatric options available. Not only has it been touted as a rescue tool when DL fails, but it is also useful in difficult airway management.

VL uses a laryngoscope blade with a video camera at the tip to enhance visualization of the larynx in situations in which direct visualization may be difficult or unobtainable. The two main steps are exposure of the larynx and advancement of the ETT. View–tube discrepancy can occur when the laryngeal view is good, but the anesthesia provider encounters difficulty advancing the ETT through the vocal cords. This is commonly due to the angle of the stylet and can be addressed by hyperangulating the stylet to improve the intubation angle. In case of extreme difficulty advancing the ETT, a hybrid technique of VL and flexible bronchoscopy is an option, which is discussed later in the chapter.

Unlike DL, VL does not require the alignment of the oral, laryngeal, and tracheal axes due to direct visualization with a camera. The use of a traditional Mac or Miller blades with video technology allows for both direct visualization via a

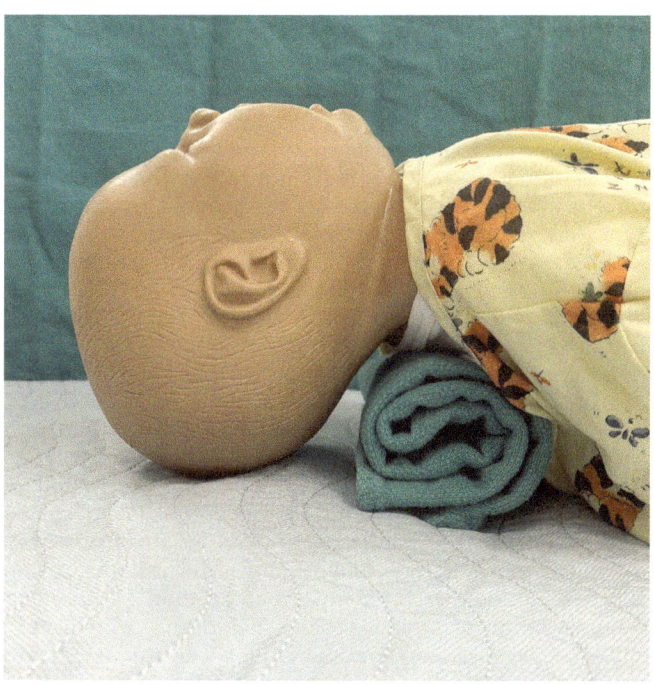

Figure 6.9: Proper infant positioning.
The use of a shoulder roll can facilitate proper head and neck alignment for this age group.

traditional DL and indirect visualization via a camera. The Storz C-Mac® and McGrath® VLs are two examples of this type of technology.[18] The Storz C-Mac® has blades available in Miller 0-1 and Mac 0-2 blade configurations, with a hyperangulated PED D-blade as well. The McGrath's smallest size available is equivalent to a Mac 2 blade, so it is only suitable for older children.[19] Using these blades in potential difficult airway allows for the use of standard DL with immediate backup of the VL if direct visualization is not possible. This is also a valuable teaching tool to aid in instruction and placement of ETTs. The clinical educator can use the video feature to observe ETT placement, while the trainee uses the blade via DL, without the guidance of the video feature.[18]

Another type of VL includes laryngoscopes with hyperangulated blades, such as the GlideScope. The GlideScope is one of the most popular and widely used VL devices in pediatric airway management and offers sizes from neonates to adults.[19] The hyperangulated blade has a 60-degree curve to improve glottic exposure and visualization and requires minimal head and neck manipulation. The sizing of the GlideScope hyperangulated blades is weight-based. To perform VL, the hyperangulated blade is placed midline into the vallecula. They do not require sweeping of the tongue, and midline placement helps prevent intraoral injury, specifically to the tonsillar pillars.[20] Due to the extreme shape of the blade, a stylet is required to ensure the ETT curves in the direction of the blade. A "hockey stick" contour is often referred to when shaping the stylet for use. Other hyperangulated laryngoscopes, such as the Pentax® and Airtraq®, provide a guide channel for the ETT. The ETT is preloaded onto the laryngoscope, making the use of a stylet unnecessary. These blades tend to be small and portable and, without the need for a stylet, make them ideal for field airway management.[18] Both the Pentax and Airtraq come in sizes from neonates to adults.[19]

Flexible Bronchoscopy

The flexible bronchoscope, commonly referred to as fiberoptic, flexible fiberoptic, or fiberoptic bronchoscope, is a useful tool for difficult airway management. Flexible bronchoscopes were originally created using fiber optic technology, and they retain the common name of "fiber optic" in clinical practice. However, the majority of newer flexible bronchoscopes now use video technology, which is preferable from a cost, processing (cleaning and storage), and an image quality standpoint. Flexible bronchoscopes for the smallest infants still use fiberoptic technology due to the size of the embedded video camera. Good planning and the presence of experienced providers are critical to the success of this advanced airway management technique. Basic strategies for successful flexible bronchoscopy will be introduced here; further discussion on more advanced techniques appears later in the chapter.

As with all airway management strategies, selecting the appropriately sized equipment is important. Currently, the smallest bronchoscope is 2.2 mm in diameter and can fit an ETT with a 2.5-mm ID.[3] To ensure the correct size has been selected, confirm that the tube fits onto the bronchoscope. This will provide stability when guiding the ETT into the glottis and will prevent tissue entrapment.[21] Prior to using the bronchoscope, test the lighting and functionality. Use of an antifogging solution is helpful to aid in visualization, especially if the patient is spontaneously breathing.

Once the bronchoscope has been prepared for use and an appropriately sized ETT has been loaded, ensure that the patient is in the optimal position. Flexible bronchoscopy requires minimal head and neck movement for successful intubation. The head should be flat on the table with slight extension of the neck; this will help prevent the epiglottis from obstructing the view of the vocal cords.[3] With the patient in the proper position, pass the bronchoscope midline. Several techniques can be utilized to aid in glottic visualization. A jaw thrust and/or manual traction on the tongue can open the posterior laryngeal space by displacing pharyngeal tissue.[3] The use of an intubating oral airway, such as an Ovassapian airway, can ensure that the scope stays midline while displacing the tongue. The intubating oral airway is also advantageous when intubating an awake patient as it protects the bronchoscope from potential damage. Gentle external laryngeal pressure can also be utilized when a partial glottic view is obtained. As the bronchoscope is advanced, be sure to maintain identifiable structures. If visualization is lost, withdraw until structures become recognizable; redirect the bronchoscope and advance again. Once the glottis is visualized, advance through the vocal cords. Do not advance the ETT until tracheal rings are seen, and it is clearly determined that the bronchoscope is in the trachea. Advance ETT, with the bevel facing downward, into the trachea and verify placement via bronchoscopic visualization, bilateral breath sounds, and confirmation of end-tidal CO_2.[3]

Nasal Intubation

Nasal intubation can be useful in certain pediatric procedures. A cuffed nasal RAE is most often used to aid in placement and ventilation when nasal intubation is necessary. Nasal intubation ensures the ETT will not hinder surgical exposure of the oral cavity or mandible. Nasal intubation may also be preferred when long-term intubation in the intensive care unit (ICU) is anticipated, as it is more comfortable, thus decreasing sedation requirements. It should be noted that a standard ETT may be used, however, it may not be long enough and may be more prone to kinking as it does not account for the shape of the nasal cavity.

Nasal intubation requires planning and specialized equipment to ensure smooth placement. Nasal intubation may be performed under DL, VL, or flexible bronchoscopy. Ensure all of the following necessary equipment is available: warm sterile water to soften the ETT, water-based lubricant, multiple-sized nasopharyngeal airways, a topical nasal vasoconstrictor, such as oxymetazoline nasal spray, and Magill forceps. Using a stylet is not possible for nasal intubation, therefore Magill forceps are utilized. Magill forceps are specially shaped forceps designed to grasp the tip of the ETT in the oropharynx and are used to guide the ETT into the glottis. They are available in different sizes to accommodate the infant to the adult airway and are commonly used during DL and VL nasal intubation techniques.

Once anesthesia has been induced and IV access has been obtained, many providers apply a vasoconstrictor to both nostrils, such as oxymetazoline to reduce the risk of poor visualization due to blood in the airway. Oxymetazoline, a topical sympathomimetic causes direct vasoconstriction via its direct effect on alpha-adrenergic receptors. Positioning of the bottle in the inverted position can lead to inadvertent overdose, as it is designed to be administered in the upright position and deliver a fine mist of medication.[22] Options for administration of oxymetazoline include transferring to a tuberculin syringe and administering via an atomizer device or soaking a cotton swab and gently placing in the nares for approximately 30 seconds. Once the nares have been appropriately decongested, the next step is to place a lubricated nasopharyngeal airway into the nare intended for placement of the ETT. Confirm the OD of the first nasopharyngeal airway is smaller than the ETT selected.[17] If the nasopharyngeal airway does not pass easily, try the other nostril. Prior to placement of the ETT, attempt to pass a nasopharyngeal airway that has an OD the same as, or larger, than that of the intended ETT. Although this step is not always performed, it is a good indicator of how easily the tube will pass through the nasal cavity. Due to the friability and narrowed nasal passages, it may be helpful to select a cuffed ETT that is a half-size smaller than the age-appropriate ETT, keeping in mind that a smaller tube will also be shorter.[17]

Depending on the technique selected, placement of the nasal ETT will vary. If a DL or VL technique is chosen, insert the ETT bevel facing medially into the nare in a downward direction. The tip of the ETT should move along the nasal septum to avoid causing trauma to the nasal turbinates. If resistance is encountered, withdraw and rotate the ETT. Some gentle force may be required to advance the tube, but caution should be exercised as too much force can create a false passage, causing major trauma.[17] Once the tip of the tube has been advanced into the oropharynx, a laryngoscope or video laryngoscope may be inserted into the mouth. Perform DL or VL, per normal procedure, to obtain a view of the glottis. Once an adequate view is attained, use Magill forceps to advance the ETT toward and through the vocal cords, being careful not to damage the cuff of the ETT. It can also be helpful to have a second provider administer gentle pressure on the proximal end of the ETT as it is being advanced through the vocal cords with Magill forceps.

If flexible bronchoscopy is the chosen strategy, nasal technique resembles that of an oral bronchoscope intubation. A jaw thrust can be helpful in obtaining a good view of the glottis. As with oral intubation, nasal intubation can cause some noteworthy complications, with epistaxis being the most common complication. The nasal cavity is prone to bleeding, which is why the use of a nasal vasoconstrictor, a smaller ETT, and lubricant is an important step to take when performing nasal intubation. Other notable complications are sinusitis, edema, which can lead to middle ear issues, and superficial necrosis, usually seen in long-term intubations.[23] Nasal intubation is contraindicated in the presence of suspected epiglottitis, midface instability, coagulopathy, and suspected basilar skull fractures.[24] If flexible bronchoscopic nasal intubation is required due to trauma, it may be more difficult due to swollen and friable tissues.

Rapid-Sequence Intubation
Rapid-sequence intubation (RSI) becomes necessary when there is risk of aspiration of a foreign body or gastric contents prior to securing an airway. For an RSI, planning and preparation are key. Ensure necessary equipment for the initial airway plan and a backup plan, such as VL, are available and ready. Multiple sizes of equipment should be open and accessible. The use of a cuffed ETT is indicated for RSI airway management, as the cuff may help protect the lungs from aspiration. Functioning suction should be readily available as the risk of aspiration is high and the need to quickly clear the airway may become necessary. Prior to performing an RSI, IV access must be established prior to induction. Once IV patency has been confirmed, begin preoxygenation. Preoxygenation is a vital step in this process, as it helps to prevent rapid desaturation during intubation and avoidance of positive pressure ventilation. Children often do not tolerate the mask for complete preoxygenation, and this step is cut short due to lack of patient cooperation. Careful and judicious premedication with anxiolytic medications as appropriate for patient condition can facilitate preoxygenation. Atropine may be used as a premedication as well, as desaturation and use of succinylcholine can precipitate bradycardia, particularly in infants and small children.[25]

Induction of anesthesia for an RSI requires an IV induction agent (such as propofol, ketamine, or etomidate), followed immediately by IV succinylcholine. If succinylcholine is contraindicated, the use of high-dose IV rocuronium may be administered.[25] Cricoid pressure, or a Sellick maneuver, is performed just prior to induction. Appropriate pressure should prevent aspiration by way of compressing the esophagus. The use of cricoid pressure, however, has been debated in recent years. It can distort anatomy and make for less-than-ideal intubating conditions. If performed too early, cricoid pressure can cause emesis and lead to aspiration. If the pressure exerted is too much, it can compress the trachea, hindering intubation.[26] When utilized, however, it should not be released until after end-tidal CO_2 is confirmed.

MANAGEMENT OF A PATIENT WITH A TRACHEOSTOMY

At times, it may be necessary to anesthetize an infant or child with a tracheostomy. A cuffed tracheostomy tube is preferred to provide effective positive pressure ventilation. If an uncuffed tracheostomy tube is in place, consider exchanging to a cuffed tracheostomy tube or ETT, standard or reinforced, both one-half size smaller. When exchange necessitates insertion of a different brand, note that the OD may be larger, even with a smaller size, making placement difficult or impossible. Ensure multiple sizes are available. Be sure that the stoma is healed prior to exchange; the incidence of airway complications, such as a false track, is greatest in the first week of creation. It should also be noted that reinsertion of a tracheostomy tube or ETT is not always smooth with a mature stoma.[26] This highlights the importance of preparedness with multiple-sized tubes and ensuring the availability of an obturator.

DIFFICULT AIRWAY MANAGEMENT

Pediatric patients with a difficult airway differ from their adult counterparts in numerous ways. The risk factors, physical features, and management techniques of a pediatric difficult airway are unique and require a refined skill set specific to the age group. *Difficult airway* can be defined in a variety of ways but is generally understood to mean a patient with difficult laryngeal exposure via conventional DL who may also be difficult to ventilate with a bag mask. Hypoxemia is the leading cause of anesthesia-related morbidity and mortality in children, so management of difficult airways and the surrounding events influences outcomes for these children.[27,28]

PREVALENCE AND PREDICTORS OF DIFFICULT PEDIATRIC AIRWAY

The majority of factors associated with difficult airway are observable and measurable preoperatively allowing the clinician to plan ahead. Benchmarking research from the Pediatric Difficult Intubation Registry (PeDI Registry) suggests that approximately 2 to 5 in 1,000 pediatric intubations are difficult, with 80% of those being anticipated in advance.[27] Micrognathia, or short thyromental distance, is the most common physical examination finding in infants

Table 6.4	Congenital Abnormalities Associated With Pediatric Difficult Airway	
Congenital Abnormality	**Associated Syndrome**	
Maxillary/mandibular hypoplasia	• Achondroplasia • Apert syndrome • CHARGE syndrome • Cornelia de Lange syndrome • Cri du chat syndrome • Crouzon syndrome • DiGeorge syndrome • Goldenhar syndrome • Hallermann Streiff syndrome	• Moebius syndrome • Pierre–Robin sequence • Pfeiffer syndrome • Saethre–Chotzen syndrome • Smith–Lemli–Opitz syndrome • Stickler syndrome • Treacher Collins syndrome • Turner syndrome
Subglottic abnormalities	• Laryngeal web • Laryngocele • Laryngomalacia	• Subglottic stenosis • Tracheal stenosis • Tracheomalacia
Large tongue	• Beckwith–Wiedemann syndrome • Congenital hypothyroidism	• Hemangioma • Trisomy 21
Abnormalities of the entire airway	• Epidermolysis bullosa • Mucopolysaccharidoses	
Limited mouth opening	• Freeman–Sheldon syndrome	
Limited neck mobility	• Achondroplasia • Arthrogryposis	• Klippel–Feil syndrome • Noonan syndrome

Source: From Burjek NE. The difficult pediatric airway. In: Jagannathan N, Fiadjoe JE, eds. *Management of the Difficult Pediatric Airway.* Cambridge University Press; 2020:8–19; and Fiadjoe JE, Litman RS, Server JF, et al. The pediatric airway. In: Cote CJ, Lerman J, Anderson B, eds. *A Practice of Anesthesia for Infants and Children, Sixth Edition.* Saunders-Elsevier; 2019:297–339.

who are difficult to intubate.[2] The most important predictors of difficult intubation in a pediatric patient are an age younger than 1 year old and a weight less than 10 kg.[2] Difficult intubation is also associated with American Society of Anesthesiologists (ASA) Physical Status Classification III or IV and smaller body habitus.[29] Additional predictive factors include ICU admission, obesity, the presence of a craniofacial syndrome with associated facial dysmorphia, and presentation for cardiac, oromaxillofacial, or otolaryngologic surgery.[2,30]

CONGENITAL AND ACQUIRED AIRWAY ABNORMALITIES

Conditions associated with a difficult pediatric airway can be divided into congenital and acquired abnormalities of the airway as outlined in Table 6.4 and Box 6.2, respectively. The congenital abnormalities consist of syndromes and congenital physical malformations. While these syndromes are rare, patients with these diagnoses often present with a multitude of procedures requiring anesthesia throughout their lifetime. The acquired conditions are often found in otherwise healthy children and are typically the grounds for their presentation to the healthcare arena. Many of these conditions progress rapidly and require early expert airway management to provide ventilatory support, airway protection, and preparation for surgical intervention.[2]

DIFFICULT AIRWAY ANESTHESIA INDUCTION

Anesthesia induction for the patient with a difficult airway aims to preserve spontaneous ventilation until the success of bag-mask ventilation can be confirmed. In a difficult airway that is anticipated, it is recommended to obtain IV access preoperatively regardless of the anesthesia induction technique.[31] Small doses of IV induction agents and/or inhalation induction agent can preserve spontaneous ventilation throughout the induction process. Once successful bag-mask ventilation has been established,

> **BOX 6.2 ACQUIRED ABNORMALITIES ASSOCIATED WITH DIFFICULT PEDIATRIC AIRWAY**
>
> • Adenoid and tonsillar hypertrophy
> • Airway masses and tumors
> • Airway trauma and burns
> • Anaphylaxis
> • Cervical spine immobility or instability
> • Infections: epiglottitis, croup
> • Juvenile rheumatoid arthritis
> • Peritonsillar abscess
> • Postintubation edema/granuloma/stenosis
> • Presence of foreign body
> • Vascular ring
>
> *Source:* From Burjek NE. The difficult pediatric airway. In: Jagannathan N, Fiadjoe JE, eds. *Management for the Difficult Pediatric Airway.* Cambridge University Press; 2020:8–19; and Fiadjoe JE, Litman RS, Server JF, et al. The pediatric airway. In: Cote CJ, Lerman J, Anderson B, eds. *A Practice of Anesthesia for Infants and Children, Sixth Edition.* Saunders-Elsevier; 2019:297–339.

there is a choice to preserve spontaneous ventilation throughout airway manipulation or control ventilation via anesthesia depth or muscle paralysis with nondepolarizing muscle relaxants (NDMRs). Spontaneous ventilation has traditionally been viewed as the safest option as it can help to maintain oxygen saturation and airway tone. However, the PeDI Registry found no difference in severe complications (i.e., cardiac arrest, severe airway trauma, aspiration, and death) between spontaneous and controlled ventilation during intubation.[32] Nonsevere complications (i.e., mild hypoxia, minor airway trauma, and laryngospasm) were higher in the spontaneous ventilation group.[32] The drawback to having a spontaneously breathing patient is the risk of light anesthesia as a contributing factor to difficult airway management. It should also be noted that there are patient populations that should never receive NDMRs. These include patients with large head and neck masses, mediastinal tumors, profuse airway bleeding, and poor tissue compliance. If an aminosteroid-based neuromuscular blocker is used during difficult airway management, ensure sugammadex is readily available. Sugammadex is a newer drug that offers immediate reversal of aminosteroid-based neuromuscular blockers and has been used to emergently rescue from neuromuscular blockade (16 mg/kg). There are limited data in the pediatric population, but there has been favorable experience with the use of sugammadex in children and neonates.[33]

DIFFICULT BAG-MASK VENTILATION

While difficult tracheal intubation is an important part of difficult airway management, DBMV may go under appreciated. In fact, the PeDI Registry found no association between DBMV and difficult tracheal intubation.[27] In healthy children, the following factors have been associated with DBMV: ear, nose and throat (ENT) surgery, the use of neuromuscular blocking agents, and obesity.[30,34] Obesity should be given special attention, particularly in otherwise healthy older children, as a risk factor for perioperative adverse respiratory events, specifically intraoperative hypoxemia, difficult mask ventilation, and bronchospasm.[30]

When faced with DBMV, it is important to distinguish between anatomical/mechanical versus functional airway obstruction as the interventions differ depending on the cause.[35] Anatomical/mechanical airway obstruction is generally caused by improper patient positioning and oropharyngeal obstruction.[35] The source of functional airway obstruction can be above or below the glottis and is commonly caused by insufficient depth of anesthesia, laryngospasm, opioid-induced glottic closure, or bronchospasm.[35] Functional airway obstruction is often relieved with pharmacologic interventions. Tables 6.5 and 6.6 show the different causes of airway obstruction and their treatment.

OXYGENATION STRATEGIES

During management of the difficult airway, providers should deliver supplemental oxygen throughout the process of airway management. Preoxygenation, apneic oxygenation, and transnasal humidified rapid insufflation ventilatory exchange (THRIVE) are three strategies that can be used to prolong the safe apneic oxygenation period postinduction to allow for more time to safely establish a secure airway. The goal of preoxygenation is to increase oxygen reserve in the lungs and increase the duration of apnea without desaturation. While this practice is routine in adult airway management guidelines, it is not often a realistic option in children who are uncooperative. Judicious administration of an anxiolytic medication, however, may help overcome anxiety potentially improving compliance in the anxious child. Preoxygenation is effectively achieved with tidal volume breathing of 100% oxygen via a sealed facemask for 3 minutes or eight deep breaths of 100% oxygen with a goal of end-tidal oxygen concentration of 90%.[36] It should be noted that even with preoxygenation, the onset of oxygen desaturation is age-dependent, with neonates desaturating more rapidly due to their unique respiratory physiology.

Apneic Oxygenation

Apneic oxygenation is the act of delivering oxygen to an apneic patient. During apnea, blood absorbs oxygen from the functional residual capacity faster than the outflow of carbon dioxide. This ultimately produces a negative pressure gradient of 20 cmH$_2$O allowing oxygen to continue to flow from the upper airways to the alveoli.[36] Oxygen can be provided to the patient via nasal cannula, face mask, or an ETT placed in the oropharynx. Using this technique in conjunction with preoxygenation has shown to increase the duration of apnea without desaturation.[36] An important limitation of apneic oxygenation is the steady increase of carbon dioxide that occurs without ventilation for extended periods. This can

Table 6.5	Causes and Treatment of Anatomical and Mechanical Airway Obstruction
Causes	**Treatment**
Poor mask technique	Head tilt, chin lift, jaw thrust, two-hand/two-person mask ventilation
Inadequate head position	Repositioning, placement of shoulder roll
Large adenoids/tonsils/pharyngeal obstruction	Oropharyngeal/nasopharyngeal airway, SGA placement
Blood/foreign body/secretions	Suction, removal, antisialagogue

SGA, supraglottic airway.

Source: From Engelhardt T, Machotta A. Universal algorithms and approaches to airway management. In Jagannathan N, Fiadjoe JE, eds. *Management for the Difficult Pediatric Airway.* 2020;20–25. Cambridge University Press.

Table 6.6	Causes and Treatment of Functional Airway Obstruction
Causes	**Treatment**
Inadequate anesthesia	Deepen anesthesia—increase inhaled volatile anesthetic gas, administer IV medications such as propofol, benzodiazepines, and/or narcotics
Laryngospasm	Jaw thrust, positive pressure, and muscle relaxant
Muscle rigidity	Muscle relaxant
Bronchospasm	Deepen anesthesia (sevoflurane and ketamine) inhaled beta-2 agonists, IV/IM beta-2 agonists, such as epinephrine and terbutaline, and IV steroids

Source: From Engelhardt T, Machotta A. Universal algorithms and approaches to airway management. In Jagannathan N, Fiadjoe JE,. eds. *Management for the Difficult Pediatric Airway.* Cambridge University Press; 2020;20–25.

result in hypercapnia and severe respiratory acidosis, which can ultimately lead to arrythmias and cardiac arrest.

High-Flow Nasal Cannula

THRIVE is an oxygenation technique that uses rapidly insufflated, heated, humidified gases administered via a high-flow nasal cannula (HFNC) to achieve apneic oxygenation and ventilation.[37] HFNC provides oxygen at flow rates higher than the patient's inspiratory flow demands and creates a distending alveolar pressure of up to 7 cmH$_2$O, which prevents airway collapse and atelectasis.[37] The fraction of inspired oxygen can be titrated from 0.21 to 1, and flows can be titrated up to 2 L/kg/min with 60 L/min typically being the maximum amount of flow. While THRIVE prolongs the safe apnea time in healthy children, it is a form of apneic oxygenation and therefore has no effect on carbon dioxide clearance, which is a limiting factor in its use.[28] Complications related to THRIVE are rare and include abdominal distention, pneumothorax, pneumomediastinum, and pneumocephalus. To provide protection against excessive lung distention and barotrauma, the nasal prongs should not exceed more than 50% of the nasal diameter to allow for air egress.[36] A patent upper airway is required for THRIVE to be effective, so this is not a rescue technique for the cannot intubate cannot ventilate situation.

ANTICIPATED DIFFICULT AIRWAY MANAGEMENT

When a difficult airway is anticipated, as is the case for the majority of difficult pediatric airways, the clinician has time to optimize the patient and develop a safe anesthesia plan including the type of anesthesia, anesthesia induction technique, and the airway instrumentation method. While tracheal intubation is usually easily accomplished by conventional DL in the pediatric population, difficult airway management requires the expertise and advanced skill set of an experienced pediatric anesthesia provider. When difficulty is anticipated, decreasing the number of attempts to intubate can decrease the overall risk of harm. It has been demonstrated that greater than two tracheal intubation attempts and greater than three DL attempts before transitioning to an indirect technique are both associated with an increased risk of airway complications.[2]

SGA devices, flexible bronchoscopy, and VL are the three main tools that the anesthesia provider can utilize, alone or in combination with one another, to successfully intubate the difficult pediatric airway. Table 6.7 provides a comparison of the pros and cons of flexible bronchoscopy and VL. Other options for intubation management include the use of transillumination via optical stylets and light-guided equipment, intubating bougies, and rigid bronchoscopes.

Flexible Bronchoscopy

Flexible bronchoscopy for placement of an ETT can be used in patients with a difficult airway. For details about this technique, refer to the flexible bronchoscopy section earlier in the chapter. Difficult airway management requires increased skill with the flexible bronchoscope and utilization of other adjuncts to increase the probability of success.

Flexible Bronchoscopy via Supraglottic Airway

The role of the SGA device in routine airway management and in difficult airway algorithms is well established. In addition to being a potential lifesaving device in patients who are difficult to mask ventilate, the SGA device can be used as a conduit for tracheal intubation. Overall, the use of a flexible or fiberoptic bronchoscope for intubation via supraglottic

Table 6.7	Indirect Intubation Techniques
Fiberoptic Intubation	**Video Laryngoscopy**
Pros	Pros
• Useful in limited mouth opening • Nasal or oral • Can be used with SGA	• Easy-to-acquire skill • Portable • Panoramic magnified view • Proven efficacy in difficult airway
Cons	Cons
• Steep learning curve—technically difficult • Expensive • Suboptimal view with blood and secretions • No suction port of pediatric fiberoptic bronchoscopes	• Moderate degree of mouth opening needed • View can be obstructed by blood or secretions • Time to intubate can be longer than direct laryngoscopy

SGA, supraglottic airway.

airway (FOI-SGA) and VL have similar rates of first-attempt success in difficult airways. In children younger than 1 year old, FOI-SGA is more successful than VL with fewer intubation attempts.[2] There is no difference in complication rates for flexible bronchoscopy or FOI versus VL techniques.[2]

The most commonly used intubating SGA device is the air-Q. It was designed with many unique features that make it suitable for SGA device tracheal intubation, which are illustrated in Table 6.8. The LMA Classic can also be used as an intubating device but is limited by its length, which makes it challenging to remove the LMA without dislodging the ETT, the presence of aperture bars that must be cut to fit an ETT through the SGA, and the airway connector that is not wide enough to accommodate a pilot balloon of a cuffed ETT.[38] The steps of FOI-SGA device are outlined in Box 6.3. It is important to use an appropriately sized flexible bronchoscope. If the bronchoscope is too small, it increases the risk of the ETT getting caught on the posterior arytenoids rather than advancing into the trachea. If the view of the larynx is not optimal, visualization can be improved with a jaw thrust, head and neck extension, and/or advancement or withdrawal of the SGA device.[38] It is not recommended to perform a blind intubation through an SGA device as there is a high incidence of epiglottic downfolding, which could lead to laryngeal trauma or esophageal intubation. Hypoxemia is less common during FOI-SGA when continuous ventilation is used during intubation attempts.[39] The technique to provide continuous ventilation during FOI-SGA is outlined in Box 6.4 and illustrated in Figure 6.11.

A novel technique for intubation in neonates, particularly those in which bag-mask ventilation will be of uncertain success, as in the case of Pierre–Robin sequence, is the placement of awake SGA. Neonates tolerate awake SGA device placement well. Infants with an intact gag reflex require topicalization of their oropharynx to tolerate awake SGA placement. This can be achieved with 2% lidocaine via a gloved finger or with viscous lidocaine applied directly to the SGA device.[38] After the SGA device is placed, the anesthesia provider has the option to proceed with an awake flexible bronchoscopy or FOI or to induce anesthesia with sevoflurane in a spontaneously breathing patient.

Table 6.8 Beneficial Features of air-Q® for SGA Device-Assisted Tracheal Intubation

Feature	Benefit
Oval-shaped mask with ridges	Improves the seal of the cuff in oropharynx
Removable 15-mm circuit adapter	Eliminates the narrowest portion of the device
Raised mask heal near the ventilating orifice	Prevents epiglottic obstruction of the airway tube
Wide shaft	Able to accommodate a larger tracheal tube
Shorter shaft	Improves ease of removal of SGA device after successful tracheal intubation

SGA, supraglottic airway.

Source: From Olomu PN, Hsu G, Lockman JL. Hybrid approaches to the difficult pediatric airway. In Jagannathan N, Fiadjoe JE, eds. *Management for the Difficult Pediatric Airway.* 2020;118–128. Cambridge University Press.

BOX 6.4 FOI-SGA TECHNIQUE WITH CONTINUOUS VENTILATION

- Remove 15 mm circuit adapter from the SGA device.
- Partially insert an appropriately sized lubricated cuffed endotracheal tube into the shaft of the SGA device.
- Inflate the endotracheal tube cuff, creating a seal.
- Attach a bronchoscope swivel adapter to the proximal end of the endotracheal tube.
- Perform tracheal intubation via fiberoptic bronchoscope while maintaining ventilation.
- Deflate the endotracheal tube cuff and advance into the trachea.

Source: From Olomu PN, Hsu G, Lockman JL. Hybrid approaches to the difficult pediatric airway. In: Jagannathan N, Fiadjoe JE, eds. *Management for the Difficult Pediatric Airway.* Cambridge University Press; 2020;118–128.

FOI-SGA, fiberoptic intubation-supraglottic airway.

BOX 6.3 PROCEDURAL STEPS FOR FIBEROPTIC INTUBATION VIA SGA

- Place appropriately sized SGA.
- Disconnect anesthesia circuit from SGA and remove 15-mm circuit adapter (if using air-Q®).
- Insert fiberoptic bronchoscope loaded with an appropriately sized endotracheal tube with cuff deflated through SGA.
- Advance the fiberoptic scope past the vocal cords until carina is visualized.
- Advance the endotracheal tube and confirm placement via bronchoscopy.
- Remove the bronchoscope carefully, attach the circuit to the endotracheal tube, ventilate the patient, and further confirm placement via end tidal carbon dioxide and auscultation.
- To remove the SGA, disconnect the tracheal tube from the anesthesia circuit.
- Remove the 15-mm circuit adapter on the endotracheal tube.
- Insert the disposable air-Q® removal stylet, laryngeal forceps, the fiberoptic bronchoscope, or an airway exchange catheter into the proximal end of the endotracheal tube to stabilize it.
- Withdraw the SGA.
- Reconnect the 15-mm circuit adapter to the endotracheal tube and connect to the anesthesia circuit.
- Reconfirm endotracheal tube placement with fiberoptic bronchoscopy.

Source: From Olomu PN, Hsu G, Lockman JL. Hybrid approaches to the difficult pediatric airway. In: Jagannathan N, Fiadjoe JE, eds. *Management for the Difficult Pediatric Airway.* Cambridge University; 2020: 118–128.

SGA, supraglottic airway.

Video Laryngoscopy

VL for placement of an ETT can be used in patients with difficult airway. For details about this technique, refer to VL section earlier in the chapter. Difficult airway management requires increased skill with the VL, including using it in conjunction with a flexible bronchoscope and other adjuncts to facilitate intubation.

Video Laryngoscopy–Assisted Flexible Bronchoscopic Intubation

VL-assisted flexible bronchoscopy or FOI is a valuable skill that can be utilized in difficult airway management. The combination of these two devices maximizes individual advantages of each and has been shown to improve intubation success rates in patients with a difficult airway.[38] VLs have a wide-angle view (40–80 degrees) and provide a magnified, indirect image of the glottis. Flexible bronchoscopes have a narrow-angle view and can be used as a controllable and maneuverable stylet. Additionally, the VL displaces soft tissue and provides an oropharyngeal pathway for the flexible bronchoscope. This

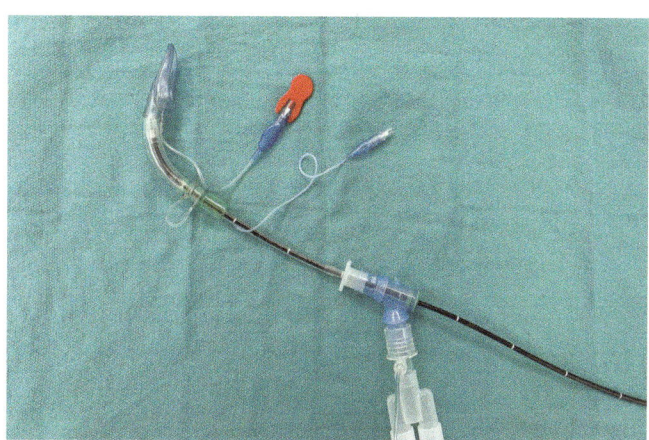

Figure 6.11: Continuous ventilation setup for FOI-SGA.
FOI-SGA, fiberoptic intubation-supraglottic airway.

> **BOX 6.5 VIDEO LARYNGOSCOPY–ASSISTED FIBEROPTIC INTUBATION PROCEDURAL STEPS**
>
> - Preload the fiberoptic scope with the appropriately sized endotracheal tube.
> - Select the appropriate video laryngoscope blade based on patient size.
> - Perform gentle video laryngoscopy.
> - After the best possible view is obtained, move the video laryngoscope blade slightly left of midline.
> - Insert the fiberoptic scope into the mouth towards the glottic opening, past the vocal cords and into the trachea.
> - Advance the endotracheal tube into the trachea with video laryngoscopic guidance ensuring that the endotracheal tube does not get caught on the arytenoids.
> - Confirm final endotracheal tube placement with fiberoptic bronchoscope, end-tidal carbon dioxide and bilateral breath sounds.
>
> *Source:* From Olomu PN, Hsu G, Lockman JL. Hybrid approaches to the difficult pediatric airway. In Jagannathan N, Fiadjoe JE, eds. *Management for the Difficult Pediatric Airway.* Cambridge Unversity Press; 2020:118–128.

technique is particularly valuable when rescuing a failed intubation that has been attempted with a VL or flexible bronchoscope alone, in patients with a fixed or unstable cervical spine, or during a tracheal tube exchange in a patient with a known difficult airway.

The technique for intubating with VL-assisted flexible bronchoscope or FOI is outlined in **Box 6.5**. It is important to have a second anesthesia provider to perform this technique as it is essential to have another set of skilled hands to operate either the VL or the flexible bronchoscope. If difficult ventilation is anticipated, moderate to deep sedation with airway topicalization should be considered. It is imperative to avoid airway trauma as bleeding and secretions can render both the VL and flexible bronchoscope unusable. To prevent glare, the brightness of the flexible bronchoscope may need to be reduced when the scope is in the oropharynx with the VL. The flexible bronchoscope should never be advanced blindly as this can lead to bleeding and airway trauma.[38]

UNANTICIPATED DIFFICULT AIRWAY

When presented with an unanticipated difficult airway, it is important for the anesthesia provider to remain calm and methodical. The first step is to call for help and notify other medical and nursing staff in the room of the difficulty in airway management. Using a difficult airway algorithm can help provide optimum care by following a stepwise, evidence-based approach. As long as the patient can be oxygenated via bag-mask ventilation, there is time to think carefully and create a stepwise plan for success. Depending on practice setting (surgery center, gastroenterology clinic, etc.), it may be prudent to emerge the patient from anesthesia and create a plan for safe management of the difficult airway in a controlled setting in which all advanced instrumentation equipment and additional personnel are available. As discussed earlier, multiple unsuccessful attempts are unwise and harmful and can lead to an escalating situation.

DIFFICULT AIRWAY ALGORITHM

In the event of an airway crisis, a pediatric patient can rapidly deteriorate becoming hypoxic and bradycardic within seconds. A pediatric difficult airway algorithm and the tools to successfully carry out the algorithm must be readily available to prevent significant morbidity and mortality. Pediatric airway algorithms are relatively new in comparison with well-established adult difficult airway algorithms. There are numerous different pediatric airway algorithms from various pediatric and airway societies around the world. **Figure 6.12** illustrates a practical algorithm for the anticipated and unanticipated difficult airway. Important characteristics of a chosen algorithm include simple and intuitive, easy to memorize and practice, and applicable to all situations.[35] Two important commonalities amongst the algorithms include calling for help immediately and limiting the number of attempts at laryngoscopy.[31] Emergency front of the neck airway, such as a cricothyrotomy, is a last resort solution to rescue a scenario where oxygenation/ventilation is not possible.[35] It should only be performed if otolaryngology is not available to perform a tracheostomy or rigid bronchoscopy as success rates for anesthesia providers performing either scalpel cricothyrotomy or cannula cricothyrotomy are extremely poor and especially challenging in smaller pediatric patients.[31]

EXTUBATION

Extubation, or removal of the ETT, is elective and concludes nearly all anesthetics. Plans for extubation should be considered during anesthesia planning and further evaluated after tube securement.[3] Unique conditions must be considered when extubating the pediatric patient. The anesthesia provider must understand criteria for the varying pediatric patients. Deep versus awake extubation techniques should be based on the patient, anesthesia provider, and surgical procedure. Experience plays an important role in management of a successful extubation. Planning for extubation requires consideration of neuromuscular blockade, analgesics, and other sedation medications.[40] Positioning, temperature, hemodynamic stability, and metabolic state should all be optimized to facilitate successful extubation.[40] Readiness of extubation can be assessed by confirmation of strength verified by objective means (e.g., train-of-four monitoring), a return of regular spontaneous ventilation and respiratory efforts, adequacy of tidal volumes, a return of protective airway reflexes, a capacity to manage secretions, and the ability to maintain oxygenation. Following antagonism of neuromuscular blockade, strength can be demonstrated by cough and achieving acceptable tidal volumes.[3] In infants, strength can be confirmed by hip flexion.[40] Brow furrowing and nonauditory crying both also express a readiness to extubate.

The anesthesia provider should be aware that airway dynamics may be altered postprocedure due to possible trauma from airway instrumentation, secretions, fluid shifts, and potential for respiratory compromise related to anesthesia medications. The surgical procedure itself may also directly affect the airway. In this case, discussion with the surgeon and careful consideration of immediate postsurgical airway changes should be assessed before extubation is attempted. The anesthesia provider should be prepared to emergently reinstrument the airway if the patient is unable to meet the goals of oxygenation and ventilation after extubation. It is

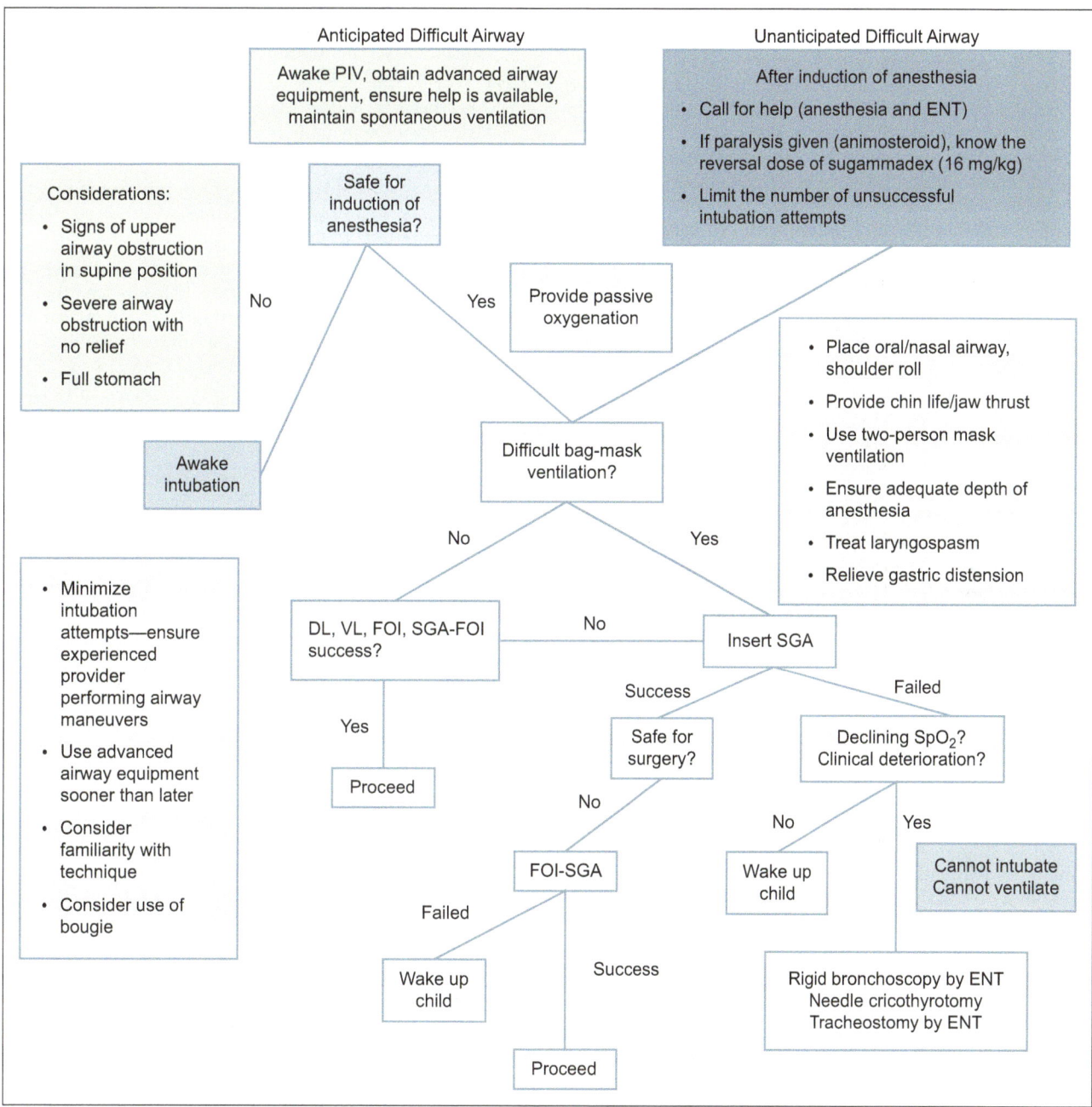

Figure 6.12: Difficult airway algorithm.

DL, direct laryngoscopy; FOI, fiberoptic intubation;

Source: From Huang AS, Hajduk J, Rim C, Coffield S, Jagannathan N. Focused review on management of the difficult paediatric airway. *Indian J Anaesth.* 2019; 63(6):428–436. doi: 10.4103/ija.IJA_250_19.

essential to have the equipment needed to perform successful bag-mask ventilation and tracheal intubation immediately available. This is important at the time of planned extubation and for the duration of an anesthetic in the untoward event of accidental extubation. As with any extubation, one must be prepared to manage the airway if complications arise (e.g., desaturation, obstruction, apnea, laryngospasm, and bronchospasm). Postextubation obstruction, specifically subglottic edema, is one of the more common complications following extubation of the pediatric airway.[41] Prior to transport to either the postanesthesia recovery unit or the ICU, adequate ventilation, oxygenation, a patent airway, and sufficient respiratory efforts should be confirmed.[3]

Extubation of the Patient With a Difficult Airway

In children with difficult tracheal intubation, special consideration should be taken with regard to safe extubation practices. The majority of anesthesia providers would agree that children with a difficult airway should be extubated awake, once spontaneous ventilation, sufficient muscle strength, and appropriate airway reflexes have returned with the goals of extubation being to maintain adequate oxygenation and ventilation.[42] If the preceding criteria are unable to be met, the anesthesia provider should have a low threshold to keep the child intubated, with a plan to extubate at a later time with anesthesia and otolaryngology surgical assistance if necessary.

When preparing to extubate the child with a difficult airway, it is important to follow the same basic principles of positioning, neuromuscular blockade reversal, pain control, maintenance of normothermia, and optimization of cardiovascular, neurological and metabolic status that are routinely followed for the patient with a nondifficult airway.[40] Additionally, alveolar recruitment maneuvers may be helpful as well as continuous oxygenation via nasal cannula or HFNC placed prior to extubation or immediately after extubation.[40] Prior to an extubation attempt, the entire surgical care team should be aware of the plan of action if extubation is not successful.

Airway exchange catheters are a valuable tool designed to maintain a guide to reintubate a patient with a difficult airway while allowing for oxygenation via a face mask or nasal cannula. The smallest airway exchange catheter is the Cook airway exchange catheter and is 2.7 mm (8 Fr) in diameter.[40] This technique is more practical in slightly older or larger children, while small infants may not have the luminal capacity for these catheters.

Several medications serve a variety of roles in the anesthetic care and extubation plan for children with difficult airways. Small infants and those whose airway required significant and perhaps traumatic manipulation for tracheal intubation are at risk of airway swelling and postextubation croup. The administration of dexamethasone IV after airway manipulation can help reduce airway swelling. Racemic epinephrine nebulizer applied immediately postextubation can also help reduce airway swelling and potential stridor. Medications such as remifentanil and dexmedetomidine can be used as infusions designed to smooth emergence and allow for assessment of suitability for extubation without causing distress or coughing and gagging on the ETT. The use of caffeine citrate in preterm infants can reduce the risk of apnea and improve extubation conditions. As appropriate, the use of regional anesthesia will allow the safe reduction in narcotic pain medications, which can lower respiratory drive and delay extubation.

Clinical circumstances are dynamic; thus, there is no standard approach for the management of all pediatric airways. How the anesthesia provider ultimately decides to approach the airway is dependent on individual patient disease, review of successful and unsuccessful airway attempts from previous anesthetic records, available equipment and drugs, and comfort with available airway tools.

KEY TAKEAWAYS

- A careful preanesthetic evaluation and clinical assessment are the pillars of pediatric airway management.
- Unanticipated difficult airway in pediatrics is rare.
- Syndromes are commonly associated with difficult airway.
- Age younger than 1 year, weight less than 10 kg, and mandibular hypoplasia are the three main features that correlate with difficult airway in children.
- Preparedness and availability of properly sized airway equipment are paramount in the safe administration of pediatric anesthesia.
- Anesthesia providers should be familiar with the pediatric airway management equipment their institution provides.
- Mask management, one of the most important airway skills, can be complex in pediatrics. Multiple strategies can be used to optimize mask management.
- Supraglottic airways are safe in children of all ages and sizes. They have a lower failure rate in children than adults and can be used as a primary airway instrumentation technique as well as a conduit to intubation.
- Appropriate endotracheal tube leak is 20 to 25 cmH$_2$O. An oversized endotracheal tube can cause airway complications, such as edema, postextubation croup, and, in worse cases, tracheal stenosis.
- A skilled and experienced anesthesia provider should be present for pediatric difficult airway management. Familiarity with difficult airway algorithms is paramount.
- When faced with a difficult airway, it is vital to call for help immediately and to limit the number of attempts at laryngoscopy.
- Extubation of the difficult airway should be done in a controlled setting, with an airway exchange device if possible. Advanced airway equipment should be present in the room, particularly the technique that was used to successfully intubate the patient.

KEY REFERENCES

Complete references for this chapter are online and available at https://connect.springerpub.com/content/book/978-0-8261-3875-0/part/part02/toc-part/ch006.

3. Fiadjoe JE, Litman RS, Server JF, et al. The pediatric airway. In Cote CJ, Lerman J, Anderson B, eds *A Practice of Anesthesia for Infants and Children, Sixth Edition*. Saunders-Elsevier. 2019:297–339

7. Huang AS, Sarver A, Widing A, et al. The design of the perfect pediatric supraglottic airway device. *Paediatr Anaesth*. 2020;30(3):280–287. doi:10.1111/pan.13785

10. Jagannathan N, Ramsey MA, White MC, Sohn L. An update on newer pediatric supraglottic airways with recommendations for clinical use. *Paediatr Anaesth*. 2015;25(4):334–345. doi:10.1111/pan.12614

27. Fiadjoe JE, Nishisaki A, Jagannathan, N, et al. Airway management complications in children with difficult tracheal intubation from the Pediatric Difficult Intubation (PeDI) registry: a prospective cohort analysis. *Lancet Respir Med*. 2016;4(1):37–48. doi:10.1016/S2213-2600(15)00508-1

38. Olomu PN, Hsu G, Lockman JL. Hybrid approaches to the difficult pediatric airway. In: Jagannathan N, Fiadjoe JE, eds. *Management for the Difficult Pediatric Airway*. Cambridge University Press; 2020:118–128.

CHAPTER 7

Ventilation Management

Saundra L. Smalley

LEARNING OBJECTIVES

- Define tidal volume and anticipated normal values.
- Understand normal respiratory rates in different-age pediatric patients.
- Define inspiratory-to-expiratory (I:E) ratio.
- Understand different ventilation modes.
- Discuss the rationale for dead-space reduction.
- Discuss the difference between intensive care unit (ICU) ventilators and anesthesia machine ventilators.

INTRODUCTION

One of the most important aspects of anesthesia practice is managing the patient's airway, which includes ventilation while under general anesthesia. Ventilation is not only important for maintaining oxygenation but also key in eliminating carbon dioxide (CO_2) as well. Ultimately, anesthesia providers are charged with maintaining adequate ventilation while anesthetizing any patient as hypoventilation can lead to decreased oxygenation, as well as an excess of CO_2 leading to respiratory acidosis. There are many approaches to ensuring adequate ventilation, with different modes and ventilation strategies readily available to ensure the delivery of safe, effective care to the patient during the surgical procedure.

Anesthesia providers must also consider the influence of developmental differences between the adult and pediatric patients when considering ventilation. Pulmonary maturation continues through 8 years of age. During this period, there is significant variance that impacts ventilation. Infants and children have far fewer alveoli compared to adults, with the size of each individual alveolus being much smaller in children. This markedly decreases the surface area available for a gas exchange. As the patient grows, the airways enlarge both in length and diameter. This growth, however, lags behind that of the proximal airways early in life, which can result in increased peripheral airway resistance. Likewise, developmental influences, such as horizontally aligned ribs in young infants or a soft and compliant chest wall precluding the ability to generate negative intrathoracic pressure, impact respiratory mechanics. For additional information regarding key aspects of airway and respiratory system development, please refer to Chapter 1, "Anatomy and Physiology of the Pediatric Patient" and the Respiratory System and Renal System sections.

There are a variety of ventilators and anesthesia machines commonly employed in pediatric anesthesia, all of which offer a host of differing functions and nuances, making it important for anesthesia providers to familiarize themselves with proper operation and utilization of the ventilator prior to anesthetizing a patient. This includes exploring the default mode of the ventilator and the appropriateness of this mode for the patient being anesthetized. This chapter focuses on the different ventilation modes commonly encountered in anesthesia practice and key parameters. It also identifies the difference between the anesthesia machine ventilator and those commonly used to ventilate patients in the Intensive care unit (ICU).

VENTILATION PARAMETERS

TIDAL VOLUME

Tidal volume is the amount of air that enters and exits the lungs while breathing. In pediatric anesthesia, the target tidal volume typically ranges from 5 to 8 mL/kg, regardless of the mode of ventilation utilized. The ability to achieve this volume, however, depends on the mode of ventilation and the patient's physiology. For example, when controlled ventilation (CV) is utilized, the tidal volume desired is programmed into the ventilator, whereas chest wall compliance determines the tidal volume when pressure-controlled ventilation (PCV) is employed (Figure 7.1). Anesthesia providers should be aware that high tidal volumes associated with high-end inspiratory pressure have a negative impact on outcomes in the critically ill child. Likewise, low tidal volumes may promote atelectasis, increase pulmonary shunting, and foster ventilator-associated lung injury. The ensuing hypercapnia predisposes the patient to increase in intracranial pressure, pulmonary hypertension, and impaired myocardial contraction. Thus, it is imperative that anesthesia providers ensure the delivery of adequate volumes to preclude negative sequelae due to poor ventilation.

RESPIRATORY RATE

Respiratory rate is the number of times a minute the patient breathes either spontaneously or via the ventilator. Knowing the age of the child helps determine the age-appropriate respiratory rate necessary to allow for adequate ventilation of the child. Table 7.1 provides the normal respiratory rates for children.

INSPIRATORY-TO-EXPIRATORY RATIO

I:E ratio indicates inspiration to expiration ratio. Most anesthesia machine ventilators default to 1:2, which allows for an expiration time twice as long as that offered for inspiration. When a patient requires a higher pressure to ventilate adequately, there are times that the I:E ratio needs to be altered to allow for better ventilation. For example, in a patient with cystic fibrosis, lower ventilation pressures are suggested to decrease the incidence of pneumothorax.

PEAK INSPIRATORY PRESSURE

Peak inspiratory pressure (PIP) is the maximum pressure at inspiration. A child with decreased chest compliance will need a greater PIP to adequately ventilate the lungs. This child may have a chronic lung disease, asthma, or bronchospasm. Positioning the patient prone or in lithotomy may also decrease the chest compliance, thereby increasing the PIP. In

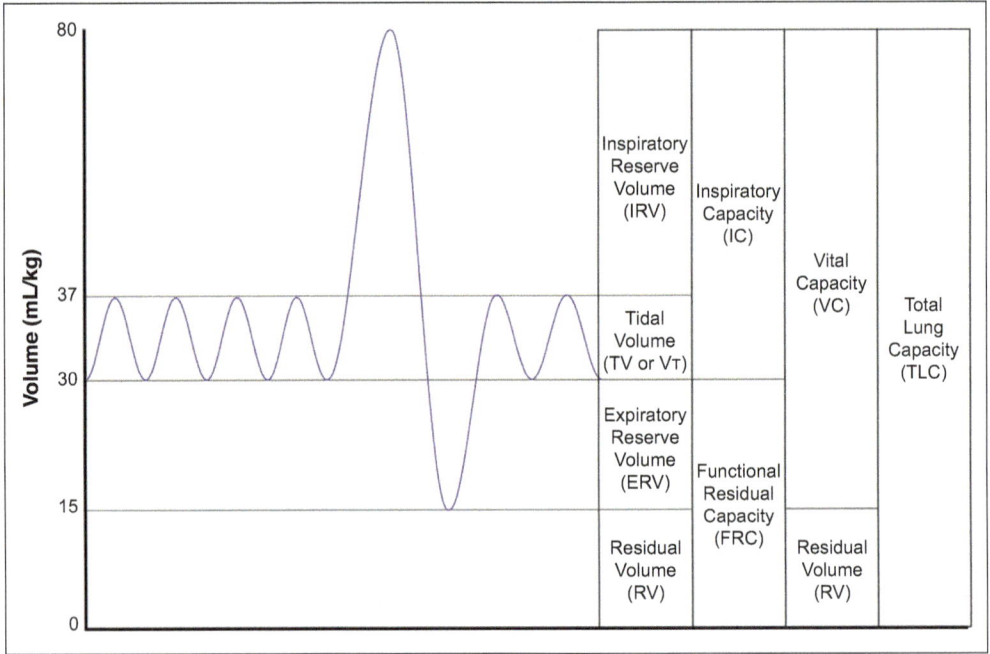

Figure 7.1: Tidal volume.

Source: ERV, expiratory reserve volume; FRC, functional residual capacity; IC, inspiratory capacity; IRV, inspiratory reserve volume; RV, residual volume; TLC, total lung capacity; TV or VT, tidal volume; VC, vital capacity.

Table 7.1	Normal Pediatric Respiratory Rates	
Age Category	**Age Range**	**Normal Respiratory Rate**
Infant	0–12 months	30–60 per minute
Toddler	1–3 years	24–40 per minute
Preschooler	4–5 years	22–34 per minute
School Age	6–12 years	18–30 per minute
Adolescent	13–18 years	12–16 per minute

order to adequately ventilate this child, the anesthesia provider may need to increase the respiratory rate to decrease the end-tidal CO_2 (ETCO$_2$). A child with increased chest compliance will have greater tidal volumes with less pressure. Many factors will affect the PIP, and it is important for anesthesia providers to remain mindful of these factors while anesthetizing the pediatric patient.

POSITIVE END-EXPIRATORY PRESSURE

Positive end-expiratory pressure (PEEP) plays several key roles during ventilation. The addition of PEEP improves oxygenation by recruiting collapsed lung spaces and preventing alveolar collapse. In an ill child, PEEP is necessary to restore end-expiratory lung volume and improve respiratory system compliance. This is especially true in patients with severe lung injury or disease. PEEP can also be used to stent open floppy airways. Excessive PEEP, however, can preclude venous return and negatively affect hemodynamics. Therefore, anesthesia providers must understand that PEEP should be titrated to achieve the optimal balance between hemodynamics and oxygenation.

END-TIDAL CARBON DIOXIDE

ETCO$_2$ measurement is a key parameter in determining the adequacy of ventilation. Normal ETCO$_2$ values range from 30 to 40 mmHg. On the anesthesia machine, the ETCO$_2$ sample line is connected to the circuit.

DEAD SPACE

A humidifying filter placed inline that protects the anesthesia machine from viruses the patient may have. The use of a humidifying filter, however, creates dead space that can be detrimental to ventilation. As there are many filters available, it is imperative that anesthesia providers know how much dead space is in the filter being utilized. There are some filters that have 30- to 50-mL dead space. For a 50- to 70-kg person whose tidal volume is 500 to 700 mL, this would be less than 10%, thus not significant to the ventilation of this child. In a 3-kg patient, however, 30 mL may equate to the patient's entire tidal volume. If the entire tidal volume is within the filter, delivery of volatile anesthetic agents will be impeded, as will the delivery of oxygen and removal of CO_2. Fortunately, there are dead space reducers available for use with pediatric patients and small heat and moisture exchanger (HME) filters that allow the 3-kg patient to adequately ventilate and humidify while on the anesthesia ventilator. **Figure 7.2** depicts a dead space reducer and small HME filter. For more information regarding the use of HME filters, please refer to Chapter 4, "Equipment and Monitoring."

VENTILATION MODES

SPONTANEOUS VENTILATION

Spontaneous ventilation is associated with many physiologic benefits, including intact respiratory tone, improved ventilation–perfusion matching, maintenance of distal airway patency, prevention of atelectasis, improved functional residual capacity, and improved hemodynamics. In addition, knowing the innate respiratory rate conveys information regarding the depth of anesthesia and adequacy of analgesia. For surgical procedures that are short in duration and the patient is over a year of age, many anesthesia providers allow the patient to spontaneously ventilate without ventilatory support. If, however, the procedure is greater than 1 hour or the patient is younger than 1 year of age, it is best to place the patient on the ventilator and use the PSV-PRO mode if available. This ventilator mode can be used with a mask, laryngeal mask airway (LMA), or endotracheal tube (ETT).

MECHANICAL VENTILATION

Mechanical ventilation is necessary during many surgical procedures due to the surgery scheduled, the length of the surgery, or the patient's presenting medical history. Invasive positive pressure mechanical ventilation, however, is not without consequence (see Table 7.2). Hence, anesthesia providers should be careful of the specific ramifications associated with the various modes of mechanical ventilation commonly employed.

Default Mode

Anesthesia providers should be aware that some anesthesia machines have a default mode. When an anesthetic is complete, the patient is removed from the anesthesia ventilator and transported to the postanesthesia care unit (PACU) or ICU, and the machine will alarm until placed in standby mode. Place the machine in standby mode inherently restores the ventilation mode to one set in the factory. The specific settings are vendor- and model-specific;

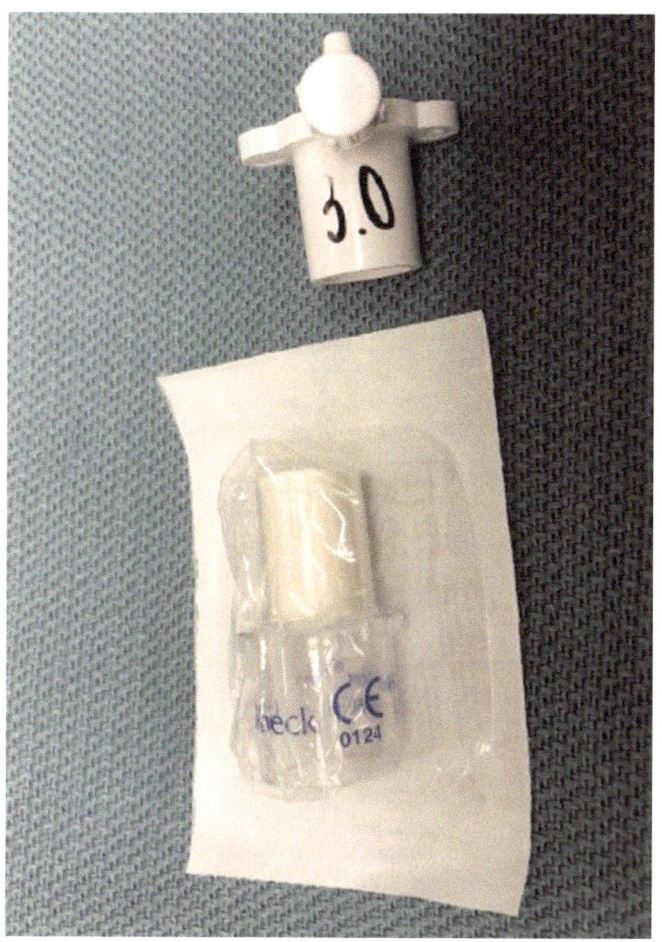

Figure 7.2: Dead space reducer.

Table 7.2	Adverse Effects of Invasive Positive Pressure Mechanical Ventilation		
System	**Adverse Effects**		
Respiratory	Upper airways	Nasal trauma	
		Nasopharyngeal and pharyngeal trauma	
		Laryngeal trauma (e.g., vocal cord fixation/paralysis)	
		Subglottic edema/stenosis	
	Lower airways	Air leak	
		- Pneumothorax	
		- Pneumomediastinum	
		- Pulmonary interstitial emphysema	
		Atelectasis	
		VARI	
		- VAP	
		- VAT	
		- Nosocomial sinusitis	
		Ventilation-associated lung injury	
Cardiovascular	Decreased venous return		
	Increased pulmonary vascular resistance		
Central Nervous System	Increased intracranial pressure		
Renal	Decreased urine output (direct and indirect effect)		

VAP, ventilator-associated pneumonia; VARI, ventilation-associated respiratory infection; VAT, ventilator-associated tracheobronchitis.

however, the setting may not be well tolerated by all pediatric patients and may have the potential to induce barotrauma or ventilator-associated lung injury. Having a sound understanding of the default mode associated with the anesthesia machine being used in clinical practice is key to protecting the patient.

Pressure-Controlled Ventilation

PCV is the mode most commonly used in pediatric anesthesia and is especially useful with neonates and small infants in which measurement of the tidal volume is inherently inaccurate. This mode of ventilation should only be used when an ETT is in place. With PCV, the breath is delivered at a set rate with a decelerating flow pattern and is terminated when a preset PIP is realized. The child's chest compliance ultimately determines the tidal volume the patient will receive in a single breath. Therefore, by setting the pressure desired, the incidence of barotrauma is reduced. PCV has also been reported to be associated with decreased work of breathing, improved oxygenation at lower peak pressures, and better patient outcomes.

When utilizing this mode of ventilation, the anesthesia provider also chooses the respiratory rate and I:E ratio the child should receive. The main concern with PCV is the tidal volume and minute ventilation by the patient's respiratory mechanics. Should these worsen, the ability to deliver adequate tidal volumes will decline.

Volume-Controlled Ventilation

During volume-controlled ventilation (VCV), a preset volume is delivered with each breath via a constant flow pattern, terminating at a preset time or after delivery of the preset tidal volume. Variations in tidal volume delivery, due to leaks in the system or inaccurate measurement, limit the utility of this mode in the neonate or young infant. Additionally, higher peak pressures may be encountered as the preset volume is being delivered. This can result in overdistention and/or ventilator-associated lung injury.

Controlled Ventilation

CV involves delivery of breath at a preset interval, irrespective of the patient's effort. This is more commonly reserved for use with adults or older children. However, if a child is not tolerating the ventilator due to physiologic or surgical factors, anesthesia providers may consider utilizing this mode even in a small child to improve ventilation.

When utilizing this mode of ventilation, the anesthesia provider determines the tidal volume, respiratory rate, and I:E ratio the child should receive. The anesthesia provider will also select the maximum PIP the ventilator should achieve when delivering a breath; typically this is around 35 to 40 cmH_2O. If the ventilator PIP reaches 35 to 40 cmH_2O, the ventilator will stop delivering the breath regardless of the tidal volume that has been delivered. This mode of ventilation is not the first choice when providing anesthesia to a small child as barotrauma could result. This mode of ventilation should also only be used with an ETT in place.

Synchronized Intermittent Mandatory Ventilation

Synchronized intermittent mandatory ventilation (SIMV) is a mixed ventilatory mode that allows both mandatory and spontaneous breathing to occur. The mandatory breaths delivered can be either pressure- or volume-regulated. In addition, the spontaneous breaths have the option of being pressure supported with the ventilator supporting negative pressure inspiration. With this mode, anesthesia providers can determine the minimum number of breaths they want the patient to receive over a minute, thereby ensuring the patient receives a mandatory amount of breaths per minute whether the patient initiates a breath or not. This mode can be used to support respiratory effort intraoperatively or when attempting to get the patient to breathe without allowing long periods between breaths. This mode of ventilation may be used with LMA or ETT.

Pressure Support Ventilation

Pressure support ventilation (PSV) augments only spontaneous breaths in an effort to reduce the work of breathing experienced by the patient. When a breath is initiated and the ventilator is triggered, flow is delivered to achieve a preset inspiratory pressure. The respiratory rate, inspiratory time, and tidal volume are all determined by the patient. PSV modes, such as PSV-PRO, incorporate the use of PEEP to decrease the incidence of atelectasis. This ventilator mode can be used with an LMA or ETT.

ICU VENTILATORS

Ventilators found in the ICU have the ability to generate greater inspiratory pressures than the ventilators found on anesthesia machines, which is useful when caring for an acutely or severely ill patient. This includes patients with pulmonary issues requiring higher PIPs or PEEPs to adequately ventilate the patient. These ventilators are often more efficient in delivering adequate volumes to neonates and young infants. If a patient requiring high-pressure support needs to be transported to the operating room for a procedure, it is prudent the anesthesia provider trial ventilation with a Jackson Rees Mapleson or Ambu bag prior to leaving the ICU to see how well the patient tolerates ventilation. If the patient does not tolerate this transition, they may require the use of the ICU ventilator intraoperatively. This would necessitate the use of a total IV anesthetic as the ICU ventilators do not have or accommodate vaporizers.

In contrast, there are times that a patient will need to be maintained on an anesthesia machine in ICU due to status asthmaticus. These patients are intubated and placed on an inhaled anesthetic agent. The agent used most is sevoflurane. In many institutions, the ICU attending and/or RN communicates with the anesthesia department regarding anesthesia machine maintenance. There are protocols that need to be followed in terms of anesthesia rounding on the patient, changing of the anesthesia circuit, and filling of the vaporizers. This patient requires a team approach in order to overcome the episode, and communication is key.

KEY TAKEAWAYS

- Tidal volume should be 5 to 10 mL/kg.
- Respiratory rate norms decrease as the patient ages.
- PCV is most commonly used in pediatrics.
- Patients weighing less than 5 kg require a dead space reducer.
- ICU ventilators generate more pressure for acutely ill patients.

REFERENCES

1. *ACLS Medical Training.* (n.d.). https://www.aclsmedicaltraining.com
2. Dosch MP, Tharp D. (n.d.). *The Anesthesia Gas Machine.* http://healthprofessions.udmercy.edu/programs/crna/agm
3. Keegan MT. Intraoperative management of the critically ill patient. *Curr Rev Nurse Anesth.* 2013;36(16):195-203. https://www.currentreviews.com/dlfile.cfm
4. Butterworth JF, Mackey DC, Wasnick JD. *Morgan & Mikhail's Clinical Anesthesiology.* McGraw Hill Education. 2018.
5. Pardo M, Miller RD, Miller RD. *Basics of Anesthesia.* Elsevier. 2018.

CHAPTER 8

Fluids, Electrolytes, and Transfusion Therapy

Christopher A. Allphin, Fernando Franco Cuadrado, and Joseph W. McSoley

LEARNING OBJECTIVES

- Understand the basic energy requirements of the pediatric patient as it relates to daily fluid requirements.
- Recognize the importance of the patient's fluid deficit and how to calculate/replace this deficit safely and effectively.
- Describe the most commonly used crystalloids, including the benefits and drawbacks of each.
- Explain the importance of dextrose-containing solutions in the neonate.
- Recognize when blood transfusion is necessary and which products are available.

INTRODUCTION

Pediatrics does not deal with miniature men and women, with reduced doses and the same class of disease in smaller bodies, but… has its own independent range and horizon.
— Dr. Abraham Jacob

There are many different IV fluids and blood products administered to the pediatric patient in the perioperative setting. The replacement of preoperative fluid deficits, management of ongoing maintenance requirements, the assessment of fluid losses, and the treatment of anemia and coagulation disturbances must be considered with treatment tailored appropriately to each patient intraoperatively. This chapter aims to introduce these topics and provide the most current information to enable the anesthesia provider to effectively treat ongoing changes in fluid homeostasis in the pediatric patient.

PHYSIOLOGICAL CONSIDERATIONS AND NORMAL FLUID REQUIREMENTS

While it has been said many times before, neonates are not small adults. During the first few days to months of life, major physiological changes will occur. More specifically, the rapid development of organ systems poses a great challenge when approaching fluid and electrolyte management in the pediatric patient.

In all living species, energy is constantly being burned to maintain and sustain life. This energy is often measured as calories and/or a caloric requirement. Holliday and Segar described caloric requirements in pediatrics in their 1957 paper.[1] Their work is often cited to this day. Their approach to calculating caloric requirement is based on an estimation of a child's basic metabolic requirements while at rest as related to their weight in kilograms. Table 8.1 demonstrates these requirements.

From this understanding, Holliday and Segar were able to determine that one's water requirement mirrored that of total energy expenditure (i.e., 1,000 mL of water is required

Table 8.1	Daily Caloric Requirements in Children (Based on kg)
Weight	Daily Caloric Requirement
0–10 kg	1,000 kcal/kg/day
11–20 kg	1,000 kcal + 50 kcal/kg/day for each kg over 10
21–70 kg	1,500 kcal + 20 kcal/kg/day for each kg over 20

for every 1,000 kcal expended). With the understanding that water maintenance requirements parallel that of energy metabolism requirements, the "4–2–1 rule" that is commonly referenced was created to more easily calculate daily maintenance needs.

As mentioned, under normal circumstances, 1 mL of water is required to actively metabolize 1 kcal in the pediatric patient. In general, as the size of the child decreases, there will be a subsequent increase in water requirement comparatively. This increase in water requirement is secondary to many factors. Specifically, there is a higher metabolic rate in the neonate along with a higher evaporative loss due to a greater ratio of body surface area to weight. These physiological differences are further accentuated in the premature infant, as their evaporative losses continue to be inversely proportional to gestational age. This increase in water requirement is due to an increase in thermal conductance; thinner, more permeable skin; a more vascularized skin bed; and a higher respiratory rate.

FASTING GUIDELINES AND SUBSEQUENT PREOPERATIVE DEFICITS

The goal of preoperative fasting is to minimize the volume of gastric contents and thereby decrease the risk of regurgitation of stomach contents and subsequent aspiration during the induction of anesthesia. While strict NPO guidelines are important in the adult patient, they are often deemed to be more critical in the pediatric patient. This is due to the often-used inhalational induction technique that carries a variable amount of induction time, subsequently increasing the risk of regurgitation, compared to a standard IV induction. While an appropriate NPO time may reliably decrease the patient's gastric contents, and thus the risk of aspiration, this risk must be weighed against the possibility of dehydration and hypoglycemia in the pediatric patient.

The American Society of Anesthesiologists (ASA) task force on preoperative fasting originally published guidelines in 1999. These guidelines have since been revisited in 2011 and again in 2015.[2] As the guidelines were created and revised, the recommendations from the ASA continue to be based on the analysis of current literature, expert opinion, open forum, and clinical data. Current recommendations are illustrated in Table 8.2. Recommendations include the appropriate fasting times for elective procedures requiring general anesthesia, regional anesthesia, or procedural sedation.

Table 8.2	Current ASA NPO Guidelines to Reduce the Risk of Pulmonary Aspiration
Content	Time (hours)
Clear liquids	2
Breast milk	4
Infant formula, light meal without fat content	6
Full meal, intake of fried foods, fatty foods, or meat/eggs	8

The ASA preoperative fasting guidelines are intended for healthy patients undergoing elective procedures requiring anesthesia/sedation. Coexisting disease and chronic illnesses must be considered. Certain disease processes specifically affect gastric emptying and gastric fluid volume, thus increasing the risk of regurgitation and aspiration with the induction of general anesthesia. While the ASA does provide these recommendations as a guideline, individual clinical assessment and preoperative planning must be considered to minimize the risk of aspiration.

Abiding by the appropriate ASA NPO guidelines will help reduce the risk of pulmonary aspiration and in turn will also produce some degree of fluid deficit in the pediatric patient. An appropriate and thorough preoperative assessment can help assist in the evaluation of the patient's current volume status. While a fluid deficit in the adult patient may produce patient-reported symptoms, such as lightheadedness, blurry vision, and diaphoresis, the pediatric patient's volume status is more difficult to assess due to the inability of the patient to verbalize and communicate the presence of these symptoms. Understanding and recognizing the patient's fluid deficit are paramount in providing quality anesthetic care. The importance of a thorough history and appropriate physical examination prior to surgery cannot be overstated. Certain physical examination findings, such as capillary refill, skin turgor, heart rate, and blood pressure, can assist the clinician in assessing the patient's current volume status. In addition, caregivers can also assist the anesthesia provider in developing a global picture of the patient's current volume deficit by extracting information, such as NPO time, normal feeding schedule, and the production of wet diapers. See Chapter 3, "Preoperative Evaluation and Testing," for further information regarding preoperative assessment.

While clear liquid ingestion is recommended and encouraged up to 2 hours prior to the induction of anesthesia to decrease the volume deficit, it is likely that the patient's fasting period will occur over a longer period of time. A prolonged fasting time coupled with the natural vasodilation associated with general anesthesia and expected intraoperative fluid/blood loss, often necessitates replacing the fluid deficit from the beginning of the anesthetic to maintain adequate perfusion and hemodynamic stability. An understanding of the patient's preoperative fluid deficit must be considered, along with the knowledge of age-related norms for heart rate and blood pressure (see Table 8.3).

Comprehending these two assessments allows the anesthetist to make guided clinical decisions in terms of intraoperative fluid administration.

INTRAOPERATIVE FLUID MANAGEMENT

Due to the difficult nature of placing an IV catheter in an awake child, most pediatric anesthesia providers will obtain IV access after an inhalation induction of general anesthesia if the patient is appropriately NPO and has no other comorbidities that would put the patient at increased risk of complications. Selection of appropriately sized IV catheter along with semipermanent venous lines, such as peripherally inserted central catheters (PICCs) and central venous catheters (CVCs), is covered further in Chapter 36 of this text.

Intraoperative fluid administration is aimed at providing basal metabolic requirements, compensating for the preoperative fluid deficit, and replacing losses from the surgical field. Replacing the fasting deficit should be a priority. To adequately replace this deficit, the hourly maintenance fluid requirement (based on the 4–2–1 rule) can be calculated, and then multiply that number by the number of fasted hours. Traditionally, 50% of this deficit should be replaced in the first hour, with the additional 50% replaced over the next 2 hours. Replacing the fluid loss over a prolonged period allows the body to acclimate to the new IV volume and reduces the chance of fluid overload.[4]

In addition to the ongoing metabolic needs of the patient, three physiological processes will begin to occur with the induction of anesthesia. The relaxation of sympathetic tone that occurs with the induction of general anesthesia will increase capacitance of the vascular system, thus leading to a relative state of hypovolemia. With any surgical procedure there is always the potential, and sometimes expected loss of blood/fluid volume. And finally, with the induction of anesthesia and the insult of surgical trauma, the potential for capillary leak of isotonic fluid into the interstitial space begins to occur immediately, also referred to as "third spacing."

Table 8.3	Age-Related Heart Rate and Blood Pressure Ranges		
Age	Mean Heart Rate Range (beats per minute)	Mean Systolic (mm Hg)	Mean Diastolic (mm Hg)
Premature	120–170	55–75	35–45
0–3 months	100–150	65–85	45–55
3–6 months	90–120	70–90	50–65
6–12 months	80–120	80–100	55–65
1–3 years	70–110	90–105	55–70
3–6 years	65–110	95–110	60–75
6–12 years	60–95	100–120	60–75

Source: From *Pediatric Vital Signs Reference Chart*. 2020. http://www.pedscases.com/pediatric-vital-signs-reference-chart.

Replacement of ongoing blood loss can be difficult to assess, specifically in the neonate, as their circulating blood volume leaves little room for error. This topic is covered more thoroughly later in the chapter. While all patients can physiologically handle some degree of blood loss, remaining diligent and proactive in managing such losses remains key to successful management of the pediatric patient. In general, replacing 1 mL of colloid, whether that be blood or 5% albumin, for every 1 mL of blood loss continues to be the standard to managing ongoing blood loss and maintaining hemodynamic stability.

The loss of intravascular volume due to the third spacing of crystalloid fluid also presents a challenge. The degree of third-space loss is oftentimes attributed to the amount of tissue trauma incurred with the surgical procedure. Minor procedures with little to no surgical trauma have been shown to produce a third-space loss of about 1 mL/kg/hr. As the invasiveness of the surgical procedure increases, so does the potential for intravascular volume loss and thus increased requirement for additional fluid administration. Surgical procedures with minor to moderate trauma often require 5 to 7 mL/kg/hr of fluid administration, while large abdominal procedures in the infant may incur losses of 10 mL/kg/hr or more.[5]

The ongoing balance of fluid replacement in the pediatric patient to maintain hemodynamic stability and maintenance of intravascular volume must be weighed against the potential overload of fluid that remains a possibility in the infants, developing organ systems. The potential damage that can be incurred if fluid administration goes unchecked cannot be overstated. Postoperative pulmonary edema, ongoing bowel swelling, anasarca along with airway edema can all occur if fluid administration is not carefully calculated and titrated to the individual needs of the patient and subsequent procedure. Therefore, different methods can be employed to help prevent potential fluid overload. In infants, volumetric chambers are often utilized in order to limit the amount of fluid that can be administered and to prevent the administration of excess fluid. In addition, many anesthesia providers have seen great benefit from the use of an infusion pump, which allows the anesthesia provider to actively control the volume and rate of administration of their selected fluid throughout the duration of the anesthetic.

CRYSTALLOIDS

The question remains, which fluid type should the pediatric anesthesia providers use to replace such losses? Many considerations must be made when selecting the appropriate fluid, specifically how the fluid will affect intravascular volume, the coagulation cascade, microcirculation, and the possibility for allergic reaction. In general, intraoperative fluid replacement and maintenance should be achieved with the use of isotonic (tonicity similar to plasma) crystalloid solutions; the mainstay of isotonic solutions are 0.9% NaCl (normal saline [NS]) and lactated Ringer's (LR). Intraoperatively, the loss of whole blood and third-space fluid is seen as isotonic losses, therefore replacing such losses with a similar solution is deemed physiologically safe and appropriate. When hydrating the patient with solutions that contain near-physiological serum levels of sodium and chloride, along with low concentrations of bicarbonate, calcium and potassium are the most appropriate replacement fluids to administer in order to maintain physiological homeostasis. These two crystalloids have become the mainstay of therapy due to their low cost, lack of effect on coagulation, absence of anaphylactic reaction and isotonic nature, and the absent risk of infectious agent transmission.[6] One of the many goals when it comes to intraoperative fluid administration in the pediatric patient is to administer a solution that is similar in osmolarity to that of the body's normal physiological state (Table 8.4).

Lactated Ringer's

LR solution remains one of the most commonly used fluids intraoperatively in the pediatric patient. Although LR is hypotonic compared to NS, for instance, providing 100 mL of free water per liter and a lower sodium (130 mEq/L) compared to the patient's physiological serum, LR will generally have minimal effect on extracellular fluid composition. LR remains the most physiologically stable solution when large volumes are required.[7] Of course, the use of LR does not come without risk and is not appropriate for all patient populations.

LR contains, among other ions, 28 mEq/L of lactate along with 4 mEq/L of potassium (K+). In the otherwise healthy patient, this lactate is taken up by the liver and converted to bicarbonate, which can be exhaled via the respiratory system or excreted via the kidneys. In patients with normal-functioning organ systems, LR continues to be the crystalloid of choice. Caution must be exercised in the patient with damaged or absent renal function due the patient's inability to regulate bicarbonate and potassium excretion/reabsorption. This dysfunction has the potential for producing significant metabolic derangements, including the potentially fatal hyperkalemia. In addition, when caring for a patient with hepatic dysfunction/failure, caution must be used due to the patient's inability to metabolize the lactate within the crystalloid solution. This inability of lactate metabolism can be catastrophic due to the buildup of lactate

Table 8.4	Composition of Extracellular Fluid and Common IV Solutions						
Fluid	pH	Na+ (mEq/L)	Cl- (mEq/L)	K+ (mEq/L)	Ca2+ (mEq/L)	Other	mOsm/L
Extracellular fluid	7.4	142	103	4	5	-	280–300
LR solution	6.5	130	109	4	3	Lactate 28 mEq/L	275
0.9% NaCl (NS)	5.5	154	154	0	0	0	308
Plasmalyte	7.4	140	98	5	0	27 acetate and 23 gluconate	294
Dextrose 5% (D5)	4.5	0	0	0	0	Dextrose 50 g/L	285
Dextrose 5% LR	5	130	109	4	3	Dextrose 50 g/L	275
Dextrose 5% NS	4	154	154	0	0	Dextrose 50 g/L	308

LR, lactated Ringer's; NS, normal saline.

within the body and potential for lactic acidosis and subsequent effect on all major organ systems.

Normal Saline
Much like the use of LR, NS provides both benefits and drawbacks when used intraoperatively. NS, or 0.9% NaCl, is slightly hypertonic to the body's physiological serum. While the extracellular fluid of normal physiological serum carries an osmolarity ranging from 280 to 300 mOsm/L, NS's osmolarity is recognized to be 308 mOsm/L. This increased osmolarity is due to the high sodium concentration (154 mEq/L), and elevated chloride concentration (154 mEq/L), respectively. While this increased osmolarity has little to no detrimental effects to an otherwise healthy surgical patient when given in maintenance-level increments, the concern arises when major fluid resuscitation is necessary. With NS administration, the risk of hyperchloremic metabolic acidosis is a considerable risk in larger volumes.[8] This acidosis is associated with the increased chloride ion concentration and an overall alteration in the strong ion difference. The subsequent metabolic derangement can have deleterious effects on overall cardiac and renal function, leading to both intraoperative and postoperative complications.

Plasma-Lyte
A third option as a balanced isotonic salt solution is the administration of Plasma-Lyte. Like the use of NS and LR solutions, Plasma-Lyte also has a low relative cost, no effect on coagulation, and does not produce an allergic response with administration.[8] Overall, Plasma-Lyte is more physiologically similar to serum than either 0.9% NS or LR solution due to its both isotonic nature and balance with respect to plasma base. The osmolality of Plasma-Lyte is 294 mOsm/L, which approximates normal serum osmolality as compared to LR. Plasma-Lyte also has a reduced sodium concentration (140 mEq/L) as compared to NS, closely resembling normal serum concentrations. In addition, its lower chloride composition (98 mEq/L) also more closely resembles that of physiological serum.[8]

Although NS is still recommended for kidney transplantation by the Kidney Disease: Improving Global Outcomes transplantation guidelines, its overall safety has come into question when compared to other solutions. Hence, interest in the use of balanced salt solutions, such as Plasma-Lyte, is rising.[9] A commonly cited drawback of Plasma-Lyte administration centers on the presence of acetate within the solution. The administration of acetate within Plasma-Lyte, much like the administration of lactate within LR, must be considered in certain populations. While lactate metabolism is almost entirely dependent on hepatic function, acetate is metabolized mainly within the peripheral tissue and only partially within the hepatic system.[10] In addition, acetate metabolism occurs more rapidly than lactate metabolism and can begin to act as a buffering ion within 15 minutes of metabolism. Like all fluid administration, there are certain pitfalls to consider, such as a global understanding of the patient and their fluid balance, and the procedure must be considered when selecting the appropriate crystalloid solution.

Glucose-Containing Fluids
With fluid administration comes the question of glucose management in the pediatric and neonatal population. While it was once considered mandatory to include dextrose within the IV solution in the surgical setting to avoid hypoglycemia, this no longer holds true. The risk of hyperglycemia secondary to ongoing surgical stress and the subsequent risk of hyponatremia due to the hypotonic nature of the solution have shown to be more deleterious to the safety and well-being of the patient as compared to the risk of hypoglycemia.[8] While the risk of hypoglycemia remains in certain intraoperative populations, specifically malnourished children, neonates, and infants younger than 6 months of age, it is no longer recommended to include dextrose in all intraoperative fluids. It has been shown that the stress of surgical stimulation produces a natural hyperglycemic response, with the resulting influx of glucose into the bloodstream being enough to prevent tissue catabolism.[5] Recent studies have shown hyperglycemia as being more of a clinical concern, primarily due to the increased risk of intraoperative infection, osmotic diuresis leading to electrolyte disturbances, and the possibility of poor wound healing postoperatively.[5]

The pediatric populations at the greatest risk of fluctuations in blood glucose levels are the hospitalized neonates and the premature infants. Due to the inherent lack of glycogen reserves, these patients are at risk of quickly developing hypoglycemia if additional sources of dextrose are not provided. Recognizing hypoglycemia in the neonate can be challenging but must be at the forefront of the pediatric anesthesia provider's mind in order to prevent long-term neurological damage. Therefore, in the at-risk population, it is commonplace to provide a 1% to 5% dextrose solution at the infant's basal maintenance rate while not in the operating room. In the intraoperative period, it is recommended that the infusion rate of dextrose-containing fluids be reduced to half in anticipation of the hyperglycemic response to surgical stress. The stress of surgery and the hyperglycemic response can vary among patients; therefore, vigilance is recommended and anesthesia providers should monitor the patient's glucose level, at minimum, every hour during the intraoperative period while providing fluid replacement with an isotonic solution.

COLLOIDS
Crystalloid solutions are not the only option for resuscitation, as many anesthesia providers choose to administer colloid solutions. Colloids are often divided into two categories: natural colloids and synthetic colloids. Albumin is a natural colloid, as it is derived from human plasma. It is available in 5% and 25% concentrations. Many anesthesia providers use 5% albumin as a volume expander as it has a similar osmotic concentration as human plasma. The 25% solution is five times more concentrated, so five times less volume is needed for volume expansion when compared to the 5% solution. The cost of albumin is higher than that of crystalloid solutions, which should be considered when selecting a solution for fluid replacement.[11] In the pediatric populations, the continued use of albumin for fluid resuscitation has come into question. While many consider albumin as the gold standard in neonates and infants to maintain intravascular osmotic pressure, others choose alternative solutions, such as crystalloids or synthetic colloids.

Anesthesia providers should be aware that the use of a 25% solution can cause fluid translocation from the interstitial space to the intravascular compartment because of the high concentration of proteins. Additionally, either concentration of albumin may worsen edema in patients with damaged or highly permeable capillaries, such as in cases of sepsis, burns, or trauma. This is due to the albumin leaking across the capillaries and out of the intravascular compartment, causing fluid to accumulate in the interstitial space. Other side effects of albumin administration include allergic reactions and adverse effects on blood clotting. The administration of albumin may lead to inhibition of platelet aggregation and effects on antithrombin III that are similar to the effects of heparin on antithrombin III. When the administered volume of albumin is less than 25% of the patient's total blood volume, these effects are not clinically significant. In addition to these side effects, some data suggest that albumin administration may be harmful in the patients with traumatic brain injury.[5]

Synthetic colloids include hydroxyethyl starches (HES), gelatins, and dextrans. Pediatric studies involving synthetic colloids are varied and scarce. HES colloids contain modified polysaccharides, making them resistant to hydrolysis, thereby allowing them to have a prolonged effect. The role of HES is plasma volume expansion, with effects lasting 2 to 6 hours. Side effects include pruritus, hypocoagulation, and renal toxicity. Gelatins are produced by degrading bovine collagen into polypeptides. They have decreased colloid oncotic effects and have been shown to have a negative effect on thromboelastography (TEG) values. While gelatins are the least expensive of the synthetic colloids, they are not available in the United States due to the history of hypersensitivity reactions with their administration. Dextrans are polysaccharides synthesized from sucrose by bacteria. They can remain intravascularly for 3 to 6 hours, depending on the formulation. Dextrans have high potential for anaphylactic reactions and negative coagulation effects.[5]

BLOOD

Blood Management

The estimation of blood loss is generally difficult to assess in the operating room. The challenges are further compounded in specific types of procedures (e.g., solid organ transplantation and orthopedic surgery), trauma, and small circulating blood volumes. Special consideration should be given to neonates given the impact of small volume losses in the context of total blood volume and hemostatic system immaturity that develops throughout infancy up until 6 months to 1 year of age.[12] Limited resources exist for the standardization of transfusion practices in pediatric patients compared to adults. Patient blood management (PBM) protocols have been described in the adult population with questionable applicability in pediatric patients in specific clinical scenarios.[13] While the evidence of blood transfusion effectiveness is relatively abundant for adults, the same level of evidence is lacking in pediatrics. Barriers to the creation and standardization of blood management protocols in the younger population include the physiological differences within the different age groups, the smaller number of large pediatric centers, and the limited literature available.[13,14]

Prior to surgery, useful tools available as part of a preanesthetic evaluation help determine the estimated blood volume (EBV) of the patient. EBV is often estimated based on the patient's age and weight (Table 8.5). Using EBV values can determine how administered fluid and blood volumes individually influence homeostasis in the patient. It may also allow the clinician to estimate the maximum allowable blood loss (MABL) for individual patients. The MABL is determined using the following equation:

$$MABL = EBV \times [(Starting\ hematocrit - Target\ hematocrit) \div Starting\ hematocrit]$$

Estimating how much blood the patient can lose during the procedure allows the clinician to tailor therapy and set intraoperative thresholds that best fit changing clinical scenarios.

Table 8.5	Estimated Blood Volume
Age	Estimated Blood Volume (mL/kg)
Premature infant	90–100
Full-term infant	80–90
Children 3 months–1 year	70–80
Older children	70
Adult males	70
Adult females	65

These tools, when combined, allow each clinician to make an informed decision of whether to transfuse or not transfuse. Once the hematocrit reaches the target value, the provider should begin transfusing the patient with packed red blood cells (pRBCs). The target hematocrit will be different for each patient, depending on their age or coexisting disease.

The overarching goal of blood transfusion is to optimize tissue oxygen delivery. While blood oxygen-carrying capacity is only one of the pillars in which tissue perfusion rests on, its importance is accentuated in certain scenarios, such as in cardiac mixing lesions or situations in which cardiac output is suboptimal, such as in heart failure. In general, oxygen requirements for neonates and children are higher than that of adults on a per kilogram basis, and the maintenance of oxygen delivery is a key intraoperative goal in this population. Transfusion thresholds in children vary when a hemoglobin level is used as a marker. Specific thresholds exist only as guidelines given that clinical judgment is crucial and greatly influenced by the disease process.

For critically ill children, several studies support the practice of blood transfusions when the hemoglobin level falls below 5 g/dL.[15–17] The benefits of blood transfusion in these patients are further increased when respiratory symptoms, such as dyspnea, are present.[18] Transfusion should be considered when the hemoglobin falls below 7 g/dL in stable critically ill children and in children older than 28 days who do not have cyanotic heart disease. A hemoglobin level of 7 g/dL can also be used as a guide in children with sepsis. As demonstrated in the TRIPICU trial, a transfusion threshold of 7 g/dL may lead to a decrease in blood transfusions with minimal adverse outcomes in children with sepsis.[19] In children with cyanotic heart disease, the recommended threshold for transfusion is a hemoglobin of 9 g/dL.[20] A more cautious approach is suggested in cancer patients in regard to blood administration. Blood transfusion in cancer patients can result in immune and inflammatory changes that may lead to proliferation and spread of cancer cells. A hemoglobin threshold of 9 g/dL in surgical oncology adult patients was associated with minimal exposure to blood cells and fewer major adverse outcomes.[21] However, a threshold of 7 or 8 g/dL is a common practice among pediatric hematologists, oncologists, and transplant physicians for stable nonsurgical pediatric patients.[22]

It is important to understand the factors influencing intraoperative decision-making regarding blood transfusion. Determining threshold values for individual patients may be helpful prior to surgery as part of a thorough preanesthetic plan. Hemoglobin levels are only one marker to help guide clinicians improve oxygen delivery in changing clinical scenarios. The data available to guide decision making when caring for pediatric patients is comparatively limited among surgical patients, trauma patients, and patients undergoing combined procedures due to the lack of studies specific to these populations.

Blood Components, Alternatives, and Special Factors

Packed Red Blood Cells

Packed red blood cells (pRBCs) increase oxygen-carrying capacity and total intravascular volume while simultaneously leading to volume expansion by mobilization of extracellular fluid into the intravascular space. pRBCs consist of mostly red blood cells after the majority of the plasma has been removed by apheresis or centrifugation of whole blood for a final hematocrit in the range of 65% to 80%. Leukoreduction is common, and the addition of additive solutions in addition to refrigerated storage between 1°C and 6°C can achieve a shelf life between 35 and 42 days.[23]

Red blood cells can be administered with or without any dilution with a crystalloid or a colloid. Not all crystalloid solutions are truly compatible given that the presence of Ca2++ can lead to clotting, hypotonic solutions can lead to cell lysis, and excessive dilution can lead to hemodilution and volume overload during transfusion. Although usually diluted with crystalloid solutions, such as NS, LR are also an acceptable alternative.[24] After pRBC units are issued by the blood bank, transfusion is recommended to occur within a 4-hour window, and rapid administration should be avoided whenever possible to prevent volume overload and perhaps increase the likelihood of early detection of transfusion reactions.

Platelets

Platelets are available as random donor platelets or single donor platelets. Both types are generally available in most blood banks. Platelet administration primarily is aimed at treating thrombocytopenia and is used for a number of additional indications. Thrombocytopenia can be absolute, a total low number or absence of platelets, or it can be functional, due to impaired platelet function. However, indications for platelet administration hinge on the overarching goal of restoring or optimizing coagulation and clot formation due to thrombocytopenia, whether functional or absolute.

Random donor platelets are generally issued in smaller volumes (50 mL), while apheresis units come in larger volumes (250 mL) for a higher total number of platelets given per transfusion.[23] Platelets have important differences compared to other blood components. Storage at room temperature (20°C–24°C) highlights the risk of infection given optimal conditions for bacterial growth. Bacterial sepsis after platelet administration has been described, and a high index of suspicion is warranted during and after administration. Although bacterial sepsis is a risk with administration of any blood component, platelets remain at the forefront of infection risk.[25,26]

Cryoprecipitate

Cryoprecipitate is most commonly used in the clinical setting to replete von Willebrand factor (vWF) and plasma proteins, more specifically fibrinogen. Cryoprecipitate can only be obtained from fresh frozen plasma (FFP), and it is the insoluble portion emerging from the process of thawing and centrifugation of FFP. Cryoprecipitate typically consists of small volumes (5–20 mL) and is given more rapidly compared to pRBCs or FFP for example. Cryoprecipitate may have variable amounts of plasma proteins, but in general they are present in low concentration. Nevertheless, cryoprecipitate is commonly administered as an ABO-compatible blood product. Cryoprecipitate is a poor volume expander, but given its relatively high fibrinogen concentration, it is considered the optimal blood component for the repletion of fibrinogen. Additionally, cryoprecipitate is an important component of balanced transfusion strategies.

Fresh Frozen Plasma

FFP is used to treat factor deficiencies and is an essential part of massive transfusion protocols and balanced transfusion strategies for both adult and pediatric patients. Administering FFP will also result in an increase in intravascular volume given its commonly shared characteristics with physiological plasma. Rapid administration is avoided whenever possible mainly to prevent fluid overload, especially in heart failure. In contrast to cryoprecipitate, FFP contains all the clotting factors. FFP is plasma frozen to a minimum temperature of −18°C that be stored for up to a year and thawed prior to administration. Although FFP is part of a balanced transfusion strategy, ASA guidelines recommend checking coagulation tests in patients with excessive bleeding prior to transfusion of FFP.[13] FFP administration is not without potential harm, including transfusion associated lung injury, transfusion-associated volume overload, and allergic reactions, and less common risks, such as infection. In neonates, the utility of FFP administration is questionable. FFP is not an optimal source of factor VIII and factor V, and longer storage times may increase risks of its use in neonates.[27]

Whole Blood, Desmopressin, Antifibrinolytic Agents, and Recombinant Factors

Blood transfusion can be tailored to address a multitude of clinical scenarios by administering individual components (FFP, cryoprecipitate, pRBCs, and platelets). However, there is renewed interest in whole blood administration for trauma patients.[28] In contrast to blood components, whole blood is characterized by the absence of high concentrations of preservative solutions with their effects magnified in high transfusion volumes such as in the treatment of the trauma patient.

Blood transfusions serve an important role in therapy, whether it is whole blood for transfusion or a combination of blood components. Other methods to minimize perioperative blood loss have been described. Some include desmopressin, factor concentrates, and antifibrinolytic agents.

Desmopressin is a vasopressin analog that acts by increasing the concentration of vWF from the endothelium. Factor VIII and tissue plasminogen factor are also released from platelets and endothelium after administration of desmopressin. The use of desmopressin is most commonly associated with treatment of bleeding disorders, such as von Willebrand's disease, hemophilia A, and platelet disorders. Its clinical use has been reported to reduce bleeding and blood product administration requirements in surgical patients.[29] Desmopressin is commonly given to patients with von Willebrand's disease preoperatively.

Factor concentrates and recombinant factor concentrates, such as prothrombin complex concentrates (PCCs) and recombinant activated factor VII (rFVIIa), increase the concentration of specific factors while minimizing the risks associated with donor-derived sources in case of recombinant factors (such as FFP or cryoprecipitate). Factor concentrates are most commonly used to reverse the effects of warfarin in the case of PCC and treat acquired factor deficiency from inhibitors to factor VIII or IX. The use of recombinant factor concentrates in surgery is an active area of investigation, and their widespread use is limited by the lack of data regarding their effectiveness. Although the utility of recombinant factors in addressing intractable bleeding has been described, administration of these for intractable bleeding is normally done after other causes are ruled out. Monitoring of coagulation and blood loss is especially important as part of the decision-making when recombinant factors are considered. Because of the risk of arterial thromboembolic events, dosing of recombinant factors should be done cautiously.

Antifibrinolytic agents prevent clot dissolution by plasmin. Agents include the lysine analog tranexamic acid and epsilon aminocaproic acid. Both are part of the armamentarium of agents available to minimize blood loss in the perioperative period. Although promising in their utility to prevent blood loss, their use is limited by patient selection, availability of evidence, and prothrombotic risk. The most common applications include spine surgery, orthopedics, and cardiac surgery.

A myriad of emerging technologies is currently under investigation to increase oxygen-carrying capacity, potentially minimize allogeneic blood transfusions, and decrease the need for transfusions with its potential risks. Oxygen-carrying capacity molecules represent a number of technical challenges in vivo, including nephrotoxicity, short half-life, cost, and overall benefit compared to standard blood transfusions. Several approaches exist including the production of synthetic molecules, such as Fluosol-DA, Oxygent, and Oxycyte, for example.[29,30,31] Other approaches aim to replicate the physiological properties of hemoglobin and are based on modifications of the hemoglobin molecules from different sources. The clinical application of these technologies remains limited and clinical trials are still underway; however, their true potential cannot be overstated.

Blood Conservation

Administering a blood product is not an entirely benign intervention, and analysis of risks versus benefits is paramount. This is especially true in the pediatric population, which may have lifelong acute and chronic processes starting early in life, increasing their exposure to blood products and perhaps needing lifelong treatment.

Significant adverse effects of blood product administration include allergic reactions, transfusion-related acute lung injury, transfusion-associated circulatory overload, and infection.[32] Moreover, emerging data suggest that blood product administration can lead to changes in the immune response influencing interactions with cancer cells. It is important to develop a blood conservation strategy for each patient, which may include the preoperative, intraoperative, and postoperative periods (Table 8.6).

Preoperative Optimization
Strategies to avoid transfusion include the preoperative optimization of the patient's blood status. This includes optimizing hemoglobin, as preoperative anemia is a risk factor for the need for intraoperative blood transfusion.[33] The World Health Organization has established guidelines for the classifications of anemia for different age groups (see Table 8.7).

Treatment options for increasing hemoglobin level prior to surgery include iron and erythropoietin. Ideally, strategies aiming to increase hemoglobin levels preoperatively must be initiated in advance in order to allow for adequate time for the treatment to work. Iron has been shown to be effective in adults at reducing the need for blood transfusions.[35] A recent systematic review and meta-analysis in adults showed a decrease in allogeneic blood transfusions with the preoperative administration of erythropoietin. It also showed no change in the incidence of thromboembolic events.[36] The data available in infants and children are relatively lacking, but the administering erythropoietin may also decrease the need for allogeneic blood transfusion in children as well.[37]

In addition to evaluating for anemia, the early detection of preexisting coagulation disorders and intraoperative coagulopathy should take place. This may include a medication reconciliation for account for blood-thinning agents, antiplatelet medications as well as a thorough history of bleeding diathesis.

It is particularly important to limit blood draws in the perioperative period, as this can be an unnecessary source of blood loss for the pediatric patient and the need is inversely related to age. Timing of blood draws should be optimized to enhance their utility as well as coordination with line access. Whenever appropriate, any unneeded blood or waste should be returned to the patient, such as in arterial blood sample or central venous sample draws, for instance.

Table 8.7	World Health Organization Classifications of Anemia
Population	**Anemia**
Children 0.50–4.99 years	<11.0 g/dL
Children 5.0–11.99 years	<11.5 g/dL
Children 12.0–14.99 years Nonpregnant women ≥15.0 years	<12.0 g/dL
Pregnant women	<11.0 g/dL
Men ≥15.0 years	<13.0 g/dL

Source: From https://www.who.int/vmnis/indicators/haemoglobin.pdf.

Table 8.6	Blood Conservation Strategies	
Preoperative	**Intraoperative**	**Postoperative**
Evaluation and treatment of anemia	ANH	Close management of postoperative bleeding
Evaluation of coagulopathy	Cell salvage	Cell salvage
Limitation/coordination of blood draws	Tolerance of anemia	
Stimulation of erythropoiesis (erythropoietin)	Antifibrinolytic agents	
PAD	Deliberate hypotension	
Establishment of transfusion thresholds	Factor concentrates	
	Topical hemostatics	
	Point-of-care testing	

ANH, acute normovolemic hemodilution; PAD, preoperative autologous donation.

Intraoperative Management
Strategies for blood conservation should continue through the intraoperative management period. Techniques for intraoperative management include preoperative autologous donation (PAD), acute normovolemic hemodilution (ANH), cell salvage, and deliberate hypotension.

Preoperative Autologous Donation
PAD is the donation and storage of autologous blood prior to elective surgery. PAD allows the anesthesia provider the ability to transfuse the donated blood during surgery to avoid allogeneic blood transfusion. This method of blood conservation is not well studied in the pediatric population, and it is not commonly employed.

Acute Normovolemic Hemodilution
ANH is the strategy of removing one or more whole blood units prior to surgery while replacing the removed blood with crystalloid or colloid solution. The provider then readministers the whole blood at the end of the surgery. This strategy has been shown to be beneficial in adults, but few studies have been done in children. Of the studies done in children, ANH has been shown to be safe in children.[38] A meta-analysis of 63 studies involving 3,819 patients showed a reduction in allogeneic blood transfusions,[39] and a meta-analysis of 29 randomized controlled trials for a total of 2439 patients also showed a reduction in allogeneic blood transfusions.[40]

Cell Savage
Cell salvage is a technique where blood is collected from the surgical field and reinfused into the patient. It is commonly used in surgeries with significant blood loss, such as cardiac, vascular, or spine surgeries. Cell salvage has been shown to decrease the rate of allogeneic blood transfusions in posterior spine fusions for idiopathic scoliosis.[41] It should not be used in cases in which the blood is contaminated, in patients with malignancy, or in patients with hematological disorders.[42]

Deliberate Hypotension
The goal of deliberate hypotension is to maintain the mean arterial blood pressure (MAP) low in order to decrease surgical blood loss, initially described as a MAP between 55 and 65 mmHg.[43] There are no large trials in children to determine a safe blood pressure range and anesthesia providers have several different options available to augment blood pressure management, including inhalational anesthetics, beta-blockers, or vasodilatory agents.[44] Anesthesia providers must weigh the benefits of this technique with the risks, especially with coexisting disease.

MONITORING
Monitoring is a crucial component of blood therapy and fluid management in the perioperative period. Intraoperative assessment of blood loss, anemia, and coagulopathy are three of the most important tools available to aid in clinical decision-making.

Visual assessment of blood loss, although imprecise, provides insight into the status of blood loss when combined with the surgeon's assessment of hemorrhage. Evaluation of microvascular bleeding is especially difficult, and quantifying the amount of blood loss from sponges is imprecise. Using visual field estimates alone may lead to a false sense of security due to underestimation. Nevertheless, visual assessment is commonly used as a starting point as part of a more thorough assessment of blood loss.

Measurement of hematocrit and or hemoglobin can also be useful intraoperatively. Although hemoglobin levels and hematocrit are influenced by rapid intra- and extracellular fluid changes, levels can be interpreted in combination with visual assessment of the field, coagulation studies, and hemodynamic changes. Monitoring hemoglobin levels or hematocrit is most useful when a high index of suspicion for significant intraoperative hemorrhage is present.

Monitoring of coagulopathy includes a myriad of testing modalities ranging from platelet counts, coagulation tests (international normalized ratio (INR), prothrombin time test (PT), and partial thromboplastin time test (PTT)) to more advanced tests, such as TEG or rotational thromboelastometry (ROTEM). Of these, TEG provides the most thorough laboratory assessment of coagulation in real time. Its widespread adoption is limited by cost, availability, timing, and more limited experience in interpretation compared to other monitoring modalities.

No single monitoring tool has been shown to be superior to others, and interpretation of blood loss is commonly achieved with a combination of the previously mentioned methods. Visual assessment, discussion with the surgical team regarding blood loss, and monitoring of anemia and coagulopathy all provide important information regarding blood loss that will help guide clinical decision-making and planning.

KEY TAKEAWAYS

- Fluid replacement for pediatric patients is based on physiological considerations and NPO status.
- Anesthesia providers can safely use crystalloids or colloids for fluid replacement.
- The optimization of glucose is important in pediatric patients, but the prevention of hypoglycemia is especially important in the neonate and premature infant to avoid long-term neurological damage.
- The transfusion of blood products is an important aspect of fluid replacement and may be necessary to optimize tissue oxygen delivery and coagulation.
- Use of a blood conservation strategy may preclude the need for blood transfusion, thereby reducing the potential of transfusion-related risks.

KEY REFERENCES

Complete references for this chapter are online and available at https://connect.springerpub.com/content/book/978-0-8261-3875-0/part/part02/toc-part/ch008.

3. *Pediatric Vital Signs Reference Chart*. 2020. http://www.pedscases.com/pediatric-vital-signs-reference-chart

7. McCluskey SA, Bartoszko J. The chloride horse and normal saline cart: the association of crystalloid choice with acid base status and patient outcomes in kidney transplant recipients. *Can J Anaesth*. 2020;67(4):403–407. doi:10.1007/s12630-020-01578-8

8. Abdessalam S. Hypotonic versus isotonic maintenance fluid administration in the pediatric surgical patient. *Semin Pediatr Surg*. 2019;28(1):43–46. doi:10.1053/j.sempedsurg.2019.01.007

13. American Society of Anesthesiologists task force on perioperative blood management. Practice guidelines for perioperative blood management: An updated report by the American Society of Anesthesiologists task force on perioperative blood management *Anesthesiology*. 2015;122(2):241–275. doi:10.1097/ALN.0000000000000463

18. Lacroix J, Tucci M, Du Pont-Thibodeau G. Red blood cell transfusion decision making in critically ill children. *Curr Opin Pediatr*. 2015;27(3)286–291. doi:10.1097/MOP.0000000000000221
23. Ozgonenel B, Nash TA, Rajpurkar M. Blood Components for Pediatric Transfusions. *Pediatr Rev*. 2020;41(5):259–261. doi:10.1542/pir.2018-0306
31. *Safety and Tolerability of Oxycyte in Patients With Traumatic Brain Injury (TBI) - Full Text View - ClinicalTrials.gov*. 2020. https://clinicaltrials.gov/ct2/show/NCT00908063
37. Cho BC, Serini J, Zorrilla-Vaca A, et al. Impact of preoperative erythropoietin on allogeneic blood transfusions in surgical patients: results from a systematic review and meta-analysis. *Anesth Analg*. 2019;128(5):981–992. doi:10.1213/ANE.0000000000004005
41. Zhou X, Zhang C, Wang Y, Yu L, Yan M. Preoperative acute normovolemic hemodilution for minimizing allogeneic blood transfusion: a meta-analysis. *Anesthesia and Analgesia*. 2015;121(6):1443–1455. doi:10.1213/ANE.0000000000001010

CHAPTER 9

Temperature Monitoring

Dawn Elizabeth Bent and Sharifah Wilson

> **LEARNING OBJECTIVES**
>
> - Characterize physiological sites of temperature monitoring in the pediatric patient.
> - Define core body temperature.
> - Understand thermoregulatory phases of temperature distribution under anesthesia.
> - Recognize various warming devices used in pediatric operating rooms.

INTRODUCTION

Since the time of Galileo and Hippocrates, temperature monitoring has been recognized as an important aspect of care. Without question, thermoregulation and temperature monitoring remain paramount in pediatric anesthesia. Variations in development and physiology, however, account for significant differences in the approach to temperature monitoring and the management thereof when compared to the adult population.

At birth, the newborn's body temperature distinctly decreases and takes on the temperature of the environment. This poikilothermic state is largely due to radiative heat loss.[1] To counter this drop in temperature, cortisol and catecholamines are released, with the end result being the activation of brown fat, which is rich in mitochondria to create heat production by nonshivering means. The ability of the neonate to maintain normothermia can be derailed by the effects of anesthesia. Therefore, it is imperative that anesthesia providers make a concerted effort to maintain normothermia as the child's innate resources and ability to do so are limited. To do so effectively, anesthesia providers should have a sound understanding of pediatric thermoregulation and how to best monitor changes in temperature, as well as the variety of interventions available to maintain normothermia while under general anesthesia. For further information regarding pediatric thermoregulation, please refer to Chapter 1, "Anatomy and Physiology of the Pediatric Patient," the section on thermoregulation.

TEMPERATURE MONITORING

Both the American Association of Nurse Anesthetists and the American Society of Anesthesiologists recognize temperature monitoring as a basic standard of anesthetic care and assert that temperature monitoring should occur in each case in which there is an anticipated change in temperature that is clinically significant.[2,3] Depending on the location temperature monitoring occurs, body temperature will vary. A patient's core body temperature can differ by as much as 1 to 2 degrees from the peripheral temperature. Detecting changes in temperature therefore requires accurate monitoring techniques and appropriate selection of temperature monitoring sites.

CORE BODY TEMPERATURE

A patient's core body temperature represents the temperature at which internal organs, such as the brain, heart, and lungs, are maintained. Core body temperature averages 36 to 37.5°C, which is the optimal temperature at which the human body's systems function.[4] Core body temperature should not be confused with the peripheral temperature of a patient. The peripheral temperature is a skin-level temperature that can be readily measured via noninvasive sites, such as the mouth, ear, axilla, and rectum, to provide an estimation of the core body temperature. However, a patient may feel cool to the touch but in fact have a core temperature within normal range.

It is not uncommon for a patient's core body temperature to have some variability throughout the day and during various physiological aspects of human day-to-day living.[5] During the evening and nighttime hours, there is a distinct pattern in physiological functioning that results in a decrease in the core body temperature, which has been described as circadian rhythm. This circadian fluctuation is less precise in younger children.[6]

Newborns and infants are not readily able to preserve what is considered a normal body temperature as their adult counterparts. The limited ability to shiver and sweat combined with a large body surface area-to-weight ratio results in extreme variations in core body temperature when a young child is exposed to extreme temperature changes.

TEMPERATURE MONITORING LOCATIONS

From a physiological standpoint, anesthesia providers should understand the advantages and disadvantages associated with various temperature monitoring locations. While the accuracy of a patient's temperature can vary depending on the site of monitoring, anesthesia providers are charged with determining the safest, most appropriate location based on accessibility, the surgery being performed, the patient's state of health and comorbidities, and the anticipated length of time the patient will be under general anesthesia. In addition, the anticipated means of airway management plays a role in determining temperature monitoring as placing an esophageal temperature probe in patients who do not have a secured airway is not advisable.

The commonly used locations for temperature monitoring while under general anesthesia are the axilla, skin, nasopharynx, esophagus, pulmonary artery, bladder, and rectum, four of which closely resemble core body temperature. Table 9.1 describes the various sites commonly employed for temperature monitoring during general anesthesia, with numbers 3 through 6 being the sites that most resemble the core body temperature.

Axillary Temperature

The accessibility of the axilla, coupled with the low potential for risk, makes it one of the most common locations for temperature monitoring during general anesthetic. The tip of the temperature probe should be placed superficial to the axillary

134　PART II: PERIOPERATIVE ANESTHETIC CARE

Table 9.1	Common Temperature Monitoring Locations	
Location	**Advantages**	**Disadvantages**
Axilla	Easy to locate, low risk of infection	Unable to locate axillary artery, probe shifting
Skin	Multiple locations to choose from, good for shorter procedures	Environmental temperatures may alter reading
Nasopharynx	Caution with uncuffed ETT related to cool gases	Caution with uncuffed ETT related to cool gases
Esophagus	Easy to locate, resembles core temperature	Precise placement
Pulmonary artery	Accurate core temperature	Requires invasive monitoring
Bladder	Easy to place, close to core temperature	Oliguria alters accuracy
Rectum	Easy to place	Invalid related to fecal content, caution with rectal disease

ETT, endotracheal tube.

artery for best results. The patient's arm should remain adducted as the ambient temperature of an operating room or air from a forced-air warming blanket may cause variation or erroneous temperature measurement.[7] In addition, the probe may shift with patient movement or repositioning resulting in inaccurate measurement. Anesthesia providers should remember that an axillary temperature is considered skin temperature monitoring and that the placement of the temperature probe in a location other than directly on the axillary artery will render a temperature reading no more accurate than a skin temperature reading.

Skin Temperature Monitoring

The efficacy of skin temperature monitoring in the pediatric patient under general anesthesia has been challenged, as the environment and effects of general anesthesia impact younger patients to a great degree than the adult patient. The difference between the core and peripheral temperatures is dependent upon the gradient between the patient's temperature and the temperature of the environment. Skin temperature of younger pediatric patients will differ from the core temperature to a greater extent because of the exposure of the skin to the temperature of the operating room. Additionally, general anesthesia causes a redistribution of heat from the periphery to the core of the patient to preserve a constant temperature to vital organs.[5] Thus, while the skin is readily accessible, skin temperature monitoring is best suited for the adult patient as adults have the ability to conserve their core body temperature to a greater extent than do pediatric patients due to the variance in body habitus between the two populations. When used with older patients, skin temperature monitoring offers anesthesia providers the ability to follow the patient's temperature trend, which can be particularly useful during brief encounters.

Nasopharyngeal Temperature Monitoring

The accessibility of the nasopharynx makes this a widely utilized location for temperature monitoring in pediatric anesthesia. When placed correctly, the tip of the temperature probe should have contact with the nasal mucosa and lie in the posterior aspect of the nasopharynx. Because of the proximity of the nasopharynx to the internal carotid artery, nasopharyngeal temperature monitoring provides temperature measurement reflective of the core temperature.[8]

Should an uncuffed endotracheal tube be used to secure the airway, cool airway gases may alter the accuracy of temperature measurement but not necessarily the precision of the actual temperature. If an anesthesia provider utilizes an uncuffed endotracheal tube during an anesthetic, they must be cognizant of this nuance related to this mode of temperature monitoring.

Esophageal Temperature Monitoring

Like the nasopharynx, the esophagus is easily accessed and is widely utilized in pediatric anesthesia. The tip of the esophageal temperature probe should be placed at the lower (distal) one-third or one-quarter of the esophagus to provide accurate core temperature reading. In this position, temperature monitoring is least affected by airway gases that may cool the probe and provide inaccurate temperature measurements.[9]

An esophageal temperature probe may also be used in concert with, or as part of, a precordial stethoscope. A precordial stethoscope with a temperature probe allows anesthesia providers to not only continuously monitor heart tones and breath sounds but allows for temperature monitoring as well. This is especially useful as small pediatric patients are often physically distanced from the anesthesia provider due to the nature of the surgical procedure. Therefore, the utility of this combination makes it a frequently employed means of monitoring the temperature, breath sounds, and heart tones in the pediatric patient to ensure the delivery of safe, effective anesthetic care.

Pulmonary Artery Monitoring

Although the pulmonary artery is one of the most accurate of the core temperature monitoring sites, it is seldom used in pediatric anesthesia unless the patient requires a pulmonary artery catheter for the purposes of the surgical procedure. The need for accurate temperature monitoring alone does not warrant the placement of a central line as there are other less invasive means of obtaining an accurate assessment of core temperature that carry fewer potential risks and consequences.[10]

Bladder Temperature Monitoring

Bladder temperature monitoring provides an accurate measurement of core body temperature, especially when there is high urine output.[7] Low urine output states, however, decrease the accuracy of a bladder temperature monitoring. Bladder temperature monitoring can be achieved with the use of a foley catheter that has a thermistor probe incorporated in the catheter. Like a pulmonary artery temperature device, a foley catheter should not be inserted solely for the purposes of temperature monitoring during surgery as there are other temperature monitoring modalities that are more appropriate.

Rectal Temperature Monitoring

As with other modes of monitoring, rectal temperature probes are easily placed and provide a reasonably accurate means of temperature monitoring. Temperature assessment, however, may be inaccurate due to insulation by fecal matter and other organisms located in the bowel that can produce heat, such as *Clostridium difficile*.[9] If there is a suspected perforation or other malformations of the rectum, this method of temperature monitoring is contraindicated.

THERMOREGULATION DURING ANESTHESIA

Volatile agents alter the hypothalamic response to temperature changes by inhibiting central thermoregulation, with the extent of inhibition varying depending on the minimum alveolar concentration (MAC) of the agent.[11] Volatile agents also cause vasodilation, which when coupled with the impact on central regulation, increases the potential for perioperative heat loss and subsequently hypothermia.[11] Nitrous oxide also interferes with thermoregulation, although to a lesser extent than volatile agents. It should be noted that this is a bidirectional relationship as fluctuations in temperature (hypothermia or hyperthermia) impact the MAC of volatile agents, with the MAC of a volatile agent being lower when the patient is hypothermic. Conversely, if the patient's temperature is greater than 42°C, the patient will have a higher MAC of that same agent.[12] The duration of neuromuscular blocking agents is prolonged when the patient is hypothermic and should be taken into consideration when administering subsequent doses.[13]

As the body's normal thermoregulation mechanisms are inhibited during general anesthesia, hypothermia can quickly ensue as the environment cools, particularly with the pediatric patient (Figure 9.1). Considering the normal body temperature ranges between 36°C and 37.5°C, any deviation lower than the norm is considered hypothermia. Anesthesia providers, however, should make a determination on what is considered hypothermia for their specific patient. This determination will help guide care, as the more hypothermic a patient becomes, the more deleterious the effects will be during the perioperative period (see Box 9.1). Mild hypothermia should be expected, especially without active measures in place to maintain normothermia, as this often occurs inadvertently under normal circumstances.[9] There are three distinct phases of thermoregulation while under general anesthesia.

THERMOREGULATORY PHASES

Phase 1

With the induction of general anesthesia, there is a noted decline in the core temperature anywhere from 0.5°C to 1.5°C. This decline in core body temperature is a manifestation of the reallocation of blood from the core, or vessel-rich organs (heart, liver, kidneys, etc.) to the periphery.[7] This reallocation of blood is considered Phase 1 or the internal redistribution

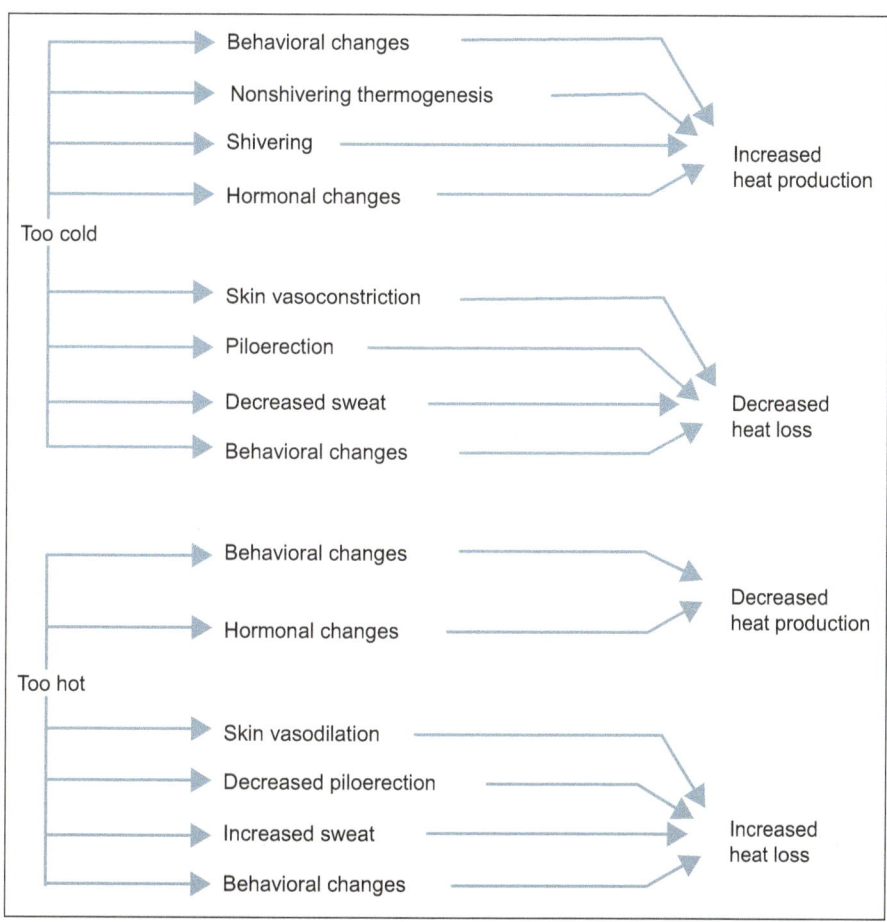

Figure 9.1: Physiological response to alterations in core temperature.

> **BOX 9.1 HYPOTHERMIA AND HYPERTHERMIA UNDER ANESTHESIA**
>
> **Takeaway Points of Hypothermia and Hyperthermia**
>
> Hypothermia causes:
> - Impaired coagulation
> - Increased wound infection
> - Increased oxygen demand
> - Changes in drug metabolism
> - Myocardial dysfunction
>
> Hyperthermia causes:
> - Mainly related to overwarming
> - Rule out infectious process
> - Malignant hyperthermia

> **BOX 9.2 THERMOREGULATORY PHASES UNDER GENERAL ANESTHESIA**
>
> **Phase 1: Internal Redistribution of Heat**
> - Widening gradient between core and peripheral temperature
>
> **Phase 2: Linear**
> - Heat loss, slow decline over time
>
> **Phase 3: Rewarming**
> - Temperature stability, active warming mitigates hypothermia

of heat.[7,14] Heat is not lost during this phase, but rather, it is redistribution throughout the body. During the internal redistribution of heat, there is a widening gradient between the core temperature and the peripheral temperature. Other contributing factors include the vasodilatory effects of volatile agents and the infusion of IV fluids that are cooler than the temperature of the child.

Phase 1 or the internal redistribution of heat occurs 30 to 90 minutes following the initiation of a general anesthetic. To combat this decline in core temperature, many anesthesia providers have adopted the practice of warming the patient prior to the start of anesthesia to prevent the reallocation of blood related to the initial decline in core temperature. While this practice varies, preemptive warming should be considered when caring for pediatric patients to stave off declines in core temperature, specifically when caring for neonatal patients.

Phase 2

Phase 2, or the linear phase of thermoregulation while under general anesthesia, consists of a slowly progressing hypothermic response due to a variety of reasons. As the physiological response to general anesthesia in Phase 1 continues, there is additional heat loss via the four mechanisms of heat loss as described in Chapter 1, "Anatomy and Physiology of the Pediatric Patient," the section on thermoregulation (radiation, conduction, convection, and evaporation). This Phase 2 or linear phase lasts for approximately 3 hours. During this phase, the metabolic rate of the heat produced by the body does not exceed the rate at which heat is lost, resulting in a slow decrease of core temperature. Additional contributing factors to progressive heat loss are the size of the patient, the patient's minute ventilation, and continued administration of anesthetics that contribute to heat loss, which may further exacerbate the degree of hypothermia.[15]

Phase 3

Phase 3 or the rewarming phase is the most intricate. As noted by the name, the rewarming phase is the phase in which the metabolic rate and heat production equalize, if not exceed, the rate of heat loss. During this phase, the patient's core body temperature reaches a level of stability. It is prudent for the anesthesia provider to acknowledge the need to actively warm the patient during this time in an effort to avoid progression of hypothermia. During this phase, neonates and infants have a unique response not witnessed in older children and adults. In an attempt to increase or maintain their temperature, neonates and infants will utilize brown adipose tissue to generate heat via nonshivering thermogenesis (see Chapter 1, "Anatomy and Physiology of the Pediatric Patient" for further details).[7,16] **Box 9.2** summarizes the three phases of thermoregulation under general anesthesia.

CONSEQUENCES OF HYPOTHERMIA

Core hypothermia or mild hypothermia occurs in the range between 34.0°C and 35.9°C.[7] When a pediatric patient becomes hypothermic, a host of detrimental physiological effects can ensue. Mild perioperative hypothermia leads to impaired coagulation related to platelet function dysfunction, a higher incidence of wound infection attributed to vasoconstriction that limits delivery of oxygen to the operative site, alterations in drug metabolism, and a general increase in oxygen demand, which can result in myocardial insufficiency with a direct correlation with cardiac abnormalities and dysfunction.[7,10]

CONSEQUENCES OF HYPERTHERMIA

Outside of pathophysiological reasons for an increased temperature, such as malignant hyperthermia (refer to Chapter 126, "Malignant Hyperthermia," for further information) or neuroleptic syndrome, the most common reason for hyperthermia in a pediatric patient while under general anesthesia is overwarming of the patient by the anesthesia provider.[10] The presence of an infectious process should be taken into consideration as well when determining the cause of hyperthermia or pyrexia.

Anesthesia providers must remain cognizant that when active warming devices are utilized, hyperthermia can ensue as heat is not able to dissipate. This is especially true when the head of a neonate or small child is covered. Therefore, anesthesia providers need to be vigilant about their use of warming devices, as untoward effects or equipment malfunction can occur.

MAINTENANCE OF NORMOTHERMIA

ROOM TEMPERATURE

Pediatric patients lose heat via radiation more than any other mechanism of heat loss. According to the Association of PeriOperative Registered Nurses, temperature in operating rooms in the United States range between 20°C and 23°C.[17] When caring for a preterm or term neonatal patient, the operating room temperatures should be increased in an effort to maintain normothermia.

In most pediatric operating rooms, the anesthesia provider is responsible for controlling the temperature of the environment. It is not uncommon for the temperature in the operating room to challenge the comfort level of providers (e.g., surgeon, circulating nurse, scrub technician, and anesthesia team), but the patient is the primary responsibility of each provider. Given the deleterious effects of hypothermia, control of the environmental temperature should preferentially serve the patient. Another means of preventing radiative heat loss is covering the neonate or infants, head with a plastic heat in an effort to retain heat close to the patient.

FORCED-AIR WARMING

The use of a forced-air warming device such as a Bair Hugger® blanket is an easy and convenient way to warm patients in the operating room that has been proven to be effective in minimizing hypothermia. Such devices can also be utilized prior to the patient's arrival to the operating room as well to help create an environment that minimizes conductive heat loss. Furthermore, the use of a forced-air warming device in conjunction with a fluid warming device and warming blanket provides the optimal approach to staving off even moderate, inadvertent intraoperative hypothermia.[18] Figure 9.2 is an example of a forced-air warming system used with pediatric patients.

RADIANT WARMING DEVICES

Radiant light or heating devices are another method of keeping the pediatric patient, more specifically the neonate, warm during surgical procedures. These devices are typically used during the induction of anesthesia, as neonates are often exposed to a cool environment during this time to placement of monitors and visualization of an infant's respiratory efforts during the induction of anesthesia. It is imperative that anesthesia providers allow radiant light to be a reasonable distance from the patient to avoid overheating or burning the patient. Also, anesthesia providers should remain cognizant of their proximity to the radiant light as there have been reports of surgical hats catching fire. Figure 9.3 is an example of the use of a radiant warmer when caring for a neonatal patient.

FLUID WARMERS

Fluid warmers remain a mainstay in preventing hypothermia, not only for blood products but to warm crystalloid IV fluids as well. As the room temperature of most operating rooms is between 20°C and 23°C, there is a gradient between the environment of the patient's core body temperature (36°C–37.5°C). Infusing IV fluids at room temperature would have the potential to lower the core temperature of the patient. Having all fluids delivered via a fluid warmer lessens the temperature gradient, thereby decreasing the risk of perioperative hypothermia. Similarly, the surgical team can limit hypothermia by utilizing warm irrigation fluids, especially when the use of surgical irrigation will be extensive. Figure 9.4 is an example of a Hotline® Level One (Smiths-Medical, Nowell, MA) fluid warmer that is commonly used in pediatric operating rooms when increased volumes of fluids are necessary or for the delivery of warm blood products.

HUMIDIFICATION OF INHALED GASES

Inhaled gases are administered at room temperature with little to no humidification, resulting in heat loss. To counteract

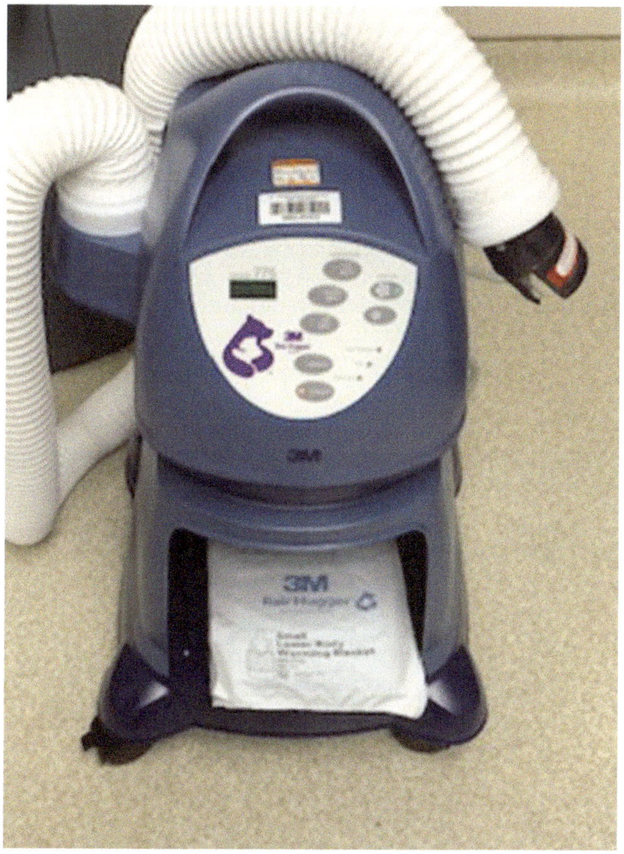

Figure 9.2: Forced-air warming blanket.

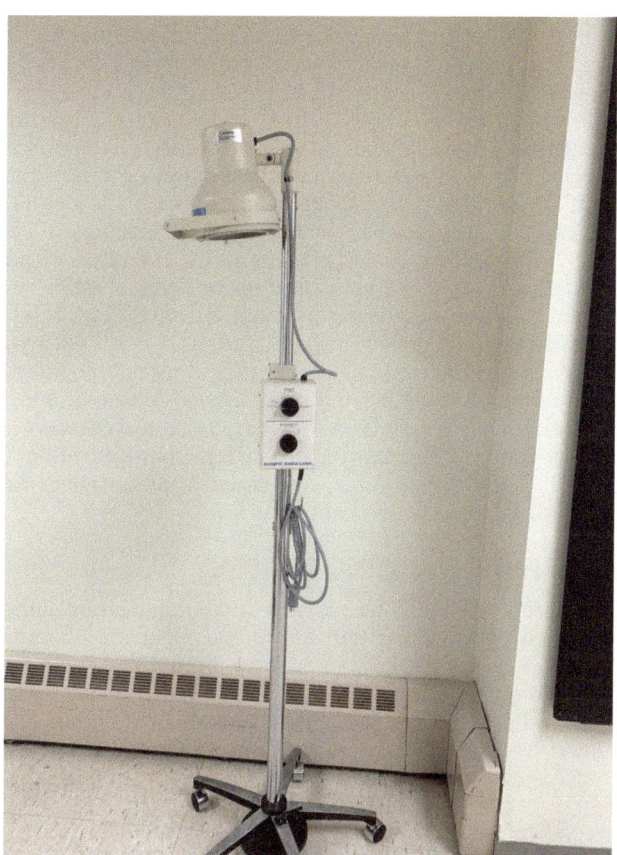

Figure 9.3: Radiant warming light.

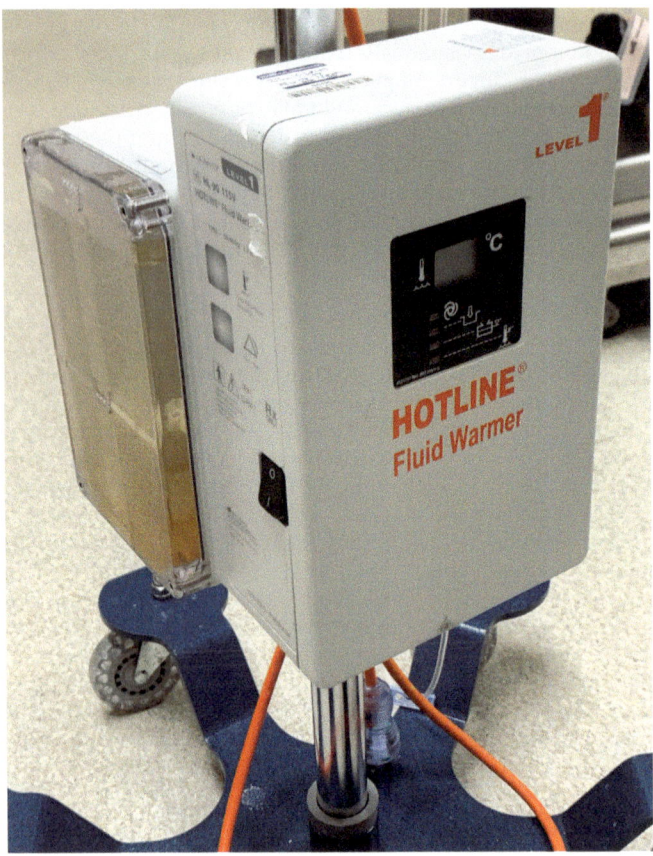

Figure 9.4: Fluid warmer.

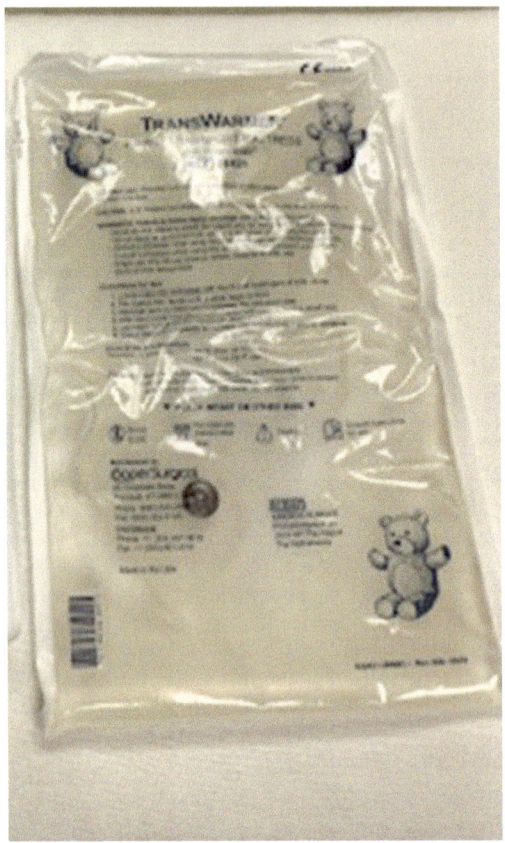

Figure 9.5: Warming infant transport mattress.

the heat loss, dry gases are humidified and warmed by the upper respiratory tract. This comes at a price, however, as humidification and warming of gases account for approximately 15% of the body's total base heat expenditure. Anesthesia providers can supplement the innate process as well with both passive and active warming techniques. Passive humidification can be achieved with the use of a heat and moisture exchanger (HME). HMEs typically contain hygroscopic material that aids in the retention of heat and moisture. Active humidification requires a water supply and external power and is more effective than passive humidification in preserving moisture and heat. A variety of active humidifiers are available, including bubble humidifiers, nebulizers, and heated humidifiers. Bubble humidifiers work by passing the fresh gas through a water reservoir. For additional information regarding humidification of inhaled gases, please refer to Chapter 4, "Equipment and Monitoring."

TRANSPORT WARMING DEVICES

Consideration should be given to maintaining normothermia when transporting patients to and from the operating room. The use of warm blankets and infant hats, and swaddling patients during transport can help keep the patient warm and prevent heat loss. Extra measures should be implemented when transporting infants to and from the neonatal intensive care unit given the potential for hypothermia due to radiative heat loss. Warming devices specifically designed to maintain heat during this time, such as a TransWarmer® (CooperSurgical, Trumball, CT), should be employed in an effort to prevent heat loss. These devices are gel-filled, chemically activated portable warming mattresses, which can be activated to release heat with the breaking or bending of a small disk within the mattress. They conform to the patient's body, reaching its maximum temperature of 40°C in a matter of 60 seconds with the ability to maintain that temperature for up to 2 hours.[19] If available, newborns can also be transported in specially designed beds with radiant warming lights built in. Figure 9.5 is an example of the TransWarmer® warming device that can be used during the transport of infants.

KEY TAKEAWAYS

- Multiple temperature monitoring sites, such as the nasopharynx, esophagus, and pulmonary artery, correlate with core body temperature.
- Neonatal patients are poikilothermic.
- Even mild hypothermia can lead to ill effects in the perioperative and postoperative periods.
- The use of warming devices should be utilized during pediatric cases.

KEY REFERENCES

Complete references for this chapter are online and available at https://connect.springerpub.com/content/book/978-0-8261-3875-0/part/part02/toc-part/ch009.

1. Elshazzly M, Anekar AA, Caban O. Physiology, newborn. In: *Stat Pearls*. Stat Pearls Publishing, 2020.
4. Lidell ME. Brown adipose tissue in human infants. *Handb Exp Pharmacol*. 2018;251:107–123. doi:10.1007/164_2018_118
5. Cheshire WP Jr. Thermoregulatory disorders and illness related to heat and cold stress. *Auton Neurosci*. 2016;196:91–104. doi:10.1016/j.autneu.2016.01.001
7. Davis, Peter J, Cladis, Franklyn. *Smith's Anesthesia for Infants and Children*. 9th ed. Elsevier Health Sciences, 2017.
9. Dorsch JA, Dorsch SE. *A Practical Approach to Anesthesia Equipment*. 2nd ed. Wolters Kluwer Health, 2012.
10. Ehrenwerth J. In: Eisenkraft JB, Berry JM, eds *Anesthesia Equipment: Principles and Applications*. Elsevier - Health Sciences Division, 2013.
17. Association of Peri-Operative Registered Nurses. eGuidelines +. *Design and Maintenance of the Operating Room*. 2019. www.aorn.org
18. Lai L, See M, Rampal S, et al. Significant factors influencing inadvertent hypothermia in pediatric anesthesia. *J Clin Monit Comput*. 2019;33:1105–1112. doi:10.1007/s10877-019-00259-2

CHAPTER 10

Postanesthetic Care

Brett J. Morey

> **LEARNING OBJECTIVES**
>
> - Describe the safe postoperative transport of pediatric patients.
> - Discuss the key elements of providing a patient handoff.
> - List the most common postoperative issues.
> - Define the criteria for safe discharge of a pediatric patient.

INTRODUCTION

Anesthesia providers are charged with ensuring the safe transition of care of a patient to a qualified healthcare provider following an anesthetic. Thus, postoperative transport and patient handoff are key components of ensuring safe, effective care. The postanesthetic phase of care is a high-risk period often associated with acute onset issues that require immediate intervention. It is imperative that anesthesia providers have the ability to recognize and treat anesthesia-related issues that may arise postoperatively. Additionally, they are responsible for ensuring a high level of patient care is continued with the transition of care.

PATIENT TRANSPORT

Transporting a pediatric patient from the operating room (OR) to the postanesthesia care unit (PACU) can present unique challenges depending on the procedure performed, general health of the patient, and plane of anesthesia or recovery. While the PACU is generally a relatively short distance away from the OR, this is a vulnerable period for the patient, mandating that anesthesia providers are ever prepared to intervene should an emergency arise. Transporting from nonoperating room anesthesia (NORA) locations to the PACU may be even more daunting as it often involves a greater distance or the need for an elevator ride between locations. Therefore, transporting with emergency medications and the proper equipment to manage an emergency is critical as laryngospasm, airway obstruction, sudden changes in hemodynamic stability, or emergence delirium (ED) may occur at any point during transport. Furthermore, the use of a transport monitor should be considered, especially if transporting over a longer distance.

SAFE HANDOFF

Upon arrival to the PACU, anesthesia providers should provide a thorough handoff report to ensure a safe transition of care. A proper handoff should include key information about the patient and the procedure performed. There are many different checklists or tools available to guide this process, with no single tool having been reported as superior or universal. In fact, handoff tools may be optimized to the setting or location to ensure key information is communicated consistently (**Figures 10.1** and **10.2**). It has been offered that the most important component of any handoff is a handoff readback, as this may highlight the need for clarification of pertinent information. Moreover, the handoff process should never be truncated due to production pressure. Ultimately, utilizing validated checklists is recommended to ensure a detailed, consistent report is given to PACU staff with each patient handoff.[1]

PACU HANDOFF CHECKLISTS

SURGERY CHECKLIST:
- [ ] PRIMARY SERVICE
- [ ] CONTACT PERSON/PAGER NUMBER
- [ ] PROCEDURE AND INCISION SITES (dressings, drains, tubes)
- [ ] SIGNIFICANT SURGICAL EVENTS
- [ ] POST OP CARE (if applicable)
  - o BP Target:
  - o Flap:
  - o Positioning:
  - o Other:
- [ ] LABS/IMAGING: CT/MRI/CXR
- [ ] DISPOSITION: INPT/OUTPT/TRANS PACU/EXT RECOVERY
- [ ] ORDERS ENTERED? PRESCRIPTION VERIFIED? MEDICATION RECONCILIATION?
- [ ] PRIMARY POST OP CONCERN
- [ ] QUESTIONS?

ANESTHESIA CHECKLIST:
- [ ] SIGNIFICANT SURGICAL/MEDICAL HISTORY
- [ ] DRUG ALLERGIES
- [ ] PACEMAKER/ICD? If Yes, needs interrogation?
- [ ] RESISTANCE/SENSITIVITY TO ANESTHETICS/SEDATION?
- [ ] DIFFICULT AIRWAY?
- [ ] OXYGENATION ISSUES?
- [ ] HEMODYNAMIC EVENTS/STABILITY
- [ ] OTHER INTRAOP EVENTS
- [ ] SPECIAL ANALGESIA (ERAS premeds, Exparel, Nerve blocks)
- [ ] SPECIAL PATIENT CONCERNS (PONV, Chronic Pain, Communicable Disease, Language, Disability, Psychosocial)
- [ ] PRIMARY POST OP CONCERN
- [ ] ANESTHESIA CONTACTS: Anesthesiologist/CRNA
- [ ] QUESTIONS?

Figure 10.1: Postanesthesia care unit (PACU) handoff checklist.

Source: An Alternative Succinct Checklist Offered for PACU Handoff Communication. Anesthesia Patient Safety Foundation. (2019, October 19). https://www.apsf.org/article/an-alternative-succinct-checklist-offered-for-pacuhandoff-communication/.

"I-PASS" Nurse to Nurse Sign-out: From IR to ICUs/PACU/floors
(Worksheet only – Do not file in Medical Record)

I	Illness Severity (Sick or Not Sick?)	(This patient is unstable, and he's full code or this is a very stable post-op patient)
P	Patient Summary	Name_____ MR# _____ Precaution_____ Age _____ Wt _____ kg Allergies_____ Diagnosis/past medical history: IR Procedure_____ Attending Radiologist:_____ Attending Anesthesiologist:_____

Procedure Info:	Access/Fluid Intake:		
Labs:	Type	Size	Site
	PIV		
	PIV		
	PICC/CVL		
	A-line		
Embolic Agents/Coils:	Total Crystalloid: Total Blood Products: Total Contrast given:		
Medications:	Output:		
	Foley	Size	ml
	Chest tube	Size	ml
	Drain	Size	ml
	Other	Size	ml
	Total Output:		

Anesthesia Issues and Plan_____

Neuro status _____

Hemodynamic status _____

Respiratory status _____

Other pertinent systems _____

A	Action List	To do list over next 12 hrs (pain needs, meds due, lines/tubes-anything to be secured/addressed, family care needs)
S	**Situational Awareness & Contingency Planning**	Summary, status, and general goals over next 12 hours
S	**Synthesis (by receiver)**	

Figure 10.2: Pediatric sedation handoff checklist.

Source: http://spsnews. pedsedation.org/do-you-know-what-i-know-patient-handoffs-in-pediatric-procedural-sedation/.

COMMON POSTANESTHETIC COMPLICATIONS

Following report, anesthesia providers should conduct a final patient before leaving the bedside, ensuring the child's airway is patent, they are hemodynamically stable, and they are free of distress.

While most pediatric patients tolerate anesthesia without incident, problems can still occur postoperatively (Box 10.1).

LARYNGOSPASM, AIRWAY OBSTRUCTION, AND HYPOXEMIA

Pediatric laryngospasm is a life-threatening event that involves blockage of the airway.[2] Laryngospasm is the forceful closure of the larynx that can quickly lead to hypoxemia if not treated immediately.[3] The incidence of laryngospasm is more common in children than adults, with an estimated range from 1 to 17.4 cases per 1,000 anesthetics.[4] Positive pressure, propofol, and

BOX 10.1 COMMON POSTANESTHETIC COMPLICATIONS

- Airway obstruction/hypoxemia
- Bleeding
- Bradycardia/tachycardia
- Emergence delirium
- Hypotension
- Hypothermia
- Laryngospasm
- Malignant hypothermia
- Pain
- PONV

PONV, postoperative nausea and vomiting

succinylcholine are commonly used to break laryngospasm. If left untreated, laryngospasm may lead to pulmonary edema, dysrhythmias, cardiac arrest, and ultimately death.[2]

The incidence of laryngospasm increases with patients who have gastroesophageal reflux disease (GERD), upper respiratory infections (URIs), and extubating in Phase 2 of anesthesia. It is important to note that extubating a child in a deep plane of anesthesia to avoid stimulation or coughing does not preclude laryngospasm from occurring as the child enters Stage 2 of anesthesia recovery. Therefore, it is important anesthesia providers transport with emergency medications if the child is extubated in a deep plane of anesthesia to facilitate swift intervention should laryngospasm occur.

Pediatric patients, especially infants and toddlers, present complex airway and respiratory challenges while emerging from anesthesia in the PACU.[5] Airway obstruction is a common problem in the PACU. Congenital craniofacial anomalies, a disproportionately large head, history of reactive airway disease, a deep plane of anesthesia postextubation, and patient positioning all may contribute to airway obstruction. Repositioning the patient may alleviate obstruction and airway maneuvers, such as a chin lift or jaw thrust, may be required for short periods. Should obstruction persist, the insertion of an oral airway or nasal trumpet should be considered to promote airway patency. As infants and young children can quickly become bradycardic when hypoxic, it is breathing, oxygen saturation, and heart rate are monitored in the PACU during the recovery period.

Hypoxemia can occur from a variety of factors. Prematurity in infants, obstructive sleep apnea (OSA), postobstructive pulmonary edema, postintubation croup, and hypoventilation from narcotics are all contributing factors.[6] Supplemental oxygen should remain on the child until they are able to meet weaning criteria. If a child cannot maintain their oxygen saturation at or above the minimum level to meet discharge criteria, further investigation is warranted to rule out aspiration, pneumonia, or pneumothorax.[4]

EMERGENCE DELIRIUM

ED is an abnormal, dissociated state of consciousness in which children may be inconsolable, irritable, uncompromising, and/or uncooperative. ED occurs soon after the emergence from anesthesia and typically lasts from 5 to 20 minutes, although symptoms may persist for an hour or longer.[7] The pathophysiology of ED is not entirely understood, but an imbalance between excitatory and inhibitory pathways, combined with the effects of anesthesia on cortical and subcortical networks, is thought to contribute to the presence of ED.[8] The incidence of ED is highest in children aged 2 to 6 years; however, it can occur in patients of all ages through adulthood.[9]

ED is especially common among pediatric patients following the administration of inhalation anesthetics, with the incidence in the pediatric population being as high as 40% when inhaled agents are the primary anesthetic.[9,10] Modern volatile anesthetic agents with low blood/gas partition coefficients contribute to ED due to their inherent short duration of action that promotes a rapid emergence from anesthesia.[8,11] The two volatile anesthetic agents most commonly associated with ED are sevoflurane and desflurane.[12] The use of inhalational anesthetics, however, is not the sole etiology of ED as it has been associated with certain surgical procedures and can be instigated by preoperative anxiety, pain, or a rapid emergence.[13] Prolonged periods of ED may lead to psychological distress of the patient or their parents. Additionally, it is associated with diminished patient satisfaction, prolonged recovery time, a longer hospital stay, and increased cost of care.[13] A number of prophylactic interventions,

such as the administration of propofol, opioids, midazolam, nonsteroidal anti-inflammatory drugs, nitrous oxide, ketamine, magnesium, alpha-2 adrenoreceptor agonists, and regional blocks, have been reported to temper the incidence and duration of ED.[7,10] Limiting exposure to short-acting volatile anesthetic agents has also been reported to decrease the incidence of ED.

POSTOPERATIVE NAUSEA AND VOMITING

Postoperative nausea and vomiting (PONV) is a significant problem following anesthesia, affecting 20% to 40% of patients despite the widespread uses of antiemetic agents, short-acting anesthetics, and minimally invasive surgical techniques.[14] The pathophysiology of PONV is complex, involving a variety of neurophysiological pathways and receptors (Figure 10.3).[14] The five primary afferent pathways involved are the chemoreceptor trigger zone, the vagal mucosal pathway in the gastrointestinal system, neuronal pathways to the vestibula system, the reflex afferent pathways from the cerebral cortex, and the midbrain afferents. The area within the brain responsible for controlling nausea and vomiting is an ill-defined region called "vomiting center," which lies within the reticular formation. Stimulation of one of the afferent pathways involved results in vomiting via activation of histamine, muscarinic, opioid, dopamine 2, or serotonin receptors.[15]

Factors that increase the incidence of PONV in children include duration of surgery >30 minutes, history of PONV, type of surgery (strabismus surgery, hernia repair, tonsillectomy and adenoidectomy, ear surgery, and laparoscopic procedures), history of motion sickness, and type of anesthetic administered.[4] Unresolved PONV can result in prolonged stays in PACU, thereby increasing healthcare-related costs and decreasing patient satisfaction.[15] PONV can also contribute to more serious medical complications including aspiration, electrolyte disturbances, dehydration, and suture damage.[16]

The use of antiemetic medications in pediatric patients has been widely studied with a wide variety of antiemetic medications readily available to anesthesia providers for the treatment and prevention of PONV. The medications commonly used for the treatment of PONV include 5-hydroxytryptamine (5-HT3) receptor antagonists, neurokinin-1 (NK-1) receptor antagonists, corticosteroids, butyrophenones, antihistamines, and anticholinergics.[14] The management strategy for each patient should be based on level of risk of PONV. Furthermore, combination antiemetic therapy employing two or more antiemetic medications acting on different receptors is more effective at preventing PONV than the administration of single antiemetic agent alone (Table 10.1).[15]

In addition to the use of antiemetic medications, anesthesia providers can utilize a number of techniques to further

Table 10.1	Antiemetic Medications
Receptor Antagonist	Antimetic Drug Examples
5-HT3	Ondansetron, granisetron, dolasetron, ramosetron, palonesetron, tropisetron, corticosteroids
NK-1	Aprepitant, cospitant, rolapitant
H1	Promethazine, perphenazine, dimenhydrinate, diphenhydramine, meclizine, chlorpromazine
Anticholinergic (M)	Scopolamine

5-HT3, 5-hydroxytryptamine; H1, histamine; NK-1, neurokinin-1.

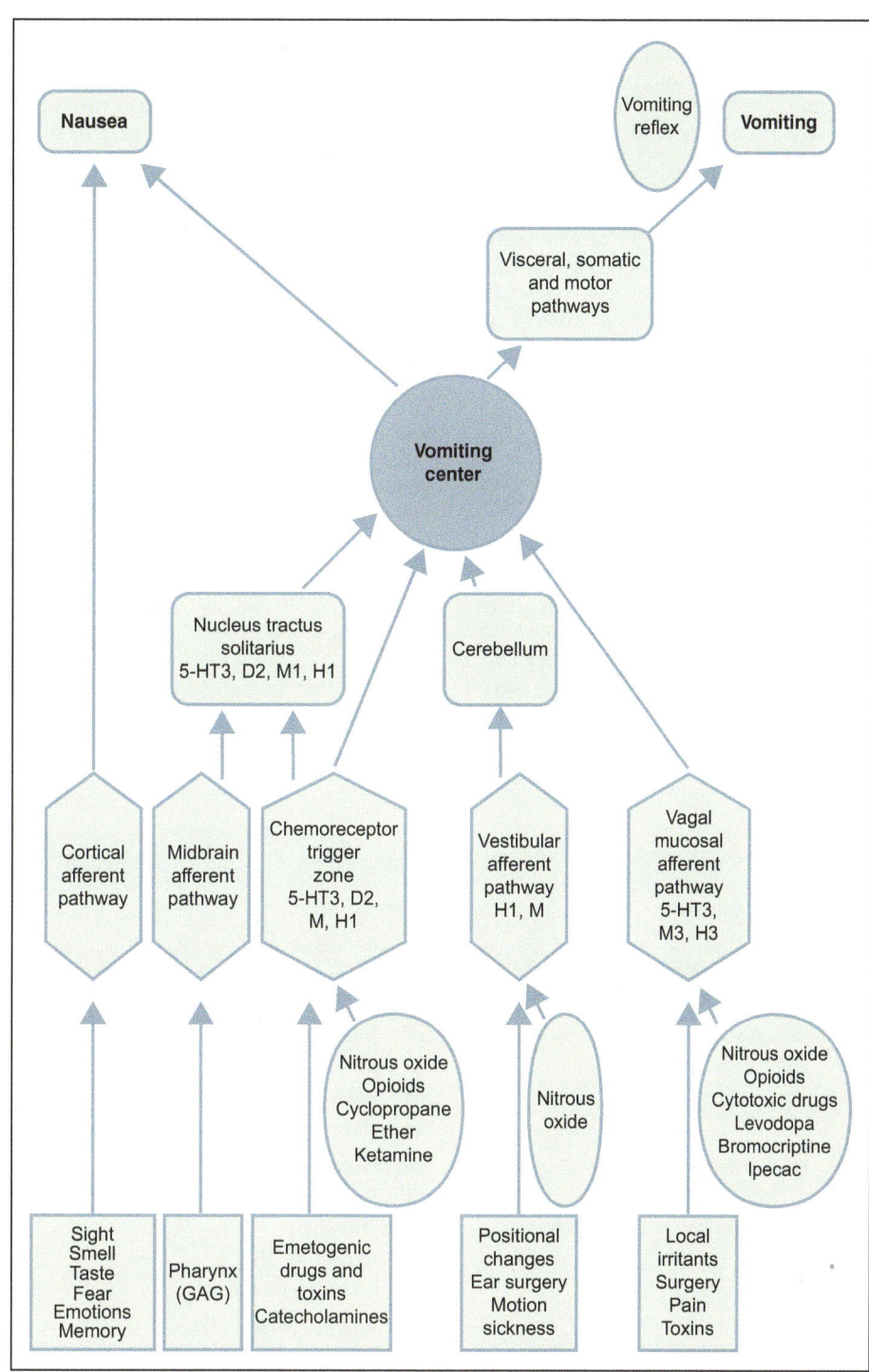

Figure 10.3: Pathophysiology of postoperative nausea and vomiting.
5-HT3, 5-hydroxytryptamine; H1, histamine.

minimize the incidence of PONV. The use of total IV anesthetics (TIVAs) without the use of inhalational anesthetics has been shown to decrease PONV. Likewise, incorporation of opioid-sparing techniques, such as regional anesthesia, and the use of acetaminophen, propofol, ketorolac, and dexmedetomidine decrease the incidence of opioid-induced PONV. Adequate hydration in children intraoperatively has been shown to improve PONV-related outcome measures as well, especially in intra-abdominal surgery.[16]

POSTOPERATIVE BLEEDING

Postoperative bleeding can be a traumatizing event that can significantly delay discharge, require additional surgery, result in unstable hemodynamics, require blood transfusions, and potentially become fatal. Tonsillectomy, with or without adenoidectomy, is one of the most common procedures performed on children worldwide, with post-tonsillectomy hemorrhage being the most common postoperative complication.[17] The rate of post-tonsillectomy oropharyngeal hemorrhage across all ages of children ranges from 2.1% to 12%.[18] Surgical technique, experience of surgeon, chronic tonsillitis, dehydration, and blood disorders all contribute to the incidence of posttonsillectomy oropharyngeal hemorrhage.[19]

Recognition and treatment of postoperative bleeding is crucial for the patient's safety and recovery. Regardless of the surgery, it is imperative that anesthesia providers and PACU staff alike monitor excessive bleeding. Tachycardia, hypotension, paleness, disorientation, and lethargy can be signs of bleeding and subsequently require further investigation. Should bleeding occur postoperatively, the PACU staff should notify the surgeon and anesthesia provider immediately as intervention should not be delayed.

POSTOPERATIVE PAIN

Appropriate treatment of postoperative pain is essential as it contributes to shorter hospital stays, decreases costs, and increases patient and family satisfaction.[20] Management of postoperative pain in the pediatric population, however, is often challenging due to the inability to clearly discern the presence or degree of pain. This, coupled with concerns related to side effects of opioid analgesics, can result in inadequate postoperative pain management in children.[20] Assessment of pain is even more challenging in the child experiencing ED.

Given the current opioid epidemic, many parents have valid concerns regarding the administration of opioids to their child. The use of narcotics, however, has proven beneficial in pain management and may be necessary depending on the procedure performed. Fentanyl, morphine, hydromorphone, and codeine are commonly used narcotics both intra- and postoperatively. For more information on opioid dosing, please refer to Chapter 2, "Pharmacological Considerations for the Pediatric Patient." For information regarding the use of nonopioid pain medications, please refer to Chapter 131, "Pediatric Pain Management."

The presence of child life specialists in the PACU offers the child and parents various means of support and they are an asset in the postoperative phase. Child life specialists possess special training that incorporates calming techniques and have access to a host of tools that can offer distraction that may help temper postoperative pain.

POSTOPERATIVE COMPLICATIONS

Variations in vital signs in the PACU can be an early indicator of postoperative complications (Table 10.2). Bradycardia, tachycardia, arrhythmias, hypotension, hypertension, decreased oxygen saturation, and extremes in temperature all warrant further immediate investigation. A head-to-toe assessment at the bedside should be conducted for obvious causes as the patient may be experiencing respiratory compromise, postoperative bleeding, hypothermia, hypovolemia, or pain.

DISCHARGE

The child can be considered for discharge from the PACU once institutional criteria have been met. Following most elective cases, children can be safely discharged home with their responsible guardian with proper instructions on postoperative care management. Prior to discharge, the child should

Table 10.2	Indicators of Postoperative Complications	
Symptom	Potential Cause	Intervention
Hypoxia	<ul><li>Obstruction</li><li>Edema</li><li>Illness</li><li>Disease process</li><li>Oversedation</li></ul>	<ul><li>Reposition</li><li>Airway maneuvers</li><li>Apply oxygen</li><li>Nasal trumpet</li><li>Breathing treatments (bronchodilator, racemic epi)</li><li>Reintubate</li><li>Treat with naloxone HCl (Narcan) or flumazenil if indicated</li></ul>
Tachycardia	<ul><li>Hypovolemia<ul><li>Under-resuscitated</li><li>Postoperative hemorrhage</li></ul></li><li>Pain</li></ul>	<ul><li>Fluid bolus</li><li>Check H/H</li><li>Transfuse</li><li>Return to OR</li><li>Provide analgesics</li></ul>
Hypertension	<ul><li>Pain</li></ul>	<ul><li>Provide analgesics</li></ul>
Hypotension	<ul><li>Hypovolemia<ul><li>Under-resuscitated</li><li>Postoperative hemorrhage</li></ul></li><li>Oversedation</li></ul>	<ul><li>Fluid bolus</li><li>Check H/H</li><li>Transfuse</li><li>Return to OR</li><li>Treat with naloxone HCl (Narcan) or flumazenil if indicated</li></ul>
Hypothermia		<ul><li>Forced air blankets/mattresses</li><li>Fluid warmers</li><li>Heat lamps</li><li>Warm blankets</li></ul>
Hyperthermia	<ul><li>MH</li></ul>	<ul><li>Monitor</li><li>Treat MH if warranted</li></ul>

MH, malignant hyperthermia; OR, operating room.

have stable hemodynamics, not require oxygen, have minimal to zero bleeding, exhibit baseline cognitive function, take fluids PO, have pain under control, and be steady on their feet (for age-appropriate children). Children should not be rushed out of the PACU. It is important that the PACU staff and responsible guardian feel comfortable with patient discharge and have a clear understanding of postoperative care.

KEY TAKEAWAYS

- A thorough handoff in PACU should include all pertinent patient- and procedure-related information.
- Anesthesia providers should have emergency medications with them when transporting to PACU.
- Despite an uneventful anesthetic, the potential for postoperative complications remains.
- It is imperative that anesthesia providers are prepared to treat airway emergencies, ED, postoperative bleeding, and pain.

KEY REFERENCES

Complete references for this chapter are online and available at https://connect.springerpub.com/content/book/978-0-8261-3875-0/part/part02/toc-part/ch010.

1. Coté CJ, Lerman J, Anderson BJ. *A Practice of Anesthesia for Infants and Children*. Elsevier; 2019.
2. Collins S, Schedler P, Veasey B, et al. Prevention and treatment of laryngospasm in the pediatric patient: a literature review. *AANA Journal*. 2019;87(2):145–151.
3. Holley D, Mendez A, Donald C. Paroxysmal laryngospasm. *JAAPA*. 2019;32(2):31–34. doi:10.1097/01.jaa.0000552724.72939.4c
5. Mamaril ME. Preoperative risk factors associated with PACU pediatric respiratory complications: an integrative review. *J Perianesth Nurs*. 2020;35(2):125–134. doi:10.1016/j.jopan.2019.09.002
8. Zou Y, Liu SH, Xue FS. Emergence agitation or delirium in children. *J Anesth*. November 19, 2020. doi:10.1007/s00540-020-02785-9.
12. Hoch K. Current evidence-based practice for pediatric emergence agitation. *AANA Journal*. 2019;87(6):495–499.
14. Cao X, White PF, Ma H. An update on the management of postoperative nausea and vomiting. *J Anesth*. 2017;31(4):617–626. doi:10.1007/s00540-017-2363-x
15. Tateosian VS, Champagne K, Gan TJ. What is new in the battle against postoperative nausea and vomiting?. *Best Pract Res Clin Anaesthesiol*. 2018;32(2):137–148. doi:10.1016/j.bpa.2018.06.005
17. Whelan RL, Shaffer A, Anderson ME, et al. Reducing rates of operative intervention for pediatric post-tonsillectomy hemorrhage. *The Laryngoscope*. 2018;128(8):1958–1962. doi:10.1002/lary.27076
20. Boric K, Dosenovic S, Jelicic Kadic A, et al. Interventions for postoperative pain in children: an overview of systematic reviews. *Paediatr Anaesth*. 2017:27(9):893–904. doi:10.1111/pan.13203

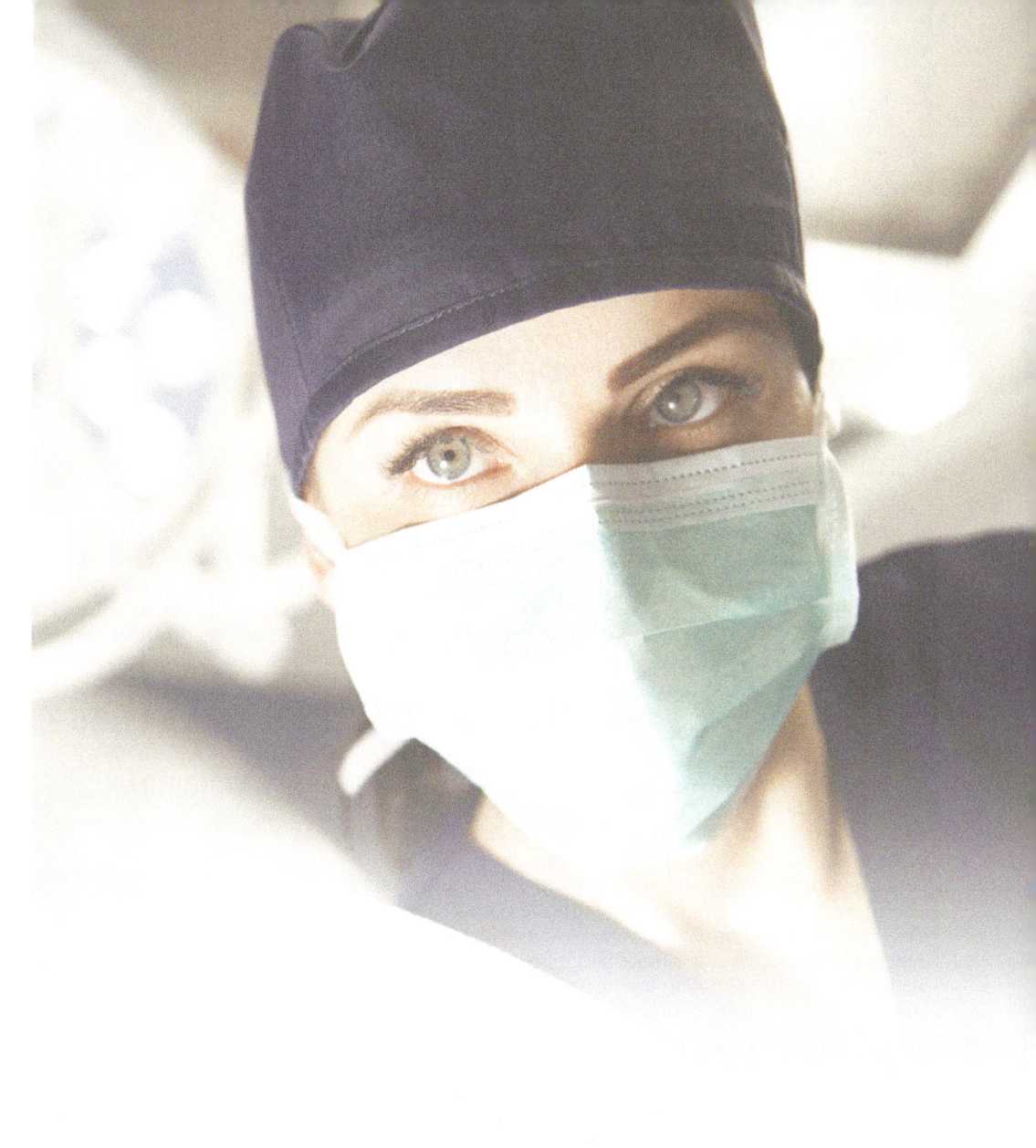

PART III

CONDITIONS, DISEASES, AND SYNDROMES IN PEDIATRIC PATIENTS

SECTION A Common Conditions and Diseases in Pediatric Patients

CHAPTER 11

The Premature Infant

Elise C. Whalen, Jamie Gilley, and Nidhy Paulose Varghese

> **LEARNING OBJECTIVES**
>
> - Explore premature births including how it is defined and specific risk factors in pregnancy.
> - Understand the importance of a comprehensive preoperative plan for infants born prematurely.
> - Review specific systems-based considerations for the premature infant.
> - Review postoperative care management recommendations including pain management concepts.

INTRODUCTION

Premature birth is a general term denoting birth prior to 37 weeks of gestation. The World Health Organization further categorizes these infants as extremely preterm (<28 weeks), very preterm (28 to <32 weeks), and moderate to late preterm (32–37 weeks).[1] Roughly 1 in 10 infants are born prematurely. Unfortunately, prematurity is one of the primary causes of death in children younger than age 5. Preventing premature birth is now a global health initiative to minimize the associated morbidity and mortality.

The current leading causes of preterm birth include multiple gestation pregnancy, maternal infection, and chronic conditions, such as diabetes or hypertension.[1] The improvement in survival translates into increased numbers of premature infants in intensive care units, inpatient floors, specialty clinics, and primary care practices. These children require additional care and monitoring as they are at higher risk of developing complex medical problems, including developmental delays, visual disturbances, and sensorineural hearing loss. They are also at higher risk of procedures involving anesthesia due to the immaturity of their organ systems, potentially complicated by associated congenital abnormalities.[2] Due to these factors, a thorough evaluation and individualized anesthesia plan should be completed preoperatively to help ensure safety in this population.[3,4]

NEURODEVELOPMENTAL CONSIDERATIONS

Intraventricular hemorrhage (IVH) or germinal matrix hemorrhage is a common neurological complication in premature infants that typically begins in the periventricular germinal matrix, which is most vulnerable in the first 48 hours of life.[5] Many infants remain asymptomatic until a screening cranial ultrasound identifies the bleed. However, some infants may demonstrate objective clinical findings, such as apnea and bradycardia events, decreased level of consciousness, decreased tone, and decreased movements. These findings could progress to more rapid deterioration including posturing, seizures, coma, or stupor.[5]

There are various degrees of bleeds, ranging from confined to the germinal matrix (grade I) to diffuse extension into the brain tissue and periventricular space (grade IV).[6] Grade I and II hemorrhages are the most common and typically result in spontaneous evolution. Grade III to IV hemorrhages are more severe and carry the risk of thrombotic obstruction of cerebral spinal fluid movement, potentially resulting in hydrocephalus.[5] For infants with germinal matrix hemorrhages/IVHs, adequate arterial blood flow, proper respiratory support, and fluid status should be ensured to prevent complications.

PULMONARY CONSIDERATIONS

BRONCHOPULMONARY DYSPLASIA

Bronchopulmonary dysplasia (BPD) is a complication of prematurity due to disrupted lung development. The definition of *BPD* is variable, without a clear consensus, although most typically it is defined as the continued dependence on oxygen at 28 days of life or at 36 weeks of postmenstrual age. The National Institute of Child Health classifies the severity of BPD into mild (oxygen use at 28 days of life), moderate (oxygen need at 36 weeks), or severe (ventilatory support at 36 weeks).[7,8] Administration of antenatal steroids and surfactant instillation are common treatments offered to minimize morbidity associated with lung immaturity. Unfortunately, pulmonary hypertension (PH) is an increasingly common complication of BPD due to vascular hypoplasia and/or dysplasia.

For the BPD infant, anesthetic considerations include adequate ventilation, oxygenation, and fluid management. Ventilator strategies for these infants can include high-frequency oscillator ventilation, high-frequency jet ventilation, conventional mechanical ventilation, nasal continuous positive airway pressure, and nasal cannula. Older infants with BPD may benefit from slower respiratory rates, larger tidal volumes, and longer inspiratory times in an effort to prevent gas trapping during mechanical ventilation. The premature infant lung is less compliant, increasing the risk of barotrauma during an anesthetic event. The converse is also possible, as general anesthesia predisposes to atelectasis, sometimes requiring higher positive end-expiratory pressure.[4] Oxygen toxicity mediated by free radicals is a real concern for the preterm infant also due to an immature antioxidant defense system.[9] Care should be taken to ensure judicious use of oxygen supplementation during the anesthetic procedure to mitigate this risk. The importance of managing ventilation and oxygenation is especially crucial for the BPD infant with PH. Even minor hypoxemia, hypercapnia, and acidosis may exacerbate vascular bed reactivity and cause an increase in pulmonary vascular resistance. Additionally, these infants are sensitive to fluid administration and have a decreased ability to clear fluid postoperatively, increasing the risk of pulmonary edema.

APNEA

Another common respiratory consideration affecting these infants is apnea. Apnea events may be central, obstructive, or mixed.[10] Apnea of prematurity, a condition affecting infants <37 weeks of gestation, is typically central or mixed. It is characterized by a period of apnea lasting 20 seconds or longer, which can lead to bradycardia, cyanosis, and/or pallor.[2] Although this is typically seen before reaching 40 weeks (corrected) of age, the risk can extend up to 60 weeks of postconceptual age.[4]

Inciting factors for apnea spells include hypoxemia, metabolic changes, temperature changes, upper airway obstruction, and certain medications like prostaglandins.[4] Management of this condition is focused on efforts to improve respiratory drive and decrease the work of breathing, including the use of respiratory stimulants, such as caffeine or theophylline, positive airway pressure to provide airway support, and prone positioning to increase chest wall compliance. Other management strategies include blood transfusions to increase the oxygen-carrying capacity of the blood, reflux treatment as needed, and hypo/hyperthermia regulation.[10,4]

AIRWAY CONSIDERATIONS

Infants with BPD may develop subglottic stenosis, tracheomalacia, and/or vocal cord paralysis/paresis due to a history of prolonged intubation. During the induction of anesthesia, the anesthesia provider should be cautioned when advancing the endotracheal tube in infants with this history and consider utilizing a smaller diameter endotracheal tube, with or without cuff, as needed.[3] Airway hyperreactivity is also common, predisposing the infant to bronchospasms and desaturation events perioperatively.[3]

CARDIOVASCULAR CONSIDERATIONS

In utero, the heart and vasculature undergo dramatic maturation during the third trimester. When infants are born prematurely, the immature heart may have persistence of cardiac shunts, such as the ductus arteriosus and foramen ovale, which may contribute to shunting of deoxygenated blood. Immaturity of the autonomic nervous system in the preterm infant can lead to wide heart rate and blood pressure instability. This instability can create a need for inotropic support, such as dopamine or epinephrine during anesthesia.[11] Other hemodynamic considerations in the perioperative period include blood loss. Preterm infants have a lower total body blood volume (~65 mL/kg), making them particularly sensitive to blood loss.[12] This is compounded by compromised baroreflexes to offset blood losses due to anesthesia.

GENERAL CONSIDERATIONS

THERMOREGULATION

The premature infant has a thinner epidermis, high ratio of body surface area to body weight, increased evaporative heat loss through the skin, and decreased brown fat metabolism, which contribute to temperature dysregulation. It is imperative that the anesthesia provider creates a warm environment, including warming devices with minimal infant handling to reduce heat loss.[4]

FLUID/METABOLIC STATUS

Fluid status maintenance is essential in these infants due to evaporative water loss and a predisposition to hyponatremia caused by alterations in sodium retention. The immaturity of the renal tubules causes abnormal responses to aldosterone and antidiuretic hormone. Serum glucose levels should also be closely monitored due to limited glycogen stores, and the risk of hypoglycemia. Caution should be taken to prevent a hyperosmolar state as this can predispose to germinal matrix hemorrhage and osmotic diuresis.[2]

PREOPERATIVE EVALUATION AND CARE

Prior to any anesthetic procedure, the anesthesia provider should review the child's antenatal and current neonatal history. A thorough review of systems should be completed, taking note of previous anesthetic events and associated complications. The patient review must also include family or individual history of malignant hyperthermia along with any bleeding disorders.

Documentation that should be incorporated into the anesthesia note includes the type of endotracheal tube, size/diameter of tube, laryngoscope blade, grade view, difficulty of intubation, number of attempts, and any complications that occurred. Infants with difficult airway syndromes, such as Pierre Robin sequence, Treacher Collins syndrome, Goldenhar syndrome, and cleft lip and palate, are at higher risk of complications during the induction of anesthesia.[3] Infants with subglottic stenosis, laryngeal atresia, laryngeal, or tracheal webs can also be difficult to intubate due to the alteration from a normal airway structure. This may require availability of an alternative airway, such as a laryngeal mask airway, in case of any complications.

Preoperative laboratory work should include hemoglobin, hematocrit, platelets, coagulation studies, serum chemistries, and glucose levels with any abnormal values being corrected prior to anesthesia. A type and screen/crossmatch should be completed for blood product availability during the procedure. A transfusion is often administered for blood loss greater than 10% of total blood volume.[4] Preoperative fasting may be required, which could increase fluid deficits if the infant has not received maintenance IV fluids. Care should be taken to replace fluids in an effort to maintain euvolemia during the procedure. Due to preterm deficiencies in vitamin K and vitamin K-related coagulation factors, these infants may also receive vitamin K or a replacement of coagulation factors prior to the procedure to prevent bleeding complications.[4]

Due to the critically ill nature of some of these infants, stability for transport from the intensive care unit to the operating room must be considered. Some infants may be too unstable to move, in which case bedside procedure may be safest. Consideration of an alternate surgical location is recommended for infants on high-frequency oscillatory ventilation, inhaled nitric oxide for PH, and/or extracorporeal membrane oxygenation.[3]

POSTOPERATIVE CARE

Up until the 1980s, infant surgery was sometimes completed with minimal to no anesthesia due to popular belief that infants do not feel pain due to underdeveloped pain receptors.[13] However, by the early 2000s, it was discovered that pain-receptive nerve pathways were developed and functioning around 24 weeks of gestation.[14] Failure to provide adequate analgesic management could potentially lead to a "rewiring" of the nerve pathways and heightened pain perception with future encounters.[14] Postoperative analgesia should be focused on recognition of pain through appropriate pain scales, minimizing pain, and preventing pain as able.[4] There are four classes of analgesics used in premature infants postoperatively as follows: local anesthetics, opioids, nonsteroidal anti-inflammatory drugs, and acetaminophen/paracetamol. Of these, opioids are the least preferred because of the risk of respiratory depression and further postoperative apnea. Administering opioids may be necessary in some conditions, and in those situations, close monitoring is required to observe for and act to respiratory compromise.[4]

KEY TAKEAWAYS

- Caring for premature infants as they undergo anesthesia can be quite challenging.
- Primary considerations to take when caring for these infants include appropriate airway management and ventilation, ensuring adequate IV access for fluid and medication delivery, ensuring a warm environment, and appropriate pain management postoperatively.[3]
- Their preliminary care should include a comprehensive preoperative evaluation and appropriate coordination with other pediatric specialists involved in their care.
- While these infants are at a higher risk of anesthetic complications, it is essential to remember the population-specific care that these infants require to ensure the safest patient outcomes.

REFERENCES

1. World Health Organization. W. Preterm birth. 2020. https://www.who.int/news-room/fact-sheets/detail/preterm-birth
2. Subramaniam R. Anaesthetic concerns in preterm and term neonates. *Indian J Anaesth.* 2019;63(9):771–779. doi:10.4103/ija.IJA_591_19
3. Frawley G. Special considerations in the premature and ex-premature infant. *Anaesthesia & Intensive Care Medicine,* 2020;21(2):92–98.
4. Taneja B, Srivastava V, Saxena K. Physiological and anaesthetic considerations for the preterm neonate undergoing surgery. 2012. https://www.ncbi.nlm.nih.gov/pmc/articles/PMC4420318/
5. Ballabh P. Intraventricular hemorrhage in premature infants: mechanism of disease. *Pediatr Res.* 2010;67(1):1–8. doi:10.1203/pdr.0b013e3181c1b176
6. Cucchiara B, Kasner S, Goddeau R. Intraventricular hemorrhage. 2020. https://www.uptodate.com/contents/intraventricular-hemorrhage
7. Jung YH, Jang J, Kim H, et al. Respiratory severity score as a predictive factor for severe bronchopulmonary dysplasia or death in extremely preterm infants. *BMC Pediatr.* 2019;19(1):121 doi:10.1186/s12887-019-1492-9
8. Jobe AH. The new bronchopulmonary dysplasia. *Curr Opin Pediatr.* 2011;23(2):167–172. doi:10.1097/MOP.0b013e3283423e6b
9. Eichenwald E, Stark A. Bronchopulmonary dysplasia: definition, pathogenesis, and clinical features. 2020. https://www.uptodate.com/contents/bronchopulmonary-dysplasia-definition-pathogenesis-and-clinical-features
10. Eichenwald EC. Apnea of prematurity. *Pediatrics.* 2015;137(1):2015–3757 doi:10.1542/peds.2015-3757
11. Fyfe K, Odoi A, Yiallourou S, et al. Preterm infants exhibit greater variability in cerebrovascular control than term infants. *Sleep.* 2015;38(9):1411–1421. doi:10.5665/sleep.4980
12. Aladangady N, McHugh S, Aitchison TC, et al. Infants' blood volume in a controlled trial of placental transfusion at preterm delivery. *Pediatrics.* 2006;117(1):93–98. doi:10.1542/peds.2004-1773
13. Rodkey E, Pillai Riddell R. The infancy of infant pain research: the experimental origins of infant pain denial. *J Pain.* 2013;14(4):338–350. https://doi.org/10.1016/j.jpain.2012.12.017
14. Davis P, Cladis F. *Smith's Anesthesia for Infants and Children.* 9th ed. Elsevier; 2017.

CHAPTER 12

Neurological Conditions

Amanda Ford and Shawn West

LEARNING OBJECTIVES

- Describe the normal flow of cerebrospinal fluid (CSF) in the brain related to the classification of hydrocephalus.
- Identify the types of Arnold–Chiari malformation, along with the associated anatomical changes.
- Define pediatric spinal cord conditions, such as tethered cord and spina bifida.
- Discuss the major types of pediatric brain tumors and their associated symptoms.
- Characterize the clinical presentation of a pediatric patient with a spinal arteriovenous malformation versus a brain arteriovenous malformation.

INTRODUCTION

Neurological diagnosis in the pediatric population is relatively common, and causes include both traumatic and nontraumatic injuries, along with congenital conditions. Some pediatric neurological conditions do not require surgical intervention (cerebral palsy), while others almost always require some degree of intervention (craniosynostosis). Many of these conditions are associated with each other or with variations of other neurological conditions (e.g., Arnold–Chiari with hydrocephalus, encephalocele with hydrocephalus, and arteriovenous malformations [AVMs] with epilepsy). While some of these conditions can be corrected, many result in multiple operative stays and/or lifelong care. These patients can present with a wide variety of symptoms, and a comprehensive assessment of baseline functional status is essential. In addition, the anesthesia provider should be proficient in a basic neurological examination, signs of increased intracranial pressure, and management during the perioperative period.

HYDROCEPHALUS

Hydrocephalus is one of the most common pediatric neurological conditions and is caused by the mismatch between CSF production and absorption. This mismatch leads to an overall increase in CSF volume in the brain. The most common cause of hydrocephalus is related to the obstruction of CSF flow or the inability of the arachnoid vili to absorb CSF. Other causes of hydrocephalus include hemorrhage, congenital blockages, trauma, infection, and/or tumors.

Hydrocephalus is typically classified as either nonobstructive (communicating) or obstructive (noncommunicating), with the classification referring to the flow of CSF. Untreated hydrocephalus overall will cause an intracranial hypertension (an increased intracranial pressure [ICP]). Clinical manifestations may vary slightly by age. Infants tend to tolerate an increased ICP better related to their unfused cranial bones. Therefore, their cranial vault has the ability to expand slightly as opposed to older children who have fused cranial bones.

Pediatric patients with hydrocephalus will demonstrate the symptoms of increased ICP, such as lethargy, vomiting, bradycardia, headache, seizures, and/or death in extreme cases. Common surgical treatments for hydrocephalus include placement of a CSF shunt (e.g., ventriculoperitoneal [VP] shunt or an endoscopic third ventriculostomy). Please refer to Chapter 50, "VP Shunt Placement and/or Externalization," for more information about the anesthetic management of VP shunt placement in the pediatric patient and Chapter 57, "Third Ventriculostomy," for more information about the anesthetic management of third ventriculostomy in the pediatric patient.

ENCEPHALOCELE

An encephalocele is a rare neural tube defect with an incidence of 1 in 5,000 live births that leads to protrusion of the brain and meninges, typically seen in the nose or posterior head/neck (occipital). The majority are occipital (70%), and all encephaloceles are associated with other congenital anomalies (60%), such as hydrocephalus, micrognathia, Chiari malformation, and renal agenesis.[1] The clinical manifestation of occipital encephaloceles is often the encephalocele itself, while nasal encephaloceles can appear as nasal polyps depending on the size. Encephaloceles are typically repaired when the patient is an infant, and prenatal ultrasound has the ability to detect many fetal encephaloceles prior to birth.

Encephaloceles can present considerable challenges for the anesthesia provider related to airway management and positioning. Nasal encephaloceles could prevent adequate ventilation with a mask and subsequent obstruction by using direct laryngoscopy for intubation. Positioning may also present a challenge for intubation, especially with an occipital encephalocele. The anesthesia provider may want to consider a lateral position, the patient's head suspended off of the bed, the head resting in a horseshoe headrest (has an open center), or a foam or gel donut under the head. The goal of positioning should be to maximize the ability to ventilate/intubate while not increasing pressure on the encephalocele itself (see **Figure 12.1**).

ARNOLD–CHIARI MALFORMATION

An Arnold–Chiari malformation is a hindbrain defect that leads to the protrusion of the medulla oblongata and fourth ventricle through the foramen magnum. It is commonly associated with myelomeningocele (see *Spina Bifida* in this chapter). There are varying degrees of compression and structure changes associated with an Arnold–Chiari malformation. Patients with this malformation may experience compression of brainstem nuclei and cranial nerves, and displacement of the cerebellar tonsils may lead to aqueductal stenosis and related hydrocephalus. **Table 12.1** summarizes the types of Arnold–Chiari malformation and their related anatomical changes with symptoms.[2] General clinical manifestations can vary widely based on the structures involved but include aspiration, vocal cord paralysis, stridor, apnea, cranial nerve deficits, and gait disturbances. Asymptomatic patients will

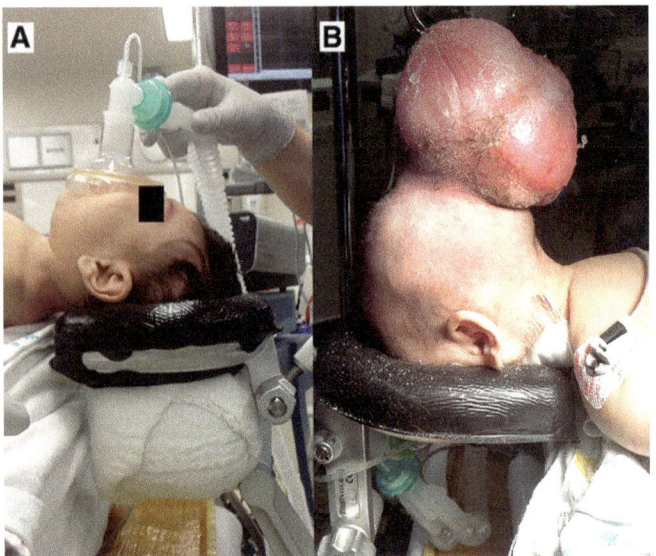

Figure 12.1: Positioning of patient with occipital encephalocele in horseshoe headrest both for intubation (A) and for surgical repair (B).

Source: Black SA, Galvez JA, Rehman MA, Schwartz AJ. Images in anesthesiology. *Anesthesiology.* 2014;120(6):1504. doi:10.1097/aln.0b013e31829f028a.

not undergo prophylactic surgical repair, but more severe clinical manifestations (e.g., apnea or vocal cord paralysis) require a prompt surgical repair.

CRANIOSYNOSTOSIS

Craniosynostosis is a congenital defect that occurs in 1 in 2,000 live births, effecting males more than females, and can also be associated with other syndromes, such as Apert and Crouzon syndromes. This defect is caused by premature closure of one or more cranial suture lines, most commonly the sagittal suture (see **Figure 12.2**). The premature closure causes a cascade of events that begin with abnormal size and shape of the calvarium/orbits/cranial base and can lead to increased ICP, structure compression, and potential neurological deficits. The severity of craniosynostosis depends on the number of sutures involved, associated syndromes, and age of repair. Repair is typically done early in life, since the skill bones and remaining suture lines are more malleable within the first year of life.[3] Please refer to Chapter 55, "Cranial Vault Reconstruction and Craniosynostosis Repair," for more information about the anesthetic management of craniosynostosis repair in the pediatric patient.

SPINA BIFIDA

Spina bifida is a result of the fetal spinal cord not closing properly in utero. Spina bifida is broken down into three subtypes as follows: occulta, meningocele, and myelomeningocele. Occulta does not have an opening on the back present. Discovery of this defect can be incidental on a radiographic exam ination since some patients can be completely asymptomatic. Occulta symptoms can include bowel/bladder dysfunction, lower extremity weakness, scoliosis, and back pain. Meningocele occurs when the layers of the spinal cord are defective and bulge through the spine. The actual spinal cord may or may not be affected. Myelomeningocele is the most common of the three subtypes and has a defect in the layers covering the spinal cord, with a portion of the spinal cord included in the defect. The defect can be covered by skin, or the defect can be completely exposed (see **Figure 12.3**). Symptoms of myelomeningocele are similar to occulta, but in severe cases, children can have complete paralysis below the area of the defect. Please refer to Chapter 56, "Myelomeningocele Closure," for more information about the anesthetic management of myelomeningocele closure in the pediatric patient.

TETHERED CORD

Tethered cord syndrome is associated with tissue attached to the spinal cord that limits the movement of the cord. Diseases that are commonly associated with tethered cord syndrome include spina bifida occulta, myelomeningocele, and lipoma. Another common cause is adhesion from previous surgical repair of spina bifida. Tethered cord repair usually requires a neurosurgeon to surgically release the tissue restricting the spinal cord and free the cord of the "tethering." Typically, the tissue that causes the tethering is the filum terminale. Symptoms usually include issues with control of bowel, bladder, and lower extremity coordination or weakness. One of the classic signs that patient will present with is toe walking. For diagnosis, children will present for an MRI for definitive diagnosis.

TUMORS

Aside from leukemia, brain tumors are the most common forms of cancer in children. Tumor location can be divided into supratentorial, infratentorial, midbrain, and choroid plexus tumors. Infratentorial masses are more common in children and usually located in the posterior fossa. When tumors are in the posterior fossa, it is common for children to exhibit signs of increased ICP due to an obstruction of CSF flow. Diversion of CSF using a VP shunt or external drain (EVD) will be required until the tumor creating the obstruction can be excised.

Table 12.1	Types of Arnold–Chiari Malformations, Associated Characteristics, and Clinical Manifestations
Type	**Characteristics and Clinical Manifestations**
Type 1	Tonsillar herniation >5 mm below foramen magnum, no brainstem herniation; mild symptoms (headache, hypotonia, and/or neck pain); low risk of hydrocephalus
Type 2	Herniation of brainstem/vermis/4th ventricle; associated with myelomeningocele; hydrocephalus, apnea, and vocal cord issues are common
Type 3	Occipital encephalocele (contains dysmorphic cerebellar and brainstem) present; severe symptoms and high long-term disability risk (associated with high mortality)
Type 4	Hypoplasia or aplasia of cerebellum, large posterior fossa CSF spaces; survival is rare

CSF, cerebrospinal fluid.
Source: Davis PJ, Cladis FP. *Smith's Anesthesia for Infants and Children.* Elsevier; 2017.

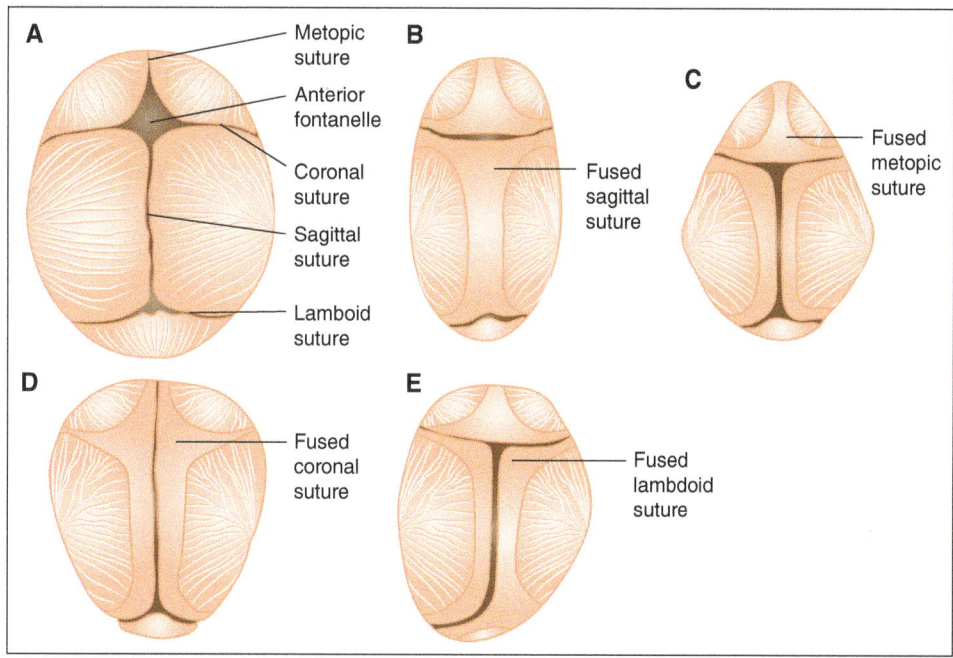

Figure 12.2: Examples of single suture craniosynostosis defects. (A) Normal skull of the newborn. (B) Fused sagittal suture. (C) Fused metopic suture. (D) Fused coronal suture. (E) Fused lambdoid suture. The most common form is sagittal craniosynostosis.

Supratentorial tumor symptoms are usually associated with seizures or focal deficits, which is why these patients commonly require antiepileptic drugs. Choroid plexus tumors are rare and affect children usually under the age of three years.[2] Tumors affecting the choroid plexus result in increased production of CSF and obstruction of CSF flow resulting in hydrocephalus and symptoms of increased ICP. Midbrain tumors are commonly associated with hormonal imbalances related to tumors affecting the hypothalamus and pituitary. Common symptoms are related to irregularities of growth, endocrine abnormalities, and visual disturbance from the compression of the optic nerve. One of the more common endocrine abnormalities is diabetes insipidus (DI). DI can occur preoperatively, intraoperatively, and/or postoperatively.

ARTERIOVENOUS MALFORMATIONS

An AVM occurs when there is direct communication between arteries and veins (there is typically a capillary network between the two). AVMs are usually congenital and can be located in the brain or spinal cord, as well as other areas of the body. They can potentially cause damage, such as hydrocephalus, hemorrhage, mass effect, and/or local ischemia.[4] Clinical manifestations of brain AVMs include seizures, headache, and vomiting. Spinal AVMs typically present as sudden and severe back pain, weakness in the extremities, and paralysis. The vessels that make up an AVM are fragile and lack the ability to autoregulate. Accordingly, vigilance is key to prevent sudden increases in ICP or hemodynamics that can be devastating.

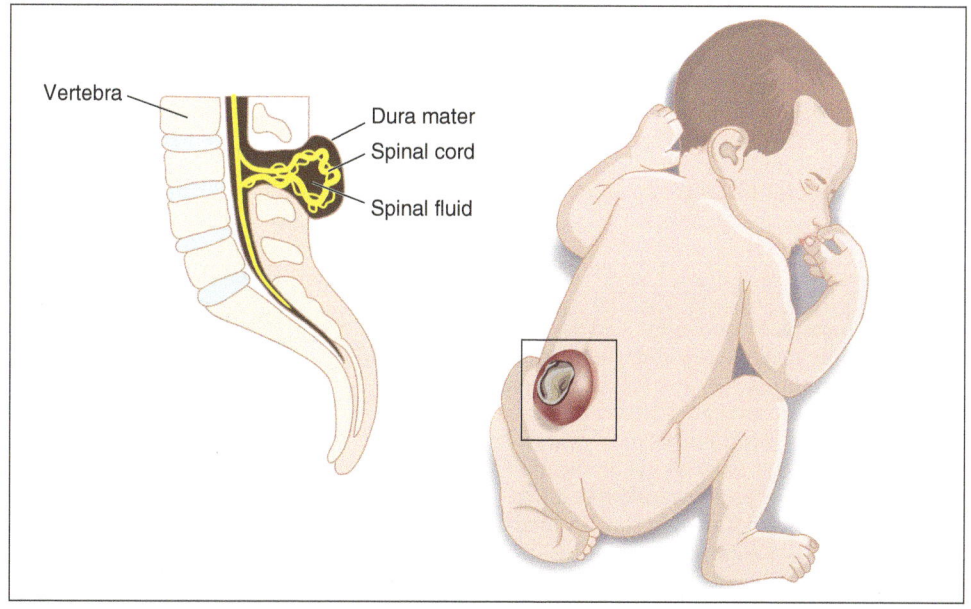

Figure 12.3: Spina bifida/myelomeningocele.

Table 12.2	Surgical Management Options for Epilepsy in Patients Resistant to Medication Therapy Procedure
Management Option	**Description**
ATL	Resection of the anterior temporal lobe with some degree of hippocampal resection, most common in adult epilepsy surgery; complications include visual field and verbal disturbances
SAH	Less radical surgical resection than ATL (spares dominant hemisphere); approaches include transsylvian, transcortical, or subtemporal, not frequently used in pediatrics
Temporal lesionectomy	Used frequently in pediatric temporal sclerosis, cortical dysplasia, and vascular lesions
Extratemporal resection	Lower rates of success (measured as freedom from seizures) compared to ATL, SAH, and temporal lesionectomy; includes electrode implantation procedures with staged monitoring followed by resection
Hemispherectomy	Disconnection of the cerebral hemisphere, patient with diffuse seizures, can be functional or anatomic disconnection
Neurostimulation	Most common palliative procedure for epilepsy; VNS and DBS are types of neurostimulation
Corpus callosotomy	Transection of the corpus callosum is treatment for severe, intractable epilepsy, seen commonly in Lennox–Gastaut patients
Minimally invasive therapy	Stereotactic radiosurgery and laser ablation therapy are the most common

ATL, anterior temporal lobectomy; DBS, deep brain stimulators; SAH, selective amygdalohippocampectomy; VNS, vagal nerve stimulators.
Source: Guan J, Karsy M, Ducis K, Bollo R. Surgical strategies for pediatric epilepsy. *Transl Pediatr.* 2016;5(2):55–66. doi:10.21037/tp.2016.03.02.

CEREBRAL PALSY

Cerebral palsy is the most common disability in childhood with an incidence of 2 in 1,000 live births. Cerebral palsy is related to a central nervous system insult that can occur during pregnancy or childbirth (or shortly after birth). It is a mixed disease, meaning that it includes a mix of spasticity, dystonia, and ataxia. The symptoms are the effect of damaged upper motor neurons in the brain or spinal cord, leading to tone dysfunction and dysfunction with coordination and movement. Cerebral palsy can also be associated with seizures, aspiration, chronic pulmonary issues, obstructive sleep apnea, varying degrees of cognitive dysfunction, and visual/hearing impairment. There is no specific surgical repair to treat cerebral palsy; however, anesthetic providers will encounter pediatric patients with cerebral palsy for a variety of procedures (e.g., dental rehab, Nissen/G-tube placement, spinal fusion, baclofen pump placement, tracheostomy and botox injections). Procedures such as baclofen pump placement and dorsal rhizotomy can be performed in an attempt to reduce spasticity. Please refer to Chapter 54, "Dorsal Rhizotomy," for more information about the anesthetic management of dorsal rhizotomy in the pediatric patient.

Regardless of the procedure, it is important for the anesthesia provider to understand the patient's baseline neurological and functional status to allow for full consideration of the anesthetic options.

EPILEPSY

Epilepsy in children has a variety of etiologies and is estimated to affect nearly 10.5 million children worldwide. Drug-resistant epilepsy is relatively common (20%–40%), and even those patients with positive seizure outcomes from medications frequently encounter side effects from those medications.[5] Therefore, epilepsy treatment can vary from single medication therapy to multiple medication therapy and surgical procedures. Surgical options for those patients who are resistant to medication therapy for their epilepsy are described in **Table 12.2**.

Anesthesia providers should also recognize that there are several syndromes/disorders that are associated with epilepsy. Examples include metabolic disorders, fevers (febrile seizures), recent head trauma, AVMs, tuberous sclerosis, Sturge–Weber syndrome, encephalitis, and/or Lennox–Gastaut syndrome.[6] Patients with a history of epilepsy could come to the operating room for unrelated procedures or for surgical procedures for epilepsy treatment. Please refer to Chapter 51, "Stereotactic Grid Placement and Removal," for more information about the anesthetic management of stereotactic grid placement in the pediatric patient and Chapter 53, "Epilepsy Surgery," for more information about the anesthetic management of epilepsy surgery in the pediatric patient.

> ### KEY TAKEAWAYS
>
> - Patients with Arnold–Chiari malformation may not undergo surgical repair if they are asymptomatic, but if vocal cord or apnea symptoms are present, surgical intervention is required.
> - Craniosynostosis is associated with other syndromes (Apert, Crouzon), and repair is performed early in life while suture lines are still relatively malleable.
> - There are three types of spina bifida, with myelomeningocele as the most common. Spina bifida occulta and myelomeningocele are also associated with tethered cord.
> - Brian tumors are the second most common type of pediatric cancer. Infratentorial tumors (typically posterior fossa) usually present with symptoms of increased ICP-related CSF flow obstruction. Midbrain tumors are associated with hormone imbalances, such as CSF.
> - AVMs are typically congenital in nature, and the vessels that form the AVM are fragile with no ability to autoregulate.

KEY REFERENCES

Complete references for this chapter are online and available at https://connect.springerpub.com/content/book/978-0-8261-3875-0/part/part03/toc-part/ch012

1. Black SA, Galvez JA, Rehman MA, Schwartz AJ. Images in anesthesiology. *Anesthesiology*. 2014;120(6):1504. doi:10.1097/aln.0b013e31829f028a
2. Davis PJ, Cladis FP. *Smith's Anesthesia for Infants and Children*. Elsevier; 2017.
5. Gadgil N, LoPresti M, Muir M, et al. An update on pediatric surgical epilepsy: part I. *Surg Neurol* Int. 2019;10:257. doi:10.25259/SNI_417_2019
10. El-Ghanem M, Kass-Hout T, Kass-Hout O, et al. Arteriovenous malformations in the pediatric population: review of the existing literature. *Interv Neurol*. 2016;5(3–4):218–225. doi:10.1159/000447605
11. Mahajan C, Rath GP, Dash HH, Bithal PK. Perioperative management of children with encephalocele. *J Neurosurg Anesthesiol*. 2011;23(4):352–356. doi:10.1097/ana.0b013e31821f93dc

CHAPTER 13

Ear, Nose, and Throat Conditions

Anita Deshpande, Carol Li, and Charles M. Myer, IV

LEARNING OBJECTIVES

- Describe common ear, nose, and throat (ENT) conditions.
- Identify common ENT procedures for which antibiotic prophylaxis is recommended.
- Review procedure-specific anesthesia considerations for common ENT procedures.

INTRODUCTION

Otolaryngologic conditions, such as otitis media and tonsillitis, are seen frequently in the pediatric population and frequently require operative intervention. The procedures used to treat these conditions vary in complexity, with each having unique anesthetic considerations. For example, children undergoing tympanostomy tube placement are routinely mask-ventilated throughout the case and do not require intubation or IV line placement. Conversely, a child undergoing thyroidectomy will benefit from intubation with a special endotracheal tube (ETT) that allows for recurrent laryngeal nerve monitoring. Due to the need for neuromonitoring, anesthesia providers must be aware of the importance of avoiding long-acting paralytic medications. In addition, while rare, a goiter can lead to difficult intubation depending on size. Given the variety of otolaryngologic conditions that can present for procedural intervention, and the incidence of otolaryngology conditions in the pediatric population, a general understanding of the pathophysiology of the common disorders, potential association with any systemic manifestations, and the general health of the child is important in planning a safe and effective anesthetic.

ANESTHETIC MANAGEMENT

PREOPERATIVE EVALUATION

Prior to any anesthetic, a thorough history should be ascertained. Details should be taken regarding the otolaryngologic condition, including specific symptoms, duration, and treatment history. Although many otolaryngologic conditions are isolated, there is an increased incidence of certain otolaryngologic conditions as part of congenital syndromes. In these cases, anesthesia providers must be aware of other associated comorbid conditions, and care must be taken to ensure that these comorbidities are addressed as part of the preoperative evaluation and intraoperative management.

Airway management should always be an important consideration as many otolaryngologic conditions either directly or indirectly affect the airway or are in association with a syndrome that may have airway manifestations. Patients and families should be queried regarding symptoms of airway involvement, such as dyspnea, exertional limitation, noisy breathing, and history of recurrent croup. In children who have undergone prior airway surgery, procedure notes as well as previous airway records should be reviewed. In children who have a tracheostomy, anesthesia providers should be aware of the reason the tracheostomy was placed and if the patient can be mask-ventilated or endotracheally intubated in the case of tracheostomy tube dislodgement. In some instances, children are not able to be intubated via rigid bronchoscopy or conventional laryngoscopy and require flexible fiberoptic transnasal intubation. A prime example of this scenario is the child with a history of tracheostomy and subglottic stenosis, which can result in potential difficulty with endotracheal intubation or mask ventilation.

PHYSICAL EXAMINATION AND ASSESSMENT

Prior to consideration of procedure-specific details, anesthesia providers should perform risk stratification and ensure that the pediatric patient is safe to undergo anesthesia from a cardiopulmonary standpoint. It is important to note that cardiopulmonary evaluation should be specifically guided by the patient's underlying conditions and risks related to general anesthesia. With few exceptions, the cardiopulmonary status of the patient and risk of general anesthesia are not secondary to the otolaryngologic conditions.

Therefore, auscultation of heart and lungs is a key component of the physical examination and assessment. Based on the patient's presenting symptoms or comorbidities, an electrocardiogram (ECG) or echocardiogram preoperatively may be warranted. Likewise, the pulmonary evaluation may mandate evaluation of a chest x-ray prior to anesthesia.

When performing a comprehensive head and neck examination, special attention should be given to features that may suggest difficult intubation or ventilation. These include specific craniofacial anomalies (i.e., micrognathia, cleft palate, and macroglossia), trismus or ankylosis of the temporomandibular joint (TMJ), and maxillary or mandibular hypoplasia. Physical examination should also include assessment of respiratory effort. Stridor, stertor, and retractions may all indicate evidence of airway obstruction.

The presence of a neck mass should prompt further consideration of airway evaluation and management. Large neck mass may cause direct airway obstruction or an inability to mask-ventilate. Neck masses with extension into the chest, such as venolymphatic malformation or substernal goiter, may cause tracheal deviation and portend difficult ventilation when under anesthesia, even when intubated. Similarly, mediastinal lymphadenopathy may also cause tracheal obstruction and difficulty with ventilation. In cases where a head and neck malignancy, such as lymphoma, is suspected, a chest radiograph should be considered. Cross-sectional imaging, such as computed tomography (CT) or magnetic resonance imaging (MRI) scans, may be useful to assess the location and severity of potential airway involvement for larger neck mass and those masses with concern for chest extension or mass effect on the distal airway.

ANESTHETIC PLANNING

It is imperative that an airway management plan be established for every otolaryngology patient prior to procedural intervention. For many procedures, such as otologic or sinus surgeries, standard airway management and intubation are acceptable. However, this is not always the case as the location of the pathology alters airway management, either due to the need for surgical access or due to the effect of the pathology on the airway. It is critical that airway management plan is discussed between the surgical and anesthesia teams prior to the induction of anesthesia, notably in those patients in whom an airway abnormality is suspected.

EAR CONDITIONS

OTITIS MEDIA

Otitis media is a broad term encompassing the following conditions: chronic otitis media with effusion (COME), as well as persistent or recurrent acute otitis media (AOM). AOM and otitis media with effusion (OME) are distinct diseases with different treatments. AOM involves signs and symptoms of middle ear inflammation, such as bulging and erythema of the tympanic membrane, otalgia, and fever, accompanied by middle ear effusion. OME is defined as middle ear effusion without signs or symptoms of acute inflammation.[1] Certain congenital conditions, such as Down syndrome, craniofacial disorders, including cleft palate and Treacher Collins syndrome, and the mucopolysaccharidoses may predispose a patient to otitis media. When evaluating patients with these conditions, the physical examination should include assessment of other coexisting anomalies, such as cleft palate, bifid uvula, or other distinctive craniofacial features, and anesthesia providers should be aware of the effect of the comorbid condition on airway management.

Tympanostomy tube placement is the most commonly performed ambulatory surgery on children in the United States[2] and is the primary surgical intervention for otitis media. This procedure involves the creation of a myringotomy, or an incision in the tympanic membrane, followed by placement of a tympanostomy tube through this incision to ventilate the middle ear space.[2] Tympanostomy tubes have been shown to produce large short-term improvements in the quality of life for children and their caregivers with the largest degrees of improvement reported with caregiver concerns, physical suffering, and emotional distress and moderate improvement occurring with hearing loss, speech impairment, and activity limitations.[3]

Anesthetic Considerations

In children, tympanostomy tube insertion is generally performed as an outpatient procedure under general anesthesia. When performed as an isolated procedure, pediatric patients usually receive an inhalational mask induction with mask ventilation throughout the procedure. In most instances, there is no need to intubate the patient or insert a peripheral IV catheter. When tympanostomy tube insertion is performed in conjunction with other procedures, intubation and IV catheter insertion may be necessary.

Anesthetic complications during tympanostomy tube insertion are rare but do occur. A study of over 3,000 children found that fewer than 9% experienced minor adverse events, which included upper airway obstruction, prolonged recovery longer than 30 minutes, emesis, and persistent agitation.[4] Major events, which included laryngospasm, bradycardia, stridor, decreased oxygen saturation, and dysrhythmia, occurred in 1.9% of children.[4] This study found a significantly higher prevalence of adverse events in patients with concurrent medical conditions compared to children with no concurrent medical conditions. All children were discharged the same day with no admissions, consultations, or deaths occurring during the study period.

When a patient has a retained tube or residual patent tympanostomy following tympanostomy tube placement, a paper patch or Gelfoam myringoplasty may be undertaken to remove the tube and close the tympanic membrane. In the healthy patient, a similar anesthetic approach to tympanostomy tube placement may be utilized, entailing a general anesthetic with mask ventilation or laryngeal mask airway (LMA) placement.

Tympanostomy tube placement is considered a clean-contaminated or contaminated otologic procedure, depending on the status of the middle ear. Despite the frequent presence of inflammation, perioperative antibiotic use is not recommended as it has not been found to reduce postoperative complications.[5,6] Please refer to Chapter 58, "Myringotomy and Pressure Equalization Tubes," for additional information regarding the anesthetic management of tympanostomy tube placement.

CHRONIC EAR DISEASE

Otitis media may progress, and the terminology of chronic ear disease encompasses tympanic membrane perforation, middle ear atelectasis, adhesive otitis media, ossicular erosion or fixation, and cholesteatoma, which may be complicated by mastoiditis, labyrinthitis, or facial paralysis.[7] Long-standing eustachian tube dysfunction can lead to middle ear atelectasis and tympanic membrane retraction onto the promontory and ossicles. A cholesteatoma, or epidermal inclusion cyst of the middle ear or mastoid, can form within this retraction pocket. Cholesteatomas can be congenital or acquired. Due to the propensity to erode bone, including the ossicles, they frequently result in conductive hearing loss. Further bony erosion and extension may lead to other complications, including labyrinthine fistula, facial nerve paralysis, or erosion of the skull base with intracranial infection.

Congenital and acquired cholesteatomas are both treated with surgical management, with the initial goal to eradicate disease and then later to reconstruct hearing. Surgical procedures are tailored to the specific patient and presentation of cholesteatoma. This may range from an entirely endoscopic transcanal procedure without external incision, to a larger procedure including a postauricular incision. The tympanic membrane perforation or retraction should be repaired at the initial procedure; however, timing of ossicular chain reconstruction may vary, and a revision procedure to ensure complete disease removal is common.

Anesthetic Considerations

Tympanoplasty and mastoidectomy are performed under general anesthesia and generally require the patient to be endotracheally intubated. Facial nerve monitoring is often performed; hence, it is crucial long-acting paralytics are avoided. This is especially imperative in mastoidectomy performed for cholesteatoma, in which bony erosion of the facial nerve canal can occur. Mastoidectomy under local anesthesia with sedation[8] and nerve block[9] has been described. In this setting, the branches of the auriculotemporal nerve, auricular branch of the vagus nerve, the great auricular nerve, and the lesser occipital nerve are anesthetized.[9] However, this is rare in the pediatric population, and the majority of mastoidectomies are performed under general anesthesia.

Postoperative nausea and vomiting (PONV) is a common complaint after middle ear surgery. Prophylaxis with ondansetron has been shown to reduce PONV and need for antiemetics after middle ear surgery performed under general anesthesia.[10] Transdermal scopolamine has also been shown to be effective in reducing PONV, and vertigo, although this is typically reserved for patients 12 years of age or older.[11] Prophylactic IV administration of dexamethasone has been shown to reduce postoperative dizziness and nausea but has little to no effect on postoperative pain.[12]

A Cochrane review classified tympanoplasty (including stapedectomy) and mastoidectomy as clean.[6] Procedures performed on ears with the presence of cholesteatoma or otorrhea are considered clean-contaminated (seromucous effusion) or contaminated (purulent effusion).[5,6] Antibiotics are not recommended in clean otologic surgery, but short perioperative dosing may be considered in the setting of cholesteatoma and draining tympanic membrane perforation.[5]

SENSORINEURAL HEARING LOSS

Hearing loss involving dysfunction of the inner ear or auditory nerve is referred to as sensorineural (SNHL) and can be associated with a wide variety of etiologies, including genetic, infectious, vascular, neoplastic, toxic, iatrogenic, and traumatic. Assessment should include a thorough medical history, surgical history (including head trauma), and family history of hearing loss. Physical examination should evaluate not only the ear but also the cranial nerves, as well as investigate for manifestations of systemic disease or congenital anomalies that may be associated with hearing loss. Comprehensive audiologic testing should be performed to quantify the degree of hearing loss. Imaging should be considered on an individual basis, based on the type and pattern of hearing loss. For example, MRI can be considered in patients in whom a retrocochlear lesion, like a vestibular schwannoma, is suspected; whereas a CT scan should be considered in the evaluation for labyrinthine anomalies, temporal bone fractures, and other bony abnormalities.[13]

A large range of hereditary hearing loss patterns have been identified, including autosomal-dominant, autosomal-recessive, and X-linked. SNHL may be present at birth, manifest in childhood, or present during adulthood. Some genetic syndromes associated with SNHL include Waardenburg syndrome, Alport syndrome, and Usher syndrome. If a syndrome has been identified, anesthesia providers should be aware that expression of the syndrome may be progressive and variable, and they should familiarize themselves with the nonotologic characteristics, which may factor into anesthetic considerations. Examples of these can include end-stage renal failure, which can be seen in Alport syndrome, or prolonged QTc interval seen in Jervell and Lange-Nielsen syndrome.

Inner ear anomalies associated with SNHL involve dysplasia that may be inherited, sporadic, or due to chromosomal abnormalities, and included Schiebe dysplasia (cochleo-saccular dysplasia involving the membranous labyrinth), Mondini dysplasia (dysplasia of bony and membranous labyrinth), and common cavity deformity (otocyst-like labyrinth without clear cochlear or vestibular organs).[14]

An extensive cataloguing of the etiologies leading to hearing loss is beyond the scope of this chapter. Once SNHL has been diagnosed, hearing aids may be fitted. In the case of profound hearing loss, cochlear implantation (CI) may be pursued. Pediatric criteria for CI include the following: (a) 12 months of age or older, (b) profound SNHL, (c) minimal benefit from hearing aids, (d) no evidence of auditory lesions or lack of auditory nerve, and (e) no contraindications for surgery.[15] Furthermore, CI is usually pursued after 3–6 months of hearing aid use, counseling of family members to ensure realistic expectations, and enrollment in a postoperative rehabilitation program. However, if cochlear ossification is noted on imaging or anticipated, as in the case of SNHL due to meningitis, CI is performed on a more rapid timeline.

Anesthetic Considerations

Mastoidectomy is a crucial step in cochlear implant insertion, and the considerations for this are identical to those mentioned earlier. As in mastoidectomy performed for chronic ear disease, mastoidectomy performed for cochlear implantation is typically performed under general anesthesia with endotracheal intubation. Long-acting paralytics should again be avoided, as facial nerve monitoring is routinely performed. The bone of the facial recess, located between the facial nerve and chorda tympani, is removed to facilitate the electrode entry into the cochlea, and monitoring is helpful for nerve localization at this step.

Local anesthesia with conscious sedation has been described as a safe, efficient, and cost-effective alternative for cochlear implant patients considered unfit for general anesthesia.[16] Disadvantages to this approach, however, include the unfeasibility of facial nerve monitoring and minor detrimental effect on training, as well as patient reporting of vertigo triggered by electrode insertion, pain during the round window approach, and distress during the use of the drill.[17]

Antibiotic prophylaxis is recommended, even with a lack of randomized controlled studies, due to the significant and potentially devastating risks of infection, which include meningitis.[5] Given the increased risk of pneumococcal meningitis with cochlear implants, the Centers for Disease Control and Prevention (CDC) recommended that all patients receive age-appropriate pneumococcal vaccination according to the Advisory Committee on Immunization Practices (ACIP) schedules.[18] Please refer to Chapter 61, "Cochlear Implant Surgery," for additional information regarding the anesthetic management of cochlear implant surgery.

NASAL CONDITIONS

NASAL OBSTRUCTION

Obstructed nasal breathing is typically a result of an anatomic obstruction limiting air passage through the nose. Although external nasal deformity may impact nasal respiration, more frequently the obstruction is at or posterior to the internal nasal valve, the name given to the space defined by the inferior nasal turbinate, upper lateral nasal cartilage, and anterior nasal septum. Obstruction of the nasal choanae, most frequently secondary to adenoid hypertrophy, is a frequent cause of nasal obstruction in children. Less common etiologies include nasolacrimal duct cysts, pyriform aperture stenosis, choanal atresia in infants, and nasal septal deviation and turbinate hypertrophy in older children.

The diagnostic evaluation for nasal obstruction starts with a thorough physical examination of the nose, initially focusing on size and symmetry of the external nose. A prior nasal fracture may cause external asymmetry or palpable step-offs. The nostrils should be examined for narrowing and collapse. Examination of the anterior nasal passage with anterior rhinoscopy allows for assessment of the inferior turbinate size and septal position. This evaluation should be performed prior to application of any medications that may lead to mucosal decongestion. Nasal endoscopy with a rigid endoscope allows for more thorough evaluation of the sinonasal structures and will allow the physician to evaluate for polyps, intranasal masses, adenoid size, and the presence of purulent drainage from sinus ostia, all of which can lead to nasal obstruction. CT scanning may also be useful to help further delineate bony anatomy, including the pyriform aperture and choanae.

Choanal atresia, one of the most common congenital nasal defects, results from a persistence of the bucconasal membrane. Most frequently associated with CHARGE syndrome, choanal atresia may be associated with several other congenital anomalies, including craniofacial syndromes, and associated airway abnormalities, including laryngomalacia, tracheomalacia, and subglottic stenosis.[19]

Nasal septal deviation is a common cause of nasal airway obstruction and may result from nasal or midfacial trauma. Microfractures caused during minor trauma can lead to bending of the cartilage away from the site of injury as they heal.[20] Mucosal turbinate hypertrophy can also lead to nasal obstruction, usually occurring bilaterally, and be relieved with topical decongestants. Bony turbinate hypertrophy also occurs bilaterally, but obstruction is usually constant. If turbinate hypertrophy presents in conjunction with septal deviation, correction of the septal deviation and turbinate reduction should be performed together, as straightening of the septum only will result in ongoing obstruction due to large turbinates, especially on the side on which obstruction was not previously perceived.[20]

Nasal septal deviation is corrected through septoplasty. Although most commonly performed for posttraumatic obstruction and nasal airway obstruction, other indications include infection, or hematoma, frequently an acute complication of nasal trauma.[21,22] It is not performed as frequently in children as it is in adults and is frequently deferred until the child is older to allow for completion of nasal development when possible.[21] Septoplasty is typically performed as an endonasal surgery to remove the deviated septal cartilage, restoring normal anatomy and nasal patency. Similarly, turbinate reduction is performed as an endonasal procedure to reduce the size of the turbinates, either resecting the hypertrophic submucosal tissue or performing a more extensive procedure to remove a portion of the turbinate.

Anesthetic Considerations

Septoplasty and turbinate reduction are usually performed under general anesthesia with endotracheal intubation. Often, the surgeon stands on the patient's right side; therefore, the ETT should be taped to the patient's left lower lip. Infiltration with lidocaine with epinephrine is usually performed to obtain hemostasis and optimize visualization, and in the case of septoplasty, achieve mucoperichondrial flap elevation through hydrodissection.[23] Nasal pledgets soaked in epinephrine or oxymetazoline are placed in the nasal cavities to further decongest mucosa and reduce bleeding. Septoplasty is rarely performed under local anesthesia with sedation or under pure local sedation,[24,25] although is uncommon in pediatric patients.

Both septoplasty and turbinoplasty are considered clean-contaminated procedures, with no antibiotic prophylaxis recommended.[5] Antibiotic therapy should be considered if nasal packing or splints are planned to be in place for at least 48 hours, as these may serve as a nidus for local or systemic infection.[5] A single dose of dexamethasone given intravenously during induction has been shown to decrease pain and PONV.[26] Please refer to Chapter 68, "Septorhinoplasty," for additional information regarding the anesthetic management of septoplasty.

SINUSITIS

Sinusitis is defined as an infection of a paranasal sinus. Obstruction of the outflow tract from the affected sinus, typically from viral upper respiratory infection, allergy, or anatomic factors, leads to mucostasis and secondary infection by bacteria. Chronic rhinosinusitis in children is defined as 12 weeks or longer of sinonasal inflammation characterized by two or more symptoms, including nasal blockage, obstruction, congestion or nasal discharge, and cough or facial pain or pressure. To make the diagnosis, objective evidence of sinonasal disease, as determined by nasal endoscopy or CT scan, must also be determined.[27] Commonly implicated organisms include alpha-hemolytic Streptococci, *Staphylococcus aureus, Streptococcus pneumoniae, Haemophilus influenzae,* and *Moraxella catarrhalis*.[28,29] Comorbid conditions[30] can include allergic rhinitis,[31] asthma,[32,33] gastroesophageal reflux disease,[34] primary ciliary dyskinesia,[35] and cystic fibrosis.[36,37]

The preoperative evaluation should include a thorough head and neck examination, as well as anterior rhinoscopy. Nasal endoscopy allows for visualization of the middle meatus, adenoids, and nasopharynx. Nasal polyps should raise the suspicion of cystic fibrosis, as they are unusual in children. If purulent drainage is present, a culture should be taken to allow for targeted medication therapy. Depending on the medical history, it may also be prudent to proceed with further testing, such as allergy skin or serologic testing, immunodeficiency testing, sweat chloride or genetic testing, and ciliary evaluation.[30] A CT scan of the paranasal sinuses is the initial imaging test of choice and can guide eventual surgical intervention.[38]

Endoscopic sinus surgery is usually pursued after a patient has failed maximal medical therapy. The definition of maximal medical therapy can vary; however, it usually includes a prolonged course of antibiotics, intranasal and/or systemic steroids, and nasal saline irrigation.[30] Surgical goals include opening of the ostia to restore aeration and promote mucous drainage, including the removal of nasal polyps if present.

Anesthetic Considerations

Endoscopic sinus surgery is most often performed under general endotracheal anesthesia, with the ETT taped midline or to the left lower lip. As in septoplasty and rhinoplasty, the surgeon will usually stand on the patient's right side. Placement of the patient in 20-degree reverse Trendelenburg position has been shown to be a safe, simple, and cost-free method to decrease intraoperative blood loss without compromising surgical technique.[39] Often, infiltration of lidocaine with epinephrine is performed. Topical epinephrine or oxymetazoline can also be applied to assist with hemostasis. Infrequently, topical cocaine may be applied intranasally.

Endoscopic sinus surgery is considered a clean-contaminated procedure as it involves sinonasal mucosa. There is limited data to guide the use of preoperative and intraoperative antibiotic use.[5] Several randomized controlled trials have shown no difference in symptoms, endoscopic findings, or infection rates when placebo is compared to various antibiotics, including cefuroxime,[40] amoxicillin/clavulanate,[41] or amoxicillin.[42] Prophylactic antibiotics are not routinely recommended for endoscopic sinus surgery.[5] However, if skull base surgery is performed, intraoperative and postoperative (longer than 24 hours) antibiotic use is recommended to avoid the risk of intracranial complications.[5] Again, if nasal packing or splints are to be used (as may be the case if concurrent septoplasty is performed), longer duration of antibiotic therapy can be considered.

THROAT CONDITIONS

PHARYNGOTONSILLITIS

Pharyngotonsillitis is most commonly caused by a viral pathogen and is commonly associated with other upper respiratory infection symptoms, such as rhinorrhea and nasal congestion. The most common cause of bacterial pharyngotonsillitis is group A beta-hemolytic *Streptococcus*.[43] Acute bacterial pharyngotonsillitis presents with fever, throat pain, and odynophagia. Physical examination may reveal erythema of the oropharyngeal mucosa, tonsillar hypertrophy, tonsillar exudates, palatal petechiae, and anterior cervical lymphadenopathy.[44] Complications of acute pharyngotonsillitis include abscesses of the peritonsillar and parapharyngeal space. Patients with recurrent, culture-positive tonsillitis, and/or suppurative complications are candidates for adenotonsillectomy.[45]

SLEEP-DISORDERED BREATHING

Sleep-disordered breathing (SDB) represents a spectrum of upper airway obstruction that encompasses snoring, upper airway resistance syndrome, obstructive hypoventilation, and obstructive sleep apnea (OSA). In the pediatric population, caretakers are often the first to notice symptoms, which can include snoring, gasping, apneas, restless sleep, insomnia, increased fatigue, or hyperactivity. Long-term untreated SDB in pediatric patients can lead to detriments in neurocognitive function, as well as cardiopulmonary disorders, such as hypertension.[46] While SDB can be diagnosed based on history and physical examination, polysomnography is the gold standard for the diagnosis of OSA in children, with the apnea–hypopnea index used to categorize the severity of disease. The first-line treatment of OSA in children is adenotonsillectomy. For additional information regarding the care of children with SDB, please refer to Chapter 69, "Care of Children With Sleep Disorder Breathing."

Anesthetic Considerations

The majority of adenotonsillectomies are performed under general anesthesia with endotracheal intubation for both adult and pediatric patients. The ETT is usually placed over the tongue and taped to the midline lower lip, allowing it to fit into the groove of the mouth retractor. Unless contraindicated, as in patients with Down syndrome or cervical spine instability, a shoulder roll is placed, the neck extended, and the retractor suspended from a Mayo stand. Monopolar cautery is often used, so the fraction of inspired oxygen (FiO_2) should be ensured to be kept to the lowest possible level to avoid airway fire. Other options for tonsillectomy, including cold steel or radiofrequency ablation (coblation), minimize the risk of airway fire by removing the ignition source of the fire triad.[47,48]

Tonsillectomy in adults under local anesthesia has been described, with no significant differences found in bleeding rates and with the cohort undergoing local anesthesia found to have significant reduction in cost and duration of surgery.[49] It should be noted that a suprazygomatic maxillary nerve block would provide only partial analgesia to both the palatine tonsils and adenoids, as blockade of the glossopharyngeal nerve, which is partially responsible for innervation of both the palatine tonsils and adenoids, would be spared. Careful perioperative patient selection is crucial if tonsillectomy under local anesthesia is to be attempted, as it can be challenging in patients who are obese or have maxillofacial deformities as this can lead to poor visualization of the oropharynx.

Perioperative antibiotics are not recommended for routine tonsillectomy, which is considered a clean-contaminated procedure.[5] Antibiotic therapy has not been shown to reduce pain significantly and consistently, reduce the need for analgesics, or reduce secondary hemorrhage rates.[50] Please refer to Chapter 62, "Adenotonsillectomy," for additional information regarding the anesthetic management of pediatric patients presenting for adenotonsillectomy.

HEAD AND NECK CONDITIONS

THYROIDECTOMY

Thyroid disorders in children can involve functional diseases, such as hyperthyroidism and hypothyroidism, or benign and malignant thyroid tumors. Because the thyroid gland controls body metabolism, disorders can manifest in all bodily functions. Constitutional symptoms of hyperthyroidism include tachycardia, palpitations, anxiety, fatigue, increased bowel movements, heat intolerance, and weight loss.[51] Affected patients may exhibit a tremor, moist and warm skin, eyelid retraction, exophthalmos, and an enlarged thyroid gland.

Although Graves' disease, an autoimmune disorder that manifests with hyperthyroidism, is most common in middle-aged women, it can occur in children and is most commonly associated with a diffusely enlarged thyroid gland. Medical treatment for Graves' disease includes antithyroid medications, such as methimazole and propylthiouracil, and radioactive iodine. Additionally, beta-blockers are utilized to alleviate the sympathetic overdrive effects of hyperthyroidism, such as tachycardia and tremors. In children and adolescents who are being evaluated for radioactive iodine, negative side effects, such as gonadal damage and secondary thyroid malignancies, should be considered. Surgical therapy, such as a total or subtotal thyroidectomy, is also an effective treatment for Graves' disease. Patients for whom surgery is indicated include those who have adverse reactions to antithyroid medications, those with very large thyroid glands and nodular disease, and those of childbearing age who wish to become pregnant or are lactating.[51] Another relative indication for thyroidectomy is significant Graves' ophthalmopathy, which may be exacerbated by the administration of radioactive iodine.[52] Preoperative management of patients with Graves' disease is aimed at preventing thyrotoxicosis upon induction of general anesthesia and with manipulation of the thyroid gland during surgery. This includes the administration of antithyroid medications for several weeks prior to surgery as well as inorganic iodine for a week prior to surgery.[53]

Representing 5% of all pediatric head and neck malignancies, thyroid cancer is the most common pediatric endocrine neoplasm.[54] Compared to adults, the risk of malignancy in a pediatric thyroid nodule is higher and children are more likely to have larger tumor burden, as well as locoregional and distant metastases.[55,56] Papillary thyroid cancer is the most common thyroid malignancy and often presents as an asymptomatic mass incidentally detected by the patient, caregiver, or physician. In young children, papillary thyroid cancer can also present as a diffusely enlarged thyroid due to invasion of unencapsulated tumor. Treatment involves a total thyroidectomy with or without central and lateral neck dissection, depending on the stage of the tumor.[57] Please refer to Chapter 88, "Pediatric Thyroidectomy and Parathyroidectomy," for additional information regarding the anesthetic management of the pediatric patient presenting for thyroidectomy and/or parathyroidectomy.

HYPERPARATHYROIDISM (PARATHYROIDECTOMY)

Single glandular enlargement is the most common cause of primary hyperparathyroidism, accounting for more than 80% of patients overall.[58] Symptoms of hyperparathyroidism include bone disease, kidney stones, malaise, constipation, abdominal pains, and muscular weakness. More commonly, however, hyperparathyroidism is now detected incidentally during health screening or evaluations for other issues.[59] Many patients are asymptomatic or minimally symptomatic at presentation and only exhibit an elevated serum calcium level. The decision to proceed with surgical exploration and parathyroidectomy is made to avoid long-term complications from prolonged hyperparathyroidism and hypercalcemia. Accordingly, specific indications for surgery include (a) serum calcium greater than 1 mg/dL above the upper limit of normal, (b) age-based creatinine clearance is reduced by greater than 30% than normal, (c) 24-hour urinary calcium greater than 400 mg/dL, (d) patients less than 50 years of age, (e) T-score less than −2.5 on bone mineral density measurements, and (f) those who are unable to undergo long-term disease surveillance.[60] Intraoperatively, parathyroid hormone levels can be monitored and in the case of a single adenoma that is discovered and removed, a decrease in serum parathyroid hormone greater than 50% of baseline provides confirmation of successful removal of hyperfunctional parathyroid tissue.

SALIVARY GLAND DISEASE

Salivary gland disorders in children are more commonly inflammatory or infectious in etiology rather than neoplastic. Acute suppurative sialadenitis manifests with a tender, erythematous, firm swelling of the affected gland with or without associated expression of purulent discharge from the salivary duct. Conditions that can lead to dehydration or salivary stasis, such as the presence of a sialolith, often predispose to infection.[61] Cultures taken from the secretions are often polymicrobial, with *Staphylococcus aureus* being the most commonly isolated bacterium. Treatment often involves medical management with hydration, sialogogues, pain medications, frequent gland massage, and systemic antibiotics.[61] Progression of the infection can lead to the formation of abscesses, which may require incision and drainage. Abscesses and infections that involve the submandibular gland may extend beyond the submandibular space and lead to Ludwig angina. In this case, urgent intravenous antibiotic therapy as well as establishment of a secure airway, often via elective, awake fiberoptic nasotracheal intubation in the operating room, is advisable.

Salivary gland tumors are rare in children, with hemangiomas being the most common nonepithelial salivary gland tumor. The second most common vascular anomaly of the salivary glands is a lymphatic malformation. Pleomorphic adenoma is the most common epithelial tumor in the pediatric population, while mucoepidermoid carcinoma is the most common salivary gland malignancy.[62] Compared to adults, solid tumors of the salivary glands in children are more likely to be malignant. Treatment often involves surgical excision, with the extent specified by the type of tumor.

NECK MASSES

Pediatric neck masses can be categorized into congenital or acquired. Congenital neck masses include branchial cleft cysts, which will present with laterality at a depth, which is associated with the specific type of branchial cleft involved. Second branchial cysts are the most common and often manifest high in the neck, deep to the anterior sternocleidomastoid muscle. Midline, congenital neck masses are most commonly thyroglossal duct cysts, which present as a midline mass, which can elevate with tongue protrusion or swallowing. Most thyroglossal duct cysts present near the level of the hyoid bone but can occur anywhere along the descent tract of the thyroid diverticulum, which starts at the foramen cecum of the tongue and travels to below the level of the larynx. Other congenital lesions include vascular tumors, teratomas, and dermoid cysts. Congenital neck masses are most commonly managed with surgical excision, with the exception being lymphovascular malformations, which may be responsive to medication or sclerotherapy.[63]

Acquired neck masses in children are commonly infectious or inflammatory in nature. Viral lymphadenopathy can arise from upper respiratory tract infections and will present as bilateral cervical lymphadenopathy associated with other respiratory symptoms. Bacterial lymphadenitis is most commonly caused by *Staphylococcus aureus* or group A beta-*streptococcus*.[63] Treatment includes empiric antibiotic therapy or incision and drainage in the case of failed antibiotic therapy and development of an abscess cavity.

The most common pediatric neck malignancy is lymphoma, which presents as an enlarging neck mass, often in the posterior cervical or supraclavicular regions. Other associated symptoms may include constitutional issues, such as fever, night sweats, fatigue, and weight changes. While overall treatment will involve chemoradiation, an incisional or excisional biopsy under anesthesia is frequently required for definitive diagnosis and to guide therapy.[63]

Anesthetic Considerations

Thyroidectomy, parathyroidectomy, salivary gland excision, and neck mass excision, including neck dissections, are typically performed under general endotracheal anesthesia. Both the surgical and anesthesia teams must be aware of the potential for difficult ventilation and intubation in the case of a neck mass causing significant airway deviation or compression, as in the case of substernal goiter or mediastinal lymphadenopathy. Cross-sectional imaging, such as CT or MRI scan, should be obtained and reviewed prior to operative intervention to determine location of potential airway compromise and establish a plan to secure the airway, such as awake flexible fiberoptic intubation. In selected cases, a procedure under local anesthesia may be considered to maintain airway protection.

Electrophysiologic recurrent laryngeal nerve (RLN) monitoring during thyroidectomy and parathyroidectomy has gained widespread acceptance and is commonly used to map the RLN in the paratracheal region, aid in dissection, and assist in prognostication of operative neural function and lesion site identification.[64] Electrodes are either needle-based or endotracheal tube-based. There is a risk of vocal cord or laryngeal trauma during placement of needle-based electrodes. Endotracheal tube–based surface electrodes should be placed under direct visualization during intubation, as with a GlideScope. The surgeon may desire to perform repeat laryngoscopy to assess positioning of the ETT after optimal patient positioning has been achieved. In the case of parotid and submandibular gland excision, the facial nerve is monitored intraoperatively, either using electrophysiologic systems or clinically with visual inspection of the face for movement during surgical dissection. To allow for neuromonitoring, use of long-acting neuromuscular blocking agents should be avoided, as electromyography (EMG) data from cranial nerve stimulation will be negatively affected.[64] If short-acting neuromuscular blocking agents are used during intubation, the goal should be for return within minutes of spontaneous respiration and muscle twitch activity.

These are all considered clean procedures. Studies analyzing the use of cefazolin,[65] cefuroxime,[66] and sulbactam/ampicillin[67] have not demonstrated a significant difference in postoperative infection rates in clean head and neck surgery when comparing cases with and without single intraoperative antibiotic use. Intraoperative and postoperative (less than 24 hours) antibiotic therapy can be considered for neck dissection, as data are discordant and there is a lack of data from randomized controlled trials[5] but is not indicated for other clean head and neck procedures.

There have been studies describing thyroidectomy performed in awake patients with local anesthesia[68] or patients under conscious sedation.[69,70] In the latter, the procedure was performed using monitored IV sedation with propofol and local anesthesia with a 50:50 mixture of 0.5% lidocaine and 0.25% bupivacaine used to achieve a regional C2 to C4 superficial cervical and local field block. Contraindications for performing thyroidectomy under local anesthesia include patient preference for general anesthesia, language barrier, allergy to local anesthetic, recurrent laryngeal nerve paralysis, known retroesophageal or retrotracheal goiter, concomitant cervical lymphadenectomy, and known or suspected locally invasive cancer.[70] Parathyroidectomy has also been described with local anesthesia and IV sedation in patients with image-guided, well-localized single-gland disease (i.e., solitary parathyroid adenoma).[71]

KEY REFERENCES

Complete references for this chapter are online and available at https://connect.springerpub.com/content/book/978-0-8261-3875-0/part/part03/toc-part/ch013.

1. Casselbrandt M, Mandel E. Acute otitis media and otitis media with effusion. In: Flint P, Haughey B, Lund V, et al., eds. *Cummings Otolaryngology Head and Neck Surgery*. 6th ed. Elsevier Saunders; 2016:3019–3037.
15. Wackym P, Tran, A. Cochlear implantation: patient evaluation and device selection. In: Flint P, Haughey B, et al., eds. *Cummings Otolaryngology Head and Neck Surgery*. 6th ed. Elsevier Saunders; 2016:2428–2443.
20. Kridel R, Sturm-O'Brien A. Nasal septum. In: Flint P, Haughey B, Lund V, et al. eds. *Cummings Otolaryngology Head and Neck Surgery*. 6th edn. Elsevier Saunders; 2016:474–492.
30. Baroody, F. Pediatric chronic rhinosinusitis. In: Flint P, Haughey B, Lund V, et al., eds. *Cummings Otolaryngology Head and Neck Surgery*. 6th ed. Elsevier Saunders; 2016:3038–3044.
39. Gan EC, Habib AR, Rajwani A, Javer AR. Five-degree, 10-degree, and 20-degree reverse Trendelenburg position during functional endoscopic sinus surgery: a double-blind randomized controlled trial. *Int Forum Allergy Rhinol*. 2014;4(1):61–68. doi:10.1002/alr.21249.
42. Liang KL, Su YC, Tsai CC, et al. Postoperative care with Chinese herbal medicine or amoxicillin after functional endoscopic sinus surgery: a randomized, double-blind, placebo-controlled study. *Am J Rhinol Allergy*. 2011;25(3):170–175. doi:10.2500/ajra.2011.25.3610. PMID: 21679528.
59. Darr E, Sritharan N, Pellitteri P, et al. Management of parathyroid disorders. In: Flint P, Haughey B, Lund V, et al., M, eds. *Cummings Otolaryngology Head and Neck Surgery*. 6th ed. Elsevier Saunders; 2016:1929–1956.
61. Jackson N, Mitchell J, Walvekar R. Inflammatory disorders of the salivary glands. In: Flint P, Haughey B, Lund V, et al., eds. *Cummings Otolaryngology Head and Neck Surgery*. 6th ed. Elsevier Saunders; 2016:1223–1237.
63. Rizzi M, Wetmore R, Potsic W. Differential diagnosis of neck masses. In: Flint P, Haughey B, Lund V, et al., eds. *Cummings Otolaryngology Head and Neck Surgery*. 6th ed. Elsevier Saunders; 2016:3055–3064.

> **KEY TAKEAWAYS**
> - Pediatric patients, particularly neonates and infants, have different characteristics in terms of anatomy, physiology, pharmacology, and psychology from adults.
> - When caring for pediatric patients, airway management should be a key consideration as many otolaryngologic conditions either directly or indirectly affect the airway.
> - Communication preoperative planning between otolaryngology and anesthesia providers is essential for the delivery of safe, effective care.

CHAPTER 14

Ophthalmic Conditions

Kathleen Anulao

LEARNING OBJECTIVES

- Understand ophthalmic anatomy and physiology.
- Appreciate full range of visual acuity from no light perception, legally blind, visually impaired, to normal visual acuity.
- Demonstrate a general understanding of ophthalmology and the different subspecialties within ophthalmology.
- Name common ophthalmic intraoperative noninvasive and diagnostic testing.
- Identify most common pediatric ophthalmic diagnoses, procedures, and anesthetic considerations.

INTRODUCTION

Over 600,000 children in the United States younger than age 18 are blind and/or are visually impaired.[1] The familial, educational, and socioeconomic implications of a blind child are immeasurable. Combining nonsurgical (glasses, patching, and medication) and surgical interventions can help maximize every child's visual potential. The purpose of this section is to obtain a general overview of common pediatric ophthalmic conditions.

VISUAL ACUITY

Vision is best understood as a continuum (see Table 14.1) that ranges from perfect vision at 20/20 to completely blind (inability to detect light). The measurement of vision is what the examinee can see compared to what the average person can see at 20 feet. The numerator is what the average person can see from 20 feet. The denominator is what the examinee can see. For example, if a patient's visual acuity is 20/80, the patient can see at the letter line at 80 feet while most people can see it 20 feet away. Legal blindness in the Unites States is defined as best corrected visual acuity (BCVA) 20/200[2] of the better seeing eye.

There are times when surgery is recommended for patients who have poor vision. Although no surgery is without risk, eye surgery can preserve or improve vision, and ocular health, and have a positive impact on a patient's quality of life.

AMBLYOPIA

Amblyopia is a problem of decreased visual acuity in one or both eyes due to interruption in visual input to the eye. This can be due to refractive error, strabismus, visual deprivation (e.g., cataracts, and ptosis), or structural abnormalities (coloboma, and optic nerve hypoplasia).[3] The brain chooses to ignore the amblyopic eye and that eye will begin to drift and is sometimes described as a "lazy eye." Interventions to improve vision must be implemented as soon as possible as any delay may result in permanent vision loss. As the child gets closer to school age and older, the window for any visual improvement closes. Treatment options range from glasses, contact lenses, patching, eye drops, and surgery.

INTRAOCULAR EYE CONDITIONS

ANTERIOR SEGMENT CONDITIONS

The anterior segment of the eye includes cornea, iris, and lens. Examples of anterior segment pathology include cataracts, corneal scars, glaucoma, Peter's anomaly, refractive error, and trauma. The two most common pediatric anterior segment conditions include cataract and glaucoma.

Cataract

A cataract is an opacification of the lens in one or both eyes. Cataract occurs in approximately 3 out of 10,000 children.[4] Pediatric cataracts can be congenital/infantile or acquired/juvenile.[5] Congenital/infantile cataracts are often due to genetic mutations or intrauterine infections, such as rubella, varicella-zoster virus, syphilis, or toxoplasmosis. Acquired/juvenile cataracts occur after birth due to a variety of causative factors, including steroid usage, trauma, chronic intraocular inflammation, resulting in a uveitic cataract, or as a result of another eye procedure (laser or vitrectomy).

Patients may be referred to ophthalmology due to a lack of red reflex during routine screening, decreased visual behavior, or strabismus. In some cases, the cataract is obvious and can be seen by the naked eye without dilation. Infants with bilateral cataracts should have their first surgery within the first 2 to 3 months of life.[6]

Table 14.1	Visual Acuity Continuum
Visual Classification	**Subjective Measurement (Best Corrected Vision)**
Blind	No light perception
Legally blind	Light perception
	Hand motion
	Count fingers at 1 foot
	20/400
	20/200
Moderate visual impairment	20/160
	20/100
	20/80
Mild visual impairment	20/60
	20/50
	20/40
No visual impairment	20/20

Glaucoma

Glaucoma is a group of eye diseases that exhibit high intraocular pressure (IOP), which causes damage to the optic nerve and results in visual loss. High IOPs are usually secondary to an abnormal trabecular meshwork that precludes the outflow of fluid from the eye, thereby creating a buildup of fluid, which causes increased IOP.[7] There are several types of pediatric glaucoma, with the most common being primary congenital glaucoma (PCG) and juvenile glaucoma. PCG is usually diagnosed between 3 and 9 months of age. Children will present with buphthalmos (enlarged eyes), tearing, light sensitivity (photophobia), and blinking eyes (blepharospasm). On clinical examination, corneal edema, cupping of the optic nerve, optic nerve damage, and corneal enlargement are all readily appreciated, and the IOP will be elevated beyond the normal range of 10 to 20 mm Hg. Surgery to correct glaucoma includes goniotomy, trabeculotomy, tube shunt, and laser correction (Yag or Diode).[7]

POSTERIOR SEGMENT CONDITIONS

The posterior segment of the eye includes the vitreous, retina, fovea, macula, and the optic nerve. Pediatric retina diseases range from congenital pathology, oncological processes, to retinal detachments. Following an examination under anesthesia (EUA), several noninvasive interventions can be performed, such as photocoagulation, cryotherapy, and intravitreal injections. Please refer to Chapter 75, "Retinal Surgery," for more information about the anesthetic management of retinal surgery in the pediatric patient.

Retinopathy of Prematurity

A normally developed and vascularized retina releases vascular endothelial growth factor (VEGF), which is a key signaling protein that promotes the growth of new vessels. Retinopathy of prematurity (ROP) is caused by abnormal and undeveloped retinal blood vessels in premature infants. Infants who are at risk of ROP include those born at 30 weeks or less of gestational age and those who weigh less than 1500 grams at birth.[8] As the retinal vasculature is undeveloped at the time of birth in premature infants, it predisposes infants to ROP and potentially permanent blindness. If the retina vessels grow incorrectly, the treatment plan includes inhibition of VEGF. Most ROP resolves without causing damage to the retina. In severe cases, ROP that is allowed to progress can cause a retinal detachment (RD) that can lead to permanent vision loss.

Retinoblastoma

Retinoblastoma (RB) is a rare intraocular tumor affecting the retina. About 200 children in the United States are diagnosed with RB each year.[9] RB can affect one or both eyes and in rare cases extend to the brain. The majority of cases affect children 2–3 years of age, altoguth patients have been diagnosed in the neonatal period. RB can present as leukocoria, strabismus, or a lack of red reflex. Parents often will describe seeing a "glow" in the eye or "cat's eye." Fortunately, the survival rate of RB is above 98%. As RB is such a rare disease, most hospitals and surgical centers will not have an RB service. Throughout treatment and evaluation, it is not uncommon for patients to have up to 40 EUAs by the time they are 5 years old.

Retinal Detachment

While dislocation of the lens is an anterior segment problem, the surgical removal of dislocated lenses is performed through a posterior approach. Dislocated lenses are commonly associated with Marfan's syndrome. Therefore, patients presenting with RD with no identifiable cause or no formal diagnosis of Marfan's syndrome should be referred for genetic testing and/or cardiology for further evaluation.

EXTRAOCULAR EYE CONDITIONS

EYELIDS AND ORBITS

Blepharoptosis

Blepharoptosis (also called ptosis) is dropping of the upper eye lid.[10] If progressive and uncorrected, blepharoptosis has the potential to occlude the pupil, placing the child at risk of amblyopia. Anesthesia providers should be aware that congenital ptosis may be associated with a syndrome that may have anesthetic implications. Please refer to Chapter 76, "Ptosis Repair," for more information about the anesthetic management of blepharoptosis in the pediatric patient.

Nasolacrimal Duct Obstruction

Nasolacrimal duct obstruction (NLDO) occurs when lubricating tears cannot pass through the lacrimal duct. Children of 12 months old and younger are typically affected by NLDO. Congenital NLDO occurs in newborns and can affect one or both eyes. Less than half of NLDO can resolve on its own with warm compresses, lacrimal massage, and antibiotics. Nasolacrimal duct probing should be considered if excessive tearing continues. Nasolacrimal duct stent, balloon catheter, or endoscopic dacryocystorhinostomy (DCR) can be considered in more complicated cases.[11] Please refer to Chapter 74, "Nasolacrimal Duct Probing, Irrigation, and Dacryoplasty," for more information about the anesthetic management of nasolacrimal duct stent placement, balloon catheter placement, or endoscopic DCR in the pediatric patient.

Strabismus

Strabismus is the misalignment of ocular muscles and will present as asymmetric eye movement. Surgery is indicated if other noninvasive methods fail to improve strabismus. Non-surgical management of strabismus can include glasses, contact lenses, patching, and medication. The correction of strabismus is not only to improve the cosmetic appearance of the eyes but, in some cases, also prevent amblyopia.[4] Please refer to Chapter 76, "Ptosis Repair," for more information about the anesthetic management of eye muscle surgery in the pediatric patient.

OCULAR TRAUMA

While a variety of mechanisms can lead to eye trauma, the most common injuries are dog bites, penetrating injuries (knives and scissors), and blunt trauma (balls and falls). Trauma can range from eye lid lacerations to perforating injury of the eye. It is not uncommon for patients to require more than one surgery to repair the eye if the injury is extensive. Ocular trauma is more common in males, and the median age of onset is 11 years old.[12]

OPHTHALMIC SURGICAL PROCEDURES

Many ophthalmic procedures have similarities that apply across the spectrum of surgeries. The majority of pediatric ophthalmic cases do not require specific laboratory work, antibiotics, or steroids for healthy patients. Exceptions include trauma patients who may need antibiotics, steroid pulse for patients' ophthalmic inflammatory disorders, or request for genetic laboratory draw while a child is under anesthesia. It is imperative that anesthesia providers make a concerted effort to limit patient coughing, gagging, bucking, and vomiting in an effort to maintain a low IOP in the patient. This is especially important during intraocular procedures (e.g., cataract and vitrectomy cases) where instruments are inside the eye. Another common practice is to turn the surgical table necessitating that the patient's airway be secured by the anesthesia provider.

EYE EXAMINATION UNDER ANESTHESIA

An EUA is a common diagnostic test, performed either alone or in conjunction with other ophthalmic procedures. For example, children diagnosed with RB have serial EUAs as the primary part of their treatment. In other scenarios, surgical interventions can be better delineated, changed, or aborted based on EUA findings. Additional tests are summarized in Table 14.2.

COMMON SYNDROMES ASSOCIATED WITH OPHTHALMIC CONDITIONS

Common syndromes associated with ophthalmic conditions are summarized in Table 14.3.

Table 14.2	Eye Examination Under Anesthesia and Possible Additional Tests	
EUA Procedures	**Description**	**Anesthetic Considerations**
Eye examination	Inspection of anterior and posterior part of the eye; may include dilated fundus examination	May require preoperative/intraoperative mydriatic eye drops and additional intraoperative dilation time
Refraction	Measurement of eye for glasses	n/a
Fundus photos	Photography of the retina using the Ret Cam	n/a
Fluorescein angiogram	Injection of fluorescent dye to assess retinal blood vessels	Anesthesia to inject fluorescein dye Dosage is 7.7 mg/kg[13] Be sure to coordinate with surgeon as dye injection is time-sensitive
IOP	Glaucoma check	Sevoflurane, propofol, and remifentanil decreases IOP[14]; IOP check to be done after induction and before intubation
SD-OCT	Cross-section imaging of retina	n/a
Ultrasound	Ultrasonography of lens, vitreous, retina, choroid, sclera, and orbit	n/a
ERG	Measurement of electrical activity of the retina in response to light stimuli	Patient will be under drapes during procedure Dark adaptation May be asked to not use sevoflurane[15]
Eye prosthetic removal		n/a

ERG, electroretinogram; EUA, examination under anesthesia; IOP, intraocular pressure; SD-OCT, spectral domain optical coherence tomography.

Table 14.3	Conditions/Syndromes Associated With Ophthalmic Conditions		
Diagnosis	**Condition/Syndrome**	**Description**	**Anesthetic Consideration**
Ptosis	Noonan syndrome[16]	Genetic disorder with multi-systemic involvement	Heart problems, high-arched palate, bleeding disorder
	Smith–Lemli–Opitz syndrome[17]	Genetic disorder associated with altered ability to make cholesterol	Cardiac and/or pulmonary malformation; hypotonia
	Rubinstein–Taybi syndrome[18]	Genetic disorder associated with short stature, irregular facies	Cardiac defects, kidney defects, high palate, micrognathia
Strabismus	Moebius syndrome[19]	Neurological condition that affects muscles in the face. Inability to smile, frown, raise eyebrows	Micrognathia, microstomia, cleft palate, hypotonia, hearing loss, developmental delay
	Cerebral palsy[19]	Musculoskeletal disorder that affects muscle tone	Developmental delay, premature birth

(continued)

CHAPTER 14: OPHTHALMIC CONDITIONS | 165

Table 14.3	Conditions/Syndromes Associated With Ophthalmic Conditions (*continued*)		
Diagnosis	**Condition/Syndrome**	**Description**	**Anesthetic Consideration**
Strabismus (cont.)	Craniosynostosis syndromes		
	Apert and Crouzon syndromes [19]	Fusion of facial bones	Cardiopulmonary problems, spinal bone fusion, cleft lip, upper airway issues
	Apert and Crouzon syndromes [16]	Facial dysmorphia, hypertelorism	Cardiac disease, pulmonary valve stenosis
	Trisomy 21 [4]	Extra chromosome at chromosome 21	Large tongue, obstructive sleep apnea, cardiac disease, obesity
Cataract, glaucoma	Lowe syndrome [1-3,14]	X-linked genetic disorder	Developmental delay, hypotonia
	Trisomy 21	Extra chromosome at chromosome 21, lesion	Large tongue, obstructive sleep apnea, cardiac disease, obesity
Retina	Sickle cell	Coagulopathy	Coagulopathy
	ROP	Premature birth <30 weeks; gestational age and birth weight <1500 g	Cardiac prematurity; chronic lung disease prematurity
	Marfan's syndrome	Connective tissue disorder that can result in dislocated lenses	Cardiomyopathy

ROP, retinopathy of prematurity.

Table 14.4	Anesthetic Management of Common Ophthalmic Procedures*		
Procedure	**Preoperative Evaluation/Requirements**	**Intraoperative Management**	**Postoperative Care**
EUA		**ERG:** May be asked to not use sevoflurane **IOP check:** To be done after induction and before intubation	
Nasolacrimal duct probing		Consider endotracheal tube if surgeon expects copious drainage	
Ptosis	**Associated syndromes:** Smith–Lemli–Opitz [17], Rubinstein–Taybi, [18] Noonan, [16] Trisomy 21		
Strabismus	**Associated syndromes:** cerebral palsy, Apert syndrome [19], Noonan, Trisomy 21, Moebius, Crouzon syndrome [19]	Ocular cardiac reflex may be stimulated during manipulation of extraocular muscles. Notify surgeon to pause/relax tension to stop stimulation [20]	Increased risk of nausea and vomiting
Cataract/glaucoma	**Associated syndromes:** Lowe syndrome, Trisomy 21 [4]		Limit coughing, sneezing, vomiting
Retina	**Sickle cell:** Needs hematology recommendations and clearance; first/early case **ROP:** Needs preoperative anesthesia clearance; may need pulmonary/cardiac clearance; first/early case **Marfan's syndrome:** Requires cardiac clearance if positive for cardiac history	**Scleral buckle:** Ocular cardiac reflex may be stimulated during manipulation of extraocular muscles. Notify surgeon to relax tension and heart rate will return to normal **Vitrectomy:** Patient may need to be face down or side-lying once stable in recovery room	May require postoperative admit Can be painful Limit coughing, sneezing, and vomiting
Enucleation		Possible stimuli of ocular cardiac reflex	Can be painful
Trauma		May require intraoperative antibiotics	Limit coughing, sneezing, and vomiting

*Perioperative anesthetic management of common ophthalmic conditions. Note that the diagnoses are associated with more conditions/syndromes than those listed. Only the conditions/syndromes that have an impact on anesthesia management are listed.
ERG, electroretinography; EUA, eye examination under anesthesia; IOP, intraocular pressure; ROP, retinopathy of prematurity.

KEY TAKEAWAYS

- Understanding ophthalmic anatomy and physiology and ophthalmology and its subspecialties is helpful in understanding the purpose of diagnostic testing, invasive and noninvasive procedures.
- Visual acuity is not binary, and an appreciation of the full range of visual acuity enhances understanding of timing of ophthalmic procedures.
- The most common ophthalmic noninvasive procedure performed is an eye EUA. Prior to the start of an EUA case, the surgeon and anesthesia provider should discuss if an IOP reading should be done after induction and prior to intubation. If an electroretinogram (ERG) is being performed, the surgeon may ask sevoflurane not be used.
- The most common ophthalmic surgical procedures are cataract removal, chalazion removal, and strabismus surgery.

ANESTHETIC MANAGEMENT OF COMMON OPHTHALMIC PROCEDURES

The anesthetic management of common ophthalmic procedures is summarized in Table 14.4.

KEY REFERENCES

References for this chapter are online and available at https://connect.springerpub.com/content/book/978-0-8261-3875-0/part/part03/toc-part/ch014.

1. Centers of Disease Control and Prevention. Vision Health Initiative. Fast facts of common eye disorders. 2020. https://www.cdc.gove/visionhealth/basics/ced/index/html
3. Wallace DK. Amblyopia. In Wilson ME, Saunders RA, Trivedi RH, eds. *Pediatric Ophthalmology*. Berlin, Hedielberg: Springer-Verlag; 2009:33–46.
4. American Association for Pediatric Ophthalmology and Strabismus. Cataract. 2017. https://aapos.org/HigherLogic/System/Download
5. Wilson ME. Pediatric cataracts: overview. American Academy of Ophthalmology. 2015. https://www.aao.org/disease-review/pediatric-cataracts-overview
6. Trivedi RH, Wilson ME. Pediatric cataract: preoperative issues and considerations. In: Wilson ME, Saunders RA, Trivedi RH, eds. *Pediatric Ophthalmology*. Springer-Verlag; 2009:311–324.
9. Dimaras H, Corson TW, Cobrinik D, et al. Retinoblastoma. *Nat Rev Dis Primers*. 2015;1(1):15021. doi:10.1038/nrdp.2015.21
11. Petris C, Liu D. *Probing for Congenital Nasolacrimal Duct Obstruction*. Cochrane Database System Review. The Cochrane Collaboration. John Wiley & Sons; 2017.
12. Gise R, Truong T, Parsikia A, et al. A comparison of pediatric ocular injuries based on intention in patients admitted with trauma. *BMC Ophthalmol*. 2019;19(1):37. doi:10.1186/s12886-018-1024-7
15. Garcia-Filion P, McCulloch D, Cytros A, Flotildes K, Contractor D, Borchert M. A direct comparison of sevoflurane and propofol anesthesia for paediatric electroretinograms and visual evoked potentials. *Invest Ophthalmol Vis Sci*. 2020;61(7):764.
19. Wiwatwongwana A, Lyons CL. Eye movement control and its disorders. In: *Handbook of Clinical Neurology*. Elsevier; 2013;113:1505–1513.

CHAPTER 15

Oral, Maxillofacial, and Dental Conditions

AnnMarie Matusak

LEARNING OBJECTIVES

- Review tooth development which begins as early as 4 to 6 weeks in utero.
- Describe the process of dental caries development and consequences of leaving dental decay untreated.
- Define disturbances in utero that can cause changes to teeth and craniofacial complex.
- Discuss those differences in dentition, malocclusion, trauma, and craniofacial complex that impact the delivery of anesthetic care.

INTRODUCTION

Oral, maxillofacial, and dental conditions cover a wide berth of topics. This chapter begins with osteogenesis and continues to topics of malocclusion, craniofacial anomalies, and trauma. The restoration of dental decay and trauma are a few reasons that a pediatric patient may require the need for general anesthesia. This chapter gives insight to the many ways pediatric anesthesia may be influenced by oral, maxillofacial, and dental conditions.

TOOTH DEVELOPMENT AND ERUPTION

ODONTOGENESIS

The development of a tooth, known as odontogenesis, begins at approximately 8 weeks in utero. Neural crest cells migrate into the first pharyngeal arch, which leads to development of the craniofacial complex.[1]

Morphological development can be separated into the dental lamina, bud, cap, and bell stages. The dental lamina forms on the inside of the dental arch and grows into the underlying ectomesenchyme. The dental lamina is the foundation on which tooth germs will eventually form. The entire human primary dentition is initiated by 8 weeks in utero.

The bud, cap, and bell stages are named for the shape of the tooth bud during the respective stage. The bud stage begins in the eighth week in utero. Tooth buds are formed from swellings on the dental lamina. The cap stage encompasses the multiplication of cells in the tooth bud, giving rise to the tooth germ. This stage brings mesoderm into the structure. The mesoderm ultimately forms the dentin and pulp, and the ectoderm becomes the enamel. The tooth germ consists of the dental organ (which produces enamel), the dental papilla (which produces the dentin and pulp), and the dental sac (which produces the cementum and periodontal ligaments).[2] The cap stage generally occurs in the 9- to 11-week-old fetus.

Histodifferentiation and morphodifferentiation of the teeth occur during the bell stage and begins in the 14 week in utero. Histodifferentiation corresponds to the action of a single cell type changing into multiple different and distinct types of cells. The undersurface of the enamel organ deepens with the dental papilla inside, creating a bell shape. During histodifferentiation, the cells of the enamel organ fall into four cell groups based on their morphology and function: the inner enamel epithelium, stratum intermedium, stellate reticulum, and the outer enamel epithelium.[1] As morphodifferentiation occurs, the final shape and size of the tooth crown are determined. Abnormal size (microdontia or macrodontia) occurs when there is a disruption of the tooth formation during the morphodifferentiation stage.

At the end of the bell stage, the only remaining dental lamina is that directly adjacent to the developing primary tooth. This dental lamina continues to grow to the lingual side of the primary tooth, where the permanent tooth begins to develop.[2] Permanent molars, which do not replace an exfoliated primary tooth, are formed from a posterior extension of the epithelium behind the second primary molar.[3] The late bell stage also brings about the deposition of mineralized tissue consisting of enamel and dentin created by ameloblasts and odontoblasts, respectively. Clinically, this is significant in that damage to a primary tooth has the potential for interrupting development or the permanent tooth still in nascent development.

Eruption of Teeth

Eruption of the tooth appears to be directly related to the root formation of the tooth. After the clinical crown is completed, the inner and outer epithelia, now called Hertwig's epithelial root sheath, continue to grow. This is responsible for the shape and size of the root, and the eruption of the tooth.[2] Teeth generally emerge into the oral cavity when approximately half to two thirds of the root has formed. Complete root formation of both primary and permanent teeth occurs after the tooth has reached its final eruptive position in the mouth.[2] Damage to the tooth bud during development may result in an aberrant eruptive pattern

Table 15.1 Primary and Permanent Teeth Formation and Eruption

Primary Dentition	Calcification Begins	Formation Complete	Eruption		Exfoliation	
			Maxillary	Mandibular	Maxillary	Mandibular
Central incisors	4th fetal mo	18–24 mo	6–10 mo	5–8 mo	7–8 yr	6–7 yr
Lateral incisors	4th fetal mo	18–24 mo	8–12 mo	7–10 mo	8–9 yr	7–8 yr
Canines	4th fetal mo	30–39 mo	16–20 mo	16–20 mo	11–12 yr	9–11 yr
First molars	4th fetal mo	24–30 mo	11–18 mo	11–18 mo	9–11 yr	10–12 yr
Second molars	4th fetal mo	36 mo	20–30 mo	20–30 mo	9–12 yr	11–13 yr

Permanent Dentition	Calcification Begins at	Crown (Enamel) complete at	Roots Complete at	Eruption*	
				Maxillary	Mandibular
Central incisors	3–4 mo	4–5 yr	9–10 yr	7–8 yr (3)	6–7 yr (2)
Lateral incisors	Maxilla: 10–12 mo Mandible: 3–4 mo	4–5 yr 4–5 yr	11 yr 10 yr	8–9 yr (5)	7–8 yr (4)
Canines	4–5 mo	6–7 yr	12–15 yr	11–12 yr (11)	9–11 yr (6)
First premolars	18–24 mo	5–6 yr	12–13 yr	10–11 yr (7)	10–12 yr (8)
Second premolars	24–30 mo	6–7 yr	12–14 yr	10–12 yr (9)	11–13 yr (10)
First molars	Birth	2.5–3 y	9–10 yr	5.5–7 yr (1)	5.5–7 yr (1)
Second molars	30–36 mo	7–8 yr	14–16 yr	12–14 yr (12)	12–14 yr (12a)
Third molars	Maxilla: 7–9 yr Mandible: 8–10 yr			17–30 yr (13a)	17–13 yr (13a)

*Figures in parentheses indicate order of eruption. Many otherwise normal infants do not conform strictly to the stated schedule.

Source: From Logan WHG, Kronfeld R. Development of the human jaws and surrounding structures from birth to the age of fifteen years. *J Am Dent Assoc.* 1933;20(3):379–427.

that requires further intervention; for this reason, extra care must be taken to avoid tooth damage during intubation/extubation.

Table 15.1 summarizes a typical timeline of tooth formation from calcification through exfoliation of primary teeth and calcification through eruption of permanent teeth.

DENTAL CARIES

Dental caries is an infectious and communicable disease that affects people of all ages, races, and gender. When the continuous dynamic process of demineralization and remineralization of the tooth is imbalanced toward demineralization, tooth decay results.[4] In 2000, the U.S. Surgeon General reported that dental caries is the most common chronic childhood disease. In children aged 5 to 17 years, the incidence of dental caries is five times that of asthma and seven times that of hay fever.[5] The impact dental caries have on the pediatric population is significant, including loss of school days, diminished ability to learn, high treatment costs, emergency department visits and hospital admissions, inability to eat, unwillingness to smile, and possibly the need for general anesthetic.

The American Academy of Pediatric Dentistry defines early childhood caries (ECC) as "the presence of one or more decayed (noncavitated or cavitated lesions), missing (due to caries), or filled tooth surface in any primary tooth in a child under the age of 6." It goes on to define severe childhood caries (S-ECC) as "any sign of smooth-surface caries in a child younger than three years of age, and from ages three through five, one or more cavitated, missing (due to caries), or filled surfaces in primary anterior teeth or a decayed, missing, or filled score of greater than or equal to" the age plus one.[6] The U.S. Surgeon General's report from 2000 reported that in children aged 5 to 9 years, 51.6% had at least one carious lesion or filling. That number jumps to 77.9% in 17-year-olds.[5]

INITIAL INFECTION

Dental caries is a complex process that requires three main components: a host, bacteria, and a food source. The host is the tooth in the oral environment. Many strains of bacteria, including mutans streptococci (MS) and *Lactobacillus* species, survive in the low pH environment that is created during the breakdown of the substrate of fermentable carbohydrates.[7] A biofilm, also referred to as plaque, is created by saliva, bacteria, and substrate and adheres to the tooth. The bacteria in the biofilm create acid as a byproduct as it uses the substrate as nutrients. As the pH reaches 5.5, the enamel begins to dissolve, leaching calcium from the surface. The saliva will buffer the pH and provide minerals to replenish the enamel.[4] If the balance of this process spends more time in the acidic environment, the result is cavitation of the tooth and progression of dental caries. Aside from the biological mechanism, there is a proposed socioeconomic overlay in which access to pediatric providers, socioeconomic status, parental education, and prematurity can contribute to the acquisition and progression of cariogenic bacteria.[8]

Initial colonization of oral bacteria in infants has been shown to be predominantly by vertical transmission of MS from the mother as early as 3 months of age.[4,9] However, the "window of infectivity" is generally thought to be between 19 and 31 months of age.

PROGRESSION OF CARIES

The initial stage of dental caries is referred to as a white spot lesion. In this phase, the calcium from the enamel surface is lost and the surface has a white, chalky appearance. At this point, the lesion is not cavitated and can be reversed and remineralized by improving oral hygiene to remove the biofilm, changing dietary habits, and increasing the use of fluoride products. When reversed, the lesion remains white; however, it takes on a smooth, glossy appearance.[7]

As the carious lesion progresses past the initial stage of the white spot lesion, the enamel becomes cavitated. If left unchecked, the caries will advance through the enamel and into the dentin. Dissolution of the minerals in the dentin occurs at a much higher pH.[4] Dental decay at this stage is generally brown/tan in color and is soft to the tactile touch. Dental caries can continue onward through the enamel to infect the pulp of the tooth. If left untreated, the tooth could form a localized abscess or progress to a facial cellulitis or infection.

With changes in oral hygiene and diet and the use of topical fluoride and antimicrobial agents, it is possible to arrest the progression of the carious lesion. When the lesion is arrested, it will take on a dark brown to black color and be hard when touched.

FACIAL CELLULITIS/INFECTION DUE TO CARIES

Facial cellulitis of odontogenic origin represents a diffuse infection of soft tissue that originates from a tooth (either primary or permanent)[1] or supports tooth structures. The infection often has its origin in untreated dental caries that, after progressing through the enamel and dentin, makes its way into the pulp and gradually spread via systemic circulation. Cellulitis differs from an abscess, which is often a localized infection surrounded by a fibrous capsule. The systemic manifestations of cellulitis include fever, trismus, lethargy, and mental confusion. The potential for cellulitis to spread through the fascial spaces of the head and neck is extremely worrisome as it has the potential to oppress and strangulate the airway if untreated. The most dramatic example of this is "Ludwig's angina," which represents a bilateral infection of the submandibular, sublingual, and submental spaces, resulting in elevation of the tongue and restriction of paratracheal tissues.[10]

Definitive treatment of a dental infection involves immediate management of the source of necrotic or infected tissue. Therefore, a tooth extraction or extirpation of the pulp tissue will be required. Anesthesia providers should be aware that antibiotics serve as an adjunct but do not provide definitive treatment of a dental infection. True resolution will only be gained through surgical intervention.

During the course of diagnosis and treatment, it is important to determine if the etiology of cellulitis is odontogenic or nonodontogenic (NOd), as a NOd infection could be related to systemic pathology including malignancy or inflammatory lesions. Understanding the fascial spread of cellulitis is critical, as displacement of fascia will ultimately displace anatomic structures. Posterior displacement of the tongue secondary to odontogenic cellulitis can quickly result in a critical situation should vocal cord visualization be impeded, which may ultimately make securing the airway ever more challenging.

In the assessment and progression of facial cellulitis, there are certain fascial spaces that present greater risk than others (Figure 15.1). The masseteric, parapharyngeal, pterygomandibular, and infratemporal spaces are among those considered to be high-risk secondary fascial spaces.[11]

PERIODONTAL CONDITIONS

The health of the gingiva and periodontium in children and adolescents should be assessed during all dental visits. Microbial spectrum, local host factors, and environment are the three major determinants of periodontal health in an individual. Microbial determinants include supragingival plaque and the biofilm composition found in subgingival spaces.

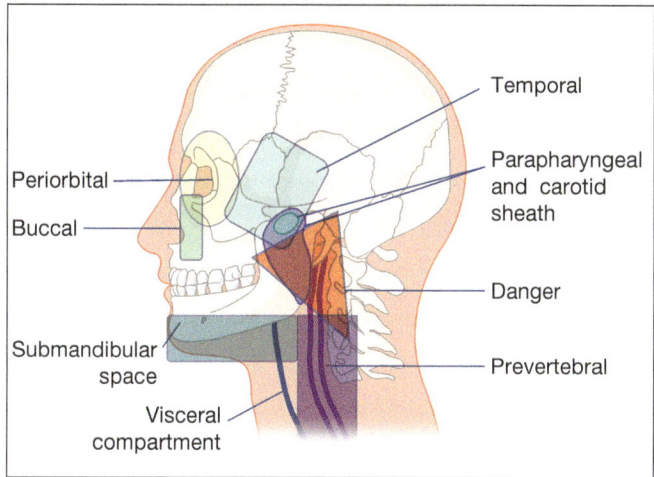

Figure 15.1: Fascial spaces at high risk with the progression of facial cellulitis.

Host determinants include local factors (periodontal pockets, dental restorations, root anatomy, and tooth position) and systemic factors (immune function, systemic healthy, and genetics). Finally, smoking, medications, stress, and nutrition are several factors that constitute environmental factors.[12]

A healthy gingiva is often described as pink, firm, and stippled, with the marginal gingiva having a knife edge.[13] The color of the gingiva can be impacted by the color of the complexion of the individual. Healthy periodontium includes minimal gingival sulcus pocket depths of 1 to 2 mm, no bone loss, no gingival recession or mucogingival defects, and periodontal ligament space that is consistent and narrow around the root.

GINGIVITIS

Gingival inflammation with no loss of periodontal attachment or bone is classified as gingivitis. Gingivitis can be seen in approximately 50% of the population at age 4 or 5 years. This increases to nearly 100% by puberty.[14] Signs of gingivitis include edema, redness, bleeding on probing, and soreness. Gingivitis is a reversible condition and generally responds well to measures aimed at removing plaque and calculus and improving overall oral hygiene.

The American Academy of Periodontology and the European Federation of Periodontology jointly held the World Workshop on the Classification of Periodontal and Peri-Implant Diseases and Conditions in 2017. It was at this workshop that gingivitis was divided into the two categories of gingivitis: dental biofilm-induced and gingival diseases–nondental biofilm-induced.[15] Included in the dental biofilm-induced category is gingival overgrowth that is related to systemic medications. The anticonvulsant phenytoin, immunosuppressant cyclosporin, and calcium channel blockers are several medications that can induce gingival overgrowth. The progression of gingival size is slow and painless, resulting in fibrous, firm, pale pink gingival tissue that tends not to bleed. Overall, oral hygiene and genetics seem to play a role in gingival overgrowth. Surgical intervention may be necessary if the appearance becomes unacceptable or if the gingival overgrowth interferes with normal function and the health of the area cannot be maintained.[14]

PERIODONTITIS

Periodontitis differs from gingivitis in that it involves the loss of periodontal attachment. It is a multifactorial, microbially associated, host-mediated inflammatory disease characterized by gingival pocket formation and alveolar bone loss.[12,13]

The 2017 meeting previously mentioned defined the three forms of periodontitis: necrotizing periodontal diseases, periodontitis as manifestation of systemic diseases, and periodontitis. The third category, periodontitis, incorporates a stage and grade rubric adopted from the field of oncology.[15]

Systemic diseases which may have a periodontal component include hematological disorders, such as acquired neutropenia and leukemias. Cyclic neutropenia, Down syndrome, leukocyte adhesion deficiency syndrome, Papillon–Lefèvre syndrome, Chédiak–Higashi syndrome, histiocytosis syndromes, and glycogen storage disease are all genetic disorders that may play a role in periodontal disease in young people.[13]

Treating periodontitis in the young population consists of many modalities. Often, several forms of treatment will be necessary to treat the condition in one individual. In all cases, patient education and removal of supragingival and subgingival plaque are required. Additional courses of treatment could include, but are not limited to, chemotherapeutic agents, surgical procedures for resection or regeneration, occlusal therapy, tooth extraction, orthodontics, and systemic disease management.[16]

ORTHODONTICS

Teeth do not exist as singular units; rather, they function as part of a larger group classified by location (maxillary vs. mandibular) or function (incising vs. chewing). The first description of orthodontics (the alignment of teeth) can be traced to the 1850s with Norman Kingsley.[17] However, descriptions of "straightening" teeth in the context of facial esthetics goes back to at least 1000 BCE.

MALOCCLUSION

The current system of malocclusion was defined by Edward Angle in 1890. Dr. Angle established that the mesiobuccal cusp of the maxillary first molar resting in the buccal groove of the lower mandibular first molar was the foundation of a "normal occlusion" and all other relationships were a form of "malocclusion."[17] Additionally, Dr. Angle described a "line of occlusion," in which a smooth curve passed through the central fossa of each tooth and the cingulum of canine and incisor teeth (Box 15.1).

It is important for anesthesia providers to understand that during childhood and into adolescence, the face "grows'" down and forward; thus, the relationship between the jaw and teeth changes over time. A Class II, or brachycephalic, growth pattern often results in a flat mandibular plane, with excessive overjet. A Class III, or dolichocephalic, growth pattern often results in a steep mandibular plane, with a potential for an open bite. This can also impact anesthesia related care as the growth of jaws can contribute to repositioning of the airway. Alterations in growth patterns have the potential to contribute to repositioning of the airway, with exaggerated anterior repositioning making visualization of the airway challenging.

BOX 15.1 ANGLE'S CLASSIFICATION OF MALOCCLUSION

Class I: normal relationship of molars, but line of occlusion is incorrect due to malposed teeth, rotations, etc.

Class II: lower molar distally positioned relative to the upper molar, line of occlusion not specified

Class III: lower molar mesially positioned relative to the upper molar, line of occlusion not specified

TOOTH IMPACTION

Dental positioning or skeletal (jaw) positioning can contribute to malocclusions. Skeletal malocclusions may preclude maximal mouth opening due to positioning of condyle. Dental malocclusions (where the tooth is in an eccentric position) are associated with a higher risk of injury during intubation as teeth may have compromised periodontal support. Tooth impaction can best be summarized as blockage in the path of eruption of a tooth, resulting in noneruption. This blockage can be secondary to alterations in the bone, tooth, or other pathology. Often tooth impaction results in the need for multidisciplinary care between the orthodontist and the oral surgeon.

Craniofacial Anomalies

An area where tooth impactions are particularly notable is in craniofacial anomalies. There is a myriad of craniofacial anomalies that should all be consulted on prior to anesthesia. We focus in this chapter on cleft lip and palate (CLCP). The incidence of CLCP can reach up to 3.7 per 1,000 live births globally. There are many prenatal teratogenic influences that can result in the development of CLCP. Veau established the classification for CLCP in 1931 based on location (**Box 15.2**).

For more information regarding the anesthetic management of CLCP repair, please refer to Chapter 81, "Cleft Lip and Cleft Palate Repair."

DENTAL TRAUMA

Estimates are that the annual U.S. expense related to dental trauma approaches $5 million per one million people.[19] The age of the patient, the nature of trauma, and the developmental status of the tooth all play critical roles in long-term prognosis and short-term management. Dental trauma has the potential to interrupt tooth development and can result in premature loss of tooth. This can have a devastating effect to the child's psychosocial development, as well as with speech and eating.[20]

Anesthesia providers must be intimately aware of several key aspects when treating patients with dental trauma: primary/permanent dentition, the nature of injury (luxative vs. nonluxative), and the ability to follow up. A dental provider may not always be readily available to provide care when other traumatic injuries are being stabilized, and the anesthesia provider's decisions can have lifelong ramifications for the patient.

PRIMARY VERSUS PERMANENT DENTITION

The overriding concern with dental trauma is always injury to the permanent teeth. Current literature demonstrates that cohorts of children who lose primary incisors early (due to caries or trauma) are very likely to catch up with their nonaffected peers in terms of speech by the age of 8.[21] Therefore, the concern related to primary teeth is in relation to the permanent tooth buds. Dental trauma that results in impaction of primary teeth into developing tooth buds (via intrusion) may affect the permanent tooth's ability to form. Additionally, untreated primary tooth trauma with open pulp or risk of necrosis may contribute to an abscess, which can limit development of the permanent tooth bud. It is common to sacrifice the primary tooth with a questionable prognosis to spare the permanent tooth from injury and infection.

The permanent tooth, conversely, will be treated with all manners of heroics to avoid extraction. Long-term speech, psychosocial interactions, eating, and self-esteem may be significantly impacted.[20] Additionally, the use of long-term prosthetics, such as crown and bridge or osseointegrated implants, will be dependent on alveolar bone level (ABL). ABL is impacted by presence of the tooth, with loss of a tooth resulting in atrophy of bone levels. Often, bone graft will be required to reestablish a healthy periodontium in concert with restorative treatment.

It should also be noted that dentists treating traumatic injuries will need to assess and base treatments off of apical (root) development of the immature permanent tooth. While a tooth may erupt at 7 years of age, the full root/apical development will typically not be completed until about 3 years posteruption. A tooth with an incomplete root development will have what is termed a "poor crown-root ratio," and this will make the tooth poorly serviceable as a long-term replacement.

NATURE OF INJURY

A luxative injury refers to displacement of the tooth within the alveolar bone and periodontal supporting structures. Luxative injuries can be defined as the direction in which the tooth is displaced. Intrusion equates to *into bone*; extrusion equates to *out of bone* but not out of mouth; lateral is displaced to either side, or palatally/lingually or facially/buccally. Avulsion is complete disarticulation of the tooth from the socket. The major sequelae from a luxative injury is damage to the neurovascular bundles supplying vitality to the tooth.

Almost immediately following a luxation-type injury the body begins a natural healing and recovery process with organization of a blood clot and bony healing with approximated borders. Therefore, the priority in a luxation-type injury is to get the tooth into its preinjury housing of bone/gingivae and blood supply as soon as possible. The longer after-injury return of the tooth to its preinjury housing is attempted, the more organized the healing response will have been potentially necessitating "reinjury" of bone and blood clot to replace the tooth. In extrusive/intrusive injuries, there may be irreversible damage to the nerve supply of the tooth, resulting in pulpal and periapical necrosis if there is no intervention (pulp removal and root canal initiation). Additionally, there may be loss of supporting bone due to injury. For this reason, the tooth may have increased mobility and may have to be splinted to unaffected healthy teeth to allow periodontal healing. Splinting is often accomplished through use of a fishing line (40 lb. test), which allows for stability within physiological movement. For more significant injury involving maxillary or mandibular bony plates, the use of more rigid stabilization, through a stainless steel archwire, may be required. See Chapter 80, "LeFort Osteotomy," for more information regarding the anesthesia management of a LeFort osteotomy.

Avulsed teeth present their own set of challenges, as they should be replaced within 15 minutes of avulsion to preserve periodontal ligament cells. Should the avulsed tooth not be

---

BOX 15.2 CLEFT LIP AND PALATE CLASSIFICATION

Class I: unilateral notching not extending into the lip, limited away from vermillion border

Class II: unilateral notching of vermillion border with cleft extending into the lip but not to the floor of the nose

Class III: unilateral notching/clefting extending from the vermillion border through the lip into the floor of the nose

Class IV: any bilateral clefting involving any structures from the vermillion border (including notching) to the floor of the nose

replaced within 30 minutes, it is less likely the tooth will be "received" by the immune system and more likely resorption (either inflammatory or replacement, in which root structure is replaced with alveolar bone) will occur.

With all these considerations, it should be noted that studies have demonstrated that even with a poor prognosis and questionable restorability, parents and patients often want an avulsed or luxated tooth replaced to reestablish some sense of normalcy following the trauma. Anesthesia providers should not underestimate the psychological value of reimplantation of a tooth.[22]

ORAL PATHOLOGY

Oral pathology for anesthesia providers is based more on understanding variations from normal rather than providing a definitive diagnosis during the anesthetic episode. As with any healthcare provider, a general survey is part of an anesthetist provider's preparation. The overall low frequency of oral pathology in a healthy pediatric patient can make diagnosis challenging, particularly in the absence of a genetic syndrome or other medical overlay.[23] For the purposes of this section, the approach will be to present areas that anesthesia providers should consider when performing an oral exam and what types of variations should be noted.

Specific considerations include[24]

1. **Lips**: examination of texture and notice of any irregular swellings. These may include but are not limited to the following:
   a. Lip biting leading to traumatizing of minor salivary glands and appearance of mucocele or other fluid-filled lesion.
   b. Discolorations suggestive of malignant changes such as squamous cell carcinoma. These will be typically related to unusual color, irregular or eroded borders, ulceration, purulence, or pain.
   c. A common appearance in the lip mucosa is a cobblestone appearance consistent with focal epithelial hyperplasia (aka Heck's disease) that often requires no treatment.
2. **Buccal mucosa**: appearance of pigmented lesions should be noted. Additionally, Fordyce granules appear as small white–yellow multifocal lesions.[23] These represent sebaceous glands and can be present in up to 30% of prepubertal children.
   a. In immunosuppressed children, a white appearance or glossy red appearance may be suggestive of candidiasis (thrush), particularly if the lesion does not wipe away.
3. **Gingiva**: ulcerations or blunting of gingival papillae may be suggestive of a viral illness (either active or resolving). Particular care must be given in the child with an active, shedding viral lesion as aerosolization of lesions can accompany use of a handpiece, and so elevated personal protective equipment is recommended if the case needs to be completed (if there is urgency associated with the case).
4. **Tongue**: while there are certain genetic associated variations of the tongue (e.g., Down syndrome associated macroglossia), the majority of tongue-associated pathology will be related to consistency and color.
5. **Uvula**: a bifid uvula is strongly predictive of a submucous cleft, and so caution should be taken into account when planning for anesthesia treatment. Additionally, in patients with a poor medical history such as children with a history of foster care, and/or international adoption it may be suggestive of previous, undocumented cleft repair.[24]
6. **Salivary gland**: a careful palpation of the submandibular and sublingual areas should be considered when planning any anesthetic. Deviations from normal here may represent cystic lesions such as cystic hygroma or thyroglossal duct cyst. Patients with a history of radiation therapy or salivary gland ligation due to sialorrhea may present with a thick, mucous heavy saliva that may impede visualization of the airway without pharmacological intervention (such as use of glycopyrrolate).

It is expected that any deviation from normal, or any suspicion of pathology, is documented in the preanesthetic examination and shared with the surgical team for clinical follow-up. Please refer to Chapter 78, "Dental Rehabilitation," for more information about the anesthetic management of dental rehabilitation for the pediatric patient.

KEY TAKEAWAYS

- Dental caries is an infectious and communicable disease that affects people of all ages, races, and gender.
- Microbial spectrum, local host factors, and environment are the three major determinants of periodontal health in an individual.
- Teeth do not exist as singular units; rather, they function as part of a larger group classified by location or function.
- Dental trauma has the potential to interrupt tooth development and can result in premature loss of tooth.

KEY REFERENCES

Complete references for this chapter are online and available at https://connect.springerpub.com/content/book/978-0-8261-3875-0/part/part03/toc-part/ch015.

1. Kwon H, Jiang R. Development of Teeth. *Reference Module in Biomedical Sciences*. Elsevier; 2018.
2. Gross E, Nowak A. The dynamics of change. In: Nowak A, Christensen J, Mabry T, Townsend J, Wells M, eds. *Pediatric Dentistry Infancy through Adolescence*. 6th ed. Saunders; 2019:181–199.
6. American Academy of Pediatric Dentistry. Policy on early childhood caries (ECC): Classification, consequences, and preventive strategies. *The Reference Manual of Pediatric Dentistry*. American Academy of Pediatric Dentistry, 2020;71–73.
7. Tinanoff N. Dental caries In: Nowak A, Christensen J, Mabry T, Townsend J, Wells M, eds. *Pediatric Dentistry Infancy through Adolescence*. 6th ed. Saunders; 2019:169–179.
12. American Academy of Pediatric Dentistry. Classification of periodontal disease in Infants, children, adolescents, and individuals with special healthcare needs. *The Reference Manual of Pediatric Dentistry*. American Academy of Pediatric Dentistry; 2020:387–401.
14. Stenberg W. Periodontal problems in children and adolescents. In Nowak A, Christensen J, Mabry T, Townsend J., Wells M, eds. *Pediatric Dentistry Infancy through Adolescence*. 6th ed. Saunders; 2019:371–378.
15. Caton J, Armitage G, Berglundh T, et al. A new classification scheme for periodontal and peri-implant diseases and conditions – introduction and key changes from the 1999 classification. *J Clin Periodontol*. 2018;45(Suppl. 20):S1–S8. doi:10.1111/jcpe.12935
22. Flaitz C. Differential diagnosis of oral lesions and developmental anomalies. In: Nowak A, Christensen J, Mabry T, Townsend J, Wells M, eds. *Pediatric Dentistry Infancy through Adolescence*. 6th ed. Saunders; 2019:8–49.
24. Feka P, Banon J, Leuchter I, La Scala G. Prevalence of bifid uvula in primary school children. *Int J Pediatr Otorhinolaryngol*. 2019;116:88–91. doi:10.1016/j.ijporl.2018.10.026

CHAPTER 16

Endocrine Conditions

James S. Furstein and Aimee Langley

> **LEARNING OBJECTIVES**
>
> - Review common endocrine disorders seen in the pediatric population.
> - Discuss key aspects of various endocrine disorders that may impact anesthetic planning.

INTRODUCTION

A variety of glands throughout the body produce hormones that are collectively responsible for regulating a host of bodily functions, such as growth and development, metabolism, electrolyte balances, and reproduction. Unfortunately, endocrine disorders are common comorbid conditions in children presenting for surgery. Autonomic dysfunction is commonly encountered in many endocrine disorders, such as diabetes or adrenal disease, making it imperative anesthesia providers complete a thorough preoperative assessment and consider the unique implications of any coexisting endocrine disorders when developing the anesthetic plan to ensure the delivery of safe, effective care.

DIABETES MELLITUS

Diabetes mellitus (DM) affects as many as 20% of patients scheduled for surgery and requiring anesthesia and is the most frequently encountered endocrine disorder during the perioperative period.[1] DM is a metabolic disease entailing inadequate control of blood levels of glucose. It occurs when the pancreas does not produce enough insulin or when the body cannot effectively use the insulin produced. Within the pancreas, the islets of Langerhans are composed of two main subclasses of endocrine cells: insulin-producing beta cells and glucagon-secreting alpha cells. Normally, beta and alpha cells alter the degree of hormone secretion based on the glucose level of the environment. With DM, the balance between insulin and glucagon is skewed as insulin is either absent or has impaired action, which results in hyperglycemia.

There are several forms of DM; however, type 1 and type 2 are most commonly seen in the pediatric population. Type 1 DM is characterized by an absolute insulin deficiency. This is often the result of an immune-mediated destruction of the pancreatic beta cells. In contrast, type 2 DM is characterized by a combination of insulin deficiency and insulin resistance. This type of DM is often familial in nature and most often seen in the obese patient population. Unfortunately, due to the high prevalence of obesity in the pediatric population, the incidence of type 2 DM is increasing.[2]

There are many preoperative anesthetic considerations when caring for a patient with DM, and preoperative consultation with an endocrinologist is highly recommended.[3] Control of glucose levels is the most important preoperative consideration. While perioperative blood glucose concentrations of 90 to 180 mg/dL are recommended to reduce the risks of metabolic acidosis, infection, and hypoglycemia, acceptable ranges are patient-dependent. In addition to glucose control, a full assessment of serum electrolytes, glycated hemoglobin (HbA1c), and ketones is recommended for all patients undergoing elective surgery. Currently, there are no recommendations for HbA1c cutoff and perioperative risk. If glycemic control is poor, however, it is recommended to cancel or delay any elective surgeries.[4] Confirmation of metabolic control should occur at least 10 days preoperatively to avoid surgical delays. To avoid a prolonged period of fasting, patients with DM should be scheduled as the first case of the day when possible.[5]

Surgery will trigger a complex neuroendocrine stress response that will lead to the suppression of insulin and an increase in stress hormones, such as cortisol and catecholamines. Anesthesia providers must carefully consider the use of certain anesthetics that have the potential to contribute to perioperative hyperglycemia.[6] This is discussed in further detail later in this chapter.

DIABETIC KETOACIDOSIS

Diabetic ketoacidosis (DKA) is a complication of decompensated diabetes mellitus. With DKA, insulin deficiency causes the body to metabolize triglycerides and amino acids instead of glucose for energy. Subsequently, serum glycerol and free fatty acid levels rise secondary to unrestrained lipolysis. The increase in production of ketoacids (hydroxybutyrate, acetoacetate, and acetone) creates an anion-gap metabolic acidosis. Likewise, alanine levels rise because of muscle catabolism. Glycerol and alanine provide the substrate for hepatic gluconeogenesis, which is stimulated by the excess of glucagon that accompanies insulin deficiency. Glucagon also stimulates mitochondrial conversion of free fatty acids into ketones, which is normally blocked by insulin. Ultimately, hyperglycemia due to insulin deficiency causes an osmotic diuresis that leads to marked urinary losses of water and electrolytes. In addition, urinary excretion of ketones obligates additional losses of sodium and potassium.

The signs and symptoms of DKA include symptoms of hyperglycemia with the addition of nausea, vomiting, and, particularly in children, abdominal pain. This is primarily the result of abnormalities in carbohydrate and fat metabolism. Episodes of DKA occur more commonly in patients with type 1 DM and are often precipitated by infection or acute illness. Treatment of DKA includes repletion of the patient's circulating volume, insulin therapy, electrolyte replacement, and the treatment of any underlying precipitating event.

INSULINOMA

An insulinoma is a neuroendocrine tumor, deriving mainly from pancreatic beta cells that hypersecrete insulin. While rare, they are the most common cause of hypoglycemia resulting from endogenous hyperinsulinism and usually occur as an isolated finding, although they may present as part of multiple endocrine neoplasia syndrome type 1. The main symptom of an insulinoma is fasting hypoglycemia, with diagnosis confirmed by a 48- or 72-hour fast followed by measurement of glucose and insulin levels. Although only about 10% of insulinomas are malignant, all cause fasting hypoglycemia and subsequently require treatment.

THYROID DISEASE

The thyroid gland secretes hormones that control the body's metabolic rate. Hormones secreted by the thyroid stimulate the production of proteins and increase cellular oxygen consumption. In children, thyroid hormones also play a key role in growth and development. The thyroid produces two principal hormones: thyroxine (T4) and triiodothyronine (T3). The primary hormone secreted by the thyroid gland is T4, which has a minimal effect on overall metabolic rate. T4, however, is converted to T3 in the liver, which is the more active hormone. Thyroid disease is common and can result in either over- or underproduction of T4 and T3 hormones. The function of the thyroid gland is regulated by a feedback mechanism involving the pituitary gland and hypothalamus. As such, disorders of these tissues can also affect thyroid function.

Hypothyroidism is the most common thyroid disorder in children. It is characterized by elevated thyroid stimulating hormone (TSH) levels with normal concentrations of T4 and T3.[7] Since thyroid hormone affects all metabolically active cells, hormone abnormalities can result in a variety of systemic problems. Classic signs of hypothyroidism include short stature, fatigue, weight gain, and coarse facial features. Myxedema coma is a severe manifestation of hypothyroidism and can occur in those exposed to extreme stress, such as anesthesia.[8] Hyperthyroidism, not as frequently seen, is often the result of Graves' disease. It presents with decreased TSH concentrations resulting from negative feedback by the increased concentrations of T4 and T3.[9] Classic signs of hyperthyroidism include tachycardia, palpitations, dyspnea, tremor, heat intolerance, weight loss, and development of a goiter.

HYPOTHYROIDISM

Congenital Hypothyroidism

Congenital hypothyroidism (CH) occurs in approximately 1 in every 2,000 to 4,000 live births and is one of the most common preventable causes of intellectual disability worldwide. CH is defined as a thyroid hormone deficiency present at birth. Most cases of CH are sporadic, making it challenging to predict which infants are likely to be affected.

CH is classified into permanent and transient forms, which are then further divided into primary, secondary, or peripheral etiologies. Thyroid dysgenesis accounts for 85% of permanent, primary cases of CH, while inborn errors of thyroid hormone biosynthesis account for 10% to 15% of the cases. Secondary CH commonly is associated with congenital hypopituitarism. The underlying etiology of CH typically will determine whether hypothyroidism is permanent or transient; primary, secondary, or peripheral; and whether there is involvement of other organ systems. Transient CH most commonly occurs in preterm infants born in areas of endemic iodine deficiency.

The clinical manifestations of CH are often subtle or not present at birth due to transplacental passage of the maternal thyroid hormone. Common symptoms include decreased activity and increased sleep, feeding difficulty, constipation, and prolonged jaundice. On examination, patients also often have myxedematous facies, large fontanels, macroglossia, a distended abdomen with umbilical hernia, and hypotonia.

Hashimoto's Thyroiditis

Hashimoto's thyroiditis (HT) is an autoimmune disorder characterized by thyroid-specific autoantibodies. It is the most common cause of goiter and acquired hypothyroidism in children and adolescents. While the exact etiology has not been fully elucidated, it is thought to have genetic, environmental, and epigenetic influences. The interaction between HT and certain genes has been reported, and a genetic predisposition to thyroid autoimmunity is suggested by observations in twins.

Clinically, HT is characterized by systemic manifestations of thyroid gland destruction. Diagnosis of HT is clinical and based on clinical manifestations, in addition to the presence of serum antibodies against thyroid antigens (thyroid peroxidase and thyroglobulin), and lymphocytic infiltration on cytologic examination. Treatment focuses on management of symptoms with substitution therapy. While the clinical course is variable, spontaneous remission may occur in adolescence.

HYPERTHYROIDISM

Hyperthyroidism occurs secondary to a hyperfunctioning thyroid gland, resulting in excessive secretion of active thyroid hormones. Most cases of hyperthyroidism result from one of three pathologic processes: Graves' disease, toxic multinodular goiter, or a toxic adenoma.

Graves' Disease

Graves' disease is an autoimmune disease resulting in nonsuppressible overproduction of thyroid hormones. It is the most common cause of hyperthyroidism. While the etiology is unknown, there is a genetic predisposition to the disease, often with a family history of both Graves' disease and autoimmune thyroiditis.

Graves' disease results in production of thyroid-stimulating immunoglobulins (TSIs), which are antibodies to the TSH receptors of the thyroid follicular cell. Activation of TSH receptors by TSIs induces the intracellular production of cyclic AMP, resulting in excessive thyroid hormone secretion.

The presentation of Graves' disease in children varies with age. In the antenatal period, there is marked intrauterine growth retardation, fetal tachycardia, premature birth, and intrauterine death. In the neonatal period, the presenting symptoms often include arrhythmias, systemic and pulmonary hypertension, heart failure, hepatosplenomegaly, prolonged neonatal jaundice, flushing, fever, diaphoresis, diarrhea, vomiting, failure to thrive, goiter, and ophthalmic manifestations (lid lag, exophthalmos, and stare). As children age, they may present with marked weight loss despite enormous appetite, enlarged thyroid gland with bruit, tachycardia, hypertension, high output cardiac failure, tremors, nervousness, sweating, heat intolerance, diarrhea, hyperactivity, fatigue, behavior disturbances, poor concentration, hyperreflexia, and ophthalmic manifestations.

The diagnosis of Graves' disease is based on clinical features, as well as elevated levels of T4 and T3, low or undetectable levels of TSH, and the presence of TSI. Treatment entails the use of antithyroid drugs to normalize thyroid hormone production, destruction of the thyroid using radioactive iodine, or surgical removal of the thyroid.

Thyroid Storm

Thyroid storm, or thyrotoxic crisis, is an uncommon condition that is characterized by compromised organ function. It is a severe manifestation of hyperthyroidism and must be treated immediately.[10] Thyroid storm most commonly presents in patients with Graves' disease following thyroidectomy due to a thyrotoxic state. Thyroid storm may also occur in poorly managed patients with hyperthyroidism following trauma, infection, or severe medical illness.

Anesthesia providers should be aware that the presentation of thyroid storm can be like that of malignant hyperthermia (hyperpyrexia, tachycardia, and hypermetabolism), making it challenging to differentiate between the two. Nonetheless, mortality rates approach 10% to 20%, necessitating prompt recognition and intervention. Treatment includes the administration of glucose-containing crystalloid solutions, active cooling measures to counter hyperpyrexia, administration of beta-blockers to limit tachycardia and the administration of dexamethasone or cortisol to decrease hormone release and the conversion of T4 to T3. Antithyroid drugs may also be considered. The use of vasopressors may be required if circulatory shock is present. In most instances, serum thyroid hormone levels return to normal within 24 to 48 hours, and recovery occurs within 1 week.

GOITER

A goiter, or thyromegaly, is an enlargement of the thyroid gland. A goiter can be indicative of an underactive or overactive thyroid gland, though most patients presenting with a goiter are euthyroid. The etiology of a goiter can vary and may be secondary to neoplasm (either benign or malignant), autoimmune disease (such as Graves' or Hashimoto's disease), inflammation, infection, iodine deficiency, or food and/or drug allergies. Congenital goiter most commonly occurs in neonates born to mothers with known thyroid disease especially Graves' disease. The most common causes of euthyroid goiter in childhood are chronic lymphocytic thyroiditis and a colloid, or simple, goiter.

Morphologically, goiters may be diffusely smooth or nodular, though thyroid nodules are relatively common in adolescents. In some cases, the thyroid gland grows so large it causes breathing or swallowing problems.

Preoperatively, the assessment should focus on the patient's thyroid status, predictors of difficult airway, and potential sequelae secondary to the goiter such as dyspnea, dysphagia, superior vena cava obstruction, Horner's syndrome, and recurrent laryngeal and phrenic nerves neuropathy. Pemberton's sign, which can be elicited by having the patient elevate both arms until they touch the sides of the head, is indicative of thoracic inlet obstruction secondary to a goiter when the maneuver results in facial congestion, flushing, and cyanosis. Airway management in patients with a large goiter may be difficult due to compression of the airway in the supine anesthetized patient. Hence, anesthesia providers should be prepared to manage a difficult airway and have a fiberoptic bronchoscope in the room prior to the induction of anesthesia.

PARATHYROID DYSFUNCTION

The parathyroid glands are located on or near the thyroid gland in the neck. There are typically four parathyroid glands in total. Although the thyroid and parathyroid glands are physically near each other and are both part of your body's endocrine system, their functions are unrelated. The parathyroid glands' only purpose is to release parathyroid hormone (PTH). PTH is a peptide hormone that is the primary regulator of the levels of calcium and phosphorus stored in the bones and circulated in the blood. PTH has the ability to induce either an anabolic or catabolic effect to regulate bone turnover. In addition to mobilizing phosphorus and calcium in bone, PTH can also increase phosphate excretion, resulting in a net lowering of phosphate concentrations in the bloodstream.

Parathyroid disorders lead to abnormal levels of calcium in the blood that can cause brittle bones, kidney stones, fatigue, weakness, and other problems. While hypocalcemia is not uncommon in pediatric practice, hypercalcemia is.

PRIMARY HYPERPARATHYROIDISM

Primary hyperparathyroidism is uncommon in infants and children, with an incidence estimated to be two to five in 100,000 and without an apparent sex predilection. Childhood primary hyperparathyroidism can stem from multigland hyperplasia resulting from germline mutations in a variety of genes or can be secondary to either single parathyroid adenomas or multiple adenomas. Most cases, however, will result from a single benign parathyroid adenoma.

Childhood primary hyperparathyroidism often presents with vague symptoms, such as bone and abdominal pain. Primary hyperparathyroidism in children can have greater morbidity when compared to adults, however, as most children will have symptomatic hypercalcemia or complications such as kidney stones, abdominal pain, and skeletal fragility. Fortunately, surgery is curative in most pediatric with primary hyperparathyroidism, although patients may require more than one surgery if the surgical approach employed with the initial parathyroidectomy is conservative.

HYPOPARATHYROIDISM

Hypoparathyroidism results from defective synthesis or secretion of PTH, end-organ resistance, or inappropriate regulation due to activated or antibody-stimulated calcium-sensing receptors. As a result, the circulating levels of calcium become too low. In infancy, hypoparathyroidism can occur due to a transient problem. This may also be an acquired problem, often secondary to damage to the parathyroid glands during surgery, or due to a genetic or congenital syndrome, such as DiGeorge syndrome, Kenny–Caffey syndrome, Barakat syndrome, or Sanjad–Sakati syndrome.

Severe hypocalcemia presents with seizures, stridor, prolonged QTc, and tetany. Autoimmune-related hypoparathyroidism increases the risk of Addison's disease and pernicious anemia later in life.

HYPOTHALAMIC–PITUITARY–ADRENAL AXIS

Key among the hormone secreting endocrine glands are the hypothalamus, pituitary gland, and adrenal glands. The hypothalamic–pituitary–adrenal (HPA) axis is a complex, interactive neuroendocrine system of neuroendocrine pathways and feedback loops that function to maintain physiologic homeostasis (Figure 16.1). For the body to function properly, homeostasis among the hormones secreted by these glands must be maintained.[11] The underproduction or overproduction of hormones can impact normal physiology and therefore cause anesthetic implications that are important to consider.[12]

There are several developmental stages key to the proper function of the HPA axis. Development of the HPA axis begins early in the fetal stages. Within the first month of gestation, regions of the central nervous system are already formed and differentiated, with prolific neurogenesis following soon after. Throughout development, the HPA axis

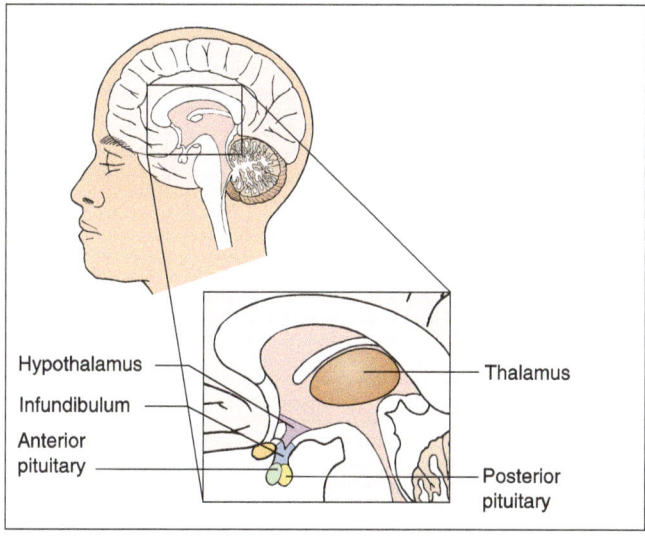

Figure 16.1: Hypothalamus and pituitary gland anatomic location.

Source: From Yedinak C, Hurtado CR, Leung AM, et al. Endocrine system. In: Tkacs NC, Herrmann LL, Johnson RL, eds. *Advanced Physiology and Pathophysiology: Essentials for Clinical Practice.* Springer; 2020:Fig. 17.06.

remains vulnerable to a variety of influences that can severely impact function. Early life exposure to excess fetal glucocorticoid (GC) hormones or environmental perturbations, such as maternal stressors, can alter normal neuropeptide synthesis and disrupt the normal development of the HPA axis. Derangements in HPA development also have the potential to be detrimental later in life due to the abnormal physiologic function that ensues. In addition, the HPA axis will become sexually dimorphic due to differing levels of gonadal hormones as puberty begins. A variety of pathologic conditions that may occur later in childhood, such as metabolic and cardiovascular disease, hypertension, obesity, osteoporosis, altered gastrointestinal and immune function, sleep disturbances, and affective disorders, that have the potential to result in HPA axis dysregulation.

When a hormone imbalance occurs, endocrine conditions such as diabetes mellitus, hyper- or hypothyroidism, adrenal insufficiency and hypercortisolism can occur. When a child presents with derangements in endocrine function, it is imperative anesthesia providers consider the ramifications the disease process may have on the patient's perioperative course to ensure the delivery of safe, effective care.

HYPOTHALAMUS DISORDERS

The hypothalamus is a subcortical collection of nuclei that monitor, modulate, and regulate physiology and behavior including feeding, thirst, reproduction, temperature regulation, sleep, and emotional behaviors, such as fear and aggression. Anatomically, the hypothalamus is organized in the sagittal plane into three main regions: the anterior, middle, and posterior regions. The anterior region contains five nuclei: preoptic, paraventricular, supraoptic, suprachiasmatic, and anterior hypothalamic nucleus. The middle region of the hypothalamus is situated directly above the tuber cinereum and the infundibulum and contains three nuclei: the arcuate nucleus, ventromedial nucleus, and dorsomedial nucleus. The posterior region contains two nuclei: the posterior hypothalamic nucleus, and the mammillary nucleus in the mammillary bodies. Each of the hypothalamic nuclei serves different physiologic functions while collectively working to maintain homeostasis.

The primary function of the hypothalamus is to maintain homeostasis by stimulating or inhibiting major bodily functions via the secretion of releasing and inhibiting hormones. It consolidates signals derived from upper cortical inputs, autonomic function, environmental cues such as light and temperature, and peripheral endocrine feedback. The hypothalamus itself contains several types of neurons that release different hormones including thyrotropin-releasing hormone (TRH), gonadotropin-releasing hormone (GnRH), growth hormone-releasing hormone (GHRH), corticotropin-releasing hormone (CRH), somatostatin, and dopamine. Once released, these hormones are transported by the hypophyseal-portal system to the anterior and posterior pituitary, which then prompts the release of secondary hormones that influence most endocrine systems in the body by targeting such organs as the adrenal glands, the gonads, the thyroid, the parathyroid, and the pancreas.

There are numerous causes of hypothalamic dysfunction, including brain tumors, brain surgery, radiation, chemotherapy, traumatic brain injury, brain aneurysm, paraneoplastic disorders, genetic disorders, nutritional deficiencies, infection, and inflammatory disease. Hypothalamic hamartomas are rare, tumor-like malformations that occur during fetal development and are present at birth. They are nonprogressive lesions and grow in proportion to normal brain growth; thus, the size of the lesion relative to the rest of the brain remains the same. Treatment ranges from medical management to surgery. Idiopathic hypothalamic dysfunction is a rare disorder that presents between 3 and 7 years of age and is thought to be autoimmune in nature. Unfortunately, treatment is often unsuccessful with brainstem dysfunction resulting in death in 25% of patients.

Disorders of the hypothalamus can result in appetite, temperature, and sleep disorders. Hypothalamic obesity occasionally develops in response to major hypothalamic injury or damage affecting the centers of appetite regulation and energy balance. Hypothalamic obesity is characterized by an uninhibited eating disorder that often results in morbid obesity and can be associated with other obesity-related complications such as diabetes, dyslipidemia, obstructive sleep apnea, mood disorder, and others. Disorders involving both the hypothalamus and anterior pituitary can also result in hypopituitarism, including adrenal insufficiency, hypothyroidism, hypogonadism, growth hormone deficiency, and prolactin deficiency.

PITUITARY DISORDERS

The pituitary gland is located at the base of the brain, just beneath the optic nerve housed in the sella turcica. Its function is regulated by the hypothalamus and is often called the "master gland" as it produces several hormones that regulate other hormone glands in the body. The lobes of the pituitary gland are connected to the hypothalamus by a stalk that contains blood vessels and nerve axons. The hypothalamus controls the anterior lobe by releasing hormones through the connecting blood vessels. It controls the posterior lobe through nerve impulses.

The anterior and posterior lobes of the pituitary gland each have a distinct function. The anterior lobe of the pituitary gland secretes seven hormones that stem from one of five anterior pituitary cells. The posterior lobe of the pituitary gland is responsible for the release of oxytocin and antidiuretic hormone (ADH).

Table 16.1	Disorders of the Pituitary Gland	
Parts Involved	Hyperactivity	Hypoactivity
Anterior pituitary	Gigantism Acromegaly Acromegalic gigantism Cushing's disease	Dwarfism Acromicria Simmond's disease
Posterior pituitary	Syndrome of inappropriate antidiuretic hormone secretion	Diabetes insipidus
Anterior and posterior pituitary		Dystrophia adiposogenitalis

Noncancerous pituitary tumors are the main cause of pituitary disorders, although head injury, bleeding near the pituitary gland, certain medications, and radiation have all been implicated as causes of pituitary disorder. Pituitary disorders are classified as being either secretory tumors or nonsecretory tumors. Secretory tumors are functioning adenomas that affect hormone production, leading to either hypersecretion or hyposecretion. Nonsecretory tumors are nonfunctioning adenomas that do not affect hormone production. Pituitary gland dysfunction can result in a host of disorders, each with unique sequelae and consequences (Table 16.1).

Acromegaly and Pituitary Gigantism

Acromegaly and pituitary gigantism are rare disorders of growth that are a result of persistent secretion of growth hormone from the pituitary gland. The conditions stem from the same mechanism, with the sequelae determined by the timing of the onset of the disorder. Acromegaly refers to the overproduction of growth hormone after the fusion of the epiphyseal growth plates in adults. Pituitary gigantism is also the overproduction of growth hormone but occurs in children and adolescents before the fusion of their epiphyseal growth plates.

Excess growth hormone can originate from excess hypothalamic growth hormone-releasing hormone, excess growth hormone production by the pituitary somatotroph cells, and rarely due to an ectopic source of either growth hormone or growth hormone-releasing hormone. Excess growth hormone leads to excess secretion of insulin-like growth factor from the liver, which then mediates growth-promoting effects in skeletal muscle, cartilage, bone, liver, kidneys, nerves, skin, and lung cells and regulates cellular DNA synthesis.

Children and adolescents with pituitary gigantism present most often with a rapid abnormal increase in height concurrent with rapid weight gain. Other less common features include large hands and feet, macrocephaly, coarsening of the facial features, and excessive sweating. Anesthesia providers should also be aware that the patient may have unstable serum glucose levels and hypertension.

Cushing's Disease

Hypercortisolemia causes Cushing syndrome, most often when a pituitary adenoma produces an excess amount of adrenocorticotrophic hormone (ACTH), resulting in Cushing disease. The most common cause of Cushing's disease in children over 5 years of age is an ACTH-secreting pituitary corticotroph adenoma. Excess ACTH can result in a variety of symptoms, including weight gain (especially in the abdominal area), change in facial appearance, high blood pressure, thinning of the skin, and easy bruising. These signs and symptoms are usually slow to progress and may be intermittent in nature, making diagnosis challenging. It should be noted that Cushing's disease is only due to ACTH secretion and thus can be classified into two groups: ACTH-independent and ACTH-dependent causes. Prolonged treatment with GCs can result in iatrogenic Cushing's syndrome.

Diagnosis is confirmed by examining urinary free cortisol excretion over a period of 3 days, a serum cortisol circadian rhythm study, or by a low-dose dexamethasone suppression test. Magnetic resonance imaging may also be used to detect the presence of an adenoma if Cushing's disease is suspected. Treating Cushing's disease includes surgery, medication, and radiation therapy. Surgical removal of the pituitary adenoma is currently the only long-term cure of Cushing's disease.

If the tumor cannot be surgically excised and does not respond to medication or radiation, a bilateral adrenalectomy may be indicated.

Syndrome of Inappropriate Antidiuretic Hormone Secretion

Syndrome of inappropriate antidiuretic hormone secretion (SIADH) is a condition defined by the unsuppressed release of ADH from the pituitary gland or nonpituitary sources or potentially secondary to continued action on vasopressin receptors.

SIADH is a rare in children but may be seen in children with central nervous system disease, such as meningitis or brain tumors. Other potential causes of SIADH include cancer, especially certain lung cancers, psychosis, lung disease, head trauma, Guillain–Barré, secondary to certain medications, damage to the hypothalamus or pituitary gland during surgery, thyroid or parathyroid hormone deficiencies, or hereditary causes. Sometimes, the exact etiology remains unknown, with the cause being idiopathic in nature. Despite its low incidence among pediatric patients, SIADH remains the leading cause of hyponatremia

SIADH is characterized by a euvolemic or slightly hypervolemic state, with hyponatremia occurring due to increased antidiuretic actions of arginine vasopressin (AVP). Increased concentrations of ADH lead to activation of V2 receptors located in the renal tubules, which mediates the concentration of urine, with relative water excess in plasma leading to hyponatremia.

Diagnosis of SIADH should include ruling out other possible causes for increased ADH secretion, including true volume depletion via gastrointestinal or renal losses, decreased tissue perfusion due to low cardiac output or cirrhosis, or cerebral salt wasting (CSW). While CSW may also occur secondary to subarachnoid hemorrhage, its clinical management is different than that for SIADH, making it imperative the proper diagnosis is made (Table 16.2).

Treatment includes fluid restriction with administration of hypertonic saline, urea, and demeclocycline. Recently, vasopressin receptor antagonists such tolvaptan have been introduced as specific and direct therapy of SIADH; however, its use in pediatric patients is still very limited.

Diabetes Insipidus

Diabetes insipidus (DI) is a heterogeneous clinical syndrome of hereditary or acquired polyuria and polydipsia diseases in which the kidneys pass large amounts of water irrespective of the body's hydration state. With DI, the renal tubular collecting ducts cannot concentrate urine due to either ADH deficiency or an underlying resistance to ADH. As a result, the body lacks the ability to conserve water through reabsorption in the collecting duct, thereby depriving the body of water without affecting sodium levels. This results in extremely

Table 16.2	SIADH Versus Diabetes Insipidus versus Cerebral Sale Wasting				
	Mechanism	Serum Sodium Concentration	Urine Output	Urine Sodium Concentration	Volume Status
Cerebral salt wasting	Excess secretion of sodium and water	Decreased	Increased	Increased	Hypovolemia
Diabetes insipidus	Free water loss due to decreased ADH	Increased	Normal	Decreased	Hypovolemia
Syndrome of inappropriate antidiuretic hormone secretion (SIADH)	Water retention due to elevated ADH	Decreased	Increased	Increased	Normovolemic or hypervolemia

ADH, antidiuretic hormone.

dilute urine output and hypernatremia, followed by polydipsia as the thirst mechanism is stimulated.

In children, there are three primary mechanisms that drive polyuria and polydipsia: central DI, nephrogenic DI, and primary polydipsia. Central DI is caused by defective vasopressin synthesis and/or secretion. Nephrogenic DI is caused by defective renal tubular response to vasopressin action. Primary polydipsia is due to psychogenic or dipsogenic causes. The most common etiologies of DI in children include head trauma, tumors, a variety of neurosurgical procedures, and congenital derangements. Nephrogenic DI is more common than central DI and is often acquired, whereas central DI usually has an acute and sudden onset.

Children with DI often present with nonspecific symptoms, such as poor feeding, failure to thrive, and irritability. They may also present with a fever due to dehydration. Constipation and excessively wet diapers are not uncommon in infants. Older may be irritable, which can be suggestive of dehydration, polyuria, nocturia, and polydipsia. Hypotension is a late-appearing sign.

Diagnosis is based on the presence of high plasma osmolality and low urinary osmolality with significant water diuresis. A water deprivation test with vasopressin challenge may be done to further differentiate central DI and nephrogenic DI. Treatment goals are primarily to reduce polyuria and decrease the thirst mechanism. This is achieved by providing free access to water, dietary management, treatment with a vasopressin analogue such as desmopressin for central DI, treatment with drugs to enhance water reabsorption for nephrogenic DI, and treatment of the underlying cause.

ADRENAL DISORDERS

The adrenal glands are primarily responsible for the stress response in the human body secondary to physical or emotional stimuli. There are two adrenal glands, each of which is pyramid-shaped organs located directly anterior to the kidneys and behind the peritoneum. Each adrenal gland consists of two distinct portions: an inner medulla and an outer cortex. While each portion has differing structures and hormonal functions, they are interrelated.

Adrenal disorders can result in adrenal insufficiency or hypercortisolism. The adrenal gland produces three types of steroids: mineralocorticoids, GC, and sex steroids. Adrenal disorders can result in adrenal insufficiency. Autoimmune adrenal insufficiency is the most common cause of adrenal insufficiency and is the result of both mineralocorticoid and GC deficiencies. Adrenal insufficiency manifests as weight loss, nausea and vomiting, poor appetite, and skin hyperpigmentation. Hypercortisolism results in muscle wasting, truncal obesity, moon facies, hyperglycemia, and hypertension. Iatrogenic hypercortisolism is the most common in pediatric patients, whereas Cushing's disease or syndrome is rare.

Hyperaldosteronism

While rare, primary hyperaldosteronism, or Conn's syndrome, is the most common cause of mineralocorticoid excess. Conn's syndrome is due to unilateral or bilateral adrenal gland hyperactivity. Unilateral adrenal gland hyperactivity is usually caused by an aldosterone producing adenoma (benign tumor) and less commonly by adrenal cancer or hyperplasia, whereas bilateral adrenal gland hyperactivity is usually secondary to hyperplasia.

The syndrome is characterized by increased aldosterone, low renin level, and arterial hypertension, with hypertension being the sole presenting symptom. Diagnosis is confirmed via assessment of aldosterone and renin levels, a captopril suppression test, measurement of 24-urine excretion of aldosterone, of a saline suppression test.

If the underlying cause of hyperaldosteronism is an adenoma, an adrenalectomy is curative. Hypertension in patients presenting with Conn's syndrome due to bilateral hyperplasia can be difficult to manage and is often refractory to treatment. If not managed properly, severe complications, such as impaired vascular smooth muscle function secondary to increased aldosterone, endothelial dysfunction, deterioration of left ventricular functions, acute effects on the cardiovascular system, and proteinuria, may ensue.

Addison's Disease

Primary adrenal insufficiency, or Addison's disease, occurs secondary to adrenal gland defects that result in the inability to produce adequate amounts of GC, mineralocorticoid, and adrenal androgens, despite an increased concentration of ACTH. This can be due to adrenal dysgenesis, adrenal gland defect, adrenal destruction, or infection.

Adrenal dysgenesis refers to congenital adrenal structural developmental defects. An example is mutation in the dosage-sensitive sex reversal adrenal hypoplasia gene 1 (*DAX-1*), which can cause an X-linked form of congenital adrenal hypoplasia (CAH). This form of CAH typically presents as a life-threatening adrenal crisis in males during the newborn period and hypogonadotropic hypogonadism later in adolescence. Adrenal gland defects refer to disorders of cholesterol or steroid biosynthesis. CAH from 21-hydroxylase is the most common cause of adrenal insufficiency in early infancy. Adrenal destruction refers to pathologic processes that damage the adrenal gland. Autoimmune destruction of the adrenal cortex is the most common cause of Addison disease beyond infancy; however, destruction can also occur secondary to infection, metabolic and infiltrative or metastatic diseases, and the effects of drugs. Historically, tuberculosis (TB) was the leading cause of Addison's disease.

Autoimmune damage to the adrenal gland may be isolated or can occur in the context of autoimmune polyendocrine syndrome

Unfortunately, symptoms and signs of Addison's disease are nonspecific in the early stages and can mimic a gastrointestinal disorder, with nausea, vomiting, and abdominal pain, or a psychiatric disorder, especially depression. Consequently, the clinical diagnosis of very difficult and the first presentation is often an acute and potentially life-threatening adrenal crisis in the ED. Most children who have Addison's disease experience ill-defined fatigue, generalized muscular weakness, loss of appetite, poor weight gain, and hyperpigmentation. Some patients crave salt. Teenagers may notice loss of pubic and axillary hair.

Diagnosis can be confirmed via a stimulation test with synthetic ACTH. If autoimmune Addison's disease is suspected, the possibility of other endocrine gland dysfunction should be evaluated and ruled out as possible causes. Similarly, the possibility of hypogonadism should be investigated.

The long-term treatment of Addison's disease entails GC and mineralocorticoid replacement. Hydrocortisone is the drug of choice for the GC replacement in children as its short half-life allows for best control. Adrenal androgen replacement is being studied in adults; however, no data are available for children and adolescents.

Secondary adrenal insufficiency can also occur secondary to suppression of the HPA axis. This occurs when secretion of CRH from the hypothalamus or of ACTH from the pituitary leads to hypofunction of the adrenal cortex. Unlike in Addison's disease, there is only a GC deficiency as mineralocorticoids and sex steroids are unaffected. In most cases the cause is iatrogenic, such as pituitary surgery, pituitary irradiation, or, most commonly, the use of synthetic GC.

Pheochromocytoma

Pheochromocytoma is a rare chromaffin cell tumor that secretes catecholamines. Eighty-five percent of pheochromocytomas are in the adrenal glands, with the rest developing in the extra-adrenal parasympathetic and sympathetic paraganglia. Approximately 10% of intra-adrenal and 40% of extra-adrenal pheochromocytomas are malignant. The overall prevalence of hypertension has risen from 2% to 4.5% in the pediatric population, which has been largely attributed to obesity-induced hypertension.

Pheochromocytomas become symptomatic from the increased secretion of norepinephrine, epinephrine, and dopamine. Norepinephrine is the predominant catecholamine secreted in children. The clinical presentation is variable, with approximately 60% to 90% of children presenting with sustained hypertension as their primary sign, which may be severe enough to cause encephalopathy or cardiac failure. It should be noted that children are less likely than adults to present with the classic triad of tachycardia, headache, and diaphoresis. Ultimately, symptomatology depends on the type of hormone being secreted. Children with epinephrine secreting tumors can present with hypoglycemia and hypotensive shock due to excess catecholamine production and circulatory collapse. Children with dopamine-secreting tumors are usually asymptomatic, delaying diagnosis until the mass effect of the tumor is apparent

The gold standard for diagnosis is via the measurement of plasma-free metanephrines, with imaging studies to aid with identification of metastatic lesions for surgical resection. Surgery is the preferred treatment option, although tumor resection should not be attempted without preoperative medical preparation. Preoperative therapy with alpha-blocking agents and beta-blockers help ensure safe pre-, intra-, and postoperative courses. Once alpha-adrenergic blockade has been obtained, beta-adrenergic blockade is instituted to blunt reflex tachycardia. Beta-adrenergic antagonists never should be started alone as blockade of the vasodilatory effects of beta-adrenergic receptors will lead to unopposed alpha-adrenergic activity and worsening hypertension. Alternative regimens for preoperative management include administration of calcium channel blockers and tyrosine hydroxylase inhibitors to inhibit catecholamine synthesis. These agents are typically reserved for patients who have refractory hypertension

POLYCYSTIC OVARIAN SYNDROME

Polycystic ovary syndrome (PCOS) is a common disorder characterized by hyperandrogenism and disordered gonadotropin secretion. The clinical manifestations of PCOS often emerge during childhood or in the peripubertal years, suggesting that the syndrome is influenced by fetal programming or early postnatal events.

There remains no consensus regarding the diagnosis and management of PCOS in the pediatric population. In adolescents, PCOS is largely a diagnosis of exclusion that hinges on evidence of ovulatory dysfunction and androgen excess. The clinical evaluation of girls suspected of having PCOS should focus on excluding other causes of androgen excess and menstrual dysfunction. While the presence of polycystic ovary morphology is included as a key diagnostic criterion of PCOS in adults, it is currently not recommended for the diagnosis in adolescents.

Treatment should be individualized to the presentation, needs, and preferences of each patient. Ultimately, the goal of treatment is to improve quality of life and long-term health outcomes. This may entail lifestyle modifications, the use of combined oral contraceptives, spironolactone to improve menstrual irregularities, and electrolysis. As PCOS often modulates both hormonal and metabolic processes and is frequently associated with insulin resistance, metformin is also indicated as part of the treatment regimen.

ANESTHETIC CONSIDERATIONS

DIABETES MELLITUS

Familiarity with the prescribed insulin and antihyperglycemic medications is critical to helping develop a perioperative plan. Various regimens for managing perioperative insulin therapy have been proposed; however, not one is superior. It is essential anesthesia providers verify the patient's usual insulin regimen and to confirm the dose and time of the last insulin administration. On the morning of surgery, no inulin should be administered unless the blood glucose is greater than 250 mg/dL.[13] Type 2 diabetic patients should hold metformin for 24 hours before major surgical procedures due to the risk of lactic acidosis.[14]

Postoperative nausea and vomiting prophylaxis, initiated preoperatively, can aid in normal resumption of postoperative oral intake. Dexamethasone can be used to manage Postoperative nausea and vomiting (PONV); however, it should be used with caution in patients with DM as it can cause undesirable hyperglycemia.[15] There are suggestions in the literature to withhold preoperative sedation from diabetic patients to avoid masking the signs and symptoms of hypoglycemia; however, preoperative sedations is still recommended.[16]

THYROIDECTOMY OR GOITER

Children should be euthyroid prior to proceeding with surgery to minimize complications and avoid precipitation of myxedema coma or thyroid storm. If a large goiter is present, the possibility of airway compromise should be considered. Additional airway equipment may be necessary to avoid an airway emergency.

In patients with hyperthyroidism, the precipitation of thyroid storm can occur from the insult of surgery. This may be difficult to differentiate from malignant hyperthermia and therefore, anesthesia providers must be aware of the differential diagnoses: neuroleptic malignant syndrome, pheochromocytoma, and malignant hyperthermia. Thyroid storm is an endocrine emergency and must be treated immediately with beta blockers, methimazole or propylthiouracil, GCs, and antipyretics.

SURGERY-INDUCED STRESS

Surgery induces an increase in GC production that correlates with the intensity of the surgical procedure. In general, an increase in total plasma cortisol begins in the immediate postoperative period and returns to its presurgery baseline on postoperative day 2. The extent of variation in total plasma cortisol levels is proportional to the extent of surgery, with minor procedures having little to no impact on the increase in cortisol levels.

SEPSIS

Sepsis is an inflammatory condition associated with elevated cortisol levels. With sepsis, ACTH levels rapidly decrease within 3 to 5 days, despite an initial rise in plasma levels. This results in a dissociation between ACTH and cortisol levels. Ultimately, adrenal function may be disturbed, and exogenous ACTH may result in little or no cortisol synthesis.

Relative adrenal insufficiency has been defined as an insufficiently high cortisol level in the context of physiologic stress, such as septic shock. The 2013 guidelines of the Surviving Sepsis Campaign recommend the use of a hydrocortisone stress dose in patients with septic shock with a poor response to vasoconstrictors. Of note, a cosyntropin stimulation test is not recommended.

ANESTHETIC IMPACT ON THE HPA AXIS

Several commonly used anesthetic agents have the potential to affect the HPA axis. The main effects are reported in **Table 16.3**.

Table 16.3 Impact of Anesthetics on the HPA Axis

Anesthetic	Enzyme Inhibition	Hormonal Effect
Ectomidate	11β-hydroxylase P450scc 17α-hydroxylase 16 α-hydroxylase	↓↓↓Cortisol (in vivo, in vitro)
Midazolam	21-hydroxylase 17α-hydroxylase 11β-hydroxylase P450scc	↓↓Cortisol (in vivo, in vitro) ↓CRF (in vitro) ↓Aldosterone
Propofol	?	↓Cortisol (in vitro, not in vivo)
Ketamine	?	Contradictory results
Barbiturates	?	↓Cortisol (in vitro, not in vivo)
Halogeneted gases	?	↑Cortisol (in vivo)
Dexmedetomidine	?	↓Cortisol (in vitro, not in vivo)
Opioids	?	↓ACTH (in vivo) ↓Cortisol (in vivo)
Local anesthetics	?	Contradictory results

ACTH, adrenocorticotrophic hormone; CRF, corticotropin-releasing factor; HPA, hypothalamic-pituitary-adrenal; P450scc, P450 side-chain cleavage.

Source: Besnier E, Clavier T, Compere V. The hypothalamic–pituitary–adrenal axis and anesthetics: a review. Anesth Analg. 2017;124(4):1181–1189. doi:10.1213/ANE.0000000000001580.

PART III: CONDITIONS, DISEASES, AND SYNDROMES IN PEDIATRIC PATIENTS

KEY TAKEAWAYS

- Endocrine diseases are common comorbid conditions in surgical patients.
- DM involves absence of insulin secretion (type I) or peripheral insulin resistance (type II), causing hyperglycemia. Type 1 diabetes is one of the most common childhood diseases.
- The airway is a key consideration in patients undergoing thyroid surgery.
- Parathyroid disease can have a profound impact on the regulation of bone turnover and serum calcium concentrations.
- The hypothalamic–pituitary–adrenal (HPA) axis is essential for human adaptation to stress. Drugs commonly used in anesthesia have the potential to modulate HPA axis activity.
- The primary function of the hypothalamus is to maintain homeostasis by stimulating or inhibiting major bodily functions.
- The implications of growth hormone excess and adrenal steroid excess should be considered when preparing a child for pituitary surgery.
- Patients with pheochromocytoma require careful preoperative preparation.
- Patients with polycystic ovary syndrome may be insulin-resistant.

KEY REFERENCES

Complete references for this chapter are online and available at https://connect.springerpub.com/content/book/978-0-8261-3875-0/part/part03/toc-part/ch016.

2. American Diabetes Association. 13. Children and adolescents: standards of medical care in diabetes—2020. *Diabetes Care.* 2020;43(Suppl. 1):S163–S182. doi:10.2337/dc20-s013
4. Jefferies C, Rhodes E, Rachmiel M, et al. Ispad clinical practice consensus guidelines 2018: management of children and adolescents with diabetes requiring surgery. *Pediatr Diabetes.* 2018;19:227–236. doi:10.1111/pedi.12733
9. Mitchell AL, Pearce SH. Subclinical hyperthyroidism: first do no harm. *Clin Endocrinol.* 2016;85(1):15–16. doi:10.1111/cen.13070
15. Tien M, Gan, TJ, Dhakal I, et al. The effect of anti-emetic doses of dexamethasone on postoperative blood glucose levels in non-diabetic and diabetic patients: a prospective randomised controlled study. *Anaesthesia.* 2016;71(9):1037–1043. doi:10.1111/anae.13544
17. Aronson S, Murray S, Martin G, et al. Roadmap for transforming preoperative assessment to preoperative optimization. *Anesth Analg.* 2020;130(4):811–819. doi:10.1213/ane.0000000000004571

CHAPTER 17

Cardiovascular Conditions

Brian J. Gronert, Peace C. Madueme, and Karen S. Bender

LEARNING OBJECTIVES

- Describe common pediatric cardiovascular conditions.
- Recognize the pathophysiology of common cardiovascular conditions from anatomic/structure, electrophysiologic, and myocardial muscle perspectives.
- Discuss pulmonary hypertension and the anesthetic implications.
- Review preanesthetic assessments for patients with congenital heart disease.
- Identify risk factors and develop a cardiac lesion-specific anesthetic, including premedication, invasive monitoring, and need for postanesthesia intensive care.

INTRODUCTION

Congenital heart disease (CHD) is the most common congenital anomaly affecting .7% to .8% of live births.[1] Although the incidence of CHD has remained stable worldwide, the age standardized mortality rate of CHD in developed countries has declined substantially over the past three decades.[2]

Due to innovations in surgery, anesthesia, and cardiopulmonary bypass, 85% of all children born with congenital heart defects are now long-term survivors, resulting in many patients with repaired or palliated heart anomalies present for noncardiac surgery.[3] Except for the simplest of completely repaired lesions (atrial septal defect [ASD], ventricular septal defect [VSD], and patent ductus arteriosus [PDA]), these patients carry a burden of residual cardiac pathophysiology and decreased cardiovascular reserve that increases anesthesia risk (**Figure 17.1**).

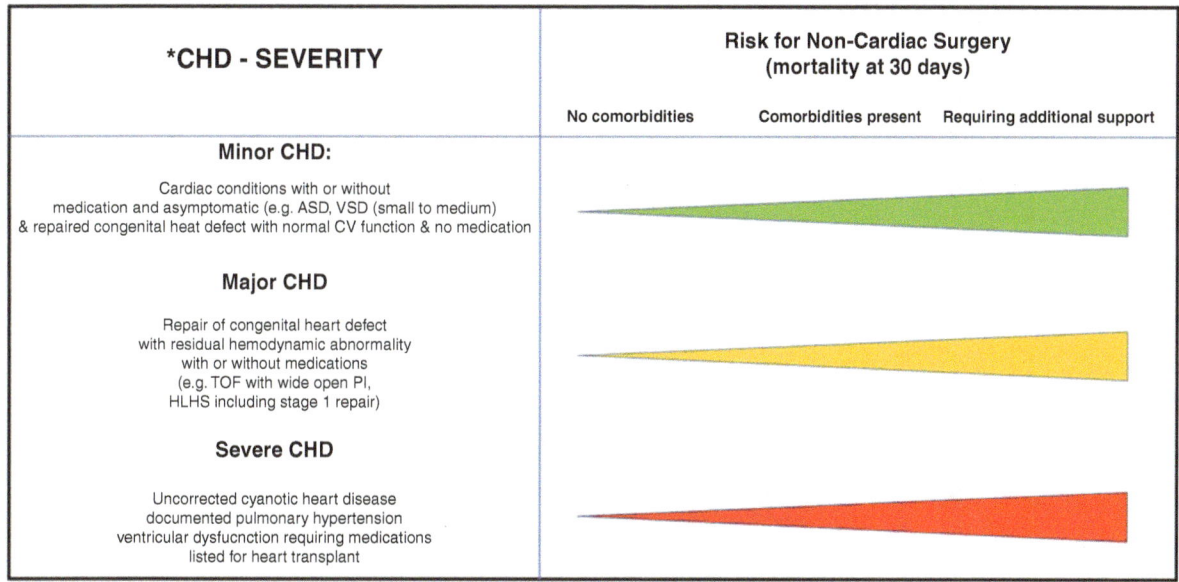

Figure 17.1: Stratification of patient risk for children with CHD undergoing noncardiac surgery. The risk is lowest in children with minor (green) CHD when compared to those with major (yellow) and severe (red) CHD. The 30-day noncardiac surgical mortality risk increases with presence of comorbidities and need for mechanical or inotropic support. *CHD + comorbidities = prematurity, chronic lung disease, acute or chronic kidney injury, sepsis, and emergent procedure; additional support = inotropes, mechanical ventilation, and preoperative CPR.

ASD, atrial septal defect; CHD, congenital heart disease; CPR, cardiopulmonary resuscitation; CV, cardiovascular; HLHS, hypoplastic left heart syndrome; PI, pulmonary insufficiency; TOF, tetralogy of Fallot; VSD, ventricular septal defect.

Source: Benjamin K, Skubas N, Belani K. Risk prediction in children with congenital heart disease: business as usual-or not? *Anesth Analg.* 2020;131(4):1080–1082. doi:10.1213/ANE.0000000000005042, p. 1081.

LEFT-TO-RIGHT SHUNTS

Congenital heart defects with left-to-right shunts make up more than 40% of all CHDs. They include VSD, ASD, PDA, and atrioventricular septal defects (AVSDs). Operative and transcatheter treatment of VSD, ASD, and PDA is curative. Catheter delivered devices to close ASDs and PDAs are more common than for VSDs. AVSD surgical repair is often problematic and associated with ongoing valvular abnormalities that require long-term medical therapy and reoperation. Endocarditis prophylaxis is indicated in the first 6 months after surgical or device closure of a congenital heart defect.[4]

> **BOX 17.1 TYPES OF VENTRICULAR SEPTAL DEFECTS**
>
> - Perimembranous (also called membranous, param-embranous, and conoventricular), most common
> - Muscular, usually closes spontaneously
> - Outlet (also called doubly committed subarterial, subpulmonary, supracristal, or infundibular)
> - Inlet (also called canal type), most common in atrioventricular septal defect

VENTRICULAR SEPTAL DEFECT

VSD occurs in 15% to 20% of all patients with CHD. A VSD can occur anywhere along the interventricular septum inlet, membranous, muscular or outlet. Approximately 30% to 40% of VSDs close without intervention, most of which are small muscular and small perimembranous VSDs (**Box 17.1** and **Figure 17.2**). VSDs can be an isolated defect or part of a more complicated lesion like tetralogy of Fallot (TOF). The aortic valve (AV) can be affected by a subarterial VSD. Turbulent flow can cause prolapse of the AV leaflet through the VSD and aortic insufficiency (AI).

Pathophysiology and Clinical Manifestations

Shunting from a VSD is from the higher pressure left ventricle (LV) to the lower pressure right ventricle (RV), producing a left-to-right shunt. This left-to-right shunt leads to increased pulmonary blood flow and left atrial (LA) and LV volume overload. Shunting will vary according to the pulmonary arterial pressure. Pulmonary pressure is high at birth and then decreases. As pulmonary pressure decreases and left-to-right shunting increases, the infant may develop congestive heart failure (CHF). Small VSDs (less than one third the size of the normal AV) are well tolerated with normal weight gain. Moderate to large VSDs are associated with poor feeding and poor weight gain, symptoms of CHF. A moderate VSD presents some resistance to flow with the LV pressure remaining higher than that of the RV, whereas a large VSD produces equal pressure in the LV and RV. Infants with CHF are treated with diuretics and afterload reduction prior to surgical repair. Echocardiogram (ECHO) can diagnose the position and size of the VSD (**Figure 17.3**). Cardiac catheterization is rarely necessary.[5] Physical examination reveals a harsh holosystolic murmur that can be best heard at the lower left sternal murmur.

Shunting is quantified using pulmonary blood flow (Qp) to systemic blood flow (Qs) ratio. A normal Qp:Qs ratio is 1:1, with Qp equaling Qs. In the presence of a VSD, the left-to-right shunt causes more blood to flow out the pulmonary artery than the aorta, resulting in the Qp:Qs ratio being greater than

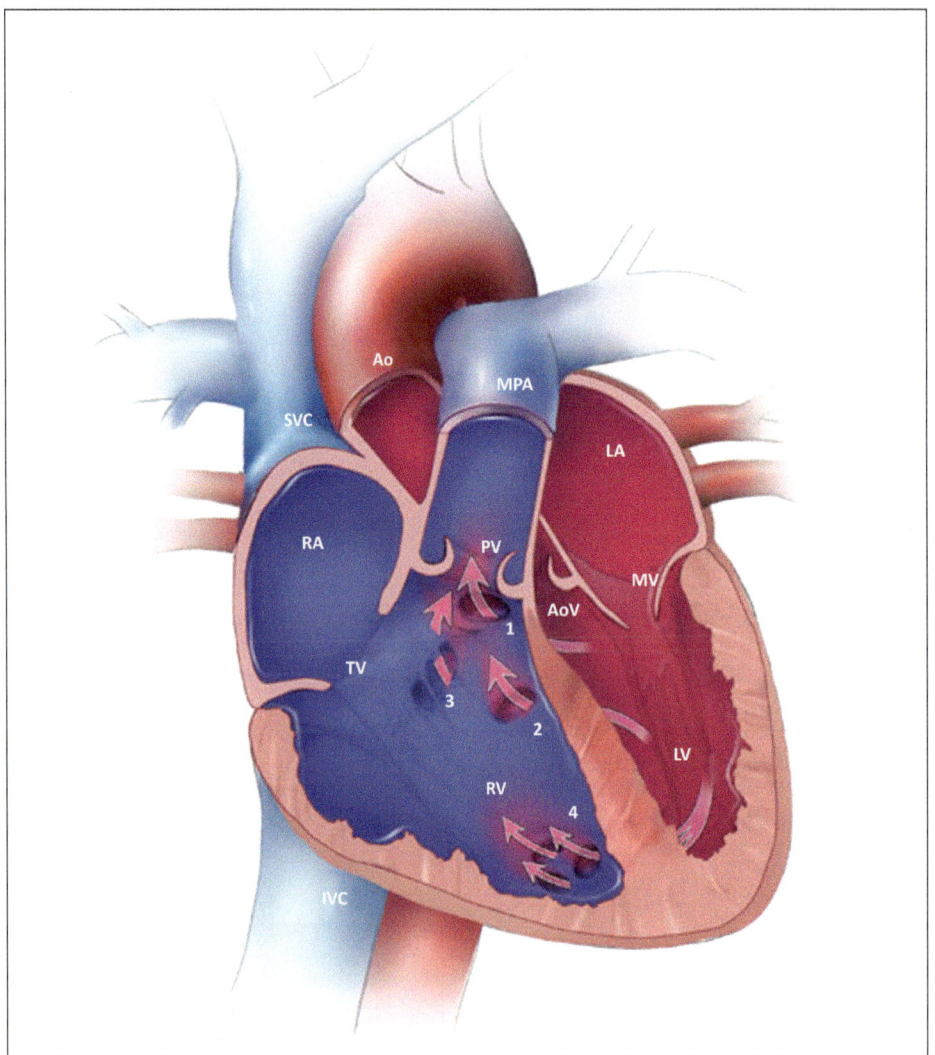

Figure 17.2: Names and locations of the different VSDs. Ventricular septal defect. (1) conoventricular, malaligned; (2) perimembranous; (3) inlet; (4) muscular.

Ao, aorta; AV, aortic valve; IVC, inferior vena cava; LA, left atrium; LV, left ventricle; MPA, main pulmonary artery; MV, mitral valve; RA, right atrium; RV, right ventricle; SVC, superior vena cava; TV, tricuspid valve

Source: Courtesy of the Centers for Disease Control and Prevention. Flamm KL, Granger M, Gawlik K, et al. Evidence-based assessment of the heart and circulatory system. In: Gawlik KS, Melnyk BM, Teall AM, eds. *Evidence-Based Physical Examination: Best Practices for Health and Well-Being Assessment.* Springer Publishing Company; 2021. Fig. 6.51.

1:1. This is often referred to as "pulmonary overcirculation." Surgery is indicated for a Qp:Qs ratio of greater than 1.5:1. Classically, the Qp:Qs ratio is measured by cardiac catheterization; however, this invasive procedure is rarely performed for simple VSDs. The Qp:Qs ratio can also be measured noninvasively by cardiovascular MRI (CMR).

Infants with a VSD that has not decreased in size who also develop CHF requiring medical treatment will undergo elective surgical repair between 6 months and 1 year of age. Elective closure of a VSD may be performed via a transcatheter or surgical approach. While the transcatheter approach avoids sternotomy and cardiopulmonary bypass with a shorter length of hospital stay, it is associated with a similar risk of complete heart block. If the VSD is associated with AI, it should be repaired regardless of size or symptoms. Of note, VSDs located in the inlet or outlet portion of the ventricular septum do not close spontaneously, are not amenable to transcatheter closure due to proximity to the heart valves, and require surgical closure.

A patient with a large VSD that is left untreated will develop fixed pulmonary hypertension. Shunting will reverse to a right to left shunt causing cyanosis. This is called Eisenmenger syndrome. Once this occurs, surgical repair is not possible, because the pulmonary hypertension is fixed. If the VSD is closed, the RV will be unable to pump blood through the pulmonary circulation and fail acutely leading to LV failure and death.

The exact anesthetic management in patients with an unrepaired VSD, in terms of induction technique, invasive monitoring, plan for extubation and postanesthesia care, depends on the degree of CHF. In general, keeping the pulmonary vascular resistance high and the systemic resistance low will help minimize left-to-right shunting. Avoid hyperventilation, excessive oxygen delivery, and causes of systemic

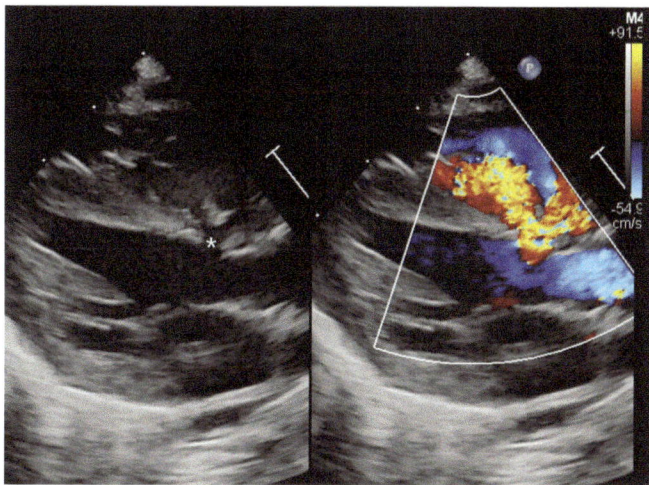

Figure 17.3: Echocardiogram image of ventricular septal defect. Parasternal long-axis view of small outlet ventricular septal defect (*) with left-to-right shunting.

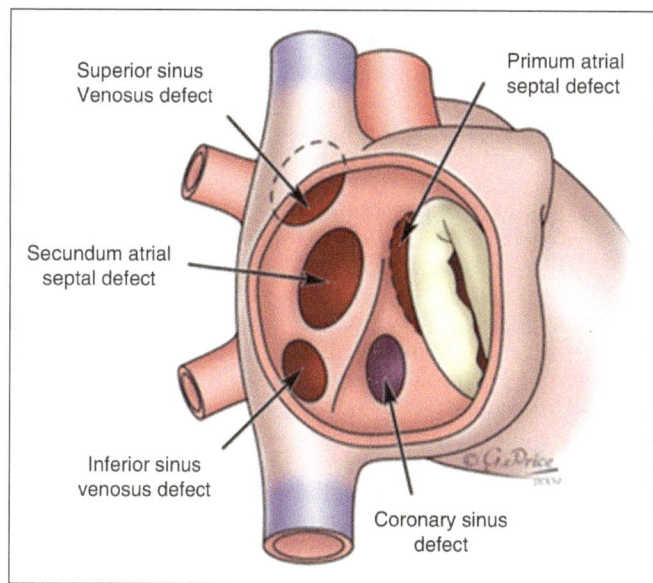

Figure 17.4: Locations of atrial septal defects along the atrial septum.
Source: Sridharan S, Price G, Tann O, et al. Transposition of the great arteries: arterial switch operation. In: *Cardiovascular MRI in Congenital Heart Disease*. Springer; 2010. doi:10.1007/978-3-540-69837-1_36.

vasoconstriction like hypothermia and intense sympathetic stimulation. IV lines need to be carefully prepared to remove any air bubbles. When using the line for fluid, blood, or drug administration, avoid introducing air. Please refer to Chapter 89, "Cardiac Surgery: On-Pump," for more information regarding the anesthetic management of children undergoing cardiac surgery with cardiopulmonary bypass.

Postsurgical Repair Assessment

A thorough preoperative evaluation should focus on identifying the presence of a residual VSD and the extent of shunting. The atrioventricular (AV) node can be damaged during repair of a perimembranous VSD resulting in third-degree heart block. An epicardial pacemaker may be present and should be interrogated prior to an elective procedure. The patient with a complication-free VSD repair does not require special considerations other than antibiotics in the first 6 months after closure to prevent infective endocarditis.

ATRIAL SEPTAL DEFECT WITH OR WITHOUT PARTIAL ANOMALOUS PULMONARY VENOUS RETURN

ASD occurs in 5% to 10% of all patients with CHD, with a female preponderance of 2:1. There are four types of ASDs (Box 17.2 and Figure 17.4). Shunting is from the left atrium (LA) to the right atrium (RA), except in an unroofed coronary sinus, which results in volume overload of the RA and RV thereby increasing pulmonary blood flow. In an unroofed coronary sinus, desaturated blood from the heart or the systemic circulation if associated with a left superior vena cava (LSVC) returns to the LA and creates a right-to-left shunt.

Pathophysiology and Clinical Manifestations

Patients with ASD are usually asymptomatic and do not develop CHF unless the defect is very large or associated with other CHDs. A patient with ASD can remain asymptomatic until the third or fourth decade of life.[6] ECHO findings for an ASD will show the shunt and the size and position of the defect on the atrial septum (Figure 17.5). Eighty percent of ASDs are 3 to 8 mm in size (measured by ECHO) and will close spontaneously by 18 months of age.[7] On physical examination, a murmur is heard at the left upper sternal border with a fixed split S2.

Closure of an ostium secundum ASD can be performed in the cardiac catheterization lab using a catheter delivered

---

BOX 17.2 TYPES OF ATRIAL SEPTAL DEFECTS

- Ostium secundum, most common
- Ostium primum, associated with atrioventricular septal defect
- Sinus venous, associated with partial anomalous pulmonary venous return
- Unroofed coronary sinus with or without left superior vena cava

---

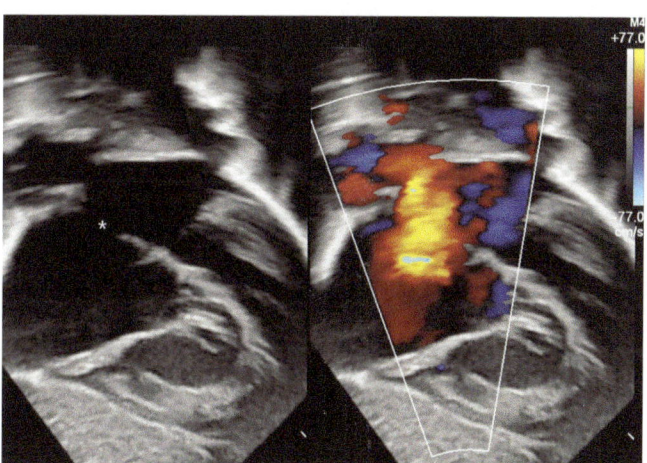

Figure 17.5: Echocardiogram image of atrial septal defect (ASD). Subcostal coronal view of a moderate sized secundum ASD (*) with left-to-right shunting.

device. This requires an adequate rim of tissue for device anchoring. The defect cannot be larger than 32 mm. Surgical closure is required for ostium primum ASD, sinus venosus defects, unroofed coronary sinus, and some large secundum ASDs. Closure of an ASD is indicated for Qp:Qs greater than 1.5:1 even in the absence of symptoms. Surgery for ASDs not amenable to device closure is usually performed at 2 to 4 years of age unless CHF is a problem.[7] Please refer to Chapter 91, "Cardiac Catheterization Laboratory," for more information regarding the anesthetic management of a child in the cardiac catheterization laboratory.

Partial anomalous pulmonary venous return (PAPVR) occurs when some but not all pulmonary veins connect to either the RA, a systemic vein (superior vena cava [SVC], inferior vena cava [IVC], and left innominate vein), or the coronary sinus. Right pulmonary veins are more commonly involved than left pulmonary veins. Scimitar syndrome is a rare form of PAPVR involving the right pulmonary veins connecting to the IVC–RA junction in association with right lung hypoplasia. The anomalous vein creates a curvilinear density on chest x-ray (CXR) adjacent to the right heart border resembling a scimitar or Turkish sword.[8]

As with simple ASDs, children are usually asymptomatic with PAPVR. While performing a transthoracic ECHO is diagnostic, it is not sufficient for surgical planning. CMR delineates the anomalous pulmonary anatomy and avoids the need for more invasive cardiac catheterization. Surgical closure is performed at 2 to 5 years of age. If CHF is a problem, the defect should be repaired sooner. As with VSDs, anesthetic management before repair focuses on minimizing left-to-right shunting by avoiding hyperventilation, excessive oxygen delivery, and causes of systemic vasoconstriction like hypothermia and intense sympathetic stimulation.

Postsurgical Repair Assessment

A thorough preoperative evaluation focuses on the type of ASD repaired. The most recent ECHO will evaluate the heart for residual shunts or stenosis (PAPVR repair can lead to SVC or pulmonary vein stenosis), the type of ASD and nature of the repair (surgical vs. transcatheter device). A patient with a surgically repaired ostium secundum ASD and no residual shunting will not require special considerations when planning an anesthetic except for antibiotics to prevent infective endocarditis in the first 6 months following repair. These patients do not require lifelong cardiology care.

A child with a transcatheter device will be prescribed aspirin for 6 months after placement. Elective noncardiac surgery should be postponed for these 6 months to avoid the risk of endocarditis. Patients with a history of sinus venosus ASD, scimitar syndrome associated ASD and coronary sinus ASD may have ongoing problems. Repair of sinus venosus ASD with PAPVR to the SVC requires interatrial baffling or transecting and reimplanting the distal SVC to the RA more laterally before patching the ASD to direct the pulmonary flow to the LA. Stenosis of the SVC, pulmonary vein stenosis, and sinus node dysfunction are possible complications.[9]

PATENT DUCTUS ARTERIOSUS

Patent ductus arteriosus (PDA) accounts for 5% to 10% of all patients with CHD, excluding premature infants. In premature infants under 1750 g at birth, it occurs in 45%, with CHF in 15%. In infants born with a birth weight under 1200 g, 80% have a PDA, with CHF diagnosed in 40% to 50%. PDA is the result of failure of the ductus arteriosus to close after birth, the connection between the pulmonary artery and the aorta (Figure 17.6). The size and length of the PDA and the level of pulmonary resistance determine the magnitude of the left-to-right shunt.

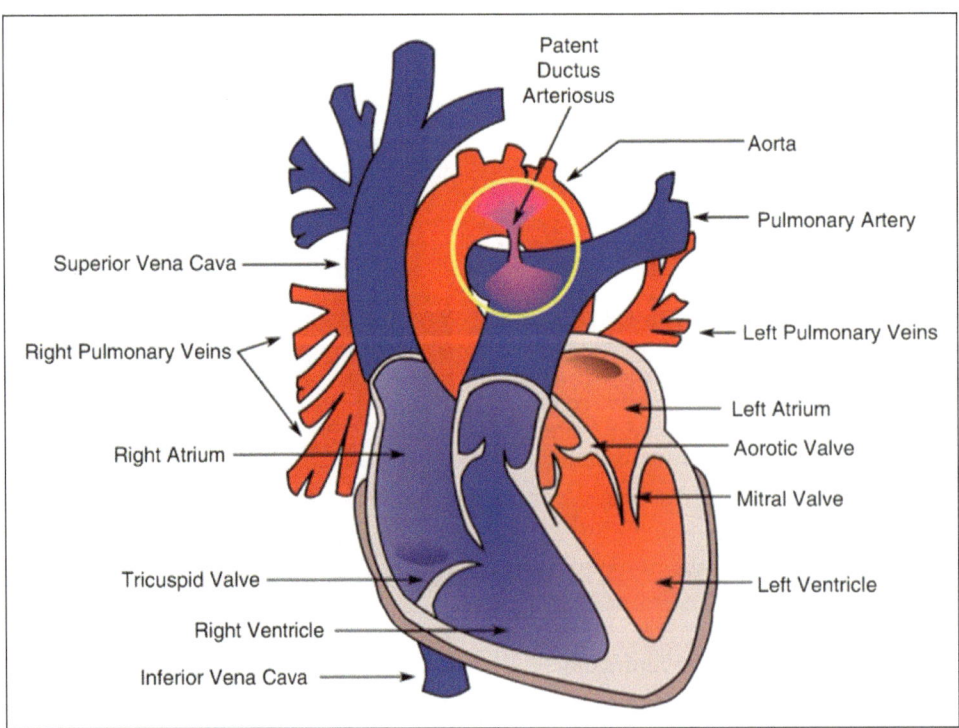

Figure 17.6: Patent ductus arteriosus.

Source: Carabuena JM. Patent Ductus Arteriosus (PDA). In: Mankowitz S. ed. *Consults in Obstetric Anesthesiology*. Springer; 2018. doi:10.1007/978-3-319-59680-8_120.

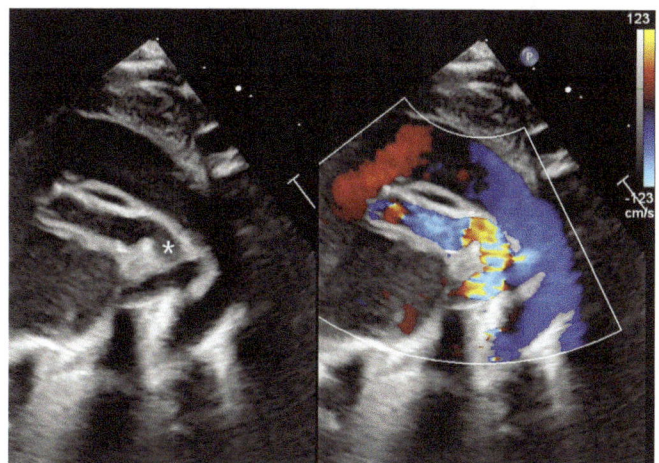

Figure 17.7: ECHO image of patent ductus arteriosus (PDA). Suprasternal long-axis of large reverse oriented ductus arteriosus (*) with systemic to pulmonary shunting.

Table 17.1	Types of Atrioventricular Septal Defects	
Partial	Single AV valve annulus	Two orifices with ostium primum ASD
Transitional	Single AV valve annulus	Two orifices with ostium primum ASD and small inlet VSD
Intermediate	Single AV valve annulus	Two orifices with ostium primum ASD and large unrestricted VSD
Complete	Single AV valve annulus	One orifice with ostium primum ASD and large unrestricted VSD

ASD, arterial septal defect; AV, atrioventricular; VSD, ventral septal defect.

Pathophysiology and Clinical Manifestations

Small PDAs are asymptomatic. A large PDA is associated with CHF. On physical examination, there is a continuous "machinery" type of murmur heard best at the upper left sternal border. In a small to moderate PDA, ECG findings are either normal or demonstrate left ventricular hypertrophy (LVH). Biventricular hypertrophy is present on ECG with a large PDA. CXR may show cardiomegaly with increased pulmonary vascular markings. ECHO is excellent for diagnosing a PDA and defining the hemodynamic significance (Figure 17.7).

Medical treatment of PDA in preterm infants has evolved with advances in ventilator strategies, use of antenatal steroids, exogenous surfactant, and medical management of pulmonary overcirculation while waiting for spontaneous closure. Fluid restriction and diuretics are first-line treatment for premature infants with symptomatic PDAs followed by pharmacologic treatment with indomethacin, ibuprofen, or acetaminophen.[10]

If medical treatment to close the PDA fails and CHF persists, the next step is surgical or transcatheter closure. Surgical closure of PDA via a left thoracotomy has been the standard in premature infants for decades. Although percutaneous catheter closure of PDA is well established in older infants and children, recent advances in transcatheter closure device miniaturization (Medtronic Microvascular Device and Abbott Amplatzer Piccolo) has resulted in infants weighing less than 2 kg successfully treated without complications.[11]

Postsurgical Repair Assessment

A thorough preoperative evaluation should include a review of the ECHO for a residual PDA. If there is no residual PDA and no comorbidities, give endocarditis prophylaxis for the first 6 months after repair; otherwise, anesthetic management is routine. Children who are born prematurely will often have ongoing medical issues (e.g., developmental delay, chronic lung disease, tracheomalacia, pulmonary hypertension). The chronic pulmonary disease will often be the most important preanesthetic consideration.

ATRIOVENTRICULAR SEPTAL DEFECTS

AVSDs account for approximately 4% of all CHDs. There is a well-recognized association of AVSD with trisomy 21, as 30% of children with AVSD also have Down syndrome.[12] There are four forms of AVSDs, all of which have deficient AV septum as the cause of the defect (Table 17.1). Previously, this group of anomalies was called "AV canal" or "endocardial cushion" defects. Despite the differences, each type of AVSD shares the following features: right and left AV valves insert at the same level in the heart (normally mitral is higher); the aortic valve is unwedged, displaced anteriorly with elongation of the left outflow track (creating a gooseneck deformity); and the left AV valve has a cleft. Partial AVSD (ostium primum ASD) and complete AVSD (ostium primum ASD and large, unrestrictive inlet VSD) are the two main forms. Two other subtypes are also described, transitional AVSD, a variant of partial AVSD, and intermediate AVSD, a variant of complete ASVD.

Pathophysiology and Clinical Manifestations

The left-to-right shunting for complete and intermediate AVSD is similar in physiology to a large VSD and ASD. Transitional and partial AVSD physiology is similar to an ASD (Figure 17.8). It should be noted that trisomy 21 children are at higher risk of developing pulmonary hypertension and may require surgery sooner to prevent pulmonary vascular disease.

Common physical examination findings are a hyperactive precordium with a holosystolic murmur. There are often signs of CHF and failure to thrive in infants with a large shunt. ECG shows a superior QRS axis (−40° to −150°), and a prolonged PR interval is common. CXR shows cardiomegaly with increased pulmonary vascular markings. ECHO allows

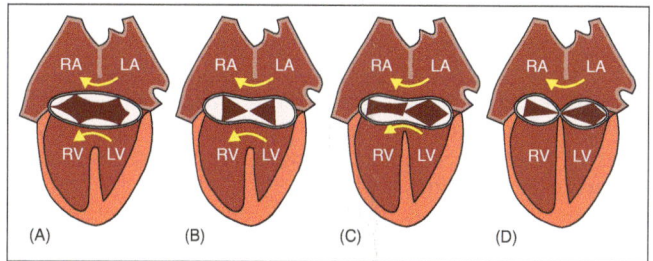

Figure 17.8: Classification of atrioventricular septal defect. (A) Complete, (B) intermediate, (C) transitional, and (D) partial. A and B share similar physiology (i.e., large ventricular septal defect (VSD) and arterial septal defect), while C and D share similar physiology (i.e., arterial septal defect and no defect or small VSD).

LA, left atrium; LV, left ventricle; RA, right atrium; RV, right ventricle.

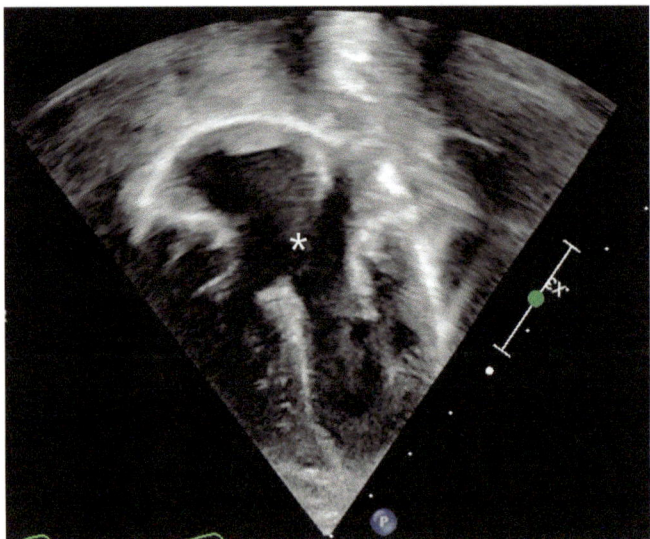

Figure 17.9: Echocardiogram (ECHO) of atrioventricular septal defect (AVSD). Apical four-chamber ECHO image showing a common AVSD with absence of the crux of the heart (*) due to a primum defect, a ventricular septal defect, and a common atrioventricular valve.

imaging of all components of AVSD and assessment of the hemodynamic severity (Figure 17.9). CHF management is often required while awaiting cardiac surgery. If a child with AVSD requires surgery prior to repair, avoid making the left-to-right shunt greater and worsening CHF. Carefully titrate anesthesia and avoid excess ventilation and inspired oxygen. Surgical closure of the ASD, VSD and reconstruction of AV valves occurs at 2 to 4 months of age, as it is difficult to perform AV valve surgery on very small infants.[13]

Postsurgical Repair Assessment

AVSD requires closure of atrial and/or ventricular shunt, and AV valve repair. After surgery, the AV valves can have residual regurgitation or stenosis. Preoperative review of ECHO and review of cardiology notes will help guide anesthetic planning. Left ventricular outflow tract obstruction is the most common indication for late reoperation following repair of partial AVSD.[14] Late reoperation for complete AVSD occurs most commonly due to left AV valve regurgitation.[14]

COARCTATION OF THE AORTA

Coarctation of the aorta (CoA) is a discrete stenosis of the thoracic descending aorta at or in close proximity to the insertion of the ductus arteriosus (Figure 17.10). Four out of every 10,000 babies are born with CoA, accounting for 7% to 10% of all congenital heart defects.[15] CoA and other congenital left heart obstructive lesions occur more often in males. When CoA occurs in females, it may be associated with Turner syndrome.[16] CoA is also associated with other intracardiac and extracardiac anomalies (Box 17.3).

Pathophysiology and Clinical Manifestations

The severity of the CoA, the extent of arterial collaterals to the distal aorta, and the presence of other defects, in particular arch hypoplasia and VSD, influence the timing and severity of clinical presentation. If the ductus arteriosus is crucial for distal perfusion (severe coarctation with few arterial collaterals), a prostaglandin E1 (PGE1) infusion will be started after birth to maintain ductus patency and to prevent

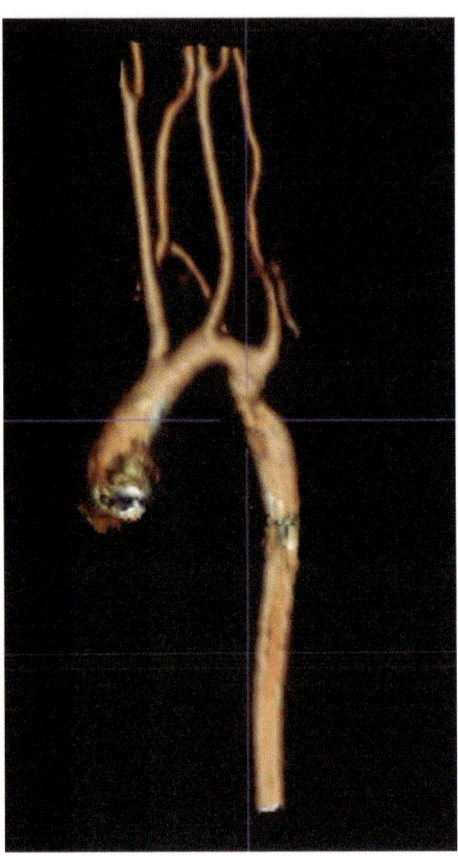

Figure 17.10: MRI of unrepaired coarctation of the aorta. Three-dimensional reconstruction of a discrete coarctation by cardiac magnetic resonance imaging (CMR).

LV dysfunction and end organ injury until surgical repair. Even with the use of prenatal ultrasound, newborn pulse oximetry screening, and four-extremity blood pressure monitoring, some neonates with severe coarctation remain undiagnosed and present in extremis after the ductus arteriosus closes at a few days or weeks of age. These infants develop symptoms of CHF (poor feeding, tachypnea, and lethargy) which are nonspecific and often missed, progressing to cardiogenic shock with profound acidosis and renal and hepatic dysfunction. Treatment is with PGE1, inotropes, mechanical ventilation, and diuretics. After stabilization, surgical repair is by left thoracotomy for an isolated CoA or median sternotomy to correct CoA with associated arch hypoplasia. A neonate with CoA and duct-dependent lower body perfusion may require anesthesia for noncardiac surgery, reliable IV access for delivering the PGE1 infusion separately from the IV used to bolus medications or fluids during the procedure is paramount.

If the patient tolerated ductal closure without problems in infancy, an evaluation of an asymptomatic systolic heart murmur, best heard over the child's back, or systemic hypertension in a young child can lead to the diagnosis of CoA (Figure 17.11). A delay in the femoral pulse compared to the right radial pulse is an important sign of CoA on physical examination. Older children and adolescents with an undiagnosed CoA may develop symptoms of fatigue, chest pain, dyspnea, headaches, epistaxis, pain, or weakness of the legs, prompting a cardiology consultation. Although these children and adolescents tolerated ductus arteriosus closure after birth, the area of narrowing becomes more significant as the rest of

BOX 17.3 ANOMALIES ASSOCIATED WITH CoA

Cardiac
- Bicuspid aortic valve (75%–80%)
- Ventricular septal defect (particularly if conal septum displaced posteriorly)
- Diffuse hypoplasia of the transverse aortic arch and/or isthmus
- Dextro-transposition of the great arteries
- Double outlet right ventricle (Taussig–Bing)
- Mitral stenosis
- Shone's complex (multiple left sided obstructive lesions)
- Atrioventricular canal defect
- Hypoplastic left heart syndrome
- Extracardiac vascular
- Saccular aneurysms in the circle of Willis ("berry" aneurysm)
- Aberrant right subclavian artery arising below the CoA with subclavian steal syndrome (reversed flow in vertebral artery)
- Stenotic origin of the left subclavian artery
- Arterial collaterals from internal mammaries, epigastric, thyrocervicals, intercostals
- Musculoskeletal
- Scoliosis

Syndrome
- Turner syndrome (15%–20% have CoA)
- Posterior fossa abnormalities, hemangioma of the face and neck, arterial cerebrovascular anomalies, cardiac defects, eye anomalies syndrome (PHACE)
- Jacobsen syndrome
- Kabuki syndrome

CoA, coarctation of the aorta.

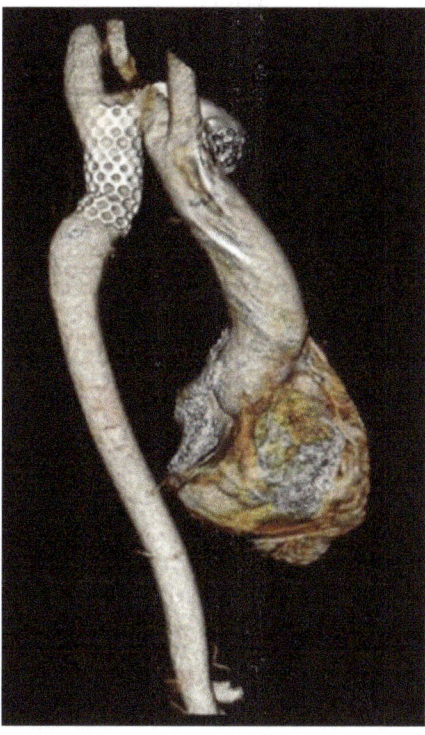

Figure 17.12: Computed tomographic image of a tortuous aortic arch with a stent in the proximal descending aorta.

the aorta grows with the child. The gradient between upper and lower extremity blood pressure depends on the degree of arterial collateralization and does not necessarily predict the severity of the CoA. Repairing CoA is still usually surgical in these age groups, although balloon angioplasty and stenting are an alternative (Figure 17.12).

Postsurgical Repair Assessment

Long-term survival after CoA repair is excellent, but patients do require lifelong cardiology follow-up. Chronic hypertension is the most common long-term complication, reported in 30% to 50% of patients, and potentially related to the increased stiffness of the repaired aorta irrespective of a residual stenosis.[17] Recoarctation occurs in 20% of patients repaired in the neonatal period, 10% to 15% repaired as infants and 5% of childhood repairs.[18]

Before elective procedures, review a recent ECG, ECHO, any advanced imaging studies, medication list, and cardiology office note with attention to the blood pressure measurement in the arms and legs along with the measured gradient across the repair on the imaging studies. The primary cardiologist should address significant stenosis, defined as a gradient of 20 mm Hg or greater at rest. Balloon dilatation is the procedure of choice for treatment of recoarctation. In addition to looking for residual cardiac pathophysiology, assess for airway abnormalities. Damage to the recurrent laryngeal nerve is a possibility after CoA repair, and patients may have symptoms of hoarseness, noisy breathing, choking/coughing while swallowing, or a history of a vocal cord injection in addition to syndrome-related airway abnormalities.

VASCULAR RINGS AND SLINGS

Vascular rings are abnormalities of the aortic arch that can lead to compression of the trachea and/or esophagus.[19]

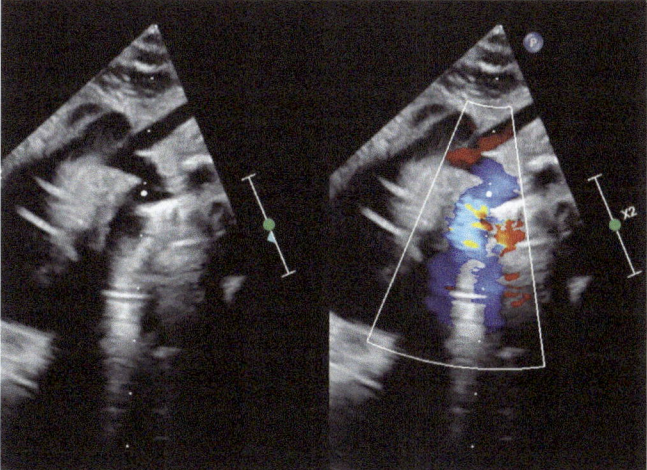

Figure 17.11: Echocardiogram of unrepaired coarctation of the aorta (CoA). Suprasternal long-axis ECHO side-by-side image showing a juxtaductal coarctation with associated flow acceleration..

> **BOX 17.4 TYPES OF VASCULAR RINGS**
>
> - Complete ring
> - Double aortic arch, most common form
> - Right aortic arch with mirror image branching and aberrant left subclavian artery arising from diverticulum of Kommerell
> - Incomplete ring
> - Left aortic arch and aberrant right subclavian artery
> - Left aortic arch with aberrant innominate artery origin leftward compressing trachea

Vascular rings form in the second month of fetal life when the two dorsal aortas do not undergo the normal pattern of regression and migration (Box 17.4). They make up less than 1% of CHD and are associated with wheezing, cyanosis, and swallowing difficulties. The tracheal compression may also cause tracheomalacia. Double aortic arch is the most common vascular ring. The two arches completely encircle the trachea and esophagus. The other abnormality associated with a complete vascular ring is a right aortic arch (RAA) and mirror image branching with aberrant left subclavian artery. The RAA gives off left carotid, then the right carotid artery, then the right subclavian artery, and, finally, the aberrant left subclavian. The aberrant left subclavian often arises from a retroesophageal diverticulum, called the diverticulum of Kommerell. The left ligamentum arteriosum (remnant of PDA) completes the ring.

Pathophysiology and Clinical Manifestations

Although anatomically not a complete vascular ring, patients with a left aortic arch and aberrant right subclavian can have swallowing and breathing difficulties. Another variation of an incomplete vascular ring is an innominate artery that is leftward in origin and compresses the trachea anteriorly. Not all patients with incomplete rings are symptomatic. Aortic arch anomalies are associated with genetic disorders such as 22q-microdeletion, CHARGE, and Down syndrome.

A pulmonary vascular sling is another cause of tracheal and esophageal compression. The anomalous left pulmonary artery (LPA) arises from the right pulmonary artery (RPA) coursing over the proximal right mainstem bronchus, then behind the trachea and in front of the esophagus, causing both respiratory (coughing, wheezing, stridor, and apnea) and feeding problems (difficulty swallowing). LPA sling is often associated with significant tracheal stenosis including complete tracheal rings, and maldevelopment of the bronchial tree.[20]

Surgical repair depends on the severity of symptoms. Vascular ring surgery is via a thoracotomy with ligation and division of the appropriate part of the ring. A leftward innominate artery and LPA sling surgery involve median sternotomy. For the LPA sling, the use of cardiopulmonary bypass facilitates dissection and reimplantation of the LPA on to the main pulmonary artery. In the patients with LPA sling and tracheal stenosis, surgical repair will also involve tracheal reconstruction and LPA division and reimplantation to the main PA.

Postsurgical Repair Assessment

Outcomes after vascular ring division[21] and LPA sling repair[22] are excellent, even with tracheomalacia. Airway management is the primary concern, not cardiac. Infants who had severe respiratory symptom and airway obstruction may have persistent airway symptoms for weeks or months after surgery. Evaluation of the trachea and bronchi will be important to review. Tracheomalacia will cause intrathoracic airway collapse during exhalation. Positive pressure ventilation with positive end-expiratory pressure will help stent open the airway. A smaller sized endotracheal tube may need to be considered and available. If the patient has any preoperative respiratory symptoms, consider observation in the ICU.

CYANOTIC CONGENITAL HEART DEFECTS

Cyanotic congenital heart defects are a group of diverse cardiac malformations with reduced oxygen saturation (SpO_2, Box 17.5). Fifteen percent of all congenital heart defects fit into this category.[23] Anesthesia providers should be aware that a low SpO_2 does not necessarily mean reduced pulmonary blood flow, as high Qp:Qs is a salient feature of many of these cyanotic defects.

The widespread use of prenatal ultrasonography and mandatory newborn pulse oximetry screening for critical congenital heart defects (CCHD) has led to earlier recognition and a reduction in infant morbidity and mortality in children born with CCHD.[24] The anesthetic management of patients with CCHD is lesion specific. Each defect has associated pathophysiologic and hemodynamic consequences before and after repair that need to be considered before developing a comprehensive anesthetic plan. The three most common cyanotic congenital heart defects are tetralogy of Fallot (TOF) (4.7/10,000 births), Transposition of the great arteries (TGA) (2.3/10,000 births), and truncus arteriosus (TA) (1/10,000 live births).[15] Please refer to Chapter 89, "Cardiac Surgery: On-Pump," for more information regarding the anesthetic management of children undergoing cardiac surgery with cardiopulmonary bypass.

> **BOX 17.5 CYANOTIC CONGENITAL HEART DEFECTS**
>
> | |
> |---|
> | Tetralogy of Fallot |
> | Transposition of the great arteries |
> | Truncus arteriosus |
> | Total anomalous pulmonary venous return |
> | Tricuspid valve defects |
> | Tricuspid atresia |
> | Ebstein's anomaly |
> | Pulmonary atresia |
> | Critical pulmonary stenosis |
> | Single-ventricle anomalies |
> | Hypoplastic left heart syndrome |
> | Pulmonary atresia/intact ventricular septum |
> | Unbalanced atrioventricular canal |
> | Double outlet right ventricle |
> | Heterotaxy defects |
> | Double-inlet left ventricle |

> **BOX 17.6   GENETIC DISORDERS ASSOCIATED WITH TETRALOGY OF FALLOT**
>
> - 22q11.2 deletion syndrome
>   (DiGeorge, CATCH22, velo cardio facial, Shprintzen, conotruncal anomaly face syndrome)
> - Down syndrome
> - Alagille syndrome
> - Holt–Oram syndrome
> - Trisomy 13
> - Trisomy 18

TETRALOGY OF FALLOT

There are several anatomical variants of TOF. The most frequently diagnosed is TOF with pulmonary stenosis (TOF/PS). TOF/PS is associated with many syndromes; 22q11.2 deletion syndrome is the most common and diagnosed in 20% of patients (Box 17.6).[25]

Pathophysiology and Clinical Manifestations

TOF/PS is the result of anterior and cephalad displacement of the infundibular (outlet) portion of the intraventricular septum during cardiac formation. This leads to right ventricular outflow tract (RVOT) narrowing, a large VSD with the aorta overriding the intraventricular septum, and right ventricular hypertrophy that further restricts flow through the RVOT (Figure 17.13). In addition to the narrowing of the outflow tract, many patients have a small pulmonary annulus with a dysplastic bileaflet pulmonary valve, and diffuse hypoplasia of the main and branch pulmonary arteries.

The clinical manifestations of TOF/PS vary with the degree of right ventricular outflow obstruction, reduction in Qp and subsequent right-to-left shunting through the VSD. Some patients with TOF/PS have mild RVOT obstruction and are not cyanotic, commonly referred to as "pink tets." These patients are asymptomatic at birth and diagnosed by either prenatal ultrasound or the presence of a systolic ejection murmur early in life. Some pink tets may have such minimal RVOT obstruction that CHF develops at 4 to 6 weeks of age from left-to-right shunting across the VSD as pulmonary vascular resistance falls.

Infants with moderate obstruction may have a reduced arterial saturation of 85% to 90% yet remain asymptomatic and followed up as an outpatient for a few months before surgical repair. Severe obstruction with significant desaturation in the neonatal period requires immediate intervention. Life-threatening hypercyanotic episodes ("tet spells") can occur in any patient with TOF/PS prior to cardiac surgical repair. These episodes of intense oxygen desaturation and poor cardiac output are the result of dynamic narrowing of the infundibular outflow tract triggered by events, such as pain, crying, fever, feeding, stooling, awakening, and dehydration. The turbulent flow across the obstructed RVOT produces the normal systolic ejection murmur in patients with TOF/PS, and it may become very soft or even disappear during a hypercyanotic spell. The flow across the VSD does not contribute to the heart murmur.

Repair of asymptomatic patients with TOF is at 3 to 4 months of age. Some centers perform elective repair shortly after birth. The development of hypercyanotic spells usually prompts urgent surgical intervention. Patients with unrepaired TOF/PS may present for noncardiac surgery and are best cared for by anesthesia providers with experience recognizing and treating hypercyanotic spells in a setting where swift implantation of ECMO is possible. Hypercyanotic spells can lead to cardiac arrest and death if not treated rapidly and

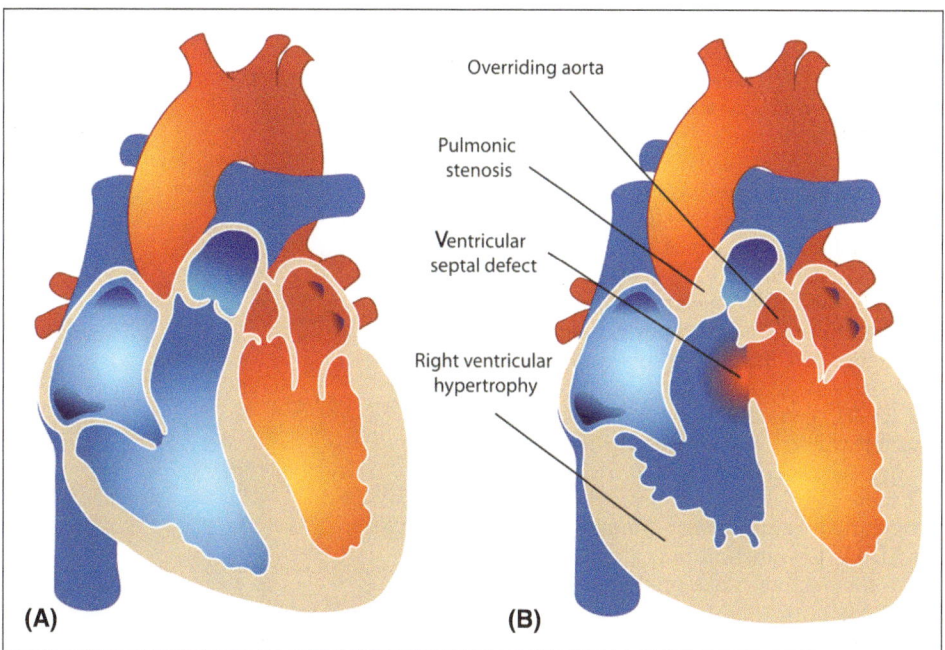

Figure 17.13: Tetralogy of Fallot. (A) Normal heart. (B) Heart with tetrology of Fallot defects.

Source: Flamm KL, Granger M, Gawlik K, et al. Evidence-based assessment of the heart and circulatory system. In: Gawlik KS, Melnyk BM, Teall AM, eds. *Evidence-Based Physical Examination: Best Practices for Health and Well-Being Assessment*. Springer; 2021:Fig. 6.5.

aggressively. Please refer to Chapter 18 in this text for more information regarding the anesthetic management of children with CHD undergoing noncardiac surgery.

The surgical repair of TOF/PS is palliative and not curative as patients with TOF/PS require lifelong cardiology care. The goal of surgery is to close the VSD and relief the RVOT obstruction by resecting obstructive muscle bundles and enlarging the outflow tract with a pericardial patch. For many years, the patch was placed across the pulmonary annulus (transannular patch) and the pulmonary valve was sacrificed, leaving the patient with severe pulmonary insufficiency. Currently, the focus is to save the pulmonary valve and accept a mild degree of right ventricular tract obstruction instead of free regurgitation. Five percent to 10% of patients with TOF/PS have an anomalous left anterior descending coronary artery. This vessel crosses the RVOT, preventing safe RVOT incision and patch placement. An alternative surgical strategy is to place an RV–to–pulmonary artery conduit. Twenty-five percent of patients with TOF/PS have an RAA and may have an aberrant left subclavian as well, leading to the need for vascular ring surgery in addition to the TOF repair if stridor or feeding difficulties occur.

Postsurgical Repair Assessment

Current survival rate to adulthood following complete repair of TOF exceeds 93%.[26] Since TOF is the most common form of cyanotic CHD and the long-term survival is excellent, it is common for patients with repaired TOF to present for noncardiac procedures. A thorough preoperative evaluation with focus on the extent of cardiac dysfunction, syndrome- related comorbidities particularly airway issues, review of previous anesthetic records, and need for subacute endocarditis (SBE) prophylaxis is key to planning a safe anesthetic. Most children remain asymptomatic for many years despite moderate to severe pulmonary insufficiency and/or residual RVOT obstruction and are seen by their cardiologist for a yearly visit, ECG, and ECHO, and, when able to cooperate, exercise testing. The development of new symptoms, such as decreased exercise tolerance, palpitations, or a syncopal episode warrants cardiology reevaluation before proceeding with an elective procedure. Review of an up-to-date ECG is important. Almost all patients with repaired TOF/PS will have a surgically induced right bundle branch block. However, a QRS duration greater than 180 seconds has been associated with ventricular tachycardia and sudden death. This may be an indication for additional cardiac interventions to reduce right ventricular size/dysfunction before elective surgery.

The ECHO is important for evaluation of right heart dilatation, hypertrophy and dysfunction (**Figure 17.14**). ECHO will reveal any residual VSD and RVOT obstruction. If a right ventricular to pulmonary artery (RV-PA) conduit is present, ECHO measures the degree of conduit stenosis and regurgitation. When RV pressure is greater than two thirds the systemic, the residual RVOT obstruction or conduit stenosis warrants a cardiac catheterization and procedure to relieve obstruction (balloon or stent). In addition to right heart pathology, the ECHO may reveal left-sided heart disease. A progressively enlarging aorta is common and dilatation of the aortic root can cause AI. LV dysfunction may develop over time from volume overload (residual VSD) or altered ventricular–ventricular interactions.

CMR is now standard for assessing right ventricular size, function, and the pulmonary regurgitant fraction after TOF repair. Serial CMR imaging begins around 8 to 10 years of age unless echocardiography reveals rapidly increasing ventricular dilatation. The goal is to intervene and place a pulmonary valve before right heart dilatation from chronic pulmonary insufficiency leads to irreversible right heart dysfunction but not too soon. Bioprosthetic valves have limited longevity (10–15 years) and increase the risk of endocarditis more than 10-fold.[27] While criteria differ from center to center, RV end-diastolic volume greater than 150 mL/m^2, right ventricular ejection fraction (EF) less than 47%, pulmonary regurgitation fraction greater than 25%, and RV systolic volume greater than 80 mL/m^2 are commonly used indicators[28] (**Figure 17.15**).

In the last 10 years, the development of a transcatheter bioprosthetic pulmonary valve (Medtronic Melody valve) has reduced the need for redo sternotomies and surgical pulmonary valve replacement in stenotic/regurgitant RV-PA

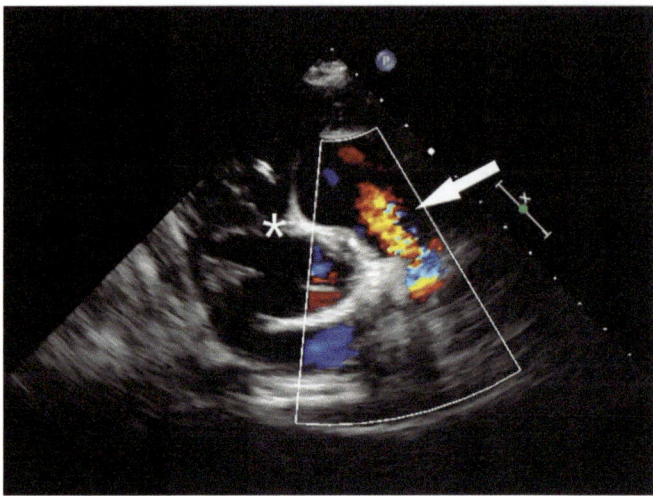

Figure 17.14: Echocardiogram (ECHO) of repaired tetrology of Fallot. Parasternal long-axis ECHO image swept to the right in a patient with tetralogy of Fallot after repair. There is diastolic flattening of the interventricular septum (*) with significant pulmonary insufficiency (arrow).

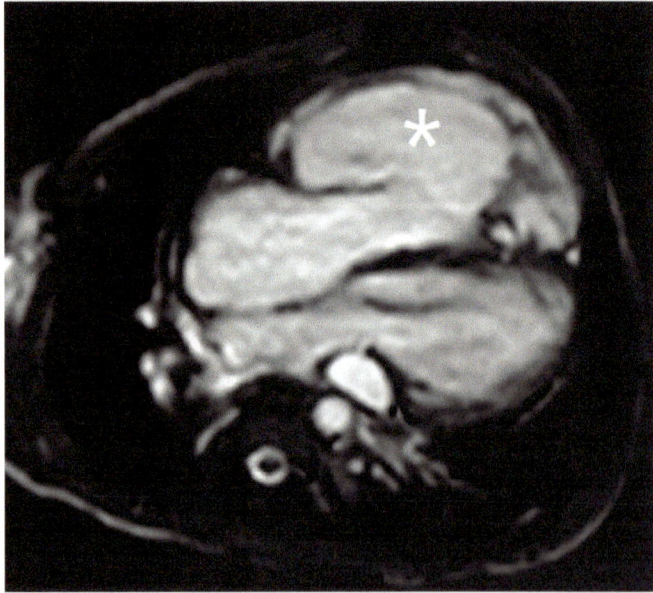

Figure 17.15: Cardiovascular MRI of right ventricle dilatation after tetralogy of Fallot (TOF) repair. Four-chamber cine image showing a severely dilated right ventricle (*) after repair for TOF.

conduits. The transannular patched native RVOT is often too large for this valve. Recent advancements in bioprosthetic valves (Edwards Sapien, Medtronic Harmony) are proving to be successful in nonconduit outflow tracts.[29] Patients with prosthetic heart valves are at risk of SBE and antibiotic prophylaxis before high-risk procedures are recommended.

TRANSPOSITION OF THE GREAT ARTERIES

Dextro-transposition of the great arteries (d-TGA) is the second-most common cyanotic congenital heart defect. Without surgical repair, it has a 90% mortality within the first year of life. The arterial switch operation (ASO), first performed in 1975, is the standard surgical approach. It replaces the original technique of redirecting blood flow by atrial baffling (Mustard or Senning procedure), which led to ventricular failure and serious arrhythmias in the second decade of life. The ASO in the first 2 weeks of life has a long-term survival rate of 96% to 99%.[30]

In d-TGA, the aorta arises from the RV and the pulmonary artery from the LV. The RA connects to the RV, LA to LV, and in their normal position. In 80% of patients with d-TGA, the aorta is to the right and anterior to the pulmonary artery, and 40% have a VSD as an additional source of mixing. Left ventricular outflow tract (LVOT) obstruction occurs in 5% to 10% of cases and correction requires a much more extensive operation than the standard ASO (Figure 17.16).

Pathophysiology and Clinical Manifestations

Survival after birth is not possible without mixing of the two parallel circulations. In the setting of the most common form of d-TGA (an intact ventricular septum and no other defects), the foramen ovale and ductus arteriosus play key roles in maintaining adequate systemic oxygenation. The severity of cyanosis varies with the adequacy of mixing at the atrial septum and the flow through the ductus arteriosus. A PGE1 infusion started immediately after birth preserves the patency of the ductus arteriosus. If there is inadequate mixing at the atrial level and severe hypoxemia persists, the interventional cardiologist performs a balloon atrial septostomy.

d-TGA is rarely associated with genetic syndromes or extracardiac malformations. The only association is with heterotaxy. It is unusual for a neonate with d-TGA to require anesthesia for a procedure other than a balloon septostomy in the catheterization lab prior to repair. Anesthesia providers trained in providing pediatric cardiac anesthesia should be involved if the situation arises.

The goals of surgery are (a) to restore ventriculoarterial concordance and (b) and close the PDA, PFO (typically large following balloon atrial septostomy), and VSD (if one is present). During the arterial switch, the surgeon divides the aorta and pulmonary artery just below the level of the pulmonary bifurcation. The surgeon then harvests the coronary arteries from the native aortic root, taking a variable amount of sinus tissue as a "button." Mobilization and reimplantation of the coronary arteries into the native pulmonary root, creating a neoaortic root, are next, taking great care not to cause distortion by stretching or kinking these small vessels. The surgeon then attaches the aorta to the neoaortic root. The last step is to reconstruct the neopulmonary root with patch material to close the defects left behind from the harvest of the coronary buttons and attach the distal pulmonary artery to the draping the pulmonary bifurcation over the ascending aorta (LeCompte maneuver, Figure 17.17).

Postsurgical Repair Assessment

Long-term outcomes after the ASO are excellent. Issues that can develop include supravalvular pulmonary stenosis (Figure 17.18) at the level of the branch pulmonary arteries (most common complication), neoaortic insufficiency related to the morphologic pulmonary valve serving as the systemic left-sided valve, and early-onset coronary artery disease.[31,32] Lifelong cardiology follow-up is required for early detection of these complications with ECG, ECHO, stress testing, Holter monitoring, CMR and coronary imaging.[33]

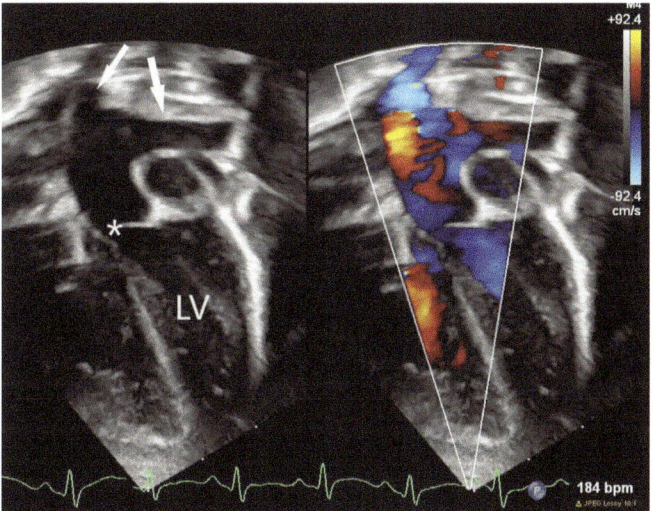

Figure 17.16: Echocardiogram (ECHO) of unrepaired transposition of the great arteries (TGA). Apical four-chamber ECHO showing TGA. The LV gives rise to the pulmonary valve (*) with visible distal branching into the right and left branch pulmonary arteries (arrows). LV, left ventricle.

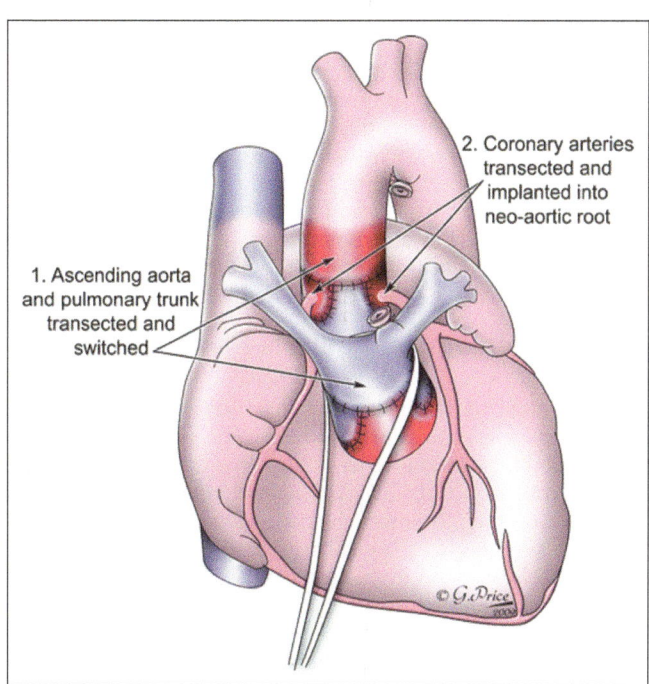

Figure 17.17: Arterial switch operation.

Source: Sridharan S, Price G, Tann O, et al. Transposition of the great arteries: arterial switch operation. In: *Cardiovascular MRI in Congenital Heart Disease*. Springer; 2010. doi:10.1007/978-3-540-69837-1_36.

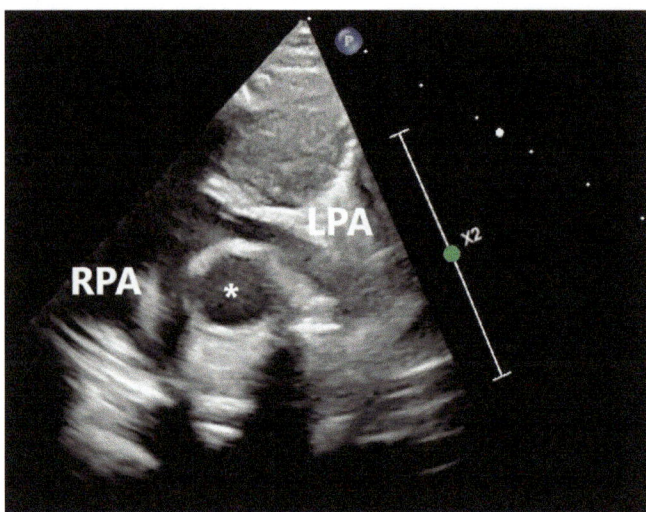

Figure 17.18: Echocardiogram of pulmonary artery stenosis after repair of transposition of the great arteries. Parasternal short-axis echocardiogram showing the orientation of the branch pulmonary arteries after arterial switch operation with a LeCompte maneuver. The branch pulmonary arteries course around the aorta (*).

LPA, left pulmonary artery; RPA, right pulmonary artery.

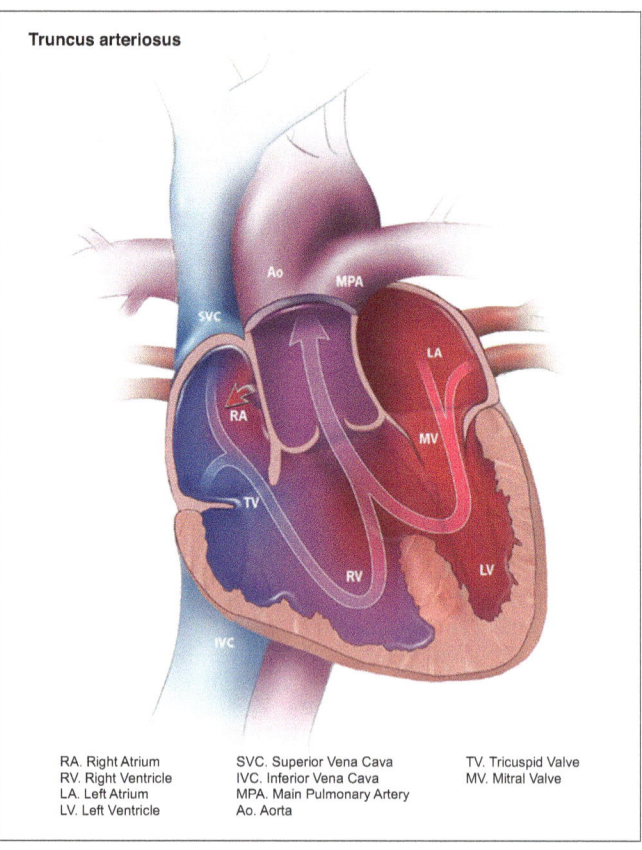

Figure 17.19: Unrepaired truncus arteriosus.

Source: Centers for Disease Control and Prevention; https://www.cdc.gov/ncbddd/heartdefects/truncusarteriosus.html.

The preanesthetic evaluation should focus on exercise tolerance, previous surgical and transcatheter interventions, and recent cardiac testing. Chest pain may not occur as a symptom of myocardial ischemia due to denervation of the great vessels, and its absence does not rule out coronary artery disease. A review of the most recent cardiac studies is crucial to assessing anesthesia risk factors and developing an anesthesia management plan keeping in mind the potential for unrecognized coronary artery disease.

TRUNCUS ARTERIOSUS

TA is a heart defect with a single vessel arising from the heart supplying pulmonary, systemic, and coronary blood flow. The trunk usually originates over both ventricles with a VSD present below the truncal valve (**Figure 17.19**). The truncal valve may consist of one to five leaflets that are often dysplastic, and the valve stenotic and/or regurgitant.[34] While there are several variations and classification schemes, the pulmonary artery takes off from the truncus above the coronaries but below the brachiocephalic artery.

Pathophysiology and Clinical Manifestations

Twenty to thirty percent of patients born with TA have a 22q11.2 microdeletion.[35] After birth, patients present with symptoms of pulmonary overcirculation and CHF. The pulmonary to systemic blood flow ratio is at least 3:1 with systemic desaturation noted on pulse oximetry. Myocardial ischemia can occur due to the low diastolic pressures and poor coronary filling from the pulmonary "run-off." Physical examination is significant for a harsh systolic ejection murmur along the left sternal murmur, audible click after the first heart sound, and a single S2.

Repair for truncus arteriosus occurs in the first week of life. The operation consists of closing the VSD, a truncal valvuloplasty if the valve is significantly stenotic or regurgitant, removing the pulmonary artery from the trunk, and connecting it to the RV with a valved RV-PA conduit. Anesthetic management can be challenging and ventricular fibrillation from coronary ischemia may occur. Few patients will present for noncardiac surgery prior to repair, and due to the complexity of the management, they are best cared for by anesthesia providers trained in providing pediatric cardiac anesthesia.

Postsurgical Repair Assessment

The RV-to-PA conduit has limited longevity, and conduit stenosis is the most common complication after repair of TA.[36] In addition, conduit regurgitation or truncal valve regurgitation may develop and require surgical intervention (**Figure 17.20**). As in the other cyanotic congenital heart defects discussed, lifelong cardiology care is required. The preanesthetic assessment should focus on obtaining an up-to-date cardiology evaluation with ECHO, ECG, and CMR. A peak conduit gradient on ECHO of 50 mm Hg or greater is an indication for surgical or transcatheter intervention. If the RV pressure is more than half-systemic, a gentle anesthetic induction is required, avoiding systemic hypotension, decreased coronary perfusion, and myocardial ischemia.

SINGLE-VENTRICLE CONGENITAL HEART DISEASE

Single-ventricle defects make up less than 1% of all patients with CHD. The most common single-ventricle defects include hypoplastic left heart syndrome (HLHS), unbalanced atrioventricular defect (AVSD), double-inlet left ventricle, and tricuspid atresia (**Figure 17.21**). These defects while diverse require a surgical approach that ultimately ends up leaving the pulmonary circulation without a dedicated pumping chamber of the heart.

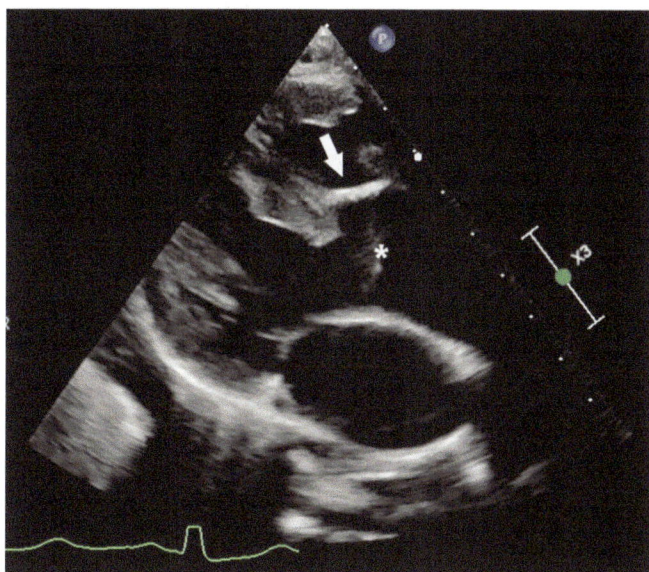

Figure 17.20: Echocardiogram (ECHO) of repaired truncus arteriosus. Parasternal long-axis ECHO of a repaired truncus. The arrow is pointing at the ventricular septal defect patch. A dilated and thickened neoaortic (formerly truncal valve) valve (*) is visible.

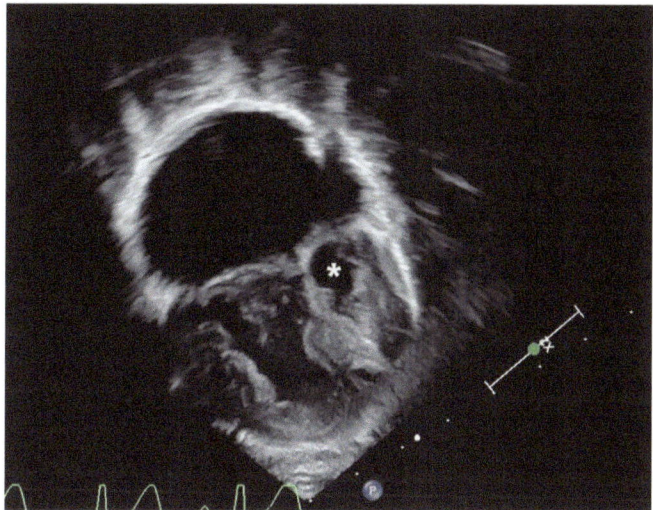

Figure 17.21: Echocardiogram (ECHO) of hypoplastic left heart syndrome (HLHS). Apical four-chamber ECHO showing HLHS with a severely hypoplastic and muscle-bound left ventricle (*).

Pathophysiology and Clinical Manifestations

In single-ventricle CHD, one of the ventricles is hypoplastic or atretic, or the ventricular septum is absent, forming a functional single ventricle (Table 17.2). There is mixing of pulmonary and systemic venous return at the atrial and/or ventricular level. Prior to palliative cardiac surgery, the PDA will need to be maintained open with PGE1 to allow for adequate pulmonary or systemic aortic blood flow, depending on the defect. The atrial septum must also allow unobstructed mixing.[37] Prior to initial palliation, the pulmonary circulation and systemic circulation need to be balanced by manipulation of pulmonary vascular resistance.

The surgical palliation of a single ventricle involves three stages. The first stage is performed during the neonatal period and involves making sure, there is unobstructed aortic blood flow and limited but adequate PA blood flow. The second stage at 3 to 6 months of age usually involves creation of a superior vena cava to PA anastomosis (bidirectional Glenn shunt) and ligation of Blalock–Taussig shunt (BT shunt) if one was placed during the first operation. The third stage at age 18 months to 3 years of age involves directing the entire systemic venous return to the pulmonary artery without an intervening ventricular pumping chamber.[38]

Postsurgical Repair Assessment

Long-term transplant free survival of patients with single-ventricle CHD has improved to 90% for single LV and 80% for single RV patients.[39] These patients require ongoing intensive medical therapy, laboratory testing, and surveillance. Interventional procedures to treat BT shunt stenosis or aortic arch obstruction and occlusion of veno–veno collaterals are common.[37]

Single-ventricle palliated patients from Stage I to Stage III repair have significant residual hemodynamic abnormalities with or without medications.[40] These are high-risk patients, particularly after Stage I repair for HLHS, and require careful coordination and planning prior to their anesthetic care. Noncardiac procedures need to be performed by a team familiar with single-ventricle physiology and in a setting with resources to manage these patients in an ICU.

CARDIOMYOPATHY

Cardiomyopathies (primary diseases of the myocardium) include hypertrophic cardiomyopathy (HCM), dilated cardiomyopathy (DCM), restrictive cardiomyopathy (RCM), arrhythmogenic right ventricular cardiomyopathy (ARVC), and left ventricular noncompaction cardiomyopathy (LVNC; Table 17.3).

HYPERTROPHIC CARDIOMYOPATHY

Pathophysiology and Clinical Manifestations

HCM is a genetic disorder usually inherited as an autosomal dominant trait and is the most common cause of sudden cardiac death in teens and young adults, especially athletes.[41] By early adulthood, most patients who inherit a disease-causing mutation will show structural evidence of HCM, such as LVH.

Table 17.2	Common Single-Ventricle Defects and Anatomical Findings
Hypoplastic left heart syndrome	Aortic and mitral valve atresia or stenosis
	Aortic atresia or hypoplasia
Unbalanced AVSD	Ostium primum ASD
	Inlet VSD
	Single unbalanced AV valve orifice
	One ventricle hypoplastic, non-functional
Double-inlet left ventricle	LV anatomic single ventricle
	Great arteries malposition (most common)
	PA valve stenosis (most common)
Tricuspid atresia	Absent tricuspid valve
	With/without VSD
	RV hypoplasia
	With/without pulmonary stenosis

ASD, arterial septal defect; AVSD, atrioventricular septal defect; LV, left ventricle; PA, pulmonary artery; RV, right ventricle; VSD, ventricular septal defect.

Table 17.3	Types of Cardiomyopathy
Hypertrophic cardiomyopathy	Common cause of sudden death in teens/young adults, especially athletes
	Avoid dehydration preoperatively
	Treat hypotension with IV fluids and IV phenylephrine
	Cardiac ischemia risk due to thick myocardium
	Automated implantable defibrillator implant malfunction due to electrocautery needs to be addressed
Dilated cardiomyopathy (DCM)	Most common form of cardiomyopathy in children
	Progression of congestive heart failure common
	Cardiac transplant free survival at 5 years is 50%
Restrictive cardiomyopathy	Least common cardiomyopathy in children
	Poor prognosis
Arrhythmogenic right ventricular cardiomyopathy	Leading cause of cardiac arrest in young people and athletes
Left ventricular noncompaction cardiomyopathy	Usually asymptomatic
	May require antiplatelet therapy or anticoagulation to prevent thromboembolism

The clinical course of disease and the risk of sudden death is not usually predictable based on the disease-causing mutation. One exception, lysosome-associated membrane protein-2 (LAMP2) cardiomyopathy, is associated with a lethal natural history and survival uncommon beyond 25 years of age despite an implantable defibrillator. These patients need consideration for early heart transplantation. There are published guidelines regarding the workup and treatment of HCM (Box 17.7).

LVH occurs in many anatomic segments (Figure 17.22). The wall thickening in HCM is usually asymmetric so that one or more segments of the heart are thicker than other areas.[42] While the HCM heart has enhanced systolic function, the hypertrophied muscle causes diastolic dysfunction and impaired filling. LVOT obstruction can occur from asymmetric septal hypertrophy of muscle and/or by dynamic means. Inotropic agents, such as epinephrine, underfilling of the LV from dehydration or blood loss, or low systemic vascular resistance can cause worsening LVOT obstruction. The thickened myocardium is also at risk of subendocardial ischemia and ventricular arrhythmias.

Anesthetic Considerations

Physical examination findings for patients with HCM are variable and related to the degree of hypertrophy and hemodynamic status. Patients with LV obstruction have a systolic ejection murmur. The ECG may show increased voltage, suggestive of LVH, and ST-T wave changes. No particular ECG pattern is predictive of future events.[43] ECHO and CMR confirm the diagnosis of HCM. In adults, an LV thickness of >15mm or in children a Z score of >2 (relative to body surface area (BSA) is compatible with the diagnosis of HCM.

A thorough preoperative evaluation should focus on history of prior cardiac arrest, ongoing symptoms, and ECHO evaluation of function and degree of LVOT obstruction. Scheduling the patient with HCM first case of the day is a consideration to avoid dehydration. Peripheral vasodilation may cause worsening LVOT obstruction. Immediately treat hypotension with fluid administration and IV phenylephrine. Drugs that increase cardiac inotropy will worsen LVOT obstruction and hypotension. Careful induction of anesthesia, avoiding sympathetic stimulation and increased cardiac inotropy while avoiding hypotension is the goal. Invasive arterial pressure monitoring should be considered preoperatively or soon after induction of anesthesia and securing the airway. Spinal and epidural anesthesia are relatively contraindicated due to the blockade of sympathetic nervous system and possible hypotension. Cardiac ischemia is also a risk due to thick heart muscle and lower endocardial perfusion. Postoperative observation in the ICU may be necessary.

In patients with an automated implantable defibrillator (AICD) or pacemaker, preoperative evaluation of cardiac implantable electronic device (CIED) includes date of last interrogation, device type, indication for device placement,

---

BOX 17.7 AHA/ACC 2020 GUIDELINES FOR DIAGNOSIS AND TREATMENT OF HYPERTROPHIC CARDIOMYOPATHY

- Comprehensive physical examination with three-generation family history
- ECG and 24–48-hour ambulatory ECG
- Surveillance ECG every 1–2 years
- Transthoracic ECHO, if LVOT gradient < 50, provocative testing (simultaneous ECHO with Valsalva strain, amyl nitrate inhalation, or exercise)
- Surveillance ECHO every 1–2 years
- Cardiac MRI if TTE inconclusive
- Genetic testing should be offered
- First-degree relatives, clinical screening should include ECG and ECHO with periodic follow-up according to age.
- For patients with HCM with cardiac arrest or sustained VT, single-chamber transvenous or SQ implantable cardioverter is a Class I indication.
- For symptomatic patients with HCM with LVOT obstruction, nonvasodilating beta-blockers are recommended; if not tolerated or ineffective, verapamil or diltiazem is recommended.
- Mild to moderate recreational noncompetitive exercise for the purpose of leisure is beneficial.
- For symptoms refractory to all medical treatment, septal reduction therapy may be offered at a high-volume center.

ACC, American College of Cardiology; AHA, American Heart Association; ECHO, echocardiogram; HCM, hypertrophic cardiomyopathy; LVOT, left ventricular outflow tract; SQ, subcutaneous; TTE, transthoracic echocardiogram; VT, ventricular tachycardia.

Source: Ommen, et al. 2020 AHA/ACC guideline for the diagnosis and treatment of patients with hypertrophic cardiomyopathy: a report of the American College of Cardiology/American Heart Association Joint Committee on Clinical Practice Guidelines. *J Am Coll Cardiol.* 2020;76(25), e159-e240. doi:10.1016/j.jacc.2020.08.045

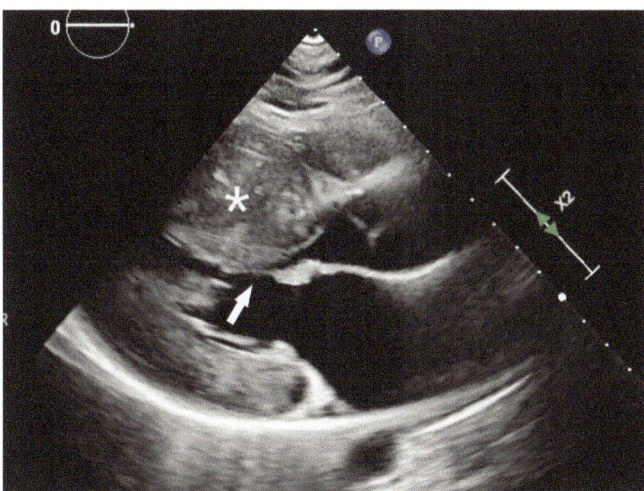

Figure 17.22: Echocardiogram (ECHO) of hypertrophic cardiomyopathy. Parasternal long-axis ECHO showing a severely thickened interventricular septum (*) with evidence of systolic anterior motion of the mitral valve (arrow) contributing to outflow tract obstruction.

battery longevity, current programming, pacemaker dependence, and magnet response.[44] Patients with pacemakers need yearly evaluations, and patients with an AICD need device interrogation every 6 months. Electromagnetic interference (EMI) in the operating room from monopolar electrocautery needs to be prevented. An EMI source within 6 inches of the device pulse generator can inhibit pacing or cause inappropriate tachyarrhythmia therapy by sensing the EMI interference as cardiac electrical activity. If it is not possible to separate the generator from the EMI source, this will necessitate discussion with the patient's cardiologist and surgical team to consider reprogramming and suspending antitachyarrhythmic device therapy.[45] To minimize EMI from the cautery, place the grounding pad so the current pathway does not pass through or near the device pulse generator or implanted cardiac leads. Underbody grounding pads do not prevent device EMI interference (Box 17.8). A magnet should not be routinely be used on the pulse generator. The CIED response to the magnet will vary depending on the type of device, age of battery, and device programming. Magnet application to an AICD will turn off the tachyarrhythmia functions but not turn off the pacemaker function.

DILATED CARDIOMYOPATHY

Pathophysiology and Clinical Manifestations

DCM is the most common form of cardiomyopathy in children.[46] About half of the time, the cause is unknown. Other causes are myocarditis, neuromuscular disease (muscular dystrophies, e.g., Duchenne, Becker, Emery–Dreifuss, Limb Girdle, and myotonic dystrophy), toxic exposure to anti-neoplastic agents (doxorubicin with chest irradiation), and ischemia, volume or pressure overload due to CHD. Starting at 6 to 7 years of age, patients with muscular dystrophies are screened for DCM. Early treatment prolongs the interval to florid heart failure.[47]

Physical examination findings will vary, depending on how the heart has compensated. Symptomatic heart failure may manifest as gallop heart rhythm, mitral regurgitant murmur, tachypnea with rales, and tachycardia. Infants and children

> **BOX 17.8 PACEMAKER/AICD DEVICE AND EMI CONSIDERATIONS**
>
> - Pacemaker patients require yearly evaluations.
> - AICD patients require interrogation every 6 months.
> - EMI source needs to be kept 6 inches away from device.
> - Bipolar electrocautery is not a problem because electrical current is small and between the tips of the forceps.
> - Place grounding pad so current pathway is not through or near device.
> - Underbody grounding pads do not prevent device interference from EMI.
> - Have temporary pacing equipment and external defibrillation equipment readily available.
> - Use short (less than 10 seconds), intermittent, and irregular bursts of monopolar electrocautery at the lowest possible energy level if bipolar electrocautery is not possible.
> - If any programming changes were made, the cardiac implantable electronic device should be reprogrammed back to the original settings immediately after the procedure.
>
> AICD, automated implantable defibrillator; EMI, electromagnetic interference.
>
> *Source:* Thompson et al. Perioperative management of cardiovascular implantable electronic devices (CIEDs). *Curr Anesthesiol Reports.* 2013;3(3):139–143. doi:10.1007/s40140-013-0026-5.

rarely have peripheral edema. The liver maybe enlarged. ECG may show sinus tachycardia and T-wave inversion in multiple leads with LVH. CXR will show cardiomegaly with pulmonary vascular congestion. ECHO is the imaging modality most used to make the diagnosis (Figure 17.23). Criteria for diagnosis include LV end-diastolic dimension >2 *SD*s above normal for BSA, combined with depressed systolic function, such as shortening fraction (SF) or EF of <2 *SD*s below normal for age.[48] Pericardial effusion or intracardiac thrombus may also be seen.

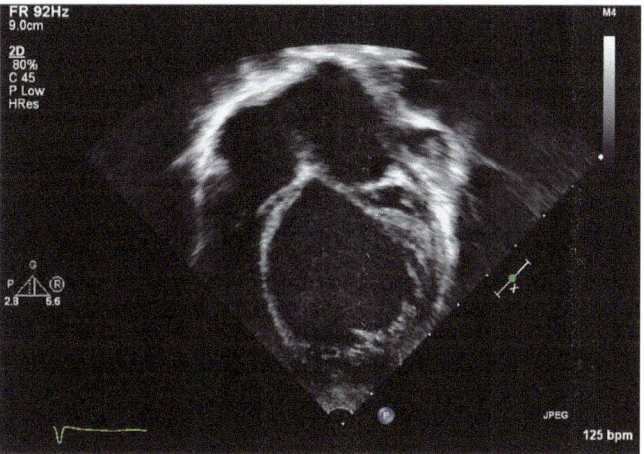

Figure 17.23: Echocardiogram (ECHO) of dilated cardiomyopathy. Apical four-chamber ECHO showing a severely dilated left ventricle.

The progression of CHF is the rule. Patients with Pediatric cardiomyopathy have a greater mortality, length of hospital stay, and hospital charges when hospitalized for heart failure compared to adults.[49] CHF is treated with digoxin, diuretics (furosemide and spironolactone), angiotensin-converting enzyme inhibitors (captopril and enalapril), and activity restriction. Patients may take daily aspirin to prevent thrombosis formation in the heart. Amiodarone is commonly administered to treat arrhythmias.[50] Cardiac transplantation is an option for children who fail medical therapy. In the Pediatric Cardiomyopathy Registry, the transplant free survival at 5 years was 50%.[46]

Anesthetic Considerations

A thorough preoperative evaluation should focus on current medical therapy, ECHO results, and patient symptoms. The goal of anesthetic management is to avoid myocardial depression and sudden increase in afterload, especially on induction and emergence. When hypotension occurs, treat with positive inotropic drugs such as calcium gluconate or epinephrine if there is severe hypotension.

An infusion of low-dose dopamine (3–5 mcg/kg/min) may minimize cardiac depression and low cardiac output during the procedure. Invasive pressure monitoring (arterial and central venous pressure) is helpful for early recognition of hemodynamic changes. These patients may need admission to the cardiac ICU postoperatively for close observation during recovery.

RESTRICTIVE CARDIOMYOPATHY

Pathophysiology and Clinical Manifestations

RCM is the least common cardiomyopathy in children. It maybe idiopathic, or associated with systemic disease such as scleroderma, amyloidosis, and sarcoidosis. Metabolic disorders with specific enzyme deficiencies, Hurler syndrome, Gaucher disease, Fabry disease and glycogen storage diseases can also result in RCM. Stiff ventricular walls cause abnormal diastolic function and filling.[51]

Clinical manifestations include a history of exercise intolerance, weakness, and dyspnea. Physical examination findings commonly include gallop rhythm, loud P2, hepatomegaly, ascites, and edema. ECG is abnormal 98% of time with RA and/or LA enlargement and ST-T wave abnormalities. CXR shows cardiomegaly and pulmonary venous congestion. ECHO is diagnostic, showing markedly dilated atria and normal size and function of the LV (Figure 17.24). Cardiac catheterization is important to distinguish between RCM and constrictive pericarditis. Overall, RCM has a poor prognosis.[52] Medical treatment alleviates symptoms but does not improve survival.

Anesthetic Considerations

A thorough preoperative evaluation with focus on ongoing medical treatment and ECHO results is important. Anesthetic management is particularly challenging in children with RCM. General anesthesia causes myocardial suppression, vasodilation and reduced venous return, which will not be well tolerated in a patient with RCM. As in other cardiomyopathies, assess the need for arterial and central venous monitoring as well as the need for observation in the ICU after the procedure.

ARRHYTHMOGENIC RIGHT VENTRICULAR CARDIOMYOPATHY

Pathophysiology and Clinical Manifestations

The most common clinical presentation of ARVC is palpitations or syncope associated with sports. It is a leading cause of cardiac arrest in young people and athletes.[53] Sudden death maybe the first clinical manifestation.

ECG screening can detect 80% of children with ARVC. ECG often shows increased P waves in lead II, T-wave inversion in V1 to V4. Ventricular arrhythmias range from frequent premature ventricular beats to ventricular tachycardia triggered or worsened by sympathetic stimulation. ECHO shows RV enlargement, extreme thinning of RV free wall with RV akinesia, dyskinesia, or aneurysm.[53] CMR is diagnostic because it combines evaluation of structural and functional ventricular abnormalities. Treatment consists of restriction from intense sports and beta-blockers. Catheter ablation of ventricular arrhythmias is not curative due to the high frequency of developing new sites of arrythmogenicity, although an implanted AICD is effective.

Anesthetic Considerations

A thorough preoperative evaluation needs to focus on ECG and ECHO results. The main goal of anesthetic management is to prevent or reduce the risk of arrhythmias. Patients need to continue their antiarrhythmic medications until just before the procedure. In a patient with an AICD, external defibrillation pads need to be attached prior to or just after induction of general anesthesia, because the AICD may need to be programmed off to avoid EMI interference (see HCM section for more details). Postprocedure observation in the ICU should be considered.

LEFT VENTRICULAR NONCOMPACTION

Pathophysiology and Clinical Manifestations

Most patients with LVNC are asymptomatic. The patient's ECG will show LVH and intraventricular conduction delay, especially left bundle branch block (LBBB).[54] ECHO shows an excessive meshwork of muscle bands and deep valleys called trabeculation in the LV. LV dysfunction may occur due to mechanical dyssynchrony between the noncompacted and compacted parts of the myocardium.[55]

Symptoms determine the medical management. Patients with CHF will require diuretics and afterload reduction. Due to deep recesses in LVNC, antiplatelet therapy with aspirin is recommended. If atrial fibrillation occurs or thrombosis detected, warfarin is recommended.[56]

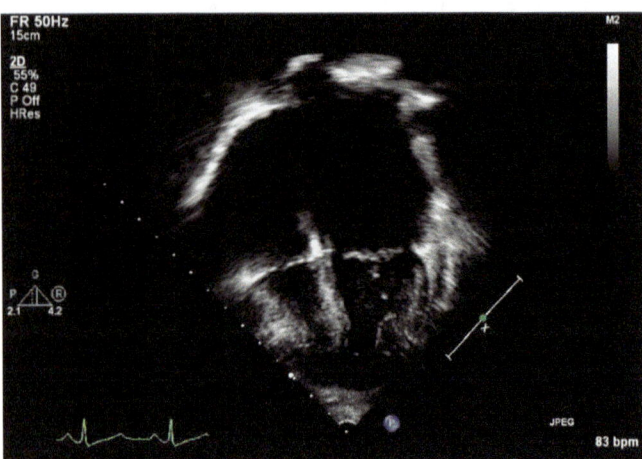

Figure 17.24: Echocardiogram (ECHO) of restrictive cardiomyopathy. Apical four-chamber ECHO of severe bilateral atrial dilatation in the setting of restrictive cardiomyopathy.

Anesthetic Considerations

A thorough preoperative evaluation should focus on the ECG and ECHO results. Managing antiplatelet and/or anticoagulation therapy will need to be discussed preoperatively with the pediatric cardiologist and surgeon. If the patient has normal cardiac function, it is safe to proceed with a routine anesthetic. In LVNC patients with LV dysfunction, an IV induction of anesthesia is preferred. As in the other cardiomyopathies reviewed, assess the need for arterial and central venous monitoring, as well as the need for observation in the ICU after the procedure.

ACQUIRED CARDIAC DISORDERS FROM INFECTIOUS DISEASES

MYOCARDITIS

Myocarditis is usually caused by infectious agents but may also be associated with autoimmune disease, hypersensitivity reactions and toxins.[57] In the United States and developed countries, viral myocarditis is most common. The viral infections associated with myocarditis range from Coxsackie B, the most recognized cardiotoxic virus, to adenovirus, parvovirus, and in 2020, severe acute respiratory syndrome coronavirus (SARS-CoV-2).[58,59] In Central and South America, parasitic infection with *Trypanosoma cruzi* (Chagas disease) is the most frequent cause of myocarditis. In parts of the world without widespread immunization, diphtheria causes myocarditis.[60] Although the immune response is important to eliminate the pathogen, if the response is excessive, it can lead to immune-related chronic tissue damage as in the case of Kawasaki disease, rheumatic fever, and SARS-CoV-2-related multisystem inflammatory disease syndrome (MIS-C).[59]

Pathophysiology and Clinical Manifestations

Myocarditis is often proceeded by a history of a non-specific infection days to weeks prior to the development of cardiovascular symptoms. Symptomatic children will show signs of CHF or develop arrhythmias. The most common presentation is shortness of breath.[61] Physical examination may reveal tachypnea, tachycardia, hepatosplenomegaly, and abnormal lung findings. The ECG is virtually always abnormal. ECG abnormalities vary widely from low-voltage QRS complexes to ST-T wave changes.[57] CXR demonstrates cardiomegaly. ECHO may show enlarged chambers and decreased function. CMR is useful to evaluate the myocardium for edema, hyperemia, and scarring, the hallmarks of myocarditis. It is the primary tool for noninvasive assessment of myocardial inflammation in patients with suspected myocarditis.[62] Acute treatment of myocarditis includes high-dose IV immunoglobulin (IVIG) and corticosteroids, along with supportive care.

Patients should be restricted from sustained aerobic activity.[57] Pharmacologic management of heart failure and LV dysfunction have a role in the supportive care. The American Heart Association guidelines suggest angiotensin-converting-enzyme inhibition for the acute phase if there are ECHO findings of reduced LV function, adding beta-blockade with selective aldosterone antagonists if symptomatic heart failure, and the use of inotropic agents with mechanical ventilation and ECMO for a patient in cardiogenic shock.

Anesthetic Considerations

A thorough preoperative anesthetic evaluation should focus on how long patient has had myocarditis, cause of myocarditis, and treatments. ECHO, CMR, and the cardiology assessment of the patient will help guide your anesthetic plan. If the patient is within the first 6 months of the myocarditis diagnosis or has ongoing medical treatment for myocarditis, directly communicate with the pediatric cardiologist and surgical team before proceeding.

MULTISYSTEM INFLAMMATORY DISEASE SYNDROME

MIS-C is associated with SARS-CoV-2 that emerged in December 2019. Initial reports indicated that children typically had mild or no SARS-CoV-2 symptoms. However, in early May, the United Kingdom and several European countries reported the occurrence of a hyperinflammatory process in children that had features similar to Kawasaki disease (KD). In New York State, the emergence of MIS-C coincided with widespread SARS-CoV-2 transmission.

Pathophysiology and Clinical Manifestations

This hyperinflammatory syndrome presents with gastrointestinal symptoms (80%), dermatologic (62%), lower respiratory manifestations (40%), and myocarditis (53%), diagnosed by ECHO and either elevated troponin levels or proBNP levels. Thirty-two percent had hypotension at admission; 62% received vasopressor support, and 80% were admitted to an ICU.[59] Patients with MIS-C are commonly treated with IVIG, glucocorticoids, and vasopressors.

Anesthetic Considerations

A thorough preoperative anesthetic evaluation should focus on the patient's SARS-CoV-2 disease course, severity of symptoms, and treatment. The timing of elective surgery after recovery from SARS-CoV-2 utilizes both symptom- and severity-based categories (Table 17.4).

KAWASAKI DISEASE

KD is often preceded by upper respiratory or gastrointestinal symptoms.[63] The onset of KD is associated with a high fever, rash, bilateral conjunctivitis, and "strawberry tongue," diffuse erythema of hands and feet, and cervical adenitis. It is now one of the leading causes of acquired cardiovascular disease in young children, although the etiology of the disease is still unknown. Most cases occur in children younger than 5 years old. Coronary artery aneurysms are the most concerning complication.

Table 17.4	Timing of Elective Surgery After Recovery From SARS-CoV-2 Infection
4 weeks	Asymptomatic patient or only mild, non-respiratory symptoms without hospitalization
6 weeks	Symptomatic patient (e.g., cough and dyspnea) who did not require hospitalization
8–10 weeks	Symptomatic patient requiring hospitalization or with comorbidities (diabetic and immunocompromised)
12 weeks	Symptomatic patient admitted to intensive care unit due to SARS-CoV-2 infection

Source: From https://www.apsf.org/news-updates/asa-and-apsf-joint-statement-on-elective-surgery-and-anesthesia-for-patients-after-covid-19-infection/.

Pathophysiology and Clinical Manifestations

The physical examination findings for acute disease as noted are high fever, rash, and diffuse erythema of hands and feet. The ECG, during the acute illness, may show an arrhythmia, including sinus node and AV node functional abnormalities, prolonged PR interval, nonspecific ST and T-wave changes, and low voltage if there is myocardial or pericardial involvement.[64] ECHO is the primary imaging modality for cardiac assessment because it is noninvasive and has a high sensitivity and specificity for the detection of abnormalities of the proximal coronary artery segments (Figure 17.25). If positive for KD, the cardiologist will repeat the ECHO within 1 to 2 weeks and again 4 to 6 weeks after treatment.[64]

Acute treatment of KD is high-dose IVIG along with acetylsalicylic acid. This initial treatment is to reduce inflammation and arterial damage, and to prevent thrombosis in those with coronary artery abnormalities. Long-term follow-up is risk stratified. Patients with no coronary involvement or dilation that has returned to normal do not need additional cardiology assessment. Patients with any size aneurysm require cardiology assessment every 6 months to 1 year.

Anesthetic Considerations

A thorough preoperative anesthesia assessment should focus on the extent of the coronary dilation and/or aneurysms. If the patient is within the first 6 months of the diagnosis of KD or has ongoing medical treatment for coronary aneurysm/dilation, directly communicate with the pediatric cardiologist and surgical team before proceeding. The benefit of aspirin continuation for the prevention of coronary thrombosis needs to be weighed against the risk of bleeding with the proposed procedure.

ACUTE RHEUMATIC FEVER

Acute rheumatic fever (RF) is the delayed sequela of group A hemolytic streptococcal infection of the pharynx. In developing countries, RF is the most common cause of acquired cardiac disease in children and young adults. The cardiac disease after acute RF is called rheumatic heart disease. Over the past 50 years, most developed countries have seen a significant decline in the incidence of RF.[65] There are major and minor criteria used to diagnose RF. Rheumatic carditis occurs in 30% to 70% of cases. Mild carditis disappears rapidly in weeks, while severe carditis may last for months. Treatment of acute rheumatic carditis should include an antibiotic to eradicate pharyngeal streptococci, bed rest, and anti-inflammatory treatment.

PATHOPHYSIOLOGY AND CLINICAL MANIFESTATIONS

The physical manifestations may include arthritis involving large joints (knees, ankles, elbows, wrists) and chorea. Cardiac examination may be positive for tachycardia, murmur, and a friction rub (pericarditis). The ECG may show first-degree block. A chest x-ray may demonstrate cardiomegaly. ECHO is able to diagnose the severity of valvular heart disease.

Anesthetic Considerations

A thorough preoperative anesthesia assessment should focus on the ECHO results for valve regurgitation/stenosis and heart chamber size and function. If the patient has atrial fibrillation, the patient may be taking an anticoagulant that needs to be held. In the setting of acute RF, if the patient has arthritis alone, activity is restricted for 4 to 6 weeks. Elective surgery and anesthesia need to be scheduled after this period of observation. If there are signs and/or symptoms of carditis, discuss the proper timing of elective surgery with the cardiologist and surgical team.

PULMONARY HYPERTENSION

Patients with pulmonary hypertension (PH) have 20-fold or greater increased risk of anesthesia-related cardiac arrest and death.[66-68] The 6th World Symposium on Pulmonary Hypertension (WSPH) in 2018 redefined PH as a resting mean pulmonary artery pressure (mPAP) of ≥20 mm Hg (2 SDs above the mean) after 3 months of age.[69] The previous definition of PH used for many years was mPAP ≥25 mm Hg.

Pathophysiology and Clinical Manifestations

Like in adults, PH in children is associated with a diversity of diseases. The World Health Organization (WHO) classifies the diverse etiologies of PH into five groups.[70] Group 1 includes all causes of pulmonary arterial hypertension (PAH). The unifying mechanism in group 1 is endothelial dysfunction resulting in vasoconstriction and remodeling of the pulmonary arterioles leading to obstruction, thrombosis, and eventual obliteration. Group 1 includes conditions such as idiopathic PAH, hereditary PAH, PAH associated with connective tissue disorders (lupus and scleroderma), HIV, end-stage liver disease, drug/toxin-induced (e.g., diazoxide for treatment of hyperinsulinemia in newborns), and simple congenital heart defects with left-to-right shunts. Eisenmenger syndrome is in this category as is persistent PH of the newborn (PPHN).

Group 2 includes pulmonary hypertension due to left heart inflow or outflow obstruction. This category includes pulmonary vein stenosis, mitral stenosis, aortic stenosis, and cardiomyopathy with an elevated left ventricular end-diastolic pressure. These disorders have in common pulmonary postcapillary bed obstruction.

Group 3 consists of pulmonary hypertension due to lung disease, developmental lung disorders and hypoxia. Bronchopulmonary dysplasia (BPD) and congenital

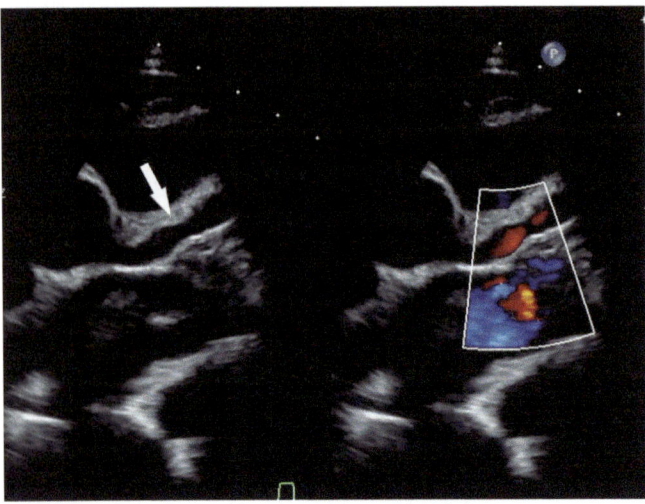

Figure 17.25: Echocardiogram (ECHO) of coronary aneurysm in KD. Parasternal short-axis ECHO demonstrating fusiform coronary aneurysms (arrow) resulting in a beaded appearance that can be often seen in KD. KD, Kawasaki disease.

diaphragmatic hernia are the most frequent diagnoses in group 3. Rare disorders such as surfactant protein deficiencies, alveolar capillary dysplasia, and pulmonary alveolar proteinosis also fall in this category.

In group 4, pulmonary artery obstruction is the key mechanism and includes chronic thromboemboli, tumor emboli, and congenital pulmonary artery stenoses. Group 5 covers conditions with unclear and multifactorial causes of PH such as chronic hemolytic anemia, sickle cell disease, metabolic disorders (e.g., Gaucher disease, glycogen storage disease, neurofibromatosis, and sarcoidosis), and complex CHD (e.g., single-ventricle physiology). In patients with single-ventricle physiology and nonpulsatile flow to the pulmonary arteries (Glenn, Fontan stages) the pulmonary artery pressure may not be elevated, but pulmonary vascular disease is present and leads to increased morbidity and mortality (plastic bronchitis, protein-losing enteropathy, failing Fontan circulation). Groups 1 and 3 are most common in children (Table 17.5).

Clinical manifestations of PH are nonspecific. In infants and young children, symptoms include poor growth, easy fatigability, tachypnea, tachycardia, diaphoresis, and irritability. Older children and adolescents report shortness of breath, tiredness, dizziness, or chest pain. Syncope or seizures are signs of advanced disease.

ECHO evidence of PH includes an increased tricuspid regurgitant jet, right atrial enlargement, right ventricular dilatation and hypertrophy, flattening or leftward bulging of the interventricular septum and decreased right ventricular EF. Parameters used to evaluate and monitor PH include Doppler estimation of the pulmonary artery and RV pressure using the tricuspid regurgitant jet, tricuspid annular systolic plan excursion (TAPSE), RV:LV systolic ratio at end systole and tissue Doppler imaging. With severe PH, bidirectional or right-to-left flow occurs in existing shunts (e.g., patent foramen ovale (PFO), PDA). Suprasytemic PH is a predictor of major complications.[71] CXR may reveal cardiomegaly and darkened lung fields from reduced Qp. Chest computed tomography angiography (CTA) is another useful tool to assess the pulmonary vascular tree. Measurement of brain natriuretic peptide (BNP) or its terminal end, N-terminal pro-brain natriuretic peptide (NT-proBNP), is one way to assess disease severity and follow response to therapy. The ventricles secrete BNP in response to increased wall stress.

Anesthetic Considerations

While PH is a relatively uncommon diagnosis, the improved survival of extremely premature infants has dramatically increased the number of children presenting with Group 3 PH for surgery and diagnostic procedures requiring anesthesia. With ECHO screening, approximately 25% of premature infants with BPD meet the criteria for the diagnosis of PH.[72] Pulmonary vein stenosis is emerging as an important ECHO finding in these infants, and while the etiology is unclear, it is a significant contributory factor for PH. In terms of heart disease and PH, with advances in the treatment of children with congenital heart defects, Eisenmenger syndrome in childhood and adolescence is rare.

Anesthesia providers should have experience in the anesthetic management of patients with PH, and the patient should be cared for in a setting that can initiate ECMO rapidly. Acute severe changes in PVR can lead to a pulmonary hypertensive crisis during anesthesia. PA pressure can exceed systemic pressure resulting in acute right heart failure, cardiac arrest and death. Early signs of a pulmonary hypertensive crisis in anesthetized patients include bradycardia, decrease in End-tidal carbon dioxide ($ETCO_2$), oxygen desaturation, hypotension, and arrhythmias. Bradycardia is often an early signal and the result of decreased coronary perfusion of the sinus node. As PAH increases and RV EF decreases, the interdependence of the two ventricles leads to LV dysfunction.

Anesthesia providers should be prepared with nitric oxide and inotropic support (e.g., isoproterenol, epinephrine, and dopamine) readily available. Consider placement of an arterial line for continuous blood pressure monitoring. Avoid interruption of medications for PH and avoid dehydration (early case of the day, admit for overnight hydration). If a decision is made to give a premedication to prevent anxiety mediated increases in PVR, careful monitoring is required. Induction and emergence are periods with potential for hypoxia, hypercarbia, changes in SVR and rapid increases in PVR. Hypothermia and an inadequate plane of anesthesia also can trigger a spike in PVR. The treatment of a pulmonary hypertensive crisis includes mild hyperventilation with 100% oxygen and initiation of nitric

Table 17.5	WHO Classification of Pulmonary Hypertension (Modified in 2018 by WSPH in Nice)
Group 1: Pulmonary artery hypertension	Idiopathic PAH, familial PAH, drug and toxin-induced PAH, PAH associated with connective tissue disease, portal hypertension, HIV, CHD simple with left-to-right shunts, Eisenmenger, schistosomiasis, pulmonary capillary hemangiomatosis, PPHN
Group 2: Congenital left heart inflow or outflow obstruction	Pulmonary vein stenosis, mitral stenosis, aortic stenosis, cor triatriatum, obstructed total anomalous pulmonary venous return, coarctation of the aorta, elevated left ventricular end diastolic pressure from left heart disease
Group 3: Lung disease	Lung disease-restrictive/obstructive/mixed, developmental lung disorders (BPD, congenital diaphragmatic hernia, Down syndrome, alveolar capillary dysplasia with misalignment of veins, surfactant protein abnormalities), hypoxia without lung disease
Group 4: Pulmonary artery obstruction	Chronic thromboembolic PH, malignant tumors (sarcoma, renal cell, uterine carcinoma, testicular germ cell tumors), congenital pulmonary artery stenoses, parasites
Group 5: Unclear or multifactorial mechanisms	Chronic hemolytic anemia, myeloproliferative disorders, histiocytosis, Gaucher disease, glycogen storage disease, neurofibromatosis, sarcoidosis, chronic renal failure, complex CHD–single ventricle, scimitar, pulmonary atresia with VSD and multiple aortopulmonary collaterals, pulmonary artery of ductal origin, absent pulmonary artery

BPD, bronchopulmonary dysplasia; CHD, coronary heart disease; PAH, pulmonary arterial hypertension; PPHN, persistent pulmonary hypertension of the newborn; VSD, ventricular septal defect; WHO, World Health Organization; WSPH, World Symposium on Pulmonary Hypertension

Source: Rosenzweig EB, Abman SH, Adatia I, et al. Paediatric pulmonary arterial hypertension: updates on definition, classification, diagnostics and management. *Eur Respir J.* 2019;53(1):1801916. doi:10.1183/13993003.01916-2018.

oxide, with vasopressors often needed as well. Overnight observation in an intensive care setting should be arranged in patients with significant pulmonary hypertension.[67]

COMMON CONDUCTION SYSTEM DISTURBANCES

SUPRAVENTRICULAR TACHYCARDIA

Supraventricular tachycardia (SVT) refers to a tachyarrhythmia (nonsinus) originating above the bifurcation of the bundle of His. Most SVTs are narrow QRS tachycardias, but if the rhythm conducts retrograde through the AV node, the QRS can be wide. This can be confused with ventricular tachycardia. SVT is triggered by a reentry circuit or enhanced automaticity. Reentry is the most common mechanism and is caused by an accessory pathway atrioventricular reentrant tachycardia (AVRT), parallel pathways in the bundle of fibers in the AV node with different conduction velocities and refractory periods Atrioventricular nodal reentry tachycardia (AVNRT), or differences in the refractory period of atrial tissue leading to macro reentry circuits (atrial flutter and atrial fibrillation). The other mechanism, enhanced automaticity, involves a cell or group of cells in the atrium, which depolarize faster than the sinus node, leading to arrhythmias, such as ectopic atrial tachycardia, multifocal atrial tachycardia, and junctional ectopic tachycardia.

In the pediatric population, SVT is the most commonly diagnosed arrhythmia.[73] Accessory pathways account for most cases. These pathways are muscular connections between the atrium and ventricle that usually disappear before birth. Wolf–Parkinson–White (WPW) syndrome, described in 1930, is the most common accessory pathway SVT and occurs in .1% to .3% of the population.[74] The accessory pathway in WPW quickly conducts the electrical signal from the sinus node to the ventricles; the AV node conduction then follows. This leads to the characteristic WPW preexcitation pattern on ECG: a short PR interval and slurred QRS upstroke (delta wave, Figure 17.26). In addition, the QRS is longer than normal for age and ST-T waves can be abnormal due to the differing rates of depolarization and repolarization. Only 40% of patients with the WPW preexcitation pattern on ECG develop SVT (WPW syndrome), consequently, preexcitation may be first diagnosed on a screening ECG for either initiation of medication to treat attention deficit hyperactivity disorder, or as part of a sport physical. Not all accessory pathways conduct antegrade; thus, SVT can develop in the absence of preexcitation on ECG.

Pathophysiology and Clinical Manifestations

While patients with congenital heart defects can present with SVT, most children have a structurally normal heart.[75] Approximately 50% to 60% of pediatric patients with episodes of SVT are infants at time of diagnosis.[76] Symptoms of SVT in infants include irritability, poor feeding and pallor. Since these symptoms are nonspecific, parents are unlikely to suspect a heart arrhythmia and check the pulse. Therefore, infants are more likely to present with tachycardia-induced cardiomyopathy and CHF. By 1 year of age, 50% to 75% of infants with SVT no longer have recurrent episodes. However, in 30% of these infants, episodes of SVT will recur between 6 and 8 years of age.[76] Teenagers with SVT report episodes of palpitations, chest pain, fatigue, and lightheadedness. The episodes usually occur at rest; the onset is abrupt and of variable duration.

Anesthetic Considerations

Beta-blockers are effective for infants with recurrent SVT and continued for the first year of life. Refractory SVT may require treatment with sotalol or flecainide. Beta-blockers may increase the risk of hypoglycemia during fasting and prevent the heart rate acceleration needed to maintain cardiac output in the setting of vasodilatation, hypovolemia, and myocardial depression during anesthesia. Older children and adolescents are candidates for electrophysiology studies and ablation. Infants and young children rarely undergo catheter ablation for SVT due to a greater risk of cardiac perforation and femoral vein injury except when arrhythmias are incessant and unresponsive to medical management. Ablation in older children and teenagers is very successful with a 5 % recurrence rate.[77]

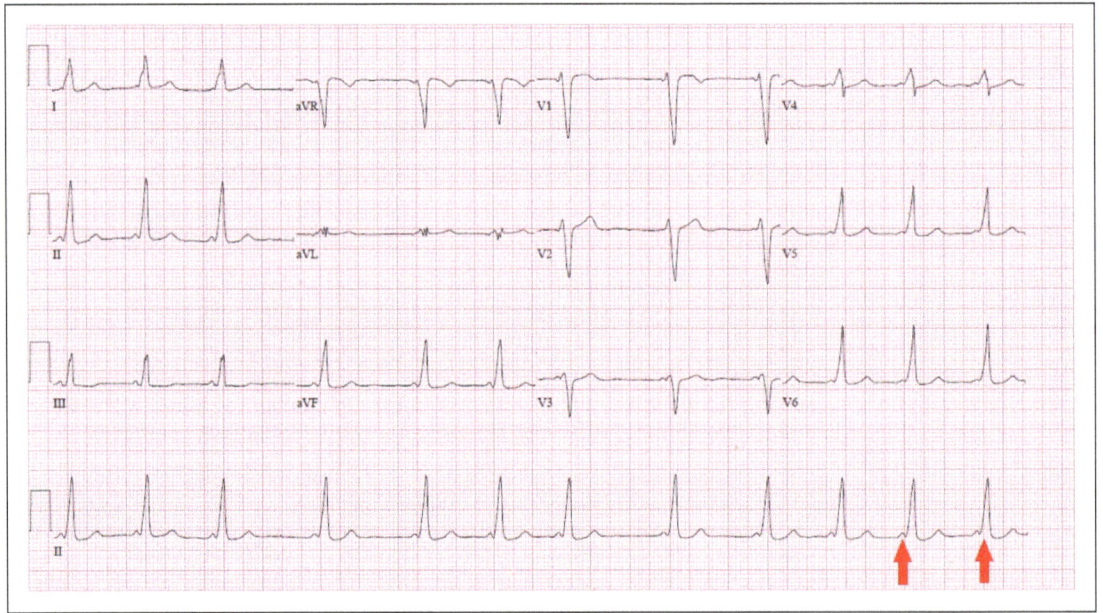

Figure 17.26: ECG of Wolff–Parkinson–White syndrome. Electrocardiogram demonstrating classic short PR intervals with a delta wave (arrows) consistent with preexcitation.

The preanesthetic evaluation should include the following questions: When did the last episode of SVT occur? Is ablation an option before other elective procedures requiring anesthesia? Are there anesthetic implications of the prescribed daily medications to help prevent episodes of SVT? For example, SVT refractory to beta-blockers is treated with amiodarone or sotalol. Both of these medications prolong the QT interval and increase the risk of polymorphic ventricular tachycardia.[78] An ECHO is part of the workup for SVT and should be reviewed to rule out tachycardia-induced cardiomyopathy and structural heart disease.

Prior to the induction of anesthesia, adenosine should be readily accessible. Administration of adenosine requires rapid IV push followed immediately with a bolus of saline to be effective (5 mL in infants, 10 to 15 mL in children, and 20 mL in adolescents). Having two stopcocks in-line with the adenosine syringe and saline syringe preattached allows for the rapid IV delivery needed. If SVT is associated with hemodynamic instability or fails to respond to escalating doses of adenosine (100, 150, and 200 mcg/kg to a maximum single dose of 18 mg), synchronized cardioversion with .5–1 joule/kg is appropriate. Adenosine can cause bronchospasm, carefully monitor peak airway pressure and the $ETCO_2$ trace.

SVT occurs during times of stress, and the first episode of SVT can arise during an anesthetic. If a strip recorder is available during treatment of an episode of SVT, continuously record and save the ECG for later review by a cardiologist. Preexcitation may be visible for only a few beats after the tachyarrhythmia converts to sinus rhythm.

CONGENITAL LONG QT SYNDROME

Pathophysiology and Clinical Manifestations

Long QT syndrome (LQTS) is a major cause of syncope and sudden cardiac death in the pediatric population. LQTS can be congenital or a drug-induced abnormality of cardiac ion channels leading to prolongation and increased dispersion of ventricular repolarization. In LQTS, the QT measured on a surface ECG is prolonged and since the QT interval varies with heart rate, calculation of the heart rate corrected QT (QTc) by the Bazett formula is standard. A QTc greater than 460 ms suggests LQTS. Patients with LQTS are at risk of a distinctive form of polymorphic ventricular tachycardia known as torsades de pointes (TdP) that can quickly degenerate into ventricular fibrillation (Figure 17.27). In TdP (French for twisting

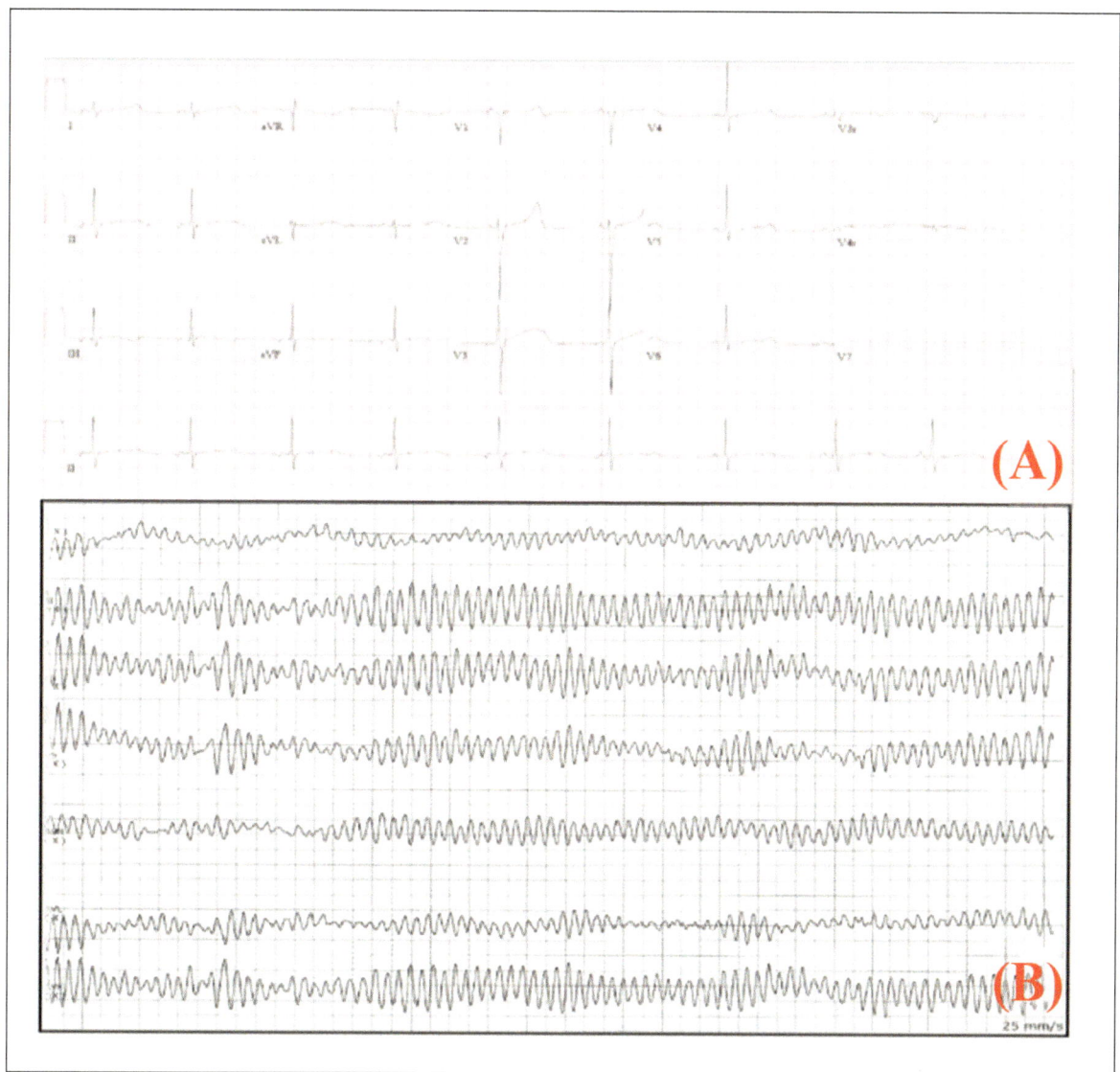

Figure 17.27: Corrected QT prolongation and torsades de pointes(TdP). (A) top image of ECG with long QT syndrome (LQTS) type 1 with a corrected QT interval of 540 milliseconds. (B) Bottom image demonstrating torsades de pointe.

of the point), the QRS vector alternates between positive and negative twisting around the isoelectric line.

In congenital LQTS, genetic mutations of ion channel proteins involved in conducting the action potential cause prolongation of myocardial repolarization. There are now many subtypes of congenital long QT identified by genetic testing with LQT1, LQT2, and LQT3 representing 90% of the cases.[79] The T-wave morphology helps in determining the subtype while awaiting genetic testing. LQT1 and LQT2 are disorders of potassium channel proteins and LQT3, the sodium channel. Increased sympathetic stimulation can TdP in LQT1 and LQT2. Bradycardia triggers TdP in LQT3. The cornerstone of prevention of TdP in LQT1 and LQT2 is daily medication with a beta-blocker. In patients with LQT3, beta-blockers are contraindicated, with sodium channel blockers being the preferred medication (e.g., mexiletine, flecainide, and procainamide). In addition to daily medication, the patient may have a CIED or undergone a left cardiac sympathetic denervation as a bridge to CIED placement. Although the prevalence of LQTS is not much different from malignant hyperthermia, it receives little attention in the anesthesia literature.[80]

Anesthetic Considerations

Review the baseline ECG with attention to the QTc interval and T wave before proceeding with anesthesia. The T-wave interval from its peak to end (Tp-e) measures the time to repolarization across the myocardium, the transmural dispersion of repolarization. This interval is prolonged in LQTS, and the degree of prolongation closely correlates with the risk of TdP. Normal Tp-e in children is 65 ms.

Instruct patients to take their usual cardiac medications on the day of the planned anesthetic. If a CIED is in place, interrogation before the procedure to check battery life and functionality is indicated. It is important to understand the device and plan for appropriate intraoperative management if electrocautery will be used (Box 17.8). While there are no definitive guidelines on how to prevent TdP and other malignant ventricular arrhythmias during anesthesia, using agents with minimal prolongation of the QTc and Tp-e is prudent[78] (Table 17.6). Preparation for the treatment of a malignant arrhythmia is key. Magnesium sulfate 40 mg/kg to a maximum of 2 g should be on hand and defibrillator pads should be placed on the patient prior to induction.

Premedication prevents sympathetic stimulation related to anxiety and fear in LQT1 and LQT2. Loud noise can trigger TdP in LQT2, so a quiet environment is important. In LQT3, sleep triggers TdP, so careful monitoring is crucial if premedication is given. Midazolam is a good choice, as it does not influence the length of the QTc.

All inhalational agents can prolong the QTc and some anesthesia providers avoid mask induction, choosing propofol, which does not prolong the QTc, for induction and maintenance. Nitrous oxide has been used safely but does have a small effect on the QTc. Since sevoflurane has a greater effect on the QTc than isoflurane, isoflurane may be the preferable inhalational agent for maintenance of anesthesia.[81] In general, light anesthesia and sympathetic stimulation may lead to TdP. Many anesthesia providers avoid sympathetic stimulating agents such as ketamine. Anticipating and maintaining an adequate depth of anesthesia at times of increased stimulus is important. Intubation and particularly extubation are periods of abrupt swings in sympathetic stimulation with increased risk for a malignant ventricular arrhythmia. Care must be taken to minimize stimulation during airway manipulation; IV lidocaine, a short-acting beta-blocker (although not in LQT3), and additional analgesia have been used to reduce this risk.

Table 17.6 Suggestions for Anesthesia and Long QT Syndrome			
Commonly Used Anesthesia Medications	**Preferred**	**Exercise Caution**	**Avoid**
Sedatives	Midazolam	Dexmedetomidine (safe use varies with LQTS subtype)	
Volatile anesthetics	Isoflurane	Sevoflurane Nitrous oxide	
IV anesthetic agents	Propofol	Etomidate	Ketamine
Opioids	Fentanyl Morphine Remifentanil Alfentanil		Sufentanil Methadone Meperidine
Neuromuscular blockers	Rocuronium Vecuronium Cisatracurium		Pancuronium Succinylcholine
Reversal agents	Sugammadex	Anticholinesterase–anticholinergic reversal agents	
Antiemetics	Dexamethasone	Ondansetron (5HT3 antagonists)	Droperidol
Local anesthetics	Bupivacaine Lidocaine Ropivacaine		Adding epinephrine to the local anesthetic

Source: O'Hare M, Munro J, Sorajja D, et al. Perioperative management of patients with congenital or acquired disorders of the QT interval. *Br J Anaesth*. 2018;120(4):629–644. doi:10.1016/j.bja.2017.12.040.

When giving muscle relaxants, it is preferable to avoid succinylcholine as it prolongs the QTc and causes acute potassium shifts. Of the nondepolarizing agents, only pancuronium might affect the QTc as it is a vagolytic agent. Adverse events have occurred at emergence after anticholinergic/anticholinesterase administration and ondansetron.[82] Reversal with sugammadex is the recommended choice as it does not cause QTc prolongation.

Regarding narcotics, fentanyl, morphine, remifentanil and alfentanil do not alter the QTc. Sufentanil, methadone and meperidine should be avoided.[83] Dexmedetomidine reduces the sympathetic outflow from the locus coeruleus and is useful in LQTS1 and LQTS2 but is not safe in LQT3 as lower heart rates predispose to TdP. Regarding antiemetics, 5HT3 antagonists (ondansetron, dolasetron, granisetron) may lengthen the QTc. Dexamethasone is the safest choice for an antiemetic.

Do not add epinephrine to local anesthetics as it prolongs the QTc. Regional anesthesia has been used without triggering TdP, although spinal anesthesia may prolong the QTc. The Valsalva maneuver lengthens the QTc, so avoid sustained high airway pressures. Hypothermia also prolongs the QTc, and keeping patients warm is important. Electrolyte abnormalities (hypokalemia, hypocalcemia, and hypomagnesemia) increase the risk of TdP and should be treated promptly.

ECG monitoring in two leads can aid in differentiating TdP from monomorphic ventricular tachycardia. Continue ECG monitoring until the patient is fully emerged and the QTc is at baseline. Have a low threshold for admission and overnight monitoring especially if the scheduled outpatient procedure will cause ongoing pain. The website www.crediblemeds.org is a regularly updated database that can assist families and health care professionals in choosing the safest medications in LQTS.

KEY TAKEAWAYS

- Congenital heart defects are the most common of all congenital anomalies.
- Eighty-five percent of all children born with congenital heart defects survive long term; a significant subset of these patients will require anesthesia for ongoing medical and surgical treatment.
- Understanding the pathophysiology of common congenital heart diseases will provide a basis to evaluate these patients for anesthetic care.
- With this knowledge, you will be able to choose the appropriate location, proper timing, and the best-suited anesthesia team to quickly recognize and respond to abnormal physiologic responses and mitigate risk.

KEY REFERENCES

Complete references for this chapter are online and available at https://connect.springerpub.com/content/book/978-0-8261-3875-0/part/part03/toc-part/ch017.

4. Wilson W, Taubert KA, Gewitz M, et al. Prevention of infective endocarditis: guidelines from the American Heart Association: a guideline From the American Heart Association Rheumatic Fever, Endocarditis, and Kawasaki Disease Committee, Council on Cardiovascular Disease in the Young, and the Council on Clinical Cardiology, Council on Cardiovascular Surgery and Anesthesia, and the Quality of Care and Outcomes Research Interdisciplinary Working Group. *Circulation.* 2007;116(15):1736–1754. doi:10.1161/CIRCULATIONAHA.106.183095

11. Backes CH, Ball MK, Cheatham SL, et al. Percutaneous Patent Ductus Arteriosus (PDA) closure in very preterm infants: feasibility and complications. *Am Heart J.* 2016;5(2):e002923. doi:10.1161/JAHA.115.002923

24. Glidewell J, Grosse SD, Riehle-Colarusso T, et al. Actions in support of newborn screening for critical congenital heart disease - United States, 2011–2018. *MMWR. Morb Mortal Wkly Rep.* 2019;68(5):107–111. doi:10.15585/mmwr.mm6805a3

25. Pierpont ME, Brueckner M, Chung WK, et al. Genetic basis for congenital heart disease: revisited: a scientific statement from the American Heart Association. *Circulation.* 2018;138(21):e653–e711. doi:10.1161/CIR.0000000000000606

29. Benson LN, Gillespie MJ, Bergersen L, et al. Three-year outcomes from the harmony native outflow tract early feasibility study. *Circulation.* 2020;13(1):e008320. doi:10.1161/CIRCINTERVENTIONS.119.008320

40. Kloesel B, Skubas NJ, Belani K. Risk prediction in children with congenital heart disease: business as usual-or not? *Anesth Analg.* 2020;131(4):1080–1082. doi:10.1213/ANE.0000000000005042

45. Schulman P, Treggiari M, Yanez N, et al. Electromagnetic interference with protocolized electrosurgery dispersive electrode positioning in patients with implantable cardioverter defibrillators. *Anesthesiology.* 2019;130(4):530–540. doi:10.1097/ALN.0000000000002571

59. Dufort EM, Koumans EH, Chow EJ, et al. Multisystem inflammatory syndrome in children in New York State. *N Engl J Med.* 2020;383(4):347–358. doi:10.1056/NEJMoa2021756

67. Chau DF, Hartke LP, Gangadharan M, et al. The post-anesthetic care of pediatric patients with pulmonary hypertension. *Semin Cardiothorac Vasc Anesth.* 2016;20(1):63–73. doi:10.1177/1089253215593179

68. Latham GJ, Yung D, Arnold P, Ramamoorthy C. Current understanding and perioperative management of pediatric pulmonary hypertension. *Paediatr Anaesth.* 2019;29(5):441–456. doi:10.1111/pan.13542

96. Sridharan S, Price G, Tann O, et al. Transposition of the great arteries: arterial switch operation. In: *Cardiovascular MRI in Congenital Heart Disease.* Springer; 2010. doi:10.1007/978-3-540-69837-1_36

CHAPTER 18

Gastrointestinal Conditions

Kahleb Graham and Khalil El-Chammas

> **LEARNING OBJECTIVES**
>
> - Review the pathophysiology of a variety of gastrointestinal conditions.
> - Discuss the clinical manifestations of various gastrointestinal conditions.
> - Highlight existing medical and surgical treatment options for different gastrointestinal conditions.

INTRODUCTION

Various gastrointestinal (GI) conditions require a pediatric gastroenterologist to perform endoscopic procedures which are critical for both diagnostic evaluation and therapeutic intervention. It is important anesthesia providers have a sound understanding of these conditions given the unique preoperative, intraoperative, or postoperative management decisions that may be made related to a patient's underlying GI condition.

ESOPHAGEAL CONDITIONS

ESOPHAGEAL DUPLICATIONS

Esophageal duplications can appear as cysts, diverticula, and/or tubular malformations. They lie within the wall of the esophagus and are defined by their location. Depending on size and location they may be benign and symptomatic, or cause more significant clinical sequelae such as respiratory distress, dysphagia, regurgitation of undigested food, frequent aspiration, noisy deglutition (gurgling), halitosis, voice changes, or esophageal wall erosion secondary to presence of acid-producing gastric mucosa.

Duplications are identified using imaging such as contrast swallow studies (esophagram or upper GI), esophagogastroduodenoscopy (EGD), or chest CT. The management is typically surgical excision.

ESOPHAGEAL STENOSIS, STRICTURES, WEBS, AND RINGS

Intrinsic luminal narrowing of the esophagus can be congenital or acquired secondary to inflammation (e.g., peptic strictures, Crohn's disease, and eosinophilic esophagitis), scarring (e.g., secondary to caustic ingestions or medications), fibrosis, or neoplasia. Congenital abnormalities consist of webs, which are typically found in the proximal mid-esophagus, rings (e.g., Schatzki ring) found in the distal esophagus, fibromuscular stenosis, or due to cartilaginous tracheobronchial remnants. Narrowing of the esophagus can be benign in nature with slow and insidious progression or malignant with a more rapid progression. Benign strictures are by far the most common, with peptic strictures accounting for 70% to 80% of all causes of esophageal strictures. Patients present with dysphagia, food impaction, odynophagia, chest pain, and/or weight loss.

EGD and contrast swallow studies are the mainstays of the initial workup and diagnosis. The management varies based on the underlying cause of the narrowing, and conditions that are due to inflammation may be amenable to acid suppression from a proton pump inhibitor (PPI) or H2 blocker, and/or anti-inflammatory medications, such steroids or biologics. Meanwhile, other conditions may require esophageal dilation or surgical excision. Please refer to Chapter 106, "Endoscopy and Colonoscopy," for more information about the anesthetic management of endoscopy for the pediatric patient.

ESOPHAGEAL ATRESIA/TRACHEA ESOPHAGEAL FISTULA

Esophageal atresia is a congenital condition that occurs when the proximal and distal portions of the esophagus do not communicate. The proximal segment is a dilated blind pouch while the distal end is typically narrow. In addition, esophageal atresia typically presents with a trachea esophageal fistula (TEF), which is an abnormal communication between the trachea and the esophagus. There are five types of TEF abnormalities, with the most common being an upper esophageal atresia with a distal fistula. Most patients will have other non-GI congenital abnormalities as well. Patients typically present with a prenatal history of polyhydramnios, absent to small gastric bubble, increased secretions requiring frequent suctioning, cough, emesis, recurrent pneumonia, choking or respiratory distress while feeding, the inability to pass a nasogastric (NG) tube into the stomach. Esophageal atresia/TEF is diagnosed with radiographic evidence of an NG coiled in the esophagus with intestinal air, or direct visualization via endoscopy, bronchoscopy, or contrast swallow study. Treatment consists of surgical closure of the fistula and reconnection of the proximal and distal esophageal segments. There are multiple short- and long-term postoperative complications, including anastomotic leak stricture, recurrent fistula, esophageal dysmotility, gastroesophageal reflux disease (GERD), and Barrett's esophagus. Please refer to Chapter 95, "Trachea Esophageal Fistula," for more information about the anesthetic management of TEF repair for the pediatric patient.

ESOPHAGITIS

Esophagitis is an inflammation caused by conditions including, but not limited to, peptic disease, eosinophilic esophagitis, infections, Crohn's disease, medication, caustic ingestion, radiation, or graft-versus-host disease. The consequence of acute and/or chronic esophageal inflammation depends on the underlying etiology. These changes include tissue friability, edema, furrowing, plaque formation, ulcerations, microabscesses, cellular hyperplasia or metaplasia, necrosis, scarring, trachealization of the esophagus, fibrostenosis leading to stricture formation, and even esophageal wall perforation. Patients with esophagitis can present with dysphagia, odynophagia (particularly with eating), reflux, chest pain, emesis, hematemesis, drooling, food impaction, and/or weight loss. Diagnosis is typically made with endoscopic visualization combined with histological confirmation. Treatment for esophagitis may include acid suppression with H2 blocker or PPIs, mucosal protectants (like sucralfate), anti-inflammatory medications, antimicrobials, and initiation of hypoallergenic diets.

ESOPHAGEAL ACHALASIA

Esophageal achalasia is the absence of peristalsis and absent or incomplete relaxation of the lower esophageal sphincter (LES), with swallows resulting in a functional obstruction. The causes of achalasia are idiopathic, infectious, autoimmune, or related to genetic disorders (like Allgrove's syndrome). Patients present with vomiting, regurgitation, weight loss, dysphagia, odynophagia, and chest pain. Evaluation includes chest radiograph, esophageal contrast study, and esophageal manometry study. The management of achalasia includes endoscopic LES botulinum toxin injection, endoscopic pneumatic balloon dilation, and endoscopic or surgical myotomy. Please refer to Chapter 107, "Manometry Placement, Esophageal Dilation, Botox Injection," for more information about the anesthetic management of manometry placement, esophageal dilatation, and botulinum injection for the pediatric patient.

FOREIGN BODY INGESTIONS AND FOOD IMPACTIONS

Foreign body ingestions in children usually involve common objects found in the home environment, such as coins, magnets, toys, batteries, and food boluses. Patients can present with symptoms such as stridor, odynophagia, drooling, fussiness, chest pain, abdominal pain, fever, feeding refusal, wheezing, or respiratory distress. They may also be asymptomatic but brought in seeking medical attention after a witnessed ingestion. Objects that typically warrant endoscopic retrieval include button batteries, magnets, sharp/pointed objects, food impactions, coins/blunt objects, and superabsorbent objects. Objects in the esophagus are almost universally removed endoscopically due to risk of aspiration, perforation, and potentially death. During retrieval it is important for the airway to be protected with an endotracheal tube. The timing of the removal depends on multiple factors, including the patient's clinical status, time of last oral intake, type of ingestion, and location of the object within the GI tract (Table 18.1).

GASTRIC CONDITIONS

GASTRITIS AND GASTROPATHY

Gastritis and gastropathy are characterized by injury to the gastric mucosa with or without the significant presence of inflammatory cells, respectively. They are classified into two predominant groups: erosive and/or hemorrhagic gastritis/gastropathy and nonerosive gastritis/gastropathy (see Box 18.1). Endoscopic and histological evaluations are both

Table 18.1 Timing of Endoscopic Intervention in Pediatric Foreign Body Ingestion

Type	Location	Symptoms	Timing
Button battery	Esophagus	Yes or no	Emergent
	Gastric/SB	Yes	Emergent
		No	Urgent (if age <5 years and button battery ≥20 mm)
			Elective (if not moving on serial x-ray)
Magnets	Esophagus	Yes	Emergent (if not managing secretions, otherwise urgent)
		No	Urgent
	Gastric/SB	Yes	Emergent
		No	Urgent
Sharp	Esophagus	Yes	Emergent (f not managing secretions, otherwise urgent)
		No	Urgent
	Gastric/SB	Yes	Emergent (if signs of perforation, then with surgery)
		No	Urgent
Food impaction	Esophagus	Yes	Emergent (if not managing secretions, otherwise urgent)
		No	Urgent
Coin	Esophagus	Yes	Emergent (if not managing secretions, otherwise urgent)
		No	Urgent
	Gastric/SB	Yes	Urgent
		No	Elective
Long object	Esophagus	Yes or no	Urgent
	Gastric/SB	Yes or no	Urgent
Absorptive object	Esophagus	Yes	Emergent (if not managing secretions, otherwise urgent)
		No	Urgent
	Gastric/SB	Yes or no	Urgent

Notes: Timing: emergent <2 hours from ingestion regardless of NPO status; urgent <24 hours from ingestion, following standard NPO guidelines; elective >24 hours from ingestion, following standard NPO guidelines).

SB, short bowel.

Source: From Kramer RE, Lerner DG, Lin T, et al. Management of ingested foreign bodies in children: a clinical report of the NASPGHAN Endoscopy Committee. *JPGN.* 2015;60(4):562–574. doi:10.1097/MPG.0000000000000729.

> **BOX 18.1 CAUSES OF GASTRITIS AND GASTROPATHY**
>
> **Erosive and/or Hemorrhagic Gastritis or Gastropathy**
> - Alcohol gastropathy
> - Bile gastropathy
> - Corrosive gastropathy
> - Chronic varioliform gastritis
> - Exercise-induced gastropathy or gastritis
> - Nonsteroidal anti-inflammatory drug gastropathy
> - Neonatal gastropathies
> - Other medication causing gastropathy
> - Portal hypertensive gastropathy
> - Radiation gastropathy
> - "Stress" gastropathy
> - Traumatic gastropathy
> - Uremic gastropathy
>
> **Nonerosive Gastritis or Gastropathy**
> - Allergic gastritis
> - Celiac gastritis
> - Collagenous gastritis
> - Crohn's gastritis
> - Cytomegalovirus gastritis
> - Eosinophilic gastritis
> - *Helicobacter pylori* gastritis
> - Gastritis of autoimmune disease
> - Graft-versus-host disease
> - Menetrier's disease
> - "Nonspecific" gastritis
> - Non–*H. pylori* infectious gastritis
> - Other noninfectious granulomatous gastritis
> - Pernicious anemia
> - Phlegmonous and emphysematous gastritis
> - Proton pump inhibitor gastropathy

critical in determining an underlying etiology of gastritis and/or gastropathies. Patients present with epigastric or generalized abdominal pain, reflux, emesis, hematemesis, nausea, vomiting, and/or weight loss. The management is variable and may include using acid suppression with H2 blocker or PPIs, mucosal protectants (like sucralfate), anti-inflammatory medications, antimicrobials, initiation of hypoallergenic diets, or elimination of the insulting agent.

GASTROPARESIS

Gastroparesis is a delay in the emptying of the stomach without evidence of mechanical obstruction. The most common cause of gastroparesis is idiopathic, but additional causes include postsurgical, post infectious, drug-induced, or diabetes mellitus. Patients typically present with nausea, vomiting, early satiety, abdominal pain, weight loss, and/or postprandial fullness. Evaluation may include an upper contrast study, 4-hour solid-phase gastric emptying scintigraphy, and antroduodenal manometry. In many cases symptoms self-resolve without intervention. Medical management includes prokinetics, antiemetics, endoscopic intrapyloric botulinum toxin injections with or without pyloric dilation, or surgically implanted gastric electrical stimulators.

GI BLEEDING

GI bleeds (GIBs) can occur anywhere along the GI tract. GI bleeding is classified based on its location. Upper GI bleeds (UGIBs) occur proximal to the ligament of Treitz. They are characterized by bright red or "coffee-ground" hematemesis, melena, and in rare cases hematochezia if there is a large volume upper tract bleeding source. In most cases, hematochezia indicates the presence of a lower GIB. Lower GIBs occur distal to the ligament of Treitz (see **Box 18.2**). GIBs are further stratified into two categories: nonvariceal and variceal bleeds. Patients can present with overt signs of blood loss, hemodynamic instability, abdominal pain, and/or acute or chronic anemia.

Initial management of GI bleeding is focused on airway and hemodynamic stabilization, volume repletion with intravenous fluids, or blood transfusions. Evaluation of GI bleeding includes assessment of complete blood count, liver function test, coagulation labs, electrolytes and blood type and crossmatching, and appropriate imaging studies. In some cases, occult blood testing is indicated when the presence of bleeding is uncertain. Additional NG lavage is occasionally used when determining the presence of an active upper GI bleeding. IV PPIs are standard in patients with UGIBs, and in some cases the use of octreotide is warranted in patients with liver disease.

While many GIBs can be managed conservatively, endoscopy remains critically important for diagnostic evaluation and achieving hemostasis through various therapeutic interventions. Nonvariceal bleeding can be controlled by injecting sclerosing agents or epinephrine, using thermocoagulation, applying hemostatic clips, and/or using argon plasma coagulation. Three methods are used to control variceal bleeding: (a) endoscopic variceal ligation with elastic bands, (b) endoscopic sclerotherapy injections into the varix, and (c) balloon tamponade. In other cases, the bleeding source can be decompressed, excised, or reduced either endoscopically, surgically, or fluoroscopically.

SMALL BOWEL CONDITIONS

CHRONIC DIARRHEA

Chronic diarrhea in children can be nonspecific or due to epithelial defects, macronutrient malabsorption, or electrolyte malabsorption. It is also associated with intestinal failure, recent antibiotic use, small bowel bacterial overgrowth, allergic enteropathy, immunodeficiency state, autoimmune enteropathy, inflammatory bowel disease (IBD), celiac disease, irritable bowel syndrome, Hirschsprung's disease, pseudo-obstruction, and/or neuroendocrine tumors. Diarrhea is classified into two groups: secretory and osmotic. Each of these groups is further divided based on whether the diarrhea presents with or without failure to thrive (FFT). Dietary challenges, assessment of stool volume, pH levels, presence of reducing substances, infectious stool studies, and electrolytes are critical to determining the type of diarrhea. Endoscopy with intestinal biopsies is needed to identify the cause of chronic diarrhea.

BOX 18.2 CAUSES OF UPPER AND LOWER GI BLEEDING IN PEDIATRIC PATIENTS

Upper GI Bleed
- Aortoesophageal fistula
- Coagulopathy
- Duodenitis
- Esophagitis
- Foreign body
- Gastritis
- GI anastomosis
- GI duplication
- Mallory–Weiss tear
- Neoplasm
- Prolapse gastropathy
- Stress ulcer
- Swallowed maternal blood
- Thrombocytopenia
- Toxic ingestion
- Vascular malformation
- Varices

Lower GI Bleed
- Aortoenteric fistula
- Anal fissure
- Allergic proctocolitis
- Coagulopathy
- GI anastomosis
- Hemolytic uremic syndrome
- Hemorrhoid
- Henoch–Schonlein purpura
- Hirschsprung's enterocolitis
- Infectious colitis
- Inflammatory bowel disease
- Intestinal duplication
- Intussusception
- Ischemic colitis
- Lymphonodular hyperplasia
- Meckel's diverticulum
- Necrotizing enterocolitis
- Neoplasm
- Polyps
- Pseudomembranous colitis
- Radiation enteritis/colitis
- Rectal prolapse
- Solitary rectal ulcer
- Swallowed maternal blood
- Vascular malformation
- Vasculitis
- Volvulus

CELIAC DISEASE

Celiac disease is an immune-mediated disorder triggered by gluten and related prolamins present in wheat, barley, and rye that occurs in genetically susceptible individuals who have the human leukocyte antigen. It is characterized by an inflammatory enteropathy, along with a wide range of GI and systemic symptoms. Patients present with abdominal pain, distention, diarrhea, steatorrhea, malnutrition, constipation, and in some cases a protein-losing enteropathy. In addition, patients can have various extraintestinal manifestations such as delayed puberty, anemia, dermatitis, fatigue, and headaches. In some cases, patients are asymptomatic. Initially screening can be done with serological testing, but the diagnosis is confirmed with endoscopy and histological findings of duodenal biopsies showing flattened villi, crypt hyperplasia, and intraepithelial lymphocytes. Strict exclusion of gluten within the diet (gluten-free diet [GFD]) and avoidance of nonfood gluten sources such as cosmetics or pet food are the required treatments.

MALNUTRITION OR FAILURE TO THRIVE

Malnutrition or FTT is a state of undernutrition due to inadequate caloric intake, inadequate caloric absorption, or excessive caloric expenditure. Malnutrition can be defined as acute or chronic in nature. Acute malnutrition is characterized by muscle weakness, muscle loss, and/or loss of lean body mass or weight. Chronic malnutrition presents with growth stunting, evidence of macronutrient or micronutrient deficiencies, and Tanner stagnation in preteens and adolescents. The most common cause of malnutrition/FTT is inadequate caloric intake; however, it is important to assess for evidence of organic causes of the malabsorption, which may include endoscopy of upper and lower GI tract. Video capsule endoscopy and single/double-balloon enteroscopy can be used for deep visualization of the small bowel in areas unable to be seen, but the standard EGD is used to identify obscure small bowel inflammation, polyps, lesions, and tumors.

COLONIC AND ANORECTAL CONDITIONS

INFLAMMATORY BOWEL DISEASE

IBD is a subset of conditions triggered by a complex interplay of environmental, genetic, and immunological factors that lead to chronic and acute inflammation of the GI tract (not due to infection). It is primarily separated into three different phenotypes: Crohn's disease (CD), ulcerative colitis (UC), and IBD-unclassified (IBD-U). The phenotypes have different but overlapping clinical, mucosal, and histological features.

The clinical features of CD can be found anywhere along the GI tract, and include, but are not limited to, abdominal pain, diarrhea, nocturnal diarrhea, hematochezia, perirectal disease (skin tags, perianal fissures, abscesses, and fistulae), weight loss, anorexia, growth failure, nausea, vomiting, odynophagia, dysphagia, fever, and fatigue. Patients with CD may also have extraintestinal manifestations affecting other areas outside of the GI tract. UC patients present with many of the same symptoms as those with CD; however, hematochezia is more common, growth failure and upper GI tract symptoms are less common, and patients typically have a normal perianal examination, along with fewer extraintestinal manifestations.

The use of radiographic imaging studies (abdominal radiographs, contrast studies, magnetic resonance imaging [MRI], abdominal CT, magnetic resonance enterography [MRE], MRI of the pelvis, and/or ultrasound) is valuable in assessing the presence of small bowel disease, colitis, abscesses, fistula, strictures, or perforations, all of which can be seen in IBD. The distribution of inflammation seen when performing EGD, colonoscopy, and terminal ileoscopy is critical in determining the accurate phenotype. Endoscopy findings seen in CD anywhere along the GI tract include erythema, exudates, superficial or deep ulceration, tissue friability, nodularity, cobblestoning, fistula, strictures, stenosis, and skip areas with normal-appearing mucosa. The typical distribution of inflammation in UC includes pancolitis, predominately left-sided colitis with a small area of cecal inflammation after a large area of normal-appearing colon, although it can be limited to proctosigmoiditis. Less commonly compared with CD, patients with UC may have milder upper GI tract disease or backwash ileitis. Endoscopy findings seen include diffuse erythema and tissue friability, ulcers of various sizes, and continuous inflammation extending from the rectum. In contrast, IBD-U has confounding features of both CD and UC, such as the inability to differentiate ileocolonic CD from backwash ileitis seen with UC, patchy colonic inflammation, pancolitis with anal fissures or skin tags, and colitis with growth failure.

Classic histological features of CD include transmural chronic or chronic active inflammation, presence of granulomas, discontinuous inflammation with intervening zones of normal bowel, a fissuring ulceration stricture and fistula formation, and small bowel involvement not consistent with backwash ileitis. In contrast, classic histological findings of UC include chronic and active chronic inflammation limited to the mucosa or submucosa, and continuous colonic inflammation.

The management of IBD includes medical management with 5-aminosalicylates (5-ASAs), corticosteroids, immunomodulators (thiopurines and methotrexate), biologics (infliximab, adalimumab, vedolizumab, and ustekinumab), calcineurin inhibitors (tacrolimus and cyclosporine), nutritional therapy, and antibiotics. In addition, it is not uncommon for patients with IBD to undergo surgical resection (such as colectomy) and require ostomies, stricturoplasty, fistulotomy, incision and drainage, and/or transanal dilation.

NONINFLAMMATORY BOWEL DISEASE COLITIS

There are a variety of inflammatory conditions of the colon that can be differentiated from IBD by their clinical, endoscopic, and histological characteristics. These conditions include infectious colitis, microscopic colitis, ischemic colitis, diversion colitis, radiation proctitis, chemical/medication-induced colitis, eosinophilic colitis, graft-versus-host disease, neutropenic colitis, solitary rectal ulcer, and Behcet's disease. Clinical presentation includes chronic, watery diarrhea, abdominal pain, and intermittent rectal bleeding. Evaluation includes infectious stool studies, radiographic studies (CT scan or MRI), and a colonoscopy with colonic biopsies. Treatment varies from anti-inflammatory medications, corticosteroids, antimicrobials, initiation of hypoallergenic diets, elimination of the insulting agent, and/or surgery.

INTRACTABLE FUNCTIONAL CONSTIPATION

Intractable functional constipation is a constipation occurring in the absence of evidence of organic pathology, medication, or anatomical cause and unresponsive to optimal conventional therapy for at least 3 months. Patients present with hard stools, painful stools, bright red blood in stools, anal fissures, abdominal pain, distention, decreased oral intake, and encopresis. Evaluation may include a detailed history and physical examination, digital rectal examination, colonic transit studies, water-soluble contrast enema, anorectal manometry, and/or colonoscopy with colonic manometry. Treatment includes dietary interventions, use of oral osmotic or stimulant laxatives, prokinetics, chloride channel activators, rectal disimpactions with enemas or suppositories, anal sphincter injections of botulinum toxin, biofeedback therapy, behavioral modification, and less commonly surgical therapies, including placement of a cecostomy/appendicocecostomy for antegrade colonic enemas, sacral nerve stimulator, colonic diversion, or colonic resection.

HIRSCHSPRUNG'S DISEASE

Hirschsprung's disease is a congenital condition characterized by the absence of intestinal ganglion in the rectum and extending to variable lengths of the bowel. In the vast majority of patients, intestinal aganglionosis is limited to the rectum and sigmoid colon. Patients present with chronic constipation, neonatal distal obstruction, growth failure, Hirschsprung's-associated enterocolitis, explosive stool, abdominal distention, and emesis. Diagnostic evaluation includes water-soluble contrast enema, anorectal manometry, and confirmation with a rectal biopsy. The management is surgical; however, given that postsurgical bowel issues are common, frequently patients will require a colonoscopy with colonic manometry to assess underlying colonic dysmotility.

ANORECTAL DISEASE (HEMORRHOIDS, FISSURES, ABSCESSES, AND FISTULA)

Hemorrhoids, anal fissures, perianal abscesses, and fistula are considered benign anorectal diseases. Hemorrhoids are engorged submucosal veins either proximal to the dentate line (internal) or distal to the dentate line (external) that become symptomatic with the deterioration of tissues that support the anal fibrovascular cushions, causing abnormal downward displacement and venous dilation. Hemorrhoids are typically worsened by lifting, straining, prolonged sitting, and constipation. They can present with painful or painless rectal bleeding, prolapse, mucus drainage, perianal fullness, tender perianal mass, perianal itching, mild fecal incontinence, and painful skin irritation. Anoscopy and colonoscopy are typically necessary to visualize internal hemorrhoids. Treatment varies from conservative medical management, rubber band ligation, sclerotherapy, or surgical treatment.

Anal fissures are linear tears in the anal mucosa. They are caused by trauma secondary to hard stools, diarrhea, and IBD. Patients present with anal pain and painful bleeding with bowel movements. The diagnosis is made clinically during a perianal examination. Treatment consists of stool softeners, fiber supplementation, sitz baths, topical lidocaine, nitrate or steroids, injection of botulinum toxin into the internal anal sphincter, or surgical interventions.

Perianal abscess is an infection in the anal canal within the muscular, perianal, or submucosa spaces. Perianal abscess can be due to hidradenitis, furuncles, pilonidal disease, or CD. Perianal fistula is a persistent epithelialized tract from the anal canal to the perianal skin. Fistulas are most often secondary to congenital defect, radiation, malignancy, or infection. Patients present with fever, pain, tenderness, erythema, fluctuance, and purulent or feculent drainage. Clinical examination, radiographic imaging via CT scan, pelvic MRI, or endorectal ultrasound can be critical for fistula mapping and localization of the abscess. Treatment includes antibiotics, biological therapy, incision and drainage, placement of a seton, and staged fistulotomy.

COLONIC POLYPS

A polyp is a mass protruding into the lumen of the GI tract. Most polyps in children are benign and can be solitary or related to a familial polyposis syndrome. Polyps are classified into four general histological categories: hamartomatous polyps, adenomatous polyps, inflammatory polyps, and mixed polyposis syndromes. Polyps present with painless rectal bleeding, prolapsing rectal mass, abdominal pain, intussusception, or mucopurulent stools. Colonic polyps are diagnosed via visualization during a colonoscopy. The indications for performing a polypectomy include screening for dysplasia, anemia, and hematochezia.

DISORDERS OF THE BRAIN–GUT AXIS

PAIN-PREDOMINANT FUNCTIONAL GI DISORDERS

Functional gastrointestinal disorders (FGIDs) are prevalent in the pediatric population and make up more than 50% of GI outpatient visits. They arise from the complex interactions of various biopsychosocial factors that affect the brain–gut axis. There are four pain-predominant FGIDs: IBS, functional dyspepsia, abdominal migraine, and functional abdominal pain. The symptoms associated with FGIDs, including nausea, early satiety, vomiting, constipation, abdominal pain, bloating, and diarrhea, can significantly impact a patient's well-being and quality of life. Although the diagnosis is made based on a detailed history and thorough physical exam, a limited evaluation is recommended due to the chronicity and functional impairment. However, it is not uncommon for patients to have an extensive medical workup, including endoscopy of both the upper and lower tract. The goals of management for these disorders are to improve functioning and achieve symptom reduction. The therapies fall under three domains: pharmacological, dietary modification, and nonpharmacological.

KEY TAKEAWAYS

- There are a variety of gastrointestinal conditions that involve diagnostic and/or therapeutic procedures requiring general anesthesia.
- The specific diagnostic and/or therapeutic procedures for the various gastrointestinal conditions may guide the type of anesthesia and airway management needed.

KEY REFERENCES

Complete references for this chapter are online and available at https://connect.springerpub.com/content/book/978-0-8261-3875-0/part/part03/toc-part/ch018.

4. Kramer RE, Lerner DG, Lin T, et al. Management of ingested foreign bodies in children: a clinical report of the NASPGHAN Endoscopy Committee. *JPGN*. 2015;60(4):562–574. doi:10.1097/MPG.0000000000000729
6. Adegboyega T, Rivadeneira D. Lower GI bleeding: an update on incidences and causes. *Clin Colon Rectal Surg*. 2020;33(1):28–34. doi: 10.1055/s-0039-1695035
7. Dohil R, Hassall E, Jevon G, Dimmick J. Gastritis and gastropathy of childhood. *JPGN*. 1999;29(4):378–394. doi:10.1097/00005176-199910000-00004
9. Zella GC, Isreal EJ. Chronic diarrhea in children. *Pediatr Rev*. 2011;33(5):207–218. doi:10.1542/pir.33-5-207
12. North American Society for Pediatric Gastroenterology, Hepatology, and Nutrition; Colitis Foundation of America; Athos Bousvaros et al. Differentiating ulcerative colitis from crohn disease in children and young adults: Report of a Working Group of the North American Society for Pediatric Gastroenterology, Hepatology, and Nutrition and the Crohn's and Colitis Foundation of America. *JPGN*. 2007;44(5):653–674. doi:10.1097/MPG.0b013e31805563f3
14. Tabbers MM, DiLorenzo C, Berger MY, et al. Evaluation and treatment of functional constipation in infants and children: evidence-based recommendations from ESPGHAN and NASPGHAN. *JPGN*. 2014;58(2):258–274. doi:10.1097/MPG.0000000000000266

CHAPTER 19

Hematologic Conditions

Marika Highberger, Lindsay Johnson-Bishop, Brandi M. Runnels, and Heather Soni

> **LEARNING OBJECTIVES**
>
> - Describe common hematologic disorders found in the pediatric population and some of the challenges they can pose in regard to anesthetic management.
> - Identify preoperative considerations for various pediatric hematologic conditions.
> - Discuss factors to consider in the anesthetic management of pediatric patients who have these hematologic conditions.

INTRODUCTION

Hematologic diseases are varying disorders of the blood and blood-forming organs which afflict millions of Americans.[1] Considerations in the setting of anesthetic management are vital as 7% of all deaths among children with sickle cell disease (SCD) were related to surgery.[2]

DISSEMINATED INTRAVASCULAR COAGULATION

Disseminated intravascular coagulation (DIC) is an acquired hematologic syndrome characterized by a disproportionate activation of the body's coagulation mechanisms, resulting in both hemorrhaging and thrombosis in a patient simultaneously. This occurs often without a specified trigger or source and may even be multifactorial in insult of origin. There is damage to the microvasculature that can result in tissue injury and ultimately organ dysfunction if severe enough.[3] DIC occurs due to an underlying disease or initial insult that causes excessive stimulation of coagulation, followed by excess production of thrombin, and which in turn results in incapacitation of the body's anticoagulant control mechanisms. This overwhelming coagulopathy allows thrombosis to occur without restriction and initiates the competition between superfluous thrombin and uncontrolled hemorrhage from the decreased platelets and a lack of coagulation factors.[4]

DIC manifests clinically as increased thrombosis and microvascular occlusion resulting in tissue ischemia and multiorgan dysfunction syndrome, in combination with hemorrhaging caused by platelet depletion, the body consuming coagulation factors unnecessarily, and the accelerated formation of plasmin. This is how both uncontrolled bleeding and thrombosis may occur in a patient simultaneously.[5] The clinical manifestations of DIC in an acute setting are commonly fatigue, alteration in mentation, development of petechiae or purpura without major trauma source, bleeding of the skin or oral mucosa, or alterations in hemodynamics, most commonly hypotension.[6] There is no single test or diagnostic indicator for DIC, and the diagnosis is made with a combination of comprehensive medical history, symptom history, laboratory testing, and clinical presentation.[7]

In the preoperative evaluation of patients presenting with DIC, it is imperative anesthesia providers elicit a thorough health history. The health history should include questions regarding any past hematologic concerns or previous problems during procedures, including history of anemia or thrombocytopenia, history of abnormal coagulation studies, any history of cancer, or previous hematopoietic stem cell transplant. There is no single factor to isolate in laboratory screening to assess the risk of bleeding in a child with DIC; however, it is imperative to optimize coagulation if able. The abnormalities that may be demonstrated in what is described as "consumption coagulopathy" are prolongation of activated partial thromboplastin time (aPTT) and prothrombin time test (PT)/international normalized ratio (INR), a decrease in fibrinogen, decreased platelet count, and a subsequent increase in the products responsible for fibrin degradation, most notably an elevated D-dimer in a patient.[7]

The pharmacotherapeutic treatment during the preoperative period includes short-term treatment of bleeding to replete the deficits elicited in the laboratory testing. If the patient has an INR of greater than 1.5, fresh frozen plasma (FFP) should be administered. If the patient has a platelet count of less than $50 \times 10^9/L$, platelet transfusion should be administered. If the patient has a fibrinogen of less than 100 mg/dL, it would be beneficial to administer cryoprecipitate. If the patient presents with a hematocrit of less than 21%, a transfusion of red blood cells would be warranted. Most important, anesthesia providers should be investigating the underlying source or inciting factor of the DIC, and the symptom manifestations will likely resolve after the source is treated or eliminated. It is important to note that aggressive therapy in the treatment of the underlying problem is essential in order to control and correct the symptoms of DIC, as it may take up to several days for the consumed factors to be effectively replenished.[7]

In children diagnosed with hematologic disorders, the standard anesthetic management consists of a comprehensive preoperative evaluation and strict monitoring of vital signs, including respiratory rate and oxygen saturation. Induction of anesthesia can be achieved via inhalation induction or IV induction, followed by airway management appropriate for the surgical procedure. Intraoperative management of patients with DIC predominately consists of maintaining adequate levels of blood products and coagulation factors to ensure the lowest risk of bleeding. The Administration of platelets and FFP in patients experiencing active bleeding is determined based on individualized patient parameters and the clinical state of the patient.[8,9] Anesthesia providers should be aware that for patients with DIC, there is a greater risk of development of Venous thromboembolism (VTE), and it is often recommended to administer prophylactic low molecular weight heparin in the nonsymptomatic type. This is not recommended, however, in a patient with massive bleeding or hemorrhaging.[10,11]

The utilization of coagulation factor concentrates for infusion is contraindicated in patients diagnosed with DIC due to the possibility of contamination with active coagulation factors, and the concentrates of coagulation factors may not provide all the factors needed as DIC patients are deficient in all coagulation factors.[12] Finally, it is imperative to keep strict record of intake and output, specifically in regard to any volume of fluids that are administered intraoperatively. This allows for accurate evaluation of blood loss and provision of information to aid in postoperative care with repletion of volume losses and maintenance of hemodynamic stability.[4]

IMMUNE THROMBOCYTOPENIA

Thrombocytopenia is the term for a platelet count that is below the defined parameters deemed normal for age. Immune thrombocytopenia is a hematologic disorder characterized by increased platelet destruction and impaired platelet production that may be attributed to a variety of causative factors, both primary and secondary in relation to other disease processes. Thrombocytopenia may be due to deficiencies in certain vitamins, presence of infection, bone marrow infiltration, medications, or autoimmune as in the case of immune thrombocytopenia.[13] Immune thrombocytopenia is an acquired thrombocytopenia caused by autoantibodies against platelet antigens. Treatment for patients with thrombocytopenia, especially immune thrombocytopenia, should be determined based on each individual patient and their platelet count.[14]

Many patients with immune thrombocytopenia present with few, if any, clinical symptoms, especially if the patient maintains platelet counts in the 50 to 100×10^9/L range. It is not until the platelet count falls below 50×10^9/L that patients may demonstrate bruising or more frequent episodes of bleeding that is slow to resolve, such as prolonged epistaxis. When the platelet counts fall below 20×10^9/L, the patient may begin to demonstrate petechiae or purpura as bleeding under the skin occurs. There are also occasional reports of more frequent bleeding from the oral mucosa or heavy menses in females.[13]

Anesthesia providers should be aware that patients with immune thrombocytopenia who present for surgery do pose an increased risk of major surgical and anesthetic challenges in maintenance of hemostasis to ensure prevention of severe hemorrhage. There are multiple modalities for prophylactic treatment, including use of corticosteroids, various chemotherapeutic agents, and IV immunoglobulin therapy.[14]

The preoperative evaluation of patients with thrombocytopenia consists of first a thorough history and physical examination. Key questions that must be elicited during health history include any hematologic concerns or past diagnoses, increased or decreased coagulation, cancer, or a history of hematopoietic stem cell transplant. Review of pertinent labs would include a complete blood count, a reticulocyte count, peripheral blood smear, a type and crossmatch for blood products, and screening for direct antiglobulin test (DAT), HIV, or hepatitis C.[15]

There are various pharmacologic interventions for preoperative preparation in order to safely raise and maintain a patient's platelet count. Generally speaking, the life span of platelets once transfused is approximately 48 to 230 minutes, which is shortened from the normal half-life of platelets of approximately 4 days. In patients diagnosed with immune thrombocytopenia, the safe platelet thresholds may be lowered, and the indications for platelet transfusion transition away from meeting the defined parameters of normal platelet counts. Instead, the only major indications for transfusing these patients are in order to cease a severe and potentially life-threatening bleed or in preparation for surgery within 1 to 2 hours prior to the start of the procedure.[16]

In patients who present with platelet counts less than 10 to 20×10^9/L, it is common to begin first-line treatment with immunoglobulin infusion (IVIG) or corticosteroids. When proceeding with IVIG as a treatment modality, it is important to be aware that an increase in platelet count may not be seen until 2 to 3 days following initiation of treatment; however, the effects of an increased platelet count can last for approximately 1 week following infusion. This may be very useful in preoperative management and surgical planning.[17]

If the platelets continue to decline, immunosuppression may be initiated to reduce the antibody levels in the blood. If the patient fails immunosuppressive therapy, there are thrombopoietic agents such as eltrombopag or an immunotherapeutic agent such as rituximab that may be initiated. Finally, splenectomy has historically been used as a treatment for immune thrombocytopenia; however, the utilization of this procedure as treatment for immune thrombocytopenia is losing popularity due to the invasive nature of the procedure and the demonstration of patients maintaining clinical stability with much lower platelet thresholds.[13]

In children diagnosed with hematologic disorders, including immune thrombocytopenia, the standard management for anesthesia is composed of a comprehensive preoperative evaluation, monitoring of respiratory status and full vital signs, including oxygen saturation, and induction of anesthesia with inhalation or IV techniques depending on the patient's age and comorbidities. Airway management and vascular access needs are dictated by the surgical procedure being performed, as well as the patient's general state of health and comorbidities.

The major anesthetic challenge in regard to patients with immune thrombocytopenia is perioperative bleeding and risk of hemorrhage. There is an increased bleeding risk as the age of the patient increases, as well as any time the platelet count is less than 10 to 20×10^9/L.[17] Of note, the presumed prolongation of bleeding time for patients with thrombocytopenia, and the subsequent severity of bleeding, is less than what is seen in patients with similar cytopenia, such as bone marrow failure. If there is prolonged bleeding that is not controllable with transfusion, recombinant factor VIIa (rFVIIa) has been utilized in hemorrhage that is refractory to platelet-enhancing therapies.[18]

HEMOPHILIA

Hemophilia A, a factor VIII deficiency, and hemophilia B, a factor IX deficiency, are X-linked bleeding disorders caused by genetic mutations. Hemophilia primarily affects males; however, females known as "carriers" may also exhibit clinical manifestations. The incidence of hemophilia A is 1 in 5,000 to 10,000 males, whereas hemophilia B is 1 in 25,000 to 30,000 males. Although hemophilia is generally inherited, sporadic cases are not uncommon. Other less common types of hemophilia include hemophilia C, also called inherited deficiency of factor XI (factor 11) or Rosenthal's syndrome, is an autosomal recessive disorder. Acquired coagulation factor deficiencies, or "acquired hemophilia", are caused by an autoantibody (often to factor VIII). The terms *acquired factor inhibitor* or *acquired factor deficiency* are preferable to avoid potentially mislabeling the patient as having hemophilia A or B.[19]

Hemophilia A and B are classified into mild, moderate, or severe, based on the residual or baseline factor activity level; this is expressed as a percent of normal or in international units (IU)/mL. Factor levels typically correlate with the degree of bleeding symptoms. Severe hemophilia is defined as less than 1% factor activity, which corresponds to <0.01 IU/mL. Moderate hemophilia is defined as a factor activity level ≥1% of normal and ≤5% of normal, corresponding to ≥0.01 and ≤0.05 IU/mL. Mild hemophilia is defined as a factor activity level greater than 5% of normal and less than 40% of normal (≥0.05 and <0.40 IU/mL). Individuals may also be classified as having mild hemophilia despite having a factor level of ≥40% if they share a genetic variant in the relevant factor with a family member who has hemophilia.[19] Typical symptoms may include bruising, soft tissue bleeding, mucosal bleeding, muscle or joint bleeding, prolonged bleeding with injury, or surgical procedures. Individuals with hemophilia can undergo any type of major surgery, if factor replacement is given and adequate hemostasis assured.

Female carriers have variable factor levels. Those with a factor activity level near or above 50% of normal are not expected to have a clinical bleeding disorder, and carrier status is also important for potential reproductive implications (i.e., risk to male children). Other female carriers may have factor activity levels less than 50% of normal and may have greater bleeding than unaffected relatives or matched controls.[19]

It is recommended that prior to surgical procedures, patients diagnosed with hemophilia have a physical examination and laboratory evaluation including inhibitor screening to identify newly developed inhibitors and/or determine the inhibitor titer. Considerations should be made about issues related to monitoring of factor replacement, such as turnaround time for factor assays within the institution or availability of appropriate bovine substrate-based chromogenic assays for individuals receiving emicizumab. Factor activity level must be assayed using a bovine substrate-based chromogenic assay because emicizumab interferes with aPTT-based factor VIII activity assays.[19]

It will depend on the procedure type and risk of bleeding to determine the desired factor level and duration of factor replacement therapy. This should be a collaboration between surgical and hematology providers. Consideration can be made for performing pharmacokinetic studies prior to a surgical intervention to determine the intervals to give short- or long-acting factor products postprocedurally. For mild hemophilia A patients, desmopressin (DDAVP) may be considered for minor procedures. DDAVP requires a "challenge" prior to the surgical date to determine the patient's response to achieve appropriate hemostatic levels. This needs to be done prior to the day of surgery since typically levels are obtained before the infusion and at 1 hour and 4 hours after the infusion.

FACTOR CORRECTION

When determining the desired preoperative factor level for major surgery, most recommendations, including the 2020 World Federation of Hemophilia (WFH) guideline, use a desired preoperative factor level of 80% to 100% for hemophilia A and 60% to 80% for hemophilia B, with postoperative levels gradually tapering to approximately 50% until the wound is healed (typically over a period of 10–14 days).

Hemophilia A

In patients diagnosed with hemophilia A (factor VIII deficiency) without an inhibitor, treatment includes administration of an initial dose of factor VIII of 50 units/kg to raise the factor VIII level to 100%. This calculation assumes a starting factor VIII activity level close to 0%, a desired factor activity level of 100%, and a distribution that remains primarily intravascular (volume of distribution of approximately 0.5 dL/kg). The dose equals the patient's weight (in kg) multiplied by the desired rise in factor VIII level (as a whole number, such that a desired level of 100% is entered as 100) multiplied by a factor that corrects for the volume of distribution (for factor VIII, this equals 0.5). The subsequent doses are given at intervals of approximately one half-life of the infused product for that patient, which is based on peak and trough levels. A typical half-life for standard factor VIII products is approximately 8 to 12 hours. Approximate half-lives for longer lasting factor VIII products range from 10 to 20 hours. Pharmacokinetic studies are helpful in determining when to administer the first subsequent factor doses postprocedurally. The factor levels should ideally be sent stat to the laboratory to help determine the following factor dosing and timing.

Another option is to give the initial factor VIII bolus followed by a continuous infusion. A dose of approximately 4 units/kg/hr of standard half-life factor VIII concentrate will often maintain the level initially achieved by the bolus infusion. This method offers the advantage of consistent levels, less frequent monitoring, and decreased factor utilization. Factor activity levels should be checked periodically during continuous infusion, with the interval determined by the previous level, dose adjustments, and clinical bleeding. Continuous infusions should not have an attached filter, and the factor product should only be mixed with normal saline. This should be done in close collaboration with the institution's hematology physicians.[19]

Hemophilia B

In patients diagnosed with hemophilia B (factor IX deficiency) without an inhibitor, treatment includes administration of an initial dose of factor IX of 100 to 120 units/kg (except Rebinyn) to raise the factor IX level to 100%. This calculation assumes a starting factor IX activity level close to 0%, a desired factor activity level of 100%, and a volume of distribution of approximately 1 dL/kg. The dose equals the patient's weight (in kg) multiplied by the desired rise in factor IX level (as a whole number, such that a desired factor level of 100% is entered as 100) multiplied by a factor that corrects for the volume of distribution (for factor IX, this equals approximately 1).[19] For factor IX products AlphaNine, Mononine, Ixinity, and Rebinyn, no additional calculations are needed (**Box 19.1**). The prescribing information for Rebinyn lists a dose of 40 units/kg or 80 units/kg depending on the severity of bleeding.

High-Titer Inhibitor

A bypassing product is generally the first choice in a patient with hemophilia A or B who has a high-titer inhibitor and requires treatment for bleeding or surgery. Activated factor

---

BOX 19.1 DOSING REGIMENS FOR THE TREATMENT OF HEMOPHILIA B WITHOUT AN INHIBITOR

- BeneFIX: Multiply by 1.4 for children (i.e., weight in kg × desired increase × 1.4) and 1.2 for adults.
- Rixubis: Multiply by 1.4 for children and by 1.1 for adults.
- Alprolix: Multiply by 1.6 (range, 1.4–1.67) for children; no additional calculations are needed for adults.
- Idelvion: No additional calculations are needed for children; for adults, multiply by 0.77.

VII (factor VIIa) can directly activate factor X, bypassing the need for factors VIII and IX. Commonly used are recombinant human factor VII (rFVIIa; including NovoSeven, NovoSeven RT, and SevenFact) and activated prothrombin complex concentrate (aPCC), such as FEIBA (factor VIII inhibitor bypassing agent; the only aPCC available in most settings). The rFVIIa products are also appropriate in individuals with hemophilia A who have critical bleeding while receiving emicizumab.[19]

Plasmapheresis may be useful in patients with a high-titer-inhibitor to acutely lower the inhibitor titer and allow transient use of replacement factor. This approach is generally reserved for an individual with life-threatening or limb-threatening bleeding and an inhibitor titer >5 BU for whom bypassing therapy is not effective or recombinant porcine factor VIII is not available.[19]

Low-Titer Inhibitor

A high-dose factor infusion may be effective in patients with hemophilia A or B and a low titer (<5 BU) or a low-responding inhibitor, as long as the patient does not have an infusion reaction to the replacement factor (reactions are more commonly seen with factor IX). High-dose factor may also be useful in patients with high-responding inhibitors currently at a low titer or a titer lowered by plasmapheresis, with the understanding that this is only likely to be effective for a limited time period (4–7 days) and is likely to induce anamnesis.[19]

Fresh Frozen Plasma/Cryoprecipitate

Patients in resource-poor settings may not have access to these factor products. In this situation, options include FFP, or, for those with hemophilia A, cryoprecipitate. Dosing is based on the factor concentration in the product, patient weight, and the desired factor level. One bag of cryoprecipitate is made from approximately 250 mL of FFP and contains approximately 70 to 80 units of factor VIII in a volume of 30 to 40 mL (concentration of factor VIII in cryoprecipitate, approximately 3–5 units/mL). One milliliter of FFP contains one unit of factor activity. A dose of 15 to 20 mL/kg will raise the factor VIII level by approximately 30% to 40% and the factor IX level by approximately 15% to 20% (different increases are due to different volumes of distribution of factors VIII and IX).[19]

Desmopressin

Patients with mild hemophilia A may have a sufficient increase in factor VIII activity level upon administration of desmopressin (DDAVP), which is a synthetic analog of vasopressin/antidiuretic hormone that lacks pressor activity. DDAVP promotes release of endogenous factor VIII. A DDAVP test dose should be performed before use in an invasive procedure to assure an adequate hemostatic response as described earlier. Mild hemophilia B cannot be treated with DDAVP because factor IX is not stored or released. Patients with mild hemophilia B are treated with factor IX or other hemostatic therapies, such as antifibrinolytic agents and/or topical therapies.[19]

DDAVP has antidiuretic activity and can cause hyponatremia, especially with prolonged use or excess free water intake. As a result, doses are often limited to once daily for three consecutive days and water intake is restricted. The serum sodium concentration is monitored in hospitalized individuals, especially those receiving more than one or two doses of DDAVP.

DDAVP can increase the factor VIII level twofold to fourfold. A patient with a baseline factor activity of 25% who has an increase to 50% may have adequate hemostasis with DDAVP in the setting of minor bleeding or procedures and thus avoid factor infusion. Tachyphylaxis may occur; the administration should be timed to provide the maximal response at the time of greatest bleeding risk while limiting the number of doses.[19]

Antifibrotic Agents

Antifibrinolytic agents (e.g., tranexamic acid and epsilon aminocaproic acid) are very useful for oral procedures because fibrinolysis is highly active on mucosal surfaces. These can be given orally, intravenously, or as a mouthwash; mouthwash should be restricted to older children and adults because it may be inadvertently swallowed by younger children. Antifibrinolytics can also be safely combined with factor replacement. A typical regimen is to give the first dose of the antifibrinolytic agent 2 hours before the procedure and continue for up to 7 to 10 days postprocedure. This recommendation is modified depending on the risk for bleeding. Neither tranexamic acid nor aminocaproic acid should be given simultaneously with an activated aPCC, as this will increase the risk of thromboembolism. If an antifibrinolytic agent and a Prothrombin complex concentrate (PCC) are used, they should be separated by at least 12 hours. Although there is some experience using tranexamic acid and rFVIIa together in the surgical setting, consultation with a hemophilia treatment center is advised. These agents are most useful for stabilizing clots in areas of increased fibrinolysis, such as the oral or nasal cavity (i.e., dental bleeding and epistaxis) or for heavy menstrual bleeding in women with bleeding disorders. Their mechanism of action is to inhibit fibrinolysis by inhibiting plasminogen activation in the fibrin clot, thereby enhancing clot stability.[19]

There are other adjunctive hemostatic therapies that can be considered for certain procedures, including microfibrillar collagen, especially for bleeding in the oral cavity, and fibrin glue, or gelatin granules, which have been used for circumcision procedures. Use of local coagulation enhancers may also be appropriate in certain types of procedures. Wound infiltration with local anesthetic agents (lidocaine and/or bupivacaine) with an adrenaline and fibrin sealant/spray is useful to control oozing when operating in extensive surgical fields.[19]

General anesthesia has been administered to hemophiliac patients with little risk of bleeding and with appropriate correction of clotting factors. However, regional anesthesia has traditionally been considered a contraindication. There are some studies which support limited use of regional anesthesia, peripheral nerve blocks, or neuraxial techniques. For neuraxial techniques the procedure may only be acceptable if serious reasons exist against general anesthesia. It is imperative that adequate hemostatic levels are maintained while the anesthesia is being administered to minimize risk of serious side effects of potential hematoma formation within the spinal canal, which can lead to cord compression and neurological deficits. However, in general, in patients with bleeding disorders the use of central neuraxial blocks, neither spinal nor epidural anesthesia, is preferable given the high risk of serious impairment. If it is determined regional and peripheral nerve blocks are to be given in a patient diagnosed with hemophilia, it is also crucial to optimize factor levels preoperatively to 100% of the normal level, intraoperatively and postoperatively with factor product to avoid bleeding and infection complications.[19–21]

Postoperative Management

Postoperatively, agents are administered to patients diagnosed with hemophilia A without inhibitors at intervals of approximately one half-life of the infused product for that patient. This dosing regimen is based on peak and trough levels. A typical half-life for standard half-life factor VIII products is approximately 8 to 12 hours. Approximate half-lives for longer lasting factor VIII products range from 10 to 20 hours. Issues related to the use of longer lasting products for surgical procedures are essentially the same as for standard half-life products and include use of appropriate monitoring assays for levels and assurance of adequate hemostatic levels. Using longer lasting products may reduce the number of infusions needed during and after procedures, depending on the product, the patient, and the individual half-life. It is important to use an assay for factor activity that is tailored to the specific factor being used.[19]

In a patient diagnosed with hemophilia A with an inhibitor who is using bypassing therapy, there is no coagulation test that reflects clinical efficacy; therefore, laboratory monitoring of factor activity levels is not used. For pateints who have been receiving emicizumab, a bovine substrate-based chromogenic factor VIII assay must be used. In patients with hemophilia A without an inhibitor, factor infusion is recommended to maintain the factor level above the threshold determined necessary for the location and severity of bleeding. If there is unexpected postoperative bleeding, it is important to obtain an immediate factor level and consider the possibility that bleeding may be due to an anatomical or mechanical cause if adequate hemostatic factor levels are documented.

Managing breakthrough bleeding or surgery in individuals with inhibitors who are receiving emicizumab is complicated by the risk of unusual thrombotic events and thrombotic microangiopathy (TMA) when an aPCC (FEIBA) at doses >100 units/kg within 1 day or for more than 1 day was used in conjunction with emicizumab; prescribing information carries a Boxed Warning for this risk. If an aPCC is needed to treat breakthrough bleeding while receiving emicizumab, the aPCC dose should be kept below 100 units/kg in a 24-hour period; the patient should be monitored closely for thrombosis and TMA; and if one of these complications occurs the aPCC should be discontinued.[19]

In patients with hemophilia B without inhibitors the second and subsequent doses are given at intervals of approximately one half-life of the infused product for that patient, also based on peak and trough levels. A typical half-life for standard half-life factor IX products is approximately 18 to 24 hours. Approximate half-lives for longer lasting factor IX products range from 54 to 104 hours. These doses will be approximately half the initial dose and will be guided by the patient's measured factor level and the desired peak level.[19]

Another option is to give the initial factor IX bolus followed by a continuous infusion. A dose of approximately 6 units/kg/hr of standard half-life factor IX concentrate will often maintain the level initially achieved by bolus infusion. This method offers the advantage of consistent levels, less frequent monitoring, and decreased factor utilization. Factor activity levels should be checked periodically during continuous infusion, with the interval determined by the previous level, dose adjustments, and clinical bleeding. Continuous infusions should not have an attached filter, and the factor product should only be mixed with normal saline.[19]

As noted earlier, subsequent factor dosing for patients receiving bolus doses of factor should incorporate information on the patient's peak and trough factor activity levels (or steady-state levels for those receiving continuous infusion) rather than a set schedule without monitoring. This is because individual pharmacokinetics vary and can significantly impact factor half-life and ultimate hemostasis. Patient characteristics such as the volume of distribution and recovery may be altered by individual handling of drugs and body fat content.[19] The peak factor activity level should be checked approximately 5 to 15 minutes after the first dose. For major life-threatening bleeding, the trough is checked at approximately 4 to 6 hours for factor VIII and 8 to 12 hours for factor IX. Slightly longer intervals before the first trough level may be used for less serious bleeding.[19]

Patients diagnosed with hemophilia B with inhibitors vary slightly, as the WFH has no preference for the type of factor IX products used for patients with a low-responding inhibitor, but more frequent dosing is recommended due to factor IX short half-life. Also in patients with inhibitors undergoing surgery, the WFH recommends giving rFVIIa over aPCC, which can worsen allergic reactions.[21]

VENOUS THROMBOEMBOLISM

VTE is associated with surgical procedures and has been reported in patients diagnosed with hemophilia. Intensive replacement with PCC in hemophilia B can result in cumulative factors XI, VII, and X, which can be associated with higher risk of development of VTE. Mechanical thromboprophylaxis should be considered in patients at higher risk of development of VTE. There is usually no need for deep vein thrombosis prophylaxis in patients undergoing arthroplasty under factor coverage unless very high plasma levels are maintained during the postoperative period.[21]

VASCULAR ACCESS

Some pediatric patients with poor venous access may have a central venous catheter in place for their prophylactic regimen at the time of their surgical procedure. It is important that the family have sufficient supplies and training on discharge to avoid readmission for infection. Access should be a consideration if long-term factor replacement is needed in a patient postprocedure. The risks and benefits of associated with placement of a peripherally inserted central catheter (PICC) should be considered. For pediatric patients discharged from the hospital on factor replacement, if the family has not been trained or is not comfortable with venous access, home healthcare nursing needs to be arranged, or if this is not feasible then arrangements with the Hemostasis and Thrombosis Treatment Center (HTC) clinic to provide factor infusions until course is completed.

APLASTIC ANEMIA

Aplastic anemia is a rare disorder of the hematopoietic stem cells that results in hypocellular bone marrow and pancytopenia due to immune injury. This results from a variety of insults, including both congenital marrow failure disorders and acquired aplastic anemia.[22] The vast majority of cases of aplastic anemia are considered idiopathic because the primary etiology is unknown.[23] With acquired aplastic anemia, the trigger for destruction of hematopoietic stem cells is deemed to be an immune-mediated response to potential exposures in the environment, such as viruses, toxins, or certain drugs. This exposure results in anemia, neutropenia, and thrombocytopenia.[22]

If there is concern for aplastic anemia, obtaining a thorough history and physical examination is essential in the diagnosis and management of these patients, as well as in preparation for any future medical or surgical interventions that may be warranted.[22] Patients diagnosed with aplastic anemia often present with pallor, fatigue, hemorrhaging of the skin or mucosal tissue, retinal hemorrhaging, or are occasionally found to have frequent infections. Chronic anemia is typically demonstrated with fatigue, reports of decreased activity level or intolerance to exercise, or bruising resulting from minimal traumas that are slow to resolve. Clinical management of aplastic anemia is dependent on length of symptoms and severity of patient presentation.[24] Any medical or surgical intervention that is required in the management of these patients should only be done after optimization of clinical status perioperatively. Due to the rarity of the disease as well as the confounding factors of pancytopenia and the required immunosuppression, anesthetic management can be challenging in patients with aplastic anemia.[22]

Patients with aplastic anemia are at very high risk of surgical complications, especially in the perioperative period.[25] Regardless of the severity of the patient's symptoms, the presence of pancytopenia places the patient at increased risk of surgical complication and therefore increased challenges with anesthesia.[22] Preoperative optimization of the patient's clinical status is essential prior to any surgical procedure to avoid perioperative complications. Involvement of a multidisciplinary team with the inclusion of a hematologist, as well as readily available access to blood products from a well-equipped blood bank, is paramount in formulating an appropriate plan for management of these patients.

The acquisition of a thorough health history and investigation of clinical symptoms will be most beneficial in guiding the management plan of patients with aplastic anemia in preparation for procedures requiring anesthesia. Questioning the patient about a history of hematologic disorders, such as decreased or increased coagulation, anemia, thrombocytopenia, or any history of cancer or hematopoietic stem cell transplant, would be important in developing plan of care.[22] A comprehensive history of exposure to medications or environmental hazards should be taken, and if warranted any putative agent should be discontinued as quickly as able after identification. Generally speaking, there is no single screening laboratory test to assess the risk of bleeding in a child with aplastic anemia in the perioperative period.[22]

In patients with aplastic anemia, general anesthesia is deemed the only appropriate technique due to the contraindication of thrombocytopenia to regional anesthesia.[25] A laryngeal mask airway (LMA) may be utilized to avoid any trauma. Assuring that any anesthetic induction is atraumatic to prevent any possible bleeding is essential.[26]

It is paramount to adhere to strict aseptic precautions for all surgical and anesthetic components of care to prevent infection in these neutropenic patients. Any patient presenting for procedure who is deemed severely neutropenic, or with a white blood cell count of less than $0.5 \times 10^9/L$, should be placed in isolation and prophylactic antibiotic and antifungal medications should be prescribed. Patient education to promote infection prevention should also include regular oral care with antiseptic mouthwash and consumption of food low in bacterial content.[26] Postoperative management consists of providing adequate pain relief, and choice of pharmacologic agent is dependent on patient and provider preferences, although the use of IV tramadol for postoperative pain relief is a common practice.[27] Provision of adequate pain relief will allow patients to participate in airway clearance exercises, such as deep breathing and incentive spirometry, in order to avoid pulmonary complications. Successful clinical management of patients with aplastic anemia can be achieved by prevention of infection and assuring access to blood products as necessary.[27]

SICKLE CELL DISEASE

SCD is an inherited red blood cell disorder with multisystem complications, often presenting in childhood.[28] SCD affects millions of people throughout the world and approximately 100,000 Americans, occurring in about 1 in 365 Black or African American births and 1 in 16,300 Hispanic American births. This autosomal recessive sickle mutation causes a reduction, or full destruction, of the ability to produce normal beta globin and therefore results in a sickled hemoglobin (HbS). While hemolytic anemia and vaso-occlusion are major features of SCD, sickle cell anemia (SCA) is the most common and severe form.[29] The spectrum of SCD includes SCA, sickle cell/hemoglobin C (HbSC), sickle cell/B-thalassemia (HbS β-thalassemia), as well as several other uncommon variants.[30] With a number of other disease forms, the clinical manifestations of SCD in pediatric patients can present with a variety of multisystem complications.

HbS production causes the red blood cells to become hard and sticky and look like a "sickle" farm tool. These sickled cells become stuck as they travel throughout the body, causing common clinical symptoms such as pain crises, infection, acute chest syndrome (ACS), renal insufficiency, osteonecrosis, and cholelithiasis. Chronic anemia leads to long-term complications including, but not limited to, pulmonary hypertension, end-stage renal disease, and neurological disease causing significant morbidity and mortality.[2] With significant variation in severity of symptoms, every patient with SCD has a progressive clinical journey.[30] Vaso-occlusive episodes are a result of recurrent microvasculature occlusions most commonly in the phalanges, long bones, ribs, sternum, spine, and pelvis. ACS presents as acute respiratory symptoms along with a new infiltrate on chest x-ray and frequently occurs 2 to 3 days after a pain crisis. Infection is common due to immune system deficits and functional asplenia developed after splenic atrophy and dysfunction occur early in life. Stroke and other central nervous system (CNS) complications are some of the most devastating sequelae; pain crises, infection, and ACS often precipitate them. Acute and chronic renal failure may present due to renal abnormalities, such as proteinuria, hematuria, and renal tubular acidosis.

Hematologists manage patients with SCD while surgeons and anesthesia providers manage the perioperative experience (Table 19.1). Individual disease-related manifestations dictate the perioperative management. Preoperative care is individualized; however, the goal remains to maintain optimal physiologic parameters. It is imperative anesthesia providers avoid factors that may precipitate a sickle cell, optimize pain management, and consult closely with hematology and surgeons.

Pain management with judicious use of analgesics is essential since perioperative vaso-occlusive pain is common and associated with ACS. Transfusions prevent perioperative complications and allow for correction of anemia, dilution of sickled cells, compensation for blood loss, and prevention of some complications. While some patients may require exchange transfusions due to their history, a target hemoglobin concentration of 10 g/dL via simple transfusion is the goal for moderate and complicated operations.[30] Dehydration should be avoided and intravenous fluids for varying degrees of renal dysfunction should be considered, as well as use during fasting states.

Table 19.1	Perioperative Considerations in Patients With Sickle Cell Disease
Preoperative Considerations	• Screen if unknown SCD status in at-risk children • History of SCD sequelae • Neurologic assessment • History of analgesic and other medication use • Hematocrit • Oxygen saturation, chest radiograph • Pulmonary function test (when appropriate) • Practice incentive spirometry at home • Echocardiogram (when appropriate) • Neurologic imaging (for recent changes) • Renal function studies
	• Transfusion crossmatch (e.g., antibody-matched, leukocyte-reduced, sickle-negative) • Transfusion to correct anemia • Parenteral hydration when NPO • Pain management • Aggressive bronchodilator therapy • Antibiotic therapy, including presplenectomy antibiotics and immunizations
Intraoperative Considerations	• Maintain oxygenation, perfusion, normal acid–base status, temperature, hydration • Replacement of blood loss with appropriately prepared blood • Appropriate antibiotic therapy • Appropriate analgesic techniques for procedure both intra- and post-operatively • Use of tourniquets, cell save, and cardiopulmonary bypass
Postoperative Considerations	• Primary management by hematology • Monitor for complications, especially acute chest syndrome and vaso-occlusive pain crises • Prophylactic supplemental oxygen in the first 24 hours regardless of oxygen saturation, monitoring of oxygen saturation and supplementation needed • Hydration (oral plus parenteral) • Antibiotic therapy • Aggressive pain management—ensure ability to breathe deep and perform incentive spirometry

SCD, sickle cell disease.

Anesthetics management should be appropriate to the procedure and clinical status of the patient. When anesthetizing this patient population, consider the progressive vasculature damage, pulmonary hypertension, and activation of coagulation from chronic hemolysis regardless of type of procedure. Intubation may be difficult for patients with maxillofacial bony abnormalities. Techniques should avoid factors that may promote intravascular sickling: hypoxia, acidosis, hyperthermia, hypothermia, and dehydration. Some commonly used agents in general anesthesia may have altered pharmacokinetics, such as atracurium.[31] It is widely understood that inhalation anesthetics do not affect the sickling process. Sickle cell patients report more pain and use more morphine postoperatively; regional anesthesia may be effective to manage postoperative pain.[32] Adequate analgesia is an important factor, as well as early incentive spirometry use, supplemental oxygen, bronchodilator therapy, and antibiotics, to reduce the incidence of ACS.[33]

KEY TAKEAWAYS

- Discussion with the hematology provider prior to procedures necessitating anesthesia is beneficial to help anticipate the needs of pediatric patients with hematologic conditions.
- Basic preoperative bloodwork (blood counts and coagulation studies) can reveal unknown hematologic disorders worth working up prior to procedures.
- Anesthetic management and techniques that prevent bleeding are the most beneficial to this patient population.

KEY REFERENCES

Complete references for this chapter are online and available at https://connect.springerpub.com/content/book/978-0-8261-3875-0/part/part03/toc-part/ch019.

3. Thachil J. Disseminated intravascular coagulation. *Anesthesiology*. 2016;125(1):230–236.
20. Englbrecht J, Pogatzki-Zahn E, Zahn P. Spinal and epidural anesthesia in patients with hemorrhagic diasthesis: decisions on the brink of minimum evidence? *Anaethesist*. 2011;60(12): 1126–1134.
31. Akrimi S, Simiyu V. Anaesthetic management of children with sickle cell disease. *BJA Educ*. 2018;18(11):331-336. doi:https://dx.doi.org/10.1016/j.bjae.2018.08.003
32. Adams TL, Latham GJ, Eisses MJ, et al. Essentials of Hematology. In *A Practice of Anesthesia for Infants and Children*. Elsevier; 2019:217–239.e218.
34. Firth PG. Anesthesia and hemoglobinopathies. *Anesthesiol Clin*. 2009;27(2):321–336. doi:10.1016/j.anclin.2009.05.001
37. Hutton B, Burry LD, Kanji S, et al. Comparison of sedation strategies for critically ill patients: A protocol for a systematic review incorporating network meta-analyses. *Syst Rev*. 2016;5(1).
38. Sripada R, Reyes J, Sun R. Peripheral nerve blocks for intraoperative management in patients with hemophilia A. *J Clin Anesth*. 2008;20(2):120–3.

CHAPTER 20

Oncologic-Bone Marrow Transplantation Conditions

Katrina Richardson, Rachael Mohr, and Steffani Maier

> **LEARNING OBJECTIVES**
> - Provide an overview of common pediatric oncologic diagnoses, the associated complications, and the side effects of treatment.
> - Review bone marrow transplantation and associated risks and complications.
> - Offer recommendations to help guide the management of pediatric oncologic patients requiring anesthesia.

INTRODUCTION

Pediatric patients with cancer and those undergoing hematopoietic stem cell transplant (HSCT) have unique needs and often develop complications from the therapy they receive. Most treatments used in the treatment of cancer and those involved with HSCT weaken the immune system, placing these children at high risk of infections, serious side effects, and potentially life-threatening complications. It is imperative anesthesia providers have a comprehensive understanding of the various oncologic diagnoses pediatric patients may present with, as well as the complications that often develop during treatment of their disease, to ensure a safe and effective anesthetic plan is developed.

COMMON PEDIATRIC ONCOLOGIC DIAGNOSES

While a wide array of childhood cancers are diagnosed every day in the United States the most common oncologic diagnoses are leukemias and lymphomas, followed closely by the diagnosis of brain tumors and various solid tumors. The management of patients who have undergone a bone marrow transplant is discussed later in this chapter.

Leukemias and lymphomas represent roughly 35% of childhood cancers, with the most common being pre-B-cell acute lymphoblastic leukemia. Patients presenting with childhood leukemia and lymphoma often exhibit some, if not all, of the following symptoms: lymphadenopathy, fever, pallor, bone pain, limp, refusal to bear weight, bleeding, excessive bruising, or respiratory or hemodynamic symptoms secondary to the presence of a mediastinal mass. Leukemias are typically initially discovered by the presence of blast cells on a complete blood count (CBC), although additional tests employed during diagnosis may include bone marrow aspirate and biopsy, immunophenotyping by flow cytometry, cytochemistry, and fluorescent in situ hybridization (FISH) of various genetic markers of leukemia, which allows for visualization and mapping of genetic material in an individual's cells, including specific genes or portions of genes. A lumbar puncture may be performed to determine if leukemia has spread to the cerebral spinal fluid (CSF). See Chapter 110, "Lumbar Puncture," for additional information on anesthesia for lumbar puncture.

Treatment of childhood leukemia most often consists of chemotherapy, including IV, intrathecal, and oral anticancer medications. Novel therapies, such as CAR-T therapy, which employs T-cells engineered to express chimeric antigen receptors (CARs) that specifically recognize the target antigen resulting in T-cell activation, are also being used as the initial treatment of blood cancers or in relapse settings. Anesthesia providers should be aware that treatment protocols for patients diagnosed with leukemia often last up to 3 years following the initial diagnoses.[1,2]

Brain tumors represent about 25% of childhood cancers. The most common brain tumors in the pediatric population are medulloblastomas and astrocytomas (both low- and high-grade). Presenting symptoms vary depending on the area of the brain involved and the age of the patient. Symptoms commonly include headaches, seizures, cranial nerve deficits, issues with coordination, and muscle weakness.[3] Chemotherapy, surgery, and radiation (including proton therapy) are the most common therapies employed to treat brain tumors in children.

Approximately 35% to 40% of pediatric tumors are considered non-central nervous system (CNS) solid tumors. These consist of bone and soft tissue sarcomas (most commonly osteosarcoma and Ewing's sarcoma), kidney and liver tumors, neuroblastoma, retinoblastoma, and other rare tumors. Presenting symptoms are often specific to what type of area or organ the cancer is invading. Many pediatric patients with non-CNS solid tumors present with pain secondary to an injury or fracture to the bone involved, nausea, hematuria, abnormal appearance of the eye, refusal to walk/bear weight, fevers, fatigue, or anorexia. Treatment of these types of tumors can consist of chemotherapy, radiation (including proton therapy), surgery, immunotherapy, or high-dose chemotherapy with autologous stem cell rescue.

ANESTHESIA CONSIDERATIONS

STEROID ADMINISTRATION

Anesthesia providers should refrain from administration of any steroids before talking to the oncology or primary team, as administration of steroids may interfere with the treatment regimen. Conversely, some patients may already be receiving steroids as part of their treatment plan, necessitating alterations to standard dosing regimens. Glucocorticoids have many valuable roles in various chemotherapy treatment plans. In acute lymphoblastic leukemia in particular, glucocorticoids have a significant part in the treatment plan. They function by attaching to glucocorticoid receptors, which eventually inhibit cytokine production by changing the expression of oncogenes, which in turn kills the cancer cells.[1] If glucocorticoids are given prior to a lymphoblastic leukemia diagnosis, it can have a negative effect on prognosis. High-risk features—in particular, an elevated white blood cell count—could be masked by the use of glucocorticoids. There can also be a potential partial treatment response, which can result in eventual disease resistance.[2]

For children with brain tumors, the glucocorticoid dexamethasone is often used to decrease edema. Swelling can cause significant symptoms, depending on where the peritumoral edema is located. Without glucocorticoid treatment, patients can experience symptoms such as headaches, nausea, vomiting, hemiparesis, and/or aphasia.[3]

Glucocorticoids are most often used as antiemetics for patients with non-CNS solid tumors. Side effects from long-term use of glucocorticoids, as well as abruptly stopping them, can lead to adrenal insufficiency.

NAUSEA AND VOMITING

Despite the use of antiemetic medications, nausea and/or vomiting are the most common side effects of most cancer therapies, particularly chemotherapy. Chemotherapeutic agents are classified by the level of emetogenicity: minimal, low, medium, and high. This classification system can help anesthesia providers predict the severity of nausea and vomiting a patient may experience based on current treatment regimen. Patients requiring general anesthesia while being treated with chemotherapeutic agents have both a higher incidence and increased intensity of nausea and vomiting and should be considered to be at high risk of aspiration following emesis.[4]

PAIN

Pain management in patients diagnosed with childhood cancer can often be challenging as there may be multiple sites or sources of pain. Common sources of pain include pain secondary to radiation therapy, mucositis, phantom limb pain postamputation, and pain related to tumor or disease burden.[5] Narcotics are often the first-line therapy for pain treatment secondary to childhood cancer as the use of acetaminophen is avoided as it may potentially mask a fever in an immune-compromised patient or contribute to hepatic injury. Furthermore, the efficacy of nonnarcotic medications is often limited with patients presenting with cancer-related pain. Anesthesia providers should consider the current pain management regimen being employed when developing a plan to temper postoperative pain.

Neuropathic pain secondary to the administration of chemotherapeutic agents is common, especially following the administration of vincristine. Vincristine, which inhibits polymerization of tubulin, and incorporation into microtubules, thereby preventing mitotic spindle assembly and leading to extension of mitosis and apoptosis, is used in the treatment of a wide variety of diagnoses (Table 20.1). The use of vincristine leads to axonopathy, and its use is typically limited by progressive vincristine-induced neuropathy, possibly including both peripheral sensory and motor nerves, autonomic nervous functions, and the CNS.

Neuropathic pain may also be secondary to tumors compressing or invading the nerves, or due to surgical resection needed to remove tumors. This type of pain, which could be acute or chronic, is typically described as numbness, tingling, shooting sensation, and sensitivity to cold or hot. Gabapentinoids are often first-line treatment, as well as tricyclic antidepressants and serotonin–norepinephrine intake receptive inhibitors, as narcotics often prove ineffective.[5]

HEMATOPOIETIC STEM CELL TRANSPLANT

The first successful hematopoietic stem cell transplant (HSCT) occurred in 1968 on a pediatric patient suffering from severe combined immunodeficiency syndrome.[6] Since then, the use of allogeneic and autologous transplants has grown substantially. The Center for International Blood and Marrow Transplant Research (CIBMTR) reports that over 22,000 HSCTs were performed in 2017.[7] The process of

Table 20.1	Types of Vincristine-Induced Neuropathy	
Type	**Definition**	**Symptoms**
Sensory neuropathy	Sensory nerve damage	Paresthesia in the form of numbness, tingling, and pricking; pain, impaired vibration/touch sensitivity/temperature recognition
Motor neuropathy	Motor nerve damage	Motor weakness, walking difficulties, muscle cramps, weakened tendon reflexes and fine motor skills
Autonomic neuropathy	Autonomic nerve damage	Constipation, ileus, urinary retention, incontinence, hypotension
Optic neuropathy	Cranial nerve II damage	Blurred vision, color vision deficiency, transient/permanent blindness
Ocular nerve palsy	Cranial nerve III damage	Ptosis, ophthalmoplegia
Abducens nerve palsy	Cranial nerve VI damage	Ptosis, strabismus, ocular muscle paresis, diplopia
Facial nerve palsy	Cranial nerve VII damage	Limited movement of facial muscles and jaw
Acoustic nerve palsy	Cranial nerve VIII damage	Hearing loss
Ototoxicity	Cochlear damage	Decrease in frequencies, decrease of contralateral suppression amplitudes
Hypoglossal nerve palsy	Cranial nerve XII damage	Loss of tongue movement
Vocal cord palsy	Laryngeal nerve damage	Stridor, respiratory distress, persistent cough
Encephalopathy/PRES	Cerebral dysfunction	Disorientation, hemiplegia, global aphasia, seizures
SIADH	Cerebral axonal swelling	Hyponatremia, seizures, mental changes

PRES, posterior reversible encephalopathy syndrome; SIADH, syndrome of inappropriate antidiuretic hormone secretion.

Source: From Madsen ML, Due H, Ejskjær N, et al. Aspects of vincristine-induced neuropathy in hematologic malignancies: a systematic review. *Cancer Chemother Pharmacol.* 2019;84(3):471–485. doi:10.1007/s00280-019-03884-5.

HSCT involves the infusion of normal hematopoietic stem cells into a patient whose bone marrow is dysfunctional or depleted.[6] Once infused, the new cells expand in the recipient's marrow and replace the diseased or dysfunctional cells. When successful, HSCT can prolong the life of and cure those suffering from a variety of malignant and nonmalignant diseases. The donated hematopoietic cells may originate from a family member, an unrelated matched donor or a mismatched donor (allogenic donor), or the marrow can be collected from the patient and reinfused once processing is complete (autologous donor). Stem cells may be collected by a variety of methods, including bone marrow harvest, from peripheral blood draw, or from previously collected and stored cord blood.

Prior to HSCT, the recipient must go through conditioning or a preparative regimen, which may include the administration of chemotherapy, irradiation, monoclonal antibodies, or targeted therapy.[8] The purpose of conditioning is to allow for destruction of malignant cells and immunosuppression in the recipient so that engraftment can occur. The preparative regimen prescribed to the patient may involve high-dose chemotherapy with or without irradiation (myeloablative regimen) or, to reduce organ toxicity, a reduced-intensity regimen may be preferred. The type of preparative regimen the patient receives is dependent on many factors, such as the disease type (malignant or nonmalignant), comorbidities, and transplant type (allogenic or autologous). Complications and risk of HSCT are variable and are dependent on many factors.

HEMATOPOIETIC STEM CELL TRANSPLANT-RELATED COMPLICATIONS

Fever and Infection

Fever is considered an emergency for patients undergoing cancer treatment or HSCT. Infections have been found to be responsible for up to 30% of patient deaths in the first 100 days post-HSCT and up to 40% of patient deaths after day 100.[9] Invasive fungal infections account for most deaths due to infection, followed by bacterial infections.[9] There are many contributing factors that place these patients at an increased risk of infection, including profound neutropenia (absolute neutrophil count below 500), hypogammaglobulinemia, lymphopenia, prolonged use of a central venous catheter, or translocation of bacteria through injured oral and gut tissue.[9,10] In addition, oncology patients often have surgical wounds related to tumor resection, placing them at an increased risk of infection. Patients suffering from graft-versus-host disease (GVHD) related to HSCT are also at an increased risk of infection due to prolonged administration of immunosuppressive agents required for treatment.

Once a patient undergoing HSCT or chemotherapy develops a fever (defined as a temperature of >100.4 °F), prompt evaluation and management are key. Blood cultures should be collected, as well as CBC, complete metabolic panel (CMP), lactate, and procalcitonin. Broad-spectrum cephalosporins with Gram-negative coverage should be initiated. If and when bacteria are identified on blood cultures, central line removal may be pursued as a definitive treatment for sepsis. Postoperatively, it is important anesthesia providers do not administer either acetaminophen or ibuprofen without consulting the primary team. Tylenol can mask a fever, and ibuprofen may have an effect on platelet function, resulting in increased bleeding.[13]

Prophylactic Treatment of Fevers

Prophylactic anti-infective agents are administered to oncology patients receiving chemotherapy and early in the HSCT stages to minimize the incidence of neutropenic fevers, severe infections, and sepsis. Antibacterial prophylaxis with fluoroquinolones is the most common as they provide adequate Gram-negative coverage while offering a more tolerable side effect profile than other antibiotics. In some instances, oral third-generation cephalosporins may be used as an alternative to fluoroquinolones.[11] Oral trimethoprim-sulfamethoxazole may be administered for protection against *Pneumocystis jiroveci*. Patients undergoing HSCT as well as some patients with leukemia are at an increased risk of invasive fungal disease caused by yeast and molds. Infections with *Candida* and *Aspergillus* species are the most common among fungal infections.[12] Antifungal prophylaxis using oral fluconazole has been shown to decrease the risk of invasive fungal disease.[6,11]

Viral reactivation can be potentially devastating to HSCT recipients in particular and therefore, prophylactic antivirals are typically prescribed to minimize this risk. Routine monitoring of viral pathogens can be achieved through collection of blood or plasma. Quantification using polymerase chain reaction (PCR) should be monitored for viruses in which prophylactic agents are unavailable, including adenovirus, Epstein–Barr virus (EBV), and BK virus. Considerations for treatment in patients who experience severe viremias include reduction in immunosuppression, antiviral treatments such as rituximab for EBV viremia, ganciclovir or foscarnet for Cytomegalovirus (CMV) viremia, cidofovir for adenoviremia, and virus-specific cytotoxic T-cell (CTL) infusions.[11]

Sinusoidal Obstructive Syndrome

Hepatic sinusoidal obstructive syndrome (SOS), also known as veno-occlusive disease, is a potentially life-threatening complication for those undergoing HSCT and typically occurs within 4 weeks of transplant. SOS develops when injury has occurred to the liver sinusoidal endothelium, which leads to platelet activation and clot formation. Over time, this results in obstruction of sinusoidal flow and eventual tissue death.[14] SOS has been associated with patients who receive myeloablative conditioning regimens or regimens containing alkylating agents pretransplant (busulfan and cyclophosphamide are the most commonly seen agents) or with patients who have chronic medical conditions related to prior disease management, such as acute or chronic hepatitis/severe liver injury, abdominal irradiation, high-dose total body irradiation, or sepsis post-HSCT.[6,15] Clinically, the patient will complain of abdominal pain associated with new-onset weight gain, ascites, and jaundice. Lab work will demonstrate platelet refractoriness to transfusions and rising bilirubin, and hepatomegaly and reversal of portal venous flow will be witnessed on Doppler ultrasound.[6,15]

Ursodeoxycholic acid may be used to protect the liver against SOS, and in some high-risk patients intravenous (IV) defibrotide prophylaxis is employed.[6,15] Ursodeoxycholic acid is a naturally occurring hydrophilic bile acid that functions to reduce the fraction of potentially hepatotoxic hydrophobic bile acids in the hepatobiliary system. Defibrotide is a polydisperse oligonucleotide with antithrombotic, anti-ischemic, and anti-inflammatory activity at the level of the microvasculature and is the only agent with a proven efficacy for treatment of severe/very severe SOS.[14]

In addition to hepatic injury and risk of liver failure, these patients are at risk of multiorgan dysfunction or failure and have an increased risk of bleeding due to associated coagulopathy. Blood coagulation factors, hemoglobin, and platelet counts should be monitored and corrected prior to any invasive procedures; defibrotide should be discontinued at least 2 hours prior to any invasive procedure.[16] Preprocedure planning, such as ensuring irradiated blood products are ordered, processed, and ready to be transfused in case of acute uncontrolled bleeding during an operative procedure, allows for the safe care of a patient diagnosed with SOS.

Thrombotic Microangiopathy

Transplant-associated thrombotic microangiopathy (TA-TMA) is a potentially fatal complication of HSCT that can manifest as a multisystem disease after small vessel endothelial injury leads to subsequent tissue damage in different organs.[17] While the kidneys are most often affected, in patients presenting with renal manifestations such as decreased glomerular filtration rate, proteinuria, and hypertension, TA-TMA can affect the lungs, bowel, heart, and brain. TA-TMA belongs to a group of disorders that present with complement system dysregulation, which leads to uncontrolled complement activation on cell surfaces, resulting in cellular injury. Laboratory manifestations include elevated lactate dehydrogenase, schistocytes on blood smear, thrombocytopenia and anemia requiring transfusions, hypertension, proteinuria, and terminal complement activation with an elevated SC5b-9.[17]

Preoperative considerations include evaluation for anemia and thrombocytopenia and transfusion with packed red bleed cells (PRBCs) and platelets as needed. Patients with TA-TMA require aggressive blood pressure management to limit the negative impact on organ function. The cessation of antihypertensives prior to anesthesia should be discussed with the HSCT team. Patients with TA-TMA can also have pulmonary hypertension within the spectrum of clinical manifestations, which predisposes them to catastrophic cardiorespiratory compromise while under anesthesia. It is recommended echocardiography is performed in patients with TA-TMA preoperatively to ensure the patient does not have pulmonary hypertension.

Graft-Versus-Host Disease

GVHD occurs following HSCT when immune cells present in donor tissue attack the host's own tissues. The pathophysiology of GVHD has been described as a three-step process. In the first step, the conditioning regimen leads to damage and activation of the host tissues, affecting primarily the intestinal mucosa. This damage allows the translocation of lipopolysaccharide (LPS) from the intestinal lumen to the circulation, which stimulates the secretion of the inflammatory cytokines tumor necrosis factor-alpha and interleukin-1 from the host tissue. In the second step, donor T-cell activation is characterized by the predominance of T-helper type 1 (Th1) cells and the secretion of interferon gamma (INFγ), which activates mononuclear phagocytes. In the third step, the activated mononuclear phagocytes are triggered by the secondary signal provided by LPS and other stimulator molecules that leak through the intestinal mucosa that was damaged in in the first and second steps. Activated macrophages and CTLs secrete inflammatory cytokines that damage target cells. The damage from the inflammatory cytokines to the intestinal mucosa amplifies LPS release and leads to a cytokine storm that is characteristic of severe acute GVHD. The damage to tissue continues to create an inflammatory response and further release of inflammatory cytokines.[19]

GVHD is a major cause of morbidity and mortality after allogeneic HSCT and is the leading cause of late nonrelapse mortality following an allogeneic HSCT.[18] Patients are at a greater risk of developing GVHD if their donor is a human leukocyte antigen mismatched to the recipient or if they receive a myeloablative conditioning regimen or peripheral blood stem cells as their stem cell source.[20] GVHD is traditionally classified by the time of clinical manifestation, with acute GVHD occurring within the first 100 days after HSCT and chronic GVHD occurring after 100 days post-HSCT.[19] GVHD is also graded based on its effect on the organ systems, with acute GVHD often impacting the skin, liver, and gastrointestinal tract. Chronic GVHD can further affect the musculoskeletal system, contributing to fasciitis, and can lead to permanent skin changes in lichenoid and hyperkeratotic plaques of the mouth and restricted mouth opening. Skin changes can also lead to sclerosis and poikiloderma of the skin.[18] Chronic GVHD can also lead to a pulmonary complication known as bronchiolitis obliterans syndrome (BOS), which is discussed later in this chapter.

Preoperative considerations for patients with GVHD should include evaluation for anemia and thrombocytopenia and transfusion with leukocyte-reduced and leukocyte-irradiated PRBCs and irradiated platelets as needed. Patients with significant GVHD of the liver should have appropriate laboratory evaluation to evaluate for coagulopathy, including prothrombin (PT), partial thrombophlebitis time (PTT), international normalized ratio (INR), and fibrinogen, and be corrected as needed.

As the mainstay of treatment of GVHD is corticosteroids, anesthesia providers should be cognizant that prolonged treatment may lead to adrenal insufficiency. Patients at risk of adrenal insufficiency should receive stress-dose hydrocortisone intraoperatively. Patients with gastrointestinal GVHD undergo endoscopy routinely to assist with diagnosis and usually require perioperative antibiotics covering Gram-negative organisms, which should be discussed with the HSCT team. It is imperative anesthesia providers perform a thorough oral examination on patients with chronic GVHD affecting the mouth in an effort to identify potential difficulties with tracheal intubation.

Bronchiolitis Obliterans Syndrome

BOS is associated with pulmonary chronic GVHD. BOS is the result of an immune attack on the small airways, leading to fibrotic occlusion and subsequent obliteration.[21] The definitive diagnosis of BOS is based on the histologic analysis of lung biopsy tissue that shows thickening of the bronchiolar wall via inflammatory fibrosis and narrowing of the airway lumen. However, given the invasiveness of a lung biopsy, the current diagnostic criteria for BOS is based on pulmonary function test (PFT).[22] The current definition of BOS includes an forced expiratory volume in the first second (FEV_1), 75% predicted and an irreversible 10% decline in 2 years, FEV_1-to-vital capacity (VC) ratio of 0.7 or the lower limit of the 90% CI of the ratio, absence of infection, and either a preexisting diagnosis of chronic GVHD, air trapping by expiratory CT, or air trapping on PFTs by residual volume (RV) .120% or RV/total lung capacity (TLC).[21]

All patients with concerns for BOS should have an appropriate rule-out for tracheomegaly, alpha-1 antitrypsin deficiency, and invasive pulmonary infections. BOS is associated with a poor prognosis; however, early diagnosis with associated treatment and supportive strategies has improved outcomes. Improved treatment strategies, including the use of FAM therapy (fluticasone, azithromycin, and montelukast), have reduced systemic steroid exposure, which reduces the risk of life-threatening infections associated with BOS.[21,22] Ibrutinib is an irreversible inhibitor of Bruton's tyrosine kinase (BTK) and interleukin-2 (IL-2) inducible T-cell kinase and the first medication approved for treatment of chronic GVHD. Studies have reported that the use of ibrutinib can delay disease progression, increase progression-free survival, and improve pulmonary function in patients with BOS.[23]

As BOS can lead to air trapping and associated restrictive and obstructive ventilatory defects, patients with BOS should have a pulmonary consultation prior to anesthesia to discuss any necessary anesthesia and ventilation adjustments that may be required to safely manage the patient. Patients receiving ibrutinib are at a high risk of hemorrhage despite normal coagulation parameters and normal platelet counts. Given this potential risk, the anesthesia provider should discuss management with the HSCT team prior to any procedures.

KEY TAKEAWAYS

- Patients receiving chemotherapy will often experience anemia and/or thrombocytopenia.
- Due to the mechanism of many chemotherapy drugs, healthy cells and bone marrow are attacked by the medications, causing lower blood counts, which often lead to them needing transfusions.
- Extra precautions may be needed for patients with an upcoming surgical procedure.
- Prophylactic transfusions using irradiated products prior to procedures with anesthesia can help minimize the risk of complications from anemia and thrombocytopenia.
- Patients with neutropenia may have surgical procedures delayed until white blood cells are at a safe range as defined by their primary team.
- In emergent situations, anesthesia may not be delayed; therefore, specific awareness of these complications is paramount to minimize surgical complications. An understanding of the effects of cancer treatment and hematopoietic stem cell transplant is imperative to provide safe and effective anesthetic care.

KEY REFERENCES

Complete references for this chapter are online and available at https://connect.springerpub.com/content/book/978-0-8261-3875-0/part/part03/toc-part/ch020.

4. Sherani F, Boston C, Mba N. Latest update on prevention of acute chemotherapy-induced nausea and vomiting in pediatric cancer patients. *Curr Oncol Rep*. 2019;21(10):89. doi:10.1007/s11912-019-0840-0
5. Anghelescu DL, Tesney JM. Neuropathic pain in pediatric oncology – a clinical decision algorithm. *Pediatr Drug*. 2019;21(2):59–70. doi:10.1007/s40272-018-00324-4
6. Khaddour K, Hana C, Mewawalla P. Hematopoietic stem cell transplantation. In: *StatPearls*. StatPearls Publishing. 2020.
10. Dandoy C, Badia A. MBI-LCBI and CLABSI: more than scrubbing the line. *Bone Marrow Transplant*. 2019;54(12):1932–1939. doi:10.1038/s41409-019-0489-1
12. Lehrnbecher T, Fisher B, Phillips B, et al. Guideline for antibacterial prophylaxis administration in pediatric cancer and hematopoietic stem cell transplantation. *Clin Infect Dis*. 2020;71(1):226–236. doi:10.1093/cid/ciz1082
15. Nava T, Ansari M, Jean-Hugues D, et al. Supportive care during pediatric hematopoietic stem cell transplantation: Beyond infectious diseases. A report from workshops on supportive care of the Pediatric Diseases Working Party (PDWP) of the European Society for Blood and Marrow Transplantation (EBMT). *Bone Marrow Transplant*. 2020;55(6):1126–1136. doi:10.1038/s41409-020-0818-4
17. Models S, Larkin B, Dandoy C, et al. A new paradigm: Diagnosis and management of HSCT-associated thrombotic microangiopathy as multi-system endothelial injury. *Blood Rev*. 2015;29:191–204. doi.org/10.1016/j.blre.2014.11.001
19. Ferrara J, Reddy P. Pathophysiology of graft-versus-host-disease. *Semin Hematol*. 2006;43:3–10. doi:10.1053/j.seminhematol.2005.09.001
21. Williams K. How I treat bronchiolitis obliterans syndrome after hematopoietic stem cell transplantation. *Blood*. 2017;129(4):448–455. doi:10.1182/blood-2016-08-693507
23. Hill L, Alousi A, Kebriaei P, Mehta R, Rezvani K, Shpall E. New and emerging therapies for acute and chronic graft versus host disease. *Ther Adv Hematol*. 2018;9(1):21–46. doi:10.1177/2040620717741860

CHAPTER 21

Genitourinary Conditions

Hailey Silverii and Shumyle Alam

> **LEARNING OBJECTIVES**
> - Review congenital anomalies of the kidneys and urinary tract.
> - Distinguish between obstructive and nonobstructive neuropathy.
> - Briefly discuss complex urology patients at a lower risk of renal injury.

INTRODUCTION

Genitourinary surgeries are among the most encountered procedures in the ambulatory setting. Most of these procedures are elective and in general the patients are healthy, with an American Society of Anesthesiologists (ASA) classification of I or II. Urologic cases, however, range in complexity, from a simple circumcision to a complex reconstruction. In this chapter, we briefly review common pediatric genitourinary conditions, with a detailed focus on pediatric patients with congenital anomalies of the kidney and urinary tract (CAKUT) and their specific anesthesia requirements. It is important to note that even the simplest surgical procedures in vulnerable patients with underlying medical comorbidities can make providing anesthesia challenging. In this chapter and focus of the book, we feel it is important to recognize the urologic patient with chronic kidney disease (CKD) as a separate entity from other urologic patients and discuss them as such.

Many books and articles will ultimately fail to adequately demonstrate the true need for open communication with the surgeon and care team. Naming individual disease processes and quoting published statistics regarding surgical management are the standard in such reviews, but this does little to improve practice, safety, and quality. We attempt to blend the normative approach to a chapter like this with a slightly philosophical angle to illustrate the need to think about the patient in a holistic manner.

CONGENITAL ANOMALIES OF THE KIDNEYS AND URINARY TRACT

CAKUT represent a wide spectrum of diseases with an equivalent range of clinical implications. The frequency of CAKUT in the population ranged from .9% to 1.6% during mass postnatal ultrasound screening studies,[1,2] and it remains the leading cause of CKD and end-stage renal disease (ESRD) in children.[3,4] **Box 21.1** lists the associated CAKUT anomalies with their incidence and the associated risk of development of CKD. CAKUT can be classified as obstructive or nonobstructive, given that obstructive uropathy has a particular mechanism of renal injury and resultant renal dysplasia[5] as demonstrated in animal models.[6,7] The actual long-term consequences of CAKUT may be underreported as there are no clinical standards for diagnosis and follow-up. Several gene mutations have been found to be associated with CAKUT,[8–12] and given its impact on ESRD and decreased life expectancy,[13] further research is still needed in this area.

Antenatal diagnosis typically occurs with the presence of a structural anomaly on ultrasound, such as hydronephrosis or a dilated collecting system. These structural findings allow for early detection and close monitoring. In this early prenatal time frame, the development of the structural anomaly will continue through birth; however, functional assessment of the renal system is not as precise.[25] CAKUT's spectrum of anomalies may require immediate or delayed surgical intervention versus medical management with close observation. Intervention is usually guided by the degree of renal injury.

It is imperative the team caring for patients with CAKUT have a sound knowledge of the underlying condition, as renal injury at an early age can have long-lasting implications. As glomerular filtration rate (GFR) maturation continues after birth, progressive dysfunction or injury occurring during surgery can have grave long-term implications (**Table 21.1**).

OBSTRUCTIVE NEPHROPATHY

Congenital obstructions of the urinary tract can lead to dysplasia of the renal tissue and are the number one cause of renal insufficiency, leading to transplantation in children.[3] Almost half of cases of children with CKD and ESRD in the United States are due to CAKUT.[27] The degree of renal dysfunction and renal injury is often the determining factor on when intervention is indicated. Some of these individual diagnoses causing injury have been grouped as congenital obstructive nephropathy, which is defined by nephron loss from cell injury and the formation of atubular glomeruli with tubular atrophy and progressive fibrosis.[6] For a list of all congenital obstructions and the corresponding incidence, see **Box 21.1**. An unknown number of these patients will have deterioration in function over time, which can be exacerbated by surgery and anesthesia. Anesthesia providers should have a sound understanding of the disease conditions prior to the delivery of anesthesia to these vulnerable children.

Posterior Urethral Valves

Posterior urethral valves (PUV) refer to a congenital, thin membrane that extends from the verumontanum of the posterior urethra, causing obstruction.[28] PUV is often diagnosed antenatally and is associated with hydroureteronephrosis, as well as varying degrees of oligohydramnios. The severity of this condition can vary, with some neonates presenting with very mild obstructive findings and others found to have severe bilateral hydroureteronephrosis with a distended bladder on ultrasound. In some patients, the diagnosis is missed and will be delayed.

This group of patients can present with electrolyte anomalies and may be severely ill on presentation. Before being brought to the operating room, the initial diagnosis is often confirmed with a severely dilated posterior urethra on voiding cystourethrogram. With the improvements in prenatal detection and management, many institutions can appropriately plan the child's delivery, as well as any subsequent surgical

BOX 21.1 INCIDENCE OF CAKUT ANOMALIES

Obstructive
- PUV: 2 per 10,000 live male births[14]
- PBS: 4 per 100,000 live births[15]
- Ureteroceles: 1 in 5,000[16]
- Ectopic ureter: 1 in 2,000–4,000[17]
- POM: 1 in 3,000[18]
- UPJ obstruction: 1 in 1,000–1,500[19]

Nonobstructive
- VUR: prevalence of 25%–40%[20]
- Ureteral duplications: 2 in 100[21]
- Horseshoe kidney: 1/400[22]
- Cross fused renal ectopia: 1 in 1,000–7,500
- Unilateral renal agenesis: 1 in 1,300[23]
- Renal hypoplasia: 1 in 1,000[24]
- Multicystic dysplastic kidney: 1 in 1,000–4,000 live births[24]

CAKUT, congenital anomalies of the kidney and urinary tract; PBS, painful bladder syndrome; POM, primary obstructed megaureter; PUV, posterior urethral valve; UPJ, ureteropelvic junction; VUR, vesicoureteral reflux.

interventions required. Immediate management includes relieving the obstruction with a catheter, followed by valve ablation in the operating room, which will afford the primary team the time requisite for medical management and stabilization before surgery. This includes ensuring the patient is volume-replete and all electrolyte levels are normalized.

The initial surgical management includes valve ablation, followed by monitoring for postobstructive diuresis and electrolyte abnormalities postoperatively. Rarely in centers where pediatric patients are not routinely seen, there can be challenges securing the appropriate size instrumentation for ablation, mandating vesicostomy creation in the neonatal period. As a consequence of the renal injury in utero from obstruction, the kidneys can have poor concentrating ability, which results in polyuria.[29] This increases the risk of long-term renal demise;[30] therefore, preoperative stabilization, correction of fluid deficit, and correction of electrolytes before the child undergoes anesthesia are critical.

Prune Belly Syndrome

Prune belly syndrome (PBS), also known as Eagle–Barrett syndrome, is a rare congenital syndrome characterized by the triad of deficient abdominal muscles, urinary tract malformation, and bilateral cryptorchidism. PBS patients often require a large amount of surgery aimed at correction of intra-abdominal testes, abdominoplasty, and urinary tract reconstruction.[31] Anesthesia considerations specific to PBS patients include renal dysfunction or renal failure, Potter's facies secondary to oligohydramnios which may complicate intubation, and weak accessory respiratory muscles due to deficient abdominal muscles.[32] For additional information regarding the anesthetic management of patients with PBS, please refer to Chapter 42 in this text.

Congenital Ureteral Obstruction

Ureterovesical junction obstruction, ureteropelvic junction obstruction, ureterocele, and ectopic ureter are all considered obstructive congenital ureteral lesions. Isolated obstructive conditions in a CAKUT patient are not as worrisome as the aforementioned conditions as they will often have a normal contralateral kidney and thus preserved renal function.

NONOBSTRUCTIVE NEPHROPATHY

Vesicoureteral Reflux

Vesicoureteral reflux (VUR) is a descriptive term for retrograde flow of urine from the bladder into the upper urinary tracts and, just as with many other CAKUT diagnoses, represents a spectrum of severity. More important, VUR can present as a primary or secondary diagnosis. Primary VUR represents a congenital anomaly resulting from anomalous development of the antirefluxing ureterovesical junction in utero, whereas secondary VUR represents a surrogate for high-pressure voiding or high bladder storage pressures in patients with CAKUT or neurogenic bladder. Reflux is diagnosed fluoroscopically and graded based on the appearance of a contrast-filled collecting system.

Primary VUR is a common diagnosis in children. The association between reflux and urinary tract infections (UTIs) is well established, with a reported prevalence of VUR in up to 70% of children younger than 1 year of age presenting with a UTI.[33] Given the association of VUR with UTIs, renal scarring, and renal injury over time, the goal of management is prevention and relies on observation and intervention when indicated. The initial management of primary VUR consists of close observation with repeat imaging and prophylactic antibiotics. Spontaneous resolution of VUR is very common, specifically with unilateral, low-grade VUR in children diagnosed at an early age.[34] Surgery is avoided unless there is an increased risk of worsening renal injury. Should surgery be deemed necessary, reimplantation of the ureter is performed with creation of an antirefluxing ureterovesical junction. In patients with primary VUR, the probability of CKD remains 2% to 5% at 10 years after diagnosis, with an increased risk in patients with bilateral disease or contralateral renal hypoplasia.[35]

Renal Developmental Anomalies

This group of congenital anomalies is heterogeneous, with varying etiologies and clinical implications. Anomalies that commonly result in a solitary functioning kidney (SFK) are the most concerning as a solitary kidney is an independent risk factor for CKD.[36] When evaluating these patients prior to surgery, it is important anesthesia providers recognize that these patients may have decreased GFR. Compensatory hypertrophy of the contralateral kidney, as indicated by renal length, at birth is a good prognostic indicator of renal function in SFK.[37] Concomitant ipsilateral CAKUT of the SFK is a poor prognostic indicator of decreased GFR.[38] Anomalies of fusion or ascent have minimal clinical implications outside of surgical considerations

Table 21.1	Glomerular Filtration Rate (GFR) Maturation With Age	
Age	Average GFR (mL/min/1.73 m²)	Range of GFR (mL/min/1.73 m²)
0–30 days	39–47	17–68
1–3 months	58	30–84
3–6 months	77	39–114
6–12 months	103	49–157
>1 year	127	89–165

Source: From Heilbron DC, Holliday MA, al-Dahwi A, et al. Expressing glomerular filtration rate in children. *Pediatr Nephrol.* 1991;5(1):511.

> **BOX 21.2 ANOMALIES ASSOCIATED WITH A SOLITARY FUNCTIONING KIDNEY**
>
> - Renal agenesis
> - Renal hypoplasia
> - Renal dysplasia
> - Multicystic dysplastic kidney
> - Renal ectopia
> - Cross fused ectopic kidney
> - Horseshoe kidney

due to abnormal anatomy (Box 21.2). The takeaway for this group of CAKUT is that understanding the diagnosis and the associated implications helps discern which patients are at a higher risk of renal injury and development of CKD.

ANESTHESIA CONSIDERATIONS FOR CHILDREN WITH CAKUT

The preceding summary of CAKUT provides a foundation from which anesthesia providers can plan the anesthetic care for these patients, a population whose clinical vulnerability is often underestimated. It is important to be cognizant of the fact that using a diagnosis alone to guide care can fail to highlight other key aspects of care, as some children may have features of both obstructive and nonobstructive renal injury. A diagnosis-based approach to an anesthetic plan for children with CAKUT can also be myopic. For example, a child presenting for a hernia repair and circumcision may also have PUV. While they may appear as a normal infant, failure to appreciate that this child likely has a fixed urine output from pressure-related renal injury could be catastrophic. Children with a fixed urine output such as this would not likely tolerate induction of anesthesia after being NPO for several hours due to being profoundly dehydrated. The ensuing hypoperfusion to the kidneys may worsen underlying electrolyte anomalies (usually hyperkalemia from renal tubular acidosis type 4) and could result in further kidney injury. If this same child were also given ketorolac for pain control in that under resuscitated state, the degree of renal injury could be worse. Globally, this is not an aggressive theoretical discussion as there are no standards for following renal function in these patients. Adding confusion to the equation is that serum creatinine levels can underestimate the degree of renal injury in children.

COMPLEX UROLOGY PATIENTS AT LOWER RISK OF RENAL INJURY

Classic Bladder Exstrophy

Classic bladder exstrophy (CBE) and the exstrophy–epispadias complex are a rare anomaly in which the bladder and pelvis do not close during development. As a result, the bladder and the urethra are often splayed open on the outside of the body. With successful reconstruction, life expectancy and renal dysfunction are typically unaffected. Reconstruction aims at achieving continence without obstruction, with a successful primary surgery being the largest contributing factor to outcome.[39] Successful reconstruction can be achieved with a "modern staged repair of exstrophy" or "complete primary repair of exstrophy," a one-stage repair. Outcomes vary between surgeons based on experience, as these surgeries are generally done at high-volume centers of excellence.

Anesthetic considerations include adequate pain control to facilitate prolonged immobilization after surgery. A recent study reported benefits on the use of caudal epidural analgesia and early extubation, as these collectively resulted in improved outcomes.[40] Without adequate pain management and proper anxiolysis, these patients may remain unnecessarily intubated for an extended period in the early postoperative period in an effort to maintain immobilization, which is key to decreasing the risk of dehiscence when osteotomies are part of the reconstruction.[41] The discussion regarding the use of regional anesthesia, whether neuraxial anesthesia or peripheral nerve blockade, should be had prior to surgery to achieve the best possible postoperative outcomes.

NEUROGENIC BLADDER

Neurogenic bladder in children is one of the most frequently managed conditions by a pediatric urologist. Neurogenic bladder can lead to significant renal injury over time and subsequent CKD. One of the leading causes of neurogenic bladder in children is myelomeningocele. Studies pertaining to the care of this patient population make up most of the pediatric literature regarding neurogenic bladder, management, and outcomes. There are, however, multiple other causes of neurogenic bladder in pediatric patients, including spinal cord injury, cerebral palsy, pelvic surgery, anorectal malformation, cloacal anomalies, cloacal exstrophy, spinal pathologies, and neuromuscular or metabolic disease. The common anesthesia concern for all these children is proper management of fluid balance and all aspects of care impacting renal function. It is key to be cognizant that the severity of underlying renal disease is often not obvious. In addition, respiratory concerns may be present depending on the degree of spinal deformity. These children commonly undergo reconstructive surgery aimed at protecting renal function and achieving both bowel and urinary continence. Potential surgeries include genitourinary reconstruction with augmentation cystoplasty, continent catheterizable channels, or bladder outlet procedures. Anesthesia considerations for these patients include consideration of the level of the lesion, presence of comorbid conditions, increased incidence of latex allergy in these children, and decreased options for regional anesthesia given the presence of a spinal anomaly. Despite concerns surrounding epidural use in patients with spina bifida, thoracic epidurals can be safe and reduce opioid use postoperatively, as demonstrated by Roth et al. in patients with low-level spina bifida undergoing genitourinary reconstructive surgery.[42] Alternatively, quadratus lumborum (QL) blocks with indwelling catheters providing continuous infusion can be utilized for regional pain management. These blocks have established efficacy in the urologic patient undergoing abdominal surgery;[12] however, to our knowledge, there are no studies in the literature comparing QL blocks with epidural catheters in pediatric urinary tract reconstruction.

PEDIATRIC GENITOURINARY TUMORS

Pediatric genitourinary cancers include tumors of the kidneys, retroperitoneum, pelvis, and testicles. These cancers are treated with extirpative surgery and can be done both open and minimally invasive with the use of laparoscopy with or without robotic assistance. Box 21.3[3] lists the most common genitourinary tumors in pediatric patients.

NEPHROLITHIASIS

The incidence of kidney stones in the pediatric patient population is increasing with time, as demonstrated in

> **BOX 21.3 MOST COMMON GENITOURINARY MALIGNANCIES**
>
> - Wilms' tumor
> - Neuroblastoma
> - Congenital mesoblastic nephroma
> - Clear cell sarcoma
> - Rhabdomyosarcoma (bladder, prostate, paratesticular, uterine, vaginal)
> - Yolk sac testicular tumor
> - Teratoma of the testis

several recent epidemiologic studies. In 2008, the incidence was 57 per 100,000[44] and more recently was found to be 239 per 100,000 persons in a 2016 population-based study published out of South Carolina.[45] Unlike kidney stones in adult patients, pediatric kidney stones have not been shown to have an association with elevated body mass index.[46] Approximately 20% of pediatric stone formers will have greater than three recurrences prior to adulthood. Among pediatric patients presenting with a stone, approximately 22% will require an intervention, such as ureteral stent placement, percutaneous nephrostomy tube placement, ureteroscopy and laser lithotripsy, or extracorporeal shockwave lithotripsy.[47] When caring for patients presenting for stone-related surgeries, anesthesia providers should consider antibiotic prophylaxis, the need for relaxation, and postoperative pain management when developing the anesthetic plan. The risk of systemic inflammatory response syndrome response or sepsis following intervention for stones is approximately 10%,[48] so appropriate antibiotic prophylaxis is key and should be discussed with the surgeon prior to the intervention. Paralytic is not necessary for all stone procedures; however, many surgeons will request relaxation with ureteroscopy for stone treatment. Pain following stone surgery is best managed with nonsteroidal anti-inflammatory drugs if not otherwise contraindicated. Please refer to Chapter 116 in this text for additional information regarding the anesthetic management of these patients.

PENILE ANOMALIES

Some of the most commonly performed cases by pediatric urologists, and therefore pediatric anesthesia providers, are penile cases, varying in complexity from circumcision to hypospadias repairs. Following a basic circumcision, postoperative analgesia can be accomplished with either a dorsal penile nerve block or a caudal epidural blockade. A Cochrane review from 2008 did not find a significant difference in analgesia between the two techniques; however, there was a slightly increased risk of temporary motor or leg weakness with caudal epidural block.[49]

Hypospadias is a penile anomaly defined by abnormal development of the urethra, corpus spongiosum, and prepuce resulting in a proximally located urethral meatus, penile curvature, and abnormal penile skin. Hypospadias repairs can be performed via single-stage or multiple-stage repairs. These cases can last several hours based on the complexity of the repair. For more complex penile cases, such as a hypospadias repair, postoperative analgesia is generally achieved with caudal epidural blockade or dorsal penile nerve blocks.[50] For further information, please refer to Chapter 112, "Circumcision," and Chapter 113, "Hypospadias Repair."

BENIGN TESTICULAR/GROIN PATHOLOGY

Testicular torsion remains one of the few true urologic emergencies, with an incidence of approximately 3.8 in 100,000 males younger than 18 years of age.[51] Torsion repairs should be done within 4 to 6 hours of onset of pain for best chance for testicular survival. Anesthesia considerations include the urgency of the surgical procedure and postoperative pain control. Analgesia can be improved with intraoperative spermatic cord block by the surgeon.

Nonurgent testicular and groin cases include repair of a hydrocele, inguinal hernia, undescended testicle, and/or varicocele. Surgical interventions for these diagnoses are typically accomplished with open scrotal versus inguinal surgery, except for some inguinal hernia repairs and intra-abdominal undescended testicles which can be repaired laparoscopically.

Just like many penile cases, these cases are considered routine for pediatric urologists; however, the patients undergoing intervention may be some of the most complex anesthesia patients given the association of undescended testicles with numerous syndromes and other anomalies, as listed in **Box 21.4**.

> **BOX 21.4 ANOMALIES ASSOCIATED WITH CRYPTORCHIDISM**
>
> - Prune belly syndrome
> - Spigelian hernia
> - Cerebral palsy
> - Arthrogryposis
> - Myelomeningocele
> - Omphalocele
> - Anorectal malformations
> - Posterior urethral valves
> - Hypospadias
> - Trisomy 21

KEY TAKEAWAYS

- Anesthesia providers must understand that even "simple" genitourinary procedures in vulnerable patients with chronic kidney disease have the potential to place the patient at risk of renal injury when not managed appropriately.
- All patients with congenital anomalies of the kidney and urinary tract should be thoroughly evaluated before surgery.
- It is necessary to calculate the glomerular filtration rate prior to making an intraoperative hydration and pain management plan.
- If the serum creatinine underestimates the extent of renal injury, the anesthetic plan can further that same injury. Over time, especially if the same child has multiple trips to the operating room, this can result in a more rapid decline of renal function that could have been prevented.
- A holistic approach, taking into consideration all medical aspects of the child and not solely the complexity of the surgery, should be the standard of care for all anesthesia providers to ensure safety, quality, and optimal outcomes.

PART III: CONDITIONS, DISEASES, AND SYNDROMES IN PEDIATRIC PATIENTS

KEY REFERENCES

Complete references for this chapter are online and available at https://connect.springerpub.com/content/book/978-0-8261-3875-0/part/part03/toc-part/ch021.

11. Ishiwa S, Sato M, Morisada N, et al. Association between the clinical presentation of congenital anomalies of the kidney and urinary tract (CAKUT) and gene mutations: an analysis of 66 patients at a single institution. *Pediatr Nephrol.* 2019;34(8):1457–1464. doi:10.1007/s00467-019-04230-w
12. Sato M. Ultrasound-guided quadratus lumborum block compared to caudal ropivacaine/morphine in children undergoing surgery for vesicoureteric reflex. *Paediatr Anaesth.* 2019;29(7):738–743. doi:10.1111/pan.13650
13. Saran R, Robinson B, Abbott KC, et al. US Renal Data System 2019 annual data report: Epidemiology of kidney disease in the United States. *Am J Kidney Dis.* 2020;75(1 Suppl. 1):A6–A7. doi:10.1053/j.ajkd.2019.09.003
36. Kim S, Chang Y, Lee YR, et al. Solitary kidney and risk of chronic kidney disease. *Eur J Epidemiol.* 2019;34(9):879–888. doi:10.1007/s10654-019-00520-7
37. Poggiali IV, Simões E Silva AC, Vasconcelos MA, et al. A clinical predictive model of renal injury in children with congenital solitary functioning kidney. *Pediatr Nephrol.* 2019;34(3):465–474. doi:10.1007/s00467-018-4111-3
40. Okonkwo I, Bendon AA, Cervellione RM, et al. Continuous caudal epidural analgesia and early feeding in delayed bladder exstrophy repair: a nine-year experience. *J Pediatr Urol.* 2019;15(1):76.e71–76.e78. doi:10.1016/j.jpurol.2018.10.022
42. Roth JD, Misseri R, Whittaker SC, et al. Epidural analgesia decreases narcotic requirements in patients with low level spina bifida undergoing urological laparotomy for neurogenic bladder and bowel. *J Urol.* 2019;201(1):169–173. doi:10.1016/j.juro.2018.06.063
48. Mi Q, Meng X, Meng L, et al. Risk factors for systemic inflammatory response syndrome induced by flexible ureteroscope combined with holmium laser lithotripsy. *Biomed Res Int.* 2020:6842479. doi:10.1155/2020/6842479
50. Zhu C, Wei R, Tong Y, et al. Analgesic efficacy and impact of caudal block on surgical complications of hypospadias repair: a systematic review and meta-analysis. *Reg Anesth Pain Med.* 2019;44(2):259–267. doi:10.1136/rapm-2018-000022

CHAPTER 22

Musculoskeletal Conditions

Ramsey S. Sabbagh, Brian M. Grawe, Jagroop M. Parikh, and Shital N. Parikh

LEARNING OBJECTIVES

- Recognize the different subtypes of pediatric scoliosis and describe their etiologies.
- Describe the features of pediatric congenital limb deformities, including clubfoot.
- Describe the features of pediatric hip disorders, including slipped capital femoral epiphysis.
- Describe the features of sports injuries and fractures unique to the pediatric population.

INTRODUCTION

The anesthetic management of pediatric patients with musculoskeletal conditions involves complex clinical decision-making. A thorough understanding of musculoskeletal anesthesia guided by evidence-based medicine is of critical importance. This chapter reviews the etiology, pathophysiology, and clinical features of common pediatric conditions of the axial and appendicular musculoskeletal system, including scoliosis, congenital limb deformities, hip disorders, fractures, and sports injuries.

SPINAL DISORDERS

Spinal disorders in children and adolescents can encompass congenital deformities, traumatic injuries, tumors, infections, or inflammatory conditions. One of the most dreaded complications or effects of such spinal disorders is paralysis of the body below the level of spinal involvement. Scoliosis, which is defined as a three-dimensional curvature of the spine, constitutes one of the most common features of spinal disorders (Figure 22.1).

Pediatric scoliosis is a structural deformity of the spine that can present in children of any age.[1] Scoliosis affects 0.2% to 0.6% of the general population and may have a spectrum of presentations, each constituting different anesthetic needs and considerations.[2] Scoliosis is most often asymptomatic but can present with intermittent back pain or noticeable physical abnormalities, such as a prominence of the back or uneven positioning of the shoulders or waist.[3] Radiographically, scoliosis is characterized as a lateral curvature of the spine with a Cobb angle (angle between the most tilted proximal and distal vertebrae) of at least 10 degrees.[2,4] Impaired lung function is a major concern in all forms of scoliosis, as the severity, rigidity, and morphology of the thoracic curve and surrounding structures affect pulmonary function.[5]

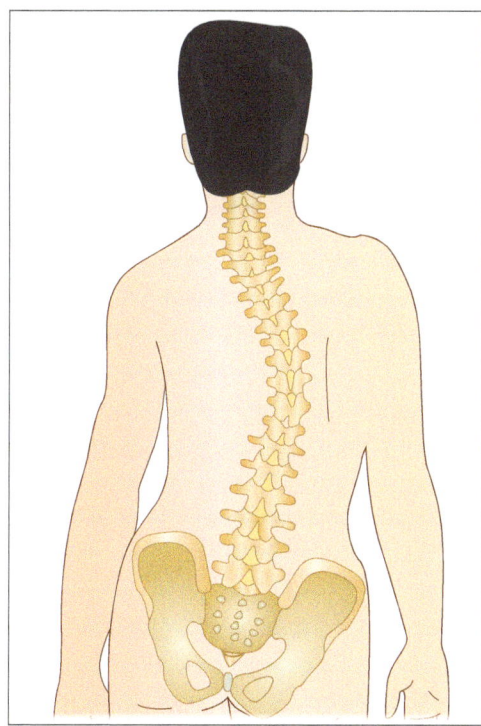

Figure 22.1: Scoliosis.

Source: From Stutzman Z, Gawlik K. Evidence-based assessment of the musculoskeletal system. In: Gawlik KS, Melnyk BM, Teall AM, eds. *Evidence-Based Physical Examination: Best Practices for Health and Well-Being Assessment*. Springer Publishing Company; 2021:434, Fig. 15.46.

IDIOPATHIC SCOLIOSIS

Idiopathic scoliosis can be cervical, thoracic, lumbar, or an S-shaped curve. The earlier the onset of the disease, the more likely the curve will worsen with time.[3] The curve progresses fastest during the adolescent growth spurt.[2,3] Idiopathic scoliosis is subcategorized into three different groups based on the time of onset: infantile, juvenile, or adolescent. Adolescent idiopathic scoliosis (AIS) has an incidence of 2% to 4%, making it the most common type of scoliosis.[6] While the etiology and pathophysiology of idiopathic scoliosis have not yet been ascertained, multiple possible genetic contributors have been identified.[2,7]

NEUROMUSCULAR SCOLIOSIS

Neuromuscular scoliosis is caused by dysfunction or injury to the central nervous system resulting in hypotonia and spasticity of the thoracic and lumbar muscles normally responsible for providing stability to the spinal column. The subsequent muscular imbalances lead to mechanical distortion of the spine, thereby causing progressive neuromuscular scoliosis.[3] Examples of underlying conditions that often lead to neuromuscular scoliosis include traumatic brain injury, cerebral palsy, stroke, spinal cord injuries, spinal muscular atrophy, Duchenne's muscular dystrophy, and spina bifida.[3,8] Evidence of neuromuscular disease may be discoverable in utero with the absence of fetal movement on ultrasound examination.[9] Early signs of neuromuscular disease in children younger than the age of 2 include diffuse hypotonia, decreased overall muscle strength, difficulty with posture changes, and a lack of spontaneous gestures.[9] Cranial nerve involvement strongly suggests a neuromuscular disorder, for which clinical manifestations include a paucity of facial expressions, poor ocular tracking, and difficulty swallowing.[9] Unlike idiopathic scoliosis, neuromuscular scoliosis is often progressive even after the end of growth.[3] About 75% of patients with cerebral palsy with a Gross Motor Function Classification Scale (GMFCS) rating of V had a spinal deformity with a Cobb angle of 40 degrees or larger by the age of 20.[10]

CONGENITAL SCOLIOSIS

Congenital scoliosis is responsible for 10% of all scoliotic deformities and is caused by defective embryogenesis resulting in spinal deformity.[11] More specifically, it involves either failure of vertebral formation, leading to a tripedicular vertebra, butterfly-shaped vertebra, or hemivertebra, or failure of segmentation resulting in a conjoined vertebra.[3,12,13] The severity of congenital scoliosis is variable and can have complex curve patterns due to simultaneous errors of vertebral segmentation and formation.[3,11,13] Importantly, congenital scoliosis is often associated with embryologic deformities in other organ systems, either as part of vertebral defects, anal atresia, cardiac defects, tracheo-esophageal fistula, renal anomalies, and limb abnormalities (VACTERL) syndrome or as an isolated abnormality.[3,13] Some of the more commonly observed malformations associated with congenital scoliosis include genitourinary abnormalities with sparing of renal function, ventricular septal defects, and neural axis abnormalities.[13]

SYNDROMIC SCOLIOSIS

In addition to having idiopathic, neuromuscular, and congenital etiologies, pediatric scoliosis may present as part of a syndrome.[3,5] These syndromic disorders include arthrogryposis, Klippel–Feil syndrome, and Marfan's syndrome, among others, and the relevant anesthetic considerations are addressed in their respective chapters of this textbook.

CONGENITAL LIMB DEFORMITIES

Several congenital deformities may affect a part or even the whole upper or lower limb. The phenotype can be varied and may include missing segments of the limb, disproportionate limbs, or limb malformation. Clubfoot is one of the most common congenital limb deformities.

Clubfoot, also known as talipes equinovarus, can be separated into three subcategories: positional, syndromic, and idiopathic (**Figure 22.2**). Smoking during pregnancy and low maternal folate levels can both contribute to congenital malformations, including clubfoot.[14] Several homeobox, apoptotic, and muscle contractile genes have also been implicated in the pathogenesis of congenital clubfoot.[14,15]

PEDIATRIC HIP DISORDERS

Pediatric hip conditions can affect children of any age. They may be present at birth (e.g., developmental dysplasia of the hip), during childhood (Perthes' disease), or during adolescence (slipped capital femoral epiphysis [SCFE]).

SCFE is a pediatric hip disorder which affects up to 0.025% of all children ages 8 to 15 years.[16,17] It involves posteroinferior displacement of the femoral head relative to the femoral neck and can occur in either a gradual or acute setting.[16] The pathophysiology is multifactorial since both genetic and environmental factors likely contribute to the development of this disease.[18,19] Foremost among these implicated factors is obesity, especially in boys, for which the relationship with SCFE has been well established in the literature.[16-21] Interestingly, children who go on to develop

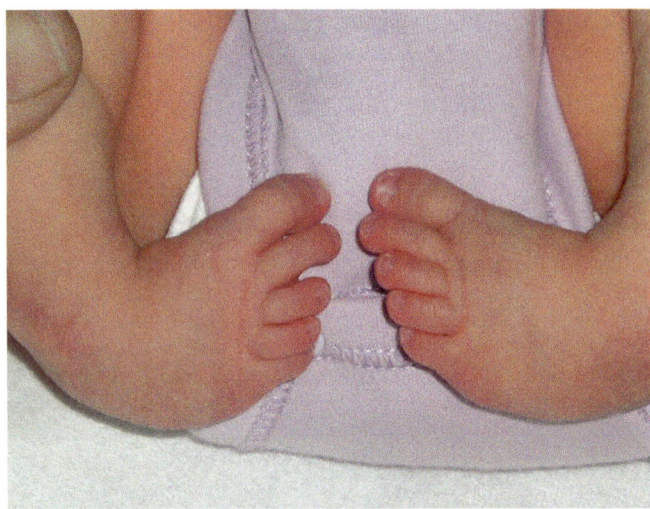

Figure 22.2: Clubfoot.

Source: From Stutzman Z, Gawlik K. Evidence-based assessment of the musculoskeletal system. In: Gawlik KS, Melnyk BM, Teall AM, eds. *Evidence-Based Physical Examination: Best Practices for Health and Well-Being Assessment.* Springer Publishing Company; 2021:434, Fig. 15.45.

SCFE in the contralateral hip tend to be younger with a higher posterior sloping angle on radiographic evaluation than children with unilateral SCFE.[22] While the majority of pediatric patients with SCFE are obese, nonobese patients tend to be older, female, and more likely to present with a severe and unstable defect.[21]

SPORTS INJURIES AND FRACTURES

The last two decades have witnessed a rise in pediatric sports-related injuries. Increased participation, competitiveness, recognition, and single sports specialization at a younger age may account for this rise. Anterior cruciate ligament tears, shoulder instability, patellar instability, meniscus tears, and osteochondritis dissecans are frequently seen in young athletes. Similarly, pediatric fractures are extremely common, occurring at least once before the age of 16 in 64% of boys and 40% of girls, and peaking between the ages of 10 and 14 years.[23,24] While pediatric orthopedic injuries historically favor nonoperative management, advancements in traumatology and fixation have shifted the general approach to fracture management in children in the direction of surgical intervention.[25]

Children have relatively pliable bones, leading to different fracture patterns than those observed in adults, primarily due to the tendency of pediatric fractures to buckle or bow under mechanical stress.[26] Excellent alignment and union are obtainable with far more angulation than in similar adult fractures due to a thick periosteum, prolific callus formation, and the high degree of remodeling that occurs in pediatric patients.[26] Fractures of the physis are of chief concern due to the risk of growth arrest in the affected extremity.[26] A high index of suspicion for nonaccidental trauma should be maintained for infants presenting with a fracture due to the prevalence and pervasive underreporting of child abuse in pediatric fracture patients.[27–29]

KEY TAKEAWAYS

- The etiology of pediatric scoliosis may be idiopathic, neuromuscular, congenital, or syndromic, each with a different constellation of clinical features and treatment challenges.
- Pediatric clubfoot is a deformity of the foot with a complex multifactorial etiology.
- Slipped capital femoral epiphysis is a pediatric hip disorder that involves displacement of the femoral head on the femoral neck and primarily affects obese adolescent boys.
- While pediatric fractures typically do not require operative intervention, fractures of the physis are of chief concern due to a high risk of growth arrest in the affected extremity.

KEY REFERENCES

Complete references for this chapter are online and available at https://connect.springerpub.com/content/book/978-0-8261-3875-0/part/part03/toc-part/ch022.

3. Sheehan DD, Grayhack J. Pediatric scoliosis and kyphosis: an overview of diagnosis, management, and surgical treatment. *Pediatr Ann.* 2017;46(12):e472–e480. doi:10.3928/19382359-20171113-01
5. Wilton NC, Anderson BJ. Orthopedic and spine surgery. In: Anderson BJ, Cote CJ, Lerman J, eds. *A Practice of Anesthesia for Infants and Children.* 6th ed. Elsevier Inc; 2019. doi:10.1016/B978-0-323-42974-0.00032-X
14. Sadler B, Gurnett CA, Dobbs MB. The genetics of isolated and syndromic clubfoot. *J Child Orthop.* 2019;13(3):238–244. doi:10.1302/1863-2548.13.190063
18. Aversano MW, Moazzaz P, Scaduto AA, Otsuka NY. Association between body mass index-for-age and slipped capital femoral epiphysis: the long-term risk for subsequent slip in patients followed until physeal closure. *J Child Orthop.* 2016;10(3):209–213. doi:10.1007/s11832-016-0731-y
21. Obana KK, Siddiqui AA, Broom AM, et al. Slipped capital femoral epiphysis in children without obesity. *J Pediatr.* 2020;218:192–197.e1. doi:10.1016/j.jpeds.2019.11.037
22. Swarup I, Goodbody C, Goto R, et al. Risk factors for contralateral slipped capital femoral epiphysis: a meta-analysis of cohort and case-control studies. *J Pediatr Orthop.* 2020;40(6):E446–E453. doi:10.1097/BPO.0000000000001482
26. Boutis K. The emergency evaluation and management of pediatric extremity fractures. *Emerg Med Clin North Am.* 2020;38(1):31–59. doi:10.1016/j.emc.2019.09.003
28. Lavin LR, Penrod CH, Estrada CM, et al. Fractures in the pediatric emergency department: are we considering abuse? *Clin Pediatr.* 2018;57(10):1161–1167. doi:10.1177/0009922818759319

SECTION B: Common Syndromes in Pediatric Patients

CHAPTER 23

Achondroplasia

Gail Shibata

PATHOPHYSIOLOGY AND CLINICAL MANIFESTATIONS

Achondroplasia is the most common short-stature skeletal dysplasia, occurring in approximately 1 in 10,000 to 30,000 live births.[1] Although, achondroplasia is inherited in an autosomal dominant pattern, approximately 80% of individuals with achondroplasia are born from two average-stature parents due to spontaneous mutations in the fibroblast growth factor receptor type 3 (*FGFR3*) gene and there is a correlation with advanced paternal age.[1] Nearly all these mutations are caused by a specific arginine-for-glycine substitution (G380R).

FGFR3, a cell-surface receptor that regulates linear bone growth, is expressed in chondrocytes and mature osteoblasts. Under normal conditions, *FGFR3* inhibits proliferation and terminal differentiation of growth plate chondrocytes. Activating *FGFR3* mutations constitutively and profoundly slow bone growth and result in structural abnormalities of the axial skeleton and those portions of the skull formed by endochondral ossification.[1]

The features of achondroplasia are well defined both clinically and radiologically (Box 23.1; Figure 23.1). Nevertheless, about 20% of affected individuals are not recognized at birth.[1,3]

Despite normal cognitive abilities overall, many children with achondroplasia have delayed motor milestones. Additional common problems include obstructive sleep apnea, middle ear dysfunction, and bowing of the legs.[1,3] Less commonly, children with achondroplasia may have a small foramen magnum, leading to compression of the brainstem and arteries at the cervicomedullary junction. Should this occur, the resulting compression of the medulla oblongata and the upper cervical cord can lead to sleep apnea, myelopathy and, in 2% to 5% of children with achondroplasia, sudden infant death syndrome.[1,2,3] Based on this, the American Academy of Pediatrics (AAP) recommends early MRI or CT studies, especially if there is evidence of central apnea by polysomnography, lower limb hyperreflexia, or clonus.[3] The clinical index of suspicion required for imaging is low, since 6% to 13.3% of all infants and children with achondroplasia will require suboccipital decompression within the first 2 years of life.[2,3,8] Increased intracranial pressure and hydrocephalus can also become a concern, and up to 13% of children with achondroplasia will require ventricular shunts by their teens.[1,2] Upper airway obstruction is common in children with achondroplasia, with 10% to 78% requiring treatment related to obstructive sleep apnea and chronic respiratory insufficiency.[4] Polysomnography may be helpful in differentiating neurological versus obstructive apnea. The causes of obstructive sleep apnea in children with achondroplasia fall into three categories: (a) midface hypoplasia resulting in relative adenoid and tonsil hypertrophy, (b) jugular foramen stenosis resulting in both muscular upper airway obstruction due to the neurological connections being compromised and progressive hydrocephalus due to jugular venous hypertension, and (c) muscular upper airway obstruction without hydrocephalus resulting from hypoglossal canal stenosis. In many cases, the definitive therapy is surgical, although patients with jugular foramen stenosis may respond to nocturnal positive airway pressure.[4]

Spinal stenosis is common in older children and complications from spinal stenosis increase by adulthood. By 10 years of age, 10% of children with achondroplasia have neurological signs of claudication and increased reflexes in their legs. Approximately one-third require lumbar laminectomy for symptomatic spinal stenosis.[3]

ANESTHETIC MANAGEMENT

Children with achondroplasia often require surgical intervention and require anesthesia for myringotomy tube placement, adenotonsillectomy, MRI or CT imaging, ventricular shunt placement, suboccipital craniectomy, and various orthopedic surgeries, including laminectomy, limb lengthening, and kyphoscoliosis correction. The unique features associated with achondroplasia require special consideration in planning anesthetic management.

PREOPERATIVE EVALUATION

Preoperative history and physical examination should focus on three key systems: airway, cardiopulmonary, and neurological status.

Airway Assessment

Pediatric patients with achondroplasia may have potential difficult airway management due to their characteristic craniofacial abnormalities of short maxilla, large mandible, large tongue, and short neck, which can lead to difficulties in obtaining an effective mask seal and ventilation. Foramen magnum stenosis and cervical instability at the atlantoaxial occipital joint may impact axis alignment for endotracheal intubation, and a careful preoperative assessment is warranted. Previous airway management records should be obtained when possible, as well as CT or MRI, if there is concern for cervical cord compression or atlantoaxial instability.

Cardiopulmonary Assessment

Restrictive pulmonary disease occurs in less than 5% of children with achondroplasia who are younger than 3 years due to their small chest, in addition to any associated chest deformity present leading to inefficient chest mechanics and increased compliance.[3] It is important to assess for severe scoliosis and rib cage deformities that could result in restrictive lung disease, pulmonary hypertension, and cor pulmonale. Chest x-ray, baseline blood gas, pulmonary function tests, and echocardiography may be indicated based on severity of the restrictive lung disease. More commonly, sleep apnea from upper airway obstruction is observed, and it is important to obtain a clinical history for upper airway obstruction, particularly for the occurrence of loud snoring, glottal stops, and

> **BOX 23.1 CLINICAL FEATURES OF ACHONDROPLASIA**
>
> **Craniofacial**
> - Macrocephaly
> - Shortened skull base
> - Protruding forehead
> - Flattened nasal bridge
> - Midface hypoplasia
> - Large tongue
>
> **Neurological**
> - Normal intelligence
> - Delayed motor development
> - Foramen magnum stenosis (cervical medullary compression)
> - Cervical myelopathy, spinal stenosis
> - Hydrocephalus
> - Hypotonia—common during infancy, improves with age
>
> **Ear, Nose, and Throat (ENT)**
> - Recurrent otitis media
> - Risk of conductive hearing loss
> - Language and speech articulation problems
> - Sleep disordered breathing, obstructive apnea, central apnea
>
> **Cardiopulmonary**
> - Restrictive lung disease, pulmonary hypertension, or cor pulmonale
>
> **Musculoskeletal**
> - Long, narrow trunk
> - Rhizomelia or short limb of the proximal segment
> - Thoracolumbar kyphoscoliosis especially during infancy; lumbar lordosis arises when walking, worsens with age
> - Genu varum varus (bowleg) or valgus (knock knee)
> - Ligamentous laxity of joints, especially of the knees and hands
> - Excess skin and SC tissues
> - Brachydactyly (short/broad fingers and toes) exhibiting a trident or three-pronged appearance at birth
>
> **Metabolic**
> - Obesity is common

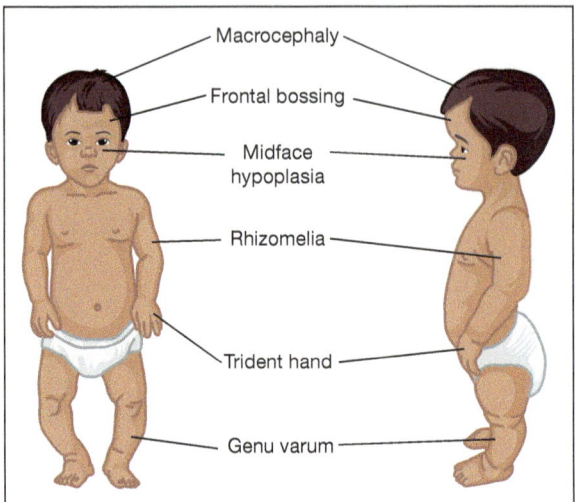

Figure 23.1: Clinical features of achondroplasia.

Specifically, stunted bone growth at the base of the skull and the spine can lead to compression of the brainstem, spinal cord, spinal nerve roots, impaired CSF drainage, and hydrocephalus. As a result, children with achondroplasia are at increased risk of central apnea, spinal myelopathy, and sudden death. Given this, baseline neurological examination is important, as well as consideration of baseline neuroimaging, especially if new neurological symptoms are present.

PREOPERATIVE PHARMACOLOGY

As in the general population, consideration of premedication with an anxiolytic medication (typically oral or IV midazolam) or parental presence for inhaled induction to assist in reducing preoperative anxiety is recommended. If an asleep fiberoptic intubation is the planned approach, an antisialagogue is recommended. Patients with history of gastroesophageal reflux disease (GERD) symptoms, which are more common in children with neurorespiratory problems, may also benefit from an H2 antagonist.

ANESTHETIC TECHNIQUE

Intraoperative Management

Special Considerations/Concerns

Achondroplasia may present challenges in airway management due to characteristic craniofacial features associated with the condition. Transient upper airway obstruction upon inhaled or IV induction is not uncommon, but this rarely leads to difficulties with mask ventilation, although an appropriately sized oral airway or laryngeal mask airway (LMA) placement may be required. Due to patients' small oral cavity size and mouth opening, supraglottic airways of various sizes and types should be available since it may not be possible to estimate the appropriate size of the supraglottic device based on weight. The challenge of tracheal intubation in achondroplasia children is complicated by concerns of risk of foramen magnum stenosis, odontoid hypoplasia, and cervical neck instability.

Neck hyperextension should be strictly avoided during both mask ventilation and endotracheal intubation due to the risk of compressing the medullar or upper cervical cord leading to potential serious neurological impairments.[6,7,8,10] For

observed episodes of apnea. Obtaining a polysomnography study can help to determine the severity and etiology, being either obstructive or central in nature or both

Neurological Assessment

Approximately 20% of all children with achondroplasia will experience a neurological impairment due to extrinsic compression of the elements of the central nervous system or impairment of cerebrospinal fluid (CSF) drainage.[1,9]

all procedures in infants with achondroplasia, the American AAP recommends careful handling of the head and neck with proper neck support and avoidance of sudden, uncontrolled head movements, which may cause compression of the brainstem and upper cervical cord.[3] Difficulties with endotracheal intubation using direct laryngoscopy are uncommon in achondroplastic patients. In two case reports, difficulties in laryngoscopy and endotracheal intubation were attributed to an inability to extend the neck (limited flexibility of the atlanto-occipital joint).[5] In-line stabilization and video laryngoscope or fiberoptic techniques are recommended for endotracheal intubation to maintain neck neutrality. The need for a smaller endotracheal tube size than would be expected for the patient's age should be anticipated, and the size of the endotracheal tube should be based on the patient's weight rather than on age.[4]

Because the head of achondroplasia children is relatively large, significant heat loss can occur during the induction phase of anesthesia, as well as during maintenance for the duration of the surgery. In addition to warming the operating room prior to induction, having a forced-air warming device and covering the head with a blanket or plastic sheet will reduce heat loss by conduction and convection.

Careful positioning and padding are essential for patients with achondroplasia as they are at high risk of intraoperative damage caused by positioning.[9] In addition, patients with achondroplasia often have ligamentous laxity, leading to loose joints, especially of the knees, which require careful positioning by avoiding hyperextension. Simultaneously, they may have flexion and extension contractures of the hip and elbow joints, requiring care in selecting appropriate protection and padding on the operating room.

Special Techniques/Equipment

Neuraxial anesthesia can be technically difficult due to narrow spinal canal and stenosis, reduced epidural space, kyphoscoliosis, and vertebral body deformities.[9] In general, the AAP recommends that spinal or epidural anesthesia should be avoided unless there are no signs of neurological compromise and neuroimaging reveals adequate space within the spinal canal.[3] Peripheral regional anesthesia may be possible, but positioning may pose challenges with access and placement of the block.

In children with achondroplasia, there are special considerations regarding monitors and IV access. Finding an appropriate blood pressure (BP) cuff size can be challenging due to their conical short arms. Alternative locations to place the BP cuff are on the forearm or the calf. Rarely, the placement of a radial arterial line is needed for monitoring BP when a noninvasive BP cuff is inadequate. Peripheral IV access may be difficult due to their short, proximal extremities, redundant soft tissue, increased SC fat, and contracted joints.[8-10] Central access in the internal jugular, subclavian, or femoral site may also be challenging due to their short neck and large head, narrow, deformed chest, and contracted hips, respectively. Access to an ultrasound or a vein viewer is recommended in anticipation of possible challenges in peripheral, central, and arterial line placement.

POSTOPERATIVE CARE

Postoperative care is dependent on the patient's preexisting conditions and the intervention. Compared with the general population, children with achondroplasia are prone to developing pulmonary complications, such as atelectasis, pneumonia, transient postoperative respiratory distress, and pulmonary edema, so closer pulse oximetry monitoring may be required.[4,9] In children with achondroplasia who have severe restrictive lung disease, severe central or obstructive sleep apnea, or other comorbidities that increase the risk of post-operative complications, intensive care monitoring should be considered.

REFERENCES

1. Horton WA, Hall J, Hect T. Achondroplasia. *Lancet*, 2007;370: 162–72. doi:10.1016/S0140-6736(07)61090-3
2. Pauli R. Achondroplasia: a comprehensive clinical review. *Orphanet J Rare Dis*, 2019; 14(1):141–49. doi:10.1186/s13023-018-0972-6
3. Hoover-Fong J, Scott C Jones M. Health supervision for people with achondroplasia. *Pediatrics*, 2020;145(6):1–19. doi:10.1542/peds.2020-1010
4. Sisk E, Heatley D, Borowski B, et al. Obstructive sleep apnea in children with achondroplasia: surgical and anesthetic considerations. *Otolaryngol Head Neck Surg*.1999;120(2):248–254. doi:10.1016/S0194-5998(99)70414-6
5. Monedero P, Rios J Pedrajas F, et al. Is management of anesthesia in achondroplastic dwarfs really a challenge? *J Clin Anesth*. 1997;9(3);208–212. doi:10.1016/s0952-8180(97)00033-0
6. Kaushal A, Haldar R, Ambesh P. Anesthesia for achondroplastic individual with coexisting atlantoaxial dislocation. *Anesth Essays Res*. 2015;9(3):443–446. doi:10.4103/0259-1162.158514
7. Veevaete L, Khalifa C, Kaminski L, Veyckemans F. Three anesthetic challenges for spinal surgery in a morbidly obese achondroplastic dwarf. *Acta Anaesth. Belg.* 2017;68:95–98. doi:10.4103/0974-8237.65483
8. Ireland P, Pacey V, Zankl A, Edwards P, Johnston L, Savarirayan, R. Optimal management of complications associated with achondroplasia. *Appl Clin Genet*. 2014;7:117–125. doi:10.2147/TACG.S51485
9. Orphananesthesia, anesthesia recommendations for achondroplasia. 2019. www.orpha.net.
10. Nisa N, Khanna P, Jain D. Anaesthetic Management of an achondroplastic dwarf with difficult airway and spine for total hip replacement: a case report. *General Medicine: Open Access*. 2016;4:2. doi:10.4172/2327-5146.1000227

CHAPTER 24

Apert Syndrome

Sarah Milligan

PATHOPHYSIOLOGY AND CLINICAL MANIFESTATIONS

First described in 1894 by S.W. Wheaton and later described in greater detail by the French pediatrician Eugene Charles Apert, Apert syndrome is a craniofacial syndrome associated with facial anomalies, syndactyly of the hands and feet, cardiac defects and craniosynostosis.[1] Apert syndrome is also referred to as acrocephalosyndactyly (ACS) type 1. All forms of ACS are characterized by craniosynostosis affecting the proper growth of the skull and head, with Apert syndrome accounting for approximately 5% of all craniosynostoses.

The incidence of Apert syndrome ranges from 1 in 65,000 to 1 in 160,000 live births.[1,2] Apert syndrome is caused by a mutation in the fibroblast growth receptor 2 (FGFR2) on chromosome 10 in 98% of patients, although there are also reports of autosomal dominant inheritance.[2] The majority of cases, however, are the result of spontaneous or new mutations in the gene encoding FGFR2. The result is abnormal osseous development that results in irregular bridging of mesenchymal tissue that eventually transforms into bone. Diagnosis most often occurs at birth based on clinical characteristics. Gene testing exploring mutations in FGFR2, as well as CT or MRI, may be employed to confirm the diagnosis or to explore the extent of associated anomalies. Apert syndrome may also be detected prenatally via ultrasound or MRI.

The cranium and distal extremities are predominately affected by the irregular bridging of mesenchymal tissue that eventually transforms into bone. The coronal sutures most commonly close prematurely, leading to a high forehead and flat facies. Other common facial features include a horizontal ridge above the supraorbital ridge, spheno-ethmoido-maxillary hypoplasia, a short nose with bulbous tip, and depressed nasal bridge. Fusion of the middle three fingers is a classic sign of Apert syndrome. The palate of a child with Apert syndrome is high and narrow.[3] Fusion at C5–C6 and cleft palate are also common findings.[4] Hydrocephalus can occur in some patients. There may be cranial nerve dysfunction because of foraminal stenosis in the base of the skull.[3] Intellectual and developmental disability in Apert syndrome is usually mild in 50% of patients but can be severe in some cases.[3,5] Infants with Apert syndrome may also present with feeding difficulties, hearing loss, synostosis of other bones, and airway abnormalities (narrow nasal passages, abnormal palate, trachea, and jaw).[5]

Apert syndrome has several characteristic hand and foot malformations, with the upper limbs more commonly being severely affected than the lower limbs. Affected individuals often have short fingers and broad thumbs and great toes that deviate outward. They may also present with partial to complete syndactyly of fingers and toes. In the feet, toenails may be partially continuous or separate. There is no curative treatment for Apert syndrome, and the prognosis depends largely on the severity of the genetic anomalies.

ANESTHETIC MANAGEMENT

PREOPERATIVE EVALUATION

Anesthesia providers should perform a thorough history and physical prior to anesthetizing a patient with Apert syndrome. Head and neck anatomy should be evaluated to plan for airway management. Neck x-rays can be helpful to determine if there is C5–C6 fusion, which could make sniffing position and airway management more difficult.[1] If a cardiac murmur is detected on auscultation, an echocardiogram is warranted due to the potential for cardiac lesions. The most common cardiac lesions in children with Apert syndrome are pulmonic stenosis and ventricular septal defect (VSD).[6]

Pertinent Labs

Lab work such as complete blood count, complete metabolic panel, and type and screen should be collected prior to surgery. Cranial vault reconstruction has a potential for large blood loss and electrolyte imbalances, and the need for blood transfusion should be anticipated.[7]

PREOPERATIVE PHARMACOTHERAPY

Premedication with anxiolytics should be used with caution in children with Apert syndrome due to the common findings of increased intracranial pressure and obstructive sleep apnea.[1] Obstructive sleep apnea is present in 50% of patients due to midface hypoplasia, and difficult airway management should be expected.[8]

ANESTHETIC TECHNIQUE

Intraoperative Management

Anesthesia providers should be prepared for a potential difficult mask ventilation and intubation. Choanal atresia is common, as is tracheal stenosis. Intubation may be difficult due to facial abnormalities and decreased neck mobility. While inhalational mask induction may be safely performed, awake intubation should be considered for the patient with a suspected or known difficult airway. It is advisable to maintain spontaneous ventilation until the patient's airway is secured.[1] In a review of 509 cases, most patients were a Cormack Lehane grade I view.[8] Supraglottic airway obstruction was most common and was managed easily with simple airway maneuvers.[8] Nonetheless, it is recommended that an appropriately sized laryngeal mask airway and fiberoptic bronchoscope be immediately available during induction.

Standard monitors, as described by the American Society of Anesthesiologist, should be employed. Should significant blood loss be anticipated, placement of an arterial line should be considered for frequent monitoring of hematocrit and hemoglobin levels. For cranial vault reconstruction procedures, placement of two large bore IV lines is prudent to facilitate blood transfusion and fluid volume resuscitation. Of note, obtaining IV access may be difficult due to limb synostosis and the use of ultrasound may be necessary to facilitate line placement. If the patient has a known cardiac defect, air bubble precautions must be utilized. Care should be taken while positioning the patient with joint synostosis. Patients with Apert syndrome commonly have proptosis and are at a high risk of corneal abrasions; thus, anesthesia providers must be vigilant in ensuring the eyes are taped and free from pressure.[8]

Close monitoring of hemoglobin and hematocrit, electrolytes, and blood glucose is imperative.[7] Cranial vault procedures have the potential for large blood loss and fluid shifts. Arterial blood samples should be drawn regularly throughout the procedure to evaluate electrolyte imbalances and blood loss. Efforts should be made to maintain normothermia during the surgical procedure, as hypothermia is not uncommon due to the need for massive transfusion.

Adequate cerebral perfusion pressure (CPP) should be maintained in patients with Apert syndrome for assumed increased intracranial pressure (ICP).[1] Anesthesia providers should avoid increasing the ICP further and ensure maintenance of adequate CPP. Ventilation should be aimed at preserving normocapnia or mild hypocapnia. In craniofacial procedures, there is a high risk of venous air embolism. For this reason, nitrous oxide should be avoided, a central line should be placed and precordial Doppler should be available throughout the procedure.[1]

POSTOPERATIVE CARE

Should the patient have tracheal or other airway abnormalities, postoperative ventilation may be necessary. The potential for airway and facial edema following craniofacial surgery also warrants postoperative intubation and ventilatory support.[1] Postoperatively, blood glucose and electrolyte levels should be monitored for at least 24 hours to assess for metabolic derangements.[7] Narcotics should be used with caution in patients with suspected obstructive sleep apnea and/or an elevated ICP.

REFERENCES

1. Bissonnette B, Luginbuehl I, Engelhardt T, eds. Acrocephalosyndactyly type i: apert syndrome. In: *Syndromes: Rapid Recognition and Perioperative Implications, 2e*. McGraw Hill; 2019. https://accessanesthesiology-mhmedical-com.ccmain.ohionet.org/content.aspx?bookid=2674&sectionid=220519985
2. Fadda MT, Ierardo G, Ladniak B, et al.; Group of Apert syndrome, Policlinico Umberto I, "Sapienza" University of Rome, Italy. Treatment timing and multidisciplinary approach in Apert syndrome. *Ann Stomatol (Roma)*. 2015;6(2):58-63. PMID: 26330906; PMCID: PMC4525098.
3. Wells RG. ed. The skull and face. In: *Diagnostic Imaging of Infants and Children*. McGraw Hill; 2013. https://accesspediatrics-mhmedical-com.ccmain.ohionet.org/content.aspx?bookid=1429&sectionid=84705838
4. Rhee L. Syndromes. In: Ellinas H, Matthes K, Alrayashi W, Bilge A, eds. *Clinical Pediatric Anesthesiology*. McGraw Hill; 2021. https://accessanesthesiology-mhmedical-com.ccmain.ohionet.org/content.aspx?bookid=2985&sectionid=250593099
5. Wenger TL, Hing AV, Evans KN. Apert Syndrome. 2019 May 30. In: Adam MP, Ardinger HH, Pagon RA, et al. eds. *GeneReviews®*. Seattle; 1993-2021. https://www.ncbi.nlm.nih.gov/books/NBK541728
6. Menser C, Hays S. Preoperative assessment of newborns and children. In: Longnecker DE, Mackey SC, Newman MF, Sandberg WS, Zapol WM, eds. *Anesthesiology, 3e*. McGraw Hill; 2017. https://accessanesthesiology-mhmedical-com.ccmain.ohionet.org/content.aspx?bookid=2152&sectionid=164216675
7. Hochhold C, Luckner G, Strohmenger U, Scholl-Bürgi S, Paal P. Intra-operative hypoglycemia and electrolyte imbalance in a child with Apert syndrome during craniosynostosis surgery. *Paediatric Anaesthesia*. 2014;24(3):352–354. doi:10.1111/pan.12344
8. Barnett S, Moloney C, Bingham R. Perioperative complications in children with Apert syndrome: a review of 509 anesthetics. *Paediatr Anaesth*. 2011;21(1):72-7. doi: 10.1111/j.1460-9592.2010.03457.x. Epub 2010 Nov 15. PMID: 21073626.

CHAPTER 25

Arthrogryposis

Michael Sikora

PATHOPHYSIOLOGY AND CLINICAL MANIFESTATIONS

Arthrogryposis is a general or descriptive term for the development of nonprogressive congenital joint contractures affecting greater than one joint prior to birth.[1] The overall prevalence of arthrogryposis is 1 in 3,000 live births.[2] Arthrogryposis is a clinical finding, not a specific diagnosis. The etiology of this disease is extremely varied and includes greater than 400 conditions. One common theme among the varied etiologies is fetal akinesia, or the inability to move joint articulations in utero.[1] This decreased mobility results in connective tissue around the joints, leading to joint fibrosis and ultimately contractures.[1] Arthrogryposis affecting two or more different areas of the body is referred to as arthrogryposis multiplex congenita (AMC).[2] AMC can be further classified into one of three subgroups: amyoplasia, distal arthrogryposis, and syndromic.

Amyoplasia is the most common form of AMC and is characterized by symmetric contractures in all four limbs in newborns, although the jaw and trunk are typically spared.[2] Although the distal joints are typically more severely affected with amyoplasia, the shoulders and hips (which are considered proximal joints) often have significant contractures. With amyoplasia, the shoulders are often internally rotated and adducted, with the elbows extended and the wrists flexed with ulnar deviation. Additionally, most children with amyoplasia have fingers that are flexed and stiff, and severe clubfoot that will require surgical release. Muscle mass is reduced in patients with amyoplasia. Anesthesia providers should be aware that approximately 10% of patients with amyoplasia have abdominal abnormalities such as gastroschisis or intestinal atresia.

In contrast, distal arthrogryposis represents a group of syndromes characterized by multiple congenital joint contractures, namely, of the hands and feet.[1] Commonly, the "windblown hand" is seen with distal arthrogryposis, which entails ulnar deviation of the digits through the metacarpophalangeal joint, stiff digits, and thumb-in-palm. Common etiologies of distal arthrogryposis include mutations in sarcomeric muscle proteins or embryonic myosin heavy chain protein.[1] Syndromic arthrogryposis may include central nervous system disorders or neuromuscular diseases. A number of syndromes, including Freeman–Sheldon syndrome, Sheldon–Hall syndrome, Shprintzen–Goldberg syndrome, whistling face syndrome, Gordon syndrome, and Dutch–Kentucky syndrome, represent possible manifestations of distal arthrogryposis.[3]

The contractures associated with arthrogryposis are present at birth. The muscles of the affected limbs are generally hypoplastic, resulting in a tube-shaped limb with a soft, doughy feeling. Soft tissue webbing may develop over the affected joints with skin dimpling. In addition to the joint abnormalities associated with AMC, patients may present with abnormally slender and fragile long bones of the arms and legs and a cleft palate. Male patients may present with cryptorchidism. Approximately one-third of patients with AMC have structural or functional central nervous system abnormalities, though intelligence may or may not be affected.

ANESTHETIC MANAGEMENT

Children with arthrogryposis require anesthetic care routinely, averaging more than five operations during childhood.[1] Expert consensus of arthrogryposis management involves early mobilization of joint contractures via physical therapy, casting, and surgical release starting during infancy.[4] The overriding feature of arthrogryposis is joint contractures, and in many cases, the anesthetic implications are consequences of managing this issue.

PREOPERATIVE EVALUATION

Careful assessment of the airway prior to an anesthetic is mandatory (Box 25.1). Limited jaw mobility results in limited mouth opening.[5] In addition, children with arthrogryposis may present with micrognathia, short neck, and/or fusion of the cervical vertebrae.[5]

Pertinent Labs

No labs are routinely required for patients with arthrogryposis requiring anesthesia, although a complete blood count, electrolytes, and renal panel may be warranted depending on the patient's comorbidities, general state of health, and the procedure scheduled. Patients with cardiac disease or severe scoliosis should have an echocardiogram. Anesthesia providers should consider obtaining pulmonary function tests for patients presenting with respiratory restrictions or anomalies.

> **BOX 25.1 KEY ASSESSMENT POINTS**
>
> Thorough airway assessment includes noting the following:
> - Abnormal orofacial musculature
> - High-arched palate
> - Limited cervical movement or cervical instability
> - Limited mouth opening
> - Micrognathia

PREOPERATIVE PHARMACOTHERAPY

Given the incidence of difficult airway is 25% among patients with arthrogryposis, sedative and anxiolytic medications should be administered with caution given the potential for difficult intubation.

ANESTHETIC TECHNIQUE

Intraoperative Management

In most circumstances, patients with arthrogryposis are not challenging to mask ventilate, allowing for the establishment of IV access after mask induction of general anesthesia. Certainly, concern for difficult airway may take precedence over challenging vascular access; however, mask induction may facilitate achieving vascular access while minimizing pain and the number of attempts needed to establish vascular access. Limb contractures can complicate positioning for IV access placement, and general anesthesia with volatile agents can partially alleviate this challenge by allowing more limb movement. If available at your facility and proficient with its use, early ultrasound utilization for IV access may decrease the number of attempts.

Depending upon the procedure, the use of a laryngeal mask airway (LMA) should be considered as placement is often successful, thereby negating the need for endotracheal tube placement.[5] Assuming continued ability to mask ventilate, many anesthesia providers will opt to electively perform a direct laryngoscopy to document ease of airway management as a means of informing subsequent anesthesia providers about airway manage given the high likelihood the patient will have multiple anesthetics. During direct laryngoscopy, limited neck mobility and mouth opening may make the airway appear "anterior"; however, cricoid pressure often allows for satisfactory airway exposure for intubation. Should direct laryngoscopy prove challenging, providers can utilize video laryngoscopes or flexible bronchoscopes to achieve endotracheal intubation. Choosing a specific technology depends on what is available at one's specific institution as well as the individual provider's experience with specific devices. Furthermore, LMAs may be utilized to support the airway as a bridge to endotracheal intubation through flexible bronchoscopy through the LMA. When attempting this technique, it is vitally important to make sure that the endotracheal tube can pass through the LMA because not all LMAs are designed for this use. Many LMAs have bars across the LMA orifice, preventing passage of the endotracheal tube.

Planned or emergent tracheotomy remains an option should intubation prove challenging despite all the aforementioned techniques. Like all medical decisions, the choice to pursue planned tracheotomy depends on carefully weighing the risks and benefits as a comprehensive care team in communication with the family and patient. Patients with a history of hypoxia or airway injury due to challenging intubation who require repeated anesthetics may benefit from tracheotomy.[1] Arthrogryposis patients with associated scoliosis or myopathy often display limited pulmonary reserve. In addition, children with arthrogryposis often present with restricted lung development. Tracheotomy allows for positive pressure ventilation postoperatively, theoretically ameliorating the risk of postoperative respiratory morbidity.[1] Finally, tracheotomy on an arthrogryposis patient with a history of challenging intubation decreases the likelihood of needing to emergently manage the airway due to over sedation or respiratory illness.[1]

Positioning during surgery can be challenging should the patient have multiple contractures. Anesthesia providers should ensure the patient is appropriately padded to decrease the risk of injury. There is historical reported concern for hyperthermia or hypermetabolic events for children with arthrogryposis who undergo anesthesia.[6] This clinical hyperthermia does not represent malignant hypothermia, or require dantrolene for management and volatile agents can be used safely in patients with AMC.[6] Active cooling alone is the primary treatment. A recent retrospective study from the Mayo Clinic including 370 discrete anesthetics did not identify intraoperative max temperature differences among patients with severe arthrogryposis, mild arthrogryposis, and control.[6]

Special Considerations
Patients with arthrogryposis commonly experience both nociceptive and neuropathic pain.[7] Stiffness due to decreased joint mobility is another factor contributing to pain in this patient population. Despite this common experience of pain, a recent scoping review of pain in arthrogryposis yielded only 21 studies that included only level II and level IV evidence, suggesting much greater research is necessary to elucidate the issue of pain in arthrogryposis.[7] This scoping review suggests that the majority of patients with arthrogryposis commonly experience pain, pain often begins during childhood, pain occurs in multiple joints, and pain is typically grater in the lower extremities than the upper extremities.[7] In addition, pain was identified, along with muscle fatigue, as a factor contributing to limitations in daily activity. Examples of activities of daily living affected by pain include walking, standing, using stairs, and sitting.[7] Without a proper pain assessment tool for arthrogryposis, comparing the effectiveness of various pharmacologic and nonpharmacologic pain relief modalities is not possible.

In addition to contractures, children with arthrogryposis are at risk for scoliosis.[1] Patients also have a high risk of vertebral column deformities, causing theoretical concern for neuraxial anesthetic techniques.[1] Despite this concern, neuraxial techniques remain a theoretical option after weighing the risks and benefits of an arthrogryposis patient's presentation and clinical scenario. A recent case presentation highlights successful combined spinal epidural anesthetic for a parturient with arthrogryposis presenting for trial of labor.[8] While attempting the procedure, the authors noted only slight loss of resistance during epidural placement but were confident in the catheter placement given presence of cerebrospinal fluid while advancing the spinal needle within the Tuohy.[8]

POSTOPERATIVE CARE

Postoperatively, patients with AMC are more susceptible to postoperative pulmonary complications due to an increased sensitivity to neuromuscular blocking agents and opioids. Furthermore, ventilation may be restrictive secondary to scoliosis or thoracic deformities. Stridor and postoperative atelectasis are also common, making it imperative that respiratory function and airway patency are monitored postoperatively.

REFERENCES

1. Isaacson G, Drum ET. Difficult airway management in children and young adults with arthrogryposis. *World J Otorhinolaryngol Head Neck Surg*. 2018;4(2):122–125. doi:10.1016/j.wjorl.2018.04.003. PMID: 30101221; PMCID: PMC6074018.
2. Bamshad M, Van Heest AE, Pleasure D. Arthrogryposis: a review and update. *J Bone Jt Surg*. 2009;91(Suppl 4):40–46. doi:10.2106/JBJS.I.00281
3. Desai D, Stiene D, Song T, Sadayappan S. Distal arthrogryposis and lethal congenital contracture syndrome: an overview. *Front Physiol*. 2020;11:689. doi:10.3389/fphys.2020.00689. PMID: 32670090; PMCID: PMC7330016.
4. Hansen-Jaumard D, Elfassy C, Montpetit K, Ghalimah B, Hamdy R, Dahan-Oliel N. A review of the orthopedic interventions and functional outcomes among a cohort of 114 children with arthrogryposis multiplex congenita. *J Pediatr Rehabil Med*. 2020;13(3):263-271. doi: 10.3233/PRM-190657. PMID: 33104047.
5. Ma L, Yu X. Arthrogryposis multiplex congenita: classification, diagnosis, perioperative care, and anesthesia. *Front Med*. 2017;11:48–52. doi:10.1007/s11684-017-0500-4
6. Gleich SJ, Tien M, Schroeder DR, et al. Anesthetic outcomes of children with arthrogryposis syndromes: no evidence of hyperthermia. *Anesth Analg*. 2017;124(3):908–914. doi:10.1213/ANE.0000000000001822.
7. Cirillo A, Collins J, Sawatzky B, et al. Pain among children and adults living with arthrogryposis multiplex congenita: a scoping review. *Am J Med Genet C Semin Med Genet*. 2019;181(3):436–453. doi:10.1002/ajmg.c.31725
8. Spooner L. Caesarean section using a combined spinal epidural technique in a patient with arthrogryposis multiplex congenita. *Int J Obstet Anesth*. 2000;9(4):282–285. doi:10.1054/ijoa.2000.0722.

CHAPTER 26

Autism Spectrum Disorder

Amanda Whippey

PATHOPHYSIOLOGY AND CLINICAL MANIFESTATIONS

Autism spectrum disorder (ASD) is the fastest growing developmental disability, diagnosed 1 in 54 children, with a male-to-female ratio of 4:1.1 ASD is a complex neurodevelopmental disorder[2] that has no single known cause, although due to the complexity of the disorder and range of symptom severity, both genetics and environmental exposures have been implicated.[3] Recent neuro-mapping studies have demonstrated cortical changes in neurotransmitter levels associated with autism severity.[4] Autism symptoms are widely ranging and fall into three categories: sensory processing, language communication skills, and strict adherence to routines or stereotypic behaviors.

The presentation of this early childhood condition characterized by difficulty in communication, social interaction, and sensory processing is widely varied from mild to severe symptoms that impact daily function. Symptoms may be observed as early as 2 to 6 months of age, but a diagnosis is rarely made before the age of 3 years. As a result, children with ASD requiring anesthesia may not have a formal diagnosis at the time of the procedure.[5,6] Recent studies have shown that 90% of children with ASD have atypical sensory processing, which may be tied to social impairment; furthermore, 33% of patients have cognitive disability (IQ <70), and concurrent psychiatric and medical disorders are common.[1,5-7] Seventy percent of children with ASD are diagnosed with a mental disorder, with 40% having two or more mental disorders. Social anxiety (29%), attention deficit hyperactivity disorder (ADHD, 28%), oppositional defiant or conduct disorder (30%), and anxiety (23%) are most common.[8]

ANESTHETIC MANAGEMENT

PREOPERATIVE EVALUATION

Due to their inability to comply with many medical interventions, children with ASD are frequent patients in the operating room. The importance of a comprehensive preoperative assessment for children with ASD cannot be overstated (Box 26.1). As this may be challenging with the child present, a phone interview or parental survey may facilitate obtaining the details needed to make an effective coping plan. Patients with ASD have higher rates of refusal of premedication, noncompliance at induction, postoperative delirium, and often exhibit flight behavior. Parental satisfaction increases when they are involved in the planning process and feel their concerns are heard.[9] They can identify known triggers (crowds, loud noises, and bright lights) and historical background that is often not found in the medical record.[10] Individualized anesthetic plans that minimize known stressors have been shown to decrease noncompliance at induction from 50% to 17%, without the use of premedication.[2] Premedication use predictably increases with autism severity, as does the use of nonconventional medications (IM ketamine).[11,12] Premedication is not always effective and can result in unwanted side effects (nausea, vomiting, and respiratory depression), require increased nursing resources and monitoring, and can delay discharge times.

Clinical pathways tailored to patients with ASD can facilitate atraumatic inductions while minimizing the use of premedication (Box 26.2). These clinical pathways include minimizing transitions and wait times, the use of quiet or sensory rooms, booking as first case of the day, avoiding changing into hospital gowns and placing name bands, and avoiding routine vitals if not indicated.[8,10,12,13] Patient and family preparation including the use of Child Life Specialists, social stories, communication boards, videos, immersive technologies, or exposure (mask desensitization) can also be effective.[14-18] Additionally, studies have shown decreased cortisol or anxiety levels with the use of service animals.[19]

Many children with ASD can be compliant when they know what to expect and what is expected from them.[16] In the hospital setting, recognizing signs of stress (often nonverbal) and having resources available that reduce stress (sensory items, music, and movement) are critical. It may be difficult for parents and healthcare providers to differentiate core symptoms of autism from perioperative anxiety or stress.[20] Many healthcare providers feel poorly equipped to care for children with ASD; programs that promote autism awareness in the perioperative setting have been met with positive results.[17,21,22] Unfortunately, significant institutional variation remains in provision of sedation for children with autism, and most formalized programs are found in the tertiary setting.[23]

PREOPERATIVE PHARMACOTHERAPY

Despite nonpharmacological interventions, premedication may be needed to facilitate a smooth transition into the operating room and induction. It can be challenging, however, for the anesthesia provider to determine the optimal medication to employ as there are insufficient data to recommend one medication over another (Table 26.1). When choosing a premedication, consider the sustainability of the plan. IM ketamine, while effective, may make the next procedural visit more challenging. Children with ASD often require higher doses than their neurotypical counterparts to achieve comparable levels of sedation. The reason for this is unclear but could in part result from higher levels of preprocedural anxiety, which is known to affect required dosing. A growing body of evidence suggests that combining multiple agents, such as midazolam + ketamine or dexmedetomidine + ketamine, provides a superior level of sedation while minimizing side effects.[24-28] For children with taste sensitivities, administering dexmedetomidine first may improve compliance with the second medication. Allowing adequate time for medication to take effect is important as onset can be variable depending on route of administration.

Benzodiazepines

Midazolam is the most used, short-acting benzodiazepine that provides a calm, drowsy state, and anterograde amnesia.

> **BOX 26.1** **PREOPERATIVE EVALUATION KEY ASSESSMENT POINTS FOR AUTISM SPECTRUM DISORDER (ASD)**
>
> **General Assessment**
> - Autism Severity Score (ASS)*
> - Anxiety: Generalized, situational
> - History of treatment noncompliance
> - Medical history: ADHD, global delay, epilepsy, genetic disorders
> - Home medications: SSRIs, alpha-agonists, cannabinoids, amphetamines†
>
> **Communication Style**
> - Nonverbal/minimally interactive
> - Beginning language
> - Communication device used
> - Interacts with others/behavior regulation
> - High functioning
>
> **Sensory Processing**
> - Loud noises—crying babies
> - Taste aversion—medication
> - Bright lighting
> - Touch
> - Commotion—multiple people
>
> **Behavioral Challenges**
> - Home medication to moderate behavior
> - Needle-phobia
> - Mask-phobia
> - Fear of hospitals/personnel
> - Panic episodes
> - Vomiting
> - Combative, self-injury
> - Flight risk
>
> **Coping Strategies**
> - Distraction: Tablet, immersive technology, toys
> - Specific motivator
> - Service animal
> - Breathing/counting/talking/singing
> - Mask scent
> - Comfort items
> - Parental presence
>
> **Induction Plan**
> - Prehospital medication
> - Premedication—anxiolysis versus sedation
> - Inhalational versus IV induction
> - Topical analgesics
>
> *ASS1—requires support; ASS2—requires substantial support; ASS3—requires very substantial support.
>
> †Selective serotonin reuptake inhibitors (SSRIs), cannabinoids and atypical antipsychotics should continue preoperatively. Rarely, atypical antipsychotics can cause hypotension during general anesthesia and can be proarrhythmic. Psychostimulants should be held as they can increase sedative dosing and lower the seizure threshold.
>
> ADHD, attention-deficit/hyperactivity disorder; IV, intravenous; SSRI, selective serotonin reuptake inhibitors.
>
> Source: Kanazawa O. Reappraisal of abnormal EEG findings in children with ADHD: on the relationship between ADHD and epileptiform discharges. *Epilepsy Behav.* 2014;41:251–256. doi:10.1016/j.yebeh.2014.09.078.

Oral midazolam is usually mixed with syrup or flavoring to conceal its bitter taste (pH 3). It also stings when administered intranasally or intramuscularly. There are reports of paradoxical reactions or disinhibition with midazolam, particularly when lower doses are used.[29] Midazolam is effective for milder forms of ASD, with ketamine typically required for more severe cases. Some studies have reported delayed emergence with midazolam; others have not with variations in intraoperative anesthetic management likely accounting for this disparity in the literature.[16] Lorazepam has a much slower onset and is usually well tolerated but can delay emergence with its much longer duration of action.

Alpha-Agonists

Clonidine and dexmedetomidine bind to the central alpha-2A adrenoreceptors, preventing further central norepinephrine release at the level of the brainstem. These drugs also mediate effects via alpha-2B adrenoreceptors, causing hypotension and bradycardia. In children, notable bradycardia has been observed though intervention is rarely necessary.[25] Importantly, clonidine and dexmedetomidine have no effect on respiration. The quality of sedation is calming and well tolerated but can be variable. Insufficient sedation may occur when peripheral catecholamines are released, and patients may rouse with loud noises and touch. This can be problematic in children with ASD and frequently dexmedetomidine is paired with another sedative in this population.[30–32] Dexmedetomidine has been shown to reduce volatile anesthetic requirement, decrease emergence delirium and analgesic use after surgery, and has been suggested as the preferred second line again to ketamine.[8,25] Dexmedetomidine has a pH of 7.1, making it well tolerated as an intranasal medication. Oral dexmedetomidine has been studied with some success; however, low bioavailability (16%) limits its use.[33]

Ketamine

Ketamine is a structural analog to phencyclidine and acts as a noncompetitive antagonist of the N-methyl-D-aspartate receptor. Ketamine is a long-standing choice of premedication particularly for uncooperative patients in whom IV or inhalational induction would be difficult given its rapid onset when given as an IM medication. It is also effective as an oral premedication, producing a dissociative state while retaining respiratory drive. Ketamine has a pH of 3.5 to 5.5 and will taste bitter to some patients with taste sensitivities. Ketamine can be used as sedative or anesthetic doses. The side effects of ketamine are the largest drawback to its use: emergence delirium, dysphoria, nausea and vomiting, nystagmus, hypersalivation, and laryngospasm and are more common in postpubescent patients, particularly females. Dysphoria and emergence delirium are not dose-dependent and can be minimized by using midazolam. Nausea and

BOX 26.2 ASPECTS OF A CLINICAL PRACTICE GUIDELINE FOR HOSPITAL ACCOMMODATION WITH AUTISM SPECTRUM DISORDER

1. **Flexible Admission Process**
   - Minimize wait times, NPO
     - Limit disruption of rigid timetables and routines
     - Food sometimes used to moderate behavior
   - Quiet room
     - Minimize sensory input (e.g., lights, crying, proximity to others)
   - Avoid hospital gowns, name bands, local anesthetic cream
     - May help to avoid early agitation
   - Preoperative vitals only when indicated
   - Communication boards, visual aid, social story
     - To address any deficit in social communication, unable to understand process of events

2. **Premedication**
   - Home medications
     - To ameliorate anxiety—may not want to enter hospital
   - Route of administration
     - Taste sensitivity—bitter tasting medications (midazolam or ketamine) intolerable, may select injection or sublingual (S/L) route
   - Anxiolysis or sedation
     - Higher levels of severity (ASS3) are more likely to require sedation versus anxiolysis

3. **Induction**
   - Transition to operating room
     - Transitions to new environment challenging—poorly recognized or understood by providers
   - Parental presence
     - Restricted communication, understanding—parent acts as translator
   - IV versus inhalational
     - Increased sensitivity to smell of inhalational agents or struggle with proximity to provider
   - Positioning
     - Anxiety may make lying down a struggle
   - Lighting
     - Fluorescent lighting can result in feeling of pain
   - Minimizing people during induction
     - Crowds of people common trigger in hospital

4. **Intraoperative**
   - Fluid replacement—saline lock (SL) intravenous (IV) at end of case
     - Increased risk for delirium, pulling out IV
   - Postoperative nausea and vomiting (PONV); prophylaxis
     - Premedication may cause nausea
   - Emergence delirium prophylaxis
     - Increased risk, unable to assimilate new environment on emergence
   - Titration of anesthetic in setting of premedication
     - Premedication can result in delayed emergence

5. **Postoperative Accommodations**
   - Quiet recovery bay
     - To ameliorate noise sensitivity (e.g., sound of crying babies)
   - Early parental presence
     - To address deficits in social communication
   - Early IV removal
     - Visual aids for pain, communication
     - Visual > verbal communication
   - Expedited discharge when possible or transfer to ward
   - Sensory hypersensitivity—recovery rooms tolerated poorly

vomiting increase at higher doses (>200 mg). Acute ketamine toxicity can rarely manifest as encephalopathy, seizures, or rhabdomyolysis.[24]

ANESTHETIC TECHNIQUE

Induction technique is based on individual preference, but flexibility is central to success. Mask inductions are most common. Although definitive data are lacking, this is a high-anxiety patient population in which parental presence at induction is thought to be helpful.[14] If the patient struggles with transitions, an IV start in a quiet preoperative room may be easier.[34] Prolonged preoperative fasting times and the wide array of sensory insults present in the operating room environment (fluorescent lights, crying children, and pungent volatile anesthetics) can be particularly problematic. Physical restraint should be a last resort as it is counterproductive, leading to mistrust in healthcare professionals. Restraint should be done by anesthesia provider who have received training and with full consent of parents.[16] Traumatic inductions can lead to negative postoperative behaviors, including sleep disturbance, nightmares, general anxiety, and social withdrawal lasting 1 month to 1 year.[35]

Induction medications requirements may be decreased if a premedication is administered and should be adjusted accordingly. If alpha-agonists are used and the patient is bradycardic, remifentanil may further lower the heart rate. Emergence delirium has been associated with both IV and inhalational anesthetics; less soluble volatiles (desflurane > sevoflurane) having the highest incidence.[36] Recent research has shown mitochondrial mutations are more common in children diagnosed with ASD (7.3% compared with 0.01% in the general population). This

Table 26.1 Commonly Used Premedication With Autism Spectrum Disorder

Medication	Dose	Peak Effect	Notes
Benzodiazepines			
Midazolam	PO/buccal 0.25–0.75 mg/kg	20–40 min	Effective in isolation or combination
	IN 0.3 mg/kg	45 min	Bitter taste difficult to conceal
	IV 0.05 mg/kg	5–10 min	
	IM 0.2–0.4 mg/kg	30 min	
Lorazepam	SL 0.1–0.2 mg/kg	60 min	Frequently a home medication, easier administration
	PO 0.1–0.2 mg/kg	60–120 min	
Clonazepam	PO 0.05–0.1 mg/kg	60–120 min	
Alpha-agonists			
Clonidine	PO 0.1 mg/kg	60–90 min	Long duration of action (4–6 hr) limits use
Dexmedetomidine	IN 2–4 mcg/kg	45 min	PO route low bioavailability
	IV 1 mcg/kg	10 min	Often paired with second agent to improve sedation
	IM 2–4 mcg/kg	5–15 min	
NMDA receptor antagonist			
Ketamine	PO 3–8 mg/kg	10–20 min	Reliable sedative, can be given IM
	IM 2–4 mg/kg	4 min	Side effects profile includes nausea/vomiting, salivation, dysphoria
	IV 1–1.5 mg/kg	<1 min	
Atypical antipsychotics			
Risperidone	PO 0.25–1 mg daily	60 min	Frequently a home medication, extra dose may be ordered pre-procedure if known to be sedating

IN, injection; SL, sublingual.

has implications for the choice of anesthetic agent in the setting of potentially decreased oxidative capacity and impaired methylation. The use of short-acting medications and avoidance of nitrous oxide, prolonged infusions of propofol, or adding B_{12} supplementation should be considered.[37] Effective and complete anesthetic plans should include analgesia, antiemetics, and fluid volume replacement as many children will have venous access removed early and not be compliant with oral medications. Rectal administration may be required for some medications. Several premedications have analgesic properties, which will reduce analgesic requirements. Avoiding long-acting opioids will help avoid oversedation postoperatively.

POSTOPERATIVE CARE

Patients should be brought sedated to the recovery room with a planned slow emergence. Fentanyl (1 mcg/kg), midazolam, dexmedetomidine (0.3–0.5 mcg/kg), and propofol (1 mg/kg) have been shown to decrease emergence delirium in a recent meta-analysis.[36] Agitation from pain or nausea may be difficult to differentiate from emergence delirium. Nonverbal communication tools, such as the face, legs, activity, cry, consolability (FLACC) scale, can be effective to increase understanding.[38] Early parental presence with comfort items (music, service animals) can assist with reorientation. IV lines should be saline locked or removed early to avoid tangling or untimely removal. Early discharge when appropriate or expedited transfer to the ward is important as the sensory experience in a typical pediatric recovery room is not well tolerated. Additionally, it is easier for parents to mobilize a slightly sedated child than an agitated, disoriented one.

KEY REFERENCES

Complete references for this chapter are online and available at https://connect.springerpub.com/content/book/978-0-8261-3875-0/part/part03/toc-part/ch026

8. Taghizadeh N, Davidson A, Williams K, et al. Autism spectrum disorder (ASD) and its perioperative management. *Paediatr Anaesth*. 2015;25(11):1076–1084. doi:10.1111/pan.12732
10. Whippey A, Bernstein LM, O'Rourke D, et al. Enhanced perioperative management of children with autism: a pilot study. *Can J Anaesth*. 2019;66(10):1184–1193. doi:10.1007/s12630-019-01410-y
13. Koski S, Gabriels, RL, Beresford C. Interventions for paediatric surgery patients with comorbid autism spectrum disorder: a systematic literature review. *Arch Dis Child*. 2016;101(12):1090–1094. doi:10.1136/archdischild-2016-310814
16. Reddy S, Deutsch N. Behavioral and emotional disorders in children and their anesthetic implications. *Children*. 2020;7(12):253. doi:10.3390/children7120253
17. Taghizadeh N, Heard G, Davidson A, et al. The experiences of children with autism spectrum disorder, their caregivers and healthcare providers during day procedure: a mixed methods study. *Paediatr Anaesth*. 2019;29(9):927–937. doi:10.1111/pan.13689

CHAPTER 27

Beckwith–Wiedemann Syndrome

Marianne S. Cosgrove

PATHOPHYSIOLOGY AND CLINICAL MANIFESTATIONS

First described by doctors Bruce Beckwith and Hans Rudolph Wiedemann in the 1960s, Beckwith–Wiedemann syndrome (BWS) was originally called EMG, based on the three clinical findings of *e*xomphalos, *m*acroglossia, and *g*igantism. BWS is the most common overgrowth disorder, occurring in approximately 1 in 10,340 live births with representation between males and females.[1,2,3] Of note, the incidence of BWS may be higher in pregnancies that benefitted from assisted reproductive technology.[3,4]

Patients with BWS often exhibit a constellaion of symptoms and physical findings including congenital anomalies, metabolic disorders, and malignant tumors. Approximately 1% of patients with BWS have a chromosomal abnormality, such as translocation, duplication, or deletion of genetic material from chromosome 11. The subsequent alterations or imprinting errors on chromosome 11p15.5 are responsible for the clinical manifestations witnessed, as chromosome 11p15.5 houses genes involved in growth regulation. Eighty percent of BWS cases occur spontaneously, with minimal familial predilection.

A diagnosis of BWS may occur either prenatally or postnatally. A BWS consensus scoring system has been established to guide the clinical diagnosis of BWS and determine the need for genetic testing. The presence of three major features associated with BWS will confirm the clinical diagnosis after ruling out clinical features of other overgrowth syndromes, such as Simpson–Golabi–Behmel, Costello, Solos, Perlman and mucopolysaccharidosis and maternal diabetes. Following a provisional diagnosis of BWS based on clinical findings, cytogenetic testing can be employed for diagnosis confirmation. Molecular genetic testing can identify epigenetic and genomic alterations of chromosome 11p15 in individuals with BWS. However, cytogenetically detectable abnormalities involving chromosome 11p15 are found in 1% or fewer of affected individuals. If testing is found to be normal, *CDKN1C* sequencing can be performed to detect any changes in the *CDKN1C* gene. Ultimately, not every patient with a clinical diagnosis of BWS will have positive confirmatory molecular test as most of the genetic and epigenetic changes that result in BWS are not present in every cell.

The most common manifestations of BWS are macrosomia (birth weight >90th percentile), macroglossia, hypoglycemia, and abdominal wall defect.[1–3,5] While there may be wide variation in presentation of BWS, two to three of these findings must exist to be considered syndromic.[3] Additional presenting features include exomphalos, visceromegaly, horizontal earlobe creases, renal medullary dysplasia, hypothyroidism, hyperlipidemia, polycythemia, hypercalciuria, and embryonal tumors. Although cardiac defects and mental retardation may occur in children with BWS, these findings are rare. Following diagnosis, BWS can be further divided into three subcategories: classic or typical BWS, atypical BWS, and isolated lateralized overgrowth. Barring sequelae from a concurrent malignancy, life expectancy for the BWS patient is normal.

ANESTHETIC MANAGEMENT
PREOPERATIVE EVALUATION

A detailed preoperative examination should occur prior to anesthetizing patients with BWS (Box 27.1). This should include assessment of the airway, cardiovascular system, urinary system, endocrine status, blood glucose, and electrolytes. Additionally, anesthesia providers should assess for any associated congenital malformations, prematurity, and interventions early in life as this has the potential to complicate anesthetic management.

Patients with BWS may present to the operating room at various points across childhood. Accordingly, there are unique age-related comorbidities that anesthesia providers must consider. In the neonatal period, surgery often focuses on establishment of the airway in the presence of obstructive macroglossia or reduction of an omphalocele, which is the most common surgical emergency in neonates diagnosed with BWS. Children with BWS ages 2 to 8 years are more likely to present for surgical resection of embryonal malignancies, such as Wilms tumor, hepatoblastoma, or neuroblastoma. School-aged to adolescent patients with BWS usually present to the operating room for cosmetic procedures and/or oral surgery to correct midface hypoplasia and malocclusion. Orthopedic procedures to correct areas of unilateral overgrowth of the upper or lower extremities are commonly performed in children with BWS from infancy through school age.[6]

Pertinent Labs

Preoperative testing is largely based on the patient's presenting comorbidities. Should there be a history of hypoglycemia, acute insulin response testing may be warranted to differentiate BWS from congenital hyperinsulinism. In addition to assessing glucose levels, anesthesia providers should review recent electrolyte, blood urea, and creatinine levels. If recent laboratory work is not available, these laboratories should be drawn and reviewed prior to surgery. All patients with BWS should be screened for hypercalciuria as this can be indicative of perioperative renal dysfunction.

If there is a history or physical finding indicative of congenital heart disease (CHD), a comprehensive cardiologic examination should occur prior to surgery, inclusive of an ECG, echocardiography, and possibly CT angiography. This is only necessary when a cardiac anomaly is suspected during clinical examination and is not indicated should there be no signs of CHD.

PREOPERATIVE PHARMACOLOGY

Given the unpredictable effect on airway patency, anxiolytics should be avoided preoperatively if there is a suspicion of possible airway compromise following sedation or in small infants with congestive cardiac failure.

BOX 27.1 KEY ASSESSMENT POINTS FOR BECKWITH–WIEDEMANN SYNDROME

Body Morphology/Abdominal Wall Defects
- Diastasis recti
- Lateralized overgrowth/asymmetry of limbs
- Macrosomia
- Omphalocele
- Umbilical hernia
- Visceromegaly

Metabolic Derangements
- Acquired von Willebrand disease
- Hyperreninemia
- Hypocalcemia
- Hypoglycemia 2° hyperinsulinemia
- Polycythemia/hyperviscosity

Craniofacial/Oropharyngeal
- Cleft palate (rare)
- Earlobe creases/pits
- Macroglossia
- Mandibular prognathia/malocclusion
- Midface hypoplasia
- Nevus flammeus
- Occipital prominence
- Ocular prominence (proptosis)/infraorbital hypoplasia

Malignancies
- Adrenocortical carcinoma
- Hepatoblastoma
- Neuroblastoma
- Rhabdomyosarcoma
- Wilms tumor (congenital nephroblastoma)

Sources: From Pappas JG. The clinical course of an overgrowth syndrome, from diagnosis in infancy through adulthood: the case of Beckwith-Wiedemann syndrome. *Curr Probl Pediatr Adolesc HealthCare.* 2015;45:112–117. doi:10.1016/j.cppeds.2015.03.001; Rare Disease Database. *Beckwith-Wiedemann Syndrome. National Organization for Rare Disorders (NORD).* 2019. https://rarediseases.org/rare-diseases/beckwith-wiedemann-syndrome; Weksberg R, Shuman C, Beckwith JB. Beckwith-Wiedemann syndrome. *Eur J Hum Genet.* 2010.18(1): 8–14. doi:10:1038/ejhg.2009.106; DeBaun M, King AA, White N. Hypoglycemia in Beckwith-Wiedemann syndrome. *Semin Perinatol.* 2000;24(2):164–171. doi:10.1053/sp.2000.6366.

ANESTHETIC TECHNIQUE

Intraoperative Management

The major anesthetic considerations in patients with BWS are abnormal airway anatomy, hypoglycemia, and the presence of cardiac anomalies. Standard monitors, as described by the American Society of Anesthesiologist, should be employed, and all patients should have at least one well-running peripheral intravenous catheter. The need for an arterial catheter or advanced monitoring is dictated by the patient's comorbidities and procedure being performed.

Macroglossia associated with BWS occurs in varying degrees of severity. Continued tongue growth and protrusion places patients at risk for obstructive sleep apnea, upper airway obstruction, and acute airway compromise. Syndromic facies can also make it difficult to mask ventilate the patient and secure the airway. Intubation via conventional direct laryngoscopy can often prove difficult. Prior to induction, anesthesia providers should ensure alternate airway management devices, such as laryngeal mask airways and fiberoptic bronchoscope, are in the room and readily available should there be difficulties securing the airway. In extreme cases, blind nasal, retrograde intubation, or tracheostomy may be required to establish a patent airway.

Despite concerns related to airway management, inhalational mask induction of general anesthesia may be considered safe depending on the presence of comorbidities. Once intubated, ventilation may prove challenging in the presence of visceromegaly or omphalocele. Visceromegaly may shift the diaphragm upward, thereby reducing functional residual capacity. Omphalocele is a protrusion of viscera at the base of the umbilicus, emanating from a failure of abdominal wall closure during embryonic development. Neonates born with this defect can be challenging to ventilate and are at high risk for increased insensitive fluid loss through evaporation, intravascular depletion, intraoperative hypothermia, and postoperative issues, such as abdominal compartment syndrome and respiratory failure.[8]

In the neonate with BWS, hypoglycemia secondary to an increased production of insulin by hypertrophic islet cells in the pancreas can be catastrophic. Sustained hypoglycemia in the neonate may lead to apnea, seizures, and permanent neurological deficits. Efforts should be made to stabilize neonatal blood glucose levels preoperatively through frequent feedings, the administration of dextrose-containing intravascular fluids, and the use of glucagon in emergent situations.[5] Perioperatively, serial glucose monitoring should occur to guide glucose management.

There is a host of pharmacologic implications anesthesia providers must consider when caring for patients with BWS. Should the use of neuromuscular blocking agents be required, it is recommended that drugs not metabolized or eliminated by the liver be used. Likewise, morphine should be carefully titrated to avoid respiratory depression and hepatotoxicity. Fentanyl can be used safely as the pharmacokinetics generally remain unaltered. In the presence of bowel obstruction or omphalocele, the use of nitrous oxide should be avoided. If the patient have CHD, drugs with a negative inotropic or peripheral vasodilating effect may be contraindicated. Additional anesthetic considerations or concerns associated with common procedures in patients with BWS can be found in **Box 27.2**.

POSTOPERATIVE CARE

Postoperatively, the primary concern is airway obstruction. It is imperative that staff monitor for edema and obstruction, especially following tongue reduction surgery. A multimodal pain management strategy should be employed to minimize opioid-induced airway compromise. Opioids, as well as anxiolytics, should be used judiciously as they have the potential to cause severe airway obstruction and hypoxemia and may precipitate a pulmonary artery hypertensive crisis in patients with CHD who have a history of pulmonary hypertension.

Hypoglycemia occurs in 30% to 50% of neonates perioperatively, most likely due to islet cell hyperplasia and hyperinsulinemia. Preventing neurological sequelae mandates a careful perioperative glucose homeostasis with infusion of glucose-containing solution in addition to hourly glucose monitoring.

BOX 27.2 SPECIAL CONSIDERATIONS/CONCERNS WITH BECKWITH–WIEDEMANN SYNDROME

Airway
- Anticipate difficult airway based on degree of macroglossia or presence of cleft palate.
- May require tracheostomy if extreme macroglossia present.
- Tongue reduction surgery may result in increased blood loss; necessitates postoperative analgesia.
- Airway competition with the surgeon.
- Limit FiO_2 to <30% to avoid airway fire.

Endocrine
- Closely monitor serum glucose, particularly in the neonatal period.
- Administer dextrose-containing solution to maintain glucose between 45 and 125 mg/dL.

Abdominal Surgery: Omphalocele
- Anticipate need for volume resuscitation.
- Focus on maintenance of normothermia.
- Surgeon may request muscle relaxation to facilitate abdominal relaxation.
- Avoid N_2O.
- Postoperative respiratory failure common due to decrease in FRC, attenuated diaphragmatic function, basilar atelectasis; continued mechanical ventilation may be required.
- Larger defects require staged reduction to avoid abdominal compartment syndrome.
  - may result in decreased hepatic perfusion/altered drug metabolism, decreased U/O, impaired venous return/swelling of lower extremities.

  *Pulse oximetry on UEs preferred.

Abdominal Surgery: Tumor Resection
- Patients may have received chemotherapeutic agents and/or radiation therapy prior to surgery; malnutrition, acute/chronic hepatotoxicity, hepatic fibrosis, SIADH, cardiac toxicity possible.
- Preoperative assessment should include cardiac echo if doxorubicin received.
- Volume status may be attenuated from malnutrition, N/V.
- Plan for large-bore IV access, invasive monitoring.
- *Hepatoblastoma*
  - May present with severe abdominal distention/mass effect.
  - Check hepatic function and coagulation profile preoperatively.
  - Anticipate coagulopathy; may require transfusion of PRBCs, FFP, platelets, and other products.

  *Plan for massive/rapid blood loss; employ fluid warmer, have rapid infuser available.
  - Potential for alterations in drug metabolism/delayed emergence.
  - Use hepatotoxic agents such as acetaminophen judiciously.
- *Wilms Tumor*
  - Check renal function preoperatively.
  - Anticipate hypertension from hyperreninemia.
  - Polycythemia/Hyperviscosity from increased erythropoietin production possible.
  - Assess U/O frequently with partial or total nephrectomy.
- *Neuroblastoma/Adrenal Tumors*
  - Anticipate hemodynamic lability with manipulation of catecholamine- or autocoid-secreting tumors.

FFP, fresh frozen plasma; FRC, functional residual capacity; N/V, nausea and vomiting; PRBC, packet red blood cell; SIADH, syndrome of inappropriate antidiuretic hormone secretion; UE, upper extremity; U/O, urinary output.

Sources: From Speath JP, Lam JE. The extremely premature infant (micropreemie) and common neonatal emergencies. In: CJ Coté, J Lerman, BJ Anderson, eds. *Coté and Lerman's A Practice of Anesthesia for Infants and Children.* 6th ed. 2019:864–865; Ross FJ, Latham GJ. Perioperative management of the oncology patient. In: CJ Coté, J Lerman, BJ Anderson, eds. *Coté and Lerman's A Practice of Anesthesia for Infants and Children.* 6th ed. 2019:245–246; Hansen TG, Henneberg SW, Lerman J. General abdominal and urologic surgery. In: CJ Coté, J Lerman, BJ Anderson, eds. *Coté and Lerman's A Practice of Anesthesia for Infants and Children.* 6th ed. 2019:683–685.

REFERENCES

1. Pappas JG. The clinical course of an overgrowth syndrome, from diagnosis in infancy through adulthood: the case of Beckwith-Wiedemann syndrome. *Curr Probl Pediatr Adolesc HealthCare.* 2015;45:112–117. doi:10.1016/j.cppeds.2015.03.001
2. Rare Disease Database. *Beckwith-Wiedemann Syndrome. National Organization for Rare Disorders (NORD).* 2019. https://rarediseases.org/rare-diseases/beckwith-wiedemann-syndrome
3. Weksberg R, Shuman C, Beckwith JB. Beckwith-Wiedemann syndrome. *Eur J Hum Genet.* 2010.18(1): 8–14. doi:10:1038/ejhg.2009.106
4. Cortessis VK, Azadian M, Buxbaum J, et al. Comprehensive meta-analysis reveals association between multiple imprinting disorders and conception by assisted reproductive technology. *J Assist Reprod Genet.* 2018;35(6):943. doi:10.1007/s10815-018-1173-x
5. DeBaun M, King AA, White N. Hypoglycemia in Beckwith-Wiedemann syndrome. *Semin Perinatol.* 2000;24(2):164–171. doi:10.1053/sp.2000.6366
6. Schultz BD, Coon D, Medina M, et al. Isolated pediatric hemihyperplasia requiring surgical debulking of the thigh. *J Ped Surg Case Reports.* 2015;3(2):53–57. doi:10.1016/j.epsc.2014.12.005
7. Cohen JL, Cielo CM, Kupa J, et al. The utility of tongue reduction surgery for macroglossia in Beckwith-Wiedemann Syndrome. *Plast Reconstr Surg.* 2020; 145(4):803e–813e. doi:10.1097/PRS.0000000000006673
8. Speath JP, Lam JE. The extremely premature infant (micropreemie) and common neonatal emergencies. In: CJ Coté, J Lerman, BJ Anderson, eds. *Coté and Lerman's A Practice of Anesthesia for Infants and Children.* 6th ed. 2019:864–865.
9. Ross FJ, Latham GJ. Perioperative management of the oncology patient. In: CJ Coté, J Lerman, BJ Anderson, eds. *Coté and Lerman's A Practice of Anesthesia for Infants and Children.* 6th ed. 2019:245–246.
10. Hansen TG, Henneberg SW, Lerman J. General abdominal and urologic surgery. In: CJ Coté, J Lerman, BJ Anderson, eds. *Coté and Lerman's A Practice of Anesthesia for Infants and Children.* 6th ed. 2019:683–685.

CHARGE Syndrome
Angela Mund

PATHOPHYSIOLOGY AND CLINICAL MANIFESTATIONS

CHARGE syndrome is a rare disorder that refers to a pattern of life-threatening congenital anomalies that affect multiple organ systems. The CHARGE acronym is derived from the first letter of the more common presenting features: *c*oloboma, *h*eart disease, choanal *a*tresia, *r*etardation of growth and development, genital hypoplasia, and *e*ar anomalies. The incidence of CHARGE syndrome in the general population is 0.1 to 1.2 per 10,000 live births, with no gender or racial predilection reported.[1] Most cases of CHARGE syndrome are sporadic, and it is uncommon to have a family history of CHARGE syndrome.

The leading cause of CHARGE syndrome is mutation of the *CHD7* gene, which is found in approximately two-thirds of patients with CHARGE syndrome, though genomic alterations in the region of chromosome 8q12.2 where the *CHD7* gene is located have been reported.[2] While no definitive causative factors of gene mutation have been identified, exposure to teratogenic substances (e.g., thalidomide and hydantoin), and maternal diabetes mellitus have been implicated.[3] Disruption in embryologic differentiation results in defects during midline development as mesoderm formation is negatively impacted.

Diagnosis is based on the clinical presentation of a combination of major and minor criteria, with none of the features in the CHARGE acronym being universally present.[4] Although many features of CHARGE syndrome are often apparent at birth, some features may not become apparent for weeks, months, or years, thereby delaying formal diagnosis. Early presenting symptoms include respiratory distress and feeding intolerance, with later symptoms typically comprised of persistent nasal drainage, failure to thrive, audiovisual defects, and developmental delay.[3] Genetic testing may be inconclusive as not all patients will have *CHD7* gene abnormalities.

Eye, ear, nose, and throat abnormalities are common features of CHARGE syndrome (Table 28.1). Colobomas, defects in areas of the eye, which may involve the iris, retina, or optic disk, are present in 75% to 90% of patients and are typically chorioretinal in nature, predisposing them to retinal detachment and visual disturbances.[2] Ear abnormalities are another common feature with both external and internal malformations and hearing loss routinely present. Externally, the ear often has a hypoplastic, overfolded helix and lobe, and the triangular concha.[2] The most common internal malformation is absence of the lateral semicircular canals leading to an altered sense of directional balance, in addition to the presence of conductive and sensorineural hearing loss. Choanal atresia is

Table 28.1	Clinical Features of CHARGE Syndrome
Major Characteristics	Minor Characteristics
Ocular coloboma	Genital hypoplasia and delayed puberty
Choanal atresia	Cardiovascular malformations
Ear abnormalities	Growth deficiencies
Cranial nerve dysfunction	Laryngomalacia
	Facial abnormalities
	Orofacial cleft
	Tracheoesophageal fistula

Source: Blake K, MacCuspie J, Hartshorne TS, et al. Postoperative airway events of individuals with CHARGE syndrome. *Int J Pediatr Otorhinolaryngol.* 2009;73(2):219–226. doi:10.4168/aard.2014.2.1.70.

present in 65% of patients with CHARGE syndrome.[2] The atresia may be unilateral or bilateral resulting on airway obstruction. Bilateral choanal atresia is deemed a surgical emergency, as neonates are obligatory nasal breathers. Further commonly witnessed airway obstruction-related issues include pharyngolaryngeal hypotonia, tracheomalacia, laryngomalacia, and subglottic stenosis.[5] The presence of a hypotonic larynx, in conjunction with hypertrophic arytenoids and uncoordinated movement of the supraglottis, have the potential to make it challenging to maintain airway patency.[5]

Cardiac malformations are found in the majority of patients with CHARGE syndrome at a rate of 75% to 85%.[2] Although a variety of congenital cardiac disorders have been reported, disorders of the cardiac outflow (conotruncal) are most common.[6] Common manifestations include the presence of an interrupted aortic arch, tretralogy of Fallot, double outlet right ventricle, and atrioventricular septal defects, with tetralogy of Fallot being the most common congenital heart disorder found in patients with CHARGE syndrome.[1]

Cranial nerve (CN) dysfunction leading to feeding and swallowing difficulties, as well as gastroesophageal reflux, often mandates insertion of a feeding tube.[2] In addition, dysfunction of CN IX and X may result in an ability to handle, thereby increasing the incidence of perioperative airway emergencies.[5,7] Should CN VII palsy be present, facial droop may occur, although this is typically unilateral in nature. Delayed cognitive ability occurs in most patients with CHARGE syndrome.[6]

Additional clinical features that may be found in this patient population include a narrow face with a very broad nasal tip, deep-set eyes with a single eyebrow, a prominent jaw, bilateral fourth and fifth toe clinodactyly.[1] Immune deficiencies, such as severe combined immunodeficiency (SCID), have also been reported, perhaps as a result of poor development of the thymus.[2] If present, immune deficiencies may result in the suppurative ear and chest infections. Diverse disorders of the endocrine system have been reported, and deficiencies in growth hormone often led to a lower percentile height for age and resultant short stature. Hypogonadotropic hypogonadism, due to impaired gonadotropin, results from the pituitary gland, results in delayed or arrested puberty, infertility, and small testes.[2] Hypothyroidism may also occur due to hypothalamic–pituitary dysfunction.

ANESTHETIC MANAGEMENT

Due to the heterogeneous nature of CHARGE syndrome, pediatric patients may present to the operating room from the neonatal period through the age of puberty. The procedures requiring anesthesia may be emergent, such as surgical correction of bilateral choanal atresia, palliation of cyanotic cardiac disorders, or repair of tracheoesophageal fistulas.[7] Patients with CHARGE syndrome also present for a variety of nonemergent surgical procedures, such as airway evaluation and treatment to placement of gastric tubes.

PREOPERATIVE EVALUATION

During the preoperative evaluation, considerations should include reviewing both the major and minor underlying health issues, as well as assessing the depth of impact of each component of CHARGE syndrome. The patient's chart should be reviewed for prior surgical intervention including tracheostomy, as these patients may have increased issues with severe saliva retention and upper airway obstruction.[5] It is important to evaluate for the presence of symptoms of obstructive sleep apnea (OSA). Although the symptoms of OSA may be tempered following adenotonsillectomy, the anesthesia provider should continue to evaluate for airway obstruction as issues with airway management are prevalent in this patient population.[4] A full airway exam should be performed preoperatively if the patient is cooperative. The use of point of care ultrasound (POCUS) may be helpful in defining the anatomy, evaluating for obstruction with inspiration and expiration, and for planning for emergent tracheostomy if necessary. Additionally, the presence of active lower respiratory tract infections should be determined. Cardiac disorders should be evaluated for whether the defect has been repaired and, if not repaired, plans should be based on the patient's underlying cardiac pathology. Consultation with a cardiologist prior to administration of anesthesia to determine the presence of an underlying or undiagnosed cardiac anomaly is recommended.[2] Further cardiac function and anatomy assessment via ECHO and/or ECG may be warranted. Patients exhibiting signs of seizure activity should have their seizures under control. Renal function should be assessed via creatinine and blood urea nitrogen measurement should renal impairments be present.

PREOPERATIVE PHARMACOTHERAPY

The administration of preoperative medications should be based on the patients presenting symptoms, surgical needs, level of anxiety and/or pain, and risk/benefit ratios. Care should be taken with the administration of sedatives due to the risk of airway obstruction and hypoxia. Preemptive multimodal pain management that is nonsedating should be considered. The anesthesia provider should consider adding an antisialagogue to mitigate increased secretions that may be problematic during induction and emergence. Additionally, chronic antiseizure medications may alter the metabolism and elimination of some drugs.

ANESTHETIC TECHNIQUE

Intraoperative Management

After reviewing the patient's history and conducting a thorough physical examination, the anesthesia provider can then make decisions for addressing the perioperative course and concerns (Table 28.2). Planning for difficult airway management should be priority. Midface hypoplasia, micrognathia,

Table 28.2	Special Considerations for the Anesthetic Management of CHARGE Syndrome
Laboratory	• No need for thyroid function testing unless the patient shows symptoms of hypothyroidism[2] • CBC for all children with CHARGE[2]
Cardiac	• Cardiology consult and possible echocardiogram • Follow recommendations for the anesthetic management of the specific cardiac disorder • Invasive monitors may be necessary
Ear, nose, throat	• Determine prior experiences with anesthesia to determine difficulty with mask ventilation and endotracheal intubation • Plan for difficult airway management • Evaluate the significance of choanal atresia versus stenosis • Assess for the presence of obstructive sleep apnea • Evaluation of level of hearing and visual dysfunction
Positioning	• Consider additional padding of the eyes and application of eye lubricant
Other	• If possible, combine more than one procedure to decrease the number of times that airway management is required as this is a considerable risk for perioperative emergencies[7] • Attention should be applied to taking measures to decrease the risk of infection

CBC, complete blood count

anterior larynx, small mouth opening, and cleft lip and palate may make face-mask ventilation and tracheal intubation difficult. During induction of general anesthesia, the presence of laryngo- and tracheomalacia may contribute to upper airway obstruction. The use of continuous positive airway pressure (CPAP) during induction and extubation may be required, and the use of ProSeal laryngeal mask airway (LMA) has been reported to be a viable means of facilitating ventilation following failed intubation attempts.[8] The use of a fiberoptic bronchoscope may be necessary for intubation and should be readily available, as well as a video laryngoscope. Management of the airway via the nares may be impossible or, at least challenging, due to the presence of choanal atresia. As the patient ages, airway management may become increasingly more challenging. Additional airway-related considerations are the requirement of a smaller than anticipated endotracheal tube secondary to subglottic stenosis and the increased risk of aspiration, even in the absence of a tracheoesophageal fistula. Consider the avoidance of muscle relaxants until the airway has been secured.

POSTOPERATIVE CARE

Appropriate airway management is a priority when planning for and managing all perioperative phases. Postoperative airway events, such as desaturation, management of excessive secretions or the need for emergent reintubation has been reported to occur 35% of the time following anesthesia for the patient with CHARGE syndrome.[7] Of note, postoperative airway issues most frequently occur following cardiac and gastrointestinal procedures and less frequently following surgeries involving the eyes. Due to this increased airway concern, anesthesia providers should consider monitoring the patient longer in the postanesthesia recovery room, especially if long-acting medications are used or following any of the higher risk procedures. Prolonged intubation and mechanical ventilation may be required due to laryngomalacia, frequent aspirations or truncal hypoplasia. As is the goal in all surgical populations, the emphasis on postoperative care should be returning the patient to a baseline or higher level of function.

REFERENCES

1. Chousou PA, Jennings A, Balmain S. CHARGE syndrome: a rare combination of cardiac and endocrine disease. *Int J Cardiol.* 2012;159(3):233–234. doi:10.1016/j.ijcard.2012.05.104
2. Hsu P, Ma A, Wilson M, et al. CHARGE syndrome: a review of CHARGE syndrome. *J Paediatr Child Health.* 2014;50(7):504–511. doi:10.1111/jpc.12497
3. Bissonnette B, Luginbuehl I, Marciniak B, Syndromes BJD. *Syndromes: Rapid Recognition and Perioperative Implications.* McGraw-Hill; 2006.
4. Trider C-L, Blake K. Obstructive sleep apnea in a patient with CHARGE syndrome. *Case Rep Otolaryngol.* 2012;2012:907032. doi:10.1155/2012/907032
5. Naito Y, Higuchi M, Koinuma G, et al. Upper airway obstruction in neonates and infants with CHARGE syndrome. *Am J Med Genet Part A.* 2007;143A(16):1815–1820. doi:10.1002/ajmg.a.31851
6. Miller-Hance WC, Gertler R. Essentials of cardiology. In: Cote CJ, Lehman J, Anderson BJ, eds. *A Practice of Anesthesia for Infants and Children.* Elsevier; 2019:355–392.
7. Blake K, MacCuspie J, Hartshorne TS, et al. Postoperative airway events of individuals with CHARGE syndrome. *Int J Pediatr Otorhinolaryngol.* 2009;73(2):219–226. doi:10.4168/aard.2014.2.1.70
8. Hara Y, Hirota K, Fukuda K. Successful airway management with use of a laryngeal mask airway in a patient with CHARGE syndrome. *J Anesth.* 2009;23(4):630–632. doi:10.12669/pjms.336.13558

CHAPTER 29

Cri du Chat Syndrome

Michael E. Conti

PATHOPHYSIOLOGY AND CLINICAL MANIFESTATIONS

Cri du chat, also referred to as Lejeune syndrome or 5p-syndrome, was first described in 1963 by the pediatrician Jerome Jean L.M. Lejeune. The name of the syndrome is derived from the characteristic, high-pitched cry in infancy, which sounds like a cat-like cry. Cri du chat syndrome is the most common human deletion syndrome, affecting females more than males. The incidence of cri du chat syndrome is approximately 1 in 15,000 to 50,000 live births, with the potential for missed diagnosis early in childhood, making it challenging to determine the true frequency of this genetic disorder.

Cri du chat syndrome occurs secondary to partial or total deletion of the short arm (p) of chromosome 5. This deletion occurs early in embryonic development and results in an anatomically abnormal larynx, which is responsible for the distinctive high-pitched, catlike cry for which the disorder is named. Most cases of cri du chat syndrome occur spontaneously (de novo), although translocation of chromosomes is responsible for approximately 10% of cases. Ultimately, the severity of the syndrome is determined by the extent of the chromosome deletion.

Diagnosis of cri du chat syndrome is based on clinical findings, in combination with chromosomal evaluation to determine the extent of variation or deletion impacting chromosome 5. Use of a fluorescent in situ hybridization test is considered the gold standard when confirming diagnosis of cri du chat syndrome.

Variation in the critical 5p15.2 region is largely responsible for most of the clinical features associated with cri du chat syndrome. Most patient present with anomalies of the larynx such as a long, curved, and floppy epiglottis, laryngeal hypoplasia, laryngomalacia, asymmetric vocal cords, and anterior approximation of the vocal cords with a large posterior commissure. However, some patients with cri du chat syndrome present .with a larynx that is structurally nomal, indicating there may also be a neurological component to the abnormal catlike cry. It should be noted that the high-pitched cry indicative of cri du chat decreases as the child ages.

Other common signs and symptoms include low birth weight, growth deficiencies, microcephaly, and distinctive facial features. Many patients presenting with cri du chat present have micrognathia, an abnormally round or plump (moon) face, strabismus, hypertolerism, palpebral fissures, epicanthal folds, low-set ears, and micrognathia. Many patients also display some degree of psychomotor and intellectual disability, and hypotonia, which later reverses to hypertonia with age. It is not uncommon for patients with cri du chat syndrome to require surgical repair of a patent ductus arteriosus (PDA), strabismus, scoliosis, club foot deformity, cleft lip and/or cleft palate, and, less commonly, syndactyly, cryptorchidism, or hypospadias.[1,2]

ANESTHETIC MANAGEMENT
PREOPERATIVE EVALUATION

As patients with cri du chat syndrome commonly present with anomalies affecting multiple body systems, including the upper airway (micrognathia, laryngeal, and epiglottic abnormalities), the cardiovascular system, and the central nervous system, it is imperative anesthesia providers perform a comprehensive evaluation prior to any anesthetic. While the focus should be on the presenting clinical symptoms and associated disorders, anesthesia providers should perform a thorough airway examination given the potential for airway anomalies.

Pertinent Labs

Should the patient have a PDA, an echocardiogram prior to surgery may be warranted to evaluate the severity of cardiac defects. A chest x-ray is also recommended for patents with a presenting history of recurrent aspiration pneumonia.

PREOPERATIVE PHARMACOTHERAPY

Preoperative anxiolytics should be used with caution in patients presenting with cor pulmonale or pulmonary hypertension due to the potential for further respiratory depression in an already hypoxic patient. Administration of an H2 antagonist and/or a prokinetic agent may be considered for a patient at risk of aspiration due to hypotonia in an effort to decrease the likelihood of aspiration pneumonitis. If fiberoptic intubation or video laryngoscopy is planned, administration of an antisialagogue preoperatively may improve visualization and optimize intubating conditions.[1]

ANESTHETIC TECHNIQUE
Intraoperative Management

While there are likely airway anomalies present, anesthesia can generally be induced via an inhalation mask induction without incident. Anesthesia providers should be prepared for upper airway obstruction during the induction of anesthesia, as well as challenges with bag mask ventilation. As cri du chat is associated with a long, curved, and floppy epiglottis, laryngeal hypoplasia, laryngomalacia, asymmetric vocal cords, and anterior approximation of the vocal cords with a large posterior commissure, intubation may prove difficult. It is recommended anesthesia providers have equipment to manage a difficult intubation, whether a videolaryngoscope, laryngeal mask airway, or both, readily available. In addition, anesthesia providers should be aware that a smaller-than-age-appropriate endotracheal tube may be necessary due to subglottic narrowing.

Given the potential for aspiration in the presence of significant gastroesophageal reflux, a rapid sequence induction may be considered. This should be determined on an individual basis, however, taking into consideration the extent of presenting airway anomalies. Moreover, the use of succinylcholine, while not contraindicated, should be done with caution as no definitive conclusions have been drawn regarding the safety of succinylcholine in this patient population. Similarly, patients with preexisting motor weakness and hypotonia may be sensitive to the effects of nondepolarizing neuromuscular blocking agents and reductions in dosing frequency or the avoidance of nondepolarizing neuromuscular blocking agents may be warranted.

Standard monitors, as described by the American Society of Anesthesiologist, should be employed. Should significant blood loss be anticipated, placement of an arterial line should be considered for frequent monitoring of hematocrit and hemoglobin levels. The requisite number of peripheral intravenous catheters is dictated by the procedure being performed, though at least one well-running peripheral intravenous catheter is necessary given the potential for airway complications.

Anesthesia providers should consider the use of active warming strategies as many patients with cri du chat have feeding difficulties and poor weight gain and subsequently have challenges maintain normothermia in a cold environment. Positioning should be done with care, as patients may present with contracture. Likewise, efforts should be made to avoid excess pressure on exposed bony prominences.

Special considerations and concerns are summarized in **Box 29.1**.

POSTOPERATIVE CARE

Patients with cri du chat should be extubated awake at the end of the procedure prior to transport to the postanesthesia care unit (PACU). Postoperative management for this population is primarily supportive, with the primary concern being ensuring adequate ventilation and maintenance of a patent airway. As a prolonged emergence or delayed PACU discharge may result from developmental/cognitive delay, use of short-acting opioids, and a multimodal analgesic strategy may be preferable. Seizures have been reported in up to 10% of patients with cri du chat; hence, padding and seizure precautions in PACU should be considered.[3,4]

> **BOX 29.1** **SPECIAL CONSIDERATIONS/CONCERNS WITH CRI DU CHAT SYNDROME**
>
> - Developmental delay may translate into a prolonged emergence.
> - High risk of aspiration may warrant an extubation when fully awake.
> - Hypo/hypertonia may necessitate the avoidance of neuromuscular blocking agents.
> - Single balloon assisted enteroscopy, if indicated

REFERENCES

1. Honjo RS, Mello CB, Pimenta LSE, et al. Cri du chat syndrome: characteristics of 73 Brazilian patients. *J Intellect Disabil Res*. 2018;62(6):467–473 doi:10.1111/jir.12476
2. Pentuik S, Mezoff A. Rare Disease Database, Cri du Chat Syndrome. National Organization for Rare Disorders. https://rarediseases.org/rare-diseases/cri-du-chat-syndrome
3. Dos Santos KM, De Rezende DC, Borges ZDd. Anesthetic management of a patient with cri du chat syndrome case report. *Rev Bras Anestesiol*. 2010;60(6):630–633, 350-351. doi:10.1016/S0034-7094(10)70078-7
4. Carmer K. Anesthetic considerations for patient with cri du chat syndrome. *Int Student J Nurse Anesth*. 2015;14:43–46.

CHAPTER 30

Crouzon Syndrome

Kimberly Hunter Olivarez

PATHOPHYSIOLOGY AND CLINICAL MANIFESTATIONS

Crouzon syndrome (CS), or acrocephalosyndactyly type II, is the most common among a constellation of fibroblast growth factor receptor (FGFR) mutations and poses numerous challenges to the anesthesia provider. Identified in 1912 by French physician, Louis Edouard Octave Crouzon, CS is characterized as a triad of symptoms: cranial vault/skull deformity, facial dysmorphism, and exophthalmos (**Figure 30.1**). CS occurs in approximately 1.6:100,0000 live births, affecting males and females equally. CS has an autosomal dominant inheritance pattern, and while often diagnosed at birth based on crouzonoid features, diagnosis may not be immediate due to variable phenotypic presentation.[1] Clinical manifestations stem from deficiencies in FGFR-2, which plays a critical role in signaling cranial suture closure during embryonic and postnatal development. Mutations in FGFR-2 increase the maturation rate of cells in the osteoblastic lineage, which leads to premature ossification and ultimately craniosynostosis.

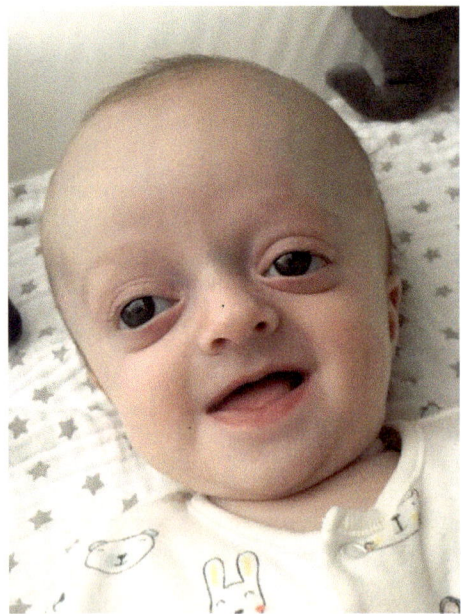

Figure 30.1: Baby with Crouzon syndrome. Note the characteristic facial dysmorphism and exophthalmos.

Source: Kate Vuk.

Table 30.1	Key Assessment Points With Crouzon Syndrome
Diagnostic studies	Polysomnography and airway imaging
	Cervical spine imaging
	ECHO, cardiac MRI
	Fundoscopic exam report
Labs	CBC ± BMP, coagulation panel, type and screen/cross with anticipated major blood loss
Physical assessment/ interview	Airway exam, including Mallampati and previous Cormack and Lehane intubation grade if available
	Neck range of motion
	Signs and symptoms of OSA/obstructive airway events
	History of tracheostomy, prolonged intubation

BMP, basic metabolic panel; CBC, complete blood count; MRI, magnetic resonance imaging; OSA, obstructive sleep apnea.

CS accounts for approximately 4.5% cases of craniosynostosis. Patients diagnosed with CS most frequently experience coronal craniosynostosis, but any cranial suture may be impacted. As normal bone growth fails perpendicular to affected sutures, compensatory bone growth occurs to allow for brain development. This causes the characteristic distorted skull morphology.[2] Other physical manifestations include brachycephaly, hypertelorism, maxillary hypoplasia, parrot beak nasal deformity, and mandibular prognathia.[3] Additionally, patients with CS may present with hydrocephalus with or without elevated intracranial pressure (ICP), Chiari malformations, obstructive airway events (obstructive sleep apnea and/or acute emergent episodes of airway obstruction), relative macroglossia, vocal cord palsy, hearing loss, C2–C3 spinal fusion, and visual impairment.[4] CS does not typically impact cognitive development; however, in extreme cases, untreated elevated ICP may cause neurodevelopmental impairment.[5] Psychosocially, older children with CS may be affected by their atypical physical appearance.[2]

ANESTHETIC MANAGEMENT

PREOPERATIVE EVALUATION

The primary focus of the preoperative evaluation in a child with CS centers on airway assessment due to the increased risk of difficult airway management (Table 30.1). Polysomnography and/or preoperative diagnostic airway endoscopy is routine in the CS patient's care and should be reviewed prior to an anesthetic as multilevel obstructive sleep apnea (OSA) and obstructive airway events are common.[6] Of note, presence of concomitant acanthosis nigricans should alert anesthesia providers to the possibility of severe OSA, should polysomnography is not be available.[4]

Midface hypoplasia and choanal stenosis/hypoplasia may contribute to difficulty with mask ventilation and preclude nasal intubation. Review of CT of airway structures is thus imperative.[7] Aforementioned diagnostic airway imaging and procedures may also reveal the presence of a tracheal cartilaginous sleeve, laryngomalacia, tracheomalacia, bronchomalacia, and subglottic stenosis.[8] The former need of a tracheostomy should be elicited as approximately 40% to 50% of patients with CS require tracheostomy early in their care and may signal the presence of subglottic stenosis.[9] Finally, cervical radiological imaging should be reviewed as spinal fusion at the level of C2–3 or C4–5 may impact patient positioning and airway management.[10]

Laboratory testing is necessary in patients with CS, particularly if significant blood loss is anticipated intraoperatively. Baseline hematological, coagulation, and electrolyte studies should be drawn preoperatively, and a type and cross should be ordered. Unveiled anemia may warrant preoperative optimization via recombinant human erythropoietin, iron therapy, or autologous blood donation.[2] Additionally, review of cardiology consults, echocardiogram, and any relevant diagnostic imaging is vital due to the uncommon but potential presence of concomitant congenital cardiac abnormalities, including, but not limited to, aortic coarctation, patent ductus arteriosus, tetralogy of Fallot, and patent foramen ovale.[11,12] Finally, due to this population being at an increased risk for ocular and optic nerve injury, it is imperative neurological and ophthalmological consults and associated imaging be reviewed as the presence of elevated ICP may impact anesthetic pharmacological selection.[5,11]

PREOPERATIVE PHARMACOTHERAPY

Anxiolytic premedication may be appropriate for patients with CS but should not be given routinely without assessment at the individual level. Administration of preoperative benzodiazepines and opiates may exacerbate difficulty with airway management, particularly in patients with OSA.[10] Ketamine and intranasal dexmedetomidine may be considered to provide anxiolysis while avoiding undue impact on respiratory tone or drive. Sedative premedication in patients with increased ICP should be used with caution.

ANESTHETIC TECHNIQUE

Intraoperative Management

Patients with CS present for primary procedures including sleep endoscopy, adenotonsillectomy, craniosynostosis repair, orthognathic surgery, and ventricular shunt creation; all of which require general anesthesia. There is no accepted standard approach to induction or intraoperative anesthetic management for patients with CS. Thus, the anesthetic plan should be tailored to accommodate the patient's comorbidities, surgical requirements, and avoidance of known potential complications. Induction may be performed via either the intravenous or inhalational route. An emergency airway cart, airways adjuncts, and personnel to perform an emergent tracheostomy should be readily available.[13] Video-assisted laryngoscopy and fiberoptic intubation equipment should be in the room prior to the induction of anesthesia should direct laryngoscopy proves unsuccessful, for those patients with cervical fusion, and to also accommodate intubation without neck extension.[11,12] In older children with anticipated or known difficult airways, maintaining spontaneous respiration for awake fiberoptic intubation is strongly recommended.[14]

In addition to standard monitors, placement of an arterial line and insertion of multiple large-gauge peripheral IV catheters may be warranted when significant blood loss is anticipated.[2] Neuraxial anesthetic techniques may be utilized in this population to bypass the postoperative airway challenges posed by narcotic administration. This may not be an option in all patients with CS due to potential spinal fusion and scoliosis.[14] Local anesthetic infiltration or peripheral nerve blocks may also aid in minimizing narcotic requirements both intraoperatively and postoperatively.[15] Regardless of pain management approach employed, awake extubation is recommended.[16]

Special Considerations/Concerns

While the primary concerns in caring for a patient with CS center around airway management, the anesthetist must also be mindful of ocular care, specific positioning considerations, and blood loss reduction (Table 30.2). Due to shallow orbital sockets and the resultant exophthalmos, patients with CS are at risk for exposure keratitis, corneal abrasion, retinal ischemia, and optic nerve ischemia. As such, careful taping and prevention of pressure on the eyes is imperative.[11] Additionally, corneal protection may be achieved in patients with severe ocular proptosis with the insertion of corneal shields or with temporary tarsorrhaphy.[17]

Atypical positioning of the patient also carries significant anesthetic implications. Utilized for surgical access during craniosynostosis repair, a modified prone position commonly referred to as "sphinx" or "sea lion" positioning may be required. This position entails prone positioning, with cervical extension and use of a horseshoe headrest to support the head. While elevation of the head promotes venous drainage thus improving the surgical field, elevation of the surgical site above the level of heart greatly increases the risk of venous air embolism. Additionally, head and neck extension may impact positioning of the endotracheal tube (ETT). Keen attention must be paid to securing the airway, and appropriate positioning of the ETT must be confirmed once patient positioning is complete.[18]

CS patients presenting for craniosynostosis repair often experience massive blood loss, with average estimates ranging from 60% to 100% of total blood volume lost.[19] In open cranial vault procedures, the need for blood transfusion should be anticipated, and available blood products should be in the room prior to incision. Blood loss may be abated via intraoperative infusion of fibrinolytics, such as tranexamic acid[12] or epsilon aminocaproic acid.[20] In addition to the prevention and response to hemorrhage, anesthesia providers must closely monitor the patient's body temperature should massive transfusion be required. Forced air warmers, fluid warmers, increased room temperature, and heat and moisture exchangers (HMEs) may aid in maintaining normothermia.[20] Large volume blood transfusion and fluid replacement may also cause airway edema, potentially delaying the appropriate time for extubation.[12] See Chapter 55, "Cranial Vault Reconstruction and Craniosynostosis Repair," in this text for information on cranial vault reconstruction and craniosynostosis repair.

Special Techniques/Equipment

Prior to induction of anesthesia in a patient with CS, assembly of airway devices is paramount. This includes, but is not limited to, multiple sized masks, ETTs, laryngeal mask airway, laryngoscope blades, and video laryngoscopes. Fiberoptic intubation equipment should be available along with both difficult airway and surgical airway carts.

Special techniques may also be utilized by the anesthesia provider to conserve blood and minimize the need for allogeneic transfusion. In older patients, acute normovolemic hemodilution may be used, in which a patient's blood is drawn and stored, with any removed volume replaced by crystalloid. This results in intraoperative blood loss being less impactful on postoperative hematocrit as fewer red blood cells are lost. The stored blood can later be used as an autologous transfusion to replace lost blood volume and to restore hematocrit. If unable to perform autologous blood donation, either due to facility restrictions or intolerance of the patient to anemia (as is the case with infants), hypervolemic hemodilution may be employed. With this technique, crystalloid is

Table 30.2	Special Considerations/Concerns With Crouzon Syndrome
Airway	Difficult airway and mask ventilation, midface hypoplasia, choanal stenosis/atresia, maxillary hypoplasia, mandibular prognathia, OSA (potentially severe), laryngomalacia, tracheomalacia, bronchomalacia, subglottic stenosis, tracheal cartilaginous sleeve
Ocular	Papilledema, exophthalmos/proptosis leading to exposure keratitis, corneal abrasion, retinal ischemia, optic nerve ischemia
Skeletal	Cervical spine fusion (C2–3, C4–5), scoliosis
Cardiac	PDA, PFO, aortic coarctation, tetralogy of Fallot
Neurological	Elevated ICP, Chiari malformation
Hematological	Major blood loss due to procedure, associated electrolyte/coagulation abnormalities, hypothermia

ICP, intracranial pressure; OSA, obstructive sleep apnea; PDA, patent ductus arteriosis; PFO, patent foramen ovale.

administered to hemodilute the patient to a predetermined hematocrit prior to incision, with the same resultant decrease in loss of blood cells with anticipated blood loss.[19] While permissive hypotension is often utilized in the adult population, it should be avoided or implemented with utmost caution in younger pediatric patients, as there are few data or evidence-based recommendations on its safety when applied to the pediatric population.[21]

POSTOPERATIVE CARE

Postoperative care for the child with CS aligns with standard postanesthetic care in a child with a difficult airway. The primary concern remains airway obstruction, thus awake extubation is recommended. Postoperative narcotics may exacerbate preexisting obstruction and should be used cautiously and in conjunction with opioid adjuvants whenever possible.[16]

KEY REFERENCES

Complete references for this chapter are online and available at https://connect.springerpub.com/content/book/978-0-8261-3875-0/part/part03/toc-part/ch030.

1. Al-Namnam NM, Hariri F, Thong MK, Rahman ZA. Crouzon syndrome: genetic and intervention review. *J Oral Biol Craniofac Re*. 2018, August 29;9(1):37–39. doi:10.1016/j.jobcr.2018.08.007
2. Pearson A, Matava CT. Anaesthetic management for craniosynostosis repair in children. *Br. J. Anaesth*. 2016;16(12):410–416. doi:10.1093/bjaed/mkw023
9. Mathews F, Shaffer AD, Georg MW, et al. Airway anomalies in patients with craniosynostosis. *Laryngoscope*. 2019;129(11):2594–2602. Wiley Online Library. doi:10.1002/lary.27589
12. Lionel KR, Moorthy RK, Singh G, Mariappan, R. Anaesthetic management of craniosynostosis repair – a retrospective study. *Indian J. Anaesth*. 2020;64(5):422–425. doi:10.4103/ija.IJA_823_19

CHAPTER 31

Down Syndrome

Jessica Storey

PATHOPHYSIOLOGY AND CLINICAL MANIFESTATIONS

In 1866, British physician John Langdon Down, for whom the syndrome is named, first described Down syndrome (DS). Today, DS is the most common chromosomal disorder, affecting approximately 12.6 per 10,000 (or 1 in 792) live births in the United States.[1] Data from the Centers for Disease Control and Prevention (CDC) indicate that nearly 200,000 people living in the United States are affected with this chromosomal anomaly. These numbers may continue to increase, as there has been a 30% increase in cases since 1979.[2] The increasing number of patients diagnosed with DS may be attributed to a higher incidence of mothers with advanced maternal age and increased access to testing and subsequent diagnosis.

DS is a chromosomally based phenomenon in which the affected patient has three copies of the 21st chromosome, also referred to as trisomy 21. The third copy of chromosome 21 occurs either by meiotic nondisjunction of the maternal chromosome 21 (96%), by translocation of an additional chromosome 21 to another chromosome (3%–4%), or by mosaicism of trisomy 21 (1%–2%). Mothers older than 40 years of age are statistically more likely to have a child born with DS compared to younger mothers.[3]

DS may be diagnosed either during pregnancy or after birth. Prenatal screening for DS can identify when a fetus is at an increased risk of being diagnosed with DS; however, it cannot definitely determine if this is the case. Similarly, prenatal ultrasound assessment can detect features common to DS, but definitive testing is necessary for a true diagnosis. Historically, diagnostic testing was invasive and increased the risk of miscarriage. Examples of diagnostic testing include chorionic villus sampling in the first trimester and an amniocentesis in the second trimester. Novel approaches to diagnostic testing are noninvasive and involve a blood draw. The current recommendation, however, is for the mother to undergo invasive testing for confirmation of diagnosis if the noninvasive test is positive. Although the foundational cause of DS is genetic in nature, phenotypic expressions of the genes, epigenetic influences, and environmental factors result in a wide variation of clinical features and presentations of the syndrome.

Universally observed characteristics of DS include facial dysmorphology, large tongue, low muscle tone, short stature, and intellectual disability (**Figure 31.1**). Facial characteristics can include a flattened midface, low nasal bridge, thin upper lip, epicanthal folds, almond-shaped eyes that slant upward, a short neck, relative micrognathia, and minor ear abnormalities.[4] Patients with DS also present with a higher incidence of cervical spine abnormalities, congenital heart defects, sleep disordered breathing, hearing impairments, visual impairments, hypothyroidism, Hirschsprung's disease, diabetes mellitus, hematologic disorders, seizure disorders, relative immunodeficiency, and obesity.[5]

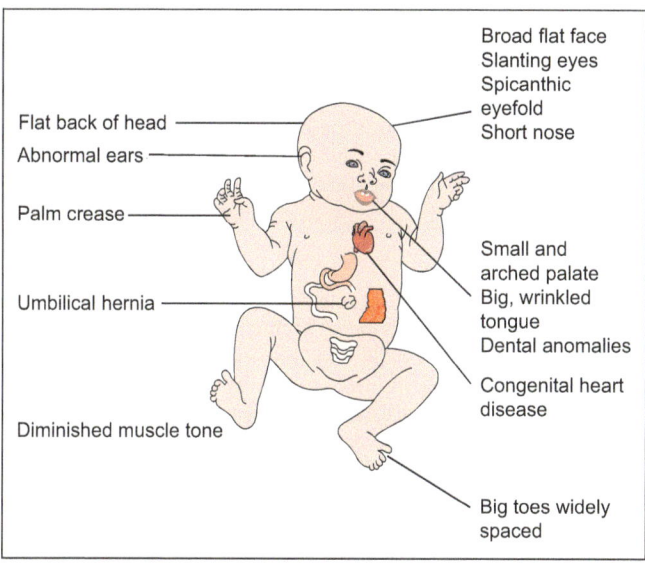

Figure 31.1: Common features associated with Down syndrome.

ANESTHETIC MANAGEMENT

PREOPERATIVE EVALUATION

DS patients have a higher incidence of medical conditions that affect health, development, and function compared to the general population that the anesthesia provider should consider when performing a preoperative assessment.

Airway Assessment

The unique facial and upper airway characteristics of DS may result in challenging airway management for anesthesia providers. Patients with DS often present with relative micrognathia and macroglossia, which are predictors of difficult exposure during direct laryngoscopy. Anesthesia providers may observe narrow upper airways related to a smaller midface and lower facial skeleton. Relatively large tonsils and adenoids may further obstruct the view of the glottis during intubation. An assessment of Mallampati score and thyromental distance is imperative to determine the need for additional airway management tools and strategies. DS patients with profound developmental delays may have poor dentition secondary to challenges with maintaining a healthy oral hygiene routine and should be assessed for the presence of caries, loose, or missing teeth if possible.

Immature and excessively pliable laryngeal cartilage causes a high incidence of laryngomalacia and collapse of the supraglottic structures resulting in characteristic inspiratory stridor and airway obstruction. Simpson, Oyekan, Ehsan, and Ingram[6] found that the incidence of obstructive sleep apnea (OSA) is 50% to 100% in childhood, nearing 100% in adulthood. Patients with DS often present with tonsillectomy, adenoidectomy, supraglottoplasty, and drug-induced sleep endoscopies related to sleep disordered breathing.

Atlantoaxial Instability

A well-known clinical feature of DS is atlantoaxial instability (AAI). Unfortunately, predicting the degree of instability in any given patient can be difficult. DS patients carry an increased risk of C1 and C2 subluxation (20%) due to laxity of the transverse ligament and malformation or absence of the odontoid process, which collectively can result in spinal cord injury during airway management. Only 1% to 2% of DS patients have a symptomatic presentation of AAI instability, so a traditional history and physical assessment may not be sufficient to predict risk.[7] Preoperative neurological assessment should be performed to assess motor and strength function at baseline. Historically, the American Academy of Pediatrics (AAP) endorsed obtaining at least one set of lateral cervical spine x-rays before proceeding with any procedure or anesthetic due to the risk of severe complications secondary to cervical spine compression. Recent studies and guidelines, however, suggest that these data may not provide meaningful practice guidance, and the need for radiologic examination should be institutionally guided for asymptomatic patients. For patients who have undergone radiologic assessment, a distance on x-ray between the atlas and odontoid process greater than 4.5 mm may indicate an increased need for cervical spine protection.[8] A new assessment tool that examines anteroposterior diameter of the spinal canal at the C1 to C4 level indicates that a C1/4 space available for spinal cord (SAC) ratio less than .8 may indicate a higher risk of developing neurological symptoms.[9] Should anesthesia providers proceed without formal evaluation, it is imperative that all individuals with DS be treated as having potential for an acute dislocation.

Cardiopulmonary Assessment

Patients with DS carry a higher rate of congenital heart defects, often stemming from embryonic defects in the endocardial cushion. Defects can include atrial septal defect (45%), ventricular septal defect (35%), patent ductus arteriosus (12%), and tetralogy of Fallot (8%). Patients with DS also carry a higher incidence and risk of pulmonary hypertension related to upper airway obstruction that can lead to right ventricular strain, and lesions that cause increased left-to-right flow triggering progressive narrowing of the pulmonary artery.[3] The assignment of risk must consider the severity of the lesions and the status of repair. A preoperative ECG and ECG are recommended to surveil potential cardiac lesions. Patients with DS also have a higher incidence of iron deficiency anemia. A complete blood count may be beneficial in those undergoing procedures that carry a high risk of blood loss.

PREOPERATIVE PHARMACOTHERAPY

Patients with DS have varying degrees of intellectual disability and may have previous individual experiences with healthcare providers that may contribute to healthcare-related anxiety. Anesthesia providers may consider pre-treatment with benzodiazepines, dexmedetomidine, or ketamine to aid in separation and transport to the operating room. Patients with DS also have a higher incidence of gastroesophageal reflux disease, so an assessment of current medications and status of control may predict the need for a rapid sequence induction. Patients may also be prescribed medications related to existing cardiac conditions. A review of these medications is imperative for appropriate anesthetic selection. In severe cases, subacute bacterial endocarditis (SBE) prophylaxis may be recommended depending on the cardiac lesion and status of repair.[10]

ANESTHETIC TECHNIQUE

Intraoperative Management

Patients with DS often have an atypical architecture of the sympathetic and parasympathetic nervous systems that can result in profound bradycardia with inhalational inductions with halogenated agents, specifically sevoflurane. Strategies to mitigate these effects are pretreatment with anticholinergic agents, such as atropine or glycopyrrolate, and a slower titration of inhalational agents during induction. In the majority of cases, the heart rate can be corrected by decreasing the volatile agent and performing airway instrumentation. IV induction is preferred whenever possible to reduce the risk of bradycardia.

Features of DS are hypotonia and reduced muscle mass. The use of succinylcholine should be judiciously considered before administering due to the risk of hyperkalemia in patients with skeletal muscle abnormalities.

Due to craniofacial abnormalities and upper airway obstruction, mask management may prove challenging. Adjunctive airway devices, such as oral airways, nasopharyngeal airways, and laryngeal mask airways, should be readily available. Preoxygenation is vital as children with DS are more prone to hypoxia during induction. Displacement of the abdomen off the chest by placing the bed in a reverse Trendelenburg position may aid in effective preoxygenation. This can also assist in aligning the tracheal and oropharyngeal axes. Cervical spine stability should always be considered whenever manipulating the patient's airway due to the high incidence of AAI and atlantooccipital instability (AOI). Cervical stability devices, such as soft collars or wedge-shaped neck supports, can be utilized to further protect cervical spine neutrality during positioning. Video laryngoscopes or fiberoptic intubation should be considered in patients with known AAI or AOI.

Patients with DS have an increased incidence of subglottic stenosis and smaller than normal tracheas. Using an endotracheal tube one to two sizes smaller than predicted for age or utilizing a microcuff tube may prevent postoperative tracheal stenosis and edema. Anesthesia providers should plan for awake extubation in patients with difficult airways.

POSTOPERATIVE CARE

Care of the patient with DS in the postoperative period should focus on respiratory and airway support. Assessment of post-intubation croup related to smaller than normal airway sizes is of importance in paients with DS. Adjunctive respiratory devices, such as continuous positive airway pressure and bi-level positive airway pressure, should be available in the postanesthesia care unit if patients use these devices at home. Supplemental oxygen may be required for longer duration as anesthetic medications are metabolized and respiratory status returns to baseline. Pain medications should be administered judiciously in an effort to limit opioid-induced airway obstruction. The use of nonopioid adjuncts should be considered if not contraindicated. A postoperative neurological assessment may ensure that acute spinal cord compression did not occur during the case.

REFERENCES

1. de Graaf G, Buckley F, Skotko BG. Estimation of the number of people with Down syndrome in the United States. *Genet Med*. 2016;19(4):439–447. doi:10.1038/gim.2016.127
2. Centers for Disease Control and Prevention. *Data and Statistics on Down Syndrome*. 2020. https://www.cdc.gov/ncbddd/birthdefects/downsyndrome/data.html
3. Bull MJ. Down Syndrome. *N Engl J Med*. 2020;382(24):2344–2352. doi:10.1056/NEJMra1706537
4. Karmiloff-Smith A, Al-Janabi T, D'Souza H, et al. The importance of understanding individual differences in Down syndrome. *F1000Res*. 2016;5:1000 Faculty Rev–389. doi:10.12688/f1000research.7506.1
5. Capone GT, Chicoine B, Bulova P, et al. Co-occurring medical conditions in adults with Down syndrome: a systematic review toward the development of healthcare guidelines. *Am J Med Genet A*, 2017;176(1):116–133. doi:10.1002/ajmg.a.38512
6. Simpson R, Oyekan AA, Ehsan Z, Ingram DG. Obstructive sleep apnea in patients with Down syndrome: current perspectives. *Nat Sci Sleep*. 2018;10:287–293. doi:10.2147/NSS.S154723
7. Meitzner MC, Skurnowicz JA. Anesthetic Considerations for Patients with Down Syndrome. *AANA J*. 2005;73(2):103–107.
8. Lewanda AF, Matisoff A, Revenis M, et al. Preoperative evaluation and comprehensive risk assessment for children with Down syndrome. *Paediatr Anaesth*. 2016;26(4):356–362. doi:10.12688/f1000research.7506.1
9. Nakamura N, Inaba Y, Aota Y, et al. New radiological parameters for the assessment of atlantoaxial instability in children with Down syndrome. *Bone Joint J*. 2016;98–B(12):1704–1710. doi:10.1302/0301-620X.98B12.BJJ-2016-0018.R1
10. Palumbo ML, McDougle CJ. Pharmacotherapy of Down syndrome. *Expert Opin Pharmacother*. 2018;19(17):1875–1889. doi:10.1080/14656566.2018.1529167

CHAPTER 32

Ehlers–Danlos Syndrome

Michael R. Everhart and Karmella M. Franic-Everhart

PATHOPHYSIOLOGY AND CLINICAL MANIFESTATIONS

The Ehlers–Danlos syndromes (EDS) are a related group of genetic disorders affecting collagen throughout the body resulting in lax ligaments, skin hyperextensibility, and fragile tissue.[1] First described in 1668, the disorder draws its name from the Danish dermatologist Edvard L. Ehlers, who presented a patient with the disorder at a meeting in Paris, France, in 1899. The incidence of the disease is estimated at 1 in 5,000 live births, inclusive of all types of EDS.[2] However, as many patients with mild joint and skin manifestations do not seek medical attention, it is difficult to determine the true frequency of EDS mutations in the general population.

EDS can be inherited as either a dominant or recessive condition. A variety of genes have been associated with EDS with some involved with encoding various subtypes of collagen (COL1A1, COL1A2, COL1A3, COL5A1, and COL5A2) and others responsible for encoding proteins responsible for processing or interacting with collagen, such as ADAMTS2, PLOD1, and TNXB. Collagen is essential in both strengthening connective tissue (e.g., bones) and providing flexibility where needed (e.g., cartilage) and is one of the major structural components of the body. Patients diagnosed with EDS experience poor strength of collagen throughout their body or lack sufficient amounts of structurally normal collagen.

Diagnosing EDS is largely based on the patient's presenting history and clinical findings. Assessments key to diagnosis focus on determining the extent of skin and joint hyperextensibility. The skin of patients with EDS is typically soft, hyperextensible, and velvety to the touch. In addition to joint hypermobility, many patients present with scoliosis and severe myopia. Once identified as having EDS, genetic testing can facilitate subtype diagnosis. Thirteen types of EDS are distinguished by the International Consortium on EDS (Table 32.1). Markers for dominant or recessive genes are diagnostic for 12 of the types. Hypermobile EDS has an unknown genetic basis and is diagnosed by physical criteria.

Table 32.1	Summary of EDS Classification
hEDS	Most common forms diagnosed using clinical criteria (Beighton system), GJH, recurrent abdominal hernias, soft velvety skin, atrophic scarring, mitral valve prolapse and aortic root dilation is common, as is chronic pain and dysautonomia
cEDS	Joint hypermobility and skin hyperextensibility
clEDS	Skin hyperextensibility, easy bruising, and GJH
cvEDS	Severe progressive cardiac valvular disease
vEDS Type IV (old nomenclature)	Vascular EDS is the most severe type with life span averaging 48 years. Patients may present in utero with dislocated hip and club feet. Collagen abnormalities in arteries, skin, and hollow organs lead to spontaneous rupture or dissection of the aorta and ruptures of the uterus and small intestine. Patients are at risk of potentially fatal arterial rupture, especially teenage boys. The PACU is also a high-risk period, possibly due to increased collagenase activity[3]
mcEDS (only 31 cases reported)	Multiple congenital deformities include micrognathia, retrognathia, pneumothorax, recurrent dislocations, large subcutaneous hematomas, and severe bleeding[4]
kEDS	Congenital hypotonia, early kyphoscoliosis, and multiple dislocations/subluxations
aEDS	Severe GJH with multiple dislocations or subluxations
BCS	Blue sclera, thin cornea, retinal detachment, deafness, hypotonia, and scoliosis
spEDS	Short stature, limb bowing, and severe hypotonia
dEDS	Extreme skin fragility, craniofacial abnormalities, severe bruising, short limbs, and growth retardation
mEDS	Congenital hypotonia or atrophy, and muscle contractures
pEDS	Severe and intractable periodontitis, and detached gingiva

aEDS, arthrochalasia EDS; BCS, brittle cornea syndrome; cEDS, classic EDS; clEDS, classic-like EDS; cvEDS, cardiac–valvular EDS; dEDS, dermatosparaxis EDS; EDS, Ehlers–Danlos syndromes; GJH, generalized joint hypermobility; hEDS, hypermobile EDS; kEDS, kyphoscoliosis EDS; mcEDS, musculocontractural EDS; mEDS, myopathic EDS; PACU, postanesthesia care unit; pEDS, periodontal EDS; spEDS, spondylodysplastic EDS; vEDS, vascular EDS.

Sources: From Brady AF, Demirdas S, Fournel-Gigleux S, et al. Ehlers-Danlos syndromes, rare types. *Am J Med Genet C Semin Med Genet.* 2017;175(1):70–115 doi:10.1002/ajmg.c.31550. Malfait F, Bloom L, Byers P, et al. The 2017 international classification of the Ehlers-Danlos syndromes. *Am J Med Genet C Semin Med Genet.* 2017;175(1):8–26. doi:10.1002/ajmg.c.31552.

Additionally, CT scanning, MRI, and echocardiography can be used to assess the presence and extent of mitral valve prolapse and aortic dilatation. Of note, prenatal diagnosis is also possible should abnormally low lysine hydroxylase enzyme activity be detected in cultured amniotic fluid cells.

Characteristic manifestations common to all mutations of EDS include joint subluxation or dislocation and skin hyperextensibility. EDS is highly associated with obstructive sleep apnea.[6] Patients within a given specific subtype of EDS share characteristics of disease beyond the common manifestations. The symptoms are wide-ranging and often unique to a specific subtype of EDS. For example, affected individuals may present with gastroparesis, spontaneous visceral rupture, uterine rupture, lung bullae, and tracheal dilation. Neurological disorders associated with EDS include idiopathic intracranial hypertension (due to pseudotumor cerebri), headache, craniocervical instability, and Chiari I malformation.[7] Mild aortic root dilation and postural orthostatic tachycardia syndrome (POTS) are common in hypermobile EDS (hEDS).[8] EDS patients are also known to frequently present with thoracic outlet syndrome.[9] Temporomandibular joint disorders (TMDs) occur in up to 70% of patients.[10] Additionally, scoliosis, kyphosis, dysautonomia, and resistance to local anesthetics are frequent findings in patients diagnosed with EDS.[2,3,11] Neonates with EDS may present with multiple, recurrent hernias.[12] Mast cell activation syndrome (MCAS) may also result in hypersensitivity reactions and rashes.[13] Unfortunately, chronic pain is common in EDS.[14]

ANESTHETIC MANAGEMENT

PREOPERATIVE EVALUATION

Prior to the initiation of anesthesia, a thorough preoperative evaluation is necessary. Special attention should be given to organ systems known to be associated with EDS. In addition, anesthesia providers should document the subtype of EDS and any current symptoms. Specific assessments should include the presence and degree of TMD and cervical instability, kyphoscoliosis, restrictive lung disease, and excessive bleeding and/or bruising even after minor trauma. It is imperative that the presence of vascular and cardiac comorbidities, such as aortic or mitral valve insufficiency or POTS, is vetted. POTS in patients aged 12 to 19 years can be identified by an increase in heart rate of 40 beats per minute within 10 minutes of standing. It is also recommended to inquire about joint laxity and document which joints are affected and the condition of the skin in the preoperative evaluation. Any complications associated with past anesthetics should be noted, especially prior difficulties with intubation.

Pertinent Laboratories

Preoperative testing is largely based on the subtype of EDS specific to the patient. Patients presenting with severe kyphoscoliosis may warrant pulmonary function tests to assess the extent of restrictive lung disease. Similarly, echocardiography may be necessary to assess the presence and extent of cor pulmonale.[15] An echocardiogram is indicated for patients with classic or vascular types of EDS and a history of aortic and/or mitral valve insufficiency. These patients are also at an increased risk of intraoperative bleeding. While coagulation studies are indicated if there is a history of abnormal bleeding or bruising, bleeding times may better identify patients with increased bleeding times.

Cross-matched blood products should be available if hemorrhage is anticipated.

PREOPERATIVE PHARMACOTHERAPY

While there are not strict pharmacologic contraindications, anesthesia providers should avoid medications that affect platelet function and coagulation. Current therapeutic regimens, such as the use of beta-adrenergic blockers to treat vascular or cardiac pathology, should be continued through surgery. Patients with a history of POTS may benefit from preoperative hydration to reduce the effects of POTS perioperatively, although vasopressors may still be necessary intraoperatively.[8]

ANESTHETIC TECHNIQUE

Intraoperative Management

The severity of symptoms and anesthetic implications are predicted based on specific disease subtype. General anesthesia with volatile anesthetic agents and use of a total IV anesthesia (TIVA) technique are both safe, effective options for patients with EDS. In patients with muscle wasting or neurological effects, the use of succinylcholine should be avoided. Adequate vascular access should be established to facilitate fluid, and blood resuscitation should intraoperative hemorrhage occur. Caution should be used in obtaining central venous access and arterial lines due to the possibility of vessel rupture and mediastinal or pleural hematoma formation. Noninvasive monitoring would be employed whenever possible. Anesthesia providers must take care when positioning patients with EDS to avoid insult to delicate skin and unintentional joint dislocation. Extra padding is recommended to reduce shear forces and external pressure to exposed tissue.

Special care is required regarding airway management as patients with EDS are at an increased risk of temporomandibular joint dislocation and cervical spine subluxation. Care must be taken during placement of a laryngeal mask airway or endotracheal intubation to avoid bruising in the airway or subluxation. Repeated attempts at intubation may result in bleeding, thus it is recommended to use a smaller endotracheal tube to decrease the likelihood of damage to the mucosa. In many instances, mask ventilation is advisable to avoid the aforementioned complications. Once a patent airway is established, it is important that patients are ventilated with low peak airway pressure to avoid pneumothorax intraoperatively.

The use of tourniquets has been associated with an increased risk of hematoma formation and compartment syndrome. This should be discussed with the surgeon prior to the start of surgery, and tourniquet inflation times should be reduced and limited in duration, if possible, to avoid complications.

Pain medications impacting coagulation should be avoided. The use of regional anesthesia has been reported, though there are several potential challenges that anesthesia providers should be aware of. Local anesthetics may have reduced efficacy in patients with EDS.[16] Peripheral nerve blocks have been reported to be unsuccessful or have reduced duration of action in as many as 24% of patients with EDS.[17] While epidural and spinal anesthesia have been used successfully for patients with EDS, the presence of scoliosis or kyphosis can make it more technically challenging to employ. The presence of Tarlov cysts, which are cerebrospinal fluid-filled perineural cysts, should be considered and may indicate meningeal involvement. This is more common with classic, hypermobile, and kyphoscoliotic types of EDS. Furthermore, the possibility of epidural hematoma in epidural or spinal-epidural anesthesia must be considered, as well as the potential for postdural puncture headache due to tissue fragility. As such, it may be best to avoid regional anesthesia in patients with vascular EDS entirely.[18]

Special Considerations/Concerns
Intraoperative bleeding is concern with patients with a history of EDS, despite normal preoperative laboratory values. The use of desmopressin (DDAVP) may aid in normalizing bleeding times in pediatric patients with EDS.[19] Additionally, tranexamic acid may reduce blood loss.[2,20]

Special Techniques/Equipment
Anesthesia providers should consider the use of video laryngoscopy or fiberoptic intubation to avoid complications due to temporomandibular joint dislocation or atlantooccipital instability.[21] The use of adequate muscle relaxation often improves intubating conditions. In addition, the use of a smaller than predicted endotracheal tube and low-cuff pressures can reduce tracheal and mucosal trauma.

POSTOPERATIVE CARE
Patients with EDS should be carefully monitored for cardiopulmonary and bleeding complications postoperatively in the postanesthesia care unit (PACU). Hemodynamic instability may occur in patients with POTS in the first several hours postoperatively. Visceral and vascular ruptures continue to be a concern, with occult bleeding often being difficult to detect. A thorough skin assessment should occur as the joints and skin continue to be at risk of injury. Patients with MCAS may have histamine release with resultant nausea. Adequate prophylaxis of postoperative nausea and vomiting is recommended as spontaneous esophageal rupture has been reported as a result of vomiting in vascular EDS. Patients with a history of chronic pain often require coordinated care with the pain management team.

KEY REFERENCES
Complete references for this chapter are online and available at https://connect.springerpub.com/content/book/978-0-8261-3875-0/part/part03/toc-part/ch032.

1. Malfait F, Bloom L, Byers P, et al. The 2017 international classification of the Ehlers-Danlos syndromes. *Am J Med Genet C Semin Med Genet.* 2017;175(1):8–26. doi:10.1002/ajmg.c.31552.
2. Chopra P, Bluestein L. Perioperative care in patients with Ehlers-Danlos syndromes. *Open J. Anesthesiol.* 2020;10(1):13–29. doi:10.4236/ojanes.2020.101002
3. Baum VC, O'Flaherty JE. Ehlers-Danlos syndrome. In: *Anesthesia for Genetic, Metabolic, & Dysmorphic Syndromes of Childhood.* 3rd ed. 2015.
5. Brady AF, Demirdas S, Fournel-Gigleux S, et al. Ehlers-Danlos syndromes, rare types. *Am J Med Genet C Semin Med Genet.* 2017;175(1):70–115 doi:10.1002/ajmg.c.31550.
14. Tinkle B, Castori M, Berglund B, et al. Hypermobile Ehlers–Danlos syndrome (a.k.a. Ehlers–Danlos syndrome Type III and Ehlers–Danlos syndrome hypermobility type): clinical description and natural history. *Am J Med Genet C Semin Med Genet.* 2017; 175(1):48–69. doi:10.1002/ajmg.c.31538
20. Wiesman T, Caston M, Malfait F, Hinnerk W. Recommendations for anesthesia and perioperative management in patients with Ehlers-Danlos syndrome(s). *Orphanet J Rare Dis.* 2014;9:109. doi:10.1186/s13023-014-0109-5

CHAPTER 33

Epidermolysis Bullosa
Kristen A. Callahan

PATHOPHYSIOLOGY AND CLINICAL MANIFESTATIONS
In 1886, Koebner applied the name epidermolysis bullosa (EB) to a collection of mechanobullous disorders. Today EB affects approximately 1 in 50,000 live births (Table 33.1). EB is characterized by protein defects in the dermal–epidermal junction, known as the basement membrane zone (BMZ). Mutations in any of at least 18 genes encoding the proteins in the epidermis, BMZ, or dermis ultimately result in the fragility of the skin and mucosa witnessed in patients with EB. Following frictional trauma, layer separation ensues, with blister and scar formation in the skin and mucosa. Patients may experience a variable phenotype depending on the level at which this separation occurs.

While most cases of EB are due to either autosomal dominant or autosomal recessive inheritance, there are rare instances in which EB presents as an acquired autoimmune disorder known as epidermolysis bullosa acquisita. While clinical diagnosis of EB is often made in the neonatal period, determination of the subtype of EB based on presentation should be avoided as all types of EB may look alike in this age group. Should EB be suspected, a skin biopsy should be obtained to confirm the diagnosis with transmission electron

Table 33.1 Incidence of EB

Subtype	All Forms	EB Simplex	Junctional EB	Dominant Dystrophic	Recessive Dystrophic
Incidence	19.6*	7.87*	2.68*	2.12*	3.05*
Prevalence	11.07*	6*	0.49*	1.49*	1.35

*Per 1 million live births.
EB, epidermolysis bullosa.

microscopy (TEM) and/or immunofluorescent antibody/antigen mapping. Additionally, genetic testing for mutations in most of the genes known to be associated with the various subtypes of EB is available.

There are four distinct subtypes of EB, which vary in presentation and severity depending on the level of the epidermal–dermal junction that is compromised. The primary subtypes of EB include EB simplex (EBS), junctional EB (JEB), and dystrophic EB (DEB). EBS is the mildest phenotype, with skin cleavage occurring within the basal keratinocytes. Blistering with EBS is typically confined to the hands and feet. While there may also be a generalized distribution of EBS, there is generally relatively mild internal involvement. Scarring is not usually witnessed with EBS, with the clinical presentation primarily being thickened calluses on the hands and feet, with thickened fingernails and toenails.

JEB involves skin separation at the level of the lamina lucida within the BMZ and DEB where skin cleavage occurs in the sublamina densa or papillary dermis. There are two major subtypes of JEB: Herlitz JEB and JEB-other. Herlitz JEB can be a very severe form of EB that may result in infant mortality due to sepsis, malnutrition, dehydration, electrolyte imbalance, or obstructive airway complications that occur secondary to the exuberant formation of granulation tissue during the healing process.

There are two major subtypes of DEB: dominant DEB (DDEB) and recessive DEB (RDEB). DDEB is typically less severe than RDEB, with blistering localized to the hands, feet, elbows, and knees, although this subtype may also be generalized (Table 33.2). RDEB is more generalized and involves mucous membranes (Figure 33.1). The cascade of manifestations can include esophageal strictures, malnutrition, anemia, webbing or fusion of the fingers and toes, development of contractures, growth retardation, malformation of teeth, microstomia, and corneal abrasions. A fourth and very rare subtype of EB is Kindler syndrome, which was identified in 2014 and involves a mixed pattern of skin cleavage (Figure 33.2).

EB can also present so mildly as to escape diagnosis with a normal life span. More severe presentations, however, are associated with much higher morbidity. Ocular complications, esophageal stricture, enamel hypoplasia and dental decay, anemia from iron deficiency and wound bleeding, growth retardation secondary to malnutrition, and even respiratory complications in JEB and dilated cardiomyopathy in RDEB can be witnessed. Exudative lesions result in constant pain and can limit activities of daily living, thereby precluding participation in sports and other activities due to the risk of injury. Alterations in activity and recurrent health complications can ultimately result in neuroplasticity as the disorder progresses.

Table 33.2 Subtypes of EB

	Subtype	Inheritance	Inheritance/Protein Affected	Severity	Presentation
EBS	EBS-WC	AD	KRT5, KRT14	Mild—hands and feet	Most common form of EB, blisters and erosions localized to mainly hands and feet. Extracutaneous signs minimal
	EBS-DM	AD	KRT5, KRT14	Severe—generalized	Generalized with a prevalence in acral areas. Oral and esophageal signs common, 2.8% mortality before age 1
	EBS-K	AD	KRT5, KRT14	Moderate to severe	Minimal scarring from blistering. Lesions predominately on extremities. Mild mucosal and nail involvement
	EBS with muscular dystrophy	AR	Plectin	Moderate to severe—associated with muscular dystrophy	Marked skin fragility milia, atrophic scarring, and nail dystrophy. Presents with significant extracutaneous signs including anemia and growth retardation. Neuromuscular symptoms consistent with limb–girdle muscular dystrophy unique to this variant

(continued)

Table 33.2	Subtypes of EB (*continued*)				
	Subtype	Inheritance	Inheritance/Protein Affected	Severity	Presentation
JEB	Herlitz	AR	Laminin 5	Most severe form of EB	Extensive extracutaneous effects including respiratory complications secondary to laryngotracheal stenosis and exuberant granulation tissue formation. Includes microstomia, ankyloglossia, enamel hypoplasia, and esophageal stricture. Epidermal atrophy occurs with blister healing
	Non-Herlitz	AR	Type XVII collagen	Similar cutaneous effects to Herlitz	Premature mortality common with an incidence of 40%–47% for both subtypes prior to age 1
	JEB with pyloric atresia	AR	α6β4 integrin	Severe	Alopecia, atrophic epidermis, enamel hypoplasia. Hemidesmosomal variant, severe and often lethal variant
Dystrophic EB	DDEB–RDEB-HS	AD–AR	Collagen VII–glycine substitution results in morphologically altered anchoring fibrils	Moderate	Extracutaneous findings minimal. Second most common form of EB presents with scarring and milia formation
	RDEB non-HS	AR	Collagen VII–PTC mutation resulting in the inability to form anchoring fibrils	Moderate	Patients present with severe and generalized cutaneous blistering and erosion at birth. Contractures and pseudosyndactyly, mitten deformity on hands and feet, microstomia and ankyloglossia are common. Chronic anemia may be present. Malnutrition and growth retardation common, secondary to increased metabolic requirements. Significant risk of squamous cell carcinoma, 7.5% by age 20, and up to 90% by age 55
Kindler EB	Kindler syndrome	AR	Kindlin-1 found in keratinocytes		Mixed pattern of skin cleavage with variable phenotypes

AD, autosomal dominant; AR, autosomal recessive; DDEB, dominant dystrophic EB; DM, Dowling-Meara; EB, epidermolysis bullosa; EBS, simplex EB; JEB, junctional EB; RDEB, recessive dystrophic EB; Kb, Köbner; WC, Weber-Cockayne.

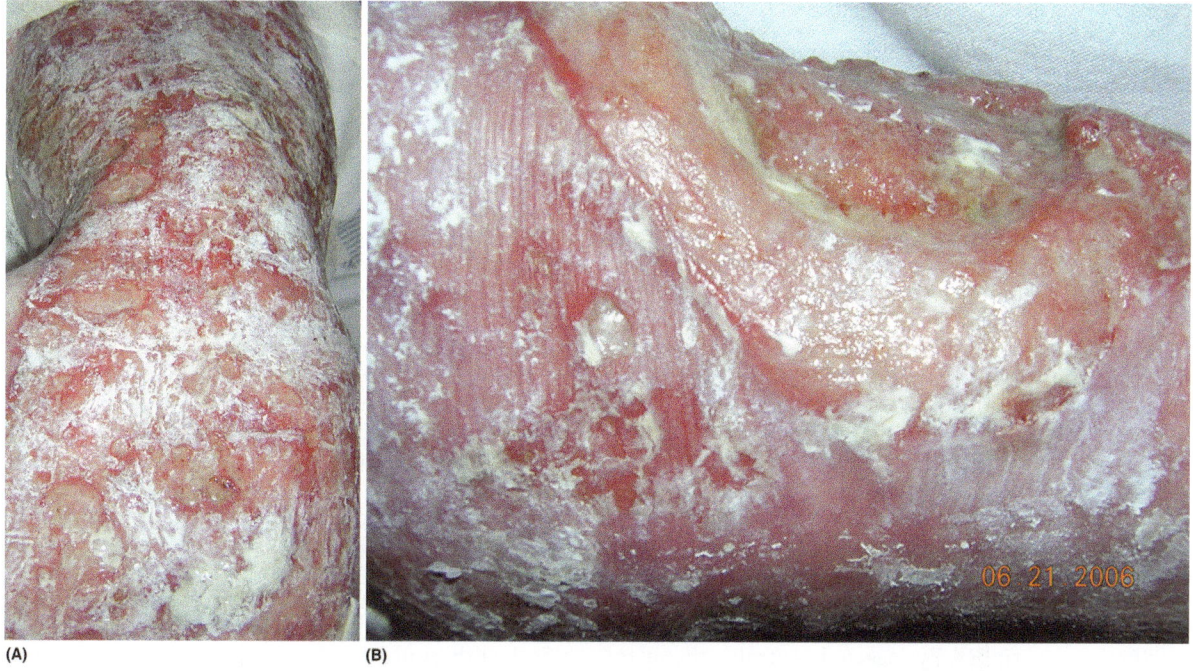

Figure 33.1: 27-year-old patient with recessive dystrophic epidermolysis bullosa. Back (A) and leg (B).

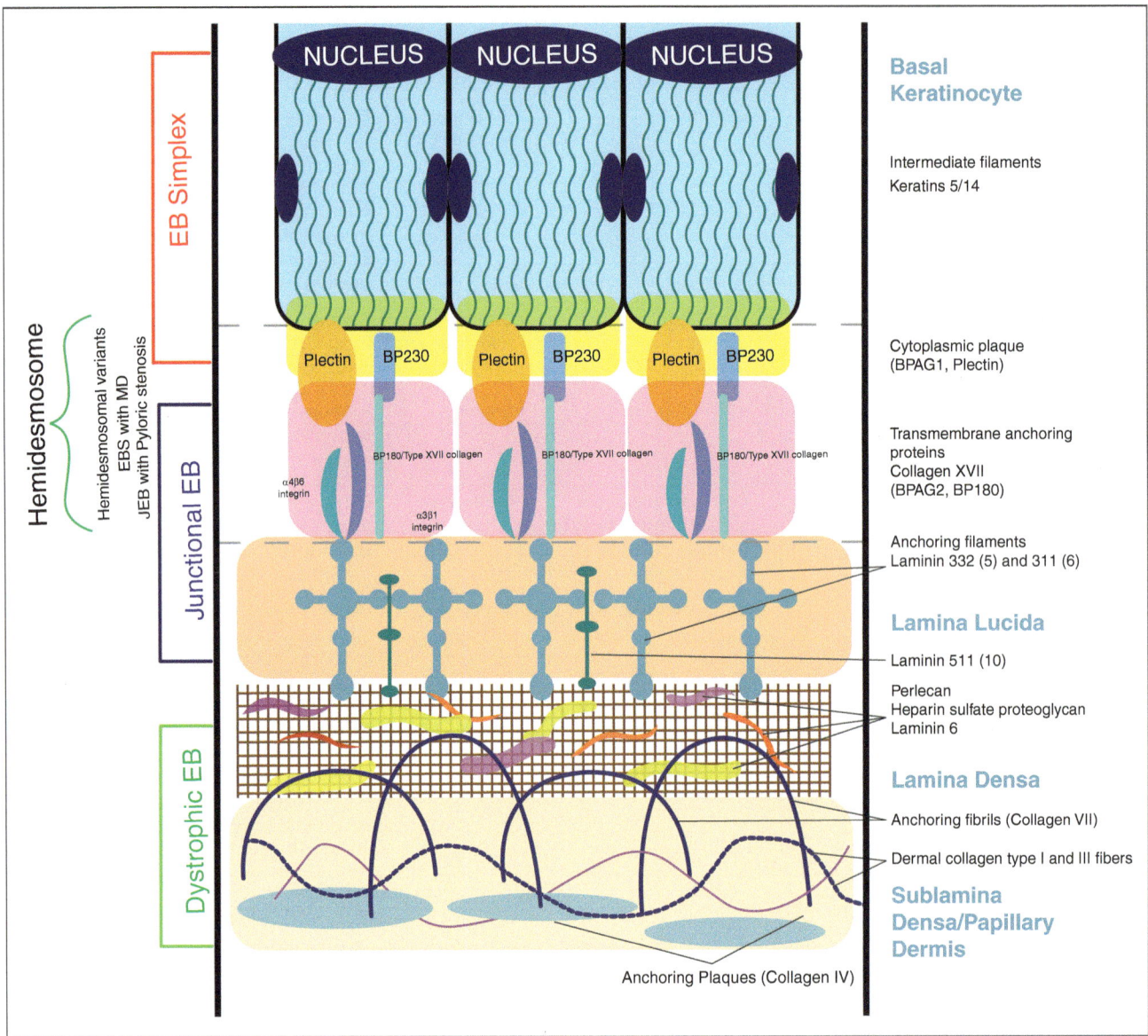

Figure 33.2: Layer of skin impacted by subtype of epidermolysis bullosa.
EB, epidermolysis bullosa; JEB, junctional EB.

ANESTHETIC MANAGEMENT

Patients diagnosed with EB often undergo multiple surgical procedures over the course of their lifetime, with patients with RDEB and JEB subtypes presenting more frequently. Contracture of the hands is a common occurrence with RDEB. Mechanical separation of the fingers to maintain function is common procedure and must frequently be done recurrently (**Figure 33.3**). Dental procedures are commonly done under anesthesia and may be combined with other procedures including esophageal dilatation. Scarring of the esophagus is a common concern in RDEB, and the need for repeated dilation at regular intervals is common. Severe cases of esophageal scarring necessitate a colonic interposition as scarring can become so severe that even liquids are unable to pass without the patient choking. Nutritional concerns as a result of both dysphagia and esophageal stricture may require insertion of a gastrostomy tube or even central venous catheter of peripherally inserted central catheter to facilitate the use of total parenteral nutrition.

PREOPERATIVE EVALUATION

Involving patients and family in discussions surrounding their care is essential. Recognizing that most EB patients are of normal intellect, including them in discussions when age appropriate is recommended. Reviewing previous anesthesia records if available can provide insight as to what techniques have been effective in providing a safe, effective anesthetic for the patient and may provide key information regarding airway management. It is imperative that anesthesia providers perform a thorough airway examination preoperatively due to the potential for difficult airway management secondary to the fragility of the skin and mucous membranes (**Box 33.1**; **Figure 33.4**). Dental decay is common and is in part due to difficult brushing secondary to oropharyngeal lesions. Mobility and mouth opening may be limited due to scarring. In addition to a standard review of systems and anesthetic complications, special attention must be paid to disease-specific health concerns. Malnutrition, anemia, and decreased immunity are common. Dilated cardiomyopathy may be

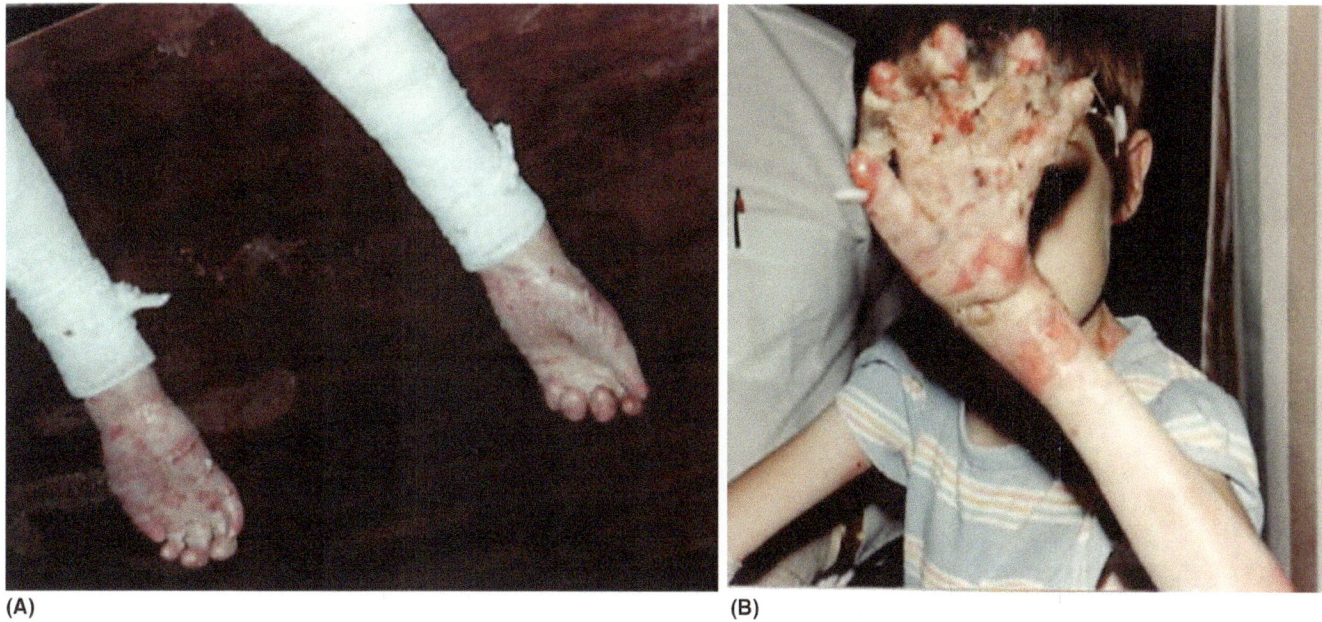

Figure 33.3: Eight-year-old girl with pseudosyndactyly. Prior to (A) and following (B) hand surgery.

> **BOX 33.1 KEY ASSESSMENT POINTS OF EB**
>
> 1. Careful airway assessment due to prevalence of microstomia and ankyloglossia. Painful sores may exist, further decreasing patient compliance and making assessment difficult. Contractures due to scars may further limit neck mobility.
> 2. Assessment of laboratory values due to chronic anemia and potential for electrolyte derangements secondary to malnutrition and dehydration. Risk of dilated cardiomyopathy, particularly in RDEB, due to carnitine deficiency.
> 3. Assessment of GERD risk, particularly in patients with a colonic interposition where the LES is no longer present.
>
> EB, epidermolysis bullosa; GERD, gastroesophageal reflux disease; LES, lower esophageal sphincter; RDEB, recessive dystrophic epidermolysis bullosa.

present, particularly in RDEB, and is thought to be related to nutritional and carnitine deficiencies. Dysphagia is a common complaint, secondary to pain and fixation of the oral cavity.

ANESTHETIC TECHNIQUE

Intraoperative Management

Premedication to prevent struggling during induction may be helpful in minimizing skin trauma. Induction of anesthesia can be accomplished in many ways. For young children, an inhalation induction followed by insertion of an IV catheter is appropriate. Insertion of an IV may be easier than expected due to the superficial location of veins. Careful mask ventilation with the use of a lubricated mask and gloves, along with application of protective silicone padding, can help to minimize friction trauma to the face. An IV induction of general anesthesia can be accomplished with standard induction agents.

A significant concern with the EB patient, particularly those with RDEB and severe JEB, is the high incidence of a difficult airway. Concerns include ankyloglossia, microstomia, and webbing of the posterior neck impairing positioning secondary to high incidence of scarring. The presence of gastroesophageal reflux (GERD) or oropharyngeal lesions further increases the likelihood of airway complications. Patients with a diagnosis of JEB are known to have a higher incidence of tracheal and laryngeal stenosis.

Anesthesia providers should consider having several tools for advanced airway management, such as a video laryngoscope and fiberoptic intubation, readily available in the operating room prior to the start of the induction process. Laryngoscope blades should be lubricated prior to insertion into the oropharynx with care taken to minimize shifting of the blade across the oropharyngeal surfaces. Nasal intubation can be done, but special care must be taken to minimize trauma. Endotracheal tube (ETT) securement can be accomplished through the use of umbilical tape and padded appropriately to prevent skin friction. Alternatives include the use of an inverted surgical mask on which the patient's head rests with the ties utilized to secure the ETT. Silicone-based adhesive tapes may also be utilized to secure an ETT if necessary. There is minimal literature regarding the use of laryngeal mask airways with patients diagnosed with EB, but due to the risk of oropharyngeal trauma, they are likely not the best choice.

Regional anesthesia can be used for pain management, but subcutaneous infiltration of local anesthetics should be discouraged to avoid the risk of skin sloughing. Careful assessment of the skin over the entry site is imperative to minimize risk of infection.

Special Considerations/Concerns

The intraoperative management of the patient with EB requires forethought and planning (Box 33.2). Positioning must be done carefully to minimize friction trauma to the skin. The patient should be placed on a foam or sheepskin

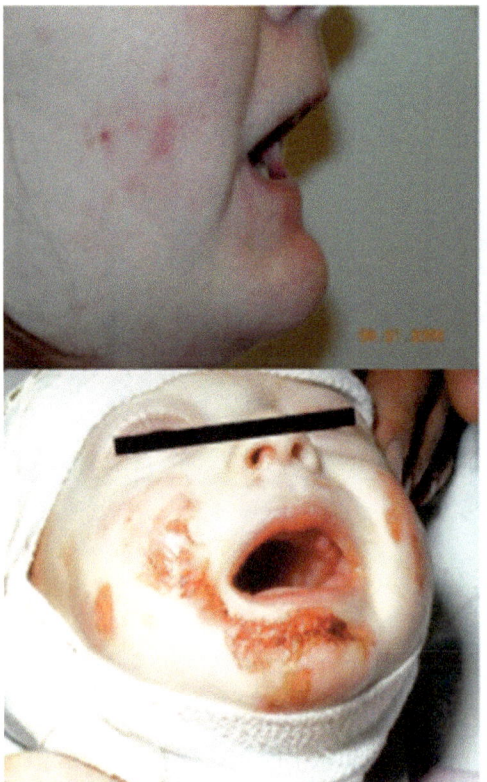
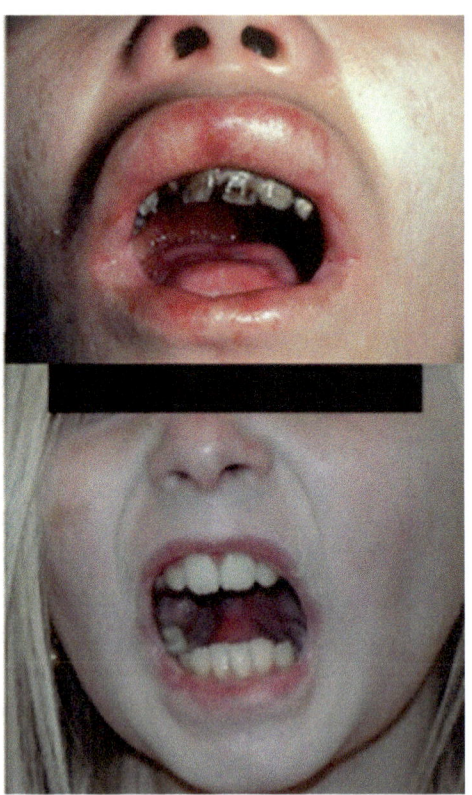

Figure 33.4: Preoperative airway evaluation.

BOX 33.2   SPECIAL EQUIPMENT/TECHNIQUES FOR EB

- Petroleum-based lubricant such as Aquaphor®
- Water-based lubricants such as KY Jelly®
- Nonadhesive pulse oximeter (clip style or cloth wrap)
- Webril® or similar padding for under BP cuff and exposed skin areas
- ECG needle electrodes or adhesive electrodes placed over thin silicone nonadherent dressings

BP, blood pressure; EB, epidermolysis bullosa.

pad while awake and then moved as a unit to minimize skin trauma. Monitoring can be accomplished by needle electrodes for ECG or skin electrodes with the adhesive portion removed, a nonadhesive pulse oximeter, and a blood pressure cuff with appropriate padding beneath. Pulse oximeter probe attachment to fingers may be difficult depending on the level of contracture of the digits. Placement of invasive lines is appropriate provided the antiseptic is dabbed on the site and not rubbed. Adhesives are inappropriate to use as subsequent removal will likely cause significant trauma to the skin and blister formation. Newer silicone-based adherent tapes and dressings (Mepitac® and Mepitel®) may be used with some patients to assist with securing lines. Use of sterile nonadherent dressings and gauze wraps can help maintain position. Ocular protection should be accomplished with the use of ophthalmic ointments.

POSTOPERATIVE CARE

An awake extubation at the completion of the procedure is encouraged to minimize risk of blood and/or secretions and the need for continued positive pressure ventilation. In the postanesthesia care unit, monitoring using the previously mentioned methods is appropriate. Including the parent in the recovery process can be helpful in decreasing anxiety and struggling in the pediatric patient. Depending on the procedure performed, the patient may be discharged home once all discharge criteria have been met.

KEY REFERENCES

Complete references for this chapter are online and available at https://connect.springerpub.com/content/book/978-0-8261-3875-0/part/part03/toc-part/ch033.

1. Bolling MC, Jonkman MF. KLHL24: Beyond skin fragility. J Invest Dermatol. 2019;139(1):22–24. doi:10.1016/j.jid.2018.08.010
2. Feinstein J, Jambal P, Peoples K, et al. Assessment of the timing of milestone clinical events in patients with epidermolysis bullosa from North America. JAMA Dermatol. 2019;155(2):196–203. doi:10.1001/jamadermatol.2018.46739
9. Has C, Bauer JW, Bodemer C, et al. Consensus reclassification of inherited epidermolysis bullosa and other disorders with skin fragility. Br J Dermatol. 2020;183(4):614–627. doi:10.1111/bjd.18921
11. Mariath, LM, Santin JT, Schuler-Faccini L, et al. "Inherited epidermolysis bullosa: update on the clinical and genetic aspects." An Bras Dermatol. 2020; 95(5):551–569 doi:10.1016/j.abd.2020.05.001
12. Martin K, Geuens S, Asche JK, et al. Psychosocial recommendations for the care of children and adults with epidermolysis bullosa and their family: evidence based guidelines. Orphanet J Rare Dis. 2019;14(1):133. doi:10.1186/s13023-019-1086-5

CHAPTER 34

Fetal Alcohol Syndrome

Jennifer McBride Schultz

PATHOPHYSIOLOGY AND CLINICAL MANIFESTATIONS

Fetal alcohol syndrome (FAS) is a toxic syndrome that is the result of maternal alcohol consumption during pregnancy. It is associated with severe birth defects, craniofacial anomalies, and growth retardation, as well as cognitive and behavioral impairments. In the United States, estimates suggest that the incidence of FAS is 0.3 cases per 1,000 live births, although data can be difficult to obtain due to limited reporting of alcohol use among expectant mothers.[1] Unfortunately, current alcohol use and binge drinking among pregnant women aged 18 to 44 years have increased slightly from 2011 to 2018 in the United States.[2] This may explain why recent studies using in-person assessment of school-age children in several U.S. communities report higher estimates, with the incidence of FAS being 6 to 9 out of 1,000 children.[3]

The onset of FAS begins during gestation as maternal consumption of alcohol freely crosses the placenta and is absorbed into fetal circulation. The fetus is unable to metabolize the alcohol due to limited functional alcohol dehydrogenase activity in the fetal liver. The inability to metabolize alcohol, coupled with the amniotic fluid storing the alcohol, causes prolonged alcohol exposure to the fetus. While noxious throughout pregnancy, such exposure to alcohol is particularly concerning during the first trimester as alcohol and its metabolite acetaldehyde are known teratogens that modify DNA and produce oxidative injury to the fetus.[4]

Diagnosis of FAS is based on presenting symptoms coupled with a history of maternal alcohol consumption during pregnancy. Fetal alcohol spectrum disorders vary and can include FAS, alcohol-related neurodevelopmental disorder, alcohol-related birth defects, and neurobehavioral disorder associated with prenatal alcohol exposure. Among the fetal alcohol spectrum disorders, patients with FAS are often the most impacted as they commonly present with central nervous system disorders, facial anomalies, cardiac defects, musculoskeletal alternations, among other physical findings.

Injury secondary to alcohol exposure in utero is irreversible and results in varying levels of impairment throughout life, with learning disabilities ranging from mild to moderate in nature. Hyperactivity and poor reasoning are common. In addition to neurological deficits, FAS contributes to defects in other systems, including cardiac, ophthalmologic, auditory, and renal. Regarding cardiac disorders, FAS may contribute to both structural defects (atrial and ventricular septal defects), as well as potentiating proarrhythmic events in individuals affected.[5] Individuals affected by FAS exhibit distinct craniofacial features, such as short palpebral fissures are common, as is ptosis, a flat midface, an upturned nose, a smooth philtrum with a thin upper lip, and microcephaly. Furthermore, they are often in the lower percentiles for height and weight and may exhibit some degree of fine motor deficit.

ANESTHETIC MANAGEMENT

PREOPERATIVE EVALUATION

Children born with FAS may exhibit distinct physical clinical features that the anesthesia provider should note during their preoperative physical assessment (Figure 34.1). The preoperative workup should also identify any potential specific system involvement and any potential intraoperative complications that might occur as a result. It is well known that FAS is associated with craniofacial anomalies (Box 34.1) as well as

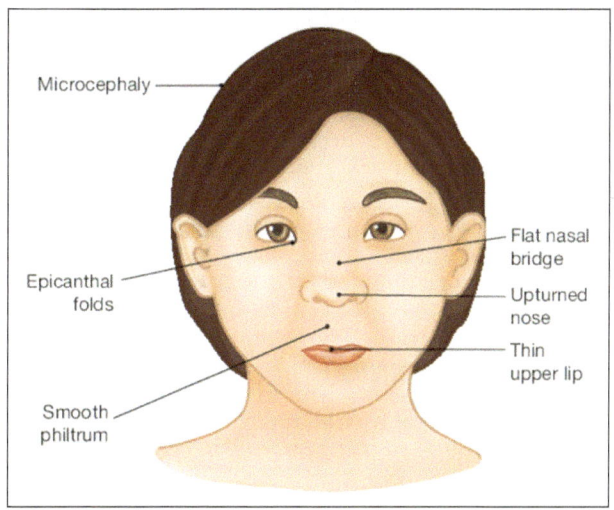

Figure 34.1: Facial abnormalities associated with fetal alcohol syndrome.

Source: From Teall AM, Gawlik K. Evidence-based assessment of the head and neck. In: KS Gawlik, BM Melnyk, AM Teall, eds. *Evidence-Based Physical Examination: Best Practices for Health and Well-Being Assessment.* Springer. 2021. Fig. 11.18.

BOX 34.1 KEY ASSESSMENT POINTS FOR FETAL ALCOHOL SYNDROME

Facial Characteristics

- Small head circumference
- Skin folds at corner of eye
- Small eye opening
- Low nasal bridge
- Short nose
- Small midface
- Indistinct philtrum
- Thin upper lip

---

multisystem anomalies including cardiovascular, ocular, auditory, musculoskeletal, renal, and neurologic. A preoperative consultation may be warranted to ensure that the patient presents with all pertinent data prior to the day of surgery. If cardiovascular abnormalities are noted during the preoperative physical examination, the provider should ensure that an ECG and echocardiogram are ordered. Concerns regarding short nose and nasolabial folds should indicate to the anesthesia provider that a nasal intubation may be contraindicated. The provider should also question what medication(s) the patient may be prescribed to help abate neurological symptoms of FAS.

PREOPERATIVE PHARMACOTHERAPY

While no medication has been approved solely as a treatment for FAS, some patients benefit from medications that help treat symptoms associated with FAS. Medications commonly used to treat FAS-related symptoms include stimulants, antidepressants, neuroleptics, and anxiolytic medications. It is important to consider the need for the FAS patient to continue taking their medication the day of surgery to facilitate lower levels of anxiety, aggression, and irritability during the perioperative and postoperative period. Additional anxiolytic medication may be required preoperatively if the patient is anxious or uncooperative. Patients exhibiting signs of seizure activity should have their seizures under control. Laboratory testing should also be performed to ensure adequate levels of antiseizure medication prior to surgery. Patients exhibiting cardiovascular anomalies may be taking medications for structural and/or electrical defects. The anesthesia provider should be informed of these medications to ensure that patients either hold their medication the day of surgery or continue taking the medication as indicated by their cardiologist.

ANESTHETIC TECHNIQUE

Intraoperative Management

The anesthesia provider should be vigilant in the intraoperative management of the FAS patient. All vital signs should be monitored with respect to the surgical procedure being performed. Care should be taken to ensure proper positioning for any range of motion limitations noted on preoperative examination. Patients presenting with ocular abnormalities might benefit from lacrimal lubricant prior to intubation to avoid corneal abrasions during the intraoperative and postoperative period. Any cardiac abnormality should be closely monitored during the intraoperative period and may necessitate invasive monitoring. Craniofacial features may make securing the airway difficult and advanced airway equipment should be available in the event of difficulty performing direct laryngoscopy. Rarely, patients with FAS will present with micrognathia and/or a short, webbed neck making direct laryngoscopy and tracheal intubation challenging.[6]

POSTOPERATIVE CARE

Emergence from anesthesia may be complicated by cognitive, visual, and auditory deficits attributable to FAS. The patient may be unable to communicate clearly and anxiety may be heightened. Anesthesia providers should consider the use of anxiolytics and sedation to avoid emergence delirium and allow for a smooth emergence and postoperative period. Parents and caregivers should be allowed in the recovery unit, when possible, to assist in facilitating a safe, trusting recovery room environment for the FAS surgical patient. If there was difficulty securing the airway during surgery, the anesthesia provider should plan to extubate the patient awake in the operating room. Should the patient not be extubated immediately following surgery, the anesthesia provider should communicate to the surgeon the need for postoperative mechanical ventilation and, if indicated, admission to the intensive care unit for extubation planning and frequent physical assessment.

REFERENCES

1. Mattson S, Bernes G, Doyle L. Fetal alcohol spectrum disorders: A review of the neurobehavioral deficits associated with prenatal alcohol exposure. *Alcohol Clin Exp Res*. 2019;43(6):1046–1062. doi:10.1111/acer.14040
2. Denny CH, Acero CS, Terplan M, Kim SY. Trends in alcohol use among pregnant women in the US, 2011–2018. *Am J Prev Med*. 2020;59(5):768–769. doi: 10.1016/j.amepre.2020.05.017
3. May PA, Baete A, Russo J, et al. Prevalence and characteristics of fetal alcohol spectrum disorders. *Pediatrics*. 2014;134(5):855–866. doi:10.1542/peds.2013-3319
4. Wozniak J, Riley E, Charness M. Clinical presentation, diagnosis, and management of fetal alcohol spectrum disorder. *Lancet Neurol*. 2019;18(8):760–70. doi: 10.1016/s1474-4422(19)30150-4
5. Onesimo R, De Rose C, Delogu AB, et al. Two case reports of fetal alcohol syndrome: broadening into the spectrum of cardiac disease to personalize and to improve clinical assessment. *Ital J Pediatr*. 2019;45(167):1–5. doi:10.1186/s13052-019-0759-y
6. Bissonnette B, Luginbuehl I, Marciniak B, Syndromes BJD. *Syndromes: rapid recognition and perioperative implications*. McGraw Hill; 2006.

CHAPTER 35

Goldenhar Syndrome

Judy Audas

PATHOPHYSIOLOGY AND CLINICAL MANIFESTATIONS

Although the features of this syndrome were first recorded in the 1800s, the syndrome was not formally recognized until 1952 when it was described by Dr. Maurice Goldenhar. The incidence of Goldenhar syndrome (GS) ranges from 1:3,000 to 1:26,500 live births, effecting males on a 3:2 when compared to females. GS falls under the oculo-auriculo-vertebral spectrum of defects and is present at birth, mainly affecting the development of the eyes, ears, and spine.[1] The etiopathogenesis of GS is not completely understood, with most cases occurring sporadically with no apparent explanation. It is thought to develop during formation of the first and second branchial arches, which form the structures of the head and neck, sometime between the third and eighth week of fetal development.[2] Interference with vascular supply and focal hemorrhage in the developing first and second branchial arches may explain the unilaterality of GS.[3] The vasculogenic theory, however, does not explain many of the extracranial manifestations seen in GS. An alternate theory suggests a defect of blastogenesis results from deficiency in migration or formation of neural crest cells and/or mesoderm formation. GS has also been attributed to exposure to environment factors during the third to eighth week of fetal development.[4] Though rare, autosomal dominant and recessive inheritance has been reported.[5]

Syndromes associated with dysmorphogenesis of the branchial arches are associated with a group of conditions known as craniofacial microsomia.[6] Eye abnormalities, such as lipoma, lipodermoid, epibulbar dermoid, or upper eyelid coloboma, in association with ear, mandibular, or vertebral anomalies (two of the three), meet the diagnostic criteria for GS.[7] The most common overall presentation of GS is unilateral hemifacial microsomia, microtia, vertebral, renal, and ocular anomalies.[6] There is unilaterality in 70% of the cases, with the right side being affected more frequently.[2] The hemifacial macrosomia may present as hypoplasia of the malar, maxillary, or mandibular regions with possible hypoplasia of the facial musculature. Figure 35.1 illustrates some of the facial features commonly witnessed with GS.

Vision or hearing may be impaired depending on the degree of ocular or middle and inner ear involvement.[2] Common and uncommon abnormalities seen in GS are shown in Table 35.1. As patients with GS tend to have a normal life expectancy, they may present for surgical repair of associated anomalies for functional or aesthetic reasons at any time throughout childhood.

ANESTHETIC MANAGEMENT

PREOPERATIVE EVALUATION

Physical assessment of a patient with GS should include a thorough history of any related criteria (see Table 23.1). Airway assessment is always a priority during a preoperative evaluation; however, this is ever important in children showing

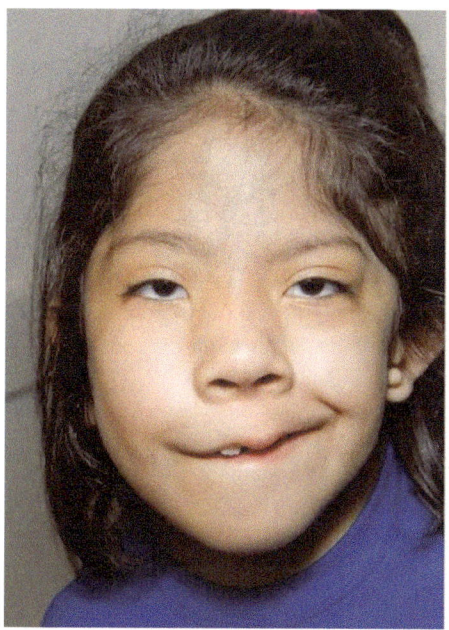 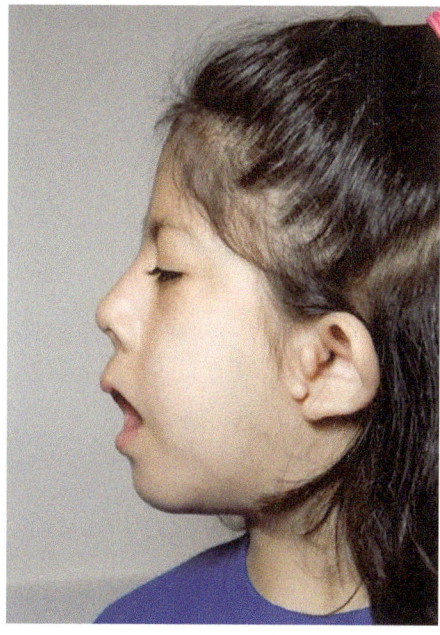

Figure 35.1: Child with Goldenhar syndrome. Note the hemifacial microsomia, macrostomia, and redundant ear tissue with preauricular tags.

Source: From De Golovine, S. Wu, S. Hunter, JV, et al, 2012. Goldenhar syndrome: a cause of secondary immunodeficiency?. *All Asth Clin Immun.* 2020;8:10. doi:10.1186/1710-1492-8-10.

Table 35.1	Goldenhar Syndrome Features and Associated Anesthetic Implications		
Anatomical Structures	**Common Abnormalities**	**Less Common Abnormalities**	**Anesthetic Implications**
Face	Malar hypoplasia Maxillary hypoplasia Mandibular hypoplasia (with TMJ involvement) Hypoplasia of facial musculature		Difficult mask ventilation Difficult intubation
Eye		Epibulbar dermoid Lipodermoid Upper eyelid coloboma Strabismus Microphthalmia Retinal abnormalities	Vision loss may necessitate alternative communication methods
Ear	Microtia Accessory preauricular tags or pits (commonly in the line from the tragus to the corner of the mouth) Redundant ear tissue Middle ear anomaly with variable deafness	Inner ear defect	Communication barrier in the presence of hearing loss Difficult mask fit with facial asymmetry
Mouth	Macrostomia (from cleft-like extension of the corner of the mouth) Soft palate malformation/dysfunction Tongue malformation/dysfunction	Cleft lip Cleft palate Dental abnormalities	Difficult laryngoscopy and intubation Risk of damage to dentition or oral cavity
Vertebrae	Hemivertebrae or hypoplasia of vertebrae (most often cervical, but can be thoracic or lumbar)	Scapular anomalies	Limited range of motion of cervical vertebrae during laryngoscopy
Central Nervous System	Hydrocephalus Arnold–Chiari malformation Occipital encephalocele Hypoplasia of septum pellucidum Enlarged ventricles Intracranial dermoid cyst Lipoma in or agenesis of corpus collosum		Risk of aspiration on induction with increased ICP Communication barriers due to neurological involvement
Cardiac		Tetralogy of Fallot VSD ASD PDA Conotruncal defects Coarctation of the aorta	Challenging balance of SVR to PVR related to fluctuations in blood pressure Risk of air emboli with cardiac shunting
Genitourinary		Ectopic or fused kidneys Renal agenesis Vesicoureteral reflux Ureteropelvic junction obstruction Multicystic dysplastic kidneys	Possible electrolyte imbalances Possible fluid management challenges
Other		Intellectual disability (13%) Speech delay Autism Branchial cleft remnants in neck Laryngeal anomaly Hypoplasia or aplasia of the lung Esophageal atresia Tracheomalacia (due to extrinsic vascular compression) Rib abnormalities	Communication challenges for patients with intellectual and speech difficulty Difficulty in ventilation and intubation Risk of airway damage with ETT cuff

ASD, autism spectrum disorder; ETT, endotracheal tube; ICP, intracranial pressure; PDA, patent ductus arteriosus; PVR, pulmonary vascular resistance; SVR, systemic vascular resistance; TMJ, temporomandibular joint; VSD, ventricular septal defect.

Source: Information on this table was derived in part from *Smith's Recognizable Patterns of Human Malformation*.[2]

features of GS. Patients with syndromes involving craniofacial abnormalities, such as hemifacial microsomia, should be evaluated for difficult intubation and airway compromise due to mandibular hypoplasia.[8] It is important to examine external facial symmetry, oral dentition, and palatal structures when considering the feasibility of mask ventilation and endotracheal intubation. The age of the patient is also noteworthy, as there is a direct correlation between age and the degree of airway difficulty.[10] Preoperative radiographic studies can provide useful information related to facial and vertebral anatomy that may make mask ventilation, laryngoscopy, and endotracheal intubation difficult. The gold standard for imaging is cone-beam CT (CBCT), which can provide three-dimensional information about facial bones and other airway structures.[11] Careful assessment of cervical range of motion, in addition to x-rays of vertebral structures, is key as some patients with GS present with cervical instability and subluxation of C1 to C2. Although less commonly seen, if cardiac defects are suspected based on physical assessment, an echocardiogram is warranted. Genitourinary abnormalities found on preliminary screening in the neonatal period can prevent long-term sequelae. If urinary concerns present during the preanesthetic period, renal/pelvic ultrasound is recommended with a nephrology consult.[12] Assessing hearing and vision deficits, as well as establishing a reliable communication plan with parents and their child, is especially important with GS patients to assure a safe and successful anesthetic. A review of previous anesthetics is a priority when formulating a plan of care.

PREOPERATIVE PHARMACOTHERAPY

Patient age and cooperation during the preoperative assessment will determine the need for preoperative sedation. Oral midazolam (0.5 mg/kg) may be helpful if a peripheral IV catheter is required prior to an "awake" fiberoptic intubation if difficult endotracheal intubation is expected. Oral midazolam may also be useful to manage separation anxiety before the child is taken to the operating room. For older children, preoperative anxiety related to esthetic procedures and perceived body image should be considered. An antisialagogue, such as glycopyrrolate (0.05–0.1 mg/kg), can be used to minimize oral secretions and optimize visualization during a fiberoptic intubation.

ANESTHETIC TECHNIQUE

If previously successful, a standard inhalation induction is acceptable, with caution used to maintain spontaneous ventilation until an IV catheter can be placed. Previous anesthesia records should have detailed information regarding ease of mask ventilation and endotracheal intubation methods. It is always best to repeat what has worked in the past unless there is a strong reason not to do so based on the planned surgical procedure. Facial asymmetry and mandibular hypoplasia may impede an adequate mask seal. Additional anesthesia providers should be available to assist with two-hand bag-mask ventilation, if necessary.

A difficult airway cart, including a fiberoptic bronchoscope (FOB) and a video laryngoscope (VL) should be present at induction of anesthesia for all GS patients. While FOB intubation has been the gold standard for managing a difficult intubation, the availability of the VL and ease of its use have replaced the FOB in many cases. If "awake" FOB is planned for intubation, a weight-based infusion of low-dose propofol (50 mcg/kg/min) and/or dexmedetomidine (0.3–1.5 mcg/kg/hr) can facilitate patient cooperation. A one-time dose of ketamine can also provide some aesthesia while maintaining spontaneous ventilation. A retrospective study of 311 patients with hemifacial microsomia by Xu, Deng, and Yan[13] showed that although FOB and VL techniques can improve intubation success rate, direct laryngoscopy (DL) with a standard technique should be the preference. In fact, DL was successful in 80% of the first-pass attempts made on expected and unexpected difficult airways.

A laryngeal mask airway (LMA) is an acceptable choice for minor surgeries not requiring muscle relaxation. An LMA may also be used to guide FOB placement of an endotracheal tube (ETT) in some circumstances. It is important to check that the appropriate ETT size will pass through the LMA opening prior to placement in the airway.

As children get older and grow, their airway typically improves naturally. If CBCT scans are available, they should be reviewed preoperatively to estimate the diameter of the glottic opening and subglottic area in order to choose the correct ETT size. Due to the possible airway narrowing from vascular compression in the airway of GS patients, it is recommended that ETT cuff pressures be checked frequently and kept below 20 mm Hg. High-dose IV dexamethasone (0.4–0.5 mg/kg) can be used to prevent airway inflammation. Awake extubation is recommended for all expected and unexpected difficult airways.

POSTOPERATIVE CARE

The priority in postoperative care of a GS patient is to manage pain without causing airway compromise. Use of nonnarcotic pain medications, such as acetaminophen, ketorolac, and local anesthesia, can prevent obstruction from oversedation. If narcotics are required, small doses of short-acting narcotics are best. It is also important to continue to assess for airway edema. If stridor is noted in the postoperative period, humidified mist can be administered to reduce mucosal edema. If stridor worsens, it can be treated with 0.05 mL/kg of 2.25% racemic epinephrine nebulized in 3 to 5 mL of normal saline. If racemic epinephrine is given, the patient should be observed for 4 to 6 hours to assure the inflammation does not return when the medication wears off.

KEY REFERENCES

Complete references for this chapter are online and available at https://connect.springerpub.com/content/book/978-0-8261-3875-0/part/part03/toc-part/ch035.

1. Goldenhar M. Associations malformatives de l'oeil et de l'oreille, en particulier le syndrome dermoide epibulbaire-appendices auriculaires-fistula auris congenita et ses relations avec la dysostose mandibulo-faciale. *J Genet Hum*. 1952;1:243–282.
2. Jones KL, Jones MC, del Campo M. *Smith's Recognizable Patterns of Human Malformation*. Philiadelphia: Elsevier; 2013.
6. Genetic and Rare Diseases Information Center. *rarediseases.info.nih.gov*. 2017. Retrieved January 12, 2021
12. Bogusiak K, Puch A, Arkuszewski P. Goldenhar syndrome: current perspectives. *World J Pediatrics*. 2017;13(5):405–415. doi:10.1007/s12519-0048-z
13. Xu J, Deng X, Yan, F. Airway management in children with hemifacioal microsomia: a retrospective study of 311 cases. *BMC Anesthesiology*. 2020;20(120):1–9. doi:10.1186/s12871-020-01038-2

CHAPTER 36

Hurler Syndrome/Hunter Syndrome

Jessica Storey

PATHOPHYSIOLOGY AND CLINICAL MANIFESTATIONS

Mucopolysaccharidosis (MPS) includes a group of genetically inherited lysosomal storage disorders that result from a total or partial deficiency of 1 of the 11 enzymes involved in the metabolism of glycosaminoglycans (GAGs), namely, heparin sulfate, dermatan sulfate, and chondroitin sulfate. These disorders are organized into seven distinct forms based on their inheritance pattern and specific enzyme deficiency. Regardless of the subtype of MPS disorder, the gradual accumulation of GAG in lysosomes of the skin, brain, heart, bone, liver, spleen, blood vessels, cornea, and tracheobronchial airway cells affects appearance, physical abilities, mental development, and organ and system functioning. The disease process is chronic and progressive with the child generally appearing normal at birth, and deteriorating as the gradual accumulation of GAGs causes permanent cellular damage to the airway, cardiac, respiratory, and skeletal systems. This chapter focuses on the two most common types of MPS: Hurler syndrome (MPS I) and Hunter syndrome (MPS II).

It is estimated that the incidence of MPS is 1 in 25,000 live births with Hurler and Hunter syndromes occurring in 1 in 100,000 live births.[1] Hurler syndrome (MPS I) is an autosomal recessive disorder caused by a mutation in the alpha-L-iduronidase (IDUA) gene. The IDUA gene provides instructions for producing an enzyme that is directly involved in the breakdown of GAGs. Hunter syndrome (MPS II) is an x-linked recessive disorder that based on its pattern of inheritance almost exclusively affects males. The IDS gene provides instructions for producing the I2S enzyme, which is directly involved in the breakdown of GAGs.

The classic symptom presentation of Hurler and Hunter syndromes develops as the child ages and GAG deposits increase in tissue. Patients generally present within the first year of life with coarse facial features, musculoskeletal alterations, cardiovascular abnormalities, neurosensorial hearing loss, enlarged tonsils and adenoids, and increased secretions (Figure 36.1). Developmental delay is generally observed between 12 and 24 months of life, and corneal opacity is observed by the third year of life. Further manifestations as the child ages are hydrocephaly and organomegaly.[2]

Outwardly noticeable signs of the disease are craniofacial aberrancies, such as a large head, bulging frontal bones, broad nose with depressed nasal bridge, enlarged tongue, enlarged and rounded cheeks, thickened lips, gapped teeth, and gingival hyperplasia. Musculoskeletal deposits result in short stature, thoracic–lumbar kyphosis, joint stiffness, limited cervical spine mobility, limited temporomandibular joint mobility, and a short immobile neck.

ANESTHETIC MANAGEMENT

Hurler syndrome and other MPS disorders have been described throughout various texts and articles as one of the most challenging airway management situations in pediatric anesthesia. Cases of MPS disorders and their disastrous anesthesia-related airway outcomes have been recorded as far back as the 1930s and 1940s when the term "gargoylism" was used to describe patients affected with this disorder due to observed coarse facial features. A review of older literature concerning these patients yields harrowing accounts of an inability to intubate and ventilate, failed emergent tracheostomies, and anesthesia-related mortality statistics as high as 4.2% even in recent history.[3] Moretto, Bosatra, Marchesini, and Tesoro[7] completed a retrospective review of the literature and found that 20% of surgical-related deaths with MPS I are directly related to airway obstruction or difficult intubations. The study found that 40% of patients had difficult intubations, and 12% of patients experienced failed intubations (p. 50). Anandan and Sharanva[1] revealed that 5% to 25% of patients experienced perioperative respiratory complications due to difficult mask ventilation, difficult or failed intubation, and airway obstruction at induction. Therefore, it is imperative that anesthesia providers place a concerted focus on airway management during the management of these complex patients.

PREOPERATIVE EVALUATION

Patients diagnosed with MPS disorders routinely present for a variety of surgical procedures but most frequently undergo otolaryngologic and ophthalmic procedures. Commonly performed procedures are myringotomy, adenotonsillectomy, tracheostomy, nasal and sinus procedures, corneal transplants, ventriculoperitoneal shunt, cardiac valve replacement, feeding tubes, hernia repair, spinal decompression, orthopedic procedures, and oral surgeries. Patients diagnosed with MPS disorders are well known for severely difficult airways and carry a significantly higher risk of airway complications compared to the general population.

Airway Assessment

While a Mallampati airway assessment is often useful in predicting a difficult airway, it may be of minimal use in this population as most MPS patients exhibit a difficult airway regardless of Mallampati scores. Therefore, preoperative testing to evaluate the extent of upper airway obstruction and predict difficulty with airway management should be obtained prior to presentation for surgery. A sleep study is useful in determining the pathophysiology resulting in airway obstruction as obstruction may occur in a ball-valve fashion related to macroglossia, adenotonsillar hypertrophy, and deposition of GAG in the pharyngeal and laryngeal walls (Figure 36.2). Likewise, a preoperative CT scan may be useful to determine the extent of supraglottic narrowing. Pulmonary function testing can more accurately help guide the anesthesia provider's decision-making related to ventilatory settings. In addition, the neck range of motion should be assessed to determine the degree of cervical immobility, and mouth opening should be assessed to determine the degree of temporomandibular joint function.

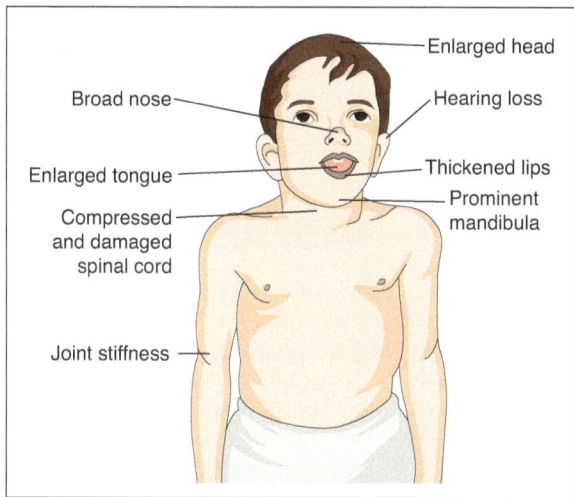

Figure 36.1: Signs and symptoms of Hunter syndrome.

Cardiopulmonary Assessment

A preoperative echocardiogram and ECG are mandatory as GAG deposits affect myocardial muscle and valvular function. Severe valvular disease (leaflet thickening), cardiomyopathy, decompensated heart failure, and significant arrhythmias may be observed on these studies in this patient population. Additionally, chronic hypoxemia and ventilation–perfusion (V/Q) mismatching may lead to pulmonary hypertension over time.

Neuroskeletal Assessment

GAG deposits accumulate in the bones, joints, and ligaments leading to short stature, abnormal body habitus, and kyphosis. Routine spine x-rays, MRI, and flexion–extension cervical film assessments may confirm the potential for atlantooccipital subluxation. Functional assessments of baseline motor and strength should be assessed as these patients are at risk of spinal cord compression. Of note, patients with MPS I (Hurler) are at a higher risk of odontoid dysplasia, subluxation of C1 and C2, and anterior dislocation of the atlas, causing spinal cord compression. Intraoperative neuromonitoring with somatosensory evoked potential evaluation is strongly recommended throughout the perioperative period to assess spinal cord integrity during intubation and positioning maneuvers.

PREOPERATIVE PHARMACOTHERAPY

Treatment options for patients with MPS disorders are limited and focus on hematopoietic stem cell transplantation (HSCT), or enzyme replacement therapy (ERT) with drugs, such as Aldurazyme and Elaprase. One study found that patients treated with HSCT had a less difficult airway than those not treated. Patients with MPS I and II treated with ERT did not have a decreased incidence of difficult airway experiences.[4] Preoperative anxiety should never be treated with opioids due to the risk of respiratory depression. Benzodiazepine administration with pulse oximetry monitoring may be used judiciously. Pretreatment with an antisialagogue and oxymetazoline may be helpful in controlling excessive secretions.

ANESTHETIC TECHNIQUE

Intraoperative Management

Due to the risk of airway complications in general anesthesia, the provider should utilize alternative methods of anesthesia and analgesia as often as possible. Regional anesthesia, when performed successfully, yields less narcotic use and subsequent respiratory depression. Smaller procedures, such as radiologic scans and lumbar punctures, may be attempted with precedex and ketamine infusions as an alternative to general anesthesia. An additional complication that may be observed is challenging IV access due to coarse skin and tissue deposits. Ultrasound

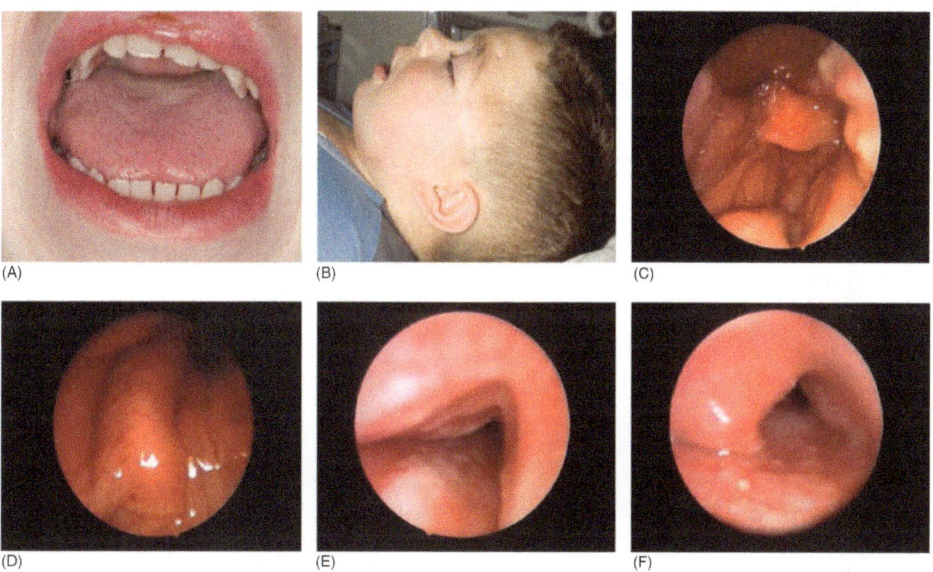

Figure 36.2: Airway assessment of Hurler syndrome. (A) Macroglossia in a child with mucopolysaccharidosis type I (MPS I). (B) Anatomical features complicating anesthesia in MPS I: large head and short stiff neck10 (written permission obtained and held by institution's medical illustration department). (C) Laryngopharyngeal deposits in MPS I. (D) Significant laryngeal obstruction in MPS I. (E) Tracheomalacia in MPS. (F) Tracheal narrowing due to MPS deposit within the tracheal lumen.

Source: From Arn P, Bruce IA, Wraith JE, et al. Airway-related symptoms and surgeries in patients with mucopolysaccharidosis I. *Annals of Otology, Rhinology & Laryngology.* 2014;124(3):198–205. doi:10.1177/0003489414550154.

IV access or providers with additional vascular access training may be necessary to obtain adequate access.[5]

In patients diagnosed with an MPS disorder, GAGs often infiltrate the connective tissues of the oropharynx and airways causing upper airway obstruction, difficult mask ventilation, and difficult intubation. Once in the airway, submucosal GAG deposits in the tongue, the floor of the mouth, the epiglottis, the aryepiglottic folds, and the tracheal wall produce a rigid airway. Patients with an MPS disorder also exhibit copious secretions that may lead to difficulty visualizing the glottis during intubation and may lead to aspiration events in periods without a protected airway. Furthering the potential for airway-related complications, a short immobile neck with limited mobility of the temporomandibular joint and cervical spine further increases the difficulty of airway management. Because this disease is chronic and progressive, patients diagnosed with an MPS disorder of an older age have a higher incidence of a difficult airway management and complications related to airway management.

Before induction, anesthesia providers should have all necessary airway equipment readily available including fiberoptic intubation equipment, traditional laryngeal mask airways (LMAs), intubating LMAs, small shoulder rolls, different-sized endotracheal tubes (ETT), and additional providers in the room. Smaller-than-predicted ETTs should be utilized to reduce the risk of postoperative subglottic stenosis and edema. Emergency tracheotomy trays should also be available in the event of an airway emergency. It should be noted that tracheostomy may be difficult due to distortion and laxity of the trachea. LMAs have proved useful in maintaining ventilation due to the ease of placement without excessive neck extension and without the use of muscle relaxant.

Inhalational induction may be preferred over IV induction due to the easier titration of depth and maintenance of spontaneous respiration during induction. Induction in the lateral position or the patient's favorite sleeping position may result in better preoxygenation efforts. Utilizing a C-MAC with a D blade is useful when a Cormack Lehane III and IV is observed due to its acutely angulate design. Displacing the tongue anteriorly by manual retraction helps access larynx when video laryngoscope is inserted.[6] Facemasks may not fit appropriately, but some studies have reported success with inverting the mask (an upside-down technique) for a better seal. Once the airway is secured, the anesthesia provider may still grapple with hypoxia and hypercarbia as lower airway deposits lead to diffusion defects in some patients. Paralytics and full-dose narcotics should be avoided whenever possible to avert postoperative airway complications. Awake extubation after a leak test should be the preferred plan for extubation, along with the coadministration of airway dose steroids to prevent laryngeal edema.[7]

POSTOPERATIVE CARE

Many patients diagnosed with an MPS disorder require continuous positive airway pressure or bilevel positive airway pressure therapy at home at baseline. Home respiratory support should be reinstituted immediately in the postanesthesia care unit due to the risk of airway obstruction. Anesthesia providers should consider multimodal analgesia to reduce narcotic dosage and the potential for respiratory depression postoperatively. Admission to the intensive care unit may be preferred to monitor for postoperative respiratory and neurological complications.

REFERENCES

1. Anandan AK, Sharanya P. Mucopolysaccharidosis and anesthetic challenges. *Indian J Anesth Analg.* 2019;6(5 (P-2):1863–1865. doi:10.21088/ijaa.2349.8471.6519.54
2. Gungor G, Bozkurt Sutas P. Overview on anesthetic management of children with mucopolysaccharidoses (MPSs). *J Res Med Sci.* 2017;1(1):30–35. doi:10.5336/worldclin.2016-50697
3. Walker RW, Garbarino J, Anesthesia risk and the mucopolysaccharidoses: a challenging and changing landscape. *J Child Sci.* 2018;08(01): e116–e123. doi:10.1055/s-0038-1667349
4. Stuart G, Pehora C, Wong G. The impact of contemporary treatments on the perioperative care of children with mucopolysaccharidoses: A case series and review of the literature. 2019.
5. Kamata M, McKee C, Truxal KV, et al. General anesthesia with a native airway for patients with mucopolysaccharidosis type III. *Pediatr Anesth.* 2017;27(4):370–376. doi:10.1111/pan.13108
6. Thakkar KD, Hrishi AP, Sethuraman M, Vimala S. Management of a difficult airway scenario in a case of Hurler's syndrome with a D-blade video laryngoscope. *JNACC.* 2020. doi:10.1055/s-0040-1714451
7. Moretto A, Bosatra MG, Marchesini L, Tesoro S. Anesthesiological risks in mucopolysaccharidoses. *Ital J Pediatr.* 2018;44(S2):116. doi:10.1186/s13052-018-0554-1

CHAPTER 37

Klippel–Feil Syndrome

Daniel Henz

PATHOPHYSIOLOGY AND CLINICAL MANIFESTATIONS

Klippel–Feil syndrome (KFS) is a rare skeletal condition that was first described in 1743 by Swiss physician Albrecht von Haller and again in 1912 by French neurologists Francois Maurice Klippel and Andre Feil. KFS is an abnormal congenital fusion of any two of the seven cervical vertebrae, resulting in shortness of the neck, limited movement of the neck, and a low posterior hairline (Figure 37.1).[1] KFS is estimated to occur in approximately 1 in every 40,000 live births throughout the world, with females accounting for 60% of all cases. While autosomal dominant and autosomal recessive inheritance does occur, most cases are thought to be sporadic.

It is believed that KFS occurs from faulty segmentation along the embryo's axis during the third and eighth weeks of development.[2,3] KFS has been found to have a high concurrence with Chiari malformation and can be part of the associated congenital anomalies that are found in the VACTERL (vertebral defects, anal atresia, cardiac defects, tracheoesophageal fistula, renal anomalies, and limb abnormalities)

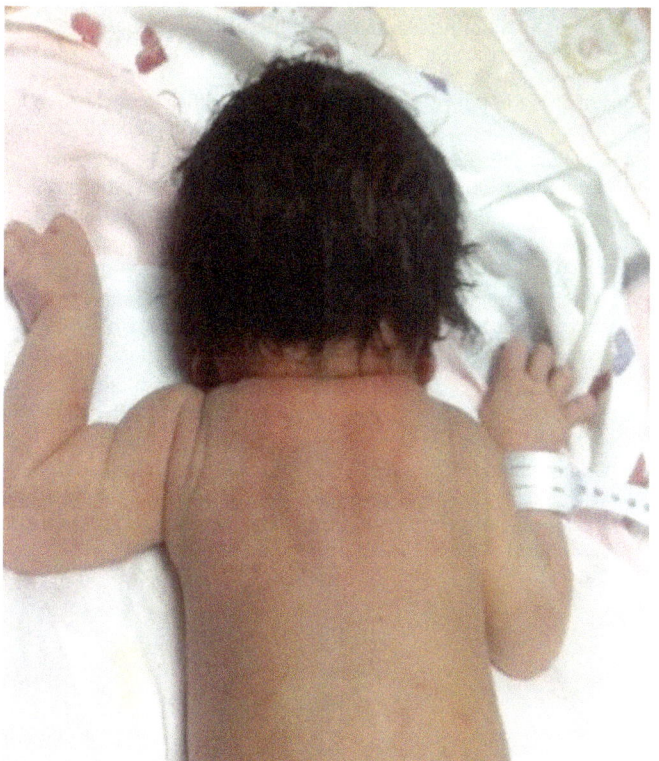

Figure 37.1: Neonate with Klippel–Feil syndrome.

Source: From Bejiqi R, Retkoceri R, Maloku A, et al. How often is Klippel–Feil syndrome associated with congenital heart disease: presentation of five cases and a review of the literature. *J Cardiol Cardiovasc Med.* 2019;4:110–116. doi:10.29328/journal.jccm.1001050.

syndrome patient population.[4] This makes it even more difficult to develop a clear genetic causation. There are at least four genetic forms of KFS that have been described, with KFS type II being the most common presentation.[3] KFS type I is characterized by extensive fusion of the cervical vertebrae and the upper thoracic vertebrae. KFS type II is characterized by fusion at one or two cervical or thoracic vertebrae, often associated with occipitoatlantal fusion and hemivertebrae. The most common cervical segments that are fused are found at C2 to 3 and C6 to 7.[5] KFS type III is characterized by fusion of vertebrae of the neck as well as vertebrae of the upper or lower thoracic or lumbar vertebrae. KFS type IV is associated with sacral agenesis.[1,3]

KFS may be diagnosed at birth based on characteristic physical findings. Diagnostic testing may include MRI, to help characterize interspaces between certain cervical and other vertebrae, the extent of abnormal vertebral union or fusion, and possible impingement of vertebrae on the spinal cord. Lateral flexion–extension x-rays of the cervical spine may be performed as well to determine the range of motion at each interspace. Additional specialized tests may also be conducted to help detect and/or characterize other abnormalities that may be associated with KFS, such as hearing impairment, congenital heart defects, renal abnormalities, or eye defects.

While the clinical triad associated with KFS is a short neck, low posterior hairline, and limited neck movement, all three clinical manifestations are present in less than 50% of cases.[3] The most common clinical manifestation of KFS is limited neck movement. Additional anomalies commonly associated with KFS include congenital heart defects, renal impairment, scoliosis, deafness, Sprengel's deformity, mental deficiencies, pulmonary impairment, mandibular hypoplasia, and cleft lip and/or palate.[6] Due to the many other underlying diagnoses, patients with KFS will sometimes be unaware of having fused cervical vertebrae.

ANESTHETIC MANAGEMENT

PREOPERATIVE EVALUATION

Preparing the patient with KFS for anesthesia should involve a thorough assessment of the airway, with a specific focus on cervical mobility. Patients with hypermobility of the upper cervical spine are at risk of neurological sequelae, such as paraplegia, hemiplegia, and cranial or cervical nerve palsies. Conversely, patients with limited mobility in the lower cervical spine are more at risk of the development of degenerative disease.

Micrognathia and mandibular anomalies may also be present that can make airway management challenging when combined with cervical immobility.[7] Radiographic imaging, specifically lateral cervical x-rays in flexion–extension, along with a thorough clinical assessment, can be very helpful in the preanesthetic evaluation and planning.

A thorough MRI evaluation should occur in patients with spinal anomalies due to the high incidence of concurrent anomalies that may occur.[4] Additionally, congenital vertebral fusion, known as block vertebra, can be distinguished from acquired fusion by a narrowing of the vertebrae at the level of the intervertebral disc with no loss of disc height resembling a "wasp waist."[8] MRI and CT imaging can also be helpful in showing the extent of spinal canal narrowing that can occur with KFS.[9] Assessment and document of neurological function and preexisting deficits are imperative.

An echocardiogram may be warranted should cardiac defects present. Additionally, pulmonary function tests may be indicated based on the extent of scoliosis and the subsequent impact on lung function.

PREOPERATIVE PHARMACOTHERAPY

Anesthesia providers may consider the administration of an antisialagogue prior to induction of anesthesia to limit the impact of secretions during intubation. Anxiolytics can be used with caution in patients with preoperative anxiety.

ANESTHETIC TECHNIQUE

Intraoperative Management

The level of cervical fusion and any cervical instability caused by the fusion of the vertebrae must be taken into consideration when deciding on the appropriate method of securing the airway. Patients with KFS should be considered to have cervical instability and are at risk of spinal cord injury during laryngoscopy, intubation, and positioning. While an awake fiberoptic intubation is theoretically the ideal approach to securing the patient's airway, this is often difficult to achieve in young children. Accordingly, inhalational mask inductions are commonly performed with the use of a fiberoptic bronchoscope to secure the airway following induction. Anesthesia providers should be aware that mask ventilation may be difficult. Every precaution should be taken while securing the airway.[10]

Using a fiberoptic bronchoscope helps limit neck movement during intubation, thereby decreasing the risk of cervical spine injury.

Anesthesia providers should be aware that due to the progressive nature of KFS, the documentation of past success in securing the airway is not always a good predictor of future success. Therefore, it is recommended having equipment for managing a difficult airway readily available and in the operating room during induction. There have been case reports of successful intubation with video laryngoscope, as well as successful use of a supraglottic airway device.

The use of standard monitors, as described by the American Society of Anesthesiologists, often proves sufficient unless the planned surgery or comorbidities dictate otherwise. The presence of associated anomalies will dictate what additional precautions must be taken during the perioperative period. For example, patients with cardiac anomalies may require antibiotic prophylaxis or patients with renal involvement may have special considerations with regard to fluid management.

Attention must be given to positioning during anesthesia as patients with KFS are prone to cervical injury from minor trauma. Additional padding and maintenance of cervical neutrality are key throughout the anesthetic to minimize the risk of injury. Syncope may be induced with sudden neck rotation at any point during the anesthetic. A neurological assessment should be documented pre- and postanesthetic to facilitate identification of changes in the integrity of the cervical spine.[2]

The use of local or regional anesthesia should be considered to limit the need for opioid analgesics that are known to promote respiratory depression. The use of epidural or spinal anesthesia in patients who have KFS is not contraindicated and has been performed successfully. It should be noted, however, that regional anesthesia can be more difficult to perform due to any spinal anomalies that may be present.[11,12]

POSTOPERATIVE CARE

Postoperatively, patients with KFS should be extubated awake at the end of surgery, with stabilization of the neck during emergence. A multimodal approach to pain management should be employed in an attempt to limit opioid-induced respiratory depression. Admission to the intensive care unit postoperatively may be indicated for monitoring after extensive surgery, as these patients are at a high risk of developing postoperative airway obstruction and respiratory failure.

KEY REFERENCES

Complete references for this chapter are online and available at https://connect.springerpub.com/content/book/978-0-8261-3875-0/part/part03/toc-part/ch037.

3. Frikha R. Klippel-Feil syndrome: a review of the literature. *Clin Dysmorphol.* 2020;29:35–37. doi:10.1097/MCD.0000000000000301.

4. Passius PG, Poorman GW, Jailai CMB, et al. Incidence of congenital spinal abnormalities among pediatric patients and their association with scoliosis and systemic anomalies. *J Pediatr Orthop.* 2019;39(8):e608-e613. doi:10.1097/BPO.0000000000001066.

7. Garcia-Marcinkiewicz, AG, Stricker PA. Craniofacial surgery and specific airway problems. *Pediatr Anesth.* 2020;30:296–303. doi:10.1111/pan.13790

10. Oliveira CRD. Pediatric syndromes with noncraniofacial anomalies impacting the airways. *Pediatr Anesth.* 2020;30:304–310. doi:10.1111/pan.13810

12. Santonastaso DP, de Ciara A, Addis A, et al. Spinal anesthesia with a low dosage of local anesthetic for urgent Cesarean delivery in a parturient with Klippel-Feil syndrome. *J Clin Anesth.* 2019;52:78–79. doi:10.1016/j.jclinane.2018.09.013.

CHAPTER 38

Mitochondrial Myopathy

Leslie Jackson and Matthew McCoy

PATHOPHYSIOLOGY AND CLINICAL MANIFESTATIONS

Mitochondrial disease is a rare genetic disorder that presents following mutation in either mitochondrial or nuclear DNA. The resulting mutation ultimately interferes with adenosine triphosphate (ATP) and energy production, with varying degrees of disruption in cellular energy production witnessed. The cellular mechanisms impacted include oxidative phosphorylation, pyruvate metabolism, carnitine metabolism, fatty acid oxidation, and cellular signaling required for homeostasis.[1] The negative impact on ATP and energy production culminates in abnormal accumulation of lactate and hypoglycemia.[2] Mitochondrial disease presents in approximately 1 in 5,000 births,[1] with 81% of mitochondrial disorders initially presenting during childhood. Unfortunately, 74% of those children die prior to 10 years of age.[3]

Mitochondrial disease is multisystemic, often involving multiple organ systems simultaneously, and can present as either a nonspecific grouping of symptoms (lactic acidosis and hypoglycemia) or as a clinical syndrome, such as Leigh syndrome, Alpers–Huttenlocher syndrome, Barth, or MELAS (mitochondrial encephalmyopathy, lactic acidosis, and stroke-like episodes), among others.[4] There are varying levels of severity with mitochondrial disease; however, common manifestations include myopathies, encephalopathy, seizures, developmental delays, sensorineural hearing loss, liver dysfunction/hepatomegaly, pancreatic insufficiency, cardiomyopathy, nephritis, renal impairment, diabetes mellitus and other growth and hormone insufficiencies, anemias, and thrombocytopenias.[4]

ANESTHETIC MANAGEMENT

PREOPERATIVE EVALUATION

As patients with mitochondrial disease often present with multiple organ system involvement, a thorough preoperative assessment should be completed with detailed exploration of any comorbidities (Table 38.1). Consultation with the primary care team is essential in estimating the likelihood of perioperative complications. The preoperative evaluation should focus on the cardiac, respiratory, hepatic, renal, and central nervous systems. A collaborative decision involving the primary care team, the surgical team, and the anesthesia providers should be made regarding what laboratory values may need to be assessed prior to surgery. In most instances, the need for preoperative testing is largely dependent on the patient's overall health status and disease progression.

Every effort should be made to schedule procedures for these medically complex patients early in the day to limit fasting as patients with mitochondrial disease are susceptible to hypoglycemia and lactic acidosis. Patients often present with elevated lactic acid levels due to anaerobic metabolism as a result of limited energy reserves. In the setting of decreased energy supplies preoperatively (fasting and hypovolemia), the patient is at risk of metabolic decompensation;[5] therefore, clear liquids containing glucose should be encouraged up to 2 hours before the induction of anesthesia.[1] For patients more severely impacted by mitochondrial disease, it may be necessary to admit the patient prior to surgery for preoperative IV hydration.

A thorough cardiac assessment is key as conduction defects or preexcitation syndromes are common in mitochondrial disorders. Assessment of activity tolerance may indicate cardiac dysfunction and warrants further evaluation via an ECG. Furthermore, ECG and chest x-ray can be reviewed to predict left ventricular dysfunction, which is not uncommon in Leigh syndrome and MELAS. If ventricular impairment is suspected or known, an echocardiogram will be necessary prior to surgery.[5]

Respiratory evaluation may benefit from review of pulmonary function testing or polysomnography (sleep study) if available. Sleep-disordered breathing is often the first indication of respiratory muscle weakness and predictive of respiratory performance in a sedated state.[5] Neurological assessment should be sure to elicit information about seizure activity, including frequency and duration, as well as current medication management. The anesthesia provider should confirm patient adherence to medication regimen and diet considerations for patients on a ketogenic diet to minimize or control seizure activity. Consulting the team managing seizure medications may be indicated to optimize seizure control preoperatively.[5]

Pertinent Laboratories

It is imperative that the anesthesia provider review baseline values for glucose, lactate levels, and liver function tests, and a basic metabolic panel should be reviewed prior to surgery as hyponatremia and hyperkalemia have been reported in patients with mitochondrial disease.[1,5] Unless recent laboratory evaluations are available, these should be redrawn and reviewed before the induction of anesthesia.

Table 38.1	Key Assessment Points: Mitochondrial Disease
System	**Testing**
Respiratory	Pulmonary function tests Polysomnography
Neurological	EEG Antiepileptic medication levels
Cardiac	ECG Chest x-ray Echocardiogram
Hepatic	LFTs
Renal	BMP
Metabolic	Lactic acid Glucose

BMP, basic metabolic panel; LFTs, liver function tests.

PREOPERATIVE PHARMACOTHERAPY

While premedication (oral or nasal versed) may be given as an anxiolytic, it should be individually adapted to prevent postoperative respiratory compromise.

ANESTHETIC TECHNIQUE

Intraoperative Management

There are no universally accepted standards of care for the anesthetic management of a patient with mitochondrial disease and currently there are no clinical trials that have studied the effects of anesthetic agents on this population (Box 38.1).[6] Despite all currently used anesthetics having an inhibitory effect on mitochondria function, they have all been used safely in this population. Propofol infusion syndrome and the accompanying lactic acidosis have been reported following the prolonged use of propofol for sedation in the intensive care unit. A single bolus of propofol or infusion of limited duration, however, has not been shown to be associated with adverse events.[1] The use of any of the potent inhalational anesthetics is acceptable as mitochondrial disease is not associated with an increased risk of malignant hyperthermia,[6] although succinylcholine should be avoided due to the potential risk of hyperkalemic cardiac arrest.[6] Neuromuscular blockade and narcotics should be used cautiously due to the likelihood of increased sensitivity.[7] Train-of-four monitoring should be utilized to assess return of neuromuscular junction intraoperatively.

POSTOPERATIVE CARE

Postoperatively, the patient with mitochondrial disease remains at risk of metabolic decompensation, as shivering, pain, tachycardia, and tachypnea can quickly deplete energy stores. In the postanesthesia care unit (PACU), the anesthesia provider should titrate pain medications slowly to avoid respiratory depressant effects.[1] Should the patient utilize respiratory equipment at baseline, such as positive pressure support (continuous positive airway pressure or bilevel positive airway pressure), due to a diagnosis of sleep-disordered breathing, the anesthesia provider should ensure the equipment is available in the postoperative setting.[5]

Similarly, it is imperative that efforts are made to avoid postoperative nausea and vomiting, temperature fluctuations, and lactic acidosis. Glucose levels should be checked while in the PACU, and hypoglycemia should be corrected. Depending on the severity of the disease, postoperative admission may be warranted to monitor for metabolic and cardiorespiratory compromise.[5]

BOX 38.1 SPECIAL CONSIDERATIONS, TECHNIQUES, AND EQUIPMENT WITH MITOCHONDRIAL MYOPATHY

- Judicious use of muscle relaxants in patients with muscle weakness, avoidance of stress response, avoiding induction agents with minimal cardiodepressive effects in patients with cardiomyopathy[2]
- Succinylcholine should be avoided
- Avoid IV fluids with lactate
- Use glucose-containing solutions (D10) without lactate
- Monitor the glucose and lactate levels prior to and throughout the case
- Avoid propofol infusions of long duration
- Avoid tourniquets
- Avoid hypo- or hyperthermia[2]

REFERENCES

1. Kloesel B, Holzman R. Anesthetic management of patients with inborn errors of metabolism. *Anesth Analg.* 2017;125:822–836. doi:10.1213/ANE.0000000000001689
2. Grier J, Hirano M, Karaa A, Shepard E, Thompson J. Diagnostic odyssey of patients with mitochondrial disease. *Neurology:Genetics.* 2018;4:1–7. doi:10.1212/NXG.0000000000000230
3. Keshavan N, Rahman S. Natural history of mitochondrial disorders: a systematic review. *Essays Biochem.* 2018;62(3):423–442. doi:10.1042/EBC20170108
4. Davison J, Lemonde H, Rahman S. Inherited mitochondrial disease. *J Paediatr Child Health.* 2019;29(3):116–122. doi:10.1016/j.paed.2019.01.009
5. Kynes M, Blakely M, Furman K, Burnette WB, Modes KB. Multidisciplinary perioperative care for children with neuromuscular disorders. *Children* 2018;5(9):126. doi:10.3390/children5090126
6. Nelson J, Kaplan R. Anesthetic management of two pediatric patients with concurrent diagnosis of mitochondrial disease and malignant hyperthermia susceptibility: A case report. *Anesth Analg.* 2017;9:204–206. doi:10.1213/XAA.0000000000000565
7. Aglio L, Lockhart B, Lunshof J, Nabzdyk C. Implications of mitochondrial dysfunction for the anesthetic and perioperative management: a case report of spinal fusion, genetic confusion, and a patient's perspective. *Anesth Analg.* 2018;10:103–105. doi:10.1213/XAA.0000000000000641

CHAPTER 39

Muscular Dystrophy

Jennifer McBride Schultz

PATHOPHYSIOLOGY AND CLINICAL MANIFESTATIONS

Muscular dystrophy (MD) comprises a group of diseases that are mediated by a genetic mutation in the skeletal muscle. This group can be further subdivided into the dystrophinopathies, of which Duchenne is the most common with approximately 1 in 3,500 males being affected. In each subset of muscular dystrophy, there is a mutation in the production and regulation of contractile proteins in the muscle.[1] This mutation occurs in the dystrophy gene for Duchenne and Becker's muscular dystrophy and in the sodium/chloride channels for Steinert dystrophy.

Approximately one-third of the cases of Duchenne MD result from spontaneous mutation, with the remainder being inherited via X-gonosomal recessive pathway.[2] Duchenne is typically diagnosed by age 3 to 5 years, as opposed to Becker's dystrophy, which presents later in adulthood. Duchenne MD affects almost exclusively males, although females can be affected.

Patients affected by MD have different clinical manifestations as the gene is completely blocked in Duchenne disease and partially blocked in Becker's disease. All forms of MD result in progressive neuromuscular weakness, which compromises respiratory, cardiac, and skeletal systems in the affected individual. The absence of dystrophin in the skeletal muscle results in the dysregulation of the sarcolemma, which leads to calcium influx into the muscle fibers. Loss of nitric oxide synthase in the muscle membrane results in destruction from vasoconstriction, which leads to muscle ischemia and necrosis of fibers within each myocyte.[3] Dystrophin functions to stabilize the muscle membrane, and the absence of dystrophin eventually leads to muscle fatigue in individuals with MD. In addition to physiological fatigue, research suggests that subjective fatigue (decreased energy and/or reported weakness and exhaustion related to sleep disturbance and depressive symptoms) is one of the strongest predictors of decreased health-related quality of life in pediatric patients with MD.[4] Identifying subjective fatigue in MD patients, and intervening appropriately, can greatly increase their quality of life as there may be modifiable risk factors associated with the reported fatigue. Taking into account the multifaceted systemic effects of MD, a multidisciplinary team provides the best approach to treatment for the MD patient.

ANESTHETIC MANAGEMENT

PREOPERATIVE EVALUATION

The preoperative clinical assessment of a patient presenting with MD should take into consideration the stage of disease for each individual. MD is a progressive disease, and anesthesia providers should be aware of the risks associated at the onset of disease, as well as the risks that present in the later stages of MD. The anesthesia provider should consider a preoperative consult to ensure that all necessary testing is done prior to the day of surgery. This should include pulmonary function tests (PFTs) to assess the degree of pulmonary impairment. Having baseline PFTs, as well as a baseline arterial blood gas (ABG), will allow the anesthesia provider to develop a safe intraoperative anesthetic plan. Patients with MD are also known to be at risk of obstructive sleep apnea (OSA). A preoperative sleep study can provide information useful to the anesthesia provider to assess the severity of each individual's level of apnea.[5]

MD patients have benefited from the use of glucocorticoids and the provider should be aware of the implications for chronic steroid use in the surgical setting. A preoperative consult should be obtained to determine the necessary steroid coverage the day of surgery to avoid complications during the intraoperative period.

To assess the degree of cardiac impairment, an echocardiogram should be performed as well as an ECG. Anesthesia providers should be aware of the potential limitations of an echocardiogram in patients with kyphoscoliosis, as well as increased adiposity of the chest wall, which may occur secondary to chronic steroid use. In these situations, cardiac MRI (CMRI) should be considered as it has been proven to provide the best assessment of ventricular function.[6] A serum creatine kinase should also be drawn to allow the anesthesia provider to carefully monitor kidney function, as rhabdomyolysis is a serious concern for the MD patient intraoperatively.

PREOPERATIVE PHARMACOTHERAPY

Patients should avoid prolonged NPO guidelines and should be admitted preoperatively to allow for IV administration of dextrose fluids during the preoperative fasting period. The anesthesia provider should be aware of the increased risk of sedation from benzodiazepines and should monitor the patient for breathing problems if benzodiazepines are indicated preoperatively and cannot be avoided. Patients with MD should be medicated with antacids and histamine blockers as indicated for potential aspiration due to muscle weakness.

ANESTHETIC TECHNIQUE

Intraoperative Management

MD patients present specific challenges during the intraoperative period. Their baseline cardiac and respiratory impairments must be considered when developing an intraoperative anesthesia plan. Communication between the anesthesia provider, the surgeon, and all staff members in the operating room should be encouraged for patient safety. All members of the intraoperative team should be aware of the potential risks and complications if general anesthesia is indicated. The anesthesia provider should alert team members ahead of time to facilitate an efficient response should the patient require an intervention during induction, maintenance, or emergence of anesthesia.

Regardless of anesthetic technique chosen or required, the MD patient is at risk of developing further complications during surgery. IV access must be inserted prior to induction for safety. Medications used for sedation, or monitored anesthesia care, present challenges due to potential respiratory depression. Smaller doses may be needed to ensure that respiratory function is not compromised and to avoid any anticipated delays in recovery time.

Special Considerations/Concerns

If general anesthesia is indicated, total IV anesthesia (TIVA) should be utilized. Propofol is the most common medication used for TIVA, but patients presenting with cardiac compromise may require the use of other agents including etomidate, ketamine, or thiopental.[6] Both volatile agents and succinylcholine should be avoided as they can precipitate a rhabdomyolysis crisis. Nondepolarizing muscle relaxants (NDMRs) can be used, but close neuromuscular monitoring is imperative. Reversal of NDMR can safely be achieved with sugamadex, and neostigmine should be avoided due to its potential to contribute to rhabdomyolysis and malignant arrhythmias.[1]

Rhabdomyolysis is a potential intraoperative complication for patients with MD. The hyperkalemia can lead to cardiac arrest and life-threatening arrhythmias. Anesthesia providers should have medications and all necessary interventions prepared for a potential crisis intraoperatively. Urine output and temperature should be continuously monitored throughout surgery.

Special Techniques/Equipment

When possible, regional anesthesia should be employed as it may provide a safer profile than general anesthetics. Caudal epidural block has been proven to be an effective and safe technique when applicable to the surgical procedure. Considerations for regional anesthesia may include using ultrasound or fluoroscopy-guided placement due to difficulty locating anatomical landmarks.[7] MD patients frequently present with osteoporosis due to treatment with glucocorticoids and regional anesthesia might be contraindicated for these patients due to the presence of vertebral fractures and long-bone fractures.

POSTOPERATIVE CARE

MD patients require monitoring for 24 hours in intensive care units (ICUs) after receiving general anesthesia. Respiratory depression from anesthesia is a potential complication, and patients may need to remain intubated postoperatively depending on the surgical procedure and anesthetic technique utilized. Managing OSA secondary to MD will need to be discussed preoperatively, and continuous positive airway pressure settings should be reported to the staff in the recovery room or ICU. The recovery team should also be aware of the potential for increased reflux and aspiration in MD patients. Postoperative analgesia is important, as it may help alleviate the work of breathing attributable to pain; however, providers must carefully titrate opiates to minimize complications from increased patient sensitivity to these medications. Vigilance during the immediate postoperative period is critical for the patient with MD, and frequent physical assessment should not be overlooked.

REFERENCES

1. Echeverry-Marin P, Bustamante-Vega A. Anesthetic implications of muscular dystrophies. *Colomb. J. Anesthesiol.* 2018;46:228–239. doi:10.1097/CJ9.0000000000000059
2. Marciniak, B., Dalens, B. J., Bissonnette, B., Luginbuehl, I. (2006). Syndromes: rapid recognition and perioperative implications. Spain: McGraw-Hill Education.
3. Gieron-Korthals, M., & Fernandez, R. (2020). New developments in diagnosis, treatment, and management of Duchenne muscular dystrophy. *Advances in Pediatrics*, 67, 183–196.
4. El-Aloul B, Speechley K, Wei y, et al. Fatigue in young people with Duchenne muscular dystrophy. *Dev Med Child Neurol.* 2020;62:245–251. doi: 10.1111/dmcn.14248
5. Birnkrant D, Bushby K, Bann C, et al. Diagnosis and management of Duchenne muscular dystrophy, part 2: respiratory, cardiac, bone health, and orthopaedic management. *Lancet Neurol.* 2018;17:347–361. doi:10.1016/S1474-44-22(18)30025-5
6. Hor K, Ling Mah M, Johnston P, et al. Advances in the diagnosis and management of cardiomyopathy in Duchenne muscular dystrophy. *Neuromuscul Disord.* 2018;28:711–716. doi: 10.1016/j.nmd.2018.06.014
7. Shafy S, Hakim M, Arce Villalobos M, et al. Caudal epidural block instead of general anesthesia in an adult with Duchenne muscular dystrophy. *Local Reg Anesth.* 2018;11:75–80. doi: 10.2147/LRA.S180867

CHAPTER 40

Pierre Robin Sequence

Heather J. Rankin, Edgar Soto, and René P. Myers

PATHOPHYSIOLOGY AND CLINICAL MANIFESTATIONS

Pierre Robin sequence (PRS) was first defined by French stomatologist Pierre Robin, who coined the term glossoptosis, which is the airway obstruction of infants created by the posterior position of the tongue.[1] PRS consists of the hallmark triad of glossoptosis, micrognathia or a small chin, and airway obstruction. The incidence of PRS varies between 1 in 8,500 and 1 in 14,000 live births in the United States.[2] If untreated, PRS can result in hypoxemia, hypercarbia, developmental delay, feeding impairment, failure to thrive, cardiopulmonary arrest, and death, with a variety of studies having reported the mortality rate of PRS patients to vary between 10% and 30%.[3]

Although the exact cause of PRS remains undetermined, genetic mutations in the DNA near the *SOX9* gene are the most common genetic cause of isolated cases of PRS. Alterations in other genes are lilkely and nongenetic influences may play a role as well. PRS may occur in isolation or be associated with a variety of other signs and symptoms (defined as syndromic PRS). Isolated or nonsyndromic PRS is when the hallmark triad is present in an otherwise healthy infant. Syndromic PRS describes the presence of the hallmark triad as a part of a genetic syndrome, such as Stickler syndrome, velocardiofacial syndrome, or Treacher Collins syndrome.[4] "PRS plus" has also been described, referring to the presence of the hallmark triad in conjunction with other congenital anomalies not indicative of a known syndrome.[5]

There is no one standard test that is routinely used to diagnose isolated PRS, though genetic testing can be used to identify mutations involving the *SOX9* gene. While a cleft palate may be a finding in some patients with PRS, not all patients with PRS present with a cleft, although it is common. Furthermore, many of the additional syndromic features do not present until later in childhood.

ANESTHETIC MANAGEMENT
PREOPERATIVE EVALUATION

Due to the complexity of and comorbidities associated with PRS, a multidisciplinary team will be involved, which includes neonatology, plastic surgery, otolarnyngology, anesthesiology, gastroenterology, geneticists, and more. The neonatology team maintains the overall disposition of the neonate in the NICU. Plastic surgery is often consulted in moderate-to-severe cases to evaluate surgical options to improve the micrognathia or airway obstruction if needed. Otolaryngology is available for airway evaluations as PRS patients may also have laryngomalacia or tracheomalacia, which can complicate their airway more; in addition, direct laryngoscopy (DL), intubations, and tracheostomies in severe cases of obstruction may also be needed. Anesthesiology is needed for support during surgical procedures or intubation.

A number of PRS patients have feeding difficulties or gastroesophageal reflux that requires gastroenterology for evaluation. If feeding difficulties are severe, a general surgery consult may be needed to resolve the feeding difficulties via a gastrostomy tube.

PRS patients have varying levels of airway obstruction severity, which leads to treatment options that have escalating interventions to adequately treat the obstruction. PRS patients are often seen in the operating room for a variety of surgical procedures related to the airway, such as diagnostic laryngoscopy and bronchoscopy, flexible bronchoscopy, mandibular distraction osteogenesis (MDO), tongue lip adhesion (TLA), tracheostomy, tonsillectomy and adenoidectomy, gastrostomy tube placement, cleft lip, and/or palate repair, and more. Findings from 46% and up to 85% of PRS patients have severe upper airway obstruction and resultant obstructive sleep apnea (OSA).[6] An apnea is defined as at least a 90% reduction in airflow from baseline over two or more respiratory cycles. The severity of airway obstruction is evaluated with polysomnography (PSG) to define the level of OSA as well as evaluate if any central sleep apnea is present. The PSG studies are performed in a supine position using standard pediatric criteria recommended by the American Academy of Sleep medicine. The OSA–apnea-hypopnea index (AHI) is a standard measure for measuring the number of OSA events, mixed apneas, central apneas, and obstructive hypopneas per hour. While there is no accepted criterion for definition of OSA in neonates, most centers define OSA as an AHI >1 event/hr, with severity criteria as follows: mild AHI 1 to <5; moderate AHI 5 to <10; and severe AHI >10 events/hr.[7]

Mild obstruction can often be treated with less invasive management, such as prone positioning or a nasal pharyngeal airway (NPA). Moderate-to-severe obstruction may include interventions, such as prone positioning, noninvasive ventilation (NIV), or surgical interventions, including MDO or TLA. See Figure 40.1 for an example of a patient requiring prone position due to moderate-to-severe obstruction when supine. NIV has been found to improve respiratory and ventilation status in infants with PRS and is less invasive than surgical interventions.[8] MDO is discussed further in Chapter 15. TLA is a surgical option that involves anterior displacement and fixation of the tongue to correct the obstruction, which advances the tongue base away from the oropharynx. TLA is only a temporary treatment in the neonatal period and must eventually be taken down to facilitate speech and dental development. Additionally, the TLA success rate is variable as there are differing techniques. TLA is a more minor procedure when compared to other surgical procedures that can be performed on PRS patients but remains an option if the facility does not perform MDO or if MDO is contraindicated.

Severe cases of obstruction or moderate or higher amounts of central sleep apnea are an indication for tracheostomy.[9] While a tracheostomy does provide a definitive airway for the infant, it does not resolve the problem of obstruction from the

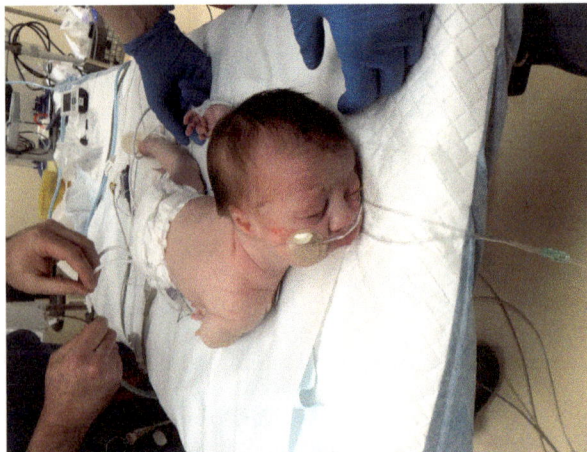

Figure 40.1: Patient with Pierre Robin sequence in the prone position due to moderate-to-severe obstruction when supine.

Source: Courtesy of René P. Myers, MD.

> **BOX 40.1   KEY ASSESSMENT POINTS: PIERRE ROBIN SEQUENCE**
>
> - Physical examination including degree of visual micrognathia present
> - Measured maxillomandibular discrepancy
> - Oxygen requirements
> - Oxygen nadir on PSG
> - Supplemental respiratory devices present, such as nasopharyngeal airway or use of CPAP
> - Degree of severity of obstruction or respiratory distress present when positioned supine
> - Results from flexible fiberoptic evaluation including other airway diagnoses, such as laryngomalacia or tracheomalacia
> - Results from rigid bronchoscopy if performed
> - Comorbidities present
> - PSG results
> - Pertinent labwork including blood gas readings
> - CT or US airway studies if available
> - Family history of anesthesia complications
>
> CPAP, continuous positive airway pressure; PSG, polysomnography; US, ultrasound.

tongue causing the difficulty breathing and has a significant degree of risk. Some individuals who require a tracheostomy may be candidates for an MDO months or years after receiving a tracheostomy given the mortality risks and poor feeding and airway outcomes longitudinally; as MDO provides an anatomic solution, if the patient is a candidate, this will be the preferred definitive treatment. In most centers, over half of PRS patients treated primarily with tracheostomy receive either a secondary MDO or TLA in an attempt to achieve normal feeding via decannulation.[10,11] That said, before TLA or MDO is attempted, the multidisciplinary team must take into account any high-risk factors, such as syndromic status and neurological impairment, in order to ensure successful decannulation in prior tracheostomy PRS patients.[12]

Preparing to optimize the difficult airway and communication between the teams is essential. Airway evaluation should consist of both a thorough physical examination as well as history of any respiratory difficulties the patient has in the past such as cyanotic events, difficulties breathing in the supine position, or respiratory difficulties with feeding (Box 40.1).[9]

ANESTHETIC TECHNIQUE

Intraoperative Management

Anesthetic management for PRS patients is a known challenge.[13] A flexible laryngoscopy is often performed by an otolaryngologist at the bedside or in the operating room to evaluate the degree of obstruction from glossoptosis as well as an overall evaluation of the airway for laryngo- or tracheomalacia. An evaluation in the operating room with a rigid bronchoscope under anesthesia may be indicated as well. The degree of obstruction can make mask ventilation in the supine position a challenge or even impossible even with anterior distraction of the tongue via suture.[14] The degree of obstruction and difficulty with mask ventilation may be increased if a cleft palate is present especially in the supine position.

In addition to difficult mask ventilation airways, the PRS patient may be difficult, and again even impossible, to intubate with conventional DL. Three different approaches to induction and endotracheal intubation for this group include an inhalation induction, an IV induction, and a combination of inhalation and IV. An advantage of an inhalation induction is the ability for the patient to maintain spontaneous ventilation; however, if the obstruction in the supine position is severe, this method may not be possible. A potential disadvantage with using solely volatile agents is it may be difficult to obtain a deep enough level of anesthesia to perform a laryngoscopy without movement or potential laryngospasm. Deep levels of volatile agent may also decrease the blood pressure significantly, especially if needed for prolonged periods of time while securing the airway. IV inductions can provide better intubating conditions, particularly if a muscle relaxant is chosen, yet risk losing a spontaneous ventilation and entering a potential cannot ventilate, cannot intubate situation. With a combination of inhalation and IV, spontaneous ventilation can be maintained with adjunct agents to enhance laryngoscopy conditions.

Depending on the presentation of the infant, those with severe obstruction may require induction in the prone or lateral position.[15] Whatever technique is chosen, a variety of equipment should be available to the anesthesia provider to provide options as needed for endotracheal intubation, and standard intubation conditions should be used, such as proper positioning of the patient and preoxygenation (Box 40.2). While traditional neutral positioning of infants and young children with DL has been found to be ideal positioning, as opposed to the sniffing position,[16] children younger than 2 years of age were shown to benefit from placement of a towel under their shoulders during airway instrumentation using C-MAC video laryngoscope (VL) Miller blades.[17] In severe cases of airway difficulties, the patient may require a surgical airway performed by an otolaryngologist, and in a controlled and elective situation, consultation and availability of an otolaryngologist are preferred with rigid bronchoscopy available.

Traditional difficult airway algorithms are typically used with PRS patients. If difficulty is present with mask airway or a traditional DL proves ineffective, a laryngeal mask

> **BOX 40.2 KEY AIRWAY EQUIPMENT: PIERRE ROBIN SEQUENCE**
>
> - Appropriately sized mask
> - Multiple sizes of endotracheal tubes
> - Variety of laryngoscope blades
> - Laryngoscope handle
> - Laryngeal mask airway
> - Stylet
> - Bougie
> - Video laryngoscope
> - Fiberoptic scope
> - Oral airway
> - Nasopharyngeal airway
> - Otolaryngologist (ENT) available with setup for rigid bronchoscopy

airway (LMA) can be inserted.[9,16] LMAs are supraglottic airway devices which have often been reported as a bridge to endotracheal intubation or rescue device with difficult mask airways. An advantage of using an LMA for the initial airway instrumentation is the ability to place successfully in an awake neonate or infant and maintain spontaneous ventilation.[14,15,18] After successful LMA placement in awake infants,[15] it showed improved intubating conditions in infants by administering muscle relaxant following an inhalation induction through the LMA, administration of relaxant, and then fiberoptic (FO) intubation. Administration of an aminosteroidal neuromuscular blocker, such as rocuronium or vecuronium, has been shown to be rapidly reversed by sugammadex and can aid in tracheal intubation. With sugammadex available as an option to reverse blockade in the event of a cannot ventilate, cannot intubate situation and a relaxant giving better intubating conditions, the anesthesia provider has additional options with induction. Sugammadex has been used safely in pediatric patients.[19,20] There are a variety of LMA sizes and brands that can be used to ventilate and bridge to intubation of neonates and infants.

FO scope intubations both with or without an LMA have been successful, traditionally are the next step in the difficult airway algorithm after LMAs, and are still seen as the gold standard for difficult airways.[13,16,21] An advantage to using a supraglottic device in conjunction with an FO scope is improved oxygenation during intubation and decreased hypoxemia.[22] In addition to FO scopes, VLs have been used increasingly to aid in intubation of known and unknown difficult airway patients. These VLs include but are not limited to the GlideScope, McGrath, C-MAC, and Airtraq. There is an increased level of competency required for swift, effective FO intubations, and FO can be challenging in the pediatric patient population and take a longer time than the use of a VL.[13] Raimann et al.[23] showed a significantly improved view of the vocal cords with indirect laryngoscopy with a VL utilizing the C-MAC 0 and 1 blades. Additional case studies and research have been reported using a variety of VL in pediatric patients with difficult airways.[24,25,26,27] While VL use continues to increase, there have been reports that while visualization improves, time to intubate using a VL is longer than a traditional DL.[24] Additional research continues using VL as this technique is relatively new compared to FO intubations and traditional DL, and more pediatric-specific blades and devices have been introduced. Having a variety of airway devices available is ideal to optimize successful airway instrumentation.

Medication adjuncts commonly used for induction and intubation are atropine, propofol, ketamine, dexmedetomidine, rocuronium, and sugammadex. Atropine is commonly given prior to induction to maintain heart rate and decrease the chance of vagal stimulation as well as dry secretions to enhance intubating conditions. Propofol will deepen the anesthetic for airway instrumentation and is a common IV induction agent IV. Dexmedetomidine, an alpha agonist, can decrease the requirement of other anesthetic agents and supports spontaneous ventilation. Rocuronium can be used for muscle relaxation with sugammadex as a reversal.[19] Ketamine is an N-methyl-D-aspartate antagonist that maintains spontaneous ventilation as well as give hemodynamic support by blocking the reuptake of catecholamines.

POSTOPERATIVE CARE

Postoperative concerns for airway complications are high, especially if the patient was difficult to ventilate, intubate, or both. Extubation ideally should occur in a controlled environment with airway experts available. If an awake extubation is planned following an anesthetic, the anesthesia provider should consider decreasing intraoperative narcotic administration and utilize adjunct medications, such as ketamine, dexmedetomidine, and nonsteroidal anti-inflammatories, to decrease the chance of obstruction and respiratory depression. Regional or local anesthesia should also be used when appropriate.

Dexamethasone administration can help decrease airway swelling if the operation was in the oral cavity or airway, if multiple intubation attempts were made, or if the intubation was traumatic. The patient may benefit from placement of an NPA prior to extubation or returning to a lateral, prone placement to decrease obstruction, or placement of a tongue suture to retract the tongue post-extubation and relieve obstruction. Planned postoperative intubation situations require discussion by the surgery team, anesthesia team, and intensivists to discuss sedation and paralytic needs. Patients who remain intubated should have reintubation equipment at bedside, including laryngoscope handle and blade, appropriately sized LMA, oral and nasopharyngeal airways, oxygen, and bag-mask ventilation sources.

KEY REFERENCES

Complete references for this chapter are online and available at https://connect.springerpub.com/content/book/978-0-8261-3875-0/part/part03/toc-part/ch040

1. Robin P. Glossoptosis due to atresia and hypotrophy of the mandible. *Am. J. Dis. Child.* 1924;48(3):541–547. doi:10.1001/archpedi.1934.01960160063005
2. Bütow K-W, Morkel JA, Naidoo S, Zwahlen RA. Pierre Robin sequence: subdivision, data, theories, and treatment - part 2: syndromic and nonsyndromic Pierre Robin sequence. *Ann. Maxillofac. Surg.* 2016;6(1):35–37. doi:10.4103/2231-0746.186134
9. Cladis F, Kumar A, Grunwaldt L, et al. Pierre Robin sequence: a perioperative review. *Anesth Analg.* 2014;119(2):400–12. doi:10.1213/ANE.0000000000000301
15. Templeton, T. W., Morris, B. N., & Bryan, Y. F. (2017). Outside is the new inside. *Journal of Cardiothoracic and Vascular Anesthesia*, 31(6), e79.
16. Walas W, Aleksandrowicz D, Kornacka M, et al. The management of unanticipated difficult airways in children of all age groups in anaesthetic practice – the position paper of an expert panel. *Scand J Trauma Resusc Emerg Med.* 2019;27(87). doi:10.1186/s13049-019-0666-7

CHAPTER 41

Prader–Willi Syndrome

Aimee Langley

PATHOPHYSIOLOGY AND CLINICAL MANIFESTATIONS

Originally described in 1956, Prader–Willi syndrome (PWS) is a rare genetic neuroendocrine disorder requiring a multidisciplinary approach to care. PWS impacts approximately 1 in 15,000 to 30,000 live births, affecting males in a 3:2 ratio compared with females. There are three specific genetic abnormalities associated with PWS, each of which leads to either changes in the genetic structure or changes in the function or expression of a gene. In 70% of patients, PWS results due to microdeletion of paternally expressed genes on the long arm of chromosome 15q11.2-13.[1] This gene mutation primarily affects the central nervous system and often involves the hypothalamus. Of the remainder, approximately 25% of the cases are secondary to maternal uniparental disomy for chromosome 15, with the rest presenting with translocation or other structural aberrations in chromosome 15.

Unexplained neonatal hypotonia is the hallmark feature of PWS and is typically the presenting symptom that initiates further testing. All infants and newborns with unexplained hypotonia and poor suck should undergo genetic testing to confirm the diagnosis and to identify the specific genetic subtype. Approximately 99% of patients with PWS can be diagnosed by DNA methylation study, which allows for examination of gene activity status in the critical region of chromosome 15 associated with PWS. Additional testing may include lung function tests, an electrocardiogram (ECG), chest x-ray, or echocardiography to assess for cardiomegaly, and/or sleep studies to assess for obstructive sleep apnea.

PWS is described as a two-stage or biphasic disorder that impacts patients differently during the infantile and childhood phases, with the most notable symptoms of each phase being hypotonia and hyperphagia, respectively. During the early infantile phase, nearly all patients with PWS exhibit hypotonia, resulting in the child feeling "floppy" when held. In addition, an infant with PWS will have a weak cry, poor feeding habits resulting in failure to thrive, neonatal asphyxia, and seizures and will experience delays in achieving milestones. Tube feeding may be required for several months. In addition, patients with PWS often have distinctive facial features, such as almond-shaped eyes, thin upper lip, a downturned mouth, a narrow bridge of the nose, a narrow forehead, and a disproportionately long, narrow head (Figure 41.1).[2,3]

By 12 to 18 months of age the disease progresses to the childhood phase and is characterized by childhood obesity due to an insatiable appetite or hyperphagia.[4] When uncontrolled, obesity can result in hypertension, pulmonary hypertension, obstructive sleep apnea, and potentially cor pulmonale due to chronic hypoxia. Additionally, it is during the childhood phase that multiple neuroendocrine abnormalities present, such as hypogonadism and diabetes mellitus. Growth hormone deficits contribute to skeletal abnormalities, resulting in short stature and small hands and feet with tapered fingers, and decrease in bone mineral density. It is important that central hypothyroidism and adrenal insufficiency not be underappreciated. Neurological manifestations prevalent during the childhood phase include global developmental delay, behavioral changes, speech delays, and seizures. Behavioral manifestations include tantrums, poor transitioning, obsessive-compulsive tendencies, autistic-like features, and skin picking.[9]

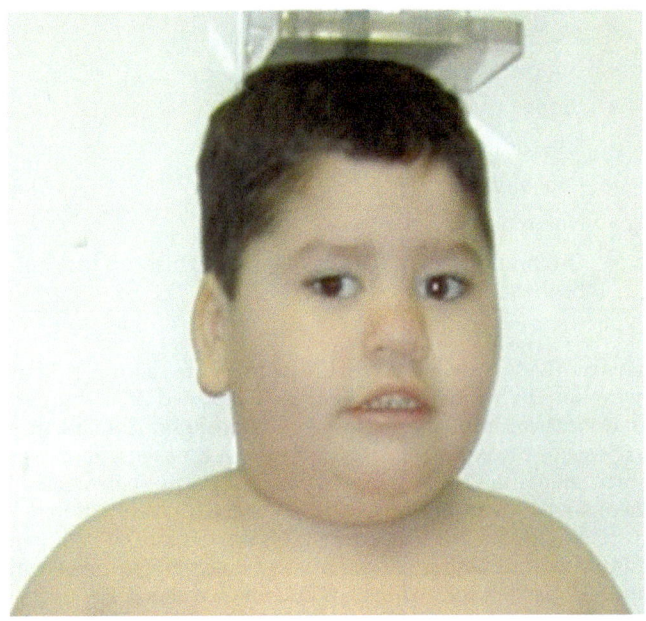

Figure 41.1: Typical facial features of a child with Prader–Willi syndrome.

Source: From Cataletto M, Angulo M, Hertz G, Whitman B. Prader-Willi syndrome: a primer for clinicians. Int J Pediatr Endocrinol. 2011;2011(1):12, Fig. 1.

ANESTHETIC MANAGEMENT

PREOPERATIVE EVALUATION

It is crucial that anesthesia providers include detailed cardiac and respiratory assessments during the preoperative evaluation of a patient with PWS.[5] A recent ECG should be reviewed, and anesthesia providers should be sure to inquire about the presence of hypertension and symptoms indicative of cardiac failure. The presence of sleep disturbances and obstructive sleep apnea should be reviewed with the patient's parents. If available pulmonary function tests should also be reviewed. Although weight loss is often advised prior to surgery, it is often not achieved. Due to hyperphagia and food-seeking behaviors, NPO status cannot be ensured, and the patient should be considered to have a full stomach. Furthermore, obesity is associated with a higher incidence of hiatal hernia, thereby placing this patient population at an increased risk of gastric aspiration.[6] Consultation with endocrinology is recommended to ensure adequate control of blood sugars in the presence of diabetes. The need for preoperative lab work is often per endocrinology recommendations. Refer to **Box 41.1**.

> **BOX 41.1 PERIOPERATIVE CONSIDERATIONS: PRADER–WILLI SYNDROME**
>
> - Unreliable NPO status.
> - Airway concerns due to obstructive sleep apnea and obesity.
> - Stress-dose steroid therapy may be indicated due to adrenal insufficiency.

PREOPERATIVE PHARMACOTHERAPY

If at all possible, preoperative sedation should be avoided due to the risk of hypoventilation, apnea, and airway obstruction. Prophylaxis against gastric aspiration with ranitidine and metoclopramide is recommended.[7] Due to the neuroendocrine effects and the increased incidence of adrenal insufficiency, preoperative supplementation of hydrocortisone is recommended if the patient is on an existing steroid therapy.[8]

ANESTHETIC TECHNIQUES

Intraoperative Management

In the presence of morbid obesity, the anesthetic management of a patient with PWS can be difficult. Children with PWS often suffer from restrictive lung disease due to hypotonia, making ventilation challenging. Furthermore, reduced functional residual capacity and higher closing capacity result in poor pulmonary reserve, which may lead to rapid oxygen desaturation. As tracheal intubation may be difficult due to obesity, it is imperative the anesthesia provider be prepared for a cannot intubate/cannot ventilate scenario, with emergency airway equipment close by prior to the induction of anesthesia. Additionally, the risk of gastric aspiration remains a concern due to obesity, failure to comply with NPO recommendations, and diabetes. Blood glucose levels should be monitored as the patient may require dextrose-containing IV fluids during the intraoperative period. See Box 41.2.

Special Techniques/Equipment

While regional anesthesia may be a viable analgesic technique, identification of anatomical landmarks may be challenging, and use of ultrasound guidance is recommended. Use of regional anesthesia as well as nonsteroidal anti-inflammatory medications may prove especially beneficial in patients with PWS as reductions in opioid requirements intra- and postoperatively may stave off postoperative respiratory complications.[7]

POSTOPERATIVE CARE

The need for supplemental oxygen in the postanesthesia care unit is not uncommon. Postoperative apnea monitoring is imperative in patients with PWS due to the increased likelihood of sleep-related respiratory complications. Patients with PWS may not tolerate lying in the supine position. While pulmonary embolism is rare in children, polycythemia may predispose the patient with PWS to deep vein thrombosis in the postoperative period. Prolonged monitoring postoperatively may be required. See Box 41.3.

> **BOX 41.3 POSTOPERATIVE CONSIDERATIONS: PRADER–WILLI SYNDROME**
>
> - Patients may require prolonged monitoring due to sleep-related respiratory complications.

REFERENCES

1. Emerick JE, Vogt KS. Endocrine manifestations and management of Prader Willi symdrome. *Int J Pediatr Endocrinol*. 2013;21:14.
2. Dearlove O, Dobson A, Super M. Anaesthesia and Prader-Willi Syndrome. *Paediatr Anaesth* 1998;8(3):267–271. doi:10.1046/j.1460-9592.1998.00689.x
3. Yatish B, Shivakumar S, Tejesh C, Vinayak P. Prader-Willi Syndrome with oculocutaneous albinism: anesthetic implicaitons and managemetn. *Natl Lab Med*. 2014;3(2):13–15.
4. Miller JL, Lynn CH, Driscoll DC, et al. Nutritional phases in Prader–Willi syndrome. *Am J Med Genet A*. 2011;*155*(5):1040–1049.
5. Mackenzie J. Anaesthesia and the Prader-Willi syndrome. *J R Soc Med*. 1991;84(4):239. doi:10.1177/014107689108400421
6. Sloan T, Kaye C. Rumination risk of aspiration of gastric contents in the Prader Willi syndrome. *Anesth Analg*. 1991;73:492–495. doi:10.1213/00000539-199110000-00023
7. Duis J, van Wattum P, Scheimann A, et al. A multidisciplinary approach to the clinical management of Prader-Willie syndrome. *Mol Genet Genomic Med*. 2019;7:e514. doi:10.1002/mgg3.514
8. De Lind van Wijngaarden, R, Otten B, Festen, D, et al. High prevelance of central adrenal insufficiency in patients with Prader-Willi syndrome. *J Clin Endocrinol Metab*. 2008;93(3):1649–1654. doi:10.1210/jc.2007-2294
9. Shilpa H, Shwetha O, Adarsh E. Prader Willi syndrome-a case report. *Indian J Clin Anaesth*. 2018;5(2):297–298. doi:10.18231/2394-4994.2018.0057

> **BOX 41.2 INTRAOPERATIVE CONSIDERATIONS: PRADER–WILLI SYNDROME**
>
> - Restrictive airway disease.
> - Be prepared for a cannot intubate/cannot ventilate scenario.
> - Limit opioid use to prevent postoperative respiratory complications.

CHAPTER 42

Prune Belly Syndrome

Daniel Henz

PATHOPHYSIOLOGY AND CLINICAL MANIFESTATIONS

Frolich first described a rare disorder characterized by the absence of abdominal wall muscles in 1839, with Parker later noting its association with urinary tract abnormalities in 1895. By 1901, Osler had coined the characteristic folds and wrinkled appearance of the abdomen associated with this rare genetic disorder as a dried plum or "prune belly" (Figure 42.1). However, the characteristic triad of deficient abdominal wall musculature, nondescended testicles, and urinary tract anomalies associated with prune belly syndrome (PBS) was not described until 1950 by Eagle and Barrett. This rare congenital syndrome is known today by a number of names, including Eagle–Barrett syndrome, Obrinsky's syndrome, abdominal wall musculature syndrome, triad syndrome, and most commonly PBS.[1,2]

The estimated incidence of PBS is 1 in every 29,000 to 50,000 live births. PBS almost exclusively occurs in males, with females comprising less than 5% of all cases. There is no specific genetic cause for PBS; however, there is an increased incidence of PBS in individuals with trisomies 13, 18, and 21.[1–3] While the etiology of this syndrome remains unknown, several theories have been offered to explain the cause of PBS, one of which is that a urinary outflow obstruction occurs in utero, causing dilation of the urinary tracts and subsequently abdominal wall distention. The abdominal wall distention results in muscle wall hypoplasia and cryptorchism. Another explanation relies on the failure of the primary mesodermal differentiation between the 6th and 10th weeks of gestation, which leads to defects on the abdominal wall and urinary tract musculature. Yet another theory offers that developmental defects of the yolk sac and the allantois, which is the fetal membrane lying below the chorion layer, are the cause of PBS.[1,4,5]

Females with PBS typically do not present with urogenital dysplasia and obviously lack the cryptorchism associated with the characteristic triad of PBS.[1,2,4–8]

Diagnosis is evident at birth, although additional testing is generally done to determine the extent of genetic abnormalities present. Testing often includes ultrasound, x-ray, and an IV pyelogram to determine the extent of genitourinary tract involvement.

In addition to the characteristic triad of PBS, as many as 75% of patients will present with pulmonary, cardiovascular, gastrointestinal, and musculoskeletal malformations.[1,2,5,8,9] Although life expectancy can be limited, with 10% to 25% of individuals with PBS dying within the first month of life and 50% within the first 2 years, it is not uncommon for patients diagnosed with PBS to reach adulthood.[2,4,9] As they grow, patients with PBS often require multiple surgeries in the early years of life to help manage renal and urological complications. Surgical intervention is frequently required to repair any outflow obstruction in an effort to prevent further dilation of the urinary tracts. Despite early surgery, patients with PBS continue to have frequent urinary tract infections (UTIs) and renal dysplasia, which can eventually lead to chronic renal failure requiring renal dialysis and possibly transplant.[1,9] Abdominoplasty, once thought to be necessary only for aesthetic purposes, helps the abdominal muscles regain normal function as the procedure strengthens the abdominal wall and creates a more defined waistline. In addition, strengthening the abdominal muscles helps improve bowel and bladder function, as well as improve pulmonary function, which is often compromised in PBS.[5,10–12]

ANESTHETIC MANAGEMENT

PREOPERATIVE EVALUATION

Ensuring safe and effective anesthetic care for a patient with PBS starts with a comprehensive preanesthetic assessment. The leading cause of postoperative morbidity after surgical intervention in this population is respiratory complication. Pulmonary hypoplasia can occur from oligohydramnios caused by in utero urinary tract obstruction, which can lead to fetal demise in the neonate.[4,13] PBS patients are often born prematurely, which also places them at higher risk of respiratory compromise.[8] Oligohydramnios can also lead to Potter's facies including micrognathia, a flattened nose, and malformed ears. It is imperative anesthesia providers thoroughly evaluate patients for potential difficulty with intubation and the need for fiberoptic or video laryngoscope to successfully intubate the patient.[7]

Recurrent UTIs are common due to residual urine in the bladder from the dilated urinary tracts and a lack of abdominal musculature to help with adequate bladder emptying.

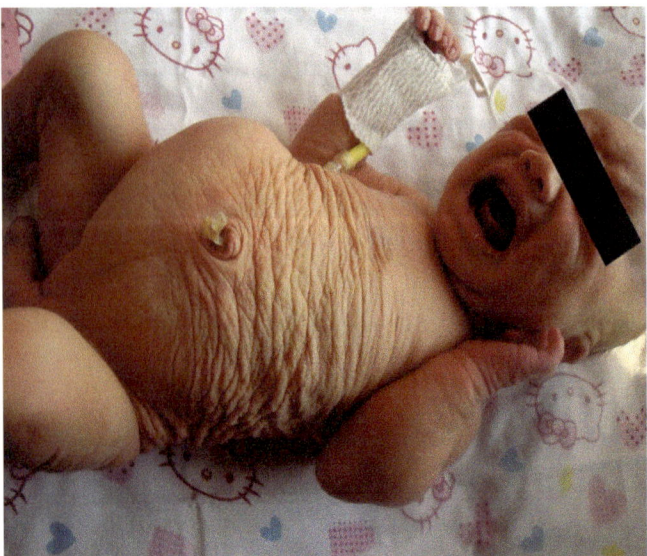

Figure 42.1: Clinical picture of a newborn showing bulging flanks, especially on the right side, and thin, flabby, wrinkled skin.

Source: From Xu W, Wu H, Wang D-X, Mu Z-H. A case of prune belly syndrome. *Pediatr Neonatol.* 2015;56(3):193–196. doi:10.1016/j.pedneo.2013.03.014.

The frequent need for catheterization is common. Hence, it is important to assess renal function prior to anesthesia. Patients with an active UTI should be treated to prevent further renal compromise.

Pertinent Labs

Blood urea nitrogen (BUN), creatinine, creatinine clearance, and electrolyte levels should be assessed prior to anesthesia to evaluate renal function. If there is significant pulmonary compromise, pulmonary function tests preoperatively may be indicated if the child is cooperative. Any history of cardiovascular insult warrants assessment of an ECG and potentially a cardiology consult.

PREOPERATIVE PHARMACOTHERAPY

Approximately 10% of patients will present with congenital cardiac anomalies. Prophylactic antibiotics for cardiac defects should be administered if present. These defects are similar to the defects found in the general population presenting with cardiac defects and can include atrial septal defects, ventricular septal defects, tetralogy of Fallot, and patent ductus arteriosis.[4,13]

ANESTHETIC TECHNIQUE

Intraoperative Management

Anesthetic management for these procedures should be tailored to the associated systems affected while being cognizant that renal impairment is most often present. Therefore, fluid management should be adjusted based on renal function. Anesthesia providers should be aware that renal impairment and the lack of muscle mass can extend the duration of muscle relaxants.[4,7] Patients who are uremic can have vomiting and regurgitation, and precautions should be taken to prevent aspiration during general anesthesia.[7] A lack of abdominal musculature may result in ventilation challenges, both intraoperatively and postoperatively. The lack of abdominal wall musculature may also decrease the need for muscle relaxation, and muscle relaxants should be used sparingly.

Opioid medications should be used sparingly. Opioids alone for pain control may cause issues with micturition after anesthesia. The lack of abdominal muscles in PBS patients can cause chronic constipation, which can be exacerbated following opioid administration due to the slowing or halting of peristalsis. Regional anesthesia for pain control has been successful and should be employed whenever possible.[6,13]

Compression of the iliac arteries by the obstructed urinary tract in utero may lead to musculoskeletal problems in the lower limbs, along with vertebral malformations. Hip dysplasia, clubfeet, and other limb deficiencies are common.[4] Lower limb malformations and hip dysplasia place the patient with PBS at increased risk of hip dislocation, and care must be taken when positioning for surgery.

POSTOPERATIVE CARE

Postoperative considerations following any surgical procedure for a patient with PBS will focus on the prevention of respiratory complications and continued monitoring of renal status to prevent renal failure. A lack of abdominal wall musculature and flattened diaphragm can make it difficult for the patient to cough postoperatively, leading to atelectasis.[4,5,13] Scoliosis, pectus excavatum, or pectus carinatum are musculoskeletal anomalies that can be present in some cases. These anomalies can also make it more difficult for PBS patients to cough and fully expand the lungs during inspiration.

REFERENCES

1. Fette A. Associated rare anomalies in prune belly syndrome: a case report. *J Pediatr Surg Case Rep.* 2015;3(2):65–71. doi:10.1016/j.epsc.2014.12.007
2. Samal SK, Rathod S. Prune belly syndrome: a rare case report. *J Nat Sci Biol Med.* 2015;6(1):255–257. doi:10.4103/0976-9668.149218
3. Ye Q, Chen Y, Zhu, J, Wang Y. Combined laparoscopic and open technique for repair of congenital abdominal hernia: a case report of prune belly syndrome. *Medicine.* 2017;96(42):e7921. doi:10.1097/md.0000000000007921
4. Bösenberg A. Anaesthesia for prune belly syndrome. *South Afr Anesth Analg.* 2004;10(2):10–11. doi:10.1080/22201173.2004.10872354
5. Panitch HB. Pulmonary complications of abdominal wall defects. *Paediatr Respir Rev.* 2015;16(1):11–17. doi:10.1016/j.prrv.2014.10.004
6. Garg C, Khanna S, Mehta Y. Quadratus lumborum block for post-operative pain relief in patient with prune belly syndrome. *Indian J Anaesth* 2017;61(10):840–842. doi:10.4103/ija.ija_246_17
7. Yoon J, Ryu J, Kim J, et al. Anesthetic experience of a patient with Prune-belly syndrome. *Korean J Anesthesiol.* 2014;67(Suppl):S94–S95. doi:10.4097/kjae.2014.67.s.s94
8. Seidel NE, Angela MA, Edwin AS, Andrew J. Kirsch clinical manifestations and management of prune-belly syndrome in a large contemporary pediatric population. *Urology.* 2015;85(1):211–215. Doi:10.1016/j.urology.2014.09.029
9. Cornel A, Duicu C, Delean D, et al. Long term follow-up in a patient with prune-belly syndrome – a care compliant case report. *Medicine.* 2019;98(33):e16745. doi:10.1097/md.0000000000016745
10. Smith EA, Srinivasan A, Scherz HC, et al. Abdominoplasty in prune belly syndrome: modifications in Monfort technique to address variable patterns of abdominal wall weakness 2017. *J Pediatr Urol.* 13(5):502.e1–502.e6. doi:10.1016/j.jpurol.2017.02.020
11. Lopes RI, Tavares A, Srougi M, Dénes FT. 27 years of experience with the comprehensive surgical treatment of prune belly syndrome. *J Pediatr Urol.* 2015;11(5):276.e1-276.e7. doi:10.1016/j.jpurol.2015.05.018
12. Woodard JR. Prune-belly syndrome: a personal learning experience. *BJU Int.* 2003 Oct;92 Suppl 1:10-1. doi: 10.1046/j.1464-410x.92.s1.8.x. PMID: 12969002.
13. Goyal S, Kumar Gupta S, Kothari N, et al. Prune-belly syndrome: anesthetic implications and management. *Indian Anaesth Forum.* 2019;20:47–49. doi:10.4103/theiaforum.theiaforum_2_19

CHAPTER 43

Pulmonary Alveolar Proteinosis

Judy Audas

PATHOPHYSIOLOGY AND CLINICAL MANIFESTATIONS

Pulmonary alveolar proteinosis (PAP) is a broad category of lung diseases characterized by an accumulation of pulmonary surfactants in the alveolar space.[1] Surfactants are a lipid–protein complex, with both hydrophobic and hydrophilic parts, that are normally synthesized and secreted into the alveolar space by type II alveolar epithelial cells. They form a membranous layer that reduces surface tension in the alveolar wall at the air–liquid interface.[2] Thus, surfactants maintain lung volumes during respiration, preventing alveolar collapse and atelectasis at end expiration.[2] Other benefits of surfactants include reduction of elastic recoil of the lung as well as aiding in the defense against microbiological pathogens that threaten invasion and infection in the alveoli.[2] Although surfactants provide many benefits in the lungs, if excess or defective surfactant material is not removed from the alveolar space, the lung's gas exchange becomes impaired, leading to reduced lung function and severe hypoxemia.[3]

PAP was originally described in 1958 by Rosen and Castleman as an ultra-rare disease involving dysfunctional alveolar macrophages.[4] Further research has shown that other factors may lead to the unfavorable accumulation of surfactants in the alveoli. It can be attributed to an alteration in surfactant production, removal, or both.[3] PAP can present at any age, and the underlying cause varies in adults and children.[5] The alveolar surfactant accumulation in PAP disorders can be broadly classified as acquired or congenital.[5] Acquired PAP is further differentiated as either primary or secondary. Primary PAP refers to hereditary or autoimmune disruption of granulocyte-macrophage colony-stimulating factor (GM-CSF) receptor signaling.[6] Impairment in the number or function of macrophages is labeled as secondary PAP.[6] Congenital PAP refers to surfactant production disorders involving mutations in surfactant proteins.[5]

The overall prevalence of PAP in the United States and Japan, where most studies were conducted, is seven cases per million annually, whereas the prevalence of pediatric PAP is 1:1,000,000 annually.[2] In the adult population, PAP is two to three times more common in males aged 30 to 50 years old.

Primary PAP represents about 90% of all PAP cases, with most cases being autoimmune or hereditary in nature.[2] Autoimmune PAP involves a dysfunction in the GM-CSF receptor signaling that leads to an alteration in macrophage and neutrophil activation, causing impaired surfactant clearance and accumulation of surfactants.[2] Autoimmune PAP is very rare in children. Recent advancements in management of autoimmune PAP include treatment with inhaled or SC GM-CSF autoantibodies, which has completely improved the prognosis for this form of PAP.[2] Rare hereditary PAP involves mutations in the GM-CSF receptor.[7] New therapies for hereditary PAP include stem cell transplantation for GM-CSF receptor mutations.

Secondary PAP represents about 10% of all PAP cases and is most commonly associated with hematological disorders, but can also be attributed to pharmacological immunosuppression, malignancies, chronic inflammatory conditions, or environmental toxin exposure.[2]

Congenital PAP is rare and is thought to occur due to mutations in genes encoding surfactant proteins on those involved in surfactant production, specifically surfactant protein B (SP-B) and surfactant protein C (SP-C), which are responsible for maintaining surface tension in the alveoli.[2] With congenital PAP, SP-B, and SP-C undergo complicated posttranscriptional processing and therefore are more likely to undergo mutations.[5] It is worthwhile noting that none of the types of PAP is associated with interstitial lung disease.[8] The underlying cause of PAP is important not only for treatment purposes but also for genetic counseling purposes.

The diagnosis of PAP is typically made with imaging and bronchoalveolar lavage (BAL) after exclusion of interstitial lung disease.[8] In PAP, BAL periodic acid-Schiff (PAS) staining shows positive endogenous surfactant.[5] There may also be an increase in foamy alveolar macrophages, granular eosinophilic material, and surface proteins A, B, and D.[9] Chest radiography in PAP (Figure 43.1A) shows a reticular pattern that is most visible in the central parts of the lung, as well as a decrease in lung translucency centrally.[4] High-resolution CT (HRCT) of the chest (Figure 43.1B) illustrates the unique radiological "crazy paving" pattern, which is characterized by interlobular septal thickening that resembles ground glass in appearance.[2] The lines in Figure 43.1B correspond to a deposition of material within the airspaces at the borders of the acini in the secondary pulmonary lobules (1), the interlobular septa (2), and intralobular septa (3).[7] Figure 43.1C shows the radiological–histopathological evaluation of a specimen from the right lung, noting amorphous eosinophilic material in the alveoli that tested positive on PAS staining. The ground-glass appearance on CT is due to the presence of this material within the alveoli.[7]

THERAPEUTIC STRATEGIES FOR PULMONARY ALVEOLAR PROTEINOSIS

In normal surfactant homeostasis, the GM-CSF receptor stimulates macrophage activation to catabolize and clear excess surfactant proteins and lipids from the pulmonary alveoli.[8] When either the macrophage itself or the GM-CSF signaling is defective (as seen in primary and secondary PAP), macrophages are unable to maintain this surfactant homeostasis, resulting in a buildup of surfactants within the alveoli.[2] Treatment with GM-CSF autoantibodies has been successful in improving macrophage function, thereby improving surfactant homeostasis. In congenital PAP, the accumulation of surfactants is as problematic as it is in the other forms of PAP. Additionally, there is a concern for alveolar collapse because alveolar surface tension is not being maintained properly (by SP-B and SP-C). As described by Laplace's law, when alveolar surface tension is imbalanced, smaller alveoli may empty into larger alveoli, leading to lung collapse.[5]

Whereas autoimmune PAP has shown improvement with recombinant and exogenous GM-CSF, a combined approach

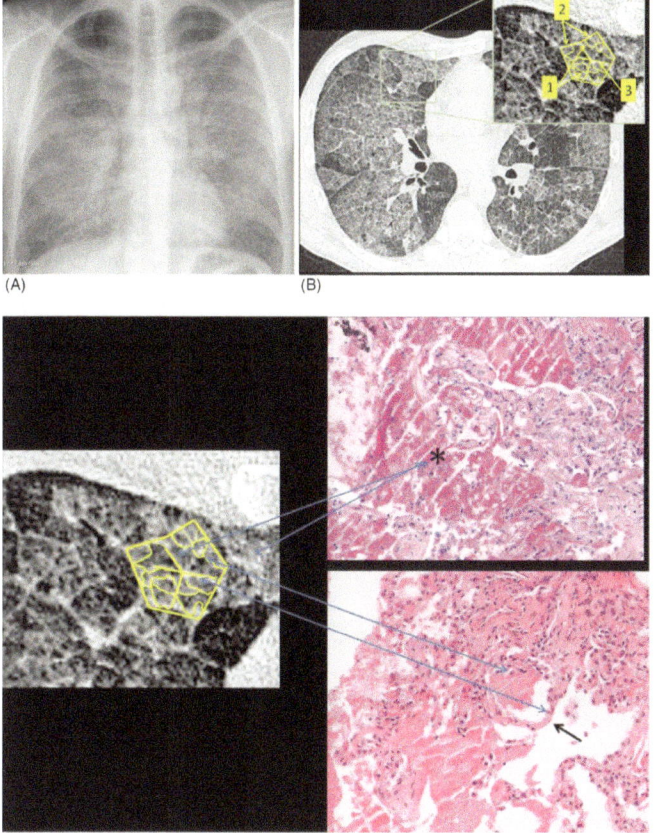

Figure 43.1: Pulmonary alveolar proteinosis radiography and histology. (A) Chest radiograph showed a reticular pattern that was most pronounced in the central parts of the lungs. There was also a decrease in the lung translucency centrally in both lungs. Heart and central vessels were normal. There was no pleural effusion. (B) On CT, a patchy distribution of a crazy-paving pattern was visible. The lines corresponded to a deposition of material within the airspaces at the borders of the acini (1) in the secondary pulmonary lobules, but also along the interlobular (2) and intralobular septa (3): the periacinar pattern. (C) Radiological-histopathological correlation.

Source: DeWever W, Meersschaert J, Coolen J, et al. The crazy-paving pattern: a radiological-pathological correlation. Insights Imaging. 2011;2(2); 117–132. doi:10.1007/s13244-010-0060-5.

with whole-lung lavage (WLL) and plasmapheresis can be used to decrease the circulating levels of GM-CSF autoantibodies, thereby restoring the alveolar macrophage catabolic functions.[1,5,8] Inhaled GM-CSF can be delivered directly to the affected lungs with fewer side effects than the SC form and has shown to have better response at a lower cost for autoimmune PAP patients.[8] Rituximab, a monoclonal antibody, can be useful in reducing the number of B lymphocytes, which in turn reduces the secretion of GM-CSF autoantibodies in autoimmune PAP patients.[1,8]

In congenital and other nonautoimmune forms of PAP, therapeutic WLL is the gold standard of care for removing the accumulated alveolar material from the lungs.[8] Bilateral, sequential WLL may be done in the same treatment session or in alternating sessions spaced 2 to 3 weeks apart.[10] Concomitant thoracic percussion can improve the quality of WLL by increasing the effluent turbidity.[8] As WLL is the most frequently encountered intraoperative presentation for PAP patients, this procedure is described in the Intraoperative Management section. In patients with severe hypoxemia, extracorporeal membrane oxygenation (ECMO) may be required for oxygenation during the WLL procedure or as a bridge to lung transplantation.[1]

Other novel approaches to treatment have been studied with some success. Lipids, mainly cholesterol, have been identified as the most abundant materials found in the accumulated macrophages in the BAL fluid of PAP patients.[2] This cholesterol accumulation leads to an alteration in the cholesterol/phospholipid ratio. Since cholesterol is critical to reducing alveolar surface tension, targeting lipid homeostasis with statin therapy could decrease cholesterol concentration and fluid turbidity in BAL fluid and alveolar macrophages.[2] Pilot studies have shown successful treatment with oral pioglitazone in autoimmune PAP patients.[8] This statin therapy seems to enhance the cholesterol efflux from macrophages, reducing cholesterol in foamy macrophages up to 40%.[2] The usefulness of statins in congenital PAP has not been studied. Transplantation of genetically corrected alveolar macrophages has shown some promise as in generating more functional macrophages in congenital PAP patients.[2]

ANESTHETIC MANAGEMENT

The indications for WLL are based on worsening dyspnea and worsening alveolar gas exchange as evidenced by lab values and lung function testing described under the Pertinent Labs section.[8] The most common lab value indicators for performing WLL are partial arterial pressure of oxygen (PaO_2) of less than 70 mm Hg on room air and alveolar–arterial (A–a) oxygen gradient of more than 40 mm Hg.[10] WLL is contraindicated if there is suspicion for bacterial pneumonia as it can lead to systemic infection and sepsis.[8]

PREOPERATIVE EVALUATION

Most patients presenting with PAP will exhibit dyspnea on exertion. Some may also present with a cough or an increase in sputum production.[2] Chronic cough and bronchitis suggest more advanced disease. Children with severe disease may require high-flow oxygen per nasal cannula or a simple mask. Other less common symptoms include fatigue and weight loss.[8] Chest pain and hemoptysis are rare symptoms that are not direct effects of PAP but may indicate other complications, such as superimposed lung infections.[8]

Pertinent Labs

Chest x-ray, HRCT, and BAL are obtained during the differential diagnostic period. Pulse oximetry is the most simple and common assessment tool to detect hypoxemia. More accurate analysis can be done with arterial blood gas sampling to determine the PaO_2 and the A–a oxygen gradient.[8] Spirometry is a useful measure of disease severity for children who are old enough to perform it properly.[1] In the early stages of PAP, lung volumes are usually within normal limits with pulmonary function testing (PFT). However, as the disease progresses, PFT may show a reduction in forced vital capacity and total lung capacity consistent with restrictive lung disease.[2] While it is notable that the diffusing capacity of the lung for carbon monoxide (D_{LCO}) is reduced, the dysfunctional alveolar gas exchange seen with increased $A–aDO_2$ is the best indicator of severity of the disease.[2,8] Oxygen desaturation with exercise, as assessed with a 6-minute walking test, has also been shown to be a reliable indicator of severity of the disease.[8]

It is recommended that patients presenting for WLL have a platelet count >50,000 and an international normalized ratio (INR) of <1.5.[10] Other laboratory blood tests may include evaluation for GM-CSF autoantibodies. Although autoimmune PAP is more common in adults, it is important to differentiate this in the rare event that a child does have this form of PAP, which can be treated with administration of GM-CSF.[1] Lactate dehydrogenase is increased in 82% of patients presenting with autoimmune PAP.[1] Serum carcinoembryonic antigen, surfactant protein A and D levels, and Krebs von den Lungen-6 (KL-6) are all markers of PAP disease activity, with KL-6 being a more specific predictor of autoimmune disease progression.[1] Genetic testing in children should include evaluation of surfactant proteins B and C, as well as the potential gene mutations of ATP-binding cassette subfamily A member 3 (*ABCA3*) and thyroid transcription factor 1 (TTF1).[1]

PREOPERATIVE PHARMACOLOGY

Preoperative anxiolytic medication should be used cautiously in children exhibiting dyspnea at rest. For highly anxious children, oral midazolam (up to 0.5 mg/kg with a maximum dose of 20 mg) or IV midazolam (0.1 mg/kg up to 2 mg total) may be used to facilitate separation from parents.

ANESTHETIC TECHNIQUE

Intraoperative Management

Successful WLL requires an experienced lavage team, including anesthesia, interventional pulmonary medicine, respiratory therapy, and nursing.[10] Because the right lung is relatively larger than the left lung, patients tend to have more hemodynamic compromise when the right lung is lavaged because the left lung is less able to manage the gas-exchange process by comparison.[14] The procedure should be performed under general anesthesia, with a recommended combination of IV propofol, short-acting opioid, and complete neuromuscular blockade throughout the procedure.[10] Inhalation agents may be helpful, especially in patients with a history of asthma or bronchospasm, but should not be the sole anesthetic agent.[10] Most centers perform WLL in separate sessions, starting with the lung demonstrating the greatest involvement via imaging and ventilation/perfusion (V/Q) scanning.[10] Once this lung has recovered, in about 2 to 3 weeks, the second lung can be lavaged more safely.[2,10]

The patient should be intubated with an appropriately sized, left-sided, double-lumen endotracheal tube (DLT), if possible, to avoid blocking the takeoff of the right upper lobe bronchus.[10] If using a single-lumen endotracheal tube (ETT), placement into the right mainstem bronchus is easier due to the less acute angle the bronchus takes off of the trachea.[11,8] If the child is too small for a DLT, two single-lumen breathing tubes can be placed, one endobronchially and one endotracheally.[12] Appropriate sizing guidelines for ETTs, DLTs, and fiberoptic bronchoscopes (FOBs) are shown in **Table 43.1**. Anesthesia providers typically use a 2.2-mm FOB to verify placement in children less than 12 years old to provide room for ventilation without occlusion of the airway while the FOB is in place.[11] Partial or complete cardiopulmonary bypass (CPB) and ECMO are options for very small children or for those with significant respiratory compromise.[13] These options would require anticoagulation and reversal per hospital protocols.

Once intubated, the patient should be carefully positioned in lateral decubitus position with the intended lavage lung up and the ventilated lung down, as shown in **Figure 43.2**, to facilitate drainage of lavage fluid with gravity.[10] By ventilating the dependent lung and lavaging the nondependent lung, blood flow is improved to the ventilated lung, thus improving the V/Q ratio.[14] The DLT, or the ETT in the lavage lung in the case of small children, should again be verified with an FOB to ensure that the cuff of the tube is appropriately placed in the bronchus of the lavage lung. A leak check should be performed by ventilating each lung separately.[10] An air leak can also be checked by venting the lavage lung ETT into a saline water seal cup while the ventilated lung is held at an airway pressure of 40 to 50 cmH$_2$O, with absence of air bubbles confirming bilateral lung isolation.[10]

Table 43.1	Recommended ETT, DLT, and FOB Sizes		
Age (mo/yr)	Single-Lumen ETT Size ID	DLT (Fr)	Largest FOB Size OD (mm)
<8 mo (if weight >3 kg)	3.0 Microcuff	-	2.8 (via ETT)
8 mo to <2 yr	3.5 Microcuff	-	2.8 (via ETT)
2 to <4 yr	4.0 Microcuff	-	2.8 (via ETT)
4 to <6 yr	4.5 Microcuff	-	3.5 (via ETT)
6 to <8 yr	5.0 Microcuff	-	3.8 (via ETT)
8 to <10 yr	5.5 Microcuff	26	2.2 (via DLT)
10 to <12 yr	6.0 Cuffed	26, 28	2.2 (via DLT)
12 to <14 yr	6.5 Cuffed	28, 32	2.2 (via DLT)
14 to <16 yr	7.0 Cuffed	35	3.5, 4.2 (via DLT)
16 to 18 yr	7.5 Cuffed	35, 37	3.5, 4.2 (via DLT)

DLT, double-lumen endotracheal tube; ETT, endotracheal tube; FOB, fiberoptic bronchoscope; ID, inner diameter; OD, outer diameter.

Source: Data from https://anestesiar.org/WP/uploads/2012/04/Microcuff-Paed-Endo-Tube.pdf; https://media.springernature.com/original/springer-static/image/chp%3A10.1007%2F978-1-4939-1610-8_22/MediaObjects/302081_1_En_22_Fig10b_HTML.gif.

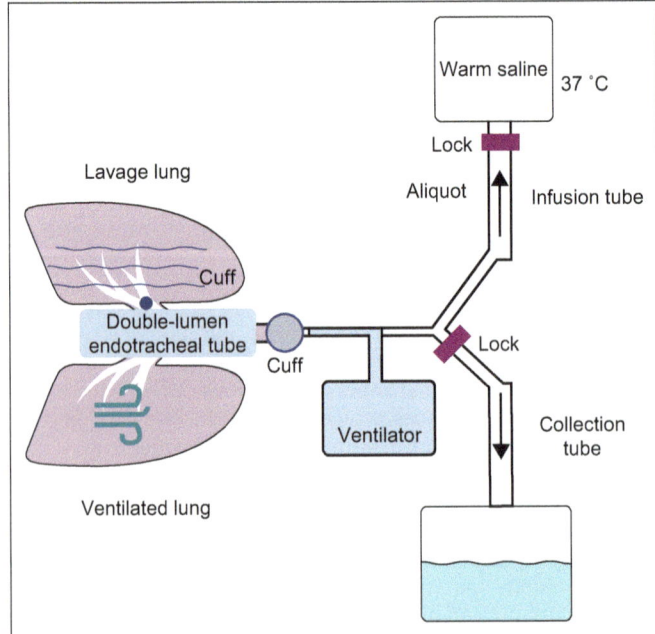

Figure 43.2: Schematic of whole-lung lavage setup.

Source: Readdy C. Whole-Lung Lavage. In: Ernst A, Herth F. eds. *Principles and Practice of Interventional Pulmonology.* Springer; 2013.

Prior to starting lavage, both lungs should be ventilated with 100% oxygen for up to 15 minutes.[10] Then the lavage lung should be disconnected from the ventilator and connected to the lavage apparatus. The setup shown in **Figure 43.2** includes a Y-connector that allows for one-way flow to be used for instillation of fluid and subsequent drainage of the fluid later. It shows the lavage fluid going through a fluid warmer (heated to 37 °C) directly into the lavage lung. The drainage limb should be closed off, and the lavage limb should be opened for delivery of warmed saline aliquots equal to the measured lung volume, usually between 250 and 500 mL at a time.[16] Total lavage fluid varies from 4 to 14 L in pediatric WLL, with an average of 250 mL/kg used.[16] The procedure is repeated until the effluent liquid is no longer cloudy.[8] Chest percussion to the lavage lung, either during the instillation or removal of fluid, can facilitate clearance of proteinaceous material.[10] Manual percussion has been found to remove more of the dense lavage fluid, while mechanical percussion has shown less postoperative discomfort.[10]

Ventilation to the nonlavage lung should be at 100% oxygen throughout the treatment. The length of treatment may be shortened by the degree of hypoxia noted during the lavage process as monitored by pulse oximetry.[10] The volume of solution instilled and recovered should be closely monitored to alert the team in the event of fluid leakage into the contralateral lung or into the pleural space.[10] A loss of lung isolation can also be monitored throughout by observing for bubbles in the lavage fluid, recognizing increased resistance to ventilation or the presence of rales or rhonchi in the ventilated lung.[14] Administering moderate positive end-expiratory pressure (PEEP) to the ventilated lung can improve ventilation and decrease hypoxia; however, high PEEP can divert the blood flow to the nonventilated lung, causing an increased shunt and desaturation.[17]

It is important to maintain normothermia throughout the procedure.[14] Increased room temperature, warmed lavage fluids, and warming blankets are all good options.

Extubation should only be done after the neuromuscular blockade is reversed and the child is fully awake. The DLT can be converted to a single-lumen ETT for emergence. ECMO or CPB patients may remain intubated in the ICU until the lung has recovered.

POSTOPERATIVE CARE

Complications of WLL are minimal if performed correctly by experienced personnel.[8] Possible complications include desaturation, pneumothorax, SC emphysema, headache, fever, cardiopulmonary edema, seizures, pneumonitis, lavage leakage to the opposite lung due to ETT dislodgment, and potential for prolonged intubation postoperatively.[8] Respiratory status should be closely monitored postoperatively for any worsening desaturation or dyspnea. Coughing is a common postoperative occurrence and should be expected. Fever and hypoxemia are the most common complications.[16] Close observation for these and other less common complications, such as wheezing, headache, pleural effusion, pneumothorax, pulmonary edema, and pneumonia, should be done for several hours after treatment.[16] A postoperative chest x-ray may be ordered to assess for lung improvement or to diagnose potential complications.[17]

KEY REFERENCES

Complete references for this chapter are online and available at https://connect.springerpub.com/content/book/978-0-8261-3875-0/part/part03/toc-part/ch043.

1. Awab A, Khan M, Youness H. Whole lung lavage - technical details, challenges and management of complications. *J Thorac Dis.* 2017;9(6);1697–1706. doi:10.21037/jtd.2017.04.10
2. Bush A, Pabary R. Pulmonary alveolar proteinosis in children. *Breathe.* 2020:16(2);200001. doi:10.1183/20734735.0001-2020
3. Campo I, Luisetti M, Griese M, et al. Whole lung lavage therapy for pulmonary alveolar proteinosis: a global survey of current practices and procedures. *Orphanet J Rare Dis.* 2016;11(115):1–10. doi:10.1186/s13023-016-0497-9
4. DeWever W, Meersschaert J, Coolen J, et al. The crazy-paving pattern: a radiological-pathological correlation. *Insights Imaging.* 2011;2(2);117–132. doi:10.1007/s13244-010-0060-5.
5. Griese M. Pulmonary alveolar proteinosis: a comprehensive clinical perspective. *Pediatrics.* 2017;140(2):1–14. doi:10.1542/peds.2017-0610
6. Jouneau S, Menard C, Lederlin M. Pulmonary alveolar proteinosis. *Respirology.* 2020;25(8):816–826. doi:10.1111/resp.13831
7. Salvaterra E, Campo I. Pulmonary alveolar proteinosis: from classification to therapy. *Breathe.* 2020;16(2):200018. doi:10.1183/20734735.0018-2020

CHAPTER 44

Treacher Collins Syndrome

Marianne S. Cosgrove

PATHOPHYSIOLOGY AND CLINICAL MANIFESTATIONS

Treacher Collins syndrome (TCS), also known as mandibulofacial dysostosis or Treacher Collins–Franceschetti syndrome, is named after London ophthalmologist Edward Treacher Collins, who first described the disorder in 1900. TCS is a rare craniofacial deformity occurring in 1:25,000 to 1:50,000 live births.[1-3] The syndrome is equally distributed between males and females.[1,4,5] Spontaneous, de novo mutations account for approximately 60% of TCS cases; 40% are genetic, with a 50% rate of transmission through an affected parent.

TCS results from a defect in neural crest development at the first and second branchial arches. The majority of transmitted cases are autosomal dominant, most commonly from mutation of the treacle ribosome biogenesis factor 1 (TCOF1) gene (73%–90%). TCOF1 is responsible for encoding treacle, a phosphoprotein, which regulates neural crest cell proliferation underlying the genesis of craniofacial and pharyngeal structures. In the absence of treacle, apoptosis is uncontrolled, disrupting neural crest cell growth. This results in underdevelopment of the bony ridges of the mid-and lateral face, the mandible, and the soft tissues of the oropharynx and nasopharynx. Less commonly, TCS may also be transmitted via autosomal recessive mutations in the RNA polymerase I subunit C (POLR1C) and RNA polymerase I subunit D (POLR1D) genes.[5,6]

The presentation of TCS can vary from mild and barely perceptible to severe.[7] Several distinctive features emanate from the underdevelopment of bones of the midface, causing a centrally convex appearance. Classic TCS manifestations result from maxillary and zygomatic hypoplasia, malar flattening, deformity of the eye sockets, micrognathia, retrognathia, and a prominent, "beaked" nose. Malformation of the external pinnae of the ears and stenosis or atresia of the external ear canals usually accompany the main elements of craniofacial dysmorphology. This anomaly contributes to conductive hearing loss, present in approximately 50% of affected patients. Anesthesia providers should remember that generally speaking, individuals with TCS are born with intact inner-ear function and are of normal intelligence.[1,2,7,8] **Figure 44.1** depicts the features common to patients with TCS.[4] In addition to the primary facial and otic anomalies, concomitant multisystemic disorders may accompany TCS. **Box 44.1** delineates other varied conditions that may be associated with TCS.

There is no cure for TCS. Due to its rarity, there remains a lack of evidence supporting a particular treatment protocol for these patients.[8] Care of a TCS patient requires a multidisciplinary approach, with involvement from various healthcare and ancillary anesthesia providers. Therapy is principally aimed at surgical intervention to alleviate the major sequelae of the syndrome. These include upper airway obstruction, feeding difficulties, and hearing deficits. Surgeries may be staged and occur at various ages throughout the pediatric and adolescent period, with initial focus on establishment of airway patency and avoidance of nutritional and developmental delays. The provision of

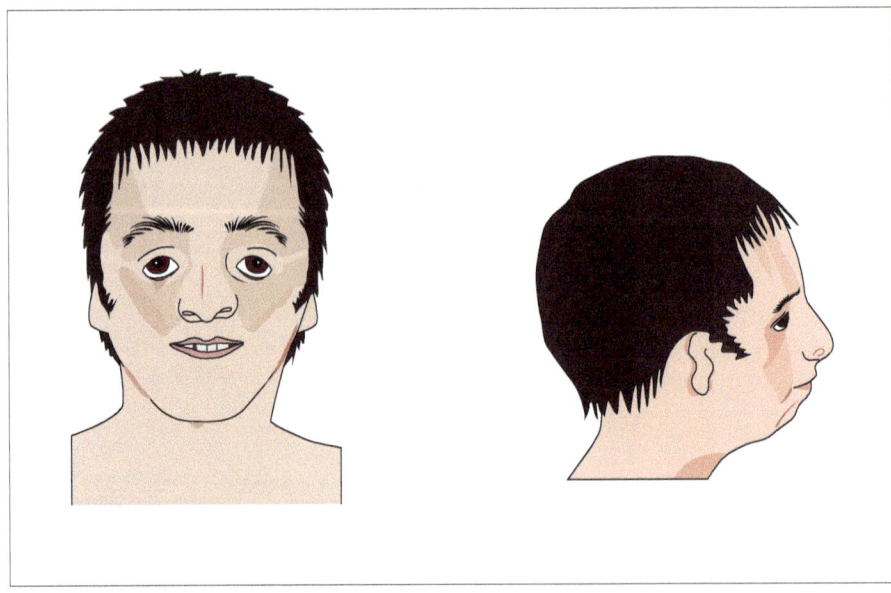

Figure 44.1: Typical features of Treacher Collins syndrome.

Source: From Cobb ARM, Green B, Gill D, et al. The surgical management of Treacher Collins syndrome. *Br J Oral Maxillofacial Surg.* 2014;52–581–589. doi:10.1016/j.bjoms.2014.02.007.

> **BOX 44.1 SYSTEMIC CONDITIONS ASSOCIATED WITH TREACHER COLLINS SYNDROME**
>
> **Ophthalmic**
> - Downward slant of palpebral fissures
> - Hypertelorism
> - Coloboma
> - Dry eye syndrome
> - Strabismus
> - Ectropion
> - Notched lower eyelids
> - Scant eyelashes (medial lower lid)
> - Visual deficits
>
> **Otic**
> - Stenosis or atresia of external ear canal
> - Fused ossicles
> - Conductive hearing loss
> - Malformation of pinnae (microtia)
>
> **Oro/Nasopharyngeal/Airway**
> - Cleft lip
> - High-arched or cleft palate
> - Macrostomia
> - Dental malocclusion
> - Collapse of the suprahyoid musculature
> - Glossoptosis
> - Choanal atresia
> - Cervical spine abnormalities (kyphosis at the cranial base)
> - Temporomandibular joint abnormality/asymmetry
> - Salivary gland hypoplasia or absence
> - Xerostomia
> - Malnutrition/failure to thrive secondary to feeding issues
> - Gastroesophageal reflux disorder
> - OSA, risk of sudden infant death syndrome
>
> **Cardiovascular**
> - Anomalies (e.g., VSD: rare)
> - Pulmonary HTN (secondary to OSA)
> - Cor pulmonale (secondary to OSA)
>
> **Developmental/Psychosocial**
> - Developmental delay secondary to hearing loss
> - Speech impediment secondary to hearing loss and malformation of the oropharynx
> - Decreased maternal/family bonding
> - Social ostracism/isolation
> - Low self-esteem
> - Depression
>
> HTN, hypertension; OSA, obstructive sleep apnea; VSD, ventricular septal defect.

rehabilitative services including physical and psychotherapy, speech pathology, psychosocial, and family-to-family support may also be indicated.[2,7]

In cases of TCS where mandibular micrognathia/retrognathia is severe, immediate intubation and/or tracheostomy may be required to avoid imminent loss of the airway. However, early establishment of a surgical airway may lead to issues such as chronic aspiration, bronchial infections, and eventual tracheomalacia or stenosis.[2,9] The tongue–lip adhesion procedure and/or mandibular distraction and advancement, usually performed at 2 to 3 months of age, also alleviate acute airway obstruction and may allow for extubation or decannulation of an existing tracheostomy. Cleft lip and palate are repaired at approximately 6 to 10 months to mitigate issues with swallowing and speech. Along with surgical airway interventions, placement of a gastrostomy tube may be necessitated to support nutritional and hydration status.[2,9,10]

Hearing deficits are addressed early on with application of banded hearing aids. Installing bone-anchored hearing aids (BAHA) is the eventual goal; however, the mastoid bones must be fully developed. Provided that there are no skull defects present, cochlear implants may be installed between 2 and 6 years of age. Ongoing craniofacial, ophthalmic, oculoplastic, and orthognathic/orthodontic procedures aimed at improving aesthetics may occur throughout the pediatric and well into the adolescent period. Cosmetic surgeries, including eyelid and outer ear reconstruction, sagittal split osteotomy/LeFort I procedure, rhinoplasty, and chin implants, are commonly performed on TCS patients.[3,10,11]

ANESTHETIC MANAGEMENT

A TCS patient may require anesthesia for staged craniofacial surgeries and ongoing otolaryngological and ophthalmic care. Anesthesia may also be indicated for diagnostic studies such as CT or MRI of the head. Ultimately, the severity of the malformation dictates the anesthetic management. Anesthetic considerations and potential concerns vary depending on the type of surgery performed and the age of the TCS patient at the time of intervention. Box 44.2 outlines key considerations for a variety of surgical procedures.

PREOPERATIVE EVALUATION

It is imperative that anesthesia providers perform a thorough preoperative examination, with an emphasis on airway and cardiovascular evaluation. Managing the airway is anticipated to be difficult in patients diagnosed with TCS; therefore, in addition to a thorough physical examination, anesthesia providers should review previous anesthesia records when available. A review of prior anesthesia may prove useful in identifying strategies that were successful or unsuccessful previously.

PREOPERATIVE PHARMACOTHERAPY

Due to the staged nature of required surgeries, the possibility of hearing and/or vision deficits, and low self-esteem, a child with TCS may be particularly fearful upon returning to the operating room. Center- and patient-specific, parental support and the aid of a child life specialist may be warranted to alleviate the anxiety that these patients may have during their perioperative visit. Depending on the surgery being performed, blood chemistry, complete blood count, and coagulation studies may be indicated.

> **BOX 44.2** **ANESTHETIC CONSIDERATIONS AND POTENTIAL CONCERNS IN PATIENTS WITH TREACHER COLLINS SYNDROME**
>
> - Difficult mask ventilation
> - Difficult direct laryngoscopy/intubation
> - Sequelae of previous tracheostomy (e.g., tracheomalacia, tracheal stenosis)
> - Risk of aspiration
> - Airway competition with surgeon
> - Local anesthetic toxicity
> - FiO_2 limited to ≤30% during airway and dental procedures
> - Excessive blood loss during craniofacial procedures
> - Venous air embolus during craniofacial procedures
> - Mandibular fixation postmaxillofacial procedures
> - Oculocardiac reflex during ophthalmic procedures
> - Corneal abrasion secondary to protruding eyes/underdeveloped eyelids
> - Enhanced effects of anesthetics secondary to malnutrition, decreased protein binding
> - Postoperative pain
> - Need for CPAP/BiPAP/ancillary airway support postoperatively
> - Occult difficult intubation in patients who have undergone cosmesis (e.g., rhinoplasty, chin implants)
> - Need for ancillary support secondary to fear/embarrassment due to appearance/social issues (e.g., child life specialist)
>
> BiPAP, bilevel positive airway pressure; CPAP, continuous positive airway pressure; FiO2, fraction of inspired oxygen.

ANESTHETIC TECHNIQUE

Intraoperative Management

Foundational to all anesthetic plans, maintenance of a patent airway is the primary concern. However, this may pose a logistical challenge in a patient with TCS. An estimated 50% of TCS patients will have a grade IV Cormack–Lehane (CL) laryngoscopic view.[11] Additionally, establishment of the airway may become increasingly more difficult as the child ages (Stricker, 2019). A variety of backup airway devices should be available prior to induction as well as anticipation of the need for emergent surgical airway. Presence of a tracheostomy may predispose the TCS patient to gastroesophageal reflux disease (GERD), posing a risk of aspiration during induction of anesthesia.[3] Laryngeal mask airways (LMAs) have been successfully used to maintain airway patency and may provide a conduit to intubate through.[12] Overall, fiberoptic intubation with careful sedation is the preferred technique to secure the airway in a TCS patient.[11] If the induction of anesthesia is preferred, maintenance of spontaneous ventilation with sevoflurane is recommended.[3]

Due to the associated aplastic/hypoplastic zygomas and midface hypoplasia, it is imperative anesthesia providers are vigilant with regard to protecting the patient's eyes during the procedure; the risk of orbital compression and perioperative blindness is also increased should prone positioning be required due to maxillary and zygomatic hypoplasia.

POSTOPERATIVE CARE

Depending on the surgical procedure performed, postoperative pain may be considerable, especially following reconstructive craniofacial surgeries. Using a multimodal pain strategy, incorporating nonopioid analgesics is advisable to avoid the risk of opioid-induced respiratory depression. Respiratory support may be required, with transfer to the ICU warranted at times to better monitor the patient's respiratory status.

KEY REFERENCES

References for this chapter are online and available at https://connect.springerpub.com/content/book/978-0-8261-3875-0/part/part03/toc-part/ch044.

1. Plomp RG, van Lieshout MJS, Joosten KFM. Treacher Collins syndrome: a systematic review of evidence-based treatment and recommendations. *Plast Reconstr Surg*. 2016;137(1):191–204. doi:10.1097/PRS.0000000000001896
2. Tolorova MM, Rohena LO. Mandibulofacial dysostosis (Treacher Collins syndrome). *Medscape*. 2018. https://emedicine.medscape.com/article/946143-print
3. Thung AK, Maranets I. Treacher Collins syndrome. In: Fleisher LA, Roizen MF, Roizen JD, eds. *Essence of Anesthesia Practice*. 4th ed. Elsevier. 2017;P 411.
4. Cobb ARM, Green B, Gill D, et al. The surgical management of Treacher Collins syndrome. *Br J Oral Maxillofac Surg*. 2014;52(7):581–589. doi:10.1016/j.bjoms.2014.02.007
6. National Organization for Rare Disorders (NORD). Treacher Collins syndrome. 2019. https://rarediseases.org/rare-diseases/treacher-collins-syndrome/#:~:text=Treacher%20Collins%20syndrome%20(TCS)%20is,to%20breathing%20and%20feeding%20difficulties
8. Alijerian A, Gilardino M.S. Treacher Collins syndrome. *Clin Plast. Surg* 2019;46(2):197–205. doi:10.1016/j.cps.2018.11.005
10. Stricker PA, Fiadjoe JE, Lerman J. Plastic and reconstructive surgery. In: Coté CJ, Lerman J, Anderson BJ, eds. *Coté and Lerman's A Practice of Anesthesia for Infants and Children*. 6th ed. Elsevier. 2019;805, 813–814.
11. Cladis FP, Grunwaldt L, Losee J. Anesthesia for pediatric plastic surgery, In: Davis PJ, Cladis FP, eds. *Smith's Anesthesia for Infants and Children*. 9th ed. 2016. Elsevier; 858–859.

CHAPTER 45

Tuberous Sclerosis

Brian DeAtley

PATHOPHYSIOLOGY AND CLINICAL MANIFESTATIONS

Tuberous sclerosis complex (TSC), also known as Bourneville–Pringle syndrome, is an inherited, progressive neurocutaneous disorder characterized by the potential for hamartoma formation in nearly every organ system, including the brain, eyes, heart, lungs, liver, kidneys, and skin.[1] The incidence of TSC is estimated to be 1 in every 6,000 to 10,000 live births, with as many as two million people worldwide believed to have the disorder.[2] This genetic disorder results from the loss of heterozygosity of two separate tumor suppressor genes (*TSC1* and *TSC2*).[3] *TSC1* usually encodes for the protein hamartin, with *TSC2* encoding for tuberin.[1] These proteins form a complex that triggers the GTPase-activating protein Rheb, which inhibits the mammalian target of rapamycin (mTOR), a highly conserved protein kinase involved in regulating cellular metabolism, differentiation, growth, migration, and protein synthesis.[4] Mutations in either *TSC1* or *TSC2* ultimately result in a loss of tumor-suppressor activity and the constitutive activation of mTOR. Consequently, abnormal cellular proliferation and differentiation ensue, with hyperactivation of the mTOR pathway, resulting in the development of hamartomatous tumors that characterize TSC.[2] Inactivation of both alleles of *TSC1* or *TSC2*, mainly through loss of heterozygosity, is required for hamartoma development. In general, alterations in the *TSC2* gene result in a more severe expression of the disorder.

The diagnosis of TSC is based on clinical suspicion, a thorough clinical evaluation, identification of hamartomatous tumors on the skin or retina, or definitive testing, such as molecular genetic testing that can detect alterations in either *TSC1* or *TSC2*. In addition, CT and MRI can be performed to evaluate the presence of tumors in the brain, kidneys, liver, or lungs. An ECG or echocardiogram can be performed to evaluate the presence of tumors in the heart. In some instances, cardiac rhabdomyoma may be detected prenatally and trigger suspicion and further testing.

TSC is a multisystem disorder with various clinical manifestations. Frequently the kidneys, skin, and central nervous system are affected (Table 45.1). Angiomyolipomas are tumors composed of fat, blood vessels, and smooth muscle cells, and usually affect the kidneys. Although they may not cause any symptoms, renal dysfunction may occur in some instances. Most patients with TSC will have hypomelanotic macules, also known as ash leaf spots.[5] Common symptoms of central nervous system involvement include seizures and intellectual disability. While patients with TSC may have normal development and cognitive function, the majority experience delays in achieving developmental milestones. The classic Vogt's triad of facial angiofibromas, intellectual disability, and intractable epilepsy occurs in approximately 30% to 40% of affected individuals.[2]

Some patients with TSC may develop multifocal micronodular pneumocyte hyperplasia (MMPH), where multiple nodules form throughout the lungs due to abnormal proliferation of pneumocytes. MMPH is usually not associated with any symptoms, although there have been rare reports of breathing difficulties and eventually respiratory failure associated with MMPH. In addition, patients with TSC are at an increased risk of repeated pneumothorax or chylothorax.

ANESTHETIC MANAGEMENT
PREOPERATIVE EVALUATION

Given the cognitive deficits and the potential for behavioral impairment, patients with TSC are likely to require anesthesia for diagnostic and therapeutic procedures. Determining the extent of neurological, cardiovascular, pulmonary/airway, and renal involvement is essential to the preoperative evaluation.[1] Obtaining medical history and information regarding

Table 45.1 Clinical Manifestations of Tuberous Sclerosis Complex

System	Sign or Symptom
Neurological	• Epilepsy • Cortical brain malformations • Tuberous sclerosis complex-associated neuropsychiatric disorder
Dermatological	• Hypomelanotic macules (ash leaf spots) • Angiofibromas (typically on the face) • Fibrous cephalic plaque (typically on the forehead) • Shagreen patch (typically on the lower back) • Confetti skin lesions • Ungual fibromas
Dental	• Dental enamel pits • Intraoral fibromas
Renal	• Renal cysts • Renal AML • Renal cell carcinoma (uncommon)
Cardiac	• Intracardiac rhabdomyomas (typically regress within the first 3 years of life)
Ophthalmological	• Retinal lesions
Pulmonary	• Lymphangioleiomyomatosis (typically in adult women) • Multifocal micronodular pneumocytic hyperplasia • Clear cell lung tumor (rare)
Other	• Extrarenal AML rarely seen in the liver, adrenal glands, pancreas, and endocrine system

AML, angiomyolipomas.

Source: From Randle SC. Tuberous sclerosis complex: a review. *Pediatr Ann.* 2017;46(4):e166–e171. doi:10.3928/19382359-20170320-01.

known triggers of seizure and behavioral outbursts from the parents will help the anesthesia provider deliver safe and effective care. If the child has had prior anesthetics, it is beneficial to ask the parents what techniques were successful previously with their child. Having the parents assist with simple tasks, such as monitor placement and premedication, can add familiarity and decrease the anxiety experienced by all parties involved.

Pertinent Labs

It is recommended that patients with TSC have the following tests performed and evaluated prior to receiving general anesthesia: chest x-ray, ECG, transthoracic echocardiogram, anticonvulsant medication levels, electrolytes, blood urea nitrogen, and creatinine.[7] Blood pressure should also be assessed to identify hypertension.

PREOPERATIVE PHARMACOTHERAPY

The administration of most medications, such as anticonvulsants, should be continued until the morning of surgery in an effort to ensure anticonvulsant levels are optimized.[8] Sedatives, such as oral or IV midazolam, can be useful in patients with TSC to help facilitate IV catheter placement and/or separation from parents, especially in the presence of anxiety, intellectual disability, or behavioral impairment. Some medications may be unsafe with increased intracranial pressure or congestive heart failure, although all potential interactions and deleterious side effects should be carefully considered prior to administration.

ANESTHETIC TECHNIQUE

Intraoperative Management

Anesthesia can be safely induced and maintained with either an inhalation mask induction or IV induction. No specific anesthetic technique or agents are absolutely contraindicated in patients with TSC.[9] The decision to intubate and the timing of extubation should be made on a case-to-case basis according to the presence of upper airway masses, severity of pulmonary disease, and type and extent of the surgery. Fiberoptic bronchoscopes and video laryngoscopes may aid in successful intubation, especially in patients who are known to be a difficult intubation. The scale of the surgery and the severity of clinical manifestations should determine the need for invasive monitors intraoperatively. The requirements for opioids and muscle relaxants may be increased secondary to chronic anticonvulsant treatment.[10] The need for inotropic and chronotropic medications, as well as the cardiovascular side effects of drugs given intraoperatively, should be considered based on the patient's history and comorbidities. Prophylactic antibiotics should be considered in patients with cardiac tumors or congenital heart disease based on the most recent recommendations. It is imperative anesthesia providers remain cognizant of preoperative renal function and make a concerted effort to maintain renal perfusion and cardiac output and avoid medications throughout the anesthetic to avoid injury to the organs.

POSTOPERATIVE CARE

Postoperative care is largely based on the surgery being performed and the patient's medical history. In most instances, the patient can be transferred to the postanesthesia care unit postoperatively for observation. At the very least, a short observation period is appropriate considering the procedure time and major organ involvement associated with TSC. Patients with significant organ dysfunction should be admitted for monitoring and treatment after more extensive procedures. Anesthesia providers should be aware that severe postoperative hypertension, bradyarrhythmias, and seizures may occur.[8] Generally, baseline medical treatment can be resumed as soon as possible, with several case-specific exceptions, such as discontinuing anticonvulsants following the placement of electrocorticography grids and strips for corticography prior to resection of a seizure focus.[8]

CHAPTER 46

Turner's Syndrome

Judy Audas

PATHOPHYSIOLOGY AND CLINICAL MANIFESTATIONS

Also known as 45,XO syndrome, ovarian short-stature syndrome, or Bonnevie–Ullrich syndrome, Turner's syndrome (TS) was first described by endocrinologist Dr. Henry Turner in 1938 as a constellation of findings in girls as a "syndrome of infantilism, congenital webbed neck, and cubitus valgus."[1] Monosomy of the X chromosome is now the most frequent genetic abnormality in females.[2] It is estimated that TS affects 25 to 50 per 100,000 females and can involve multiple organ systems throughout the life span.[3] The incidence of TS was originally underestimated due to many of the conceptions being spontaneously miscarried and subsequently not recorded. With recent developments in DNA testing, X monosomy is now reported as being present in 2% of all conceptions.[2]

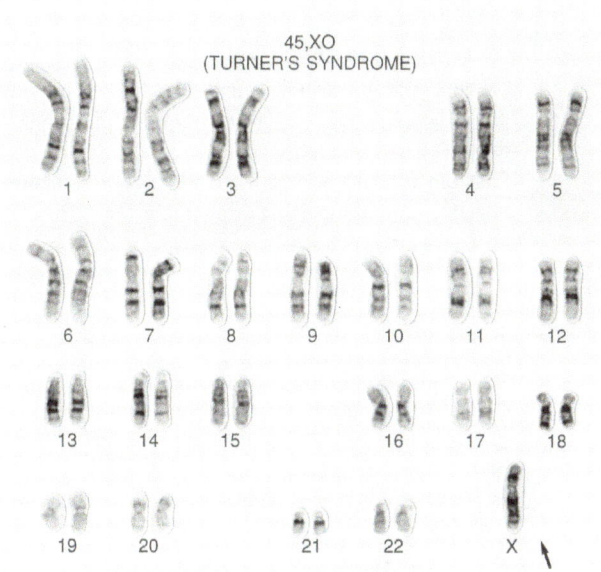

Figure 46.1: Turner's syndrome karyotype 45,XO. This female lacks the second X chromosome present in the normal karyotype.
Source: Wessex Reg. Genetics Centre/Wellcome Collection.

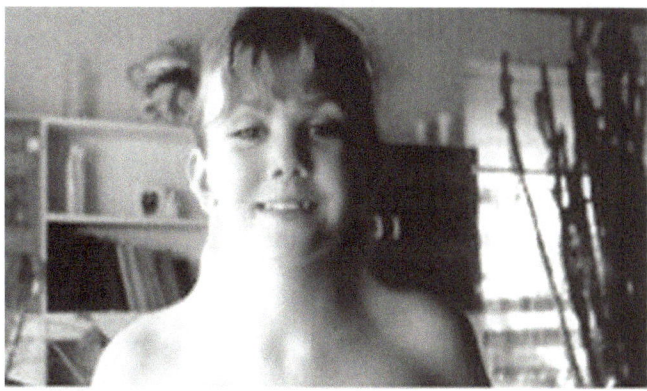
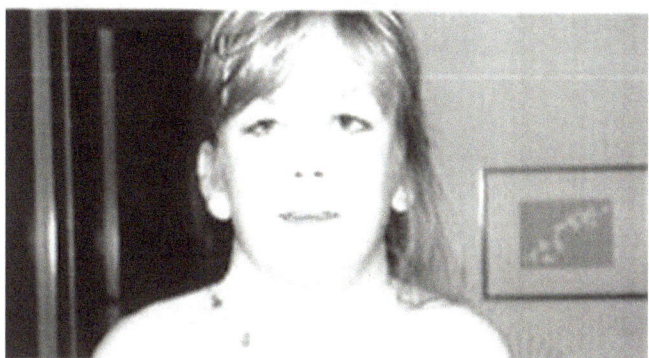

Figure 46.2: Neck of a girl with Turner's syndrome (before and after surgery).
Source: Nielson, Johannes.

The genetic origin of TS is explained as a partial or total loss of the second sexual chromosome, originally identified as 45,XO (Figure 46.1).[2] Genetically, the Y chromosome is normally responsible for determining sex, with the patient being male if the Y chromosome is present and female if the Y chromosome is absent. However, a lack of a Y chromosome alone is not sufficient to determine a female gender; two X chromosomes are necessary to maintain ovarian growth and function.[1] Hence, the lack of development of female sex organs seen in the 45,XO karyotype is due to the lack of a second X chromosome.

It has been suggested that there are epigenetic origins to TS as well. Researchers have found that several deleted genes from the X chromosome can affect various tissues, organs, and systems during embryonic development, postnatal growth, and throughout the adult life span.[2] Subsequently, there are several other karyotypes now associated with TS. While 50% of females with TS present with the 45,XO karyotype, 35% are considered to have mosaicism, with only some cells expressed as 45,XO and the remainder being normal. Of TS cases, 15% are due to structural abnormalities in the X chromosome. Nonetheless, all TS karyotypes are missing some element from the X chromosome, which explains the common features. Since the X chromosome contains over 1,000 genes, as compared with the Y chromosome, which contains approximately 200 genes, it is of no surprise that the absence of the supporting second X chromosome can present in many ways.[1]

The variety in expression of various TS phenotypes may explain the underestimation of TS diagnosis in females with mild symptoms/features. Manifestation of phenotypical features will guide treatment and anesthetic management of TS patients. Possible features include, but are not limited to, dysmorphic (facial) stigmata, short stature, gonadal dysgenesis, lymphatic obstruction, and renal, cardiac (including congenital heart disease), skeletal (including cervical vertebral hypoplasia and micrognathia), endocrine, and metabolic abnormalities.[2] Most TS patients have normal cognition; however, certain mosaic karyotypes may involve a small ring X chromosome (where X inactivation failed). These individuals may present with mild to severe cognitive impairment.[4] Early diagnosis and treatment with growth hormones have prevented many of the more devastating symptoms related to TS in females.

In addition, many patients with TS present with a bilateral webbed neck, or pterygium colli, that extends from the mastoid process to the acromion.[5] It is present in 15% of patients with TS and is most likely a remnant of the backflow of SC lymphatic obstruction around the neck during fetal development.[6] SC cysts formed on both sides cause stretching of the neck skin. This stretching, scarring, and shrinkage result in the formation of folds on the lateral sides of the neck.[6] The webbing rarely causes functional limitation in range of motion, but is aesthetically and emotionally devastating for young girls (Figure 46.2).

ANESTHETIC MANAGEMENT

PREOPERATIVE EVALUATION

The severity of TS symptoms can range from mild to severe based on the aforementioned karyotype and phenotype presentations. Anesthesia providers should be aware of the various manifestations associated with TS. Many patients with mosaic forms of TS may not display the common external features associated with TS but may have cardiovascular or other body system involvement requiring specialized anesthetic care. Table 46.1 shows the various body systems potentially affected by TS, along with key points to consider during the preanesthetic evaluation. Airway assessment should include evaluation of a short neck and micrognathia in predicting laryngoscopy and endotracheal intubation challenges.[1] A shorter neck may also indicate the patient has a shorter trachea, making endobronchial intubation more likely.

Table 46.1 Turner's Syndrome Features and Associated Anesthetic Implications

Body System	Anatomical Features of Turner's Syndrome	Perioperative Anesthetic Considerations
Skeletal/growth	• Short stature • Short neck (80%) • Abnormal angulation of radius • Scoliosis, kyphosis, vertebral fusion • Webbed posterior neck (50%) • Low posterior hairline • Broad chest with widely spaced nipples (>80%); often pectus excavatum • Cubitus valgus or other elbow anomalies (>70%)	• Possible endobronchial intubation • Possible extubation with traction on endotracheal tube • Possible difficulty with spinal and epidural punctures • Possible difficulty placing arterial line
Cardiovascular	• Bicuspid aortic valve (30%) • Coarctation of the aorta (10%) • Valvular aortic stenosis • Mitral valve prolapse • Aortic dissection (later in life)	• Thorough preoperative history with ECG, TTE, and/or CT/CMR if indicated • Consider invasive BP monitoring to maintain tight BP control • Avoid ketamine and pancuronium with aortic malformations
Facies	• Micrognathia • Narrow maxilla/palate • Relatively small mandible (>70%) • Inner canthal folds (40%) • Anomalous auricles; most commonly prominent (>80%) • Perceptive hearing impairment (>50%)	• Possible difficult mask management • Possible difficult intubation; have LMA and advanced airway equipment in room at induction (video and fiberoptic laryngoscopes) • Difficulty communicating with patient
Lymphatic	• Congenital lymphedema with residual puffiness over the dorsum of fingers and toes	• Possible difficult IV catheter placement
Renal	• Horseshoe kidney (most common) • Double or cleft renal pelvis • Collecting system abnormalities	• Use caution with renally excreted drugs
Genital	• Ovarian dysgenesis with hypoplasia to absence of gonadal structures (>90%) • Lack of breast development	• Consider medication interactions with growth hormone and estrogen home medications
Endocrine	• Diabetes mellitus • Hypothyroidism • Tendency toward obesity	• Perioperative glucose monitoring if blood sugar is labile • Possible delayed emergence with hypothyroidism
Hepatic and gastrointestinal	• Hepatic steatosis, possible liver failure • Fatty liver • Increased incidence of GERD, celiac, and inflammatory bowel diseases	• Possible coagulation abnormalities • Possible increased liver enzymes • Consider decreased liver metabolism of drugs
Psychological/cognitive	• Mild to severe cognitive impairment with some mosaic karyotypes • Anxiety and/or depression related to body dysmorphia	• Use clear, concise explanations • Consider preoperative antianxiety medication when indicated

BP, blood pressure; CMR, cardiac magnetic resonance; GERD, gastroesophageal reflux disease; LMA, laryngeal mask airway; TTE, transthoracic echocardiogram.

Anesthesia providers should be aware that approximately 50% of live females with TS have congenital cardiac malformations, with bicuspid aortic valve and coarctation of the aorta being the most prevalent anomalies.[3] Aortic dilation has also been reported in TS, with multiple case reports of dissection or rupture.[7] Both of these present most frequently in TS females with a history of congenital lymphedema and subsequent webbed neck.[1] It is also important to recognize the potential for tracheobronchial compression resulting from aortic dilation or aneurysm.[7] Airway compression of any kind necessitates careful planning for induction of anesthesia as well as patient positioning before induction with anticipated compression when supine or with loss of airway tone. Structural abnormalities of the renal system are common (30%–40%) in both 45,XO and mosaic karyotypes.

Pertinent Labs

The International Turner Syndrome (ITS) Consensus Group recommends that all infants or children with suspected TS be examined with transthoracic echocardiography (TTE) at the time of diagnosis, even if there was a prior documented normal fetal echocardiogram or other postnatal cardiac examination.[3] It is also recommended that ECG and TTE, CT, or cardiac magnetic resonance (CMR) surveillance be performed every 5 years in TS children until 16 years of age and every 10 years thereafter.[3] In TS patients with hypertension or ischemic cardiopathy, a preoperative echocardiogram is suggested.[8] Although not commonly seen in childhood years, fatal aortic dissection (especially in the thoracic region) is six times more common in the TS population, occurring at an average age of 35 years old. Overall mortality in TS patients is most likely attributed to circulatory disease 41% of the time.[1]

Preoperative assessment lab work should include a full renal panel and management should be based on patient history, with special consideration of renally excreted drugs in the anesthetic care of affected patients.[4] Hepatic and endocrine involvement is less common in TS but, when present, can complicate anesthetic care significantly. Coagulation lab values should be evaluated in patients with hepatic involvement. If liver enzymes are elevated, TS patients may also have delayed metabolism of certain drugs. Short stature is a common feature in TS, resulting from delayed intrauterine growth, progressive growth slowing in late childhood, and absence of the normal rapid growth phase associated with puberty.[9] As such approximately 90% of TS children are taking hormone-based treatments such as oxandrolone (anabolic steroid), growth hormone, and estrogen to improve stature and overall growth, as well as to promote puberty and growth of hypoplastic breast, uterus, and vagina.[9] Anesthesia providers should be aware that hormone replacement therapy medications may have effects on liver function and bone density.[9]

PREOPERATIVE PHARMACOTHERAPY

Most TS patients have normal cognition, so careful explanations of all procedures can be helpful to ease preoperative anxiety in older children. Oral midazolam (.5 mg/kg) can be given to children exhibiting preoperative anxiety or to mitigate anticipated separation anxiety. There are no specific medication contraindications in patients with TS; however, the individual patient's history and symptoms should always be considered.

ANESTHETIC TECHNIQUE

Intraoperative Management

Both general and regional anesthesia are acceptable choices for patients with TS. Induction of anesthesia can be achieved via an inhalation mask induction or IV induction. Most IV and inhalation anesthetic and adjuvant medications are considered safe for patients with TS; however, pancuronium and ketamine should be avoided in patients with aortic malformations. Should regional anesthesia be utilized, dosing of local anesthetics for neuraxial and peripheral blocks should be based on lean body weight.[9] Spinal and epidural techniques may be more challenging in patients with TS who present with scoliosis.

The presence of a short and wide neck, mandibular hypoplasia, narrow palate, and temporomandibular contractures can contribute to difficulties with endotracheal intubation.[8,9] When a difficult intubation is anticipated, it is recommended an appropriately sized laryngeal mask airway, video laryngoscope, and/or a fiberoptic bronchoscope are readily available and in the room prior to the start of induction.[8] Endobronchial intubation and accidental extubation are more likely in patients with TS due to the presence of a short neck and higher tracheal bifurcation.[8] Endobronchial intubation should be suspected with any sudden increase in airway pressure, absence of breath sounds, or decreased oxygen saturation.[8] If tracheobronchial compression is suspected from aortic aneurysm, spontaneous breathing without muscle relaxation should be maintained whenever possible to prevent loss of airway tone.[7]

In addition to potential airway concerns, patients cardiac history, assessment, and preoperative test results should guide intraoperative anesthetic management. Intraoperative fluid management should take into consideration the presence of cardiac and/or renal dysfunction. Patients with aortic involvement and older patients with TS who present with hypertension and ischemic heart disease require careful management of their blood pressure (BP) during the anesthetic. In longer and more complicated cases, invasive BP monitoring should be considered. Right radial arterial pressure monitoring will aid in monitoring perfusion to the level of the aortic arch vessels.[7]

Sugammadex may interact with steroid and estrogen medications, although, due to its short half-life, no significant growth-related effects have been reported in patients taking these medications on a long-term basis.[10] In rare instances, estrogen compounds have been known to decrease pseudocholinesterase activity, leading to prolonged muscle paralysis from succinylcholine.[10]

POSTOPERATIVE CARE

The priority in postoperative care focuses on the management of pain without causing airway compromise. Use of nonnarcotic pain medications, such as acetaminophen, ketorolac, and local anesthesia, can prevent obstruction from oversedation. If narcotics are required, small doses of short-acting narcotics are best. It is also important to continue to assess for airway edema.

KEY REFERENCES

Complete references for this chapter are online and available at https://connect.springerpub.com/content/book/978-0-8261-3875-0/part/part03/toc-part/ch046.

2. Alvarez-Nava F, Lanes R. Epigenetics in Turner syndrome. *Clin Epigenetics*. 2018;1–20. doi:10.1186/s13148-018-0477-0
3. Gravholt C, Anderson N, Conway G, et al. Clinical practice guidelines for the care of girls and women with Turner syndrome: proceedings from the 2016 Cincinnati International Turner Syndrome Meeting. *Eur J Endocrinol*. 2017;177(3):G1–G70. doi:10.1530/EJE-17-0430
4. Mashour G, Sunder N, Acquadro M. Anesthetic management of Turner syndrome: a systematic approach. *J Clin Anesth*. 2005;17:128–130. doi:10.1016/j.jclinane.2004.06.010
8. Ornek D, Aydin G, Kahveci K, et al. Anesthetic management of a child with both Marfan syndrome and Turner syndrome. *J Anesth*. 2012;26:442–444. doi:10.1007/s00540-012-1332-7
9. Maranhao M. Turner syndrome and anesthesia. *Braz J Anesthesiol*. 2008;58(1):84–89. doi:10.1590/S0034-70942008000100012

CHAPTER 47

VACTERL Association

Angela Mund

PATHOPHYSIOLOGY AND CLINICAL MANIFESTATIONS

VATER association was original described in the 1970s. At that time VATER association was explained as a statistically nonrandom group of congenital malformations that included **V**ertebral anomalies, **A**nal atresia, **T**racheoesophageal fistula, **E**sophageal atresia, and **R**adial and **R**enal dysplasia.[1] Following the original description of VATER, additional anomalies were added and *VACTERL* is now the more accepted term. The additional criteria include **V**ascular defects, **C**ardiac malformations, and **L**imb anomalies.[1] VACTERL association occurs in approximately 1 per 10,000 to 40,000 live births. Although a detailed description of the epidemiology of VACTERL is beyond the scope of this overview, Solomon[1] describes the challenges in determining its true incidence due to differing diagnostic criteria and improvements in infant survivability, the lack of evidence regarding incidence in certain parts of the world or in specific ethnicities, and the need for improved delineation of the causes of VACTERL in order to analyze clusters of cases. Additionally, VACTERL association may go undiagnosed in children with fewer problems.

While the exact cause of VACTERL association is unknown, the result is an array of malformations witnessed in the early stages of embryonic development. In contrast to CHARGE * syndrome, which can be explained by a defect on the *CHD7* gene, VATER association is considered an association as there is not a single etiology responsible for the condition. In rare instances VACTERL association has been associated with gene alterations, including duplications or deletions, and mitochondrial dysfunction. Etiological theories include errors in key signaling pathways, environmental teratogens, and maternal diabetes.[1] VACTERL association is generally not a heritable disease, with the risk of recurrence in another child from the same parents being low. VACTERL association is slightly more common in males; however, no association with a specific geographic region or ethnic group has been identified.

VACTERL association is a diagnosis of exclusion, with additional laboratory and genetic tests useful in ruling out alternative diagnoses. Some malformations seen in VACTERL association might be identified prenatally during a prenatal ultrasound. At birth, a single umbilical artery is frequent in this patient population and may be one of the first diagnostic signs of VACTERL association.[1] Most clinicians require the presence of three or more components for diagnosis. Of note, there are several syndromes that share the components of VACTERL, including CHARGE syndrome, Feingold 's syndrome, and Fanconi anemia.[2] Solomon et al.[3] describe an algorithmic approach to the identification of the components of VACTERL that may provide clinicians and researchers with a more solid foundation for differential diagnosis and the establishment of the true incidence.

Vertebral anomalies are common (60%–95%) and may also be associated with rib defects. Chen et al.[9] divide the vertebral anomalies into "(a) failure of formation, such as hemivertebra, butterfly, or wedge–shaped vertebrae; (b) failure of segmentation, such as vertebral bars, fused vertebrae, and block vertebrae; or (c) a combination of these two defects." Abnormal spinal curvatures, including scoliosis, may be indicative of VACTERL association and may warrant vertebral imaging if not done previously with initial suspicion of the diagnosis. Tethered spinal cord may occur in conjunction with other caudal malformations, such as anorectal renal malformations (ARMs), and assessment of muscle tone should be conducted.[3] The other orthopedic defect, limb malformation, is found in 10% to 50% of patients and primarily affects the radius bone, thumb, and wrist.[1,3]

Genitourinary defects and/or ARMs are associated with most cases of VACTERL association. ARMs, including imperforate anus or anal atresia, are present in 55% to 90% of patients with VACTERL association.[1] An imperforate anus is typically found in the neonate and constitutes a surgical emergency. Anal atresia may not become evident until later in infancy, typically when clinically significant obstruction occurs or if there are issues with obtaining rectal temperature. Although not all studies have found a statistical connection between ARMs and renal malformations (RMs), these two malformations are commonly found concomitantly.[1,4] In addition, Lautz et al.[6] found that patients with ARM with VACTERL association were more likely to have vertebral defects. Cunningham et al.[4] found an overall incidence of RM of 69%, with the most common type being vesicoureteral reflux (VUR) plus a structural RM (27%). RMs range in severity and can include the presence of a single kidney, cystic or dysplastic, or horseshoe kidney.[1] Cunningham and Ahn noted that these results were similar to other studies in the presence of RM.[4,5] However, a statistically significant connection between ARM and RM was not found.[4] Ahn et al.[5] noted that VACTERL patients with RM, when compared with age-matched controls, developed end-stage renal disease more frequently, had more severe issues with dialysis, and had poorer outcomes following renal transplant.

Tracheoesophageal fistulas (TEF) and esophageal atresia (EA) are life-threatening emergencies that may occur in isolation or as a component of a syndrome or association and are frequently associated with cardiac anomalies.[2,6] The literature does not delineate which type of TEF is most common in patients with VACTERL; however, in patients with VACTERL association TEFs occur at a rate of 50% to 80%.[1] Although not currently a component of VACTERL association, anesthesia providers should be aware that airway and pulmonary anomalies may occur, especially if the patient has a diagnosis of TEF/EA. These pulmonary and airway manifestations include tracheal bronchus, supernumerary bronchus, bridging bronchus, tracheal stenosis, horseshoe lung, and even pulmonary agenesis.[7] Approximately 25% of cases of TEF/EA may be found prenatally and may necessitate immediate intubation or prompt surgical procedure following birth.[6] During prenatal

---

* CHARGE is an abbreviation for several of the features common in the disorder: coloboma, heart defects, atresia choanae (also known as choanal atresia), growth retardation, genital abnormalities, and ear abnormalities.

ultrasound polyhydramnios may be noted as the fetus is unable to swallow amniotic fluid and a gastric bubble may be absent.[1,3]

Cardiac malformations occur in 40% to 80% of patients with VACTERL association.[1] The severity of the congenital heart disease (CHD) present in patients with VACTERL association varies from mild to severe. Mild defects may go undiagnosed until the patient is an adult as the symptoms often do not become apparent until the patient ages (e.g., bicuspid aortic valve). Cardiac effects commonly seen with VACTERL association include atrial septal defects, ventricular septal defects (VSD), and bicuspid aortic valve, with VSD being the most common.[8] Vascular anomalies, such as a persistent left superior vena cava (PLSVC), may also be present. With PLSVC the left subclavian drains the left side of the head and neck directly into the coronary sinus, leading to dilation of the coronary sinus.[8]

In contrast to several congenital syndromes, patients with VACTERL do not have "facial dysmorphic features, learning disabilities, or abnormalities of growth, including head circumference."[2]

ANESTHETIC MANAGEMENT

PREOPERATIVE EVALUATION

Respiratory function should be thoroughly assessed preoperatively, with the need for chest radiographs and arterial blood gas measurement if pulmonary status is compromised. If the patient has a history of recurrent pneumonia and/or respiratory difficulties, it would be prudent to examine the airway prior to laryngoscopic manipulation.[7] A chest computed tomography (CT) scan may be useful to examine for the presence of abnormal bronchi. In patients with cardiac involvement, echocardiography should be reviewed to determine the presence of CHD and the degree of anatomical anomalies. An ECG should be reviewed to rule out the presence of dysrhythmias. If the anesthesia provider is considering placing a central venous catheter (CVC), ultrasonography should be used to evaluate for the presence of a PLSVC, which may complicate the placement of the CVC. A genitourinary screening ultrasound should be included during the evaluation of suspected VACTERL association due to the clinical implications of undiagnosed RM in both the infant and the adult.[4,7] Being undiagnosed has the potential to result in renal damage, insufficiency, and ultimately failure. Furthermore, if evidence of RM exists, a nephrology consult may be necessary to provide guidance on perianesthesia management. Preoperative laboratory studies are dependent on the presence and severity of each component of VACTERL as well as the complexity of the surgical procedure.

PREOPERATIVE PHARMACOLOGY

Preoperative medication is typically unnecessary. Should an anxiolytic or analgesic be required, however, it is imperative that medications and dosing preserve spontaneous ventilation and cardiac function.

ANESTHETIC TECHNIQUE

Intraoperative Management

While a variety of approaches have been employed regarding anesthetic management, however, general anesthesia remains the most common technique used due to the complexity of this patient population and the procedures being performed. Patients with TEF and/or EA present a risk of aspiration and should be treated as such with an rapid sequence intubation (RSI), prompt intubation, and visualization of the correct endotracheal tube placement. Anesthesia providers should be prepared to manage difficult ventilation and intubation scenarios and should have emergency airway equipment on hand prior to induction of anesthesia. This should include a variety of smaller than anticipated endotracheal tubes readily available, as well as a pediatric bronchoscope in the event of a difficult intubation. In the presence of significant cardiac and tracheoesophageal defects, additional monitoring modalities are reasonable and should be based on patient condition and complexity of surgery. Two pulse oximeters should be used in the presence of CHD, with a preductal and postductal placement of oximeters. Spontaneous ventilation should be maintained until the TEF is surgically closed. In patients with genitourinary, ARM, and TEF/EA defects, the anesthesia provider should evaluate for hypovolemia and cautiously implement appropriate fluid replacement. If the ARM has not been corrected, consider nasogastric/orogastric placement to decompress the stomach and prevent aspiration until an anoplasty or colostomy is performed.[3] The inability to pass an nasogastric (NG) or orogastric (OG) should lead to the evaluation of EA in patients with VACTERL.

Regional anesthesia may be more difficult due to the presence of abnormal vertebrae and spinal curvature, and it has been argued that regional anesthesia should be avoided in the presence of vertebral anomalies or ARM. If available, anesthesia providers should review imaging studies prior to insertion of a neuraxial block or to use real-time ultrasonography during placement.

POSTOPERATIVE CARE

If the complexity of the surgery or the need for postoperative ventilation occurs, plans should be made for postoperative admission to the ICU. In addition to respiratory support ad careful monitoring of the patient's volume status, pain must be adequately managed whether it be via regional anesthesia, IV opioids, use of non-opioid adjuncts, or a combination thereof.

REFERENCES

1. Solomon BD. VACTERL/VATER association. *Orphanet J Rare Dis*, 2011;6(1), 56–56. doi:10.1186/1750-1172-6-56
2. Shaw-Smith C. Oesophageal atresia, tracheo-oesophageal fistula, and the VACTERL association: review of genetics and epidemiology. *J Med Genet*. 2006;43(7):545–554. doi:10.1136/jmg.2005.038158
3. Solomon BD, Baker LA, Bear KA, et al. An approach to the identification of anomalies and etiologies in neonates with identified or suspected VACTERL (vertebral defects, anal atresia, tracheo-esophageal fistula with esophageal atresia, cardiac anomalies, renal anomalies, and limb anomalies) association. *J Pediatr*. 2014;164(3):451–457.e1. doi:10.1016/j.jpeds.2013.10.086
4. Cunningham BK, Khromykh A, Martinez AF, et al. Analysis of renal anomalies in VACTERL association. *Birth Defects Res A Clin Mol Teratol*. 2014;100(10):801–805. doi:10.1002/bdra.23302
5. Ahn SY, Mendoza S, Kaplan G, Reznik V. Chronic kidney disease in the VACTERL association: clinical course and outcome. *Pediatr Nephrol*. 2009;24(5):1047–1053. doi:10.1007/s00467-008-1101-x

6. Lautz TB, Mandelia A, Radhakrishnan J. VACTERL associations in children undergoing surgery for esophageal atresia and anorectal malformations: implications for pediatric surgeons. *J Pediatr Surg.* 2015;50(8):1245–1250. doi:10.1016/j.jpedsurg.2015.02.049
7. Yang L, Li S, Zhong L, et al. VACTERL association complicated with multiple airway abnormalities: a case report. *Medicine (Baltimore).* 2019;98(42):e17413. doi:10.1097/MD.0000000000017413
8. Cunningham BK, Hadley DW, Hannoush H, et al. Analysis of cardiac anomalies in VACTERL association. *Birth Defects Res A Clin Mol Teratol.* 2013;97(12):792–797. doi:10.1002/bdra.23211
9. Chen Y, Liu Z, Chen J, et al. The genetic landscape and clinical implications of vertebral anomalies in VACTERL association. *J Med Genet.* 2016;53(7):431–437. doi:10.1136/jmedgenet-2015-103554

CHAPTER 48

Williams Syndrome

Sean Barclay

PATHOPHYSIOLOGY AND CLINICAL MANIFESTATIONS

First described in 1961 by J.C.P. Williams, Williams syndrome, or Williams–Beuren syndrome, is a rare genetic disorder characterized by distinctive facial features that typically become more pronounced with age, cardiac defects, varying degrees of mental deficiency, and prenatal and postnatal growth retardation. The prevalence of Williams syndrome is 1 in every 10,000 to 20,000 live births, equally affecting both males and females.

Genes located within the 7q11.23 chromosomal region are largely implicated as having a causative role in the development of Williams syndrome. This primarily includes the *ELN* (elastin) gene, the *LIMK1* (or LIM kinase-1) gene, and the *RFC2* (replication factor C, subunit 2) gene. While most cases of Williams syndrome occur sporadically, familial Williams syndrome can result from deletions of contiguous genes located on the long arm (q) of chromosome 7 (7q11.23). When this occurs, Williams syndrome is inherited as an autosomal dominant trait.

Williams syndrome is often suspected based on the presence of characteristic clinical features. The diagnosis can be confirmed with the use of fluorescent in situ hybridization (FISH), which can detect specific microdeletions as chromosome 7q11.23. Additional testing may include evaluation of serum calcium levels as hypercalcemia is common with Williams syndrome. Likewise, x-rays may demonstrate increased calcification on the skull base, periorbital area, and vertebral plates.

The primary features commonly associated with Williams syndrome are directly related to variation in the genes located within the 7q11.23 chromosomal region. These include dysmorphic facial features, ELN arteriopathy, intellectual disability, short stature, connective tissue abnormalities, infantile hypercalcemia, and a unique personality/cognitive profile. Patients with Williams syndrome often have a broad forehead, epicanthal folds, short nose with a broad tip, long philtrum, a wide mouth with a thick vermillion of the lips, and mandibular hypoplasia. A starlike (stellate) pattern in the iris of the eye is present in approximately 50% of children with Williams syndrome. Congenital heart defects (CHD) occur in approximately 75% of children with Williams syndrome, with the most frequent defect being supravalvular aortic stenosis (SVAS). SVAS is a systemic ELN arteriopathy characterized by the narrowing of the aorta above the aortic valve. Additional CHDs associated with Williams syndrome include pulmonary artery stenosis and septal defects. Children with Williams syndrome typically have a personality that is friendly, outgoing, and/or talkative, although anxiety is common.

Patients with Williams syndrome often have sensory modulation impairments, with delays noted in gross and fine motor development. In addition, the frequency of sensorineural hearing loss is high, or conversely they may be extremely sensitive to sound and may overreact to unusually loud or high-pitched sounds. The development of secondary sexual characteristics may also occur prematurely. Additional abnormalities routinely witnessed include renal abnormalities, chronic urinary tract infections, a hypoplastic thyroid gland, and the presence of umbilical or inguinal hernias.

ANESTHETIC MANAGEMENT

PREOPERATIVE EVALUATION

A preoperative anesthesia consult 1 to 2 weeks prior to surgery is recommended to allow ample time for all necessary evaluation and testing. The preanesthetic evaluation should be comprehensive and include a thorough review of all available diagnostic testing and prior anesthetic records. Cardiac assessments should screen for symptoms of myocardial ischemia, such as perspiration with feeds or dyspnea with feeding. Similarly, failure to thrive, may be present in infants with active ischemia.

It is imperative the preoperative management of children with Williams syndrome incorporates a multidisciplinary team approach. An evaluation by an endocrinologist is advisable as patients with Williams syndrome are prone to idiopathic hypercalcemia, hypercalciuria, failure to thrive, early puberty, and subclinical hypothyroidism. Additional recommended consults include cardiology, gastroenterology, otolaryngology, surgery, and possibly psychiatry and child life to assist with inherent anxiety issues commonly witnessed in patients with Williams syndrome.

Pertinent Labs

Prior to surgery, all patients with Williams syndrome should have an ECG performed, and possibly an echocardiogram depending on the severity of CHD. An ECG should be performed to rule out left ventricular hypertrophy (LVH), ST-T wave abnormalities, and prolonged QTc, all of which may be indicative of latent ischemia. An echocardiogram should be obtained to assess the degree of left ventricular hypotrophy, the severity of supravalvular aortic or pulmonary stenosis, the patency of coronary orifices, and the presence of abnormalities in wall motion. Based on the patient's medical history, a coronary angiogram may be indicated; however, the risks and benefits of an additional anesthetic should be considered.

Testing for hypercalcemia is recommended every 2 years by the American Academy of Pediatrics, and a thyroid test should be available and repeated if signs of hypothyroidism are present. Ultrasound studies of the renal arteries can be helpful in determining the extent of renal artery stenosis in patients with known renal abnormalities.

PREOPERATIVE PHARMACOLOGY

Many patients with Williams syndrome have a history of QTc prolongation. Treatment for this commonly entails beta-blocker therapy, which should be continued prior to surgery.[1] It is also recommended that adequate levels of hydration be maintained up until 2 hours prior to the induction of anesthesia to limit hemodynamic variability following induction.

Many patients with Williams syndrome present with attention deficit disorder (ADD) and anxiety. Moreover, many patients with Williams syndrome have some degree of developmental delay, which can make even painless procedures unattainable without sedation. As such, the use of a preoperative anxiolytic may be warranted.

ANESTHETIC TECHNIQUE

Intraoperative Management

While there is no contraindication to general anesthesia, it is imperative anesthesia providers are aware of the heightened incidence of sudden death in patients with Williams syndrome while under general anesthesia. The risk of sudden cardiac death in this population has been reported to be 25 to 100 times greater than that of the general population.[2] This is almost entirely due to myocardial ischemia, in conjunction with SVAS and stenosis of the coronary ostia. Although Williams syndrome is not associated with coronary artery disease, greater than 5% have coronary ostial stenosis. It has also been offered that sudden cardiac death in patients with Williams syndrome is due to an allergic coronary syndrome following exposure to anesthetics.

The most prominent risk factors for sudden death include young age, use of sedation and/or anesthesia, history of biventricular outflow tract obstruction, and presence of coronary artery stenosis. Individually, each of these risk factors contributes to decreased cardiac output, myocardial ischemia, and arrhythmias. Therefore, the goal of anesthesia providers caring for patients with Williams syndrome should be the maintenance of an age-appropriate heart rate, sinus rhythm, preload, contractility, and systemic vascular resistance, as well as pulmonary vascular resistance. Maintenance of these norms should continue throughout the preoperative, intraoperative, and postoperative period.

Several anesthetic agents are known to cause direct myocardial depression, reduced systemic vascular resistance, or increased myocardial oxygen consumption and should be avoided to decrease the likelihood of perioperative ischemia. The cardiovascular effects of common anesthetic medications are reviewed in Table 48.1. Ultimately, employing a balanced anesthetic that reduces myocardial oxygen consumption and minimize reductions in systemic vascular resistance is ideal.

Table 48.1	Cardiovascular Effects of Common Anesthetics				
Drug	SVR	Myocardial Depression	Tachycardia and Increased Myocardial Oxygen Consumption	Dysrhythmias	Respiratory Depression With Possible Reduced Oxygen Delivery
Propofol	↓↓		—	—	↓↓
Inhalation anesthetics (sevoflurane, isoflurane, desflurane)	↓↓	↓	—	—	↓↓
Barbiturates (thiopental, pentobarbital)	↓↓	↓	—	—	↓↓
Ketamine	—	—	↑↑	↑↑	—
Chloral hydrate	—	—	↑	↑↑	↓
Benzodiazepines (midazolam, lorazepam)	↓	↓	—	—	↓↓
Etomidate	—	—	—	—	↓

SVR, systemic vascular resistance.

Source: From Matisoff AJ, Olivieri L, Schwartz JM, Deutsch N. Risk assessment and anesthetic management of patients with Williams syndrome: a comprehensive review. *Pediatr Anesth.* 2015;25(12):1207–1215. doi:10.1111/pan.12775.

When possible, a peripheral IV catheter should be placed preoperatively to facilitate both preoperative hydration and IV induction. Inhalation mask inductions should be reserved for patients presumed to be at low or moderate risk of cardiovascular compromise. Standard monitors, as described by the American Society of Anesthesiologists, should be employed. Should significant extreme variability in hemodynamic parameters be anticipated, placement of an arterial line may be considered. In addition to standard resuscitation medications, vasopressors such as phenylephrine and vasopressin should be immediately available and used as first-line agents to treat hypotension and ST-T wave changes, which may be indicative of myocardial ischemia. It is essential that anesthesia providers are vigilant and promptly treat any ST-T wave changes. Furthermore, it is recommended that extracorporeal membrane oxygenation (ECMO) be deployed early should standard resuscitation measures prove inadequate or unsuccessful.

As many patients with Williams syndrome have a prolonged QTc at baseline, administration of medications that enhance QTc prolongation should be eliminated or avoided when possible. Medications capable of QTc prolongation include sevoflurane, vecuronium, and fentanyl, all of which have the potential to increase QTc during the induction phase of anesthesia.

In addition to the significant cardiac concerns, anesthesia providers should be aware that the presence of a small mandible and dental anomalies may make tracheal intubation difficult. Additionally, in older patients with progressive joint mobility limitations, positioning may be challenging and a concerted effort should be made to ensure the patient is adequately padded.

Special Considerations/Concerns

Williams syndrome is associated with an untoward cardiovascular response to general anesthesia due to ELN arteriopathy, which can cause SVAS. SVAS can result in left ventricular outflow obstruction leading to LVH. SVAS is present in approximately 70% of patients and requires surgical correction in approximately 30% of patients before the age of 5 years.[1] In addition, supravalvular pulmonary stenosis can occur with SVAS.

POSTOPERATIVE CARE

Postoperatively, patients with Williams syndrome should be extubated awake and transported to the postanesthesia care unit for continued observation. The postanesthesia disposition of same-day surgical patients with Williams syndrome remains controversial as there is no universally agreed upon protocol. However, given the potential for sudden cardiac death, patients should be monitored for at least 6 hours following anesthesia, and preferably overnight, prior to discharge. The focus of care is largely supportive, although postoperative pain should be aggressively managed to limit shivering and stave off increases in oxygen consumption.

REFERENCES

1. Collins RT, Kaplan P, Somes GW, Rome JJ. Cardiovascular abnormalities, interventions, and long-term outcomes in infantile Williams syndrome. *J Pediatr*. 2010;156(2):253–258.e1. doi:10.1016/j.jpeds.2009.08.042
2. Burch Thomas M, McGovan Jr FX, Kussman BD, et al. Congenital supravalvular aortic stenosis and sudden death associated with anesthesia: what's the mystery? *Anesth Analg*. 2008;107(6)1848–1854. doi:10.1213/ane.0b013e3181875a4d
3. Matisoff AJ, Olivieri L, Schwartz JM, Deutsch N. Risk assessment and anesthetic management of patients with Williams syndrome: a comprehensive review. *Pediatr Anesth*. 2015;25(12):1207–1215. doi:10.1111/pan.12775
4. Bird Lynne M, Billman GF, Lacro RV, et al. Sudden death in Williams syndrome: report of ten cases. *J Pediatr*. 1996;129(6):926–931. doi:10.1016/s0022-3476(96)70042-2
5. Medley J, Russo P, Tobias JD. Perioperative care of the patient with Williams syndrome. *Pediatr Anesth*. 2005;15(3):243–247. doi:10.1111/j.1460-9592.2004.01567.x
6. Twite MD, Stenquist S, Ing RJ. Williams syndrome. *Pediatr Anesth*. 2019;29(5):483–490. doi:10.1111/pan.13620
7. Williams syndrome (Williams-Beuren syndrome, WMS). In: *SpringerReference*. Springer-Verlag; 2011. doi:10.1007/springerreference_108587

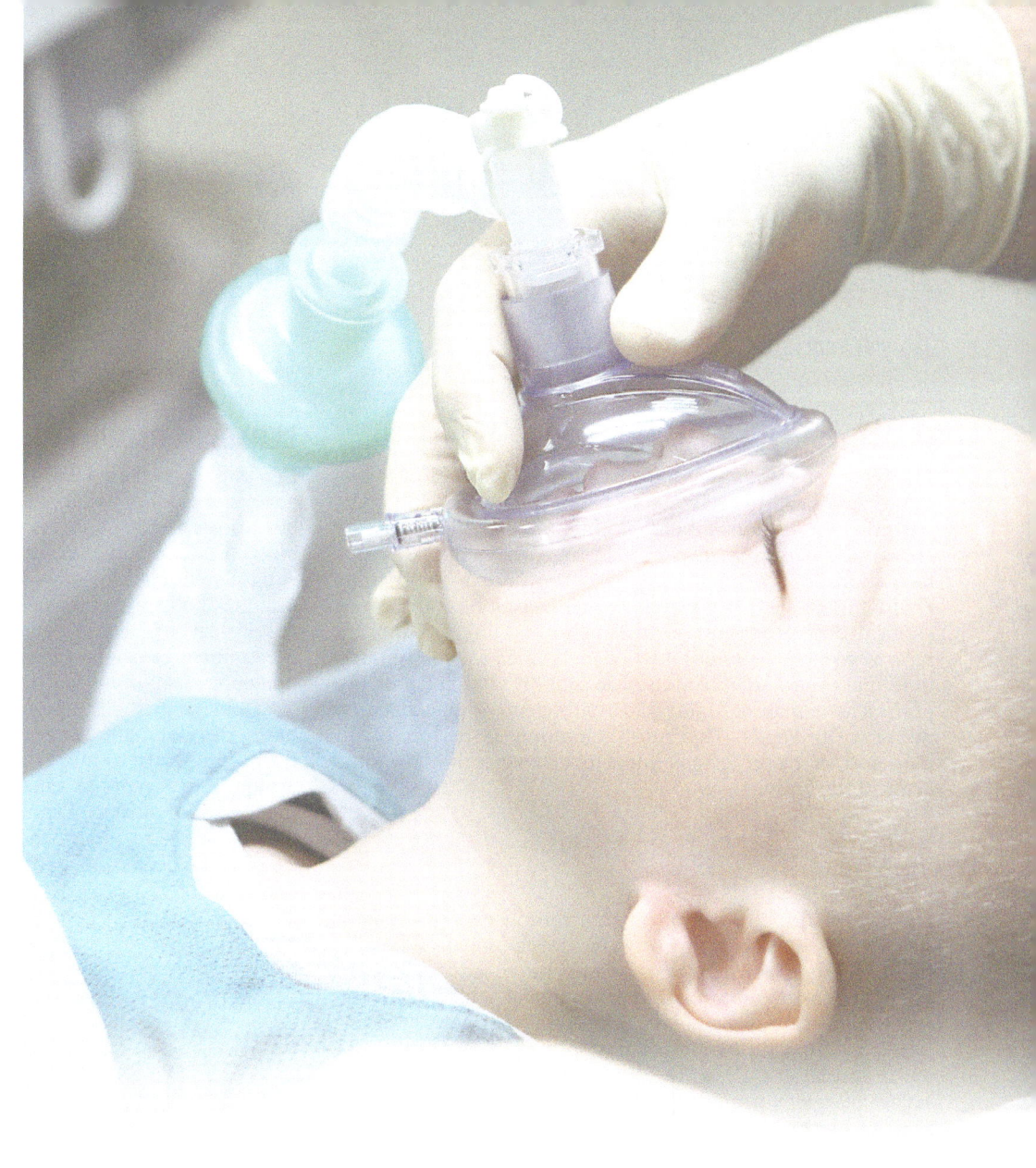

PART IV | **COMMON PROCEDURES IN PEDIATRIC ANESTHETIC CARE**

SECTION A: Neurosurgical Procedures

CHAPTER 49

Craniotomy

Jennifer Parks

INDICATIONS/CONTRAINDICATIONS

The term *craniotomy* refers to the surgical removal of a section of the skull to facilitate access to the intracranial compartment. Indications for craniotomy in the pediatric patient are wide-ranging and can include intracranial vascular formations, intracranial tumors, neurotrauma, ventricular shunt procedures, craniosynostosis correction, and craniocervical decompression (Chiari malformation).[1-4] Although rare, awake craniotomies may be performed as well to facilitate mapping and resection of lesions in vital areas of the brain where imaging is not able to sufficiently define the area necessary to resect. This most commonly is performed to map and/or resect lesions impacting the speech and motor areas of the brain.

SPECIAL CONSIDERATIONS AND CONCERNS

During the first 2 years of life, the central nervous system experiences significant growth and development. Typically, infants are born with fontanelles and cranial sutures that are open and remain so until 2 years of age at which point the fontanelles close and cranial sutures fuse.[1] The conus medullaris and dural sac also change with time, moving from L2 to L3 and S3 at birth to the adult location of L1 and S1 by 1 year of age. Normal intracranial pressure (ICP) in premature and term infants is lower than that of older children, ranging from 2 to 6 mm Hg. This increases in time reaching the normal adult range of 0 to 15 mm Hg early in childhood (**Figure 49.1**).[1]

Anesthesia providers should be aware that as the neonatal cranial vault is still developing, a slow-growing tumor or insidious hemorrhage may be masked by a compensatory rise in intracranial volume.[1] Therefore, while the fontanelles remain open and the sutures have not closed, increases in ICP occur slower than in an adult patient. However, a massive intracranial hemorrhage or an acute obstruction in cerebrospinal fluid (CSF) flow may place the pediatric patient's life in danger as the cranial vault cannot accommodate for the rapid shift in volume. Additionally, the pediatric patient has a higher ratio of brain water content, less CSF volume, and a higher ratio of brain content to intracranial capacity placing them at greater risk of herniation compared to their adult counterparts.[1]

CEREBROSPINAL FLUID

The choroid plexus is responsible for production of CSF, which is then absorbed by the body through the arachnoid villi and ependymal lining of the ventricles. As ICP increases, the rate of CSF reabsorption also increases. This process can be altered by disease states, such as intracranial tumors, infection, hemorrhage, or congenital malformations that may result in decreased CSF reabsorption leading to an elevated ICP. Of note, the volume of CSF is 4 mL/kg in infants and neonates, whereas the adult volume is 2 mL/kg.[1]

CEREBRAL BLOOD FLOW

Cerebral blood flow (CBF) is influenced by a number of mechanisms, including metabolism, partial pressure of arterial carbon dioxide ($PaCO_2$), partial pressure of oxygen in arterial blood (PaO_2), blood viscosity, and cerebral autoregulation. CBF is tightly coupled to cerebral metabolism, as well as the cerebral metabolic rate of oxygen ($CMRO_2$), at both a global and a regional level. CBF and metabolism coupling is the most crucial determinant of cerebral circulation. Thankfully, this is a phenomenon that is preserved during sleep and general anesthesia.[1]

CBF changes with age at a rate that parallels the rate of brain development: increasing in childhood and peaking during the early to mid-childhood years, before leveling off around 7 to 8 years of age.[1] Similarly, CBF accounts for 10% to 20% of the cardiac output in infants up to 6 months of age. CBF increases to 55% of the cardiac output in children aged 2 to 4 years, decreasing to the adult level of 15% by 7 to 8 years of age.[3]

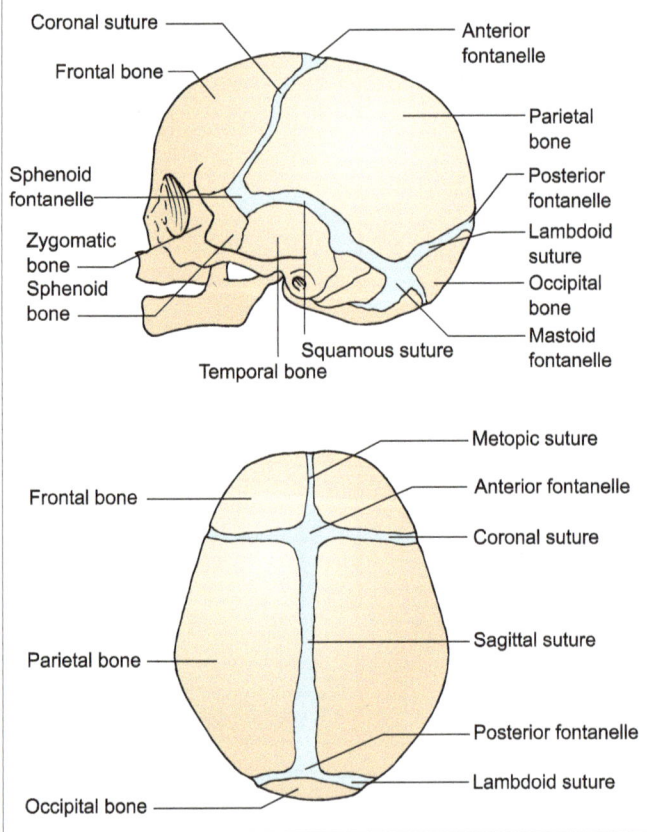

Figure 49.1: Cranial sutures and fontanelles in neonates and infants.

Source: From Bordelon C, Fanning B, Meredith J, Jnah AJ. The nervous system. In: Jnah AJ, Trembath AN, eds. *Fetal and Neonatal Physiology for the Advanced Practice Nurse*. Springer Publishing Company; 2018: Figure 3.13.

Cerebral autoregulation is maintained by dilation and constriction of arterioles over a range of blood pressures.[1] While children as young as 6 months can maintain autoregulation as well as their adult counterparts, it remains unclear if children younger than 6 months have this ability. Therefore, 6 months of age is considered the lower limit of autoregulation.[1] Anesthesia providers should be aware that a linear correlation between CBF and systolic blood pressure exists in critically ill neonates who are of low gestational age and birth weight. Therefore, close control of blood pressures in this patient population is paramount to prevent cerebral ischemia and intraventricular hemorrhage during craniotomy.[3]

ANESTHETIC MANAGEMENT

PREOPERATIVE EVALUATION

As with any surgical procedure, a complete preoperative evaluation should occur prior to inducing general anesthesia. Pediatric patients are commonly associated with cardiac and respiratory events perioperatively, making it prudent to conduct a thorough preoperative airway, respiratory, and cardiac evaluation.[3] There are several key aspects to vet in children who present for craniotomy given the breadth of indications. For example, children with congenital anomalies of facial anatomy require a thorough airway evaluation to determine the need for advanced airway techniques to ensure safe airway management. Similarly, a child with an enlarged occiput secondary to hydrocephalus may have exaggerated neck flexion when placed in the supine position. However, neurosurgical procedures in the pediatric patient may be urgent, decreasing the time available to perform assessment.

Pertinent Labs

Craniotomy procedures can be associated with significant blood loss, and it is important to evaluate the patient's hematologic status during the preoperative assessment. Anesthesia providers should consider obtaining the following labs: hematocrit, prothrombin time, and partial thromboplastin time. Patients with large tumors or with vascular malformations should have a preoperative type and screen, as well as cross-matching.[1] Patients on long-term anticonvulsant therapy may require evaluation of liver function, and an endocrinology consultation may also be helpful in patients with suprasellar lesions.[3]

CT and MRI studies are helpful in confirming the location of intracranial lesions, as well as determining the presence of hydrocephalus, midline shifts, and compressed cisterns.[1] The child with a brainstem lesion may present with respiratory distress, impaired gag and swallowing reflexes, and aspiration. Preoperative neurological evaluation should include level of consciousness (LOC), motor and sensory examination, presence of reflexes, cranial nerve function, and signs and symptoms of increased ICP.[1]

PREOPERATIVE PHARMACOLOGY

For the pediatric craniotomy patient, anesthesia providers should select medications for induction and maintenance of anesthesia that preserve cerebral autoregulation and metabolic coupling (Table 49.1). Midazolam may decrease anxiety and facilitate separation in pediatric patients presenting for craniotomy; however, it should be administered judiciously. To prevent a neurologically impaired child from becoming obtunded, preoperative sedation should be administered in a location where the patient can be closely monitored for neurological and respiratory status changes. Narcotics are not recommended preoperatively as they can promote the development of nausea and vomiting.[1]

ANESTHETIC TECHNIQUE

Intraoperative Management

The primary goal of anesthesia providers during induction is to minimize large increases in ICP. Propofol and thiopental preserve autoregulation and coupling, as well as decrease $CMRO_2$, CBF, and ICP.[1] However, in neonates, propofol may cause hypotension for up to 30 minutes after administration.[3]

Table 49.1 The Effect of Common Anesthetic Agents on Cerebral Hemodynamics

Inhaled Agents	MAP	CBF	CPP	ICP	$CMRO_2$	SSEPs Amplitude / Latency	CSF Production	CSF Reabsorption
Halothane	θ	↑↑↑	↓	↑↑	↓↓	↓/↑	θ	↓
Isoflurane	↓↓	↑	↓	↑	↓↓↓	↓/↑	θ	↑
Sevoflurane	↓↓	↑	θ↓	θ↑	↓↓↓	↓/↑	↓	↓
Desflurane	↓↓	↑	↓	↑	↓	↓/↑	θ	θ
N_2O	θ↓	↑–↑↑	↓	↑–↑↑	↑↓	↓/θ↑	θ	θ
IV Agents								
Thiopental	↓↓	↓↓↓	↑↑↑	↓↓↓	↓↓↓	↓/↑	↓↑	↑
Propofol	↓↓↓	↓↓↓	↑↑	↓↓	↓↓↓	↑/↑	↓↑	↑
Etomidate	θ↓	↓↓↓	↑↑	↓↓↓	↓↓↓	↑/↑	↓↑	↑
Ketamine	↑↑	↑↑↑	↓	↑↑↑	↑	↑/θ	↓↑	↓
Benzodiazepines	θ↓	↓↓	↑	θ	↓↓	↓ θ/↑		↑
Opioids	θ↓	↓	↓↑	θ↓	↓	↓/↑	↓↑	

↑, increase; ↓, decrease; θ, little or no change; CBF, cerebral blood flow; CSF, cerebrospinal fluid; $CMRO_2$, cerebral metabolic rate of oxygen; CPP, cerebral perfusion pressure; ICP, intracranial pressure; MAP, mean arterial pressure; N2O, nitrous oxide; SSEPs, somatosensory evoked potentials.

Source: Fom Vavilala MS, Soriano SG, Krane EJ. Anesthesia for neurosurgery. In: Davis PJ, Cladis FP, eds. *Smith's Anesthesia for Infants and Children*. Elsevier; 2017.

Subanesthetic doses of barbiturates have not been found to significantly alter CBF or cerebral metabolism.[1]

Rapid sequence induction is often recommended as neurologically compromised patients may have altered mental status and are at risk of aspiration. Succinylcholine causes increases in CBF and ICP; however, this increase may be attenuated by the administration of a prefasiculating dose of a nondepolarizing neuromuscular blocking drug.[1] In patients with neuromuscular disease states, such as central nervous system disorders, closed head injuries, cerebral hypoxia from near drowning, subarachnoid hemorrhage, encephalitis, cerebrovascular accidents, and paraplegia, succinylcholine is often contraindicated as upregulated acetylcholine receptors may cause hyperkalemia. This condition may occur within 24 to 48 hours after the injury or insult, and can last up to 2 years.[1] Additionally, these patients may be resistant to the effects of nondepolarizing neuromuscular blocking drugs and require larger doses to achieve desired muscle relaxation. The acute administration of anticonvulsants can enhance nondepolarizing neuromuscular blockade as well and can delay their reversal. Conversely, chronic administration of anticonvulsants in the pediatric patient can cause an increase metabolism of nondepolarizing neuromuscular blocking drugs secondary to the upregulation in enzymes responsible for metabolism of anticonvulsants.

Children with an enlarged occiput secondary to hydrocephalus may be obstructive or difficult to ventilate once anesthesia is induced. Thus, placing folded blankets, towels, or other support under the shoulders can improve neck alignment, improve mask ventilation, and promote visualization of airway anatomy during direct laryngoscopy.

Volatile anesthetic agents are potent cerebral vasodilators and may produce uncoupling of $CMRO_2$ and CBF, which can lead to increased cerebral blood volume and increased intracranial hypertension. Volatile anesthetic agents cause dose-dependent blunting of autoregulation, which can be mitigated by hypocapnia. In neurocompromised patients, isoflurane and sevoflurane are preferred as they decrease $CMRO_2$ in pediatric patients and maintain coupling.[1]

Opioids have not been found to significantly modify cerebral hemodynamics or ICP unless there is respiratory depression or increased $PaCO_2$. Fentanyl combined with nitrous oxide (N_2O), can decrease CBF by 47% and $CMRO_2$ by 18%; however, it can reduce the rate of CSF reabsorption by 50%. Anesthesia providers should be aware, however, that fentanyl causes dose-dependent EEG slowing, which may impact neuromonitoring.[1]

Drugs, such as sodium nitroprusside, adenosine, nitroglycerine (NTG), diazoxide, hydralazine, and adenosine triphosphate (ATP), are cerebral vasodilators and can decrease CBF and ICP.[1] Calcium channel blockers can increase CBF and ICP; therefore, ICP should be monitored during administration of these drugs during surgery. Trimethaphan, propranolol, esmolol, and labetalol do not raise CBF or ICP and are beneficial in controlling blood pressure in patients with increased ICP. Sodium nitroprusside, however, maintains CBF, brain O_2 tension, neuronal function, and brain metabolism better than trimethaphan and is the recommended agent for intraoperative blood pressure reduction.[1]

POSTOPERATIVE CARE

Postoperatively, patients will require frequent assessment and neurocognitive checks to assess for alterations in mental

---

CASE STUDY: A Female With Posterior Fossa Tumor

CLINICAL SCENARIO

Your first case of the day is a 5-year-old female patient scheduled for craniotomy for resection of a posterior fossa tumor. A preoperative anesthesia history was completed, revealing a medical history of new onset of headaches, nausea, vomiting, and ataxia. There are no known drug allergies, and the patient weighs 18 kg. Her surgical history includes a bilateral myringotomy and tube placement at age 16 months, without any complications. Upon arrival to the preoperative area, the preoperative nurse assigned to the patient communicates that the patient begins crying when "anyone dressed in scrubs" approaches her. Her vital signs are as follows: blood pressure 96/45, heart rate 111, respiratory rate 26, and temperature 36.8°C. The patient has been NPO after midnight; however, parents report nausea and vomiting this morning. A right-hand 22-gauge IV is in situ.

SPECIAL CONSIDERATIONS

Anesthetic plan: Perform a baseline neurological examination. Preoperative sedation with IV midazolam may aid in mitigating preoperative anxiety and facilitate separation from parents. Intraoperative monitoring includes standard monitors, along with consideration for arterial line and ICP monitoring. As the patient is currently experiencing nausea and vomiting, plan for a rapid-sequence induction with suction readily available. Brain tumor resection may be associated with significant blood loss. Evaluate existing IV catheter to ensure patency and consider second IV placement after induction in the event volume resuscitation is needed. Obtain and evaluate preoperative labs, including hematocrit, type and screen, and blood cross-matching, as well as any preoperative imaging. The prone position presents challenges to the anesthesia provider. Carefully pad pressure points and make sure eyes are free from pressure. Ensure endotracheal tube and anesthesia breathing circuit connections are secure. As the operating room table may be turned away from the anesthesia machine and provider, consider IV and anesthesia breathing circuit extensions.

COMPLICATIONS

While there were no complications, the patient was transported to the pediatric intensive care unit for postoperative monitoring and management.

status. It is important that the use of opioids and anxiolytics be minimized to avoid sedation precluding assessment. Radiographic studies, such as CT scans, are common to assess for bleeding or edema postoperatively. Should the patient not be alert enough, or able to comply with a neurological examination immediately following extubation, a CT scan or MRI may be performed emergently to assess hemorrhage or edema. In addition to frequent neurological assessment, it is important to assess for known complications, such as intermittent apnea, vocal cord paralysis, and an irregular respiratory pattern.[3]

REFERENCES

1. Vavilala MS, Soriano SG, Krane EJ. Anesthesia for neurosurgery. In: Davis PJ, Cladis FP, eds. *Smith's Anesthesia for Infants and Children.* Elsevier; 2017.
2. Jaffe RA, Schmiesing CA, Golianu B. *Anesthesiologist's Manual of Surgical Procedures.* Wolters Kluwer; 2020.
3. Soriano SG, McManus ML. Pediatric neuroanesthesia and critical care. In: Cottrell JE, Patel P, eds. *Cottrell and Patel's Neuroanesthesia.* 6th ed. Elsevier; 2017:337–350.
4. Rajan S, Rao S. Fluid and blood transfusion in pediatric neurosurgery. In: Prabhakar H, ed. *Essentials of Neuroanesthesia.* Academic Press/Elsevier; 2017:643–651.

CHAPTER 50

Ventriculoperitoneal Shunt Placement

Amanda Ford

INDICATIONS/CONTRAINDICATIONS

Cerebrospinal fluid (CSF) levels are typically maintained by steady rates of production and reabsorption in the brain. When an imbalance is present, an overabundance of CSF may warrant surgical intervention with placement of an external ventricular drain (EVD; see Figure 50.1) or a more permanent ventriculoperitoneal (VP) shunt. Anesthetic considerations for both procedures are similar, although an EVD can be placed emergently at bedside if the patient's condition warrants immediate action.

Common indications for an EVD include traumatic brain injury, or contraindication to a VP shunt itself (e.g., infection). Most modern shunts include one-way valves and have adjustable pressure mechanisms so that they may be easily adjusted. Manufacturers also provide the option for antibiotic-impregnated catheters that can be paired with the actual shunt mechanism.[1] Indications for VP shunt placement include hydrocephalus, Dandy–Walker syndrome, craniosynostosis, intraventricular or subarachnoid hemorrhage, and/or tumors affecting CSF flow.

An absolute contraindication for VP shunt placement is an infection at the insertion site. Relative contraindications include patient instability for operating room (OR) transport (consider bedside EVD placement) and coagulopathies.[2]

SPECIAL CONSIDERATIONS AND CONCERNS

The proximal end of a VP shunt can be placed into any ventricle (lateral, third, or fourth), with the right lateral

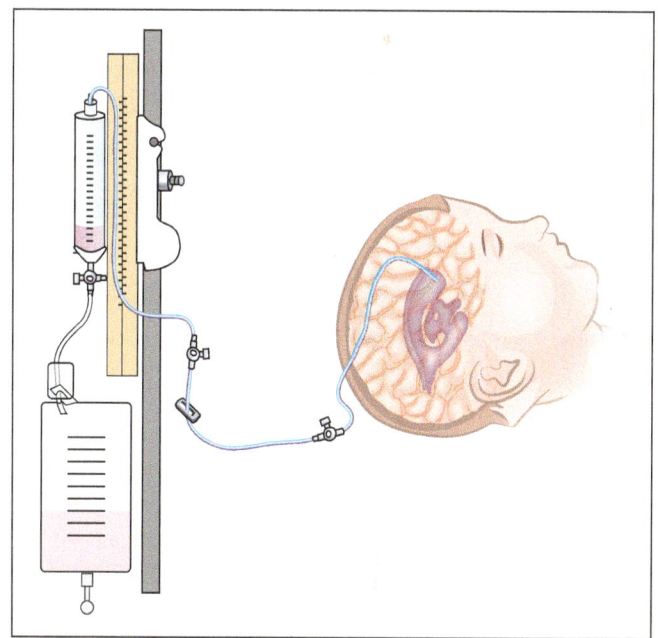

Figure 50.1: Externalized ventricular drain.

ventricle being the most common placement. The distal end is traditionally placed into the peritoneum of the abdomen, where the cells will absorb the CSF diverted from the cerebral flow tract via the shunt. Alternate distal site locations include the atrium (ventriculoatrial [VA] shunt), chest cavity, or bladder. In addition, some premature infants may require a temporary subgaleal shunt (distal end in the scalp) until they are large enough to tolerate a standard type of shunt discussed earlier.[3] Endoscopic third ventriculostomies are now also being performed by inserting a balloon tip catheter to divert CSF flow through the third ventricle into the basal cisterns.[2] For further information regarding the anesthetic management of the child presenting for a third ventriculostomy, refer to Chapter 57, "Third Ventriculostomy."

ANESTHETIC MANAGEMENT

PREOPERATIVE EVALUATION

Key preoperative assessment points are summarized in Table 50.1.

PREOPERATIVE PHARMACOLOGY

It is prudent that anesthesia providers verify administration of any anticonvulsant and/or steroid medication prior to the procedure. In addition, care should be given to the choice of fluids during the perioperative period as 0.9% normal saline is typically the preferred choice for maintenance fluid. Regardless, it is important to avoid hypotonic solutions in an effort to avoid increasing the intracranial pressure (ICP) as hypotonic solutions move water from the extracellular space to the intracellular space.

The anesthetic should be tailored to avoid increases in ICP whether that be from medication administration or an anesthetic technique standpoint. For example, consider that sevoflurane increases cerebral blood flow less than all other inhalation agents, while all inhaled agents reduce the cerebral metabolic rate. In addition, avoid ketamine due to a potential increase in ICP given the potential for increases in cerebral blood flow and cerebral metabolic rate following administration.[4] Consider preoperative patient-specific dosing of an anxiolytic, such as midazolam (oral or IV routes) after a baseline neurological examination has been completed. Midazolam can decrease cerebral blood flow and metabolic rate (and therefore ICP) but may cause an increase in drowsiness.

Table 50.1	Key Assessment Points With VP Shunts
Medications	Preoperative medications, such as anticonvulsants and/or steroids should typically be continued
Neurological Examination	Baseline neurological examination is important. Common symptoms may include headache, nausea/vomiting, drowsiness, papilledema (general increased ICP symptoms); wide age range for procedure will affect developmentally appropriate neurological examination (e.g., fontanelle assessment is essential in neonates)
Cardiovascular Examination	Caution for increased blood pressure with decreased heart rate (increased ICP—Cushing's response)
Labs	CBC with platelets, electrolyte panel (especially sodium level)

CBC, complete blood count. ICP, intracranial pressure; VP, ventriculoperitoneal.

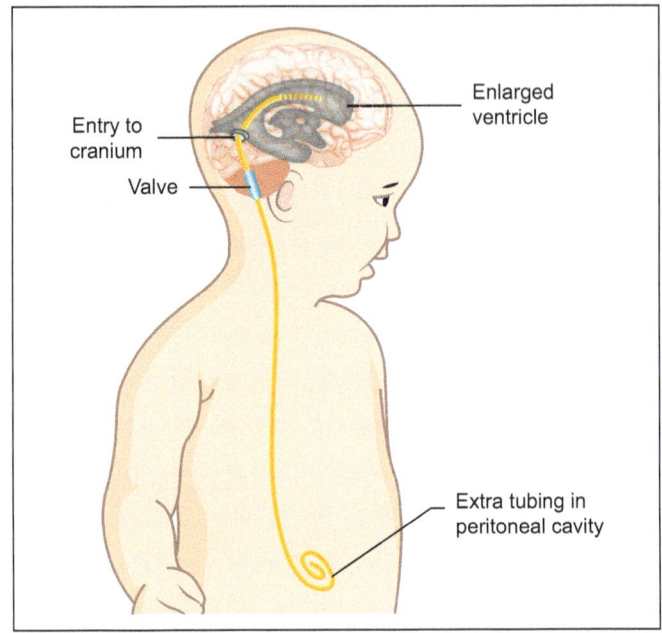

Figure 50.2: Ventriculoperitoneal shunt.

In this ventriculoperitoneal shunt placement, the valve is placed into the subgaleal space behind the ear, with the remainder of the shunt tubing tunneled down the neck and chest, where it resides in the peritoneum.

ANESTHETIC TECHNIQUE

Intraoperative Management

Induction of general anesthesia will be performed in the OR as either a standard pediatric mask inhalational induction (if no venous access is available), or standard IV induction if a

Table 50.2	Special Techniques
Mild hyperventilation	Maintain $PaCO_2$/$ETCO_2$ 30–35 mm Hg to decrease cerebral blood flow and intracranial pressure. Each 1 mm Hg decrease change in $PaCO_2$ leads to a 4% decrease in cerebral blood flow.[5]
Maintain autoregulation	Autoregulation limits for neonates are approximately 40–120 mm Hg and adults are 60–160 mm Hg. Hypertension can lead to hemorrhage, while hypotension could lead to ischemia. Remember that autoregulation remains intact at 1 MAC.[4]
Field avoidance	Ensure connections on endotracheal tube and circuit are tight since the provider will not have access to the patient's head during procedure. Consider extension tubing for anesthesia circuit.
Smooth extubation	Deep extubation is possible if patient condition warrants this technique, but be cautious of increased CO_2 with the combination of deep anesthesia and an open airway. Consider awake extubation with IV lidocaine administered prior to emergence (1–1.5 mg/kg).

$ETCO_2$, end-tidal carbon dioxide; $PaCO_2$, partial pressure of arterial carbon dioxide.

Table 50.3	Clinical Pearls
Monitoring	Standard monitors (place ECG leads on back to avoid surgical field); specific patient condition may warrant arterial line
Lines and fluid	1–2 PIVs; consider normal saline as maintenance fluid (caution not to bolus large amounts)
Antibiotics	Ceftriaxone or cefazolin
Induction	Smooth to avoid increases in ICP, tape ETT to contralateral side (if right VP shunt is placed, tape ETT to the left side of the mouth)
Position	Supine with head turned to contralateral side, shoulder roll, typically head in padded horseshoe headrest; bed will be 90 or 180 degrees so have circuit and IV extension tubing if necessary (consider straight connector on ETT), run monitor cords and lines along body as to avoid neck and abdomen; surgeon preference whether arms are tucked or remain at sides
Warming	Underbody or lower body warmer (avoid abdomen), consider fluid warmer
Emergence	Smooth to avoid increases in ICP, consider avoiding long-acting opioids

ETT, endotracheal tube; ICP, intracranial pressure; VP, ventriculoperitoneal.

peripheral or central line is already in place. Standard induction dosing for propofol and nondepolarizing muscle relaxants should be administered prior to laryngoscopy to facilitate a smooth intubation with little impact on ICP. After the endotracheal tube (ETT) is secured, the bed will be turned either 90 or 180 degrees, with the patient's head turned contralateral to the site of shunt insertion. The patient's head will be shaved, and they will be prepped from the proximal site of insertion (the head) to the distal site of insertion (e.g., chest or abdomen). Typically, the abdomen will be the distal site of insertion.

Local anesthetic is typically injected by the surgeon prior to the scalp incision and subsequent burr hole. A pocket is typically created behind the ear for the valve of the shunt to be placed, and then a tunneling device is used to tunnel a path for the shunt tubing to run, typically down the neck and into the peritoneum (Figure 50.2). Some neurosurgeons may work in conjunction with a general surgeon to prepare the abdominal site for the distal end of the shunt catheter.

Tunneling of the catheter with this device is typically the most stimulating and painful part of the procedure. Anesthesia providers should consider administering additional dosing of opioid and/or propofol at this point. Long-acting opioids should be avoided during the case as the surgeon will attempt to get a neurological examination after emergence. Fentanyl and IV acetaminophen typically provide sufficient analgesia, along with the local anesthetic infiltrated by the surgeon. At the end of the procedure, the bed should be turned back to the anesthesia gas machine to prepare for emergence. The goal of emergence should be a smooth extubation, ideally with the ability to obtain a neurological examination at the end of emergence.

Complications/Emergencies

Perioperative complications of VP shunt placement include venous air embolism (VAE), increased ICP, bowel perforation for VP shunt, and intraventricular hemorrhage. The risk of VAE can be decreased dramatically by avoiding hypovolemia and minimizing the sitting position (or minimizing the degree to which the head is above the heart). Anesthesia providers should be aware that transesophageal echocardiography (TEE) is the most sensitive method for diagnosis of a VAE. If suspected, follow previously discussed techniques in this textbook. Methods to decrease ICP are noted in Table 50.2. Postoperative complications can include device malfunction, shunt flow obstruction, and/or infection from device placement. Anesthesia providers can play a role in minimizing the incidence of these complications by ensuring an adequate depth of anesthesia to aid placement and by appropriate timing and dose of antibiotic administration.

POSTOPERATIVE CARE

Following the procedure, the patient will recover in the postanesthesia care unit (PACU) prior to transfer to their previous inpatient unit. Transfer to the intensive care unit is not typically necessary though may be indicated should there be concern about the patient's neurological status or if more frequent neurological assessments are necessary. Anesthesia providers must be careful not to administer medications that may cause excessive sedation postoperatively as neurological status and improvement in preoperative status will continue to be monitored throughout the patient's hospitalization. Acetaminophen will typically be ordered to alleviate postoperative pain.

CASE STUDY: A 2-Year-Old Child With a History of Hydrocephalus Experiencing New-Onset Neurological Symptoms

CLINICAL SCENARIO

The patient is a 2-year-old male with a known diagnosis of hydrocephalus who had a VP shunt placed 1 month ago with no initial issue per the neurology discharge notes. The father brought the child to the emergency department (ED) with headache, increased agitation, and crying. His vital signs are as follows: temperature 36.5°C (axillary), blood pressure 90/50, and heart rate 165 bpm. The patient last ate applesauce about 3 hours ago and has had no change in appetite or urinary/bowel habits. The neurology team communicates that the patient needs a VP shunt revision related to obstructed flow through the shunt. The ED staff placed an IV, and the patient is on his way to the operating room holding area from the ED.

(continued)

CASE STUDY: A 2-Year-Old Child With a History of Hydrocephalus Experiencing New-Onset Neurological Symptoms (*continued*)

SPECIAL CONSIDERATIONS

Prior to induction of anesthesia, verify that neither the ED staff nor the father has dosed any medications prior to the perioperative phase. Both the anesthesia and neurosurgery teams obtain a baseline neurological examination. Since the child has increased agitation and has an IV, consider preoperative IV midazolam. In the operating room, standard monitors and general anesthesia with a rapid sequence induction are employed given the NPO time was only 3 hours. The VP shunt revision procedure will be completed in the same manner as initial placement, but it is typically shorter in duration.

APPROACHES TO CARE

Evidence-Based Approaches to Care

VP shunt placement is one of the most common neurosurgical procedures, particularly in the pediatric population. Shunt placement also has a high first-year failure rate (31.3%), and the cost of hydrocephalus management and treatment can be over $100 million per decade in the United States.[6] In a 2016 quality metric study on preventable shunt revisions in pediatrics, they demonstrated a shunt failure rate of 21.8% within 90 days of initial placement and 69.8% within 30 days of shunt placement. Most of these cases were proximal catheter failures, and the most common reason (54.3%) of proximal catheter failure was catheter obstruction with blood, protein/debris, or choroid plexus. Since 30-day readmissions for shunt failure are reasonably common, it is worthwhile to follow and measure these metrics. Shunt readmission rates not only affect the specific patient population and facility quality and process-driven results but also can affect 30-day readmission rates (and therefore reimbursement).[7]

COMPLICATIONS

The child has an uneventful perioperative course and only required acetaminophen in the PACU. He was discharged home the morning after the procedure.

REFERENCES

1. Medtronic. Neurological - Shunts. 2020. https://www.medtronic.com/us-en/healthcareprofessionals/products/neurological/shunts.html
2. Jaffe RA, Samuels SI, Schmiesing CA, Golianu B. *Anesthesiologist's Manual of Surgical Procedures*. Wolters Kluwer Health/Lippincott Williams & Wilkins; 2009.
3. Fowler J. Ventriculoperitoneal Shunt. 2020. https://www.ncbi.nlm.nih.gov/books/NBK459351
4. Davis PJ, Cladis FP. *Smith's Anesthesia for Infants and Children*. Elsevier; 2017.
5. Miller RD. *Miller's Anesthesia*. Elsevier/Saunders; 2015.
6. Orrego-González E, Enriquez-Marulanda A, Ravindran K, et al. Factors associated with ventriculoperitoneal shunt failures in the first 30 postoperative days in pediatric patients. *World Neurosurg*. 2019;124(18):32948-32956. doi:10.1016/j.wneu.2018.12.125
7. Venable GT, Rossi NB, Jones GM, et al. The preventable shunt revision rate: a potential quality metric for pediatric shunt surgery. *J Neurosurg Pediatr*. 2016;18(1):7–15. doi:10.3171/2015.12.peds15388

CHAPTER 51

Stereotactic Grid Placement

Tiffany Jonasson and Megha Karkera Kanjia

INDICATIONS/CONTRAINDICATIONS

Epilepsy is one of the most common childhood neurological disorders. It is a disorder with a predisposition for recurrent, spontaneous seizures. A typical patient undergoing stereotactic grid placement has intractable epilepsy, possibly related to other conditions, such as cerebral palsy, tuberous sclerosis, Lennox–Gastaut syndrome, and various other neurological insults. Most children who enter the operating room for such surgical interventions have been on multiple chronic anticonvulsant medications, such as phenytoin and carbamazapine. Despite the pharmacological regimens currently available, a portion of children still experience intractable epilepsy. Surgical interventions, such as stereotactic grid placement, are aimed to assist with this condition. Stereotactic surgery is a procedure that strives to help patients seeking more definitive treatment of intractable epilepsy; it is typically performed after failing other pharmacological treatments. Stereotactic surgery is an approach using three dimensional coordinates, which allows for the localization of a specific area of the body using stereotactic equipment. By using this technique for neurosurgical procedures, important structures of the brain may be avoided while targeting the area of interest.

SPECIAL CONSIDERATIONS AND CONCERNS

INTRACRANIAL PHYSIOLOGY

The intracranial space consists of brain matter, cerebrospinal fluid, and blood. The *Monro–Kellie hypothesis* postulates that the total intracranial compartment volume is fixed, so that an increase in one component must lead to a decrease in another, unless the space is able to expand. Therefore, diseased states, such as the presence of a tumor, abscess, bleeding, or edema, may significantly alter the intracranial volume.

Cerebral blood volume (CBV) makes up approximately 10% of the intracranial space, most of which is found within the venous system. The approximate cerebral blood flow (CBF) in a healthy adult is 55 mL/100 g of brain tissue/min. In awake healthy children, there is increased CBF, of about 100 mL/100 g of brain tissue/min. The CBF is much less in neonates and preterm infants, flowing at 40 mL/100 g of brain tissue/min.

Cerebral perfusion pressure (CPP) is a measure of the pressure gradient across the brain. It can be calculated from the difference between the systemic mean arterial pressure (MAP) and central venous pressure (CVP), unless the intracranial pressure (ICP) exceeds the CVP, in which case the equation becomes CPP = MAP − ICP. Cerebral ischemia and subsequent brain injury can occur when ICP increases and CPP decreases.

There is an adaptive mechanism known as cerebral autoregulation which allows for a relatively constant CBF over a range of systemic blood pressures. In adults, this range of MAP is between 50 and 150 mm Hg (±10 mm Hg depending on the source). This adaptation is maintained by the dilation and constriction of arterioles to alter the cerebrovascular resistance. Cerebral autoregulation may effectively occur in children as young as 6 months of age.[2]

ANTICONVULSANT MEDICATIONS

Patients who are currently taking antiepileptic medication should continue therapy throughout the perioperative period, as the stress of surgery may provoke seizure activity. Antithetically, epileptologists and other team members monitoring the seizure activity during the course of the procedure may request that medications be held for a period prior to surgery based on the planning of the procedure and goals of the designated intervention.

Chronic use of anticonvulsant medications, such as phenytoin and carbamazepine, results in upregulation of hepatic P450 enzymes, leading to the rapid metabolism and clearance of neuromuscular blocking agents and opioids. Special consideration should be given to patients requiring complete paralysis during the surgery who are currently taking anticonvulsants as their dosage requirement is likely to be significantly more than that of other patients. Giving acetaminophen in conjunction with antiepileptic medications has been linked to hepatotoxicity.[3] Anticonvulsant medications, such as phenytoin and valproic acid, may also have hematological effects, such as anemia or thrombocytopenia.

HEAD FRAME

Depending on the stereotactic system being used by the neurosurgeon, a head frame may be required. A head frame introduces obstacles that anesthesia providers must consider prior to proceeding to the operating room. Once the patient is positioned and the frame attached to the operating table, head or neck manipulation will not be possible. If a wrench is used to tighten the frame in place, it should be immediately accessible in case of emergency as the presence of a head frame may present a significant barrier to airway management. Anesthesia providers should be aware that older head frames may not have an adequate opening to fit a mask underneath for mask ventilation. Fortunately, most newer head frames allow appropriate access to the airway. It is imperative that anesthesia providers confirm that the stereotactic head is MRI compatible if the patient will require intervention or imaging in the MRI scanner.

In the adult population, stereotactic procedures may be performed on awake patients. While older children and adolescents may tolerate frame application under local anesthesia with appropriate preparation, the pressure sensation may lead to significant anxiety. Thus, the majority of pediatric patients will require general anesthesia for frame placement and surgery. Head frames are typically placed following induction for ease of placement both due to pain and cooperation of the child.

MAGNETIC RESONANCE IMAGING CONSIDERATIONS

MRI often plays a major role during these procedures, which introduces a unique set of safety considerations. Anesthesia providers should ensure all necessary equipment, such as the anesthesia machine, airway and intubation devices, monitors, tubing, IV fluid pole, infusion pumps, and any other needed equipment, is MRI compatible. Pilot balloons should be taped to the circuit tubing to prevent imaging artifacts. The patient should be screened for any implanted devices, such as a vagal nerve stimulator (VNS) or ventriculoperitoneal shunts.

During scanning periods, the patient will not be immediately accessible, and it may take several seconds for the technician to stop the scan and open the door to Zone 4 of the MRI suite, so great care should be taken to plan for emergent interventions. Head frames and other surgical equipment should also be verified as being MRI compatible prior to entering the MRI scanner room. Typical operating room monitors, such as ECG leads and pulse oximeters, may need to be exchanged for MRI-compatible monitors prior to entering the MRI suite.

ANESTHETIC MANAGEMENT

PREOPERATIVE EVALUATION

Patients presenting for stereotactic grid placement often have significant comorbidities, which should be addressed preoperatively for appropriate management both during and after the surgery (Box 51.1). Patients with obstructive sleep apnea (OSA) for example are more sensitive to opioids, sedatives, and anxiolytic medications, and administration of these medications may lead to respiratory suppression and life-threatening hypoxemia. When incorporating these types of medication into the anesthetic plan, reduced dosing should be considered. If possible, the family should be asked to bring bilevel positive airway pressure (BiPAP) or continuous positive airway pressure (CPAP) equipment if applicable for perioperative use.

Consideration must also be given to ongoing respiratory conditions in patients presenting for this particular procedure as the patient is often in a challenging position in pins during the surgery and may need to be going back and forth from the MRI scanner. While this is a very important procedure, it should be advised that it is an elective procedure, and optimizing respiratory status would be prudent.

Preoperative Labs

Preoperative testing is crucial for providing integral information around the seizure foci for each individual patient. After a visit with the neurosurgeon is completed, typically a head CT scan, brain MRI, PET scan, magnetoencephalography (MEG), EEG, and electrocorticography (ECoG) are performed. These preoperative imaging tests provide information that is paramount to the surgeon's planning for the day of surgery.

PREOPERATIVE PHARMACOLOGY[4]

Benzodiazepines should be avoided if EEG monitoring is planned for the procedure as they may interfere with the readings.

ANESTHETIC TECHNIQUE

Intraoperative Management

Much of the preoperative planning revolves around the intraoperative surgical plan and the monitoring that will be required for optimal surgical results. The goal is a smooth induction that allows for blunting of the sympathetic response to laryngoscopy and skull pinning. Standard induction medications, including propofol, fentanyl, and lidocaine, can be used. Anesthetic plans may need to consider avoiding propofol if the patient will be undergoing ECoG. A discussion about paralysis should be done prior to induction to determine if a long-acting agent, such as rocuronium, can be used or if an alternative, such as cisatracurium or succinylcholine, should be considered.

IV agents do not affect cerebral autoregulation or the response to CO_2, and have varying effects on CBF and cerebral metabolic rate (CMR). Etomidate and propofol both decrease CBF and CMR. Benzodiazepines also decrease CBF and CMR, but to a lesser extent, and have anticonvulsant properties. Opioids have minimal effects on CBF and CMR; however, they can lead to hypercarbia due to respiratory depression. Ketamine is the only agent that leads to an increase in CBF by as much as 50% to 60% through cerebrovascular dilation, although it is used safely in brain injury patients without harmful effects on ICP.

Volatile anesthetics produce a dose-dependent decrease in CMR, with isoflurane having the greatest effect of up to 50% reduction. The agents cause dilation of cerebral blood vessels, leading to a generalized increase in blood flow throughout the brain and cause a concentration-dependent depression of cerebral autoregulation. However, the cerebrovascular response to CO_2 is maintained; therefore, hyperventilation can be used to blunt the volatile effects on CBF and ICP. A phenomenon referred to as circulatory steal is possible in the setting of focal ischemia in which blood flow may be increased in normal parts of the brain but not in ischemic areas, leading to a redistribution of blood flow from ischemic to non-ischemic brain tissue. Nitrous oxide has minimal effect on CBF or CMR when combined with volatile anesthetics.

The use of volatile anesthetics should also be discussed prior to the case to determine the best approach for maintenance anesthesia. If there is concern about the effect of volatile anesthetics on EEG or other neuromonitoring modalities, total IV anesthesia (TIVA) can be performed using

---

BOX 51.1　KEY ASSESSMENT POINTS: STEREOTACTIC GRID PLACEMENT

Presurgical testing
- Brain PET, MRI, MEG scan, continuous EEG monitoring

Comorbidity evaluation
- Consideration for preoperative optimization, intraoperative treatment, and postoperative planning and monitoring

Anxiety
- Midazolam, dexmedetomidine, ketamine (PO, IM, IV, intranasal); dependent upon monitoring utilized

Anticonvulsant therapy
- Consideration of medication interaction and increased requirement of other anesthetic medications

MEG, magnetoencephalography; PET, positron emission tomography.

Table 51.1 Impact of Anesthetic Agents

Volatile Agents	MAP	CBF	CPP	ICP	SSEPs Amplitude/Latency
Isoflurane	↓↓	↑	↓	↑	↓/↑
Sevoflurane	↓↓	↑	0 – ↓	0– ↑	↓/↑
Desflurane	↓↓	↑	↓	↑	↓/↑
N_2O	0 – ↓	↑– ↑↑	↓	↑– ↑↑	↓/0 – ↑
IV Agents	**MAP**	**CBF**	**CPP**	**ICP**	**SSEPs Amplitude/Latency**
Propofol	↓↓↓	↓↓↓	↑↑	↓↓	↑/↑
Ketamine	↑↑	↑↑↑	↓	↑↑↑	↑/0
Benzodiazepines	0 – ↓	↓↓	↑	0	↓0/↑
Opioids	0 – ↓	↓	↓↑	0 – ↓	↓/↑

CBF, cerebral blood flow; CPP, cerebral perfusion pressure; ICP, intracranial pressure; MAP, mean arterial pressure; N_2O, nitrous oxide; SSEPs, somatosensory evoked potentials.
Source: From Vavilala MS, Soriano SG, Krane EJ. Anesthesia for neurosurgery. In: *Smith's Anesthesia for Infants and Children.* 9th ed. Elsevier. 2017;744–772.

Table 51.2 Special Techniques and/or Equipment

Technique/Equipment	Description
ECoG	ECoG will assist with intraoperative potentials from the cortex that can be recorded and tracked during the procedure. This will assist with helping with the seizure foci and will guide resection for the maximal results. These results will guide the entire resection, which is why the anesthetic should be guided by an experienced pediatric anesthesia provider and neurosurgeon to maximize results. The goals may be different for each particular surgeon; however, if paralysis is permitted given the extent of the neuromonitoring, it is advisable to keep the patient heavily paralyzed for minimizing any movement during the procedure. If the patient moves during the procedure, the entire results of the procedure can be skewed, and the procedure may need to start over.
SSEPs	SSEPs monitor neural pathways during surgery to assess responses to the brain as it relates to touch and pressure.
MEPs	MEPs offer an opportunity to evaluate the motor system by transcranial electrical stimulation of the motor cortex and recording the subsequent muscle responses. Utilizing these monitoring systems can assist the anesthesia provider and neurosurgeon in avoiding unintended complications during the surgery. The anesthetic should be tailored carefully based on the patient's monitoring during the procedure such that appropriate signals should be elicited periodically throughout the surgery.

ECoG, electrocorticograph; MEPs, motor evoked potentials; SSEPs, somatosensory evoked potentials.

propofol; opioids, such as sufentanil or remifentanil; and other adjuncts, such as lidocaine, ketamine, and/or dexmedetomidine. Smooth emergence is desirable as coughing or bucking can elicit a sympathetic response that can result in intracerebral hemorrhage.

The brain consumes approximately 20% of total body oxygen. The rate of oxygen consumption ($CMRO_2$), about 3 to 3.8 mL/100 g/min in adults, is used to convey the CMR.[4] Many commonly used anesthetic medications have an effect on cerebral hemodynamics, as well as on EEG, somatosensory evoked potentials, and motor evoked potentials (Table 51.1).

Intraoperatively, placement of an arterial line may be indicated if a more accurate systolic and diastolic pressure measurement is necessary or if frequent blood draws during a procedure are anticipated. Like any other invasive procedure, the risks and benefits should be discussed with the patient and weighed prior to placement.

Special Techniques and/or Equipment
Special techniques are summarized in Table 51.2.

Complications/Emergencies
Complications and emergencies are summarized in Box 51.2.

BOX 51.2 COMPLICATIONS/EMERGENCIES

Seizure activity
- Administer propofol, benzodiazepines; ask surgeon to apply cool saline irrigation to brain

Venous air embolism
- Surgeon should flood surgical field, increase FiO_2 to 100%, hemodynamic support, lower head of bed if possible, aspiration of air from central line, if present

Hemorrhage
- Hemodynamic support, transfusion

Aspiration
- Suction, lower head of bed, intubation/positive pressure ventilation

Infection
- Surgical site infection secondary to implant

FiO_2, fractional inspired oxygen.

POSTOPERATIVE CARE

Admission to the intensive care unit (ICU) may be planned postoperatively depending on the patient's comorbidities and baseline neurological status. Patients who require frequent neurological assessments in the postoperative period may be better suited to be observed in the ICU rather than the floor for easier nursing staffing and care. Additionally, patients with central and obstructive sleep apnea may require respiratory support at home, and the BiPAP/CPAP settings may change perioperatively. Patients with a history of central sleep apnea may necessitate judicious use of sedative medications, especially opioids, as it pertains to apnea in the postoperative period.

REFERENCES

1. McClain CD, Soriano SG. Pediatric neurosurgical anesthesia. In *Cote and Lerman's A Practice of Anesthesia for Infants and Children.* 6th ed. Elsevier. 2019;604–628. https://www.clinicalkey.com/#!/content/book/3-s2.0-B9780323429740000264?scrollTo=%23hl0000821
2. Vavilala MS, Soriano SG, Krane EJ. Anesthesia for neurosurgery. In *Smith's Anesthesia for Infants and Children.* 9th ed. Elsevier. 2017;744–772 https://www.clinicalkey.com/#!/content/book/3-s2.0-B9780323341257000280?scrollTo=%23hl0001346
3. Ghazal EA, Vadi MG, Mason LJ, Coté CJ. Preoperative evaluation, premedication, and induction of anesthesia. In *Cote and Lerman's A Practice of Anesthesia for Infants and Children.* 6th ed. Elsevier. 2019;35–68. https://www.clinicalkey.com/#!/content/book/3-s2.0-B9780323429740000045
4. Butterworth IV JF, Mackey DC, Wasnick JD, eds. Neurophysiology & anesthesia. In *Morgan & Mikhail's Clinical Anesthesiology.* 6th ed. McGraw-Hill. 2018. https://accessmedicine.mhmedical.com/content.aspx?bookid=2444&sectionid=193560975#1161429248
5. Lee MY, Bloom MJ. Perioperative challenges during stereotactic neurosurgery and deep brain stimulator placement. In: A Brambrink, J Kirsch, eds. *Essentials of Neurosurgical Anesthesia & Critical Care.* Springer; 2020:189–192.
6. Crean PM, Tirupathi S. Essentials of neurology and neuromuscular disorders. In: CJ Cote, J Lerman, eds. *A Practice of Anesthesia for Infants and Children.* 6th ed. Elsevier; 2019:561–580. https://www.clinicalkey.com/#!/content/3-s2.0-B9780323429740000240?scrollTo=%23hl0001593
7. Butterworth IV JF, Mackey DC, Wasnick JD, eds. Anesthesia for patients with neurological & psychiatric diseases. In *Morgan & Mikhail's Clinical Anesthesiology.* 6th ed. McGraw Hill; 2018. https://accessmedicine.mhmedical.com/ViewLarge.aspx?figid=193561281
8. Cravero JP, Landrigan-Ossar M. Anesthesia outside the operating room. In: CJ Cote, J Lerman, eds. *A Practice of Anesthesia for Infants and Children.* 6th ed. Elsevier; 2019: 1077–1094. https://www.clinicalkey.com/#!/content/book/3-s2.0-B978032342974000046X?scrollTo=%23hl0000659
9. Rodichok LD, Russell GB. *Primer of Intraoperative Neurophysiologic Monitoring.* Elsevier; 1995.
10. Brown KA. Outcome, risk, and error and the child with obstructive sleep apnea. *Pediatr Anesth.* 2011;21(7):771–780. doi:10.1111/j.1460-9592.2011.03597.x
11. Rajkalyan C, Tewari A, Rao S, Avitsian R. Anesthetic considerations for stereotactic electroencephalography implantation. *J Anaesthesiol Clin Pharmacol.* 2019;35(4):434. doi:10.4103/joacp.joacp_342_18
12. Dunoyer C, Ragheb J, Resnick T, et al. The use of stereotactic radiosurgery to treat intractable childhood partial epilepsy. *Epilepsia.* 2002;43(3):292–300. doi:10.1046/j.1528-1157.2002.06501.x

CHAPTER 52

Vagal Nerve Stimulator Placement

Kelly Moon

INDICATIONS/CONTRAINDICATIONS

Epilepsy is a common neurological disorder that affects all ages, races, and socioeconomic groups. It is characterized by a lasting predisposition to develop epileptic seizure activity in an unpredictable, unprovoked fashion. In 2015, it was estimated that 3.4 million people suffered from epilepsy in the United States. Epilepsy is twice as common in the pediatric population when compared to their adult counterparts. While medical management of epilepsy with pharmacologic agents is considered first-line treatment, approximately one third of patients are unable to remain seizure-free with antiepileptic drugs (AEDs) alone. When epilepsy is resistant to drug therapies, patients are said to have refractory epilepsy or drug-resistant epilepsy (DRE). DRE can be defined as persistent seizure activity that prevents normal function or development. This diagnosis can only be made after documentation of an adequate trial of anticonvulsant medications. In patients who suffer from DRE, surgical intervention may be performed to decrease seizure activity.

In 1997, the U.S. Food and Drug Administration approved the use of a surgically implanted vagal nerve stimulator (VNS) for the treatment of epilepsy (**Figure 52.1**). Although the exact mechanism of action remains unclear, stimulation of the vagus nerve modulates the nerve pathways that are

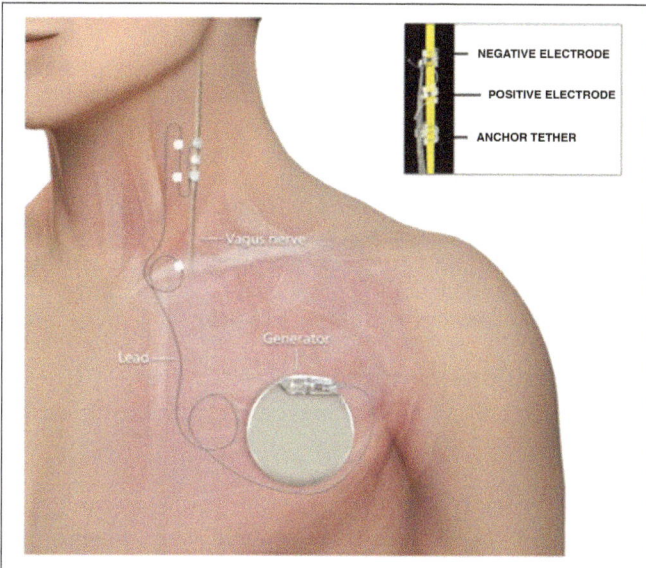

Figure 52.1: Vagal nerve stimulator placement.
Source: From Verrier R, Nearing BD, Olin B, et al. Baseline elevation and reduction in cardiac electrical instability assessed by quantitative T-wave alternans in patients with drug-resistant epilepsy treated with vagus nerve stimulation in the AspireSR E-36 trial. *Epilepsy Behav.* 2016;62:85–89. doi:10/1016/j.yebeh.2016.06.016.

CHAPTER 52: VAGAL NERVE STIMULATOR PLACEMENT

ANESTHETIC MANAGEMENT

PREOPERATIVE EVALUATION

A thorough preoperative assessment should be performed prior to anesthesia, with a specific focus on the patient's seizure history and medications. Patients requiring VNS placement generally present with uncontrolled seizures despite treatment with multiple AEDs. Current drug therapies, dosages, and times of most recent doses are important to determine. Plasma levels of monitored AEDs need to be within therapeutic levels. The patient's AEDs should be continued the day of surgery to minimize disruptions to the normal treatment regimen. If AEDs are not given prior to surgery, anesthesia providers may be required to administer them intraoperatively to decrease the likelihood of perioperative seizure activity. If the enteral route is not an option, IV medications should be used in place. A description of the patient's seizure activity regarding the type, frequency, and triggers is important to determine. An assessment of preoperative deficits, if present, should be completed to establish a baseline regarding the patient's normal function. The administration of midazolam may be of benefit before surgery in certain patients before arrival in the operating room.

Anesthesia providers should be aware that patients with a diagnosis of epilepsy may be on a ketogenic diet to help control seizures. This should be vetted in the preoperative setting as it may influence anesthetic management. Collaboration with pharmacy colleagues is essential if the carbohydrate content of any medications planning to be administered is uncertain. Medications and fluids frequently used perioperatively are not carbohydrate-free and should be avoided to maintain the patient's ketogenic diet.

Pertinent Labs

Laboratory work and preoperative testing are not routinely needed prior to this procedure. Anesthesia providers should be aware that certain AEDs may affect laboratory values. Occasionally, an ECG may be warranted if the patient has a history of cardiac conduction abnormalities. With the potential for cardiac arrhythmias during stimulation, a baseline ECG may be helpful for patient care.

ANESTHETIC TECHNIQUE

Intraoperative Management

While VNS placement can be performed under general anesthesia or regional anesthetic, it is most commonly performed under general anesthesia for pediatric patients. When performed under general anesthesia airway management can be based on the patient's specific anesthetic, requirements, with use of both an endotracheal tube and laryngeal mask airway being acceptable. If placed using solely a regional technique, a superficial and deep cervical plexus block is commonly employed.

The use of standard monitors is recommended by the American Society of Anesthesiologist. Anesthesia providers should be cognizant of keeping ECG leads out of the surgical field. Ventilation should be managed to maintain normocarbia, as hyperventilation can precipitate seizures. Additional intraoperative goals include maintenance of normothermia and euvolemia. Anesthesia providers should consider employing active warming techniques, such as warming the operating room and utilizing fluid warmers, as maintaining body temperature in this patient population can be challenging. One IV catheter is sufficient as minimal blood loss is expected under normal circumstances. Prior to surgical incision, antibiotics should be administered to stave off infection. Neuromuscular blockade is not needed for the procedure; however, its use to facilitate anesthetic management is not contraindicated.

involved in seizure activity and has been shown to decrease the frequency and intensity of seizure activity. This is not a curative treatment, but placement of a VNS often improves the quality of life in those suffering from epilepsy. Surgical placement of a VNS is associated with a low complication rate, with the benefit of effectively reducing seizures in patients diagnosed with DRE far outweighing the low incidence of complications. Contraindications to a surgical placement of a VNS include baseline cardiac conduction disorders and history of a vagotomy. As stimulation of the vagus nerve can worsen cardiac arrhythmias, this treatment option should be avoided in patients with conduction abnormalities.

Surgical placement of a VNS is currently approved by the U.S. Food and Drug Administration for treatment of epilepsy and depression; however, there is a growing body of research exploring the efficacy of VNS in treating a host of clinical disorders, such as anxiety, obesity, headaches, bipolar disorder, and Alzheimer's disease. As indications for VNS placement increase, anesthesia providers will likely see more an increase in the number of patients presenting to the operating room for this surgical procedure.

A VNS consists of a programmable generator, a subcutaneously placed lead wire, and an electrode that is wrapped around the vagus nerve. The device resembles a pacemaker and is noninvasively programmed via an external wand and software. Parameters and functional settings are patient dependent and set during placement. These parameters can be changed following placement to better manage individual needs. Patients or their guardian may also be given a magnet that can be placed in close proximity to the VNS prior to the onset of a seizure. Doing so will trigger the nerve stimulator to produce an electric impulse in hopes of lessening the severity or stopping the oncoming seizure. Batteries powering the generator typically last approximately 5 years before having to be replaced. Surgical replacement of the generator is necessary when a new battery is needed.

During surgery, the patient will be placed in a supine position with their arms adducted, with their head turned to the right. Anesthesia providers must ensure that IV access remains easily assessable after the positioning of arms. Left-sided placement of a vagal nerve stimulator is preferred due to the increased presence of efferent fibers to the sinoatrial nerve stemming from the right vagus nerve. Although rare, the left vagus nerve can innervate the sinoatrial nerve. Stimulation of these nerve fibers may lead to cardiac arrhythmias, such as bradycardia or asystole.

Surgically, two incisions will be made with one incision being a left anterior cervical incision on the neck to expose the vagal nerve. The other incision will be located in the left infraclavicular region for placement of the generator. The left vagus nerve will be isolated, and the electrode will be wrapped directly around the nerve (Figure 52.2). Prior to placement, the electrode and generator will be tested to ensure function. The surgeon should inform the anesthesia provider before testing the device as bradycardia and asystole have been observed. Should bradycardia or asystole occur, stimulation should cease immediately as this generally resolved these untoward cardiac issues. Mild bradycardia may be treated with glycopyrrolate or atropine. Severe instances of bradycardia may require the administration of epinephrine, transcutaneous pacing, and/or compressions. Intraoperative and postoperative pain should be controlled with a multimodal analgesic approach to minimize opioid requirements. Incision sites can also be infiltrated with a local anesthetic to help minimize postoperative discomfort.

Clinical Pearls

Anesthesia providers may consider avoiding etomidate and ketamine for induction, as these agents have been shown to have proconvulsant effects. Patients presenting for a VNS are often receiving multiple AEDs. Many of these medications are known to induce cytochrome P450, which may alter drug metabolism. Higher levels of neuromuscular blocking agents, benzodiazepines, and narcotics may be necessary. If neuromuscular blocking agents are used, anesthesia providers should use a nerve stimulator to assess the level of blockade and adjust the frequency of administration as needed. Patients receiving AEDs may also require a decreased dose of propofol to maintain adequate anesthesia as AEDs have an inhibitory effect on the metabolism of propofol, which reduces the amount needed and potentially prolonging emergence.

Patients are also at risk of epileptic activity occurring perioperatively. It is important to minimize disruptions to their current AED routine to lessen this risk. If a patient were to experience a seizure during the perioperative period, both propofol and midazolam can be administered as anticonvulsants. Maintaining an adequate airway and assessing the patient until seizure activity has ceased are fundamental.

All inhalation agents are appropriate to use in normal anesthetic doses. Research has demonstrated an increase in epileptogenic properties with elevated concentrations of sevoflurane. Historically, enflurane was avoided in patients with epilepsy as it can create epileptiform EEG activity and cause postoperative seizures. Meperidine, tramadol, and alfentanil should be omitted because they increase the risk of seizures. Managing patients with epilepsy can be a difficult task, and an understanding of the many potential drug interactions that can occur is essential to anesthetic management.

Complications/Emergencies

Potential complications and emergencies and their treatment are summarized in Table 52.1.

POSTOPERATIVE CARE

In addition to standard postoperative care, patients presenting for VNS placement should be monitored for nerve injury and seizure activity. Postoperative pain is usually minimal and can be treated with acetaminophen, nonsteroidal

Table 52.1	Complications/Emergencies
Complication/Emergency	Cause and Treatment
Bradycardia or asystole	**Cause:** Vagal stimulation **Treatment:** Administer glycopyrrolate, atropine, or epinephrine, transcutaneous pacing, compressions
Bronchospasm	**Cause:** Excess vagal stimulation **Treatment:** Stop stimulation, beta-2 agonist can be administered
Vocal cord paralysis / hoarseness	**Cause:** Surgical damage to the vagus nerve or its branches (recurrent laryngeal nerve or superior laryngeal nerve) **Treatment:** Close observation for airway complications
Sleep-disordered breathing	**Cause:** Stimulation of vagus nerve **Treatment:** CPAP or BiPAP, may need to adjust VNS settings
Vascular injury	**Cause:** Injury due to proximity of the carotid artery and jugular vein **Treatment:** Repair injury, monitor bleeding amount, give blood products if needed
Hematoma	**Cause:** Excessive postoperative bleeding **Treatment:** Assess for increasing neck circumference and possible airway compromise, surgical intervention if needed
Electrode fracture	**Cause:** Trauma to electrode and device site **Treatment:** Surgical removal
Infection	**Cause:** Antibiotic administration **Treatment:** Infection may require removal of the device, maintain a clean surgical site

BiPAP, bilevel positive airway pressure; CPAP, continuous positive airway pressure; VNS, vagal nerve stimulator.

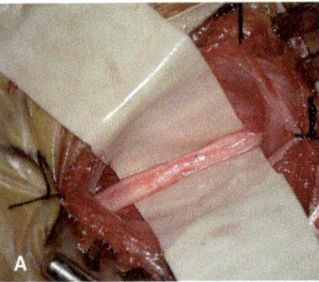 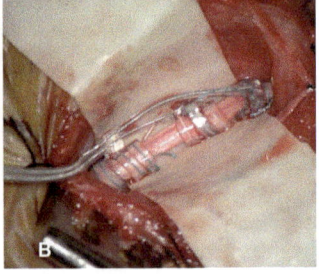

Figure 52.2: Surgical placement of vagal nerve stimulator. (A) Vagus nerve is exposed; (B) electrode is placed on the vagus nerve.

Source: From Yang J, Hoon Phi J. The present and future of vagus nerve stimulation. *J Korean Neurosurg Soc.* 2019;62(3):344–352.

anti-inflammatories, or opioids if necessary. After the placement of a VNS, patients may be at risk of sleep-disordered breathing. The exact mechanism of this phenomenon remains unknown, but it may be a result of decreased upper airway tone. Therefore, patients should be monitored postoperatively for any breathing complications. VNS is typically performed as an outpatient procedure. After surgery, the patient will return for a follow-up visit at which time the VNS settings will be assessed, with modifications made if needed.

There are several considerations for these patients moving forward. Central venous catheter placement in the left internal jugular should be avoided to ensure the vagal nerve electrode and wiring are not compromised. Also, the use of electrocautery during future surgeries should be avoided as its use may damage the generator. Grounding pads should be placed as far away as possible to prevent electrical flow through the system and unipolar cautery should be avoided. It is not recommended that the VNS is turned off for future surgeries; rather, the aforementioned considerations should be adhered to. Extracorporeal shockwave lithotripsy should be avoided as it may damage the generator. Likewise, external defibrillation may also damage the generator. If needed, defibrillation pads should be placed as far away as possible prior to a shock being delivered. MRI can cause heat production that leads to thermal injuries and may also deactivate programmable functions. Manufacturer instructions need to be reviewed before a patient has an MRI scan, and the device should be interrogated after to ensure settings have been maintained.

BIBLIOGRAPHY

The complete bibliography for this chapter is online and available at https://connect.springerpub.com/content/book/978-0-8261-3875-0/part/part04/toc-part/ch052.

Bloor M, Nandi R, Thomas M. Antiepileptic drugs and anesthesia. *Paediatr Anaesth*. 2017;27:248–250. doi:10.1111/pan.13074

Carter EL, Adapa RM. Adult epilepsy and anaesthesia. *Br J Anaesth*. 2015;15(3):111–117. doi:10.1093/bjaceaccp/mku014

Centers for Disease Control and Prevention. *Epilepsy data and statistics*. https://www.cdc.gov/epilepsy/data/index.html

Henderson J, Gigante PR, Shuer LM. Functional neurosurgery. In: Jaffe RA, ed. *Anesthesiologist's Manual of Surgical Procedures*. 5th ed. Wolters Kluwer; 2014:80–83.

Orihara A, Hara K, Hara S, et al. Effects of sevoflurane anesthesia on intraoperative high-frequency oscillations in patients with temporal lobe epilepsy. *European J Epilepsy*. 2020;82:44–49. doi:10.1016/j.seizure.2020.08.029

Perez-Carbonell L, Faulkner H, Higgins S, et al. Vagus nerve stimulation for drug-resistant epilepsy. *Pract Neurol*. 2020;20(3):189–198. doi:10.1136/practneurol-2019-002210

Revesz D, Rydenhag B, Ben-Menachem E. Complications and safety of vagus nerve stimulation: 25 years of experience at a single center. *J Neurosurg*. 2016;18:97–104. doi:10.3171/2016.1.PEDS15534

Sajko T, Rotim K. Vagus nerve stimulation for refractory epilepsy. In: Fountas K, Kapsalaki E, eds. *Epilepsy Surgery and Intrinsic Brain Tumor Surgery*. Springer; 2019:197–204. doi:10.1007/978-3-319-95918-4_18

Secen AE, Aslan A, Bulduk EB, et al. Lead fracture after vagal nerve stimulator implantation. Epilepsi. 2019;25(3):136–140. doi:10.14744/epilepsi.2018.97659

Summary of Safety and Effectiveness Data (SSED). *VNS Therapy System*. https://www.accessdata.fda.gov/cdrh_docs/pdf/p970003s207b.pdf

Yang J, Hoon Phi J. The present and future of vagus nerve stimulation. *J Korean Neurosurg Soc*. 2019;62(3):344–352. doi:10.3340/jkns.2019.0037

Zack MM, Kobau R. National and state estimates of the numbers of adults and children with active epilepsy: United States, 2015. *Morb Mortal Wkly Rep*. 2017;66(31):821–825. doi:10.15585/mmwr.mm6631a1

CHAPTER 53

Epilepsy Surgery

Jacob Stollard and Whitney Rhoades

INDICATIONS/CONTRAINDICATIONS

Epilepsy is one of the most common serious neurological disorders in childhood. It is characterized by a lasting predisposition to develop epileptic seizure activity in an unpredictable, unprovoked fashion. Epilepsy can result from a host of inciting factors, such as brain malformation, congenital conditions, genetic factors, inborn errors of metabolism, or anoxic injury during birth. The known associated conditions and genetic syndromes are numerous and include hypothalamic hamartoma, polymicrogyria, Rasmussen's encephalitis, tuberous sclerosis, Sturge–Weber syndrome, Landau–Kleffner syndrome, Dravet syndrome, Lennox–Gastaut syndrome, West syndrome, Ohtahara syndrome, infantile spasms, and epilepsia partialis continua.[1]

The impact of epilepsy can be profound as it is associated with neurological, cognitive, psychological, and social consequences. Antiepileptic drugs (AEDs) are the mainstay in treatment of epilepsy; however, they are not always effective in completely tempering seizure activity. Drug-resistant epilepsy (DRE) affects approximately 20% of children with epilepsy.

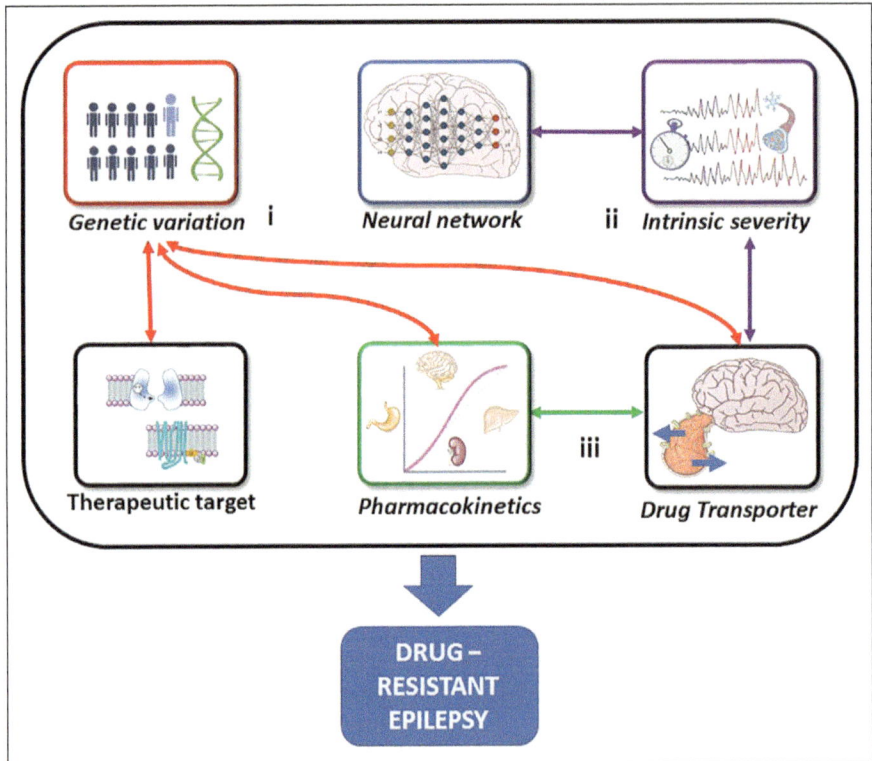

Figure 53.1: Mechanisms of drug-resistant epilepsy.

Source: From Pérez-Pérez D, Frías-Soria CL, Rocha L. Drug-resistant epilepsy: from multiple hypotheses to an integral explanation using preclinical resources. *Epilepsy Behav.* 2019:106430. doi:10.1016/j.yebeh.2019.07.031.

Resistance to drug therapy is multifactorial and can be due to a variety of mechanisms (**Figure 53.1**). Age also seems to play a role, as younger patients are less likely to achieve a seizure-free status when compared to elderly patients.

The International League Against Epilepsy defines *DRE* as failure of adequate trials of two tolerated and appropriately chosen and used AED schedules (whether as monotherapies or in combination) to achieve sustained seizure freedom.[2] If DRE is suspected, treatment should be modified to limit further disability and long-term neurological and nonneurological complications.[3] Nonpharmacological interventions, such as a ketogenic diet (high-fat, low-protein, and low-carbohydrate diet), have proved effective in decreasing seizure activity in patients with DRE. Adherence to ketogenic diets, however, can be challenging as they are restrictive and often unpleasant. Therefore, surgery should be considered as soon as patients meet the criteria for having DRE as a range of procedures are available that can potentially abate seizure activity (**Table 53.1**).

A variety of modalities, such as single-photon emission CT (SPECT), PET, magnetoencephalography (MEG), fMRI, and stereotactic EEG (SEEG) can be used in the presurgical assessment of patients with epilepsy to infer localization of epileptic foci. fMRI can identify most cerebral lesions underlying focal epilepsy, as well as the areas of the cortex that are essential for language, motor function, and memory, thereby reducing the risk of epilepsy surgery causing new morbidities. It should be noted that in children younger than 18 months of age with severe epilepsy, an fMRI may not be accurate due to the lack of contrast and immature myelination.[6] Placement of SEEG leads further aids in localizing seizure foci, with higher accuracy than the conventional methods. For more information regarding the anesthetic management of SEEG leads, please refer to Chapter 51, "Stereotactic Grid Placement and Removal."

Contraindications for epilepsy surgery include concurrent severe psychiatric illness, severe comorbidities that preclude surgery, inability to identify the epileptic foci, and when surgery may result in disabling neuropsychological deficits.[7]

SPECIAL CONSIDERATIONS AND CONCERNS

PERIOPERATIVE MANAGEMENT OF ANTIEPILEPTIC DRUGS

Patients should continue to take AEDs as scheduled on the day of surgery as missed doses, fasting, sleep deprivation, and the administration of proconvulsant anesthetics can predispose patients to perioperative seizures. Additionally, sudden discontinuation of certain AEDs, such as clobazam and clonazepam, can result in withdrawal seizures.[8]

AEDs can have a variable impact on pharmacodynamics, with some first-generation AEDs (phenytoin, phenobarbital, primidone, carbamazepine) inducing cytochrome P450 hepatic isoenzyme activity, while others (valproate) inhibit cytochrome P450 hepatic isoenzyme activity. Second-generation AEDs (vigabatrin, lamotrigine, levetiracetam, pregabalin, zonisamide) are generally associated with fewer drug interactions as they do not induce cytochrome P450 hepatic isoenzyme activity. A multitude of other interactions can occur as well that anesthesia providers should remain cognizant of (**Table 53.2**).

Table 53.1	Types of Epilepsy Surgeries
Type of Surgery	**Description and Indications**
Surgical Resection of Seizure Focus	
Resective	Surgical removal of area of brain where seizures begin (invasive) Indications: DRE
Hemispherectomy	Surgical removal or disconnection of one hemisphere of the brain (invasive) Indications: hemiplegia due to underlying cause; DRE
Hemispherotomy	Creation of a hole or multiple holes in one hemisphere of the brain Indications: DRE
Corpus callosotomy	Splitting the main connection pathway (disconnection) between the two cerebral hemispheres (invasive) Indications: DRE; drop attacks/tonic seizures; developmental delay; disabling seizures
LITT	Laser ablation of the seizure foci via burr hole. MRI is used throughout entire case Indications: DRE
Neurostimulation	
VNS	Attachment of a stimulator to the vagus nerve in the neck to decrease number and severity of seizures. Used when surgery is not an option Indications: DRE; drop attacks/tonic seizures
RNS	Generator implanted on skull with electrodes placed on area of brain where seizures arise Indications: DRE
DBS	Implantation of electrode in brain and placement of stimulator under skin of the chest. MRI is used for procedure Indications: DRE
Intracranial EEG monitoring	Placement of intracranial EEG leads (invasive). Stereotactic placement of EEG, robotic assisted (ROSA), with small burr holes for each lead (minimally invasive). Part of a two-step surgical treatment focused on epileptogenic zone and determines extent of resection needed Indications: DRE

DBS, deep brain stimulation; DRE, drug-resistant epilepsy; LITT, laser interstitial laser therapy; RNS, responsive neurostimulation; VNS, vagal nerve stimulator.

Source: From Cascino G, Britton J, Kiriakopoulos E. *Types of Epilepsy Surgery*. Epilepsy Foundation; 2018. https://www.epilepsy.com/learn/treating-seizures-and-epilepsy/surgery/types-epilepsy-surgery Jayalakshmi S, Vooturi S, Gupta S, Panigraphi M. Epilepsy in children. *Neurol. India*. 2017;65(3):485. doi:10.4103/neuroindia.ni_1033_16.

Table 53.2	Adverse Effects of Antiepileptic Drugs
Antiepileptic Drug	**Adverse Effects**
Carbazepine	Hyponatremia and leukopenia
Lacosamide	PR interval prolongation
Sodium valproate	Platelet dysfunction, thrombocytopenia
Topiramate	Metabolic acidosis
Phenytoin	May potentiate rocuronium

Source: From Bloor M, Nandi R, Thomas M. Antiepileptic drugs and anesthesia. *Pediatr. Anesth*. 2017;27(3):248–250. doi:10.1111/pan.13074.

KETOGENIC DIETS AND ANESTHESIA

Multiple medications administered during a general anesthetic contain glucose and other substances that might alter the physiological ketosis, thereby increasing the risk of seizure activity.[9] Anesthesia providers should be aware that these patients are at risk of developing metabolic acidosis during general anesthesia, particularly during prolonged surgical procedures. It is also not uncommon for children on a ketogenic diet to present in a state of mild chronic metabolic acidosis.[10] Additional considerations anesthesia providers should consider when caring for a patient on a ketogenic diet can be found in Table 53.3.

ANESTHETIC MANAGEMENT

PREOPERATIVE EVALUATION

A thorough preoperative evaluation is essential to decreasing perioperative morbidity (Table 53.4). The preoperative evaluation should focus on the patient's neurological disorder, as well as any associated neurological, cognitive, or psychological comorbidities. When reviewing the patient's current state of health, it is important to confirm the patient's current medications, as well as any changes in medications and/or dosing regimen. This is also an excellent opportunity to garner a description of seizures, prodromal symptoms, and current neurological deficits. Any physiological disturbances secondary to associated conditions or genetic syndromes should also be vetted at this time. Patients diagnosed with tuberous sclerosis, for example, often present with epilepsy due to intracranial lesions. It is imperative that anesthesia providers determine the physiologic impact

Table 53.3	Perioperative Recommendations for Children on a Ketogenic Diet
Preoperative Recommendations	• Obtain complete blood count, basic metabolic panel with serum electrolytes and glucose level on day of surgery • Avoid prolonged fasting to avoid hypoglycemia • Avoid administration of carbohydrate-containing electrolyte solutions and IV fluids • Avoid oral midazolam solution because of high carbohydrate content
Perioperative Recommendations	• Avoid carbohydrate-containing medications • Avoid high-dose propofol infusion for long duration for risk of propofol infusion syndrome • Use isotonic solutions. Normal saline is preferred over lactated Ringer's. Avoid large volumes of normal saline to prevent increase in hyperchloremic metabolic acidosis • Frequently monitor serum pH, glucose, electrolytes, and bicarbonate levels during procedures lasting more than 3 hours, and administer IV bicarbonate where necessary • Do not overcorrect hypoglycemia
Use With Caution	Etomidate, propofol, vecuronium powder for reconstitution, dexamethasone, mannitol, calcium gluconate, nitroglycerin, and plasmalyte
Avoid	Oral midazolam, IV acetaminophen injection, acetaminophen tablet/chew tablet/oral suspension, gabapentin oral solution/tablet, hydromorphone tablet, ibuprofen oral suspension/tablet, morphine oral solution, oxycodone oral solution/tablet, ondansetron oral solution/tablet, oxymetazoline nasal spray, dopamine, labetolol, milrinone, cefazolin in dextrose solution, clindamycin in 5% dextrose, and vancomycin in dextrose injection

Source: From Conover ZR, Talai A, Klockau K, et al. Perioperative management of children on ketogenic dietary therapies. *Anesth. Analg.* 2020;131(6):1872–1882. doi:10.1213/ane.0000000000005018.

Table 53.4	General Preoperative Concerns
Condition	Anesthetic Implication
Congenital heart disease	Hypoxia, arrhythmias and cardiovascular instability, and paradoxical air emboli
Prematurity	Postoperative apnea
Gastrointestinal reflux	Aspiration pneumonia
Upper respiratory tract infection	Laryngospasm, bronchospasm, hypoxia, and pneumonia
Craniofacial abnormality	Difficulty with airway management

Source: From Soriano SG, Bozza P. Anesthesia for epilepsy surgery in children. *Child's Nervous System.* 2006;22(8):834–843.

of cardiac, renal, and pulmonary hamartomatous lesions in this patient population prior to inducing general anesthesia. For all patients presenting for epilepsy surgery, it is highly recommended an anesthesia consult occurs prior to elective procedures to ensure ample time to optimize the patient prior to surgery.

Pertinent Labs

Preoperative laboratory tests should be based on the procedure being performed and the patient's medical history. At the very least, a complete blood count, basic metabolic panel with electrolytes, liver function test, and coagulation studies should be obtained. If the patient is on a ketogenic diet, a preoperative glucose should be checked. As there is a risk of rapid, significant blood loss, a type and screen should be sent prior to incision, and there should be crossmatched blood available. All available imaging studies should be reviewed to determine if the surgical area has cerebral dominance.

PREOPERATIVE PHARMACOLOGY

After consultation with the neurologist and neurosurgeon, scheduled AEDs should be administered the day of surgery to decrease the likelihood of seizure activity perioperatively. While often not an issue, the administration of benzodiazepines may interfere with intraoperative monitoring. Therefore, a discussion with the monitoring team should take place prior to administration of anxiolytics preoperatively. If the decision is made to administer an anxiolytic preoperatively, oral and IV midazolam are effective anxiolytics. If the patient is on a ketogenic diet, oral midazolam should be avoided.

ANESTHETIC TECHNIQUE

Intraoperative Management

Anesthetic management of surgical resection of epileptogenic foci without brain mapping or electrocorticography (ECoG) monitoring is similar to open craniotomy procedures (see **Box 53.1** and Chapter 49, "Craniotomy"). Assuming there are no contraindications, induction of anesthesia in infants and young children can occur via an inhalation induction. IV induction of general anesthesia with propofol is well tolerated. Proconvulsant medications, such as etomidate and ketamine, should be avoided to decrease the likelihood of seizure activity during the induction of anesthesia. Neuromuscular-blocking agents can be administered to facilitate tracheal intubation. Patients at risk of aspiration should receive a rapid sequence induction, although succinylcholine should be avoided in the presence of spinal cord injuries given the risk of sudden, catastrophic hyperkalemia. Anesthesia providers should be aware that chronic AED therapy negatively impacts the efficacy of some nondepolarizing neuromuscular-blocking agents due to the associated induced enzymatic activity that affects metabolism. Complications and emergencies are noted in **Box 53.2**.

> **BOX 53.2 COMPLICATIONS/EMERGENCIES**
>
> - Acute blood loss/hemorrhage
> - Hemodynamic instability due to fluid/blood loss or nervous system response to procedure
> - Metabolic acidosis
> - Hypothermia
> - Intraoperative seizure
> - Venous air embolism
> - Unplanned extubation/airway obstruction
> - Skin integrity issues related to length of case
> - Hyperthermia while undergoing MRI

> **BOX 53.1 CLINICAL PEARLS**
>
> - **Cranial Pins:** Administer a bolus of propofol for placement of pins to decrease sympathetic response. Avoid emerging patient prior to removal of pins.
> - **ECoG:** Use a TIVA technique.
> - **MRI:** MRI safety. Patient will be wrapped in plastic drape as heat from MRI can increase patient temperature to unsafe levels.
> - **Intraoperative Labs:** Frequently monitor Hgb/Hct for blood loss, base deficit, and electrolytes as indicated by type of surgery and health history. Antiepileptic drugs, history of ketogenic diet, and mannitol administration can all cause metabolic acidosis.
> - **Fluid/Blood Replacement:** Replace NPO volume deficit and fluid loss from mannitol administration. Transfuse blood products for acute blood loss and/or patient becomes unstable.
> - **Field Avoidance:** Patient will be turned 90–180 degrees away with head completely covered for the procedure. With procedures involving MRI, access to the airway is limited due to the MRI machine. Attention to detail with the airway is critical, and an airway plan should be discussed if issues should arise.
> - **Wake-Up Test:** Although rare in children, anesthesia providers should always be prepared to perform a wake-up test as needed.
>
> ECoG, electrocorticography; Hct, hematocrit; Hgb, hemoglobin; TIVA, total IV anesthetic.

For minimally invasive or neurostimulation procedures, routine monitoring is usually sufficient, with placement of an arterial catheter determined by the patient's overall health status, length of planned procedure, need for continuous hemodynamic monitoring, or need for frequent blood sampling. For invasive procedures, placement of an arterial catheter should be planned. Two IV catheters should be placed for all procedures should fluid or blood resuscitation be necessary. Lactated Ringer's solution should be avoided in patients on a ketogenic diet and normal saline should be used for this population.

The patient will be positioned supine with their head placed either on a horseshoe head pad or placed in cranial pins. If using a horseshoe, the anesthesia provider should confirm appropriate placement of the patient's face in horseshoe to prevent facial injuries. If cranial pins are planned, a bolus of propofol should be administered immediately prior to pin placement to limit the sympathetic response. The head may be turned or flexed to facilitate surgical access. In some instances, the patient will be positioned prone. If positioned prone, it is imperative that the anesthesia provider assess the patient's mean airway pressure before and after positioning, as well as the patient's eyes and all pressure points. Regardless of position, adequate padding with frequent reassessment is imperative to prevent compression and stretch injuries.

Maintenance of anesthesia is largely determined by the need for intraoperative monitoring, which is determined by the type of surgery and the extent of resection planned. Volatile anesthesia, IV anesthetics, and opioid analgesics all impact ECoG monitoring to varying degrees. If ECoG monitoring is required, a total IV anesthetic (TIVA) technique employing propofol and remifentanil or sufentanil infusions. Should cortical mapping or ECoG-guided resection be needed, anesthesia providers must work collaboratively with the neuromonitoring team to ensure the appropriate depth of anesthesia is being delivered.

Fluid replacement should be based on the patient's body weight and should account for insensible losses with the goal being euvolemia. Normal saline is often the maintenance fluid of choice as it is mildly hyperosmolar, which theoretically decreases the likelihood of cerebral edema. Anesthesia providers should be aware that rapid administration of large quantities of normal saline, however, can result in hyperchloremic acidosis. Additional fluid may be required depending on the extent and length of the surgical procedure, as well as the degree of exposure of the vascular beds. Mannitol is often administered per the surgeon's request to reduce brain tissue swelling and improve brain relaxation during neurosurgery. Of note, mannitol may also exhibit anticonvulsant effect via gamma-aminobutyric acid A receptor regulation.

Should cranial pins be used, it is important the anesthesia provider does not begin to emerge the patient from anesthesia until after the cranial pins have been removed. Patients are generally extubated awake at the end of the procedure to allow for a neurological assessment. Standard awake-extubation criteria for age should be used. If unable to successfully awake and extubate the patient following the conclusion of the procedure, the patient may emergently be transferred to radiology for a CT scan to rule out surgical complication versus anesthetic-related delay in emergence. In some instances, the patient may need to remain intubated in which case they will be transferred to the intensive care unit postoperatively.

Special Techniques

ECoG is an invasive version of EEG that is sometimes also referred to as intracranial encephalograph. ECoG may be used intraoperatively to confirm the location and extent of epileptic tissue using an array of grid electrodes placed on the cerebral cortex to record activity directly from the cortical brain surface.[11] Should ECoG be employed, a TIVA technique should be used with the addition of neuromuscular blockade. Anesthesia providers should be aware that depending on the dose administered, most anesthetics can have either proconvulsant or anticonvulsant effects. As the depth of anesthesia progresses to Stage III, the ratio of excitatory and inhibitory neurons changes, with high-frequency beta waves replacing the alpha waves. This ultimately progresses to high-amplitude low-frequency theta and delta waves replacing beta waves. Communication with the neuromonitoring team is essential to maintain the proper depth of anesthesia to optimize intraoperative ECoG monitoring.

POSTOPERATIVE CARE

Most often patients are transferred to the postanesthesia care unit (PACU) for recovery prior transfer to the floor. While in the PACU, the patient should be monitored for signs and symptoms of seizure activity, neurological deficit or compromise, hemodynamic stability, and pain control with interventions as necessary. Postoperative nausea and vomiting can cause sudden increases in intracranial pressure and should be treated with nonsedating antiemetic drugs as needed.

CASE STUDY: Intractable Focal Epilepsy

CLINICAL SCENARIO

An 18-year-old child with intractable focal epilepsy presented to the hospital for a minimally invasive laser ablation of the left anterior insula of the brain guided by intraoperative MRI and robotic stereotactic assistance (ROSA). The patient suffered a traumatic brain injury 5 years prior and as a result has had recurrent seizures, at least one per day, despite pharmaceutical and surgical interventions. The patient's medical history included pediatric autoimmune neuropsychiatric disease (PANDAS) and asthma. His surgical history includes a partial left anterior frontal lobe insertion of grids to monitor for ictal onset zones in the brain. This was followed by a partial left anterior grid-based resection of the ictal onset zones.

The patient arrived at the operating room and was positioned supine on the operating room table; standard MRI safe monitors were applied on the patient. Peripheral IV access was obtained, the patient was preoxygenated with 100% O_2, and induction of anesthesia was initiated with 70 mg of 2% lidocaine, 100 mcg of fentanyl, and 200 mg of propofol. Once the ability to mask ventilate was confirmed, 50 mg of rocuronium was administered and direct laryngoscopy was performed with endotracheal tube (ETT) placement into the trachea. The ETT was taped to the right, away from surgical field. After the airway was secure, a left radial arterial line and second peripheral IV catheter were placed under ultrasound guidance.

Anesthesia was maintained with a sufentanil infusion, a rocuronium infusion, and isoflurane at 1%. The rocuronium infusion was started when peripheral nerve stimulation with the train-of-four monitor returned to 4/4. The infusion was then titrated to 1/4 twitches throughout the case. Due to intraoperative MRI scanning and surgical intervention, the MRI safe operating room table must be turned 90 degrees. Once the table was in proper position and all invasive lines were in place, the surgeon performed the surgical time out. Antibiotics were given and MRI safe head pins were placed by the surgical team. The ROSA robot was then docked to the head pins.

The left anterior insula was accessed via a small opening, and fiberoptic laser catheters were placed by the surgeon directly at the abnormal region in the patient's brain. The ROSA robot and stealth guidance aid in this precise catheter placement. Following the placement of four catheters, the MRI staff arrived to go through a safety checklist to ensure all ferrous material was safely tethered or stored away. The ROSA robot was undocked from the head pins and removed from the room. Once the room was considered safe, the patient was placed in a sterile plastic drape to ensure the field was not contaminated by the MRI machine.

Laser energy was applied to the seizure-generating region of the brain to destroy the targeted area. The intraoperative MRI was imperative to protecting the normal portions of the brain from the heat generated by the laser catheters. The surgery requires multiple teams working together, which include neurosurgery, neurology, and radiology. Once the three teams determined that the targeted portion of the brain was destroyed, the MRI was removed from the room, the four catheters were removed from the brain, and they closed the small opening in the patient's skull. Thirty minutes prior to the case ending, the sufentanil drip was stopped and the isoflurane was increased to 1.2%. Communication with the surgical team was important as the closure process did not require a lot of time. The rocuronium infusion was discontinued and paralytic was reversed with sugammadex. Per the surgeon's request, 10 mg of dexamethasone was given at the end of the case to aid with inflammation in the brain caused by ablation. Following conclusion of surgery, the patient was extubated awake, with a neurological assessment completed following extubation. The patient suffered from aphasia and displayed signs of weakness on his right side. These are known complications following laser ablation surgery on the left side of the brain. The patient's language and weakness did improve prior to being discharged from the hospital.

SPECIAL CONSIDERATIONS

Positioning is a very important factor in these cases, and anesthesia providers must ensure everything is well padded and positioned prior to draping the patient. The length of the case can be as long as 10 hours, and there is very little ability to access the patient once the MRI machine is in place. Therefore, proper positioning is imperative for patient safety and avoidance of positioning-related injury.

(continued)

CASE STUDY: Intractable Focal Epilepsy (*continued*)

Another aspect of the case to consider is the patient's core temperature. As noted in the clinical scenario, the patient will be placed in plastic sterile drapes for the MRI portion of the case. This portion of the case can last several hours, and the patient's temperature will increase. The MRI safe temperature probe must be esophageal, nasopharyngeal, or rectal. Temperature urinary catheters are not MRI safe and axillary temperatures are inappropriate for this procedure as they are not as accurate. Due to the inevitable increase in the patient's core temperature, a warming device is not typically used in these cases.

Antiepileptic medications can affect multiple aspects of the anesthetic and should be reviewed prior to the start of the case. AEDs are to be taken the day of surgery unless the neurosurgeon has requested the patient to hold their medication. For this case, AEDs were taken the day of surgery. One antiepileptic drug, topiramate, is known for causing asymptomatic metabolic acidosis.[6] It is important as a provider to be aware the patient is taking this medication prior to drawing the first arterial blood gas as numbers will often be skewed. AEDs can also interfere with paralytic medications, resulting in many providers having to give significantly higher doses of paralytic throughout the case. An infusion of a paralytic, such as rocuronium, is a great alternative to constant boluses throughout the case.

The peripheral nerve stimulator is not compatible with the MRI machine, as noted on the MRI safety checklist, thus, it must be removed from the patient. Titrating to 1/4 twitches via the peripheral nerve stimulator should be completed prior to the intraoperative MRI portion of the case. The patient will remain in head pins, and the laser catheters cannot move as they are in the precise location needed to ablate the seizure-generating region of the brain. Anesthesia providers should be aware that this portion of the case can last several hours with no ability to check peripheral nerve stimulation.

APPROACHES TO CARE

Evidence-Based Approaches to Care

Laser ablation can cause severe edema to the surrounding normal brain tissue. Due to this concern, a high dose of dexamethasone is given at the end of the case to aid in decreasing edema. This high dose is continued postoperatively at a maximum sequential dose of 4 mg every 6 hours for 24 to 48 hours, followed by a taper over 5 to 7 days.[12]

AEDs can have multiple interactions with the drugs used to provide anesthesia. Chronic patient use of phenytoin and carbamazepine causes an increase in hepatic clearance of rocuronium and a decrease in duration of action.[8] This causes providers to give more paralytic throughout the case and thus supports the use of a paralytic infusion for laser ablation cases in which there is very little margin for error if the patient moves.

COMPLICATIONS

It has been noted that there are fewer complications with this procedure in comparison to other epilepsy surgeries that require open craniotomy intervention. The recovery period is known to be easier and shorter than traditional epilepsy surgeries.[13] Reported complications are rare but may include weakness in extremities, nerve damage, bleeding in the brain, aphasia, memory loss, and narrowing of vision.[11] In comparison to open surgery, cognitive function is better following laser ablation.[13]

KEY REFERENCES

Complete references for this chapter are online and available at https://connect.springerpub.com/content/book/978-0-8261-3875-0/part/part04/toc-part/ch053

1. ILAE. *Epilepsy Syndromes*. International League Against Epilepsy; 2020. https://www.epilepsydiagnosis.org/syndrome/epilepsy-syndrome-groupoverview.html
2. Wirrell E. *Drug Resistant Epilepsy*. Epilepsy Foundation; 2020. https://www.epilepsy.com/learn/drug-resistant-epilepsy
6. Kwon H, Kim H. Recent aspects of pediatric epilepsy surgery. *J. Epilepsy Res.* 2020;9(2), 87–92. doi:10.14581/jer.19010
10. Conover ZR, Talai A, Klockau K, et al. Perioperative management of children on ketogenic dietary therapies. *Anesth. Analg.* 2020;131(6):1872–1882. doi:10.1213/ane.0000000000005018
13. Koubeissi M, Bermio-Ovalle A, Schuele SU. *LITT Thermal Ablation*. Epilepsy Foundation; 2020. https://www.epilepsy.com/learn/treating-seizures-and-epilepsy/surgery/types-epilepsy-surgery/litt-thermal-ablation

CHAPTER 54

Dorsal Rhizotomy

Anne M. Que and Meghan Pursley

INDICATIONS/CONTRAINDICATIONS

While a nonprogressive condition, children with cerebral palsy (CP) often experience a progressive loss of mobility in part due to the development of spastic contractures. In addition, impaired bone and muscle development, shortening of the muscles, and deformities can result in the affected limbs secondary to chronic spasticity. Subsequently, patients affected with CP can suffer from abnormalities in gait and posture due to the damage of the motor nerve fibers that control muscle function, leading to unopposed muscular contraction and stiffness.

Surgical treatment includes osteotomies, muscle and tendon lengthening, baclofen pump insertion, and selective dorsal rhizotomy (SDR). SDR is an irreversible surgical procedure involving the division of selected sensory nerve roots, with the goal of reducing spasticity in the lower limbs and improving gross motor function and quality of life. In order to expose the spinal cord and dorsal nerve rootlets, the surgeon makes a small incision along the lumbar region and removes spinous processes and a portion of the lamina. Electrical stimulation is performed on isolated rootlets. When abnormal responses are detected, the surgeon divides that particular rootlet. This decreases electrical input to the spinal motor neurons and results in reduced spasticity. Typically, 50% to 70% of the dorsal rootlets will be sacrificed in children with spastic CP.[1]

Following SDR, patients undergo intensive physiotherapy for a period of several months. The popularity of this procedure has waxed and waned throughout the years due to improvements in oral medications and gaining interest in the baclofen pump, which continuously infuses this gamma aminobutyric acid (GABA)-agonist drug into the subarachnoid space.[2] When these modalities fail however, SDR is the next treatment of choice.

ANESTHETIC MANAGEMENT

PREOPERATIVE EVALUATION

Many children with CP also have an associated seizure disorder. During the preoperative evaluation, it is essential to investigate the frequency of the child's seizures and what anticonvulsant therapy the patient is taking. A therapeutic serum concentration of the anticonvulsant should be maintained throughout the perioperative period; therefore, the child should receive the usual dose of anticonvulsant medication the morning of surgery. If the child is scheduled to receive a dose of the anticonvulsant during surgery, the dose can be converted to the IV route, and it can be administered intraoperatively. Chronic anticonvulsant therapy affects the P450 degradation pathways, which alters the pharmacokinetics of many anesthetic drugs.[3] Increased doses may be necessary to achieve a pharmacodynamic effect.

Neurologic and neuromuscular dysfunction should be identified and documented during the preoperative period. It is imperative to have an understanding of the child's baseline neurological status to compare to when assessing for postoperative deficits. A portion of children with CP will also have some degree of impaired cognitive function. During the preoperative period, the child's developmental level should be assessed, and an appropriate means of communication should be established.

Poor oropharyngeal function, leading to excessive drooling, may be present. Along with an ineffective cough, gastroesophageal reflux is common among children with CP. As a result, children with CP are considered high-aspiration risks. The chronic aspiration of secretions and stomach acid results in damage to the pulmonary mucosa, leading to the development of recurrent pneumonia and reactive airway disease. Children with CP may also have limited respiratory muscle strength as well as restricted airways secondary to their scoliosis. Anesthesia can exacerbate respiratory pathology and perioperative dysfunction should be expected (Table 54.1).

Pertinent preoperative laboratory studies are summarized in Box 54.1.

Table 54.1	Key Assessment Points
Preoperative Consideration	**Anesthetic Implication**
Seizure disorder	Maintain therapeutic serum anticonvulsant concentration throughout perioperative period
Communication difficulty	Assess developmental level and establish means of communication
Muscle contractures	Establish baseline neuromuscular function to provide a comparison for the postoperative period
Poor oropharyngeal control	Consider child a high-aspiration risk
Gastroesophageal reflux	Consider child a high-aspiration risk
Level of hydration	Children with cerebral palsy are often chronically dehydrated. Consider preoperative IV hydration
Latex allergy	Children with cerebral palsy are at increased risk of a latex allergy. Implement latex precautions

BOX 54.1 PERTINENT LABS

- Complete blood count
- Coagulation studies
- Basic metabolic panel
- Liver function tests

PREOPERATIVE PHARMACOLOGY

Ensure the child has received any scheduled anticonvulsant medications. If the child has missed a scheduled dose, consider converting to an IV dose and administering preoperatively to maintain a therapeutic serum concentration. Preoperative sedation should be avoided in patients with reduced upper airway tone, because sedation may accentuate the problem and increase the risk of aspiration. Premedication with an antisialagogue is beneficial if excessive drooling is present. Glycopyrrolate can be administered to decrease secretions and facilitate tracheal intubation.

ANESTHETIC TECHNIQUE

Intraoperative Management

Children with CP are at a high risk of aspiration due to their poor oropharyngeal function and gastroesophageal reflux; therefore, it is safest to induce general anesthesia in these patients with a rapid sequence induction (RSI). The use of succinylcholine is controversial in children with CP due to the risk of cardiac arrest secondary to succinylcholine-induced hyperkalemia.[3] Therefore, it is best to avoid succinylcholine with this patient population. A modified RSI can be accomplished with a nondepolarizing muscle relaxant (NDMR). It is important to remember that NDMRs are less potent in patients with CP as their decreased mobility leads to an upregulation of acetylcholine receptors. Typically, high-dose rocuronium is given to safely and quickly secure the airway.

Once the airway is secured, the patient is positioned prone. Due to contractures, children with CP can be difficult to position. It is important not to force any position, which can cause skeletal or nerve damage. Extra care should be taken to ensure that pressure points are sufficiently padded to prevent pressure injuries. The head should be maintained in a neutral position, and the eyes, nose, and chin should be free from undue pressure.

In order to ensure that motor and sensory nerve monitoring can be maintained throughout the duration of the procedure, stable anesthetic conditions are important. Although an NDMR can be administered to secure the airway, muscle relaxants should be avoided after induction to facilitate monitoring of motor function of the dorsal nerve roots. Volatile anesthetic agents can safely be used; however, above a concentration of 0.5 MAC, suppression of motor evoked potential (MEP) amplitude occurs. IV anesthetics, such as propofol, are less suppressive, but still produce a dose-dependent reduction in MEP amplitude. Narcotics are the least suppressive and are generally well tolerated. A short-acting narcotic that is quickly metabolized, such as remifentanil, is ideal because other narcotics accumulate in SC tissue and can result in postoperative respiratory depression.[4]

Patients with CP frequently exhibit impaired thermoregulation. Muscular atrophy and little SC fat put them at high risk of hypothermia. Intraoperative use of warm blankets, forced-air warming devices, and fluid warmers should be used to maintain normothermia. Warming the temperature of the room at the start and end of the procedure can also help to prevent hypothermia.

Emergence can be prolonged in children with CP due to cerebral damage or the effects of anticonvulsant therapy.[5] Ideally, the child can safely be extubated once they regain their pharyngeal reflex. However, it is important to consider that this reflex may be diminished in children with CP (Box 54.2).

POSTOPERATIVE CARE

Children typically recover in the intensive care unit following dorsal rhizotomy to allow for frequent neurological checks and manage postoperative complications. Respiratory concerns following anesthesia include aspiration, diminished cough reflex, and reduced respiratory drive.[5] Patients should be monitored for hypoxemia and may require respiratory support during the immediate postoperative period. Anticonvulsant therapy should be resumed following surgery. Doses may need to be converted to the IV route if the patient is not yet able to tolerate oral medications. As children with CP have poor thermoregulation, they should be monitored for hypothermia postoperatively. Children with CP are also prone to dehydration, which can contribute to postoperative hypotension.

BOX 54.2 COMPLICATIONS/EMERGENCIES

- Postoperative hypothermia
- Hypotension
- Hypoxemia
- Seizures
- Recurrence of spasticity

CASE STUDY: A 7-Year-Old Female With Poor Oropharyngeal Control Presents for Dorsal Rhizotomy

CLINICAL SCENARIO

A 7-year-old female is scheduled for a dorsal rhizotomy at 7 a.m. She weighs 19 kg and ambulates using a walker for balance support. Her medical history includes CP and gastroesophageal reflux disease (GERD). She currently takes baclofen, ranitidine, sucralfate, docusate sodium, and glycopyrrolate. She is tube-dependent, and last received a feed at 8 p.m. last night. Her G tube is currently venting to a Farrell bag, which contains 20 mL of a tan liquid consistent with formula. A complete blood count and basic metabolic panel were drawn this morning. Her potassium is 5.0 mEq/L. All other results were unremarkable. Her airway examination is normal; however, excessive oral secretions are present.

SPECIAL CONSIDERATIONS

This patient is a high-aspiration risk due to her history of GERD and poor oropharyngeal control. A rapid sequence intubation is the safest method to secure the airway and mitigate risk of

(continued)

CASE STUDY: A 7-Year-Old Female With Poor Oropharyngeal Control Presents for Dorsal Rhizotomy (*continued*)

aspiration. The use of succinylcholine is controversial in children with CP because immobility leads to upregulation of their acetylcholine receptors, putting them at higher risk of cardiac arrest secondary to succinylcholine-induced hyperkalemia.

APPROACHES TO CARE

Evidence-Based Approaches to Care
A modified rapid sequence intubation using a 1 mg/kg dose of rocuronium can safely allow tracheal intubation of high-aspiration-risk patients.[6] High-dose rocuronium is required not only to provide intubating conditions similar to that of succinylcholine, but also because NDMRs are less potent in children with CP due to the upregulation of their acetylcholine receptors.[3]

COMPLICATIONS
In comparison to succinylcholine, rocuronium provides muscle relaxation for significantly longer duration. In the case of a dorsal rhizotomy, in which electrophysiologic monitoring of motor nerves is being conducted, muscle relaxation is contraindicated. Although the action of rocuronium is typically minimal by the time the surgeon has exposed the spinal cord and dorsal nerve roots, a dose of sugammadex may be necessary prior to the cutting of any nerves.

REFERENCES

1. Shuer LM. Surgery for spasticity. In: Jaffe RA, Schmiesing CA, Golianu B, eds. *Anesthesiologist's Manual of Surgical Procedures* (5th ed.). Wolters Kluwer; 2020:330–334.
2. Tu A, Steinbok P. Long term outcome of selective dorsal rhizotomy for the management of childhood spasticity—functional improvement and complications. *Childs Nerv Syst.* 2020:1985–1994. doi:10.1007/s00381-020-04747-8
3. Lammers C, Wyckaert C. Cerebral palsy. In: Andropoulos DB, Gregory GA, eds. *Gregory's Pediatric Anesthesia* (5th ed.). Wiley-Blackwell; 2012:769–770.
4. Lieberman J. Electromyography and evoked potentials. In: Gupta AK, Gelb AW, Duane D, Adapa R, eds. *Gupta and Gelb's Essentials of Neuroanesthesia and Neurointensive Care.* Cambridge University Press; 2018:349–356.
5. Urban MK. Cerebral palsy. In: Miller RD, ed. *Miller's Anesthesia.* 7th ed. Churchill Livingstone Elsevier; 2009:2248–2249.
6. Tran DT, Newton EK, Mount VA, et al. Rocuronium vs. succinylcholine for rapid sequence intubation: a Cochrane systematic review. *Anaesthesia.* 2017;72(6):765–777. doi:10.1111/anae.13903

CHAPTER 55

Cranial Vault Reconstruction and Craniosynostosis Repair
Anthony Prickel

INDICATIONS/CONTRAINDICATIONS

The neonate's skull is composed of multiple bony plates divided by sutures. This anatomical arrangement allows for temporary skull deformation during the physiologic birthing process as the fetus passes through the narrow birth canal. This anatomical arrangement also enables the skull to accommodate the progressive growth of the infant's brain, which will quadruple in size over the next 2 years to approximately 75% of the adult volume.[1] Structurally there are four major sutures. The metopic, coronal, and sagittal sutures conjoin to form the anterior fontanelle, palpable at the anterior midline, and immediately posterior to the forehead, respectively. The lambdoid suture intersects with the sagittal suture to form the posterior fontanelle (**Figure 55.1**).

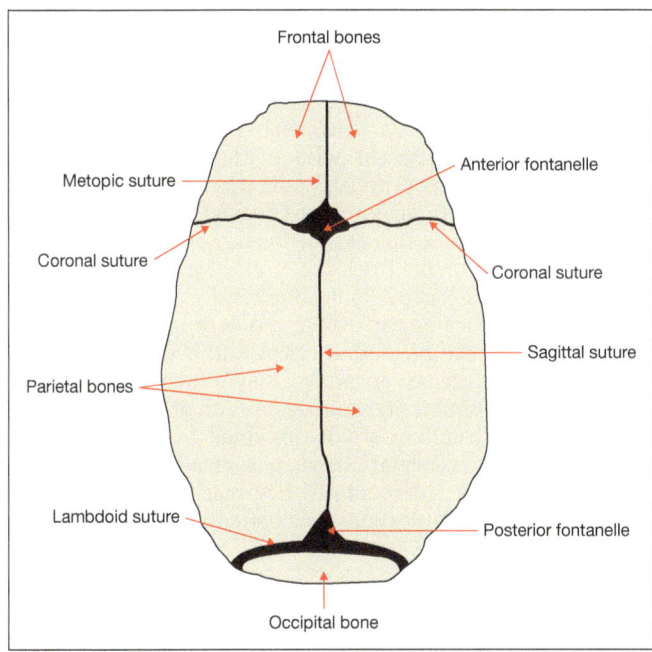

Figure 55.1: Cranial suture lines.
Source: From Barreto S, González-Vázquez AR, Cameron A, et al. Identification of stiffness-induced signalling mechanisms in cells from patent and fused sutures associated with craniosynostosis. *Sci Rep.* 2017;7:11494. doi:10.1038/s41598-017-11801-0

The calvarium, in contrast to the osseous cranial base, consists of membranous bone having no cartilaginous phase. Instead, the calvarium develops via progressive deposition of new bone along the sutures in response to the tensile forces provided by rapid brain growth.[1] Suture closure typically occurs in an organized fashion. The absence of osteoinhibitory signals from the suture(s), however, may result in the premature osseous obliteration of one or more cranial sutures.[2] This describes the congenital anomaly known as craniosynostosis, which affects approximately 1 in every 2,000 to 2,500 births globally.[1]

With the premature fusion of the cranial suture(s), skull growth is restricted perpendicular to the affected suture(s). To accommodate the growing brain, compensatory expansion of the skull occurs parallel to the affected suture. Thus, the suture(s) affected dictate(s) the resulting skull deformity.[1] Scaphocephaly (dolichocephaly), or hull-shaped skull, is the result of premature sagittal suture closure and accounts for approximately 50% of craniosynostosis cases.[1] Plagiocephaly, also known as twisted skull, is caused by synostosis of the unilateral coronal or lambdoidal sutures. Anterior plagiocephaly, premature closure of a unilateral coronal suture, accounts for roughly 20% of cases, occurring in 1 in 10,000 live births.[1] Brachycephaly is caused by bilateral coronal synostosis. It should be noted that brachycephaly is often mild and transient, presenting without sutural synostosis and occurring, rather, as a positional deformity. This form is common in infants suffering from hypotonia who are placed on their backs to sleep, so as to minimize the risk of sudden infant death syndrome.[1] Oxycephaly, or turricephaly, however, may result as a natural progression of brachycephaly, if the brachycephaly is in fact the result of bicoronal synostosis and treatment is delayed or inadequate.[1] The premature closure of the metopic suture is less common, still, occurring in approximately 1 in 20,000 live births, or just 10% of craniosynostosis cases.[1]

When multiple sutures fuse prematurely, most commonly the coronal, lambdoid, and metopic sutures, Kleeblattschädel results; also known as cloverleaf deformity. While it is a rare anomaly with fewer than 130 documented cases, Kleeblattschädel is considered the most severe form of craniosynostosis. Hydrocephalus and cognitive delays are present in nearly all affected patients.[1] Acrocephaly, known as tower skull, is caused by the combination of sagittal, coronal, and lambdoid synostosis. It is often seen in Crouzon and Apert syndromes.[1]

Craniosynostosis can be categorized as simple (nonsyndromic), involving premature closure of one suture, or complex (syndromic), involving two or more sutures. The large majority (65%–80%) of craniosynostosis cases are of the nonsyndromic type.[2] Synostosis of a single cranial suture generally occurs sporadically and as an isolated defect. There is some evidence, however, suggesting that compression of the fetal skull in utero, as in multiple pregnancies or in the presence of bicornuate uterus, can increase the incidence of craniosynostosis.[1] The remaining 20% to 35% of patients born with craniosynostosis are syndromic, with the premature closure of multiple sutures present. Anesthesia providers should be aware that with syndromic craniosynostosis, the coronal suture is most commonly involved.[2] Moreover, syndromic craniosynostosis is often related to an underlying genetic syndrome associated with various clinical anomalies, including facial dysmorphism and metabolic disturbances.[1,2] Greater than 150 associated syndromes have been described. Among the most common of these are Apert, Crouzon, Pfeiffer, Carpenter, Muenke, and Saethre–Chotzen syndromes.[3]

The complications of uncorrected craniosynostosis are synonymous with the indications for cranial vault reconstruction. Increased intracranial pressure (ICP) is both the result of numerous associative factors and the cause of severe neurological sequelae if craniosynostosis remains unrecognized and/or uncorrected. The causative factors of ICP elevation include hydrocephalus, craniocerebral disproportion—that is cranial growth restriction and direct compression of the underlying brain, thereby inhibiting brain growth and potentially resulting in airway obstruction (obstructive sleep apnea [OSA])— and/or abnormal cerebral venous drainage.[1–3] Uncorrected, these factors can lead to devastating physical, neurologic, and psychosocial consequences. Associated cognitive and neurodevelopmental impairments include global developmental delay, poor feeding and weight gain, vision, hearing, and speech deficits relative to cranial nerve involvement, poor self-esteem, and social isolation due to abnormal appearance (exophthalmos and craniofacial deformity), and negative self-image.[1–3]

Given the rapid rate of brain growth in early childhood, and because infantile brain growth shapes the skull, surgical intervention is indicated during infancy to achieve optimal outcomes both neurologically and cosmetically.[2] The specific timing of surgical correction remains controversial, however, barring an immediate threat to the airway or eyes, or the presence of increased ICP, any of which are indications for emergency surgery.[3] Advantages of early surgical intervention include the greater malleability of younger softer bone, as well as the potential for continued expansion of the cranial vault aided by active brain growth.[3] With this, however, comes the cost of performing complex surgery and anesthesia in a younger patient, the greater likelihood of complications related to blood loss, and the increased possibility of the need for reoperative surgery in the future.[3] The need for reoperative surgery is less likely in older children, and risks associated with surgery and anesthesia are generally decreased. Surgery, however, can prove to be more challenging in the older patient due to the increased severity of deformities and a thicker, less malleable cranium. A thicker, less malleable cranium may also have a diminished capacity for ossifying small defects, thereby necessitating the use of bone grafts that may have otherwise been avoidable.[3] In an effort to balance these challenges, surgery is commonly performed around 8 to 12 months of age.[3]

Provided the diagnosis is made before 6 months of age, invasive surgery for the correction of sagittal synostosis is optimally performed at a younger age, with patients typically being between the age of 3 and 6 months for the reasons discussed earlier.[2,3] Surgical correction in this instance is likely performed using an extended strip craniectomy, dividing the cranial vault into multiple segments and allowing once again for the skull to grow in conjunction with the brain. Subsequently, this surgical technique requires the patient be fit for and wear a protective helmet, a postoperative therapy that relies on continued brain growth to drive cranial remodeling.[2,3]

Total cranial vault reconstruction or reshaping is a more extensive and more invasive procedure intended to correct the prematurely fused suture, and additionally, the compensatory deformities of the calvarium preceding the diagnosis. Included in this procedure is the removal and restructuring of the cranial bones using plates and screws. Given the general complexity and more invasive nature of the procedure, an increased surgical duration is to be expected as are the risks incurred. For these reasons, total cranial vault reconstruction is usually reserved for patients until or exceeding 10 to 12 months of age.[3]

SPECIAL CONSIDERATIONS AND CONCERNS

Spring-assisted cranioplasty is a relatively new minimally invasive technique for the correction of sagittal synostosis. A midline osteotomy is performed along the fused sagittal suture, followed by the placement of two springs across the osteotomized defect, intended to mechanically separate the narrow surgical opening, gradually increasing the biparietal dimension.[2,3] Because of the more recent advent of this surgical technique, both the quality and quantity of available evidence are limited. Still, it is worth noting, early data suggest the spring-assisted cranioplasty may provide for improved outcomes regarding total operative time, intraoperative blood loss and transfusion requirement, need for intensive care unit (ICU) admission, and length of hospital stay.[2,3]

ANESTHETIC MANAGEMENT

PREOPERATIVE ASSESSMENT

A preoperative evaluation and anesthetic plan tailored to the individual patient is critical, as is a comprehensive understanding of the intended surgical procedure and the coinciding anesthetic implications. With that, the preoperative phase should be focused primarily on airway assessment, cardiac and hematologic evaluation, and the presence of an elevated ICP or related issues.[2,3] Identifying the need for intervention in these areas is of utmost importance, particularly in the presence of associated syndromes, such as those previously discussed. Most patients with nonsyndromic craniosynostosis, however, are otherwise healthy. Further evaluation may be necessary in the setting of syndromic craniosynostosis and associated congenital cardiac disease.

Associated midface hypoplasia and tonsillar hypertrophy contribute to a 50% to 70% incidence of OSA in syndromic craniosynostosis patients.[1] A thorough review of the patient's sleep study is warranted, as is consultation with ears, nose, and throat specialists if midface hypoplasia is significant and/or if OSA is present with evidence of moderate-to-severerespiratory compromise.[3] Adenotonsillectomy has been recommended in craniosynostosis patients to treat OSA preoperatively; however, this has not been shown to improve airway dimensions or the presence of airway collapse. Instead, preoperative endoscopy is recommended to evaluate the severity of midface hypoplasia and determine the likelihood of OSA persistence beyond surgical midface advancement.[1] Still, while midface advancement may alleviate the primary culprit, it cannot guarantee total resolution of OSA, and residual airway obstruction is still possible.[1] In either instance, with or without a formal obstructive airway assessment or corrective airway intervention, bag-mask ventilation may prove difficult in craniosynostosis patients, particularly those of the syndromic type.

Pertinent Labs

Prior to surgery, it is imperative that baseline hemoglobin and hematocrit (Hct) levels be assessed, as should coagulation studies. The patient's blood type should be determined, and they should be cross-matched in anticipation of the need for intraoperative blood transfusion, and blood products should be readily available.

PREOPERATIVE PHARMACOLOGY

Syndromic craniosynostosis may be associated with midface hypoplasia or retrusion resulting in OSA and other perioperative airway considerations. Therefore, the use of preoperative sedatives should be done with caution, especially in the setting of severe obstructive disease.

ANESTHETIC TECHNIQUE

Intraoperative Management

Consideration of noted midface hypoplasia or airway anomalies should play a role in determining the appropriateness of an inhalational mask induction versus an IV induction. Generally speaking, either induction route is acceptable and vastly dependent on the preferences of the anesthesia provider and the patient's parents, keeping in mind the potential for airway compromise in addition to the potential for difficult IV access in this age group—even more so in the syndromic patient population.[3] In either case, appropriate airway adjuncts should always be readily available.

Midface hypoplasia, narrow or obstructed nares, hypertrophic tonsils, and an easily collapsible upper airway can all individually or conjointly be the cause of difficult mask ventilation or upper airway obstruction during inhalation induction,[1] and/or on emergence, following extubation. Fortunately, in most instances, obstruction is quickly resolved by manually subluxing the temporomandibular joint or with insertion of an oropharyngeal airway,[1] making the potential for difficult bag-mask ventilation far less concerning. Likewise, the mandible and the temporomandibular joint are anatomically normal in most craniosynostosis patients, as are the upper airway dimensions, meaning that laryngoscopy and tracheal intubation are usually performed in this patient population with relative ease.[1] It is rare that abnormal neck mobility or mandibular hypoplasia complicate or pose challenge to either of these tasks.[1]

The type of endotracheal tube (ETT) to be used and the route of intubation should be considered in advance. Some institutions advocate for a nasal intubation due to the added stability it provides, particularly when it is sutured to the nasal septum, offering yet another measure of advanced airway security.[3] Regardless of the intubation route, however, and especially when caring for an infantile demographic such as this one, confirmation and reverification of appropriate ETT placement following intubation and with every position change are vital.[3] It is also advisable to ensure reliable tube and circuit connections after the patient is positioned and before they are draped as access to the airway will be limited once surgery has begun.[3]

Intraoperative position will depend largely on the specific sutures being addressed, with the patient being supine for correction of fused coronal and metopic sutures or prone or modified prone when addressing sagittal and lambdoid suture issues. Regardless of the position, proper padding of joints, peripheral nerves, and head is essential. Care should be taken to ensure proper eye protection. Some institutional protocols incorporate the use of corneal shields placed by the surgeon. Anesthesia providers should be aware that patients with midface hypoplasia or proptosis will require extra care to ensure the patient's eyes are adequately protected. As these are typically extensive surgical procedures that are associated with long operating times and significant amounts of volume loss/administration, temperature maintenance can be challenging. Anesthesia providers should employ such strategies as forced-air warming, blankets, and warmed fluids in an effort to maintain temperature homeostasis.

Because OSA and respiratory complications are more prevalent in this patient population, it is reasonable to limit perioperative opioid administration regardless of the patient's clinical airway interventions and findings. Being that the vast majority of craniosynostosis patients present at 24 months of age or sooner, poor airway tone and the direct effect of intraoperative opioids on the hypoglossal nucleus combine to increase both the likelihood and severity of upper airway obstruction postoperatively.[1] Many institutions utilize opioid infusions intraoperatively, such as remifentanil or sufentanil. If an agent with a short context-sensitive half time is utilized (remifentanil), a bolus of a longer acting agent prior to emergence, such as morphine, will be helpful in optimizing analgesia. The use of nonsteroidal anti-inflammatory drugs (NSAIDs), such as ketorolac, is generally avoided and is controversial in this surgical population due to the potential impact on postoperative bleeding.

Special Techniques and/or Equipment

The use of cell salvage for craniofacial surgery has grown in interest and popularity in recent years, due in part to safety concerns surrounding homologous blood transfusion (HBT), as well as the development of pediatric cell savers.[4] According to the Pediatric Craniofacial Collaborative Group (PCCG), cell saver was the second most commonly used blood conservation technique despite there being no controlled study evaluating the efficacy of cell saver as a stand-alone modality in craniosynostosis surgery.[5] Studies having evaluated cell saver as part of a multimodal blood conservation regimen for craniofacial procedures have reported variable results. Some have shown little benefit in reducing donor blood exposure due to the need for HBT before autologous blood has been processed via cell saver and made available for return, or because of insufficient blood salvage volumes.[4] However, when used in combination with other blood salvage techniques, in particular, erythropoietin (EPO), cell saver has been shown to decrease the incidence and volume of HBT.[4]

Although it does limit the number of donor exposures, directed blood donation and/or autologous transfusion has shown little evidence of improving outcomes in craniosynostosis patients. Because of the patient's age and size, autologous transfusion can prove both difficult and insufficient as a small total blood volume limits the volume that can be donated and makes it unlikely to preclude HBT during craniosynostosis repair or redo surgery.[1,4] Likewise, acute preoperative normovolemic hemodilution can be labor-intensive, and only mathematical modeling has shown the degree of blood savings with this technique to be moderate at best.[4] No clinically relevant evidence exists to show that it reduces the incidence or volume of HBT in children undergoing craniosynostosis surgery.[1] Thus, directed blood donation, autologous blood transfusion, and acute normovolemic hemodilution are rarely considered in present-day practice as a viable means of blood conservation therapy in this patient population.

Antifibrinolytic therapy has shown promising results. Administration of tranexamic acid (TXA), as the primary intervention in two placebo-controlled prospective trials, has been found to decrease both intraoperative and postoperative blood loss and transfusion requirements in complex cranial vault reconstruction.[5] Similarly, aminocaproic acid is known to reduce blood loss in cardiac and spinal procedures; however, adequate evidence supporting its effectiveness in achieving the same for craniosynostosis patients has yet to be established.[1] Despite the evidence of TXA efficacy, the PCCG reported antifibrinolytic use in just 63% of their patient population and suggested implementing the widespread use of antifibrinolytic administration as a potential improvement intervention.[5]

Controlled hypotension, defined as the deliberate induction and maintenance of a mean arterial pressure (MAP) target 10% to 20% beneath the patient's baseline, is known to decrease surgical blood loss intraoperatively and reduce operating time.[1] Inhalational agents, beta-blockers, vasodilators, and opioids have all been used to induce hypotension; however, studies demonstrating its efficacy specific to craniosynostosis surgery are lacking, presumably due to concerns regarding cerebral perfusion pressure (CPP).[1,4] Being that increased ICP is among the more prominent risk factors associated with craniosynostosis, and because inducing hypotension in the presence of increased ICP further compromises CPP, controlled hypotension should be used with caution in this patient population, and never without invasive arterial pressure (IAP) monitoring.[1,4] If controlled hypotension is used, maintenance of normovolemia and normocapnia is recommended,[1] as is maintaining a horizontal supine positioning. If a reverse Trendelenburg position is requested to decrease venous pressure at the surgical site, pay close attention to the level of the arterial line transducer. It is critical the transducer remain level with the patient's external auditory canal (EAC), or the acoustic meatus, as this most accurately reflects the level of the foramen of Monroe and therefore provides the most reliable representation of the patient's MAP in the cerebrum from which the patient's CPP can be most closely derived. Leaving the transducer below the level of the EAC will cause the patient's IAP, and therefore their CPP, to appear falsely elevated.

Complications/Emergencies

Blood Loss

Although the aforementioned surgical procedures are extradural in nature, blood loss from the scalp and cranium can be significant and pose major challenges for the anesthetist. In fact, corrective surgery for craniosynostosis is associated with an increased risk of cardiac arrest attributable to sudden massive blood loss.[1] In most cases, transfusion of erythrocyte containing blood products (ECBPs) is unavoidable. In 2017, the PCCG conducted a study with a registry query yielding 1,223 total subjects from 31 institutions and concluded that 91% of patients in the infant group (aged younger than or equal to 24 months) were transfused intraoperatively.[5] This patient population, specifically, holds the greatest risk of massive blood loss and ECBP transfusion owing to a disproportionately large head and proportionally increased cranial blood flow and volume, together creating a greater surface area and reservoir from which blood loss to occur.[3-5] Prolonged surgery duration is also associated with increased blood volume loss (BVL). This factor is more frequently encountered with syndromic craniosynostosis patients relative to the surgical complexity and invasiveness.[3,4]

While the need for intraoperative transfusion is seemingly all but inevitable, anesthesia providers should still be aware of the risk factors that give rise to massive transfusion. Among others, the specific suture(s) involved and the quantity of sutures to be repaired, the type of surgery scheduled, and the expertise of the surgeon should all be taken into consideration.[1] Additionally, anesthesia providers should be knowledgeable of the surgical stages when sudden and/or extensive blood loss is most likely to occur. Initial scalp dissection and raising of the periosteum give rise to concern for significant hemorrhage relatively early in the surgical procedure.[3,4] Communication between the surgeon and the anesthesia provider becomes critical as these and other key surgical stages are approached. Being able to predict and prepare for hemorrhage ensures appropriate intravascular fluid maintenance and prompt management of acute blood loss when it occurs.[4] Doing so may prevent patient decompensation and the need to activate massive blood transfusion protocol.[4]

While increased BVL often results in the transfusion of a greater number and volume of blood products, increased blood donor exposure is relatively limited. The PCCG reported the median number of donor exposures was just one, despite the relatively high transfusion volumes that were associated; 30% of patients in the infant group received greater than 40 mL/kg ECBPs intraoperatively.[5] This finding, however, is understandable, considering 40 mL/kg in an 8-kg infant is equal in volume to one unit of packed red blood cells (PRBCs)—320 mL.[5] Still, no single blood product administration is without the risks carried by any HBT.

Well-established risks of HBT include acute hemolytic reactions, transfusion-related acute lung injury, and infection, as well as the complications associated with massive transfusion, such as hypothermia, dilutional coagulopathy, and metabolic and electrolyte disturbances (hypocalcemia and hyperkalemia).[3,4] To alleviate and/or eliminate the need for HBT and the risks incurred, several strategies for blood conservation during craniosynostosis surgery have been proposed. Among them are preoperative recombinant human EPO, cell salvage, directed blood donation (from parents or siblings), acute preoperative normovolemic hemodilution, antifibrinolytics, and controlled hypotension.[1,4,5] Additionally, a dilute (1:400,000) epinephrine-containing solution may aid in reduction of bleeding from the scalp incision.[1] The reverse Trendelenburg position has also been suggested as a means of decreasing venous pressure and blood loss associated with the osteotomy sites. However, this comes with the increased risk of venous air embolism (VAE), thus, maintaining horizontal positioning is preferred.[1]

An increased requirement for intraoperative HBT is predicated by a low Hct preoperatively. Therefore, the diagnosis and treatment of preexisting anemia are crucial to optimize the Hct and provide for the best possible patient outcomes. SC administration of EPO for the 3 to 4 weeks preceding surgery, in conjunction with elemental iron supplementation, has been shown to improve preoperative Hct value by as much as 28% to 56% and decrease requirement for autologous blood transfusion.[1,4] In the presence of iron deficiency, iron supplementation and oral vitamin C should be started 3 weeks before EPO therapy.[1] Recombinant human EPO preoperatively, in combination with the use of the cell saver intraoperatively, has been shown to reduce transfusion requirements in children undergoing corrective surgery for craniosynostosis.[1]

Venous Air Embolism
VAE may occur in as many as 83% of cases, although significant hemodynamic concerns are rarer. The concern for VAE is significant, however, as the surgical field is above the level of the heart with open sinusoids. As the patient's central venous pressure (CVP) decreases due to hypovolemia or blood loss, air can be entrained due to pressure gradient formed between the surgical site and the right atrium. Although not commonly used, a precordial doppler is very sensitive in detecting the presence of a VAE. Should a hemodynamically significant VAE occur, this is often the result of right ventricle (RV) outflow obstruction and may be associated with hypoxemia, hypotension, decreased or absent end-tidal carbon dioxide, and cardiac arrest in extreme cases.[5]

Should a VAE be suspected, the surgeon should be notified immediately. The patient's head should be lowered, relative to the level of the heart to increase CVP, and the surgical field flooded. If a central venous catheter (CVC) is in place, efforts should be made to aspirate air from the CVC. Anesthesia providers should also make efforts to increase the patient's CVP by administering crystalloid, colloid, or blood products if available; an infusion of epinephrine may be necessary in the setting of profound or persistent hypotension.

POSTOPERATIVE CARE

Postoperatively, patients most often recover in the ICU for close monitoring. The patient may be extubated at the end of surgery though anesthesia providers may consider delaying extubation after prolonged procedures, massive transfusion, prone positioning, preoperative OSA, or airway concerns. The extent of airway edema may be evaluated by either direct laryngoscopy and assessment of the glottis and surrounding airway structures or by performing a leak test. If there is significant concern for postoperative edema or if an audible leak is not heard, the patient may remain intubated during transport to the ICU. If there are no contraindications, the administration of steroid therapy, such as dexamethasone, should be considered prior to extubation.

In addition to the airway obstruction, hyponatremia is concern postoperatively due to both the administration of hypotonic solutions or antidiuretic syndrome (SIADH). Should this occur, sequelae, such as cerebral edema, seizures, or death, may ensue; therefore, frequent monitoring of sodium levels is common in the immediate postoperative period. Similarly, serial monitoring for Hct and coagulation abnormalities occurs during the initial 48-hour postoperative period.

Fortunately, postoperative pain is not typically severe, and adequate analgesia is effectively achieved using acetaminophen in combination with carefully titrated opioids at greatly reduced doses (generally ≤50% normally prescribed doses).[1]

REFERENCES

1. Buchanann EP. Overview of craniosynostosis. In: Wesiman LE, Firth HV, eds. *UpToDate*. 2021. https://www.uptodate.com/contents/overview-of-craniosynostosis
2. Coté Charles J, Lerman J, Anderson BJ. Coté And Lerman's *A Practice of Anesthesia for Infants and Children*. Elsevier/Saunders 2013.
3. Pearson A, Matava CT. Anaesthetic management for craniosynostosis repair in children. *BJA Educ*. 2016;16(12):410–416. doi:10.1093/bjaed/mkw023
4. Hughes C, Thomas K, Johnson D, Das S. Anesthesia for surgery related to craniosynostosis: a review. Part 2. *Paediatr Anaesth*. 2013 Jan;23(1):22–7. doi:10.1111/j.1460-9592.2012.03922.x
5. Stricker PA, Goobie SM, Cladis FP, et al. Perioperative outcomes and management in pediatric complex cranial vault reconstruction. *Anesthesiology*. 2017;126(2):276–287. doi:10.1097/aln.0000000000001481

CHAPTER 56

Myelomeningocele Repair

James S. Furstein and Michael E. Conti

INDICATIONS/CONTRAINDICATIONS

Myelomeningocele represents the most severe form of spina bifida and indicates that a portion of the spinal cord has herniated through vertebral defects into a meningeal-lined sac. The incidence of meningomyelocele is approximately 1 to 6 in every 1,000 live births. While the exact cause remains unknown, genetic and environmental factors have long been implicated. Congenital anomalies, such as trisomy 13 or trisomy 18, and preconception folic acid deficiency have also been reported as possible etiologies.

Neural tube development normally occurs in the embryonic stage, with bone and muscle forming a protective barrier over the spinal cord. With myelomeningocele, normal embryological development of the neural tube is disrupted during the first month of gestation.[1] As a result, the vertebral arches fail to fuse and there is incomplete formation of the midline structures of the back. Incomplete closure of the neural tube results in a sac-like herniation of the meninges (meningocele) or a herniation of neural elements (myelomeningocele). Meningeal herniation is thought to occur secondary to cerebrospinal fluid pulsations, which progressively act to balloon the spinal cord through the bony defect.

Diagnosis often occurs prenatally due to abnormally increased levels of maternal alpha fetoprotein, reduced human chorionic gonadotropin, or reduced unconjugated estriol levels on maternal screening.[2] Imaging studies, such as fetal ultrasound, MRI, and CT, may be utilized to confirm the diagnosis, or the location and severity of the defect.

Myelomeningocele has several different presentations and can occur at any level along the neural tube. Most commonly, the neural tube fails to fuse in the middle or caudal neural groove, resulting in a thoracic or lumbosacral meningomyelocele. When the neural tube defect is more cephalad, the child will present with an encephalocele, although this is quite rare, which usually results in severe neurological deficits. Regardless of location, the presence of a myelomeningocele results in a loss of motor and sensory function below the level of lesion.

Surgical correction of myelomeningocele may be performed either antenatally or following delivery. Antenatal correction is achieved via fetoscopic surgery at a designated fetal center. This approach has been reported to be more advantageous than a postnatal repair, as prenatal correction decreases the need for a ventriculoperitoneal shunt and is associated with improved lower extremity motor functioning at 30 months of age.[3] For additional information regarding the anesthetic management of minimally invasive fetal surgery, please refer to Chapter 130 in this text.

Should surgical correction be delayed until the postnatal period, the child will be delivered via a cesarean section to negate the potential for infection and spinal cord injury associated with a vaginal delivery. It is imperative that surgical correction occur early as open communication between the neural and the environment places the child at great risk of bacterial colonization and injury to key neural structures. In most instances, surgical correction occurs within the first week of life, if not 24 to 48 hours after birth, to attenuate the long-term complications of myelomeningocele.

It is not uncommon for children born with a myelomeningocele to need multiple surgeries throughout their life to treat comorbid conditions. Conditions associated with myelomeningocele include neurogenic bladder with the potential for latex allergy due to frequent urinary catheterizations, paraparesis, scoliosis, hypotrophic lower limb development, joint contractures, pressure ulcers, and renal insufficiency. Due to meningeal and resultant cerebrospinal fluid involvement, this patient population is also at risk of the development of postoperative hydrocephalus and subsequently the need for placement of a ventriculoperitoneal shunt.

SPECIAL CONSIDERATIONS AND CONCERNS

Nearly all infants born with a myelomeningocele have supraspinal neurological manifestations of the disease process. Hydrocephalus is clinically evident at birth in 15% to 25% of all infants born with myelomeningocele, likely due to aqueductal stenosis or fourth ventricular outflow obstruction.

Likewise, children born with myelomeningocele frequently present with an Arnold–Chiari II malformation, which entails a small posterior fossa, brainstem abnormalities, and hindbrain herniation. This too can result in hydrocephalus.

As such, surgical placement of a ventriculoperitoneal shunt is required in 85% to 90% of all children with myelomeningocele to prevent downward displacement of the medulla, cerebellum, and fourth ventricle into the spinal canal. Despite the placement of a ventriculoperitoneal shunt, some children will have permanent developmental deficits secondary to the Chiari malformation.

ANESTHETIC MANAGEMENT

PREOPERATIVE EVALUATION

Children with myelomeningocele may experience life-threatening complications, though this is most often due to associated anomalies. Nonetheless, this highlights the importance of a thorough preoperative evaluation as associated comorbid conditions may necessitate further evaluation and optimization.

Anesthesia providers must be sure to vet the presence of anomalies of the cardiac, gastrointestinal, and genitourinary systems as embryologically they are formed concurrently with malformed neurological system. The most common organ anomaly involves genitourinary system, with hydroureteronephrosis and vesicoureteric reflux present in 10% to 30% of children with myelomeningocele.

As children grow older, they commonly report decreased sensation below the defect, decreased leg movement, and the inability to control the bladder and bowel function. Other associated anomalies include scoliosis, restrictive lung disease from scoliosis, tethered cord, and spinal cord syrinx. As previously mentioned, hydrocephalus is the most common comorbid condition (67.4%), followed by Arnold–Chiari II malformation (58.4%; Box 56.1).

Pertinent Labs

There are no specific labs necessary prior to myelomeningocele repair; however, if volume losses or renal insufficiency is suspected, review of serum electrolytes may be warranted. Should there be clinical suspicion of a cardiac anomaly, preoperative echocardiography may be warranted to vet the presence of congenital heart defects, such as atrial septal defect, ventricular septal defect, tetralogy of Fallot, bicuspid aortic valve, or coarctation of aorta.

PREOPERATIVE PHARMACOLOGY

Preoperative medications are not routinely indicated as this procedure typically occurs within the first 24 to 48 hours of life. The need for continuation or initiation of antibiotics should be confirmed prior to the induction of anesthesia.

BOX 56.1 ASSOCIATED CONDITIONS

- Central nervous system abnormalities
  - Chiari I malformation
  - Chiari II malformation
  - Corpus callosal agenesis
  - Hydrosyringomyelia
- Coexisting medical conditions
  - Chronic renal failure
  - Electrolyte abnormalities
  - Meningitis
  - Seizures
  - Stridor
  - Upper respiratory tract infection
- Orthopedic abnormalities
  - Congenital talipes equinovarus
  - Flat/high-arched foot/trophic ulcer
  - Scoliosis
- Urogenital abnormalities
  - Horseshoe kidney
  - Hydroureteronephrosis
  - Solitary kidney

Source: From Singh D, Rath GP, Dash HH, Bithal PK. Anesthetic concerns and perioperative complications in repair of myelomeningocele: A retrospective review of 135 cases. J Neurosurg Anesthesiol. 2010;22(1):11–15. doi:10.1097/ANA.0b013e3181bb44a9.

ANESTHETIC TECHNIQUE

Intraoperative Management

See Table 56.1. General anesthesia is typically achieved via an IV induction as most patients present with an indwelling peripheral IV catheter. Should the patient present without an IV catheter, an inhalational mask induction can be safely employed in most cases. Care must be taken when transferring the patient to the operating table for induction. Gauze, towels, or padding can be used to protect the defect and avoid excess pressure on neural structures. If the defect is unable to be supported in this fashion for induction of anesthesia, the patient may be placed in the lateral position. A roll can be placed under the patient's shoulders to facilitate axial alignment for intubation if this does not compress on the myelomeningocele.

Standard monitors, as described by the American Society of Anesthesiologists, should be employed. Invasive monitoring is generally not indicated. A single well-running peripheral IV catheter is often sufficient, however, should total IV anesthesia (TIVA) be planned due to the need for neuromonitoring throughout the surgical procedures, a second peripheral IV catheter is recommended. Blood loss is usually minimal, although may increase if a large area of skin and/or fascia is needed to achieve primary closure of the defect. Urine output should be monitored throughout the case.

As previously mentioned, care must be taken with positioning. Once positioned prone, it is imperative that anesthesia providers frequently assess the patient's eyes and face to ensure there is not excess pressure on the eyes, mouth, or bony prominences.

Table 56.1 Clinical Pearls

Special Considerations	Sequelae	Treatment
Large defect/exaggerated hydrocephalus	May be potentially difficult to mask ventilate or intubate	Have difficult airway cart available
Cerebrospinal fluid aspiration	May result in brainstem traction, bradycardia, and arrest	Have atropine and epinephrine available
Patient size and positioning	Potential for hypothermia	Warm ambient OR temperature and forced-air blanket warming

OR, operating room.

Prone positioning may also increase intra-abdominal and intrathoracic pressure making ventilation more challenging. Neonates are susceptible to hypothermia, especially when a myelomeningocele is present as autonomic function below the level of the lesion is impaired, making it essential to employ active warming strategies, such as a warm operating room, a forced-air warming blanket, and potentially warm IV fluids. Insensible fluid losses should also be considered when calculating volume repletion.

Anesthesia providers caring for older children with a history of myelomeningocele should consider avoiding the use of succinylcholine given the increased risk of hyperkalemia in the setting of motor deficits. The use of nondepolarizing muscle relaxants does not present an issue unless intraoperative neuromonitoring is planned. Narcotics should be used judiciously.

It is not uncommon for a ventriculoperitoneal shunt to be placed at the same time, although this is dependent on the surgeon and institutional protocols, as well as the patient's presenting medical history. It has been offered, however, that surgical treatment occurring in the first 5 days of life is associated with optimal patient outcomes, such as a shorter length of stay in the hospital, decreased antibiotic requirements, and lower complication rates.[3] Anesthesia providers should modify monitoring protocols on fluid management and analgesia regimen accordingly.

Complications/Emergencies

Intraoperatively, most complications are related to positioning, such as injury to the extruded neural tissue or periorbital edema, and hypothermia. It is imperative that anesthesia providers pay careful attention during patient positioning to ensure there is not excess pressure on bony prominences, the eyes, or face. Additionally, the myelomeningocele must be handled with care to avoid damage to neural structures. Active warming strategies should be employed to stave off hypothermia.

Additional concerns, albeit rare, include cardiac arrest, bradycardia, tachycardia, hypotension, arrhythmia, bronchospasm, hypoxemia, endobronchial intubation, and accidental extubation. Postoperatively, the most common complications include infection, cerebrospinal fluid leak, pseudomeningocele, hematoma, and seizures.

POSTOPERATIVE CARE

Depending on the age of the patient, institutional protocols, and the extent of surgical repair, anesthesia providers may consider keeping the patient intubated postoperatively and transferring them to an intensive care unit for monitoring and a delayed extubation. Even if extubation occurs immediately following surgery, it is essential patients are closely monitored in the immediate postoperative period as structural derangements of the postmedullary respiratory control center or the afferent and efferent pathways may lead to hypoventilation, central sleep apnea, or prolonged periods of breath holding.[4] Additionally, Arnold–Chiari malformation is often associated with an abnormal ventilatory response to hypoxia mandating judicious titration of opioid administered postoperatively.

REFERENCES

1. Yeon J, Kang J. Anesthetic implications of common congenital anomalies. *Anesthesiology Clinics.* 2020;38(3):621–642. doi:10.1016/j.anclin.2020.06.002
2. Cote C, Lerman J, Anderson B. *A Practice of Anesthesia for Infants and Children.* Elsevier; 2013.
3. Adzick NS, Thom EA, Spong CY, et al. A randomized trial of prenatal versus postnatal repair of myelomeningocele. *N Engl J Med.* 2011;364:993–1004. doi:10.1056/NEJMoa1014379
4. Singh D, Rath GP, Dash HH, Bithal PK. Anesthetic concerns and perioperative complications in repair of myelomeningocele: A retrospective review of 135 cases. *J Neurosurg Anesthesiol.* 2010;22(1):11–15. doi:10.1097/ANA.0b013e3181bb44a9

CHAPTER 57

Third Ventriculostomy

Anne M. Que

INDICATIONS/CONTRAINDICATIONS

Neuroendoscopy is becoming more routine in children of all ages. Within a broad spectrum of minimally invasive neuroendoscopic procedures, endoscopic third ventriculostomy is one that is most commonly performed to treat obstructive hydrocephalus. Hydrocephalus is the abnormal accumulation of cerebrospinal fluid (CSF) within the ventricles in the brain that occurs when there is a disruption in the formation and/or absorption of CSF. The mismatch in CSF production and absorption results in accumulation of CSF and ultimately increased intracranial pressure (ICP) if untreated (**Figure 57.1**).

Congenital causes of hydrocephalus include aquaductal stenosis, neural tube defects, arachnoid cysts, Dandy–Walker syndrome or Chiari malformation. The incidence of congenital hydrocephalus in the advanced nations has been projected to range from 0.5 to 0.8 per 1,000 live births.[1] Common acquired causes of hydrocephalus include intraventricular hemorrhage, meningitis, head injury, and brain tumors. Given the variety of potential causes of acquired hydrocephalus, the incidence of acquired hydrocephalus remains unknown. In addition to being classified as congenital or acquired, hydrocephalus can be classified as nonobstructive/communicating or obstructive-noncommunicating. With nonobstructive/communicating hydrocephalus, CSF is able to flow freely throughout the ventricular system and subarachnoid space. In obstructive-noncommunicating hydrocephalus, however, there is a physical blockage precluding the flow of CSF. While compensatory mechanisms, such as the upregulation of aquaporin channels responsible for transependymal water flow, can decrease CSF pressure to a normal range in neonates and infants, interventions, such as third ventriculostomy, are necessary if ventriculomegaly progresses or if ICP continues to rise to unsafe levels.

Unless the etiology of progressive hydrocephalus can be identified and treated, a ventricular drain or ventriculoperitoneal (VP) shunt must be surgically placed to manage rising ICP secondary to hydrocephalus. Endoscopic third ventriculostomy is an alternative to VP shunt placement in obstructive hydrocephalus secondary to aqueductal stenosis that is associated with favorable longtime results.[1,2] During endoscopic third ventriculostomy, communication is made through the floor of the third ventricle into the adjacent CSF cisterns to bypass the obstruction precluding CSF flow. Alternatively, communication may be made in the septum pellucidum to facilitate communication between the lateral ventricles. For more information regarding VP shunt placement, please see Chapter 50, "Ventriculoperitoneal Shunt Placement and/or Externalization." Contraindications to endoscopic third ventriculostomy include intraventricular hemorrhage, subarachnoid hemorrhage, and meningitis.[1]

SPECIAL CONSIDERATIONS AND CONCERNS

See **Table 57.1** for a summary of special considerations and concerns related to anesthetic management of third ventriculostomy.

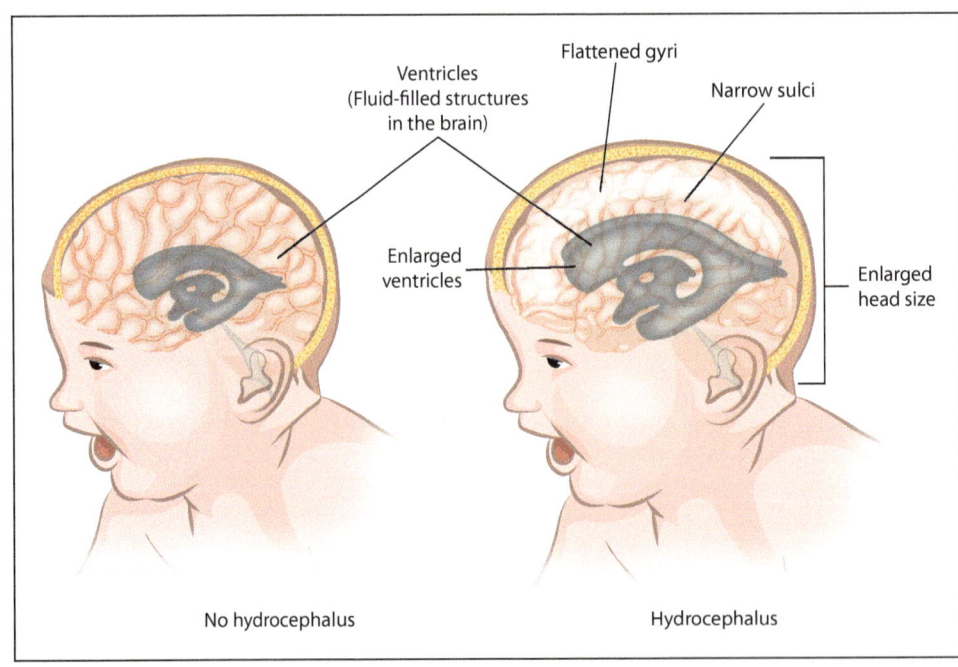

Figure 57.1: Obstructive hydrocephalus. Enlarged ventricles noted.

Table 57.1 Special Considerations and Concerns

Special Considerations	Concerns
Associated congenital malformations, such as meningomyelocele and congenital cardiomyopathies	Avoid hypotension
Avoid use of nitrous oxide	Elevation of ICP, expansion of air bubbles, VAE
Arterial line	When serious comorbidities are present
Irrigation with cold fluid	Cause bradycardia and hypothermia

ICP, intracranial pressure; VAE, venous air embolism.

ANESTHETIC MANAGEMENT

PREOPERATIVE EVALUATION

The primary focus during the preoperative evaluation is the patient's current neurological status, particularly signs of increased ICP, vomiting, and any underlying primary disease process.[3] It is important to identify the presence of bulbar palsy and sleep disturbances during the preoperative evaluation as well. Because the clinical manifestations may be part of multisystem congenital syndromes, these patients are often at high risk of urinary tract infections or impaired renal function. Likewise, dehydration and electrolyte abnormalities should be corrected prior to surgery. It is important for anesthesia providers to consider the severity and impact of additional ongoing medical conditions, as the treatment regimen may influence the anesthetic management.

PREOPERATIVE PHARMACOLOGY

Preoperative sedation is often avoided in the setting of intracranial hypertension and an altered mental status as the patient will need to be rapidly awoken postoperatively for a neurological assessment.

ANESTHETIC TECHNIQUE

Intraoperative Management

Standard monitoring is required, which includes electrocardiography, pulse oximetry, capnography, temperature monitoring, and measurement of urine output. The use of a transcranial doppler has been offered to be the fastest and most reliable method to detect fluctuations in cerebral blood flow secondary to changes in ICP. Due to practical restrictions, however, this is not routinely used in clinical practice.[2] Placement of an arterial line may be indicated based on the patient's comorbidities.

The technique for inducing general anesthesia is largely dependent on the severity of the hydrocephalus. In asymptomatic patients, inhalational induction with sevoflurane may be acceptable. Patients presenting with symptomatic hydrocephalus, however, often require an IV rapid sequence induction due to the risk of vomiting and aspiration.[2] Following placement of an endotracheal tube (ETT), a second peripheral IV catheter may be placed if blood transfusion is anticipated, although this is not a routine concern. Overall, the goal of IV fluid administration is to maintain euvolemia, and administration of hypotonic IV solutions should be avoided to prevent brain swelling.

General anesthesia can be maintained with volatile agents or by employing a total IV anesthesia (TIVA) technique with propofol and remifentanil. When volatile anesthetics are used to maintain general anesthesia, it is important to consider using <1 minimum alveolar concentration.[2] Intraoperatively, the use of nitrous oxide is discouraged as this may elevate ICP, expand ventricular air bubbles, or exacerbate symptoms in the event of venous air embolism.[2] TIVA with a propofol infusion may avoid increases in ICP, but anesthesia providers should be sure to avoid hypotension associated with higher doses. Long-acting opioids should be avoided.

The goals of general anesthesia include absolute intraoperative immobilization, cardiovascular stability, and rapid recovery to allow neurological assessment.[2] Rapid increase in ICP, which leads to fluctuations in cerebral blood flow, must be prevented, detected, and quickly managed.[2]

Maintaining normothermia intraoperatively can be challenging; however, hypothermia should be avoided. When caring for a neonate or young child, anesthesia providers should be sure the room temperature is increased, all IV fluids should be warmed, and the inspired gases should be warmed and humidified.

Complications

During endoscopic third ventriculostomy procedures in infants, bradycardia may occur when performing balloon dilatation of the ventriculostomy orifice. Bradycardia typically resolves with immediate deflation of the balloon often does not require further intervention. Irrigation may also result in abrupt bradycardia secondary to dilation of the ventricles. Toxic reactions can ensue when irrigation fluid and CSF mix, leading to fever, meningitis, headache, and increased cell count.[3] There can also be a Cushing-like response resulting in refractory hypertension and tachycardia/bradycardia. This can indicate poor brain perfusion or stimulation of the preoptic area in the brain. Vigorous irrigation can also result in neurogenic pulmonary edema. Vigilance in recognition and correction is essential, as is close communication between the anesthesia provider and surgeon, to prevent serious or irreversible injury.[4] See **Box 57.1** for a summary of complications.

Surgical complications include damage to basilar artery, which may create a pseudoaneurysm or require immediate conversion to craniotomy to control hemorrhage. Additionally, injury to the fornix while navigating the endoscope through the foramen of Monro can result in transient memory loss, personality changes, or cranial nerve injury. If the hypothalamus is injured during a lateral entry, endocrine disorders may develop postoperatively.[3]

POSTOPERATIVE CARE

Rapid recovery to allow neurological assessment is key. Typically, the surgical team will perform the first neurological examination in the operating room immediately following

> **BOX 57.1 COMPLICATIONS/EMERGENCIES**
>
> - Basal artery injury, leading to intraventricular hemorrhage, SAH, hemiparesis, and midbrain damage
> - Hypothalamus and brainstem manipulation, leading to brachyarrhythmias, hypotension, hypertension, and cardiac arrest
> - Reduction in cerebral perfusion, ischemia (from increased ICP)
> - Paralysis of III and VI nerves
> - Delayed awakening
> - Mental confusion and memory loss
> - Infection
> - Convulsions
> - Pneumocephalus
>
> ICP, intracranial pressure; SAH, subarachnoid hemorrhage.
>
> Source: From Rajesh MC. Anesthesia for endoscopic third ventriculostomy in children. Anesth Essays Res. 2017;11(1):7–9. doi:10.4103/0259-1162.186618.

emergence from anesthesia. The patient is then transferred to the postanesthesia care unit for further monitoring of their respiratory, cardiovascular, and neurological status. As CSF leak occurs in 3.6% patients, it is imperative that neurological assessments continue at predefined intervals postoperatively per institutional protocol.[3]

REFERENCES

1. Haddadi K. Pediatric endoscopic third ventriculostomy: a narrative review of current indications, techniques and complications. *J Pediatr Rev*. 2016;4(2):31–37. doi:10.17795/jpr-50742.
2. Rajesh MC. Anesthesia for endoscopic third ventriculostomy in children. *Anesth Essays Res*. 2017;11(1):7–9. doi:10.4103/0259-1162.186618
3. Meier PM, Guzman R, Erb T. Endoscopic pediatric neurosurgery: implications for anesthesia. *Pediatr Anesth*. 2014;24(7):668–677. doi:10.1111/pan.12405
4. Ozdamar D, Etus V, Ceylan S, et al. Anaesthetic considerations and perioperative features of endoscopic third ventriculostomy in infants: analysis of 57 cases. *Turk Neurosurg*. 2012;22(2):148–155. doi:10.5137/1019-5149.JTN.4118-11.15.

SECTION B: Ear, Nose, and Throat Procedures

CHAPTER 58

Myringotomy and Pressure-Equalizing Tubes

Ebone Evans and Andrew Redmann

INDICATIONS/CONTRAINDICATIONS

Myringotomy and pressure equalization tube (PET) placement are the most common otolaryngologic procedures performed in pediatric patients in the United States, most often to treat middle ear disease.[1-4] While the vast majority of cases are uncomplicated, following a few principles can lead to safe treatment of middle ear disease even in complicated patients. Given its commonness, it is important for pediatric anesthesia providers to understand the underlying basic anatomy and physiology of ear disease.

Briefly, the middle ear is defined as the space between the tympanic membrane and lateral wall of inner ear. The middle ear contents include the tympanic membrane, ossicular chain, eustachian tube, and nervous structures (CN VII, tympanic nerve of CN IX, and Arnold's nerve of CN X).[5] The middle ear amplifies airborne sound vibration by increasing vibrational amplitude through difference in surface area between the tympanic membrane and the ossicular chain. The middle ear pressure is maintained by the eustachian tube, which equalizes pressure between the middle ear and ear canal to allow the tympanic membrane to stay in a neutral position.[5]

Eustachian tube dysfunction (ETD) is the improper opening of the eustachian tube, leading to inadequate pressure equalization and drainage of middle ear fluid. ETD can be due to failure of opening mechanisms, or obstruction of the tube. In particular, inflammation during acute upper respiratory infection or tissue enlargement in close proximity to the eustachian tube orifice can cause obstruction. Consequences of ETD include accumulation of fluid in the middle ear, negative pressure in the middle ear, retraction pockets of the tympanic membrane, and conductive hearing loss. ETD is the most common underlying cause of acute otitis media (AOM) and otitis media with effusion (OME).[6]

AOM is defined as rapid onset of inflammation of the middle ear mucosa accompanied by systemic symptoms, such as otalgia, fever, and irritability. On physical examination, the patient's tympanic membrane can appear erythematous, hyper-vascular, and obscure landmarks. If an effusion is present, the tympanic membrane may bulge secondary to purulence.[3,4] AOM is typically proceeded by an upper respiratory infection, and as such, the most common microorganisms isolated are *Streptococcus pneumoniae*, *Haemophilus influenzae*, and *Moraxella catarrhalis*. The widespread implementation of pneumococcal vaccination has led to decline in *Streptococcus* pneumonia, which historically was the most common cause of AOM.[3,4]

OME is defined as a fluid-filled middle ear without signs or symptoms of an infection. The effusion present is often serous in nature. OME is classified by duration: acute being less than 3 weeks, subacute 3 weeks to 3 months, or chronic greater than 3 months. Audiograms are recommended in patients with chronic OME to evaluate for hearing loss.[3,4]

ANESTHETIC MANAGEMENT

PREOPERATIVE EVALUATION

In 2013, the American Academy of Pediatrics and American Academy of Family Physicians developed recommendations for the treatment of AOM. Observation is offered to children with nonsevere unilateral AOM in children 6 months to 23 months or nonsevere unilateral/bilateral in children 24 months and older. If symptoms fail to improve in 48 to 72 hours of observation, treatment is escalated to medical management. Antibiotic therapy (amoxicillin first line) is recommended when there are severe signs and symptoms (otalgia and fever) of AOM in children 6 months and older and to all children younger than 6 months with clinical findings of AOM. Clinical practice guidelines published by the American Academy of Otolaryngology-Head and Neck Surgery recommend surgical intervention for the indications seen in **Box 58.1**.[7]

Tympanostomy tubes benefit patients by improving hearing, decreasing number of ear infections (secondarily decreasing utilization of antibiotics), and resolution of otologic symptoms (pain and vestibular function).[7] Preoperative evaluation should be completed as for any surgical case, with special attention on the presence of syndromes that could predict difficulty with airway management (trisomy 21, CHARGE, Treacher Collins, etc.) and any history of a recent upper respiratory tract infection (URI).

A history of a recent or ongoing URI is common among patients presenting for PET placement. While patients presenting with a recent or ongoing URI may be canceled or rescheduled for most procedures due to potential airway irritability and an increased incidence of airway complications, it is not uncommon procedure for PET placement as the PETs are ultimately necessary to resolve recurrent URIs. Therefore,

---

BOX 58.1 — **AMERICAN ACADEMY OF OTOLARYNGOLOGY-HEAD AND NECK SURGERY CLINICAL GUIDELINES FOR PRESSURE EQUALIZATION TUBE SURGICAL INTERVENTION**

Surgical Indications for Pressure Equalization Tubes
Chronic bilateral OME with documented hearing loss
Chronic OME with symptoms (vestibular, poor school performance, behavioral difficulties, and ear discomfort)
Recurrent AOM with effusion (defined as four infections in 6 months or three infections in 3 months)
AOM with complications (including intracranial and extracranial complications of AOM)

AOM, acute otitis media; OME, otitis media with effusion.

a thorough respiratory assessment is key when performing the preoperative evaluation to discern the safety of moving forward with the procedure.

ANESTHETIC TECHNIQUE

Intraoperative Management

The goal of myringotomy and tympanostomy tube placement is to create a controlled perforation in the tympanic membrane to provide ventilation and drainage of the middle ear. Myringotomy and tube placement are most commonly performed in the operating room with the patient under general anesthesia. There is a recent trend to attempt in-office placement; however, this remains in the early stages and, as such, is not discussed in this chapter.

Generally, PET placement takes about 5 minutes in uncomplicated patients. Anesthesia is induced via mask with the volatile anesthetic of the anesthesia provider's choice. For uncomplicated cases, placement of an intravascular catheter may be deferred, although an IV catheter is often placed for young children, those with any medical comorbidities, and those with a history of URI. Airway management typically entails masking the patient, with general anesthesia maintained with volatile anesthetic. Postoperative analgesia can be provided by a number of medications including, intranasal or IV fentanyl, IM or IV ketorolac, PO, PR, or IV acetaminophen, intranasal, buccal, or IV dexmedetomidine, or perhaps even with a nerve block of the auricular branch of the vagus (Arnold's nerve).

The risk of anesthetic complication is quite low, with the best available data indicating that major complications (most commonly laryngospasm) occur in less than 2% of cases.[8] Complications are significantly more common in children with a recent upper respiratory illness, making a preoperative evaluation of the child by both the surgeon and anesthetist of paramount importance.

Briefly, the surgical procedure is as follows: The patient's head is rotated so that the surgical ear is up, and a binocular microscope is brought into the surgical field. An ear speculum is introduced, and the external ear canal is cleaned. The tympanic membrane is examined and an incision is made in the anteroinferior quadrant of the tympanic membrane. The middle ear effusion is aspirated through the myringotomy, and if purulent discharge is present, it may be sent for culture. An alligator forceps is used to introduce the tube into the myringotomy. Drops are then inserted in ear canal, and the tragus pumped to ensure adequate penetration of the drops; if bilateral equalizing pressure tubes are being placed, the anesthesia provider repositions the patient's head, and the procedure is repeated on the contralateral side. No preoperative antibiotics are indicated, and blood loss is minimal.

Complications/Emergencies

Few anesthetic complications are associated with myringotomy and pressure-equalizing tubes. The major complications (laryngospasm, bradycardia, stridor, decreased oxygen, and dysrhythmia) and minor complications (prolonged recovery longer than 30 minutes, emesis, and persistent agitation) are not unfamiliar in the realm of anesthetic complications.[8]

Intraoperatively, great care should be taken to avoid trauma to the external auditory canal. Minor trauma can lead to bleeding of the external auditory canal, obscuring the surgeon's vision of the PET placement and potentially plugging the lumen of the PET.[6] Although rare, the jugular bulb can be perforated during myringotomy as well resulting in significant bleeding.[9] Fortunately, this is usually controllable by packing the middle ear and aborting the procedure. Communication between the surgeon and the anesthesia provider is necessary if this rare complication occurs, especially if the child does not have IV access (which should be rapidly obtained in the event of a vascular injury).

During PET insertion, the tube may fall into the middle ear. Attempts should be made to remove the PET as leaving it behind can cause a foreign body reaction process in the middle ear. Widening the myringotomy incision can aid the surgeon in retrieving the PET. The anesthesia provider should be aware of this, which may lengthen the planned procedure.

There are a few surgical complications that should be mentioned, including tympanostomy tube blockage, otorrhea, and perforation. Approximately 3.9% of surgical cases result in early tube extrusion; tube extrusion before first postoperative visit. Early tube extrusion can be due to size of myringotomy incision or middle ear effusion pushing tube out of position. Additional surgery to place another tube may be necessary.[10] The lumen of the tube can also become blocked with postoperative blood, mucus, or granulation tissue. Office debridement can restore patency of tube, but if the tube remains blocked and middle ear effusion accumulates, tube exchange may be necessary.[10] Transient or persistent otorrhea can be present after tube insertion. Otorrhea should be treated with otic (with or without steroid) antibiotic drops. If left untreated, otorrhea can develop into a chronic suppurative otitis media.[10] Finally, persistent perforation may result once tympanostomy tube extrudes. Perforations are typically small and rarely cause significant hearing loss. However, closing perforations is beneficial in patients with persistent otorrhea (creating a safer hearing ear for the patient), and in patients with hearing loss. In patients with long-standing ETD, persistent perforations can be beneficial by acting as a natural opening for tympanostomy tube and fluid drainage.[10]

POSTOPERATIVE CARE

Following the procedure, the patient is transferred to the postanesthesia care unit for recovery. If acute ear infection is present, patients are sent home on antibiotic drops for 7 days. Follow-up is scheduled per the surgeon, generally between 1 and 3 months. After initial follow-up, the patient is seen in clinic every 6 months to evaluate if the tubes have remained in place, as well as to evaluate the health of tympanic membrane and the middle ear.

REFERENCES

1. Schilder AG, Chonmaitree T, Cripps AW, et al. Otitis media. *Nat Rev Dis Primers*. 2016;2(1):160–63. doi:10.1038/nrdp.2016.63
2. Cullen KA, Hall MJ, Golosinskiy A. Ambulatory surgery in the United States, 2006. *Natl Health Stat Report*. 2009;(11):1–25.
3. Bluestone CD, Gates GA., Klein JO, et al. Definitions, terminology, and classification of otitis media. *Ann Otol Rhinol Laryngol Suppl*. 2002;111(Suppl. 3):8–18. doi:10.1177/00034894021110s304
4. Bluestone CD, Simons JP, Healy GB. *Bluestone and Stool's Pediatric Otolaryngology*. 5th ed. Shelton, Connecticut : People's Medical Publishing House-USA, 2014.

5. Oghalai JS, Brownell WE. Anatomy and physiology of the ear. In: Lalwani AK, ed. *Current Diagnosis & Treatment Otolaryngology—Head and Neck Surgery*. McGraw Hill; 2020. https://accessmedicine-mhmedical com.ezp1.lib.umn.edu/content.aspx?bookid=2744&sectionid=229676006
6. Kesser B, Derebry M. Surgery of ventilation and mucosal disease. In Brackmann DE, Shelton C, Arriaga M, eds. *Otologic Surgery*. Elsevier;2016:59–76.
7. Rosenfeld RM, Schwartz SR, Pynnonen MA, et al. Clinical practice guideline: tympanostomy tubes in children—executive summary. *Otolaryngol Head Neck Surg*. 2013;149(1):8–16. doi:10.1177/0194599813490141
8. Hoffmann KK, Thompson GK, Burke BL, Derkay CS. Anesthetic complications of tympanostomy tube placement in children. *Arch Otolaryngol Head Neck Surg*. 2002;128(9):1040–1043. doi:10.1001/archotol.128.9.1040
9. Moore P. The high jugular bulb in ear surgery: three case reports and a review of the literature. *J Laryngol Otol*. 1994;108(9):772–775. doi:10.1017/s0022215100128087
10. Kay DJ, Nelson M, Rosenfeld RM. Meta-analysis of tympanostomy tube sequelae. *Otolaryngol Head Neck Surg*. 2001;124(4):374–380. doi:10.1067/mhn.2001.113941

CHAPTER 59

Bone-Anchored Hearing Aid Surgery

Andrew Redmann

INDICATIONS/CONTRAINDICATIONS

Bone-anchored hearing aid placement is a relatively common procedure in pediatric otolaryngology and is often performed in syndromic children. Bone-anchored hearing aids are implantable hearing devices approved for treatment of patients with single-sided deafness or those with conductive/mixed hearing loss. The procedure initially was approved for adult patients but has been performed in the pediatric population since the 1990s.[1] Specific conditions that are treated using bone-anchored hearing aids include refractory chronic ear disease, external auditory canal problems, and those with malformations of the external and/or middle ear (i.e., microtia, aural atresia, and craniofacial syndromes).

Briefly, the surgical procedure involves an incision posterior and superior to the external auditory canal, with dissection carried down to the periosteum of the skull. A small well is drilled using a specialized drill, and a titanium implant is then screwed directly into the bone of the skull. Postoperatively, a dressing is applied and the implant is allowed to osseointegrate into the skull over a period of a few weeks. After this, a processor is attached to the implant via an external post or a magnet and is activated. Hearing results across indications are very consistent, and patients are generally satisfied with the final hearing result (Figure 59.1).[2-4] In patients with conductive/mixed hearing loss, implantation allows sound to be transmitted directly to the inner ear via the skull, thus bypassing the external auditory canal and middle ear to stimulate the cochlea directly. In patients with single-sided deafness, sound is transmitted through the skull to the "good" side, allowing the potential for improved sound localization and speech discrimination in noisy situations.[5]

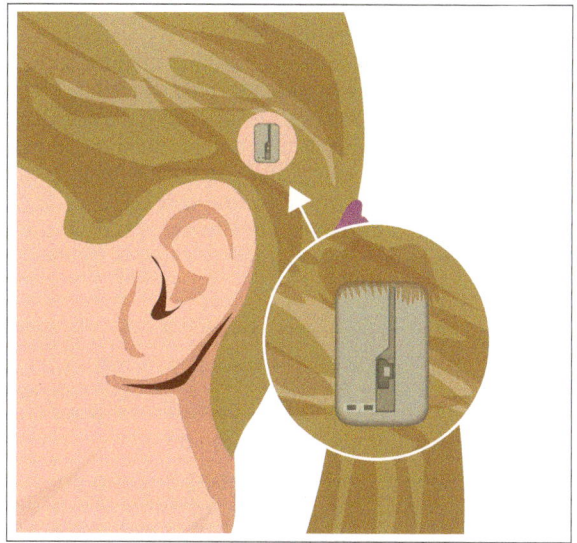

Figure 59.1: Depiction of bone-anchored hearing aid placement showing stump/implant and removable processor.

A relative contraindication to bone-anchored hearing aid placement in children is skull bone thickness of less than 2.5 mm (the length of the implant), which has U.S. Food and Drug Administration approval limited to children 5 years of age or older. This is despite evidence that children as young as 1 year old may have adequate bone thickness to accommodate an implant.[6] In patients deemed too young to undergo surgical intervention, a soft-band bone-anchored hearing aid can be used until the child is old enough to undergo implantation.

SPECIAL CONSIDERATIONS AND CONCERNS

Special considerations and concerns related to bone-anchored hearing aid placement are summarized in Box 59.1.

ANESTHETIC MANAGEMENT

PREOPERATIVE EVALUATION

The anesthetic management of children undergoing bone-anchored hearing aid placement is largely determined by the patient's underlying medical conditions. Careful consideration of anatomy and underlying physiology is important when developing the anesthetic plan for patients undergoing bone-anchored hearing aid placement. A thorough review of previous airway management should be obtained, and open communication should exist between the surgical and anesthesia teams. A number of conditions commonly found in children undergoing bone-anchored hearing aid placement have the potential to modify the anesthetic plan, including Treacher Collins, Goldenhar, trisomy 21, CHARGE,* 22q11/velocardiofacial (VCF) syndrome, and Pfeiffer syndromes. A recent paper found that 45% of 134 children undergoing bone-anchored hearing aid placement had a recognized syndrome or dysmorphism that had the potential to complicate airway management, and 16% of patients had a grade 3 or 4 view on direct laryngoscopy.[7] In addition, 17% of patients had underlying cardiac disease that required preoperative cardiac clearance.[7]

ANESTHETIC TECHNIQUE

Intraoperative Management

Induction of general anesthesia can be either inhalation or IV depending on the patient's age and comorbidities. Standard monitoring is required, which includes electrocardiography, pulse oximetry, capnography, and temperature monitoring. A single peripheral IV catheter is sufficient. Following the induction of anesthesia, the airway is secured with either an endotracheal tube (ETT) or a laryngeal mask airway (LMA), although an LMA is often sufficient to manage the airway. In the largest available study, in six out of 353 cases, placement of an LMA was not sufficient and required intraoperative conversion to an ETT.[7] Additionally, two children with severe retrognathia required elective flexible fiberoptic intubation. It should be noted that 45.5% of the children in the study had a recognized syndrome that may have affected airway anatomy. These data suggest that there should be a low index of suspicion for a difficult airway in children with syndromes who present for bone-anchored hearing aid placement, and lends itself to a number of pearls when developing the anesthetic plan.

It is reasonable to have a very low threshold to definitively secure the airway using an ETT in patients with known or suspected difficult airways. If intubation is planned, otolaryngology should be present and equipment to manage difficult intubations (video laryngoscope, flexible bronchoscope, rigid bronchoscope) should be readily available. Finally, it must be said in passing that while the majority of pediatric patients undergoing surgery require general anesthetics, select cooperative older children without a known difficult airway may also be a candidate for implantation under local anesthesia with or without conscious sedation.

POSTOPERATIVE CARE

Despite underlying comorbidities, as long as appropriate steps are taken to mitigate any potential airway difficulties, the intraoperative course is generally smooth. Immediate postoperative complications are quite rare. The most commonly documented concern is nausea/vomiting, but over 90% of patients are discharged directly from the postanesthetic care unit. There are a number of surgical complications that may develop in the weeks/months following surgery, including skin overgrowth over the implant, local wound infection, and failure of the implant to osseointegrate, which may necessitate return to the operating room.[1,3] Anesthetic management for these cases is largely identical as for primary surgery.

> **BOX 59.1 SPECIAL CONSIDERATIONS AND CONCERNS: BONE-ANCHORED HEARING AID PLACEMENT**
>
> - Blood loss is generally less than 5 mL.
> - Perioperative antibiotics covering the skin flora are prescribed to be given prior to incision.
> - Local anesthetic with epinephrine is injected around the planned incision.
> - The procedure generally takes somewhere between 30 and 90 minutes in experienced hands.

REFERENCES

1. Papsin BC, Sirimanna TK, Albert DM, Bailey CM. Surgical experience with bone-anchored hearing aids in children. *Laryngoscope* 1997;107(6):801–806.
2. Dimitriadis PA, Carrick S, Ray J. Intermediate outcomes of a transcutaneous bone conduction hearing device in a pediatric population. *Int J Pediatr Otorhinolaryngol*. 2017;94:59–63.
3. Oberlies NR, Castano JE, Freiser ME, et al. Outcomes of BAHA connect vs BAHA attract in pediatric patients. *Int J Pediatr Otorhinolaryngol*. 2020;135:110–125.
4. Doshi J, McDermott AL. Bone anchored hearing aids in children. *Expert Rev Med Devices*. 2015;12(1):73–82.
5. Kim G, Ju HM, Lee SH, et al. Efficacy of bone-anchored hearing aids in single-sided deafness: a systematic review. *Otol Neurotol*. 2017;38(4):473–483.
6. Baker A, Fanelli D, Kanekar S, Isildak H. A review of temporal bone CT imaging with respect to pediatric bone-anchored hearing aid placement. *Otol Neurotol*. 2016;37(9):1366–1369.
7. Banga R, Reid AP, Proops DW, et al. Perioperative considerations for children undergoing bone anchored hearing device surgery: an observational study. *Eur Arch Otorhinolaryngol*. 2014;271:1437–1441.

---

*CHARGE syndrome is a disorder that affects many areas of the body. CHARGE is an abbreviation for several of the features common in the disorder: coloboma, heart defects, atresia choanae (also known as choanal atresia), growth retardation, genital abnormalities, and ear abnormalities.

Tympanoplasty

Andrew Redmann

INDICATIONS/CONTRAINDICATIONS

Tympanoplasty is any surgical procedure that involves reconstruction of the tympanic membrane. It is commonly performed for chronic tympanic membrane perforations or for cholesteatoma. Cholesteatoma is a locally aggressive ingrowth of epithelial tissue that can erode surrounding structures (including the facial nerve, labyrinth, and ossicular chain) and is treated surgically (Figure 60.1). If patients have significant cholesteatoma, mastoidectomy may be performed concurrently to improve access to the middle ear space and allow visualization and removal of all the disease. Should ossicular erosion be found intraoperatively, an ossiculoplasty (placement of synthetic ossicles) may be performed in conjunction with the tympanoplasty. It is imperative both surgeons and anesthesia providers appreciate the variability associated with tympanoplasty procedures, which can range from simple to extremely complicated. A less complicated tympanoplasty may simply entail a repair of a dry perforation in an older child and can often be performed through the ear canal with either a microscope or an endoscope. Conversely, surgical revision of a cholesteatoma can be a quite complicated and extensive operation involving a postauricular incision, the need for a microscope and possibly an endoscope, and drilling of the mastoid bone.

Tympanoplasty is a common procedure performed in pediatric patients for a wide variety of indications. Due to the heterogeneity of the procedure, it is of paramount importance that the anesthesia and surgical teams communicate in the preoperative, intraoperative, and postoperative periods to mitigate any potential complications and ensure an appropriate anesthetic plan is developed.

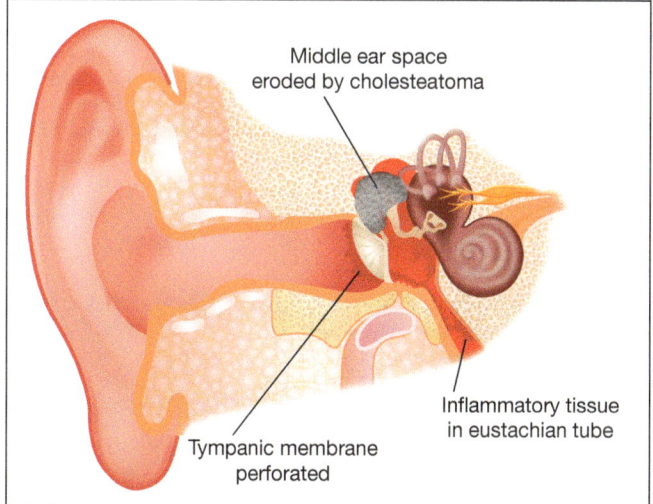

Figure 60.1: Cholesteatoma, a locally aggressive ingrowth of epithelial tissue that can erode surrounding structures.

SPECIAL CONSIDERATIONS AND CONCERNS

Surgeons use a wide variety of techniques for tympanoplasty as surgery can be performed with either a microscope or an endoscope as the primary visualization tool. Both techniques have comparable results, with surgeon preference being the primary driver of which technique is employed. Possible grafting materials include tragal cartilage, tragal perichondrium, temporalis fascia, loose areolar tissue, or a synthetic graft such as Biodesign®. The type of graft material used is based on both surgeon preference and the nature of the repair required.

Following induction of anesthesia, a facial nerve monitor is generally placed, and the patient is prepped and draped, with the head facing the anesthesia provider. The approach to the middle ear is then performed, either through the ear canal (transcanal) or behind the ear (postauricular). Depending on what the surgeon finds when entering the middle ear, the surgeon either proceeds with meticulous dissection (for cholesteatoma or removal of chronic middle ear disease), the placement of ossicular prosthesis, or placement of a graft to repair the perforation. The decision on whether mastoidectomy is necessary is usually made at this point in the operation. After all adjunctive procedures are performed, the graft material is placed to repair the tympanic membrane, and the ear is packed with Gelfoam to stabilize the graft. The patient is then returned to the care of the anesthesia provider for emergence. See Box 60.1 for a summary of special considerations and concerns.

ANESTHETIC MANAGEMENT

PREOPERATIVE EVALUATION

The anesthetic management of children undergoing tympanoplasty is largely determined by the patient's underlying medical conditions. Important factors for the anesthesia provider to consider are age (which may determine surgical technique and length of surgery, as described later), weight, medical comorbidities (including bleeding disorders), and surgical history. It is imperative the anesthesia provider inquire about a history of postoperative nausea/vomiting (PONV) as any retching in the postoperative period has the potential to disrupt the surgical repair.

INTRAOPERATIVE MANAGEMENT

The induction of anesthesia may be either inhalation or IV, with endotracheal intubation being the most common way to secure the airway during a tympanoplasty. Avoidance of paralysis is important, as in all temporal bone/middle ear surgery, given the proximity of the facial nerve to the surgical field. If necessary, to facilitate intubation, short-acting neuromuscular blocking agents should be used to allow for full reversal prior to the start of the surgical procedure. Communication with the surgeon during the preoperative

> **BOX 60.1 SPECIAL CONSIDERATIONS AND CONCERNS: TYMPANOPLASTY**
>
> - Facial nerve monitoring will occur throughout surgery, so it is imperative neuromuscular blockade is avoided.
> - Preoperative antibiotics covering the skin flora are given prior to incision.
> - Local anesthetic with epinephrine is injected at the planned incision sites.
> - Procedure takes between 1 and 3 hours in experienced hands depending on the approach used, but can vary widely depending on pathology.
> - Anticipated blood loss is less than 5 mL.

time-out should specifically acknowledge that no further paralysis will be used throughout the surgery.

One area of controversy in the intraoperative anesthesia for tympanoplasty involves the use of nitrous oxide. Traditionally ear surgeons have avoided using nitrous oxide during surgery due to its tendency to accumulate in the closed air-filled middle ear space. This theoretically means the gas has the potential to dislodge any graft material, leading to surgical failure and often the need for reoperation.[1] However, recent data suggest that the use of nitrous oxide is unlikely to impact the failure rates of tympanoplasty surgery.[2,3] Due to the controversy regarding this anesthetic agent, it is important to communicate clearly with the surgeon during the preoperative time-out to determine if they are amenable to the use of nitrous oxide during the case.

Hypertension and hypercarbia should be avoided to reduce bleeding in an effort to optimize surgeon visibility of the surgical site. The use of dexmedetomidine has also been proposed to improve hemodynamics as well as reduce narcotic consumption intraoperatively, making it a reasonable agent to consider for use.[4,5] Dexmedetomidine may also foster a smooth emergence from anesthesia, which is important following a tympanoplasty to avoid graft disruption. The use of a propofol-based total IV anesthetic (TIVA) may decrease the incidence and severity of PONV and subsequently limit retching.[6] Additional antiemetic agents, such as ondansetron and dexamethasone, should be considered as PONV is one of the most significant complications following tympanoplasty.

It should be noted that while the majority of pediatric patients undergoing surgery require general anesthetics, select cooperative older children without a known difficult airway may also be a candidate for surgery under local anesthesia with or without conscious sedation.[7] It is acknowledged, however, this is not standard of care for pediatric patients in the United States.

POSTOPERATIVE CARE

The intraoperative course during tympanoplasty is generally smooth, and immediate postoperative complications are rare. The most important immediate issue after surgery is the management of PONV. As with most surgical procedures, the use of dexamethasone has been found to decrease PONV, with or without ondansetron.[8] The author thus recommends the use of both perioperative dexamethasone and ondansetron given the potential for graft dislodgment due to PONV and the favorable safety profiles of both these medications. Most patients are discharged directly from the postanesthetic care unit, although some surgeons will admit patients undergoing mastoidectomy for postoperative observation. Rare surgical complications that may develop in the postoperative period include facial nerve weakness, postauricular hematoma, and severe nausea/vertigo due to stimulation of the labyrinth (especially in cholesteatoma cases). For this reason, it is important the anesthesia and surgical teams discuss how extensive the surgery was upon completion of the procedure to determine the risk of these complications developing. Anesthetic management for revision cases is identical to primary surgery, with the exception that in patients with known PONV more aggressive treatment with a scopolamine patch or other adjunctive antiemetics may be indicated.

REFERENCES

1. Abdelmalak B, Doyle J. *Anesthesia for Otolaryngologic Surgery*. Cambridge University Press; 2013.
2. Duzenli U, Bozan N, Turan M, et al. The effect of nitrous oxide on the outcomes of underlay tympanoplasty: a prospective study. *Ear Nose Throat J.* 2019;98(10):621–623. doi:10.1177/0145561319846460
3. Kouhi A, Hajimohammadi F, Dabiri S, et al. Effects of anesthesia with nitrous oxide on tympanoplasty outcomes: a randomized controlled trial. *Acta Otolaryngol.* 2018;138(4):363–366. doi:10.1080/00016489.2017.1388541
4. Parikh DA, Kolli SN, Karnik HS, et al. A prospective randomized double blind study comparing dexmedetomidine vs. combination midazolam-fentanyl for tympanoplasty surgery under monitored anesthesia care. *J Anaestheiol Clin Pharmacol.* 2013;29(2):173–178. doi:10.4103/0970-9185.111671
5. Kosucu M, Tugcugil E, Cobanoglu B, Arslan E. Evaluation of the perioperative effects of dexedetomidine on tympanoplasty operations. *Am J Otolaryngol.* 2020;41(6):102619. doi:10.1016/j.amjoto.2020.102619
6. Lee DW, Lee HG, Jeong CY, et al. Postoperative nausea and vomiting after mastoidectomy with tympanoplasty: a comparison between TIVA with propofol-remifentanil and balanced anesthesia with sevoflurane-remifentanil. *Korean J Anesthesiol.* 2011;61(5):399–404. doi:10.4097/kjae.2011.61.5.399
7. Sarmento KM, Tomita S. Retroauricualr tympanoplasty and tympanomastoidectomy under local anesthesia and sedation. *Acta Otolaryngol.* 2009;129(7):726–728. doi:10.1080/00016480802398996
8. Eidi M, Kolahdouzan K, Hosseinzadeh H, Tabaqi R. A comparison of preoperative ondansetron and dexamethasone in the prevention of post-tympanoplasty nausea and vomiting. *Iran J Med Sci.* 2012;37(3):166–172.

CHAPTER 61

Cochlear Implant Surgery

Nicklas Orobello and Andrew Redmann

INDICATIONS/CONTRAINDICATIONS

Congenital hearing loss (CHL) is the most common congenital sensory deficit, affecting approximately 1 in every 1,000 newborns.[1] The number of cases of CHL attributable to a genetic cause is estimated at 50%, approximately 30% of which are part of a known syndrome (see Figure 61.1).[2] Syndromes associated with hearing loss include trisomy 21, CHARGE,* Stickler, Treacher–Collins, branchiootorenal, Usher, Pendred, and Jervell and Lange-Nielsen syndromes, all of which have manifestations pertinent to the pediatric anesthesia provider (Table 61.1).

Due to the prevalence of CHL and the significant implications of delayed auditory and speech development, an emphasis has been placed on early identification of and intervention in infants with hearing loss, colloquially known within the otolaryngology community as the "1-3-6" rule. This stipulates that infants are screened for hearing loss by 1 month of age, diagnosed by 3 months of age, and offered intervention by 6 months of age.[3] Audiometric diagnosis of the etiology of hearing loss is essential for providing patients with the most appropriate means of auditory rehabilitation (e.g., conventional hearing aid vs. cochlear implant).

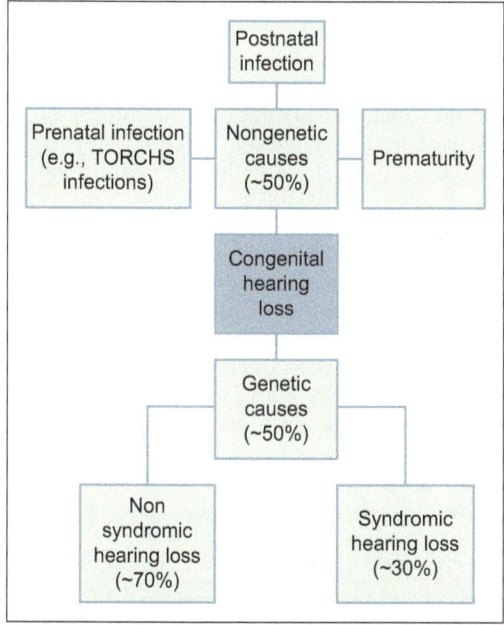

Figure 61.1: Etiologies of congenital hearing loss.

TORCH infections are a group of congenital infections that are passed from mother to child at some time during pregnancy, during delivery, or after birth. TORCH is an acronym representing infections caused by *Toxoplasma gondii*, other agents, rubella, cytomegalovirus (CMV), and herpes simplex virus (HSV).

---

*CHARGE syndrome is a disorder that affects many areas of the body. CHARGE is an abbreviation for several of the features common in the disorder: coloboma, heart defects, atresia choanae (also known as choanal atresia), growth retardation, genital abnormalities, and ear abnormalities.

Cochlear implantation provides candidates with the opportunity to receive auditory input at a young age, thus facilitating speech and language development. For those who meet the criteria, cochlear implantation can be a life-changing means of auditory rehabilitation that often allows children to progress through the mainstream education system in parallel with their normal-hearing counterparts.[4]

There are presently three corporations approved by the U.S. Food and Drug Administration (FDA) to manufacture cochlear implants, each of which is composed of three basic components: (a) a microphone, (b) a speech processor, and (c) an implanted receiver stimulator. The implant system allows auditory input to directly stimulate the cochlear nerve, thus bypassing the conductive and sensory mechanisms of hearing, to allow sound perception and higher cortical processing. As such, those with significant sensory hearing loss can obtain great benefit from cochlear implants.

Cochlear implants were first approved by the FDA in 1990 for use in children aged 2 to 17 years. The criteria for candidacy have expanded since that time, as further research has demonstrated that the original metrics used to determine candidacy were overly restrictive. A retrospective case series of 51 pediatric patients determined that nontraditional implant recipients derive significant improvements in speech recognition and auditory development.[5] Moreover, there is evidence that pediatric patients with single-sided deafness (SSD) who undergo cochlear implantation have significant improvements in objective measures of speech.[6] In light of this, the FDA recently approved cochlear implantation for patients aged 5 years or older with profound sensorineural hearing loss (SNHL) in the ear to be implanted and normal to moderate SNHL (asymmetric hearing loss [AHL]) in the contralateral ear.

As the criteria for implantation continue to expand, there is also an impetus to implant patients at younger ages to take advantage of neural plasticity in speech and auditory development. Children implanted within the first year of life have been observed to have improved speech perception and receptive language outcomes relative to those implanted between the ages of 12 and 24 months.[7-9] Due to these benefits, the FDA recently approved the use of cochlear implants in children as young as 9 months of age. These trends reflect the importance of providing auditory input at an early age, as well as the technological advances of the electrode designs and the improved overall safety profile of the procedure.

Contraindications to cochlear implantation include medical, otological, and social reasons. Otological contraindications to implantation include cochlear agenesis, vestibulocochlear agenesis (Michel deformity), and cochlear nerve agenesis. From an anesthesia standpoint, patients who are not medically fit to undergo general anesthesia for an elective procedure should not undergo implantation. Additionally, cochlear implant centers must give great consideration to patients' support systems as the auditory rehabilitation process is a long-term, multifaceted approach that requires intensive therapy and multiple follow-up appointments after implantation. As such, some centers do not implant children of families unlikely to participate in this process.

Table 61.1	Common Causes of Syndromic Hearing Loss	
Syndrome	Presentation	Pertinent Considerations
Trisomy 21	Upsloping palpebral fissures, midfacial hypoplasia, mental retardation, and micrognathia	Obstructive sleep apnea, pulmonary hypertension, atlantoaxial instability, micrognathia, and macroglossia
Treacher Collins	Microtia, downsloping palpebral fissures, cleft palate, and midfacial hypoplasia	Midfacial hypoplasia and cleft palate
CHARGE	Coloboma, cardiac anomalies, choanal atresia, developmental retardation, and genitourinary abnormalities	Congenital heart anomalies (e.g., tetralogy of Fallot, VSD, and aortic arch anomalies)
Jervell and Lange-Nielsen	Seizure disorder and syncope	QT prolongation, torsades de pointes, and risk of sudden cardiac death

CHARGE, coloboma, heart defects, atresia choanae (also known as choanal atresia), growth retardation, genital abnormalities, and ear abnormalities; VSD, ventricular septal defect.

SPECIAL CONSIDERATIONS AND CONCERNS

The presence of hearing loss itself may complicate the anesthesia provider–patient relationship in the preoperative phase. Special care and intention must be devoted to communicating with patients with hearing loss, especially in the context of bilateral hearing loss. Children who qualify for cochlear implantation, by definition, have significant hearing loss that forces them to rely on visual cues more than their normal-hearing counterparts. The anesthesia provider and the surgeon must both keep this under consideration in the preoperative setting.

ANESTHETIC MANAGEMENT

PREOPERATIVE EVALUATION

Patients considered for cochlear implantation must have a thorough history and physical examination prior to undergoing a general anesthetic. Special consideration must be given to syndromic patients, as many children with CHL who are considered for implantation have SNHL as part of a larger syndrome. Many of such patients have associated anatomical anomalies that complicate endotracheal intubation, such as cleft lip and cleft palate, mandibular hypoplasia, retrognathia, macroglossia, and atlantoaxial instability.[10] As such, a detailed stepwise algorithm for obtaining a safe airway must be prepared prior to induction of general anesthesia. Additionally, syndromes such as Down syndrome and CHARGE syndrome are associated with congenital cardiac anomalies, while Jervell and Lange-Nielsen syndrome is associated with a predisposition to prolonged QTc interval. Awareness of the associated anomalies and a team-based approach to the care of such patients are essential for good outcomes.

PREOPERATIVE PHARMACOLOGY

Short-acting benzodiazepines such as midazolam can be used to provide anxiolysis and help engage the child with the medical provider.[11,12] Depending on surgeon preference, a third- or fourth-generation cephalosporin with cerebrospinal fluid (CSF) penetrance (e.g., ceftriaxone/cefepime) can be administered for antibiotic prophylaxis, as the scala tympani (in which the electrode is inserted) has direct communication with the subarachnoid space of the posterior fossa.

ANESTHETIC TECHNIQUE

Intraoperative Management

Standard monitoring is required and includes electrocardiography, pulse oximetry, capnography, and temperature monitoring. Induction of general anesthesia can be either inhalation or IV depending on the patient's age and comorbidities. Following induction, the airway is secured with an endotracheal tube (ETT). As previously stated, many cochlear implant candidates have hearing loss as a component of a larger syndrome that may complicate endotracheal intubation. The overall prevalence of a difficult intubation was observed to be approximately 1.5% in a review of 190 pediatric patients undergoing cochlear implantation.[13] However, patients with facial dysplasia, such as those with Treacher-Collins syndrome,[14] have a higher prevalence of difficult airways that may complicate endotracheal intubation. A review of the airway management of 35 children with Treacher-Collins syndrome found a failed intubation rate of 5%.[15] Similarly, atlantoaxial instability and subluxation can be seen in approximately 20% of individuals with Down syndrome[15] and may preclude neck extension during direct laryngoscopy. In such cases, awareness of the anatomical levels that complicate endotracheal intubation is essential to obtaining a safe airway. Such patients may require fiberoptic-assisted intubation. Additional consideration to the risk of pulmonary hypertension in patients with Down syndrome and cardiac arrhythmias in patients with Jervell and Lange-Nielsen syndrome is warranted.

Cochlear implantation surgery generally takes between 2 and 4 hours in experienced hands (in cases of unilateral implantation). Expected estimated blood loss is minimal and a single peripheral IV catheter is sufficient. Long-acting paralytics should be avoided to allow the surgeon to monitor the facial nerve with the neural integrity monitoring (NIM) electromyographic (EMG) system. It is essential to ensure that the patient is properly secured and padded as otological surgery often necessitates bed rotation to optimize visualization of involved structures. Epinephrine is injected in a subcuticular plane along the course of the planned postauricular incision. While many surgeons inject lidocaine 1% with epinephrine 1:100,000, there is a theoretical risk of lidocaine mitigating the NIM's ability to monitor facial nerve activity. Care is taken to avoid lidocaine toxicity by appropriate dosing according to the patient's body weight.

The operation proceeds from exposure of the round window to implantation of the electrode and subsequent closure. Briefly, a postauricular incision is made and a pocket is formed deep to the temporalis muscle to allow placement of the device. These initial stages of the procedure are the most stimulating. A mastoidectomy is performed, exposing the facial recess, which is subsequently opened to visualize the round window niche. The electrode array is then inserted into the scala tympani in a controlled, atraumatic fashion, after which time monopolar electrocautery must be avoided. The device is placed into the preformed pocket, and attention is turned to closure in a layered fashion.

There are a few unique considerations in cochlear implantation surgery. As previously stated, the patient's head and the operative table are often rotated to optimize visualization of essential structures. As such, care must be taken to minimize the risk of accidental extubation by securing the position of the ETT prior to draping. It is also important to note that, in cases of bilateral implantation, the drapes are broken down and the patient is reprepped for contralateral surgery. Additionally, postoperative x-rays are obtained in the operating room to ensure intracochlear position of the electrode array prior to allowing the patient to wake up. Lastly, care is taken to avoid patient bucking and discomfort during the wake-up process so as to minimize the risk of increased pressure within the ear and dislodgment of the electrode. If there are no contraindications, deep extubation should be considered.

POSTOPERATIVE CARE

Patients are typically transferred to the postanesthesia care unit (PACU) for recovery and then discharged home on the same day of surgery. The postoperative course is typically uneventful, although patients may develop nausea and vomiting related to general anesthesia or stimulation of the caloric response with intraoperative irrigation of the ear. As the patient wakes up, the ipsilateral facial nerve may be found to be weak postoperatively—this is most often due to neuropraxia or temporary local anesthesia effect, but in rare cases may be due to permanent nerve injury. Regardless of the extent of injury, the surgeon should be made aware of such findings. More commonly, complications develop after discharge from the PACU. Complications include wound infection, hematoma, persistent vestibular symptoms, facial nerve paralysis, meningitis, and total device failure. However, the prevalence of major complications from cochlear implantation surgery is low, at approximately 3%.[16] The implant is typically activated 2 to 4 weeks postoperatively.

KEY REFERENCES

Complete references for this chapter are online and available at https://connect.springerpub.com/content/book/978-0-8261-3875-0/part/part04/toc-part/ch061.

1. Lalwani A, Castelein C. Cracking the auditory genetic code: non-syndromic hereditary hearing impairment. *Am J Otol*. 1999;20(1):115–132.
2. Morton, N. Genetic epidemiology of hearing impairment. *Ann N Y Acad Sci*. 1991;630:16–31. doi:10.1111/j.1749-6632.1991.tb19572.x
4. Geers A, Brenner C, Tobey E. Long-term outcomes of cochlear implantation in early childhood: sample characteristics and data collection methods. *Ear Hear*. 2011;32(1):2–12. doi:10.1097/AUD.0b013e3182014c53
5. Carlson M, Sladen D, Haynes D, et al. Evidence for the expansion of pediatric cochlear implant candidacy. *Otol Neurotol*. 2014;36(1):43–50. doi:10.1097/MAO.0000000000000607
6. Zeitler D, Sladen D, DeJong M, et al. Cochlear implantation for single-sided deafness in children and adolescents. *Int J Pediatr Otorhinolaryngol*. 2019;118:128–133. doi:10.1016/j.ijporl.2018.12.037
9. Colletti I. Long-term follow-up of infants (4–11 months) fitted with cochlear implants. *Acta Otolaryngol*. 2009;129(4):361–366. doi:10.1080/00016480802495453
10. Antoine I, Carullo V, Hernandez C, Tepper O. Anatomic approach to airway management of the syndromic child. *Int Anesthes Clin*. 2017;55(1):52–64. doi:10.1097/AIA.0000000000000131
14. Goel L, Bennur S, Jambhale S. Treacher-Collins syndrome–a challenge for anesthesiologists. *Indian J Anaesth*. 2009;53(4):496–500.
15. Hosking J, Zoanetti D, Carlyle A, et al. Anesthesia for Treacher Collins syndrome: a review of airway management in 240 pediatric cases. *Paediatr Anaesth*. 2012;22(8):752–758. doi:10.1111/j.1460-9592.2012.03829.x
16. Hata T, Todd M. Cervical spine considerations when anesthetizing patients with Down syndrome. *Anesthesiology*. 2005;102(3):680–685. doi:10.1097/00000542-200503000-00030

CHAPTER 62

Adenotonsillectomy

D. Julie Soelberg

INDICATIONS/CONTRAINDICATIONS

Tonsillectomy with or without adenoidectomy is one of the most commonly performed pediatric surgeries in the United States, with an estimated 340,000 ambulatory procedures performed annually in children <15 years of age.[1] The majority of surgeries are performed to manage symptoms of recurrent tonsillitis or obstructive sleep-disordered breathing (SDB), which is the more prominent indication among younger children in the United States.[2-4] Obstructive SDB is a group of disorders characterized by abnormal respiratory patterns or insufficient ventilation during sleep, ranging from primary snoring to obstructive sleep apnea (OSA).[5,6] For additional information regarding SDB, please see Chapter 69, "Care of Children With Sleep-Disordered Breathing."

Adenotonsillar hypertrophy is the primary cause of pediatric OSA.[2,7,8] Because untreated OSA can lead to adverse behavioral, neurocognitive, and cardiopulmonary effects, early adenotonsillectomy in children with OSA is advocated.[9-11] Accordingly, adenotonsillectomy is considered first-line treatment for adenotonsillar hypertrophy. Other indications for tonsillectomy and/or adenoidectomy are presented in **Box 62.1**. Contraindications to tonsillectomy and/or adenoidectomy include untreated hematological disorders, active infection, and uncontrolled systemic disease.[12]

Multiple surgical techniques for adenotonsillectomy have been described, although there is no clear consensus as to what approach is the gold standard.[13,14] Traditional "cold" tonsillectomy involves removal of the tonsils using metal dissecting instruments. Conversely, modern "hot" techniques employ electrosurgical instruments (diathermy or electrocautery) for dissection and hemostasis, thereby reducing intraoperative bleeding and surgical times.[4,13] While both cold and hot techniques are associated with advantages and disadvantages, the influence of technique on posttonsillectomy bleeding (PTB) and/or postsurgical pain remains unclear.[4,14-16]

SPECIAL CONSIDERATIONS AND CONCERNS

Several at-risk pediatric populations, listed in **Box 62.2**, have a higher incidence of complications following adenotonsillectomy.[5,7,12,17-20] The perioperative challenges associated with a diagnosis of OSA are well documented. Children with OSA are at higher risk of significant complications, including death and near death from anoxic or hypoxic events, following adenotonsillectomy.[4,18,21-23] Distinguishing between children with OSA and those with primary snoring or recurrent tonsillitis is therefore an imperative preoperative task.[17] The diagnostic criteria for pediatric OSA can be found in Chapter 69, "Care of Children with Sleep-Disordered Breathing."

Fortunately, for most children, major complications following adenotonsillectomy are rare—although risks do exist, even in healthy children. A meta-analysis evaluating complications in otherwise healthy children found respiratory compromise and secondary hemorrhage were the most frequent early complications, occurring 9.4% and 2.6% of the time, respectively. Older children (>10 years) more commonly experience secondary hemorrhage, with younger children (<3 years) more often experiencing respiratory complications.[18]

ANESTHETIC MANAGEMENT

Adenotonsillectomy is a highly stimulating surgical procedure requiring a shared airway. Anesthetic goals for patients undergoing adenotonsillectomy include allaying preoperative anxiety, providing smooth anesthetic induction, securing the airway, providing adequate surgical conditions, optimizing analgesia, preventing postoperative nausea and vomiting (PONV), and facilitating a safe and rapid emergence from anesthesia.[17,24] The choice of anesthetic technique during

---

BOX 62.1 INDICATIONS FOR TONSILLECTOMY AND/OR ADENOIDECTOMY

Tonsillectomy With or Without Adenoidectomy
- Sleep disordered breathing/OSA
- Recurrent tonsillitis
- Chronic tonsillitis
- Peritonsillar abscess
- Tonsillar/adenoidal mass lesion
- Periodic fever, aphthous stomatitis, pharyngitis, and adenitis

Adenoidectomy Only
- Sleep-disordered breathing from nasal airway obstruction
- Recurrent acute otitis media
- Chronic rhinosinusitis

OSA, obstructive sleep apnea.

BOX 62.2 CHILDREN AT RISK OF COMPLICATIONS RELATED TO ADENOTONSILLECTOMY

- Age <3 years
- Severe OSA documented by PSG
- Craniofacial disorders
- Neuromuscular disorders
- Trisomy 21
- Bleeding diathesis
- Sickle cell disease
- Body habitus (obesity or failure to thrive)
- History of prematurity
- Pulmonary disease
- Major heart disease

OSA, obstructive sleep apnea; PSG, polysomnography.

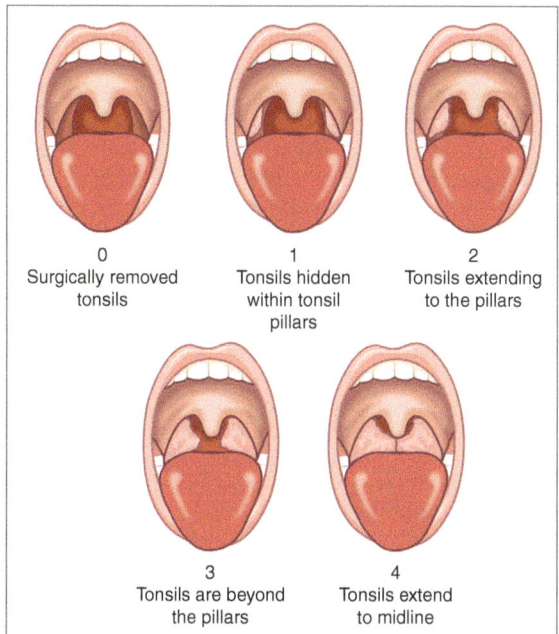

Figure 62.1: Evaluation of tonsillar size. Evaluating tonsillar size may help identify the degree of airway obstruction a child may experience during an inhalation induction. When the tonsils occupy >50% of the pharyngeal space (+3 or greater), an increased risk of airway obstruction exists.

adenotonsillectomy depends on the indication for surgery, concomitant comorbidities, provider preference, and/or institutional preference.

PREOPERATIVE EVALUATION

Preoperative considerations include evaluating the general health of the child, conducting a careful history and physical, and reviewing the indication for the procedure. As adenotonsillectomy is often performed in children who are losing their deciduous teeth, it is important to inspect for loose or missing teeth. During examination of the oropharynx, classification of tonsillar size (Figure 62.1) may predict the degree of airway obstruction during induction of anesthesia, although subjective assessment of tonsillar size or palate position is not an absolute predictor of OSA severity.[7,17,25] When available, polysomnography (PSG) should be reviewed and parental report of SDB symptoms should be elicited. In addition to identifying at-risk populations, it is important to determine if there is a recent history of upper respiratory tract infection (URI), bleeding tendencies, and the use of medications that interfere with coagulation as these all independently increase the risk of postoperative complications.[17] Available evidence supports assessing for patient/family bleeding diathesis and conducting coagulation testing as indicated by history or presence of a bleeding disorder.[26-28] The utility of preoperative complete blood count and/or coagulation profile is debated. Finally, a child with severe OSA may rarely require a preoperative cardiac evaluation or pulmonary consultation.[5]

PREOPERATIVE PHARMACOLOGY

The use of sedative premedication prior to adenotonsillectomy is not universally endorsed given the inherent loss of airway tone associated with many medications used for anxiolysis. The potential for postoperative complications is further heightened in the presence of SDB, hence the strong argument that premedication in a child with severe OSA should be avoided. If required, a short-acting agent with careful dosing and continuous monitoring by pulse oximetry and clinical observation should occur.[17,20] Oral midazolam, intranasal midazolam, and intranasal dexmedetomidine all produce adequate anxiolysis that facilitates parental separation.[29-31] The potential residual impact of sedative medications should be considered in children with SDB prior to administration and patients should be closely observed throughout their perioperative course.

ANESTHETIC TECHNIQUE

BOX 62.3 CLINICAL PEARLS: ADENOTONSILLECTOMY

Preoperative
- Assess the need for premedication; cautious use in OSA
- Elicit history and physical with focus on indication for procedure, obstructive symptoms (review PSG if available), comorbidities, bleeding tendencies, and recent URI
- Airway/oropharyngeal evaluation

Intraoperative:
Anesthesia-Related
- IV or inhalation induction
- ETT or LMA
- Airway fire precautions
- No perioperative antibiotics
- IV fluid administration
- Analgesia, including multimodal therapy; reduce opioids in OSA
- PONV prophylaxis
- Strategies to reduce emergence agitation
- Awake versus deep extubation; consider awake in OSA

Surgical-Related
- Bed turned 90 degrees
- Head extended on shoulder roll and mouth gag for oropharyngeal exposure
- Hot or cold techniques

Postoperative
- Continued analgesic and fluid management
- Monitor for respiratory complications
- NSAID (ibuprofen) generally given postoperatively, after hemostasis is achieved
- No codeine
- Inpatient admission for at-risk children
- If postoperative PTB, aggressive fluid resuscitation preinduction, RSI, and awake extubation

ETT, endotracheal tube; LMA, laryngeal mask airway; NSAID, nonsteroidal anti-inflammatory drugs; OSA, obstructive sleep apnea; PONV, postoperative nausea and vomiting; PSG, polysomnography; PTB, posttonsillectomy bleeding; RSI, rapid sequence intubation; URI, upper respiratory tract infection.

Intraoperative Management

See **Box 62.3**. An inhalation or IV induction technique is acceptable, although the latter may be preferable in a child with obesity or severe OSA.[17,20] Airway obstruction with inhalation induction is quite common in the setting of adenoid and/or tonsillar hypertrophy and desaturation may occur quickly. The anesthesia provider should be prepared to initiate airway maneuvers to promptly alleviate airway obstruction.

The anesthesia provider and the surgeon share the airway during adenotonsillectomy. Access to the airway is often limited during the procedure, with the bed turned away from the anesthesia provider. While endotracheal intubation is the standard for airway management, flexible laryngeal mask airways (LMAs) have emerged as an acceptable alternative.[32–34] Advantages and disadvantages associated with the use of flexible LMAs during adenotonsillectomy are presented in **Table 62.1**.

If an endotracheal tube (ETT) is planned, an oral Ring-Adair-Elwin (RAE) endotracheal tube or a flexible armored ETT is preferred. A cuffed ETT confers benefits of preventing an air leak and protecting the airway from blood, secretions, and risk of airway fire when electrocautery is used.[17] If required, short-acting neuromuscular blocking agents can be used to facilitate intubation, although many providers routinely intubate without muscle relaxation. Regardless of airway device used, it should be placed in the midline and secured to the chin. Adequate oropharyngeal exposure is achieved by the surgeon placing a shoulder roll to extend the neck and positioning a mouth gag. The use of a shoulder roll should be avoided if there is any concern for atlantooccipital instability, such as with a patient with Down syndrome. During insertion of the mouth gag, it is essential to watch for accidental ETT dislodgment or obstruction of the airway device.

Maintenance of anesthesia includes inhalation and/or IV agents. Adenotonsillectomies are brief procedures and the anesthetic should be planned accordingly. Spontaneous or controlled ventilation is acceptable during adenotonsillectomy.[17] Ventilation can become difficult at any stage during adenotonsillectomy and close communication between the surgeon and the anesthesia provider is essential. In the event of difficult ventilation or desaturation, the mouth gag should be released as soon as possible.[24] Desflurane may promote rapid recovery and emergence, although the benefits must be balanced with desflurane's propensity to irritate the airway. Hence, inhalation anesthetic agents with lower potential for airway irritation should be considered as children undergoing adenotonsillectomy are more likely to experience airway hyperreactivity and laryngospasm than those undergoing nonairway surgery.[17,35–37]

Parenteral opioids have been the mainstay of perioperative pain management, although multimodal, opioid-sparing techniques are now favored for a multitude of reasons to limit undesired opioid-related adverse effects.[17,38] Children with OSA have a well-documented increased sensitivity to opioids, and it is advocated that opioids be reduced by 50% in this population.[17,21] Adjuvant agents including dexmedetomidine, acetaminophen, nonsteroidal anti-inflammatory drugs (NSAIDs), and ketamine all appear to demonstrate opioid-sparing effects.[39–42] Dexmedetomidine (<2 mcg/kg) may lessen postoperative pain and decrease postoperative opioid consumption without increasing length of postanesthesia care unit (PACU) stay or causing adverse hemodynamic effects.[40,43–47] Whether or not dexmedetomidine prolongs time to extubation is still debated.

Oral and/or rectal acetaminophen have long been described as safe and inexpensive multimodal analgesic interventions in children undergoing adenotonsillectomy, although the pharmacokinetic variability associated with each route yields inconsistencies.[48–50] While IV formulations of acetaminophen produce reliable and predictable plasma concentrations, studies evaluating the effectiveness of IV acetaminophen in pediatric adenotonsillectomy patients offer mixed results.[51–54]

The use of NSAIDs has historically been associated with increased bleeding, but recent evidence suggests some NSAIDs may be safely used in children undergoing adenotonsillectomy. A multicenter randomized controlled trial (RCT),[55] Cochrane review,[56] and systematic review/meta-analysis[57] found NSAIDs did not significantly increase the risk of postoperative bleeding requiring surgical intervention in children who underwent tonsillectomy. Oral ibuprofen is advocated in the postoperative period; however, use of other NSAIDs, particularly ketorolac, remains controversial and dependent on provider preference.[4] In general, many providers avoid NSAIDs in the preoperative or intraoperative period in favor of postoperative administration, after hemostasis is achieved. Communication with the surgical team should occur prior to administering NSAIDs.

More research is necessary to understand the effectiveness of other analgesic adjuncts in pediatric adenotonsillectomy, such as magnesium and gabapentin. Additionally, while intraoperative peritonsillar infiltration of local anesthetics may reduce early posttonsillectomy pain, the risks of aspiration and other negative sequelae associated with its use often outweigh the potential benefits.[17,58]

Blood, secretions, and/or irrigation may be present in the airway when the procedure concludes and the oropharynx should be carefully suctioned.[17,24] Hemostasis and removal of surgical sponges must be assured prior to extubation. If used, neuromuscular blockade should be antagonized. Timing of tracheal extubation after adenotonsillectomy is debated. It is a challenging task to avoid coughing, breath-holding, oxygen desaturation, and laryngospasm during emergence from adenotonsillectomy, and deep tracheal extubation may avoid some of these complications.[59,60] However, respiratory complications after adenotonsillectomy are common, leading many providers to wait until the return of airway reflexes prior to extubation.[17,24] In general, the extubation strategy depends on concomitant comorbidities, intraoperative course, and provider preference. In children with OSA, the trachea is usually

Table 62.1 Advantages and Disadvantages of LMA Use During Adenotonsillectomy	
Advantages	**Disadvantages**
• Greater ease of insertion	• Unprotected airway
• Shorter extubation times	• Limited ability to deliver positive pressure
• LMA aperture may protect airway from blood/secretions	• Obstruction/kinking with mouth gag insertion or opening
• Less coughing and similar or reduced rates of laryngospasm during emergence	• Limited use in young or obese children
	• May obstruct surgical view
	• Requires surgeon comfort/experience
	• Requires anesthesia provider comfort/experience

LMA, laryngeal mask airway.

extubated when the child is fully awake.[17] At the time of extubation, the child can be placed in a lateral, head-down position ("tonsil" position) to avoid accumulation of blood and/or secretions at the laryngeal inlet.[17,61]

Complications

Adenotonsillectomy is associated with a high incidence of emergence agitation.[44,47] Perioperative dexmedetomidine may reduce the incidence of emergence agitation, with the added benefits of reducing opioid requirements and episodes of oxygen desaturation.[45,62-64] Other strategies to mitigate emergence agitation include choice of anesthetic technique, additional adjuvant drugs for pain control, and possibly acupuncture should be considered.[65]

PONV following pediatric adenotonsillectomy can occur in 30% to 70% of children when antiemetic prophylaxis is not used.[66,67] Children may experience poor oral intake, dehydration, delayed discharge, or unplanned hospital admission as a result of PONV.[68,69] Multimodal antiemetic prophylaxis is recommended and combinations of propofol, ondansetron, and dexamethasone are widely used.[17] The American Academy of Otolaryngology-Head and Neck Surgery (AAO-HHN) strongly recommends a single intraoperative dose of IV dexamethasone in children undergoing adenotonsillectomy. The optimal dose of dexamethasone is less clear, with doses ranging from .15 to 1 mg/kg.[70] Studies often suggest a dose of .5 mg/kg, but lower doses may be equally effective.[71] Dexamethasone has the added benefits of reducing pain and improving time to oral intake, presumably related to its anti-inflammatory properties.[4,70] The impact dexamethasone has on the incidence of PTB remains debated.[72-77] Other strategies to reduce PONV include fluid administration[24,67] and possibly acupuncture at the P6 point.[68,78-80] Gastric aspiration via an orogastric tube, a procedure performed by the surgeon prior to emergence, is not effective in reducing PONV.[81,82]

POSTOPERATIVE CARE

In general, the predominate postoperative issue is balancing adequate analgesia with the risk of airway obstruction or apnea. Immediate postoperative pain can be treated with IV and/or oral agents. Pain and functional limitation may last for up to 7 days following adenotonsillectomy, and the AAO-HHN endorses the use of acetaminophen, ibuprofen, or both for at-home pain control.[4,49] Oral opioids may be prescribed to mitigate postoperative pain, although codeine must be avoided in all children undergoing tonsillectomy and/or adenoidectomy due to the concern of genetic polymorphisms in isoenzyme CYP2D6, leading to heightened therapeutic effects in ultra-rapid metabolizers. Reports of deaths and near deaths in children receiving standard doses of oral codeine following adenotonsillectomy have prompted the Food and Drug Administration to place a Boxed Warning on the drug.[83-85] The Boxed Warning applies to all children undergoing tonsillectomy and/or adenoidectomy, regardless of OSA status.

Although adenotonsillectomy is most commonly performed as an ambulatory procedure, at-risk children may warrant inpatient admission. In addition, unplanned hospital admission may be required in the setting of perioperative adverse respiratory events, failure to take oral fluids, or continued vomiting. Social factors, such as living a far distance from the hospital or inadequate at-home supervision, should also be considered.[17]

Postoperative Complications: Posttonsillectomy Bleeding

One of the primary risks of adenotonsillectomy is PTB, which ranges from being self-limiting to life-threatening hemorrhage.[86,87] The average reported rate of PTB ranges from 2% to 4%.[18,86] PTB is classified as either primary (within 24 hours) or secondary bleeding (>24 hours, up to 10 days postoperatively).[4,88] Primary bleeding is generally acknowledged as inadequate surgical hemostasis, whereas secondary bleeding is attributed to disruption of the healing clot.[17] Some bleeding events require emergent surgical control, and the anesthetic management of a child with PTB differs greatly from the general management of adenotonsillectomy.

The anesthetic management of a child with PTB is complicated by anemia, hypovolemia, and a large amount of sequestered intragastric blood.[89] The reality of a second general anesthetic and surgery is often anxiety-producing for the family and the child; however, premedication is generally avoided. A brief history and physical should focus on general appearance, active bleeding, volume status, and hemodynamic stability.[88] Investigations should also include assessment of hemoglobin and hematocrit, coagulation tests, and blood crossmatching. The initial anesthetic record should be reviewed for a rough estimate of intraoperative blood loss and fluid replacement.[17] Estimating blood loss is difficult because most of the blood lost from the tonsillar area is swallowed. The spectrum of volume loss can range from mild dehydration to shock, and it is imperative to provide volume resuscitation prior to induction of anesthesia. The compensatory response to acute blood loss delays the onset of hypotension in the awake child, and profound hypotension may occur as a result of anesthesia-induced vasodilation.[17] IV access and aggressive fluid resuscitation with repeated boluses of 20 mL/kg of isotonic fluid and/or colloids should be initiated prior to induction of anesthesia and be continued throughout the perioperative period.[17,61] If bleeding is severe, it may be necessary to administer packed red blood cells.

Airway management in a child with PTB is challenging. Active bleeding or clots may obscure the airway, and edema may be present from previous airway instrumentation and/or surgery. A retrospective study of 475 children requiring surgery for PTB found 2.7% of patients to be difficult to intubate, none of whom were difficult to intubate during the initial adenotonsillectomy.[89] Airway management of the initial adenotonsillectomy should be carefully reviewed, including ETT size and any difficulties encountered. Although this is a time-sensitive procedure, preparation is essential. A cuffed ETT with a stylet, two well-illuminated laryngoscope blades and handles, and two large-bore Yankauer suction tubes must be available prior to induction.[17] Some providers opt to have two ETTs prepared: the size used previously and a half-size smaller ETT in case of laryngeal edema. There is a risk of severe hypoxemia if the larynx cannot be adequately visualized for ETT insertion, and the otolaryngologist should be available to assist with a surgical airway, if necessary.[89]

A child presenting with PTB should be presumed to have a full stomach of swallowed blood and possibly oral intake. To decrease the risk of pulmonary aspiration, an IV rapid-sequence induction with cricoid pressure is commonly practiced.[89,90] Standard doses of some induction drugs may result in significant hypotension. A hemodynamically stable induction drug (e.g., ketamine or etomidate) or a reduced dose of propofol should be considered.[88,91] Succinylcholine is most often used to facilitate tracheal intubation.[88,89,90] Nondepolarizing muscle relaxants should be used with caution, as hypoxemia associated with difficult laryngoscopy can be catastrophic if the airway cannot be secured in a timely manner.[17,21] The availability of sugammadex may influence whether rocuronium can be used. After the airway is secured, it is helpful to obtain a second large-bore peripheral IV catheter to continue volume resuscitation and/or blood administration, if indicated.[91]

The intraoperative management of a PTB should facilitate rapid recovery after surgery. Surgical hemostasis of a tonsillar bleed is generally a short surgical procedure and does not cause excessive pain.[17] Once hemostasis is achieved, the surgeon may evacuate gastric contents by placing a large-bore orogastric tube under direct visualization. The child should be fully awakened prior to extubation.[17,91] Hemoglobin and hematocrit levels may be reevaluated postoperatively. Often, the child will be admitted for observation.

KEY REFERENCES

Complete references for this chapter are online and available at https://connect.springerpub.com/content/book/978-0-8261-3875-0/part/part04/toc-part/ch062

3. Marcus C, Brooks L, Draper K, et al. Diagnosis and management of childhood obstructive sleep apnea syndrome. *Pediatrics.* 2012;130(3):576–584. doi:10.1542/peds.2012-1671
4. Mitchell R, Archer S, Ishman S, et al. Clinical practice guideline: tonsillectomy in children (update). *Otolaryngol-Head Neck Surg.* 2019;160(1):S1–S42. doi:10.1177/0194599818801757
5. Coté CJ. Anesthesiological considerations for children with obstructive sleep apnea. *Curr Opin Anaesthesiol.* 2015;28(3):327–332. doi:10.1097/ACO.0000000000000187
17. Cote C, Lerman J, Anderson B. *A Practice of Anesthesia for Infants and Children.* 6th ed. Elsevier; 2018.
24. Forsyth I, Mahendran R. Anesthesia for ear, nose and throat surgery in children. In: *A Guide to Pediatric Anesthesia.* Springer International; 2019:335–350. https://doi.org/10.1007/978-3-030-19246-4_16

CHAPTER 63

Microlaryngoscopy

Lauren Freedman

INDICATIONS/CONTRAINDICATIONS

Microlaryngoscopy involves the assessment of the larynx, which is composed of tissues situated between the trachea and the pharynx. More specifically, the larynx begins at the base of the tongue and continues to the cricoid cartilage.[1] The larynx is responsible for phonation and protection of the lower airway.[1]

Microlaryngoscopy is most often performed under general anesthesia; however, sedation may be indicated in special cases when maintenance of a patent airway is tenuous and/or the patient is too ill to tolerate a general anesthetic. During the procedure, either a flexible or a rigid bronchoscope is used to magnify the larynx and optimize visualization of the area of concern.[2] This has long been a staple among otolaryngology airway management, being first introduced in the early 1900s. As technology and understanding have advanced, so too have the indications and therapeutic utility.[3]

Pediatric patients present for microlaryngoscopy for a variety of reasons, such as noisy breathing, stridor, hoarse voice, removal of vocal cord lesions, removal of a foreign body, and difficulty swallowing.[4] While this is typically performed to diagnose an underlying problem, it can also serve as a therapeutic intervention.[4] A common therapeutic indication is foreign body removal (Box 63.1). This is often an urgent case, with the patient brought to the operating room emergently in an effort to remove the airway obstruction and stave off further respiratory complications. Microlaryngoscopy can also be performed to treat congenital or acquired tracheal lesions.

Contraindications to microlaryngoscopy are few and primarily relate to the overall health of the patient. Thus, the true contraindications include unsatisfactory management of coexisting conditions, failure to obtain clearance from other involved services, or acute illness at the time of an elective procedure.[4]

SPECIAL CONSIDERATIONS

Anesthetic management of these cases presents a unique challenge. Microlaryngoscopy is one of the few operations in which the anesthesia provider and the surgeon require access to the airway simultaneously.[1] It is imperative that there is open and constant communication between anesthesia providers and otolaryngology throughout the procedure.[1] It is highly recommended that a discussion including all stakeholders occur prior to induction to ensure safe and effective care. During this discussion, anesthesia providers should determine the otolaryngology's need to visualize vocal cord movement and periods of apnea during the procedure as this will help guide anesthetic planning.

BOX 63.1	INDICATIONS FOR MICROLARYNGOSCOPY

- Airway mass
- Airway trauma
- Chronic cough
- Foreign body removal
- Hoarseness
- Laryngotracheal infections
- Noisy breathing
- Severe hemoptysis
- Stridor
- Swallowing difficulties
- Tracheotomy surveillance
- Vocal cord lesions

ANESTHETIC MANAGEMENT

PREOPERATIVE EVALUATION

When evaluating a patient prior to microlaryngoscopy, it is imperative that anesthesia providers perform a concise history and physical examination. The history should focus on when the symptoms began and discern all exacerbating and relieving factors.[5] The physical examination should focus on physical symptoms such as stridor, retractions, and overall appearance at baseline.

Pertinent Labs

Typically, labs are not required for this procedure. However, if a patient has a history of feeding difficulty or bleeding, labs, including a complete metabolic panel and coagulation labs, should be obtained.

PREOPERATIVE PHARMACOLOGY

Preoperative medications are subject to the patient's comorbidities and physical assessment. Anxiolytics should be administered with caution given the potential impact on respiratory tone and maintenance of a patent airway. Due to the insufflation of air into the abdomen during this procedure, oral medications preoperatively should be avoided if possible.[5]

ANESTHETIC TECHNIQUE

Intraoperative Management

Anesthesia providers should plan on having the following equipment readily available for the procedure: an appropriately sized oral airway, face mask, straight laryngoscope blade, age-appropriate cuffed and uncuffed endotracheal tubes (ETT), a stylet, suction, and all appropriate pharmacological medications.

The method of induction depends on the presenting indication, current symptoms, and presence of comorbid conditions. Accordingly, inhalation mask induction may be appropriate at times, with more critical patients requiring an IV induction. Should an IV induction be utilized, medications should be titrated slowly to avoid abrupt loss of airway tone and/or patency. Standard monitors, as described by the American Society of Anesthesiologists, are often sufficient in microlaryngoscopy. At least one peripheral IV catheter should be in place, and anesthesia providers may want to consider placement of a second IV catheter if total IV anesthesia (TIVA) is planned to allow for a dedicated IV catheter for TIVA.

Anesthesia can be maintained via volatile anesthetic agents, TIVA, or a combination thereof. Regardless of the technique employed, IV propofol can be administered to provide additional anesthesia to maintain an adequate depth of anesthesia when otolaryngology is operating in the airway.[5] Adjuncts such as remifentanil, dexmedetomidine, and ketamine can be used to supplement the anesthetic, either as a bolus or as an infusion. It is important to be mindful that these procedures are usually brief in nature, frequently lasting less than 15 minutes.

Following induction and establishment of an adequate plane of anesthesia, the operating table is rotated to allow otolaryngology full access to the patient's airway. At this point, otolaryngology takes control of the patient's airway. A shoulder roll and a tooth guard are placed prior to laryngoscopy and/or placement of a Hollinger or Parsons laryngoscope for suspension. Microlaryngoscopy is frequently done without an ETT, thereby affording otolaryngology an unobscured view of the larynx. As there is no direct administration of oxygen, the likelihood of hypoxemia during the procedure is high.

Supplemental oxygenation can be administered via nasal cannula, blowby, intermittent intubation, or jet ventilation. Oxygen may also be administered via the side port of a Hollinger or Parsons laryngoscope. Administration of supplemental oxygen has been shown to decrease the degree of hypoxemia when compared with administration via a high-flow nasal cannula.[6]

The blade used for laryngoscopy varies based on otolaryngology's preference and institutional protocol. Commonly used blades include Phillips, Wis-Hipple, Miller, Hollinger, and Parsons blades, with the latter two being used for suspension (Figure 63.1). Once the laryngoscope blade is placed in the airway, a laryngotracheal topicalization anesthesia (LTA)

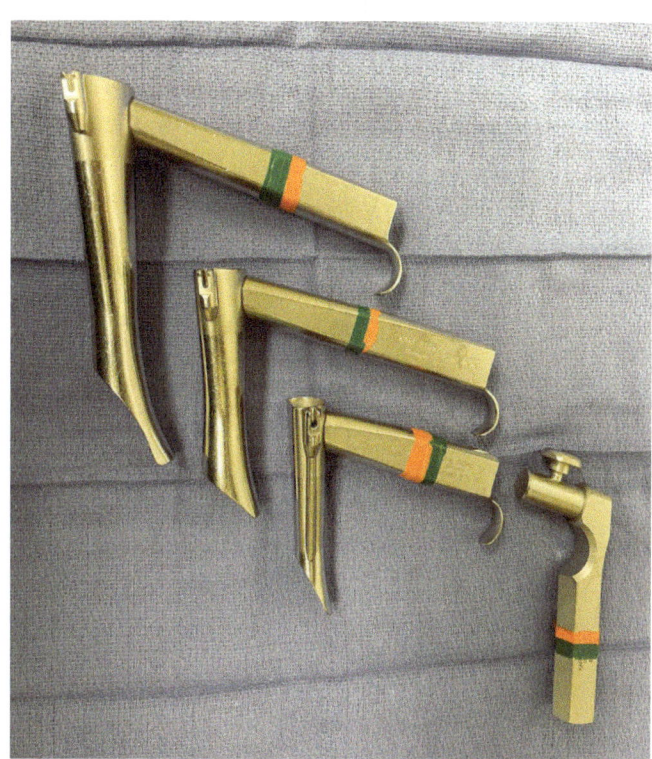

Figure 63.1: Lindholm laryngoscopes.

kit is used to deliver topical lidocaine to the larynx, with the hopes of decreasing coughing and airway irritation during the microlaryngoscopy. A rigid bronchoscope is then advanced to closely examine the larynx. Key assessments include symmetrical vocal cord movement, complete relaxation and closure of the vocal cords, and identification of a laryngeal cleft, as well as the presence of growths, nodules, or foreign bodies. Flexible bronchoscopy, and possibly esophagoscopy, is often used in conjunction with microlaryngoscopy for a more complete and comprehensive airway evaluation.[1] Otolaryngology may also size the airway with an age-appropriate ETT during the procedure for benchmarking.

Dexamethasone (.5 mg/kg) is often administered to minimize potential postoperative edema.[5] Similarly, atropine or glycopyrrolate may be administered to reduce copious secretions. Following the procedure, the bed is rotated back toward the anesthesia provider, and the patient is awoken in the operating room.

Special Techniques and/or Equipment

Jet ventilation is a method of delivering oxygen via a specialized system comprising an injector, tubing, a toggle switch, a reducing valve or regulator, and a connection to a high-pressure oxygen supply. During jet ventilation, oxygen is delivered intermittently in a high-frequency, low-tidal volume fashion, with exhalation occurring passively. This can be achieved via infraglottic, supraglottic, transglottic, and transtracheal or transluminal techniques. In microlaryngoscopy, the most commonly used is a supraglottic or transglottic catheter. TIVA in combination with profound muscular relaxation is the most common method of maintaining anesthesia during jet ventilation.

There is an increased risk of pneumothorax, pneumomediastinum, distention of the stomach and regurgitation/aspiration, damage to mucosal surfaces, and SC emphysema when using jet ventilation.[6] To avoid barotrauma, the driving pressure and the frequency of delivery must be gradually increased while checking for thoracic expansion. Also, anesthesia providers should be aware that this is not a laser-safe approach as the delivery of oxygen may cause ignition during lasering.

Clinical Pearls

Therapeutic interventions, such as removal of excess, abnormal, or damaged tracheal tissue, can be performed in conjunction with microlaryngoscopy. Removing undesired tissue can be achieved via the use of laser, shavers, or microdebriders. Should lasering be planned, it is imperative precautions be taken to keep both the patient and the staff safe as airway fires can be catastrophic. Anesthesia providers should decrease the fraction of inspired oxygen to the lowest tolerated percentage; ideally, this is close to 21% or room air. Should an airway fire occur, anesthesia providers must react quickly to extinguish the fire and limit further injury to the patient. This includes

---

BOX 63.2 MANAGEMENT OF AN AIRWAY FIRE

- Remove ETT
- Stop flow of gases
- Remove all flammable/burning materials from the airway
- Pour saline or water into the airway
- Reestablish ventilation by mask using room air if possible
- Extinguish and examine the ETT and consider bronchoscopy
- Assess the patient's condition and plan for ongoing care

ETT, endotracheal tube.

Source: From Dalesio NM, Hayward DM, Schwengel DA. Anesthesia for pediatric otorhinolaryngologic surgery. In: Davis PJ, Cladis FP, eds. *Smith's Anesthesia for Infants and Children.* 9th ed. Elsevier; 2016:Box 31–13.

Table 63.1 Laser Applications and Associated Precautions During Microlaryngoscopy

Laser	Application	Wavelength (nm)	Effect	Protective Eyewear	Tissue Penetration (mm)
CO_2	Treatment of lesions of the glottis, larynx, tonsils, and oral cavity: nodules, polyps, laryngoceles, and stenosis	10,600	Thermal	Clear	<.25
Nd:YAG	Lesions of the nose and trachea: telangiectasia, and obstructing lesions	1,064	Thermal	Clear	2–6
Dye	Vascular skin lesions	583–587	Thermal/mechanical	Blue	
KTP diode	Lesions of the nose, larynx, and oral cavity: telangiectasia, polyps, carcinomas, and sleep apnea tissue removal	532	Thermal	Orange	.5–2
Argon	Lysis of middle ear adhesions	514	Thermal	Orange	

CO_2, carbon dioxide; KTP, potassium titanyl phosphate; Nd: YAG, neodymium-doped yttrium aluminum garnet; Nd:Y3Al5O12.

Source: From Dalesio NM, Hayward DM, Schwengel DA. Anesthesia for pediatric otorhinolaryngologic surgery. In: PJ Davis, FP Cladis, eds. *Smith's Anesthesia for Infants and Children.* 9th ed. Elsevier. 2016:31–37.

removal of the ETT, discontinuing gas flows, removal of flammable or burning materials, pouring water/saline into the airway, and reestablishing ventilation (Box 63.2).

As lasers can lead to eye injury to anyone in the operating room at the time of lasering, all staff should wear protective eyewear to prevent injury. The necessary protective eyewear differs based on the type of laser being used. Typically, protective corneal shields are placed on the patient's eye if they are under general anesthesia. It is important to make sure these are removed at the end of the case and prior to emergence (Table 63.1).

Complications/Emergencies

Microlaryngoscopy is associated with both minor and major complications, ranging from throat pain to tongue numbness and pain, tooth injury, nerve damage, and laryngospasm. Coughing, periods of apnea, and intermittent oxygen desaturation commonly occur throughout a microlaryngoscopy. While throat pain following microlaryngoscopy is common, it usually resolves completely within a few hours postoperatively. Throat pain following more complex and involved procedures may last several days to weeks.[3] Intraoperative laryngospasm poses the greatest potential for harm during this procedure.

These risks are why all emergency medications and airway equipment are available throughout the procedure. In most cases, administering propofol, applying positive pressure, or administering lidocaine breaks the laryngospasm. Once the microlaryngoscopy is complete, these patients are completely awake and taken to the recovery room to ensure their airway is protected.

POSTOPERATIVE CARE

Most patients will be transferred to the postanesthesia care unit (PACU) following microlaryngoscopy. Those with tenuous airways or complicated airway needs may be transferred directly to a complex airway unit or the ICU for close observation. The primary focus postoperatively is the maintenance of a patent airway and the provision of additional airway support as indicated. Quite often these patients can develop croup, mandating that racemic epinephrine be readily available. Fortunately, this is typically not considered to be a painful procedure, with the exception perhaps being procedures involving extensive tissue debulking or lasering. Accordingly, pain can be managed effectively with acetaminophen and short-acting narcotics, such as fentanyl.

CASE STUDY: A 10-Year-Old Male With Untreated Hoarseness

CLINICAL SCENARIO

A 10-year-old male arrives at the hospital for a diagnostic microlaryngoscopy (ML). He was born full-term, and maternal labs were negative other than a history of human papillomavirus (HPV). The patient has no surgical history, and his medical history is only significant for worsening hoarseness. He denies any recent illness or sick contacts. His immunizations are all up to date. There are no significant family health problems, and there have been no family problems with anesthesia in the past. He takes no medications and has no known drug allergies. Physical examination is all within normal limits, and weight and height are in the 50th percentile.

APPROACHES TO CARE

After the appropriate NPO status was confirmed, the patient was brought to the operating room. In a preoperative discussion, the surgeon had mentioned she would like to see the vocal cord movement. The patient was placed on the operating table; monitors were applied, including ECG, pulse oximetry, and a blood pressure cuff. After a smooth, easy mask induction, a peripheral IV was started, and propofol was hooked up but not given to ensure cord mobility visualization. After adequate preoxygenation, adequate depth of anesthesia (approximately 1.3 MAC), and spontaneous respirations were achieved, a shoulder roll was inserted. The surgeon placed a tooth guard and inserted the Parsons blade and the telescope to examine the larynx. Immediately upon entering, HPV papillomas were found completely covering the vocal cords (Figure 63.2).

Evidence-Based Approaches to Care

The cause of his hoarseness was quickly identified. The concern was that the papillomas would occlude his entire airway, specifically if we had taken away his spontaneous ventilatory effort. With direct visualization of the cords by the surgeon, an uncuffed endotracheal tube (ETT) was placed and the anesthetic depth was administered using sevoflurane via the ETT. The surgeon then proceeded to use a shaver and remove as many of the papillomas as possible. The cords were then visualized and the rest of the airway was evaluated. Upon completion of the procedure and adequate hemostasis was confirmed by the surgeon, the anesthesia was discontinued and the patient was woken up completely, extubated, and taken to the recovery room.

(continued)

CASE STUDY: A 10-Year-Old Male With Untreated Hoarseness (*continued*)

Hoarseness that has a gradual presentation and is associated with a positive maternal history of HPV leads to a high suspicion for HPV papillomas. Everyone should take caution and wear appropriate filtration masks as the papillomas are removed. The removal of HPV papillomas can be accomplished by shaving, a grasper, or a laser. In the case of laser removal, everyone in the room should wear protective eyewear.

Once the patient knows that have HPV papillomas, they can help guide when they need to return for ML for removal based on ongoing symptoms, such as degree of hoarseness.

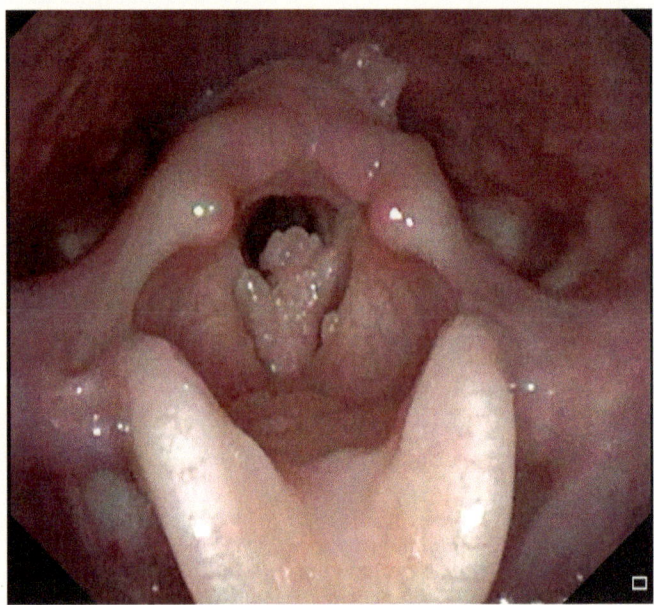

Figure 63.2: Human papillomavirus in the airway.

REFERENCES

1. Phelan E, Russell J. Pediatric airway assessment. In: *Pediatric Surgery*. Springer-Verlag; 2020. https://link.springer.com/content/pdf/10.1007/978-3-662-43588-5_21.pdf
2. Young WG, Shama L, Petty B, et al. Comparing videostroboscopy and direct microlaryngoscopy: an argument for flexible consent and operative plan. *J Voice*. 2019;33(2):143–149. doi:10.1016/j.jvoice.2017.10.005
3. Okui A, Konomi U, Watanabe Y. Complaints and complications of microlaryngoscopic surgery. *J Voice*. 2020;34(6):949–955 doi:10.1016/j.jvoice.2019.05.006
4. Nirgude A, Hemantkumar I. Anesthetic considerations in microlaryngoscopy and direct laryngoscopy. *Int J Otorhinolaryngol Clin*. 2017;9(1):10–14. doi:10.5005/jp-journals-10003-1252
5. Cote CJ, Lerman J, Todres ID. *A Practice of Anesthesia for Infants and Children*. 4th ed. Saunders; 2009.
6. Ji J, Kim E, Lee J, et al. Pediatric airway surgery under spontaneous respiration using high-flow nasal oxygen. *Int J Pedatr Otorhinolaryngol*. 2020;134:110042. doi:10.1016/j.ijporl.2020.110042
7. Dalesio NM, Hayward DM, Schwengel DA. Anesthesia for pediatric otorhinolaryngologic surgery. In: Davis PJ, Cladis FP, eds. *Smith's Anesthesia for Infants and Children*. 9th ed. Elsevier; 2016:Box 31–13.
8. Dalesio NM, Hayward DM, Schwengel DA. Anesthesia for pediatric otorhinolaryngologic surgery. In: Davis PJ, Cladis FP, eds. *Smith's Anesthesia for Infants and Children*. 9th ed. Elsevier; 2016:Box 31–7.

CHAPTER 64

Tracheostomy

Anita Deshpande and Charles M. Myer, IV

INDICATIONS/CONTRAINDICATIONS

Tracheostomy is a surgical procedure in which an opening is established in the trachea (tracheotomy) and a tube is inserted through this opening to establish an artificial airway.[1] It is performed in the pediatric population for a broad variety of indications, which can be divided into several categories.[2-4] These categories include the need for prolonged respiratory support, to bypass an anatomical obstruction, and to assist in pulmonary clearance or manage aspiration. Common indications for those who require prolonged positive pressure respiratory support include chronic lung disease of prematurity, bronchopulmonary dysplasia, and neurological insult. Anatomical obstruction requiring tracheostomy may occur in either the upper or lower airway. Upper airway obstruction may include obstructions that interfere with respiration, result in severe sleep apnea or preclude intubation. Common examples include craniofacial anomalies, head and neck tumors such as vascular malformations, and pharyngeal stenosis. Lower airway obstruction includes glottic, subglottic, or tracheal obstruction, such as stenosis or bilateral true vocal fold paralysis. Traumatic injuries involving the head and neck, which may lead to depressed neurological function, unstable airway from laryngeal or tracheal injury, respiratory compromise, and need for prolonged ventilation, can also necessitate tracheostomy to provide a secure, unobstructed, and potentially long-term airway.[5]

Few true contraindications to tracheostomy exist, although patient factors may affect the surgical procedure. Absolute contraindications would include refusal of consent and infection at the site of the planned tracheotomy.[6] Anesthesia providers should be aware that patients with poor pulmonary function or reserve requiring high ventilator requirements may be less tolerant of manipulation of the airway during the surgical procedure and the temporary interruption in ventilation when performing tracheotomy or placing the tracheostomy tube. Tumors of the head and neck may need to be debulked or removed prior to tracheostomy if they overlie the trachea and prevent access. Vascular malformations in the surgical dissection field may cause bleeding necessitating blood transfusion. Anatomical abnormalities may preclude access to the trachea and prevent tracheostomy. This includes anatomical variants of the great vessels, such as a high-riding innominate artery or aortic arch, or cervical spine abnormalities that limit the space between the larynx and the sternal notch. Anatomical variants of the trachea, such as stenosis, tracheoesophageal pouch, or severe malacia, can affect the ability to safely place a tracheostomy tube or cannula in the trachea. Because of the aforementioned concerns, it is imperative that anesthesia providers have a sound understanding of the indication for tracheostomy, the patient's pulmonary status, and any contributory anatomical factors that may prove critical in planning a safe and effective anesthetic; developing an airway management plan; and minimizing risk during surgery.

SPECIAL CONSIDERATIONS AND CONCERNS

There are several key differences between adult and pediatric tracheostomy. Children may have a shorter neck and a larger head, limiting surgical access. Accordingly, neck extension is frequently used to increase the distance between the chin and the sternum and place the airway in a favorable position. It should be noted that such maneuvers may need to be avoided in patients with certain congenital conditions that place them at risk of cervical spine instability, such as Down syndrome and mucopolysaccharidoses, or in patients with cervical spine trauma. The pleura in children can also extend into the neck, increasing the risk of injury and pneumothorax. The pediatric trachea is narrower and the cartilage softer, making the airway more prone to collapse during manipulation and more susceptible to obstruction from the mucosal edema that may develop during surgery. These age-dependent variations also make the trachea more difficult to identify during surgery, and intubation with an endotracheal tube (ETT) or bronchoscope during the operation is recommended as it improves the ability to identify the trachea by palpation.

Pediatric tracheostomy tubes also differ from adult tracheostomy tubes. Although adult tracheostomy tubes typically have an inner, or double, cannula, most pediatric tracheostomy tubes are single-lumen—that is, without a removable inner cannula. This allows for a maximal internal diameter of the tube relative to its external diameter, therefore improving ventilation and reducing the risk of plugging.[7] As a result, obstruction of the tracheostomy tube requires a complete change of the tracheostomy tube rather than only the inner cannula. When needed prior to maturation of the epithelium-lined tract from the cervical skin to the tracheotomy, the patient is at higher risk of a false passage of the tracheostomy tube into the cervical soft tissue anterior to the trachea.

The choice of tracheostomy tubes is typically based on the age and size of the patient, as well as the presence of any anatomical factors that may affect tube position or placement. Tracheostomy tubes exist in various lengths and materials, as well as with and without a cuff. A discussion between the surgical and anesthesia teams about the expected tracheostomy cannula to be used is helpful as it may affect ventilator management intraoperatively and in the immediate postoperative period.

ANESTHETIC MANAGEMENT

PREOPERATIVE EVALUATION

Prior to the surgical case, anesthesia providers should review the patient's medical history, including the indication for tracheostomy. Careful attention should be paid to current ventilator settings and the trend over the preceding days. The current ETT size and intubation history should be reviewed, as well as the operative reports of any airway evaluation, such as microlaryngoscopy, bronchoscopy, and prior airway surgeries. Physical examination should be completed, with special attention paid to factors that would affect intubation. Lab work can include complete blood count, basic metabolic panel, coagulation profile, and blood gas, depending on the clinical status of the child.

A discussion regarding airway management between the anesthesia and the operative team is essential and should occur before initiation of general anesthesia. Tracheostomy is typically performed with an airway secured by endotracheal intubation. Frequently the patient has been intubated prior to their presentation to the operating room. If any airway evaluation or manipulation is planned in addition to the tracheostomy, discussion of the timing (before or after the tracheostomy is established) and expected findings should be completed to assist in planning the anesthetic to manage the ventilatory requirements of the patient. For patients in whom intubation is not possible, adjunctive measures to manage the airway may be utilized, including placement of a laryngeal mask airway, ventilating bronchoscope, or bag-mask ventilation. Less commonly, tracheostomy may be performed under local anesthesia on an awake patient, such as in patients with obstructing head and neck or mediastinal masses.

INTRAOPERATIVE MANAGEMENT

Tracheostomy is typically performed under general anesthesia. An inhalation or IV induction technique may be employed, dependent on the patient's presenting history, degree of airway obstruction, or anticipated difficulty with airway management. Alternatively, in patients in whom induction of general anesthesia may precipitate ventilation difficulty, tracheostomy may be performed under local anesthesia,[8,9] using a low-dose superficial cervical plexus block,[10] or under conscious sedation using medications such as midazolam, dexmedetomidine, fentanyl, or ketamine, either alone or in combination.[11]

Standard monitors, as described by the American Society of Anesthesiologists, will suffice in most instances. Blood loss is typically minimal and IV access should be sufficient with a peripheral catheter. Invasive monitoring with an intra-arterial catheter is not typically necessary, nor is central venous access. However, this can be considered in patients who are at high risk of hemodynamic instability or bleeding. If needed, central venous access should be obtained via a subclavian or femoral approach to avoid the surgical field. With expected surgical time less than 2 hours and typically low-volume blood loss, urinary catheterization is not necessary. Supplies for securing the airway should be readily available in case the need for unplanned reintubation arises.

Following induction of anesthesia, the patient is positioned supine with the head toward the anesthesia provider unless an endoscopic evaluation of the airway is planned prior to the procedure. The neck is extended, if not contraindicated, by placing a rolled towel or gel pad underneath the shoulders. The patient's head is supported with the use of a foam ring. In patients who are unable to be extended or have excess cervical soft tissue, tape underneath the chin secured to the bed may be used to improve access to the neck. Removal of other indwelling monitors or tubes that traverse the cervical esophagus, such as temperature monitors and nasogastric or orogastric tubes, should be considered as these can be inadvertently mistaken for the trachea during the procedure. All pressure points should be padded, and the patient's temperature should be monitored and maintained. The patient is draped in such a fashion as to give the anesthesia provider adequate access to the patient's ETT during the procedure to ease the manipulation that occurs during surgery.

The standard surgical approach starts with a transverse or vertical cervical incision midway between the sternal notch and the cricoid cartilage. The SC adipose tissue is removed to allow for close approximation of the cervical skin and trachea, which reduces the risk of malposition of the tracheostomy tube in the postoperative period. Dissection continues until the anterior lumen of the trachea is identified and skeletonized. The surgeon will frequently palpate the trachea during the procedure to ensure midline dissection. Alterations in ventilation and oxygenation should be communicated to the surgical team as these may be secondary to the surgical manipulation and the presence of high oxygen concentrations may alter the surgical technique. If possible, the fractional inspired oxygen level (FiO_2) should be reduced to the lowest possible level during the initial stages of the operation to reduce the potential for airway fire in case of inadvertent entry into the airway during the procedure, as ETTs can be ignited in an atmosphere of 25% oxygen.[12-14]

Once the trachea is exposed and hemostasis has been confirmed, preparation for tracheotomy, entry into the trachea, is made. As there is no further anticipated need for cautery, the FiO_2 level is increased to 100% to allow for preoxygenation and increase the patient's pulmonary reserve during the change in airway. Reversal of paralytic agents and resumption of spontaneous respiration are also started as these will further assist in maintaining oxygenation during placement of the tracheostomy cannula. Traction sutures are placed in the trachea laterally alongside the planned tracheotomy incision, kept long, and are later secured, labeled left and right, to the chest until after the first tracheostomy tube change has been performed. These sutures are pulled anteriorly during tracheostomy tube placement to elevate the trachea toward the cervical skin, decreasing the chance of false passage of the cannula into the anterior soft tissue of the neck. The tracheotomy opening is matured by suturing the cervical skin to the anterior face of the trachea surrounding the tracheotomy. During placement of both the traction and maturation sutures, the ETT cuff should be deflated to avoid puncture of the cuff.

Following placement of the traction and maturation sutures, a vertical tracheotomy incision is then made in the anterior trachea at approximately the level of the second and third or the third and fourth tracheal rings. With the surgeon directly visualizing the ETT through the tracheotomy, the ETT is withdrawn by the anesthesia team to a position just proximal to the superior extent of the tracheotomy incision. By leaving the ETT in the larynx and proximal trachea, some level of ventilation can be maintained, and the ETT can be advanced distally into the trachea past the tracheotomy should there be difficulty placing the tracheostomy tube into the trachea or creating an accidental false passage. An appropriately sized tracheostomy tube is then placed into the trachea via the tracheotomy. Once the tracheostomy tube has been placed into the trachea, the cuff is inflated, and the circuit is immediately disconnected from the ETT and connected to the tracheostomy tube. Confirmation of placement into the airway is obtained with return of an end-tidal CO_2 tracing with adequate tidal volumes, appropriate chest rise and breath sounds, as well as direct visualization of tracheostomy tube placement. Only after cannula placement is confirmed should the ETT be withdrawn.

After the tracheostomy tube is in place and the patient's respiratory status is stable, the tube is checked for appropriate position endoscopically. A flexible endoscope is passed through the cannula to ensure adequate positioning above the carina and that the end of the tube is in the lumen and not angled or obstructed by the trachealis. The shoulder roll should be removed and the neck placed in a neutral position. An adapter which allows for in-line bronchoscopy may be attached between the tracheostomy tube and the circuit to maintain ventilation during this portion. During these manipulations, a surgical assistant will hold the tracheostomy tube securely in place to prevent displacement and creation of a false passage.

Following confirmation of appropriate tube selection and positioning, the tracheostomy tube is secured. Securement devices should be tight enough to prevent accidental decannulation, without being too tight as to cause pressure injury or vascular occlusion. A thin foam dressing can be applied circumferentially around the neck and under the tracheostomy flanges to help protect the skin and prevent wound complications.[15] A soft tracheostomy tube holder or twill ties are used to secure the tracheostomy tube. It is also important to indicate that the stoma is considered new (frequently described as fresh) until the first tracheostomy tube change is performed, and the stoma tract is verified intact (mature). This may include different securement devices in either type or color, suture or tape to prevent unintentional removal, or signage. Targeted interventions such as these can serve to reduce the incidence of accidental decannulation and associated morbidity.[16]

Complications/Emergencies

The anesthesia and surgical teams should be aware of potential perioperative complications associated with tracheostomy tube placement, with clear and timely communication between all team members imperative if suspected. During a tracheostomy, bleeding is typically low in volume and derived from skin edges, anterior jugular veins, thyroid vasculature, or tracheal mucosa. Large-vessel injury is rare, although can occur due to the location and anatomical variations of the innominate artery which crosses the cervical trachea. Pneumothorax can occur during dissection, as air tracks through the cervical fascial planes or through inadvertent violation of the pleura.[17]

Airway fire is a risk during the procedure given the dissection around the trachea and risk of inadvertent entry into the airway, and the tracheotomy itself, in the presence of cautery devices, which serve as an ignition source. This risk is heightened in patients who cannot tolerate a lower FiO_2 rate. Loss of the airway, either through removal of the ETT before tracheostomy tube placement, an inability to place the tracheostomy tube, or false passage of the tube during placement or in the immediate postoperative period, may occur. A false passage may occur either into the anterior cervical soft tissues or secondary to injury of the posterior tracheal wall during tracheostomy tube placement. Plugging of the tracheostomy tube may also occur after placement due to bleeding or secretions in the airway.

POSTOPERATIVE CARE

Children who undergo tracheostomy are monitored in an inpatient unit with a high level of nursing and respiratory therapy care. Typically, this correlates to admission to an ICU or step-down unit, until the tracheostomy is mature, which is determined after the first tracheostomy tube change. The patient's other comorbid conditions, including the need for invasive ventilator support, must be taken into account when selecting the appropriate postoperative destination. Unless special factors exist that make accidental decannulation or false passage more likely, patients should be allowed to recover from anesthesia and do not need continued sedation or paralysis. All patients should have continuous heart rate and pulse oximetry monitoring while the tracheostomy is immature. A chest x-ray should be obtained in the immediate postoperative period to evaluate for pneumothorax or pneumomediastinum.

Children with a tracheostomy should have the tracheostomy tube obturator, as well as an additional identically sized tracheostomy tube and a tracheostomy tube one size smaller, with them at all times to facilitate replacement in the case of decannulation or tube obstruction. The receiving unit and providers should be informed of the airway status of the child; this includes the current tracheostomy tube size, suction catheter size and insertion depth, airway exposure, and intubation history, as well as any factors that may make accidental decannulation more likely or cannula replacement more challenging. A sign relaying this information is typically placed at the bedside for quick reference in the case of emergency.

The first tracheostomy tube change is performed by the surgical team approximately 5 days after surgery. In most cases, this is performed at bedside and without any additional sedation. This serves to verify the tracheostomy is mature and the tube change is safe to be completed by other trained personnel. Following this, the traction sutures are cut and removed.

CASE STUDY: A 10-Month-Old Male With Chondrodysplasia Punctata and Genetic Disorder

CLINICAL SCENARIO

A 10-month-old male with a history of chondrodysplasia punctata and pathogenic 22q11.21 duplication underwent polysomnogram demonstrating severe obstructive sleep apnea (OSA), with an apnea–hypopnea index (AHI) of 50.3 and an oxygen nadir of 83%. His AHI improved to 33.6 on 1/4 L oxygen.

SPECIAL CONSIDERATIONS

Lateral neck x-ray was obtained, and demonstrated marked adenoid enlargement. He underwent adenoidectomy as well as an airway evaluation with the otolaryngology (ENT) and pulmonary teams, which revealed multilevel airway obstruction, including severe adenoid hypertrophy, laryngomalacia,

(continued)

> **CASE STUDY: A 10-Month-Old Male With Chondrodysplasia Punctata and Genetic Disorder (*continued*)**
>
> hypopharyngeal collapse, glossoptosis, and tracheomalacia. Repeat polysomnogram performed 2 months postoperatively demonstrated worsened OSA with AHI of 207.8 and oxygen nadir of 69%. There was no significant effect on ventilation with the addition of supplemental oxygen. He underwent revision adenoidectomy and supraglottoplasty and was trialed on a bilevel positive airway pressure (BiPAP) machine. The patient required continuous positive airway pressure (CPAP) pressures of 11 cmH$_2$0.
>
> ### APPROACHES TO CARE
> Tracheostomy was offered as a treatment option for his severe OSA, with which the family elected to proceed. The patient underwent tracheostomy at 17 months of age and is doing well with no respiratory concerns during sleep.

KEY REFERENCES

Complete references for this chapter are online and available at https://connect.springerpub.com/content/book/978-0-8261-3875-0/part/part04/toc-part/ch064.

3. Roberts J, Powell J, Begbie J, et al. Pediatric tracheostomy: a large single-center experience. *Laryngoscope*. 2020;130(5):E375–E380. doi: 10.1002/lary.28160
5. Prabhakaran K, Azim A, Khan M, et al. Predicting the need for tracheostomy in trauma patients without severe head injury. *Am J Surg*. 2020;220(2):495–498. doi: 10.1016/j.amjsurg.2019.12.018
6. Gupta S, Dixit S, Choudhry D, et al. Tracheostomy in adult intensive care unit: an ISCCM expert panel practice recommendations. *Indian J Crit Care Med*. 2020;24(Suppl 1):S31–S42. doi:10.5005/jp-journals-10071-G23184
7. Okonkwo I, Cochrane L, Fernandez E. Perioperative management of a child with a tracheostomy. *BJA Educ*. 2020;20(1):18–25. doi: 10.1016/j.bjae.2019.09.007
15. Baker LR, Chorney SR. Reducing pediatric tracheostomy wound complications: an evidence-based literature review. *Adv Skin Wound Care*. 2020;33(6):324–328. doi: 10.1097/01.ASW.0000661808.51766.9a

CHAPTER 65

Tracheal Resection

Carol Li and Charles M. Myer, IV

INDICATIONS/CONTRAINDICATIONS

Compared with subglottic stenosis, tracheal stenoses are rare in the pediatric population and are usually a congenital lesion, with complete tracheal rings being the most common cause of congenital tracheal stenosis.[1] Children with complete tracheal rings are lacking the posterior membranous portion in a segment of their trachea, as well as the trachealis muscle. Subsequently, cartilaginous rings form a complete circle smaller than the unaffected segments of the trachea.[1] Slide tracheoplasty is the surgery of choice in the operative management of complete tracheal rings; however, not all pediatric patients with this condition require surgery. In fact, a small portion of patients demonstrate adequate airway growth with time and do not ever require surgical intervention. Likewise, children with moderate obstruction do not always present immediately and can accommodate growth without episodes of respiratory distress. Children who grow at a far greater rate than their airway stenosis, however, may present more insidiously with symptoms of exercise intolerance or sleep-disordered breathing. These patients may be followed clinically over time, with surgical intervention being deemed unnecessary until they become more symptomatic. Depending on severity, children with tracheal stenosis may present acutely with respiratory distress, stridor, retractions, apneas, cyanosis, and a characteristic "washing machine respiration" or "wet" sounding airway. It is worth noting that the younger the child is at initial presentation, the higher the likelihood operative intervention such as tracheoplasty will be required.[2]

Acquired tracheal stenosis can occur as a result of endotracheal tube trauma, tracheostomy tube placement, direct airway trauma, or more rarely tumors affecting the trachea and surrounding the structures.[1] The incidence of intubation-related laryngotracheal stenosis has remained low the past few decades, ranging from 3% to 8%.[3-5] If the endotracheal tube is too large or if the cuff is hyperinflated, excess pressure imparted on the tracheal wall can result in tissue ischemia, necrosis, and subsequent scar formation and stenosis.[6] While endotracheal intubation-induced stenosis more commonly occurs in the subglottis, it can also manifest in the cervical trachea. Symptoms of acquired tracheal stenosis usually appear 1 to 3 months postextubation.[7]

Prior tracheostomy can also result in tracheal stenosis as a result of granulation tissue formation, scar formation, and/or weakness in the cartilage leading to suprastomal collapse or an A-frame deformity. Large-population studies report the rates of suprastomal collapse and stomal granulation tissue requiring intervention are between 5% and 12% in pediatric tracheostomy patients.[8,9] An A-frame deformity forms when weak or absent anterior tracheal cartilage, usually at the site of a prior tracheostomy tube, causes an inward collapse of the lateral tracheal walls. This deformity occurs approximately 34.5% of the time in pediatric patients who have undergone airway reconstruction, with 39% of patients requiring subsequent surgical intervention.[10] Anesthesia providers should be aware that this condition can arise many years following the removal of the tracheostomy tube.

Primary and metastatic tumors involving the trachea are a rare cause of tracheal stenosis necessitating a resection procedure. The most common primary tumor within the pediatric tracheobronchial tree is respiratory papillomatosis. Other rare primary tumors include infantile hemangioma, mucoepidermoid carcinoma, adenoid carcinoma, carcinoid tumor, granular cell tumor, inflammatory myofibroblastic tumor, rhabdomyosarcoma, and laryngotracheal chondroma.[11] Metastatic tumors that can invade or obstruct the trachea include lymphoma, or those arising from the thyroid, larynx, lung, esophagus, and breast.[12] Lastly, systemic inflammatory disorders, such as amyloidosis, granulomatosis with polyangiitis, and relapsing polychondritis, may also manifest within the laryngotracheal complex and cause stenosis.

The decision to proceed with open tracheal resection in patients with tracheal stenosis must take into consideration multiple factors, including the etiology of stenosis, patient-specific symptoms and comorbidities, and the length and nature of the stenosis. Children with airway stenosis who are asymptomatic or able to compensate for moderate degrees of tracheal stenosis may defer surgery in favor of ongoing airway surveillance until symptoms become more severe and surgical correction becomes essential. Tracheal resection with primary reanastomosis is indicated in cases of short-segment, circumferential stenosis, such as those involving less than one third of the trachea. In cases of long-segment stenosis, slide tracheoplasty may confer more favorable outcomes as there is less anastomotic tension with this technique. Open surgical alternatives include patch tracheoplasty using costal cartilage, pericardium, and tracheal autografts. These techniques are often better suited for upper levels of stenosis where strap muscles can provide adequate vascular supply.[13-15] Other alternatives to management of tracheal stenosis include various endoscopic techniques including laser scar excision, balloon dilation, and stenting.

Contraindications to tracheal resection include patients with severe pulmonary dysfunction, as with ventilator dependence, as the need for prolonged intubation postoperatively may compromise anastomotic healing. In these patients, a tracheostomy should be considered as a temporizing measure as the patient weans from ventilator support. Another relative contraindication includes patients on chronic steroids as these may compromise wound healing and confer an increased risk of anastomotic dehiscence. Similarly, a history of or active radiation treatments to the head and neck may also compromise wound healing and is considered a relative contraindication to tracheal resection.[16]

SPECIAL CONSIDERATIONS AND CONCERNS

In the case of a high- to mid-tracheal stenosis, a cervical approach to tracheal resection may be performed. However, over 75% of children with complete tracheal rings may have additional anomalies, including pulmonary artery sling, lung hypoplasia/agenesis, cardiac defects, or great vessel anomalies that also require surgical correction.[17] In these situations, a combined procedure through an anterior sternotomy approach may be utilized with initiation of cardiopulmonary bypass.

ANESTHETIC MANAGEMENT

PREOPERATIVE EVALUATION

Anesthesia providers should be aware that children with congenital or acquired tracheal stenosis may have other comorbidities which may necessitate cardiac anesthesia and in general can confer a higher risk of perioperative complications. For this reason, all patients should receive an anesthesia consultation and preprocedure assessment. A thorough history and physical examination should be conducted and the need for specialized anesthesia care, such as cardiac anesthesia, should be determined preoperatively. Important historical details to obtain during the patient interview include the time course and aggravation of airway obstructive symptoms. In addition to a standard, generalized physical examination, the pattern of dyspnea, if any (e.g., inspiratory vs. expiratory stridor), should be characterized. Adjunctive information, such as presence of sleep-disordered breathing, cyanosis, exercise, and feeding tolerance, is also relevant during the preoperative evaluation. Operative reports for prior airway evaluations (laryngoscopy and bronchoscopy) should be reviewed.

Pertinent Labs

Pertinent laboratory evaluation can include complete blood count and coagulation profile, as well as renal function panel.

Patients with congenital tracheal stenosis are often evaluated for concomitant cardiopulmonary and great vessel anomalies with cross-sectional imaging, such as high-resolution CT and MRI. Furthermore, these adjunct studies can provide three-dimensional reconstructions, confer more detail about the anatomy of the tracheobronchial tree, and provide insight on the length and shape of tracheal stenosis. Echocardiogram is a useful complementary study to identify cardiac anomalies, which could influence outcomes and may even need to be addressed prior to airway reconstructive surgery.

The diagnostic evaluation of children with tracheal stenosis most often will include an endoscopic evaluation (e.g., flexible or rigid bronchoscopy, under general anesthesia with a spontaneously breathing patient). This may occur on a separate day prior to the definitive surgical repair or just prior to a planned open surgery.

PREOPERATIVE PHARMACOLOGY

Preoperative management can include an anxiolytic but should not include any medications that may impede spontaneous breathing efforts as this may be required for an intraoperative airway evaluation at the beginning of the surgery.

ANESTHETIC TECHNIQUE

Intraoperative Management

General anesthesia can be induced utilizing either an inhalation or IV technique depending on the degree of airway compromise and presence of comorbidities. In addition to standard monitors, IV access should include one to two peripheral IV catheters. In more complicated patients, such as those with cardiac anomalies, an intra-arterial catheter should be considered for hemodynamic and blood gas monitoring. In patients who are considered at higher risk of hemodynamic instability, a central venous line, via a subclavian or femoral approach, may be considered for delivery of vasoactive drugs. Cannulating the internal jugular vein should be avoided due to close proximity of the surgical field. If the surgical procedure is performed under total IV anesthesia, an anesthesia depth monitor should be used.[12]

If the patient does not have a tracheostomy, endotracheal intubation should be performed with a small-caliber endotracheal tube under endoscopic guidance to pass the tube atraumatically through the area of the stenosis. Alternatively, the endotracheal tube can be placed proximal to the area of stenosis. The start of the case usually involves a rigid endoscopic evaluation of the airway prior to intubation. After the airway is secured and vascular access is optimized, the patient is typically positioned supine with the arms tucked and neck extended. As the surgical procedure involves a great deal of tracheal manipulation, complete neuromuscular blockade should be used and monitored. The average operative time is 3 hours or longer, and therefore, a urinary catheter should be inserted. Blood loss is often minimal.

If the lesion involves the proximal trachea, typically a transverse cervical incision is used for access. Distal lesions may require a midline sternotomy incision or a combined approach. Intraoperatively, the airway will be skeletonized and start to be mobilized from the surrounding structures such as the esophagus. Due to intermittent compression of the tracheal lumen during surgical manipulation and mobilization, there may be rapid changes in ventilatory function. Therefore, frequent communication between the surgeon and the anesthesia provider is essential to clarify and understand altered ventilation parameters in real time during the procedure.

Once the airway has been skeletonized, the trachea will be incised, and the endotracheal tube will be withdrawn. The distal limb of the trachea can be intubated with an armored endotracheal tube connected to a sterile circuit extension, then temporarily removed to allow for surgical dissection. Effective ventilation of the patient should be confirmed by monitoring end-tidal carbon dioxide and chest rise. If the patient has a tracheostomy distal to the level of stenosis, an armored endotracheal tube or cuffed tracheostomy tube can be used to ventilate the patient while the proximal trachea undergoes resection and anastomosis. Typically, traction sutures are placed around the tracheal rings to allow for ease of dissection and prevent the distal tracheal limb from retracting inferiorly into the thoracic cavity in the case of a cervical approach. Following resection of the diseased or stenotic trachea, the proximal and distal limbs will be anastomosed, starting with the posterior tracheal wall.

Frequent communication between the surgical and anesthetic teams is required for successful management of the shared airway during alternating periods of surgical efforts and ventilation. If there is no tracheostomy in place, prior to completing the anterior aspect of the anastomosis, the patient will be intubated orotracheally or nasotracheally with a cuffed endotracheal tube, with the cuff past the anastomosis. The anastomosis is then completed with the endotracheal tube within the lumen of the trachea. To alleviate tension on the anastomosis, a release of suprahyoid musculature is occasionally performed. Following completion of the anastomosis, a leak test is typically performed by deflating the cuff and applying a pressure of 30 cm of water to the circuit while visualizing the saline-flooded operative field for air bubbles.

Clinical Pearls

Extubation planning, including timing, postextubation respiratory support techniques, and reintubation algorithms, should take place prior to surgery but often subject to change depending on intraoperative findings and the postoperative condition of the patient. If the patient has undergone a hyoid release, is in a cervical collar, or has chin-to-chest sutures, laryngeal exposure in the postoperative period for reintubation can be affected. In the case of tracheal resection, laryngeal edema is not common but may also be a possibility, especially in cases of superior tracheal lesions or those affecting the cricoid cartilage. If present, laryngeal edema may create challenges for safe extubation, as well as successful reintubation. Thoughtful discussion between the surgery and anesthesia teams should take place to create a safe extubation plan. If extubation is delayed, careful communication should take place between surgery, anesthesia, and intensive care teams to coordinate an airway plan, including extubation timing, acceptable postextubation supportive measures, and a reintubation plan in case of respiratory failure.

COMPLICATIONS/EMERGENCIES

Potential intraoperative complications include plugging of the endotracheal tube with mucus or blood. There is also a risk of pneumothorax if the pleural space is violated during surgical dissection in the inferior neck. Although rare, large-vessel injury and consequent hemorrhage is possible given the location of the innominate artery and great vessels during dissection along the anterior trachea.

Patients should emerge from anesthesia in standard fashion following tracheal resection, with care taken to prevent excessive coughing, agitation, and head extension, which can endanger the fresh anastomosis. Neuromuscular blockade should be completely recovered to promote spontaneous breathing. Prior to extubation, the endotracheal tube should be suctioned (e.g., flexible bronchoscopy) to evacuate any residual blood clots or mucus plugs. Following the completion of the surgery, extubation may occur immediately in the operating room versus in a delayed fashion depending on the patient's overall pulmonary function and comorbidities. Frequently, patients are immobilized with a cervical collar and/or chin-to-chest sutures to prevent extension of the neck and increased tension to the tracheal anastomosis.

POSTOPERATIVE CARE

Patients who are kept intubated following the surgery should be monitored in the ICU until they meet the criteria for extubation. In the postanesthesia care unit or any other setting following extubation, patients should be monitored closely for signs of airway obstruction and have continuous pulse oximetry.

Supplemental oxygen and bronchodilators, such as nebulized epinephrine, are appropriate adjunctive treatments to improve airway swelling and work of breathing. Humidified air should be used continuously in the postoperative period to keep the airway clear and prevent mucus plug formation. Positive pressure ventilation should be kept below 30 cm of water to decrease the risk of anastomotic leak or dehiscence. Although steroids are commonly used in the periextubation setting to alleviate airway edema, their use should be limited and discussed with the surgical team prior to administration due to the negative effects on wound healing and potential risk for anastomotic breakdown.

Postoperatively respiratory support should be escalated in a stepwise manner for signs of distress and can include supplemental oxygen and noninvasive positive pressure. A laryngeal mask airway can be used for additional assistance if needed. If reintubation is required, this should be done with a smaller caliber endotracheal tube, ideally under endoscopic guidance, to protect the area of the anastomosis. Care should be taken to avoid excessive neck extension, with reintubation over a flexible bronchoscope an appropriate option. If endoscopes are not readily available, the patient can also be intubated in a shallow fashion to allow the tube to sit above the level of the anastomosis until the necessary equipment is available to allow for advancement under endoscopic guidance. Following surgery, patients are monitored in the hospital for approximately 1 week before undergoing repeat endoscopic evaluation to assess the anastomosis.

CASE STUDY: Tracheal Stenosis

CLINICAL SCENARIO
The patient is a 5-year-old male with a history of tracheostomy placed at 5 weeks of age due to meconium aspiration and respiratory failure.

SPECIAL CONSIDERATIONS
On evaluation for airway reconstruction, the patient exhibited a significant A-frame deformity at the level of his tracheostomy.

APPROACHES TO CARE

Evidence-Based Approaches to Care
The patient underwent microlaryngoscopy and bronchoscopy followed by single-stage tracheal resection and slide tracheoplasty. Following microlaryngoscopy and bronchoscopy, which confirmed the level of airway stenosis, he was intubated with an armor-reinforced endotracheal tube through the tracheostomy. During the surgery, his tracheostomy tract was removed and the airway was transected. The endotracheal tube was periodically removed and replaced within the distal limb of the trachea to provide ventilation during the procedure. After tracheal scar was resected, the proximal and distal limbs of the trachea were slid over each other and reanastomosed. The posterior trachealis was first reapproximated (**Figure 65.1**). Then, the patient was intubated orally and the endotracheal tube was advanced with the cuff distal to the anastomosis. Then, the anterior portion of the tracheal anastomosis was completed. Following closure of the cervical incision, the patient was extubated in the operating room. He was transferred to the post-anesthesia care unit (PACU) and subsequently the complex airway floor unit for further management.

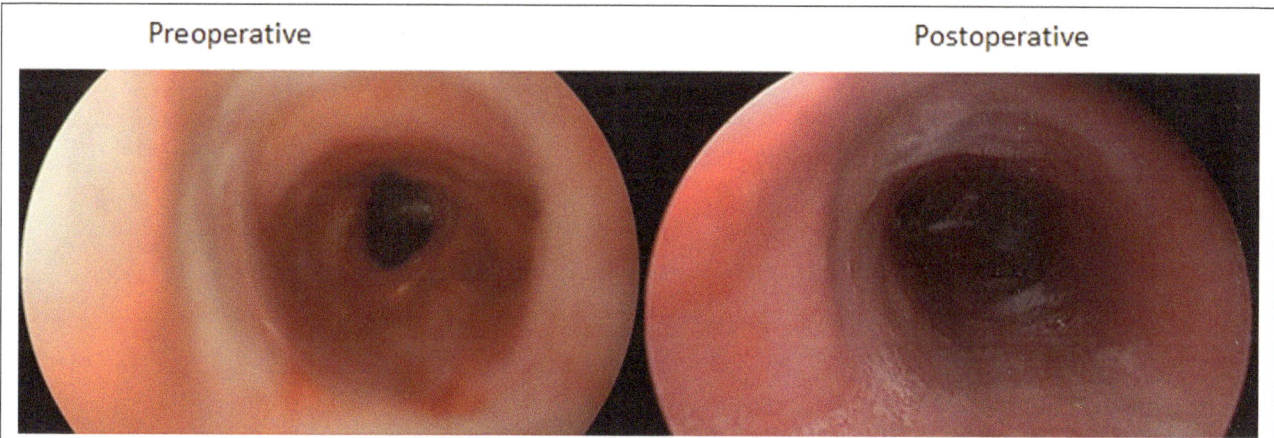

Figure 65.1: A-frame deformity. Preoperative image shows tracheal A-frame deformity at the level of the stoma. Left: Denotes the presence of tracheostomy tube. Right: Postoperative image shows widely patent tracheal lumen following tracheal resection and slide tracheoplasty.

KEY REFERENCES

Complete references for this chapter are online and available at https://connect.springerpub.com/content/book/978-0-8261-3875-0/part/part04/toc-part/ch065

1. Schweiger C, Cohen AP, Rutter MJ. Tracheal and bronchial stenoses and other obstructive conditions. *J Thorac Dis.* 2016;8(11):3369–3378. doi:10.21037/jtd.2016.11.74
8. Özmen S, Özmen ÖA, Ünal ÖF. Pediatric tracheotomies: A 37-year experience in 282 children. *Int J Pediatr Otorhinolaryngol.* 2009;73(7):959–961. doi:10.1016/j.ijporl.2009.03.020
9. Mahadevan M, Barber C, Salkeld L, et al. Pediatric tracheotomy: 17 year review. *Int J Pediatr Otorhinolaryngol.* 2007;71(12):1829–1835. doi:10.1016/j.ijporl.2007.08.007
10. Kennedy AA, Alarcon A, Tabangin ME, et al. Tracheal A-frame deformities following airway reconstruction. *Laryngoscope.* 2021 Apr;131(4):E1363–E1368. doi:10.1002/lary.28996
11. Varela P, Pio L, Torre M. Primary tracheobronchial tumors in children. *Semin Pediatr Surg.* 2016;25(3):150–5. doi:10.1053/j.sempedsurg.2016.02.013

CHAPTER 66

Parotidectomy

Michael E. Conti

INDICATIONS/CONTRAINDICATIONS

The parotid glands are the largest of the three sets of paired salivary glands, the other two pairs being the sublingual and the submandibular glands. The parotid glands are composed of superficial and deep lobes, proximal to the facial nerve (cranial nerve VII).[1] **Figure 66.1** depicts the anatomical location of the parotid gland and its proximity to the facial nerve.

Pediatric parotid masses are unusual and can represent a variety of pathological diagnoses, including malignancy. Anesthesia providers should be aware that the indications for parotidectomy differ significantly from those in adults and can generally be classified into three primary categories: congenital, infectious, and neoplastic. Of these, congenital anomalies and infections are the most common indications, with more than 80% of parotidectomies in pediatric patients performed for benign inflammatory disease or masses of the parotid gland.[2] Congenital anomalies necessitating parotidectomy include lymphatic malformations, hemangiomas, and branchial cleft anomalies. An infectious etiology is most likely attributed to atypical mycobacterial infection, and a neoplastic etiology would include pleomorphic adenomas, follicular non-Hodgkin's lymphoma, and lipoblastoma.

Despite being the least likely indication in pediatric patients, the surgical treatment of parotid tumors has witnessed great evolution over the past century. While intracapsular enucleation has long been the treatment of choice, the high incidence of recurrence (as high as 45%) led to the development of novel, improved surgical approaches. Superficial parotidectomy is now the gold standard for parotid tumor management, largely due to the incidence of reoccurrence being as low as 2%.[3]

There are three surgical approaches to parotidectomy: superficial, total, and radical. The superficial approach, most often for tumor excision, entails the excision of the parotid gland lateral to the facial nerve. A total parotidectomy involves excision of the parotid gland lateral and medial to the facial nerve, whereas a radical parotidectomy includes the lateral and medial aspects of the parotid gland in addition to the facial nerve. A radical parotidectomy also involves facial nerve reconstruction utilizing a facial nerve graft.[1]

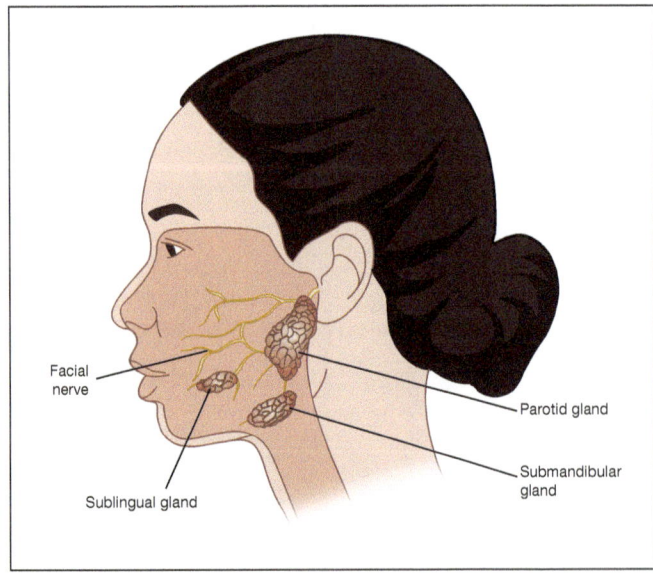

Figure 66.1: Location of the parotid gland.

Sialendoscopy is a novel, alternative approach to the management of juvenile recurrent parotitis that has gained popularity in recent years. When used in combination with conservative pharmacological treatments such as steroids and nonsteroidal anti-inflammatory drugs, sialendoscopy has the potential to negate the need for parotidectomy.[4] Pediatric sialendoscopy, which includes duct dilation and irrigation, is generally performed under general anesthesia, although it has been reported to be done successfully in pediatric patients under deep sedation. There are no apparent contraindications to parotidectomy or sialendoscopy.

SPECIAL CONSIDERATIONS AND CONCERNS

Due to the proximity of the facial nerve to the parotid glands, maintaining the integrity of the facial nerve is a primary concern for the surgeon and anesthesia providers. Prior to surgery, there should be a conversation between the surgeon and the anesthesia provider about facial nerve monitoring and the need for use of a neural integrity monitor (NIM) electromyogram tracheal tube and avoidance of neuromuscular blockade.

ANESTHETIC MANAGEMENT

PREOPERATIVE EVALUATION

Prior to surgery a thorough preanesthetic assessment should be conducted, with special attention given to airway examination. Depending on the etiology of the diseased parotid gland, patients may exhibit limited mouth opening due to discomfort or mechanical obstruction. As the majority of parotidectomies in pediatric patients are due to infection, most children undergoing this procedure are healthy, with few or no presenting comorbidities.

Pertinent Labs

Unless a comorbid condition is present, routine laboratory tests or diagnostic imaging is usually not indicated.

PREOPERATIVE PHARMACOLOGY

Depending on the age of the child, preoperative anxiolysis may be necessary to facilitate parental separation. If the preanesthetic assessment reveals a history of excessive salivation, anesthesia providers should discuss the administration of an antisialagogue, usually glycopyrrolate .01 mg/kg IV, with the surgical team.

ANESTHETIC TECHNIQUE

Intraoperative Management

Most often anesthesia is induced via an inhalation mask induction as most children presenting for parotidectomy (Box 66.1) will not have a peripheral IV catheter in place. A single well-running peripheral IV catheter is sufficient for this procedure. Standard monitors, as recommended by the American Society of Anesthesiologists (ASA), are often adequate as invasive monitoring is seldom indicated.

Intubation should be achieved without administration of a neuromuscular blocking agent, as doing so may disturb facial nerve monitoring during the surgical procedure. If facial nerve monitoring is not indicated, then a neuromuscular blocking agent may be administered. Occasionally nasal intubation may be requested if a more extensive dissection is planned secondary to neoplasm. In this scenario, it is important intubation occurs via the nares contralateral to the tumor. Nasotracheal intubation permits complete closure of the mouth, with approximation of the teeth potentially affording the surgeons improved access to deep lobe tumors that have parapharyngeal extension. Regardless of intubation technique, a throat pack is typically placed to prevent blood and secretions from entering the airway. It is imperative that this is removed at the end of the case prior to extubation.

Although considered a clean case, the interruption and retention of salivary tissue may create an environment for bacterial sialadenitis to develop. Hence, antibiotics are often administered prior to incision and possibly continued for several days postoperatively if there is a component of chronic sialadenitis present. Pain management is often achieved in a multimodal fashion. Acetaminophen may be administered preoperatively (oral) or intraoperatively (IV) in addition to administration of opioids. All narcotics should be administered judiciously to avoid opioid-induced airway obstruction postoperatively. Local anesthetics injected by the surgeon also contribute to the analgesia plan. Ondansetron can be given for prevention of postoperative nausea and vomiting (PONV).

Given the relative infrequency of parotidectomy being performed in the pediatric population, it is not uncommon for this procedure to be performed using a two-surgeon model. This approach maximizes the experience of junior surgeons as this is a relatively low-volume surgery.[2] To make room at the head of the bed, the operating table is typically rotated 90 degrees away from the anesthesia machine or simply moved farther away from the anesthesia machine to allow the surgeons access to the surgical field. Despite not being at the head of the bed, it is imperative that anesthesia providers remain vigilant throughout the surgical procedure as neck surgery is a common location for airway fires to occur.[5,6]

Potential complications and emergencies are summarized in Box 66.2.

Special Techniques and/or Equipment

If facial monitoring is indicated, the surgeon may request the use of an NIM tube and avoidance of neuromuscular blockade to direct facial nerve monitoring. Once the airway is secured and endotracheal tube placement is confirmed, the fraction of

---

BOX 66.1 CLINICAL PEARLS: PAROTIDECTOMY

Prior to surgery, discuss the need for facial nerve monitoring with the surgeon.

If an NIM tube is required, ensure the availability of a size appropriate to the patient's age.

Be aware of the potential risk of surgical fire.

Encourage dialogue with the surgeon throughout the procedure.

BOX 66.2 COMPLICATIONS/EMERGENCIES: PAROTIDECTOMY

Airway compromise

Loss of facial nerve integrity

Retained throat pack

Surgical fire

inspired oxygen should be decreased below 30% to reduce the likelihood of a surgical fire.

POSTOPERATIVE CARE

Patients undergoing parotidectomy should be extubated awake following completion of surgery and prior to transfer to the postanesthesia care unit (PACU). In the PACU, assessments should include monitoring for facial nerve deficits, such as asymmetry of facial movements, facial paralysis, or ipsilateral forehead wrinkle and eyelid closure.[7]

Patients often have a drain that will remain in situ for 24 to 48 hours postoperatively. It is important patients do not inadvertently remove the drain. In young or noncompliant patients, arm restraints or elbow cuffs may be considered.

Following parotidectomy, patients may develop Frey's syndrome, or gustatory sweating, which entails excessive sweating on the cheek, forehead, and around the ears. Frey's syndrome is a complication of parotidectomy that is thought to occur due to aberrant regeneration of the postganglionic parasympathetic nerve fibers that supply the parotid gland, with a new connection to severed postganglionic sympathetic fibers that innervate the sweat glands of the face. This can be challenging to treat, although antiperspirants or topical 1% glycopyrrolate lotion and injection of botulinum toxin A to the affected area have proved effective.

CASE STUDY: A 7-Year-Old Presenting for Parotidectomy

CLINICAL SCENARIO

A 7-year-old 23-kg male presents to the operating room with a history of right-sided facial swelling. Facial CT imaging reveals right parotid swelling. He is an otherwise healthy, American Society of Anesthesiologists physical status I pateint with no known drug allergies. Physical examination is within normal limits. A right parotidectomy is planned with general anesthesia and endotracheal intubation with right facial nerve monitoring. Preoperatively, oral midazolam 10 mg is administered to promote separation.

SPECIAL CONSIDERATIONS

- Facial nerve monitoring
- Maintenance of fraction of inspired oxygen (FiO_2) less than 30%
- Evaluation of airway patency
- Evaluation of facial nerve integrity

APPROACHES TO CARE

The child is brought to the operating room, and stand monitors are applied, including a three-lead ECG and a noninvasive blood pressure cuff. Seven liters of nitrous oxide and 3 L of oxygen are administered with an incremental addition of sevoflurane, up to 8%, to facilitate inhalation induction. Once the lash reflex is abated, the eyes are taped with paper tape, and IV access is obtained (22 ga in the left hand). Since right facial nerve monitoring will be used, the patient is intubated with administration of a neuromuscular blocking agent, relying simply on 2 to 3 mg/kg propofol and .5 mcg/kg fentanyl. A 5.0 cuffed endotracheal tube is placed and taped to the left. Confirmation of the placement is achieved via capnography and positive and equal breath sounds. Baseline facial nerve monitoring is achieved with an external nerve stimulator by the scrub nurse once the patient is prepped and draped. As airway edema is a concern, dexamethasone .5 mg IV (maximum 10 mg) is administered.

Anesthesia is maintained with 2 liters per minute (LPM) flow at .21% FiO_2, maintaining a deep plane of anesthesia since a neuromuscular blocking drug is not administered and providing adequate analgesia.

Once the parotid gland is excised and the incision is sutured and dressed, the patient will emerge from anesthesia and be extubated awake to ensure airway patency. Once awake and following commands, the integrity of the facial nerve is assessed by assessment of facial symmetry and any residual facial paralysis. On physical examination, there is facial symmetry and no facial paralysis.

REFERENCES

1. Holzman RS. *A Practical Approach to Pediatric Anesthesia.* Wolters Kluwer; 2008.
2. Carter JM, Rastatter JC, Bhushan B, Maddalozzo J. Thirty-day perioperative outcomes in pediatric parotidectomy. *JAMA Otolaryngol Head Neck Surg.* 2016;142(8):758–762. doi:10.1001/jamaoto.2016.1031
3. Kato MG, Erkul E, Nguyen SA, et al. Extracapsular dissection vs superficial parotidectomy of benign parotid lesions: surgical outcomes and cost-effectiveness analysis. *JAMA Otolaryngol Head Neck Surg.* 2017;143(11):1092–1097. doi:10.1001/jamaoto.2017.1618
4. Capaccio P, Palermo A, Lucchinelli P, et al. Deep sedation for pediatric parotid sialendoscopy in juvenile recurrent parotitis. *J Clin Med.* 2021;10(2):276. doi:10.3390/jcm10020276
5. Fisher M. Prevention of surgical fires: a certification course for healthcare providers. *AANA Journal.* 2015;34(4):271–274.
6. Muchatuta N, Sale S. Fires and explosions. *Anaesth Intensive Care.* 2007;8(11):457–460.
7. https://www.merckmanuals.com/professional/neurologic-disorders/neurologic-examination/how-to-assess-the-cranial-nerves Retrieved 7.6.2020.

CHAPTER 67

Submandibular Gland Excision

Michael E. Conti

INDICATIONS/CONTRAINDICATIONS

The submandibular glands are one of the three paired major salivary glands. They produce approximately 70% of the saliva produced in the mouth. These paired glands are in the jaw toward the back of the mouth (see Chapter 66, "Parotidectomy" Figure 66.1).[1]

As tumors are the most frequent lesions of the parotid glands, sialolithiasis and inflammatory diseases are common features of the submandibular glands. Acute inflammation of the submandibular gland, as opposed to that of the parotid, is usually due to a congenital anomaly of a salivary duct or an excretory duct obstruction.[2] Acute suppurative sialadenitis manifests with a tender, erythematous, firm swelling of the affected gland with or without associated expression of purulent discharge from the salivary duct.

Indications for removing the submandibular glands include chronic sialadenitis (inflammation or enlargement), stones within the Wharton's duct (submandibular duct), or tumor.[3,4] Of note, it is recommended that removal of the gland should not be done as a "biopsy" to rule out tumor, whether benign or malignant. Rather, a complete neck dissection is indicated as opposed to a "shell out" of the gland unless the evaluation clearly points to a nonneoplastic indication for gland removal.

Typically, a transoral surgical approach is employed to minimize the potential of remnant duct disease as the entire duct and papillae are removed. Using a transoral approach also avoids cervical scar and dissection close to the marginal mandibular branch of the facial nerve.

SPECIAL CONSIDERATIONS AND CONCERNS

As with a parotidectomy, airway fire is a concern. Once the airway is secured and endotracheal tube placement is confirmed, the fraction of inspired oxygen should be decreased below 30% to reduce the likelihood of a surgical fire.

The marginal submandibular nerve should be identified and subsequently avoided by the surgeon. Nerve stimulation can be utilized, although it is not essential.[4] Prior to surgery, there should be a conversation between the surgeon and the anesthesia provider about facial nerve monitoring and the need for use of a neural integrity monitor (NIM) electromyogram tracheal tube and avoidance of neuromuscular blockade.

ANESTHETIC MANAGEMENT

PREOPERATIVE EVALUATION

Prior to surgery, a thorough preanesthetic assessment should be conducted, with special attention given to airway examination. As most submandibular gland excisions in pediatric patients are due to infection, most children undergoing this procedure are healthy, with few or no presenting comorbidities. The presence of abscesses and infections that involve the submandibular gland may extend beyond the submandibular space and lead to Ludwig's angina. In this case, urgent IV antibiotic therapy, as well as establishment of a secure airway, often via elective, awake fiberoptic nasotracheal intubation in the operating room, is advisable. Depending on the etiology of the diseased salivary gland, patients may exhibit limited mouth opening due to discomfort or mechanical obstruction.

Pertinent Labs

Unless a comorbid condition is present, routine laboratory tests are not indicated. Diagnostic testing typically occurs en route to diagnosis. This often entails CT with or without contrast, ultrasound, sialography, and possibly a needle biopsy.

PREOPERATIVE PHARMACOLOGY

Depending on the age of the child, preoperative anxiolysis may be necessary to facilitate parental separation. If the preanesthetic assessment reveals a history of excessive salivation, anesthesia providers should discuss the administration of an antisialagogue, usually glycopyrrolate .01 mg/kg IV, with the surgical team.

ANESTHETIC TECHNIQUE

Intraoperative Management

Intraoperative management of submandibular gland excision mirrors that of a parotidectomy. Please see Chapter 66, "Parotidectomy," for further information regarding the intraoperative management of a parotidectomy (Box 67.1).

Special Techniques and/or Equipment

During submandibular gland excision, the facial nerve is monitored intraoperatively, either using electrophysiological systems or clinically, with visual inspection of the face for movement during surgical dissection. To allow for neuromonitoring, muscle relaxation should not be performed, as electromyography (EMG) data from cranial nerve stimulation will be affected by neuromuscular blockade. If short-acting neuromuscular blocking agents are used to facilitate intubation, the goal should be for return within minutes of spontaneous respiration and muscle twitch activity.

Complications/Emergencies

Potential complications related to submandibular gland excision include injury to the marginal mandibular branch of the

---

BOX 67.1 CLINICAL PEARLS: SUBMANDIBULAR GLAND EXCISION

- Prior to surgery, discuss the need for facial nerve monitoring with the surgeon.
- If an NIM tube is required, ensure the availability of a size appropriate to the patient's age.
- Be aware of the potential risk of surgical fire.
- Encourage dialogue with the surgeon throughout the procedure.

NIM, neural integrity monitor.

facial nerve, hypoglossal nerve, lingual nerve, and/or facial artery. It is not uncommon for patients to have recurrent disease in the remnant duct should a transcervical surgical approach be employed. The transcervical surgical approach can also result in an unsightly cervical scar or keloid.

POSTOPERATIVE CARE

Patients undergoing submandibular gland excision should be extubated awake following completion of surgery and prior to transfer to the postanesthesia care unit (PACU). In the PACU, assessments should focus on airway patency and pain management. Postoperatively patients often complain of pain with swallowing, eating, or neck movement. Other common complaints include tongue numbness on the side of the surgery, increased pain with eating or smelling things that illicit hunger due to stimulation of the nerves to the salivary gland, and weakness of the lower lip on the side of the surgery secondary to intraoperative retraction.

REFERENCES

1. https://www.parotidsurgerymd.com/education/articles/parotid-salivary-gland-info/?gclid=CjwKCAjw1ej5BRBhEi-wAfHyh1OFKGK3M2zCFov4WW6EJyctClrs5ccczhLZ9_gZM-RqZbTSrfK4Fy_RoCEoMQAvD_BwE
2. Ellies M, Laskawi R. Diseases of the salivary glands in infants and adolescents. *Head Face Med.* 2010;6(1):1-7.
3. https://www.parotidsurgerymd.com/education/articles/parotid-salivary-gland-info/?gclid=CjwKCAjw1ej5BRBhEi-wAfHyh1OFKGK3M2zCFov4WW6EJyctClrs5ccczhLZ9_gZM-RqZbTSrfK4Fy_RoCEoMQAvD_BwE
4. Holzman RS. *A Practical Approach to Pediatric Anesthesia.* Wolters Kluwer; 2008.

CHAPTER 68

Septorhinoplasty

Alison Henry and Lisa Wahlers

INDICATIONS/CONTRAINDICATIONS

Nasal septum reconstruction (septoplasty) combined with the remodeling of one's nasal contour (rhinoplasty) is generally considered to be both a functional and an aesthetic procedure when combined.[1] Absolute and relative indications for pediatric patients have been outlined by the otolaryngology community and categorized by their potential for functional deficits, progressive deformity, and psychosocial effect. Immediate attention should be given to severe/acute nasal trauma, septal abscess, hematoma, or malignancy. Patients with benign masses, progressive deformation, or orofacial clefting involving nasal anatomy may have surgical intervention delayed; however, it should occur prior to the adolescent growth spurt.[2] A deviated septum resulting in nasal obstruction is considered a relative indication for the pediatric population.[3] Contraindications include a large septal perforation, Wegener's granulomatosis and malignant lymphomas, or monoclonal T- or B-cell proliferations.[4]

SPECIAL CONSIDERATIONS AND CONCERNS

The timing of septorhinoplasty in children is a widely debated topic given the potential for disruption of the nasal growth pattern. There are two growth zones in the nasal septum: the sphenodorsal zone and the sphenospinal zone. Injury to either of these zones can be detrimental to the growth and development of the maxilla and nasal dorsum.[5] Animal and clinical studies have shown that conservative manipulation of the growing nose, as opposed to surgical intervention, is key in preventing severe growth inhibition.[2] Therefore, it is recommended that surgery be delayed until nasal growth has completed, approximately 14 years old for females and 15 years old for males.[6]

ANESTHETIC MANAGEMENT

PREOPERATIVE EVALUATION

Table 68.1 summarizes the preoperative assessment and pertinent laboratory studies.

PREOPERATIVE PHARMACOLOGY

Sedating medications for patients with significant nasal obstruction or known obstructive sleep apnea should be avoided or used with caution.[1] Otherwise, preoperative medications should be tailored to the child's needs (e.g., midazolam).

ANESTHETIC TECHNIQUE

Intraoperative Management

See **Box 68.1**. The child should be induced by mask induction or intravenously if IV access has been previously obtained. The airway should be secured with an endotracheal tube (ETT) to prevent blood from entering the trachea

Table 68.1	Preoperative Assessment and Pertinent Lab Studies: Septorhinoplasty
Physical assessment	• Discuss NPO status, especially if traumatic injury has occurred. • Is there baseline nasal obstruction resulting in sleep-disordered breathing or obstructive sleep apnea? • Has a diagnostic sleep study been performed?
Medications	• Sedative medications should be avoided or used with caution in the presence of neurological trauma (*Is it possible the patient also hit their head?*). • Midazolam may be appropriate for children with anxiety if they do not have obstructive pathology.
Labs	• Consider complete blood count and type and screen in a trauma setting.

> **BOX 68.1 CLINICAL PEARLS: SEPTORHINOPLASTY**
>
> **Preoperative**
> - NPO status
> - Full physical assessment, especially for trauma cases
> - History of sleep apnea or obstructive breathing
> - Need for midazolam
>
> **Perioperative**
> - Cefazolin unless contraindicated
> - Multimodal pain and PONV prevention strategies
> - Use extension tubing on circuit if needed and check connections for security
> - Ensure the eyes are adequately protected
>
> **Postoperative**
> - Oxygen delivery should not be via a nasal cannula or anything that puts direct pressure on the nose
> - Monitor for occult bleeding
>
> PONV, postoperative nausea and vomiting.

during the procedure. An oral Ring-Adair-Elwin (RAE) ETT can be used to facilitate surgical access.[1] If the procedure is being performed emergently due to acute nasal trauma, the anesthesia provider should consider performing a rapid sequence induction (RSI) as there may be blood in the esophagus and stomach. In this case it would be prudent to obtain IV access before induction if to adequately and safely perform an RSI with suction readily available. Inhalation, total IV anesthetic (TIVA), or a balanced technique may be used for maintenance of anesthesia, although the addition of a propofol or remifentanil infusion may help facilitate a smooth emergence. It is also important to note that a TIVA with propofol as the primary maintenance anesthetic has been associated with less blood loss than with volatile agents.[7] Once the airway has been secured, the bed will be turned either 90 or 180 degrees depending on surgeon preference, and local anesthetic, with or without epinephrine, will be applied to the nares for vasoconstriction. Typically, a throat pack is placed to prevent blood from entering the esophagus (Table 68.2).

After the procedure is complete, the stomach should be suctioned to remove any blood that may have entered the esophagus during the procedure as this can be irritating to the stomach. In addition, an antiemetic should be administered to help stave off postoperative nausea and vomiting (PONV). The goal of emergence is a smooth, safe extubation with minimal coughing to protect the patient from further postoperative blood loss.

Complications/Emergencies

Postsurgical occult bleeding or epistaxis can occur and puts the patient at an increased risk of aspiration when a large amount of blood is swallowed. Bleeding occurs if the patient coughs excessively during emergence. If bleeding occurs, the surgical team should be notified in case reexploration or additional nasal packing is needed. Additionally, septal perforation may occur and require future treatment or intervention.

POSTOPERATIVE CARE

Following surgery, the patient will be transferred to the postanesthesia care unit (PACU) for recovery. In the PACU, the child should be monitored for any signs of continued bleeding; however, it is normal for some oozing to occur. A moustache dressing can be placed underneath the nose to collect any drainage. Efforts should be made to reduce the incidence of PONV as retching could disrupt hemostasis. Pain can be managed with both narcotic and nonnarcotic analgesics (e.g., acetaminophen, gabapentin, or alpha-agonists). Use of ketorolac or other nonsteroidal anti-inflammatory drugs should be discussed with the surgical team before administration given their potential to increase bleeding.[8]

Table 68.2	Special Techniques to Utilize During Septorhinoplasty
Anesthetic maintenance	• Consider a TIVA with propofol to reduce the incidence of PONV. • Use of propofol is associated with less blood loss than use of volatile agents.
Field avoidance	• The bed will be rotated 90 or 180 degrees from the anesthesia provider. • Use extension tubing if needed to ensure slack on the circuit. • Check all appropriate connection sites before draping.
Smooth extubation	• IV or topical lidocaine can be used to attenuate airway reactivity during emergence. • Adjuncts such as dexmedetomidine or remifentanil can help facilitate a smooth extubation and improve pain control.[7] • A deep extubation may be amenable if the patient's current and preoperative condition allow for safe execution.

CASE STUDY: A 14-Year-Old Child With History of Nasal Septum Deviation and Obstruction

CLINICAL SCENARIO

A 14-year-old child is scheduled for septorhinoplasty. Per the electronic record, the patient has a history of obstructed nasal breathing due to a deviated septum and mild-moderate sleep apnea. The patient is otherwise healthy, and there are no other medical concerns. The patient is in the preoperative area and a thorough anesthetic interview is conducted revealing that the patient is appropriately NPO, does obstruct at times during the night (per parental report), and is slightly nervous.

SPECIAL CONSIDERATIONS

Give the state anxiety, IV midazolam is given in the preoperative area, albeit with caution due to history of nasal obstruction and obstructive sleep apnea (OSA). In the operating room, standard monitors are placed and general anesthesia is induced through the existing IV line. An oral RAE endotracheal tube (ETT) is placed to facilitate surgical access.[1] A throat pack is placed to collect blood. The operating room bed is turned 180 degrees, with appropriate circuit extensions in place.

APPROACHES TO CARE

Evidence-Based Approaches to Care

Anesthesia is maintained with sevoflurane and propofol, infusing at a rate of 100 mcg/kg/min.[1] Triple therapy antiemetics are given to prevent postoperative nausea and vomiting. Dexmedetomidine .5 mg/kg is also administered near the end of the case to facilitate a smooth extubation. Noninvasive blood pressure is maintained at 20% lower than baseline during the case in order to reduce blood loss.[1]

COMPLICATIONS

There were no surgical complications. At case conclusion, lidocaine .25 mg/kg IV was administered to reduce coughing and irritation secondary to the ETT, and glycopyrrolate .004 mg/kg was given to prevent secretions from draining on vocal cords. Prior to extubation, the oropharynx and stomach were suctioned with soft catheter and the throat pack was removed. The patient was extubated smoothly at the end of the case and nonrebreather oxygen mask applied gently to reduce pressure on the nose and allow for oxygen delivery after nasal surgery interventions.[1]

REFERENCES

1. Jaffe RA, Schmiesing C, Golianu B. *Anesthesiologist's manual of surgical procedures*. 4th ed. Lippincott Williams & Wilkins. 2009.
2. Funamura JL, Sykes JM. Pediatric septorhinoplasty. *Facial Plastic Surgery Clinic of North America*. 2014 Nov;22(4):503–8. doi:10.1016/j.fsc.2014.07.005
3. Saniasiaya J, Abdullah B. Quality of life in children following nasal septal surgery: A review of its outcome. *Pediatr Investig*. 2019;3(3):180–184. doi:10.1002/ped4.12145
4. Watson D. Septoplasty. *Medscape*. 2019. https://emedicine.medscape.com/article/877677-overview#a13
5. Bhuskute A, Sumiyoshi M, Senders C. Septorhinoplasty in the pediatric patient. *Facial Plast Surg Clin North Am*. 2016;24(3):245–253. doi:10.1016/j.fsc.2016.03.003
6. Justicz N, Choi S. When should pediatric septoplasty be performed for nasal airway obstruction? *Laryngoscope*. 2019;129(7):1489–1490. doi:10.1002/lary.27602
7. Nagelhout JJ, Plaus KL. *Handbook of Nurse Anesthesia*. 2010. Elsevier.
8. Nguyen BK, Yuhan BT, Folbe E, et al. Perioperative analgesia for patients undergoing septoplasty and rhinoplasty: an evidencebased review. *Laryngoscope*. 2019;129(6):E200–E212. doi:10.1002/lary.276169

CHAPTER 69

Care of Children With Sleep-Disordered Breathing

Pornswan Ngamprasertwong and Mario Patino

PATHOPHYSIOLOGY AND CLINICAL MANIFESTATIONS

Sleep-disordered breathing is a group of disorders characterized by abnormal respiratory patterns or insufficient ventilation during sleep. Obstructive sleep apnea (OSA) is the most severe form of sleep-disordered breathing, with the highest risk of complications.[1] OSA is characterized by prolonged partial upper airway obstruction (hypopnea) and/or intermittent complete obstruction (apnea) despite ongoing respiratory effort, leading to oxygen desaturation and disruption of normal sleep patterns.[2]

The prevalence of OSA in children is 1% to 6%.[3] The incidence of OSA is highest at 2 to 8 years of age, which corresponds with the age range in adenotonsillar hypertrophy. In adolescents, obesity is the most common significant predisposing factor. Other risk factors for OSA in children include hypotonia, craniofacial malformation, and neuromuscular disease. A high prevalence of sleep-related breathing disorders, including OSA, has been reported in children suffering from Down syndrome (57%–100%),[4] Prader–Willi syndrome (93%),[5] Duchenne's muscular dystrophy (53%),[6] Chiari malformation and myelomeningocele (60%),[7] achondroplasia (48%),[8] craniofacial anomalies such as Pierre Robin sequence (76%),[9] and craniofacial dysostosis (50%–91%).[10]

A subgroup of OSA children with Down syndrome and craniofacial syndromes may have obstruction at several anatomical sites in the upper airway.[11] Children with midface hypoplasia, micrognathia, or deformity of cranial bases often have OSA with nasal or nasopharyngeal airway obstruction. In children with Down syndrome, conditions that predispose to OSA include midface hypoplasia, macroglossia, and muscular hypotonia. In this subgroup of patients, adenotonsillectomy eliminates upper airway obstruction from adenotonsillar hypertrophy, but OSA may persist due to obstruction at other anatomical sites in the upper airway. Further interventions that might be required in patients with multiple sites of obstruction include turbinectomy, lingual tonsillectomy, uvulopalatopharyngoplasty (UPPP), or tongue reduction.

The diagnosis of OSA in children can be challenging as the disorder presents in a variety of different ways. Children with OSA may present with different symptoms from adults, and symptoms may vary by age and the developmental level of the child. Evaluating children with suspected OSA requires an extensive and thorough history. Common symptoms include snoring, intermittent pauses in breathing during sleep, and disturbed sleep. While common in adults, daytime sleepiness is uncommon in children. Children with OSA can present with neurobehavioral issues, including behavioral problems, neurocognitive impairment, attention-deficit/hyperactivity disorder, and poor school performance. Other common findings in children are headaches, enuresis, and failure to thrive.[11] Hypertension and cardiac dysfunction can develop in severe cases.[12] Parent reports alone cannot distinguish OSA from primary snoring. While the Snoring, Tiredness, Observed apnea, blood Pressure, Body mass index, Age, Neck circumference and Gender (STOP-BANG) questionnaire is one of the most widely accepted OSA screening tools for adults, there is no well-established screening tool for pediatric OSA.[13] The accuracy of clinical evaluation of OSA in children is poor, with 30% to 85% accuracy in predicting positive sleep studies. Sleep oximetry monitoring can be used to identify OSA if there are clusters of desaturation <80%.

Polysomnography (PSG) is the gold standard for diagnosis of OSA in children.[14] PSG is a sleep study with continuous monitoring of physiological variables during different phases of sleep, including electroencephalogram, eye movement, chest wall and abdominal movement, and respiratory, and hemodynamic parameters. This study distinguishes primary snoring, OSA, and central sleep apnea. In primary snoring, the PSG is normal. In central sleep apnea, there is absence of both airflow and respiratory efforts. In OSA, the respiratory efforts persist, but the airflow is obstructed. OSA-related parameters reported via PSG include the nadir of oxygen saturation and the apnea–hypopnea index (AHI). **Table 69.1** demonstrates how the relationship between the oxygen saturation (SpO_2) nadir and the number of these episodes during nocturnal oximetry can be used to determine the severity of OSA. AHI is the ratio of apnea and hypopnea events secondary to obstructive events per hour during sleep. Apnea is defined by a decrease in airflow >90% for two breaths or more. Hypopnea is defined by a decrease in airflow >50% coupled with a 3% decrease in oxygen saturation or with electroencephalographic evidence of arousal (**Table 69.2**). Even though PSG is the primary diagnostic and evaluation tool for OSA, it is expensive, time-consuming, and not readily available in all medical centers.[11]

Another challenging aspect of pediatric OSA is identification of the anatomical site of upper airway obstruction. Airway dynamic studies and examination of airway collapse during sleep facilitate planning of interventions to relieve obstruction. Measuring pharyngeal pressure via catheters at different sites in the upper airway, video endoscopy, fiberoptic bronchoscopy, cine fluoroscopy, CT and cine MRI have been used to evaluate the sites and severity of obstruction. In sedated or anesthetized OSA children, maintaining upper airway patency during spontaneous breathing without airway instrument can be difficult and complicated, especially during cine MRI. There is no consensus on the safe, acceptable lower limit of oxygen saturation during the study. Anesthetic agents suppress pharyngeal muscle tone, resulting in significant airway obstructions not seen during natural sleep. Dexmedetomidine is a preferred sedative agent for MRI sleep study in children with OSA as it creates conditions that mimic nonrapid eye movement (REM) sleep without respiratory depression or upper airway obstruction.[15]

Increased upper airway resistance during sleep is the hallmark of OSA. Upper airway resistance may be due to anatomical factors such as craniofacial abnormalities and/or soft tissue hypertrophy. These abnormalities include maxilla/mandible narrowing or retropositioning, adenotonsillar hypertrophy, and obesity. In addition to anatomical factors, upper airway stability is also dependent on

Table 69.1	The McGill Oximetry Scoring System for Obstructive Sleep Apnea			
Oximetry Score	OSA Classification	Number of Events of SpO_2 <90%	Number of Events of SpO_2 <85%	Number of Events of SpO_2 <80%
1	Normal	<3	None	None
2	Mild	≥3	≤3	≤3
3	Moderate	≥3	>3	≤3
4	Severe	≥3	>3	>3

Note: The severity of OSA is determined by SpO_2 nadir and the number of episodes during nocturnal oximetry.

OSA, obstructive sleep apnea; SpO_2, oxygen saturation.

Source: From Patino, M., Sadhasivam, S., & Mahmoud, M. (2013). Obstructive sleep apnoea in children: perioperative considerations. Br J Aneesth. 111(Suppl 1): i83–95. doi:10.1093/bja/aet371.

physiological processes. Normal ventilation during sleep requires both patent airway anatomy and intact reflexes. Upper airway patency is the result of the interaction of anatomical structures, neuromotor tone, and respiratory dynamics. Breathing is controlled by the central respiratory center in the medulla and its interaction with central and peripheral chemoreceptors. The central chemoreceptors in the medulla, pons, and cerebellum are sensitive to the pH of their environment. They mainly respond to partial pressure of carbon dioxide in the blood, changing the pH of the central nervous system. Peripheral chemoreceptors, located in the carotid bodies, primarily respond to partial pressure of arterial oxygen. Hypercapnia and hypoxia trigger the respiratory center in the medulla to increase minute ventilation.[16] The neural tone of the pharyngeal dilator muscle also plays an important role in maintenance of airway patency. In children with OSA, suppression of pharyngeal dilator muscle tone during sleep, sedation, or anesthesia leads to upper airway obstruction. This upper airway obstruction is relieved by arousal, leading to restless, interrupted sleep. In contrast, children with primary snoring often have obstructive hypoventilation, but they exhibit stable, increased respiratory effort as a compensatory neuromuscular mechanism. Consequently, children with habitual primary snoring do not exhibit the apnea, hypopnea, respiratory arousal, or gas-exchange abnormalities seen in children with OSA.[11] Pediatric OSA can lead to significant sequelae, including metabolic, cardiovascular, and neurocognitive morbidity. Chronic, recurrent episodes of hypoxemia, hypercapnia, and acidosis in children with moderate and severe OSA can result in pulmonary hypertension, right ventricular dysfunction, and cor pulmonale.[2]

These hemodynamic sequelae are usually reversible with the resolution of OSA.

ANESTHETIC MANAGEMENT

PREOPERATIVE EVALUATION

Preoperative assessment includes review of medical history and records, with a focus on clinical risk factors, and a physical examination. Physical examination should focus on body habitus, including failure to thrive, obesity, the presence of mouth breathing, tonsil size, chest wall retraction, micrognathia, macroglossia, midface hypoplasia, or presence of syndromes associated with OSA, such as those associated with craniofacial anomalies and Down syndrome (Box 69.1).

In children, the diagnosis of OSA is based mainly on clinical symptoms. Only a small minority of OSA children have a PSG to assess the severity of their OSA prior to surgery. Important information obtained from a PSG includes AHI, nadir and duration of oxyhemoglobin desaturation, and peak end-tidal carbon dioxide measurement. Patients with chronic hypoxia and hypercarbia develop persistent respiratory acidosis compensated with a metabolic alkalosis and subsequent

Table 69.2	Obstructive Sleep Apnea Severity by Polysomnography in Children and Adults	
OSA Severity	AHI Children	AHI Adults
None	0	0–5
Mild	1–5	6–20
Moderate	6–10	21–40
Severe	>10	>40

Note: OSA severity as defined by the American Society of Anesthesiologists Task Force on Perioperative Management of Patients.

AHI, apnea–hypopnea index; OSA, obstructive sleep apnea.

Source: From Patino M, Sadhasivam S, Mahmoud M. Obstructive sleep apnoea in children: perioperative considerations. Br J Anaesth. 2013;111(Suppl. 1):i83–i95. doi:10.1093/bja/aet371.

> **BOX 69.1 KEY ASSESSMENT POINTS FOR PATIENTS WITH KNOWN OR SUSPECTED OBSTRUCTIVE SLEEP APNEA**
>
> Risk factors for postoperative respiratory complications after adenotonsillectomy:
>
> - Children <3 years old
> - Severe OSA documented by PSG
> - Failure to thrive
> - Obesity
> - Cardiac involvement (right ventricular hypertrophy)
> - Down syndrome
> - History of prematurity
> - Craniofacial abnormalities
> - Neuromuscular diseases
> - Chronic lung disease
> - Sickle cell disease
>
> OSA, obstructive sleep apnea; PSG, polysomnography.
>
> Source: From Patino M, Sadhasivam S, Mahmoud M. Obstructive sleep apnoea in children: perioperative considerations. Br J Anaesth. 2013;111(Suppl. 1):i83–i95. doi:10.1093/bja/aet371.

risk of developing cor pulmonale. These patients require electrocardiography and echocardiogram as well as a cardiology evaluation prior to any elective surgery.

The most common surgery for children with OSA is adenotonsillectomy. One review of 111 cases of death or near-death following tonsillectomy in pediatric patients found that 57% of the children met the criteria for being at risk of OSA. Almost half of these events (46%) were related to apneas.[17] Accordingly, it is crucial to identify high-risk patients prior to adenotonsillectomy. High-risk patients include children <3 years of age, weight <5th percentile, craniofacial anomaly, severe OSA from a PSG, cardiac disease, prematurity, obesity (body mass index >95th percentile for age and gender), Down syndrome, and hypotonia.[1]

If a child does have a diagnosis of OSA, its severity and current management need to be assessed prior to surgery, including use of bilevel positive airway pressure (BiPAP), continuous positive airway pressure (CPAP), home monitoring, supplemental oxygen administration, and position during sleep. If noninvasive ventilatory support, such as CPAP or BiPAP, is used, settings must be reviewed. Patients should be instructed to bring their home respiratory device (CPAP or BiPAP) to the hospital with them, and devices must be immediately available during perioperative care, especially during and after anesthesia.

ANESTHETIC TECHNIQUE

Intraoperative Management

Sedative premedication should be avoided in patients with severe OSA as significant airway obstruction or severe desaturation may occur. Children with OSA that require medical sedation should have continuous clinical observation or pulse oximetry monitoring until their arrival at the surgical suite. Residual effects of sedative premedication may continue into the postoperative period, especially after short procedures.

During anesthesia, children with severe OSA and those who experienced severe airway obstruction during previous anesthesia require extreme vigilance well beyond standard anesthesia monitoring. Severe airway obstruction can occur even with light levels of anesthesia. IV general anesthesia, narcotics, and sedatives enhance upper airway muscle relaxation, reduce ventilation, and blunt respiratory reflex from sleep. Placement of an IV catheter should be completed either before induction of anesthesia or as quickly as possible after induction. Anesthesia providers should have available appropriate airway management tools prior to induction of anesthesia, including different sizes of face masks, oral airways, nasopharyngeal airways, laryngeal mask airways, laryngoscope blades and handles, and endotracheal tubes. If a difficult intubation is anticipated, fiberoptic bronchoscopes, video laryngoscopes, and a difficult airway cart should also be immediately available.

A loss of pharyngeal tone from inhaled or IV anesthetics, opioids, or muscle relaxants can contribute to postoperative airway obstruction. Respiratory depression and airway collapse are less likely to occur with ketamine and dexmedetomidine. Dexmedetomidine induces a sedative state that mimics non-REM sleep. Ketamine preserves pharyngeal and laryngeal reflexes, but its psychotropic effects limit its use. Glycopyrrolate can be administered to counteract hypersalivation, the side effect of ketamine.

It is important to realize that all surgical airway interventions, including adenotonsillectomy, lingual tonsillectomy, tongue base reduction, and supraglottoplasty, can lead to immediate postoperative swelling that could worsen airway obstruction. Following surgery, these patients should be extubated while awake, with adequate tidal volumes, appropriate oxygenation and ventilation, and full recovery of muscle strength. Even though this maximizes airway patency, significant airway obstruction and respiratory complications are still common. Airway maneuvers, including jaw thrust and nasopharyngeal airway, oral airway, or lateral positioning, may be necessary. Dexamethasone has been shown to reduce inflammation and swelling. If significant airway swelling is a concern, the patient should remain intubated and transported to the ICU.

There is no consensus on the criteria for ICU admission, but factors for consideration include significant comorbidity (including Down syndrome, Pierre Robin sequence, or neuromuscular disease), oxygen saturation on room air <90% in the postoperative care unit (PACU), oxygen requirement >40% in PACU, age <24 months, AHI >24, and intraoperative complications including laryngospasm, bronchospasm requiring medical treatment, or postoperative airway obstruction requiring nasal trumpet (Arambula et al., 2018).

Patients with OSA are very sensitive to narcotics as they depress the central response to both hypercarbia and hypoxia. If needed, narcotic administration must be carefully titrated and continuously monitored. Typically, narcotic requirements in children with OSA are roughly one half (50%) the dose required in children without OSA. When necessary, short-acting narcotics should be used for breakthrough pain whenever possible.

Opioid and narcotic sparing multimodal anesthesia regimens should be routinely employed in children with OSA, especially in patients with severe OSA. Multimodal pain regimens include intraoperative administration of IV acetaminophen, dexmedetomidine, and postsurgical administration of oral ibuprofen. During adenotonsillectomy, a single intraoperative dose of .5 mcg/kg dexmedetomidine is reported to reduce postoperative emergence delirium and improve pain scores.[18] IV administration of nonsteroidal anti-inflammatory drugs remains controversial due to the potential for bleeding. Ketorolac has been reported to cause bleeding if given before hemostasis is achieved.

POSTOPERATIVE CARE

Residual effects of anesthetic agents and administration of opioids for postoperative pain control result in changes in airway dynamics that can lead to postoperative airway obstruction. Abnormal ventilatory responses to hypoxia and hypercapnia also contribute to respiratory complications. The incidence of postoperative respiratory complications in OSA patients is as high as 27%.[19] High-risk patients should undergo surgical interventions in pediatric specialty centers with intensive care facilities.

In the PACU, patients should have continuous pulse oximetry monitoring with audible alarms for desaturation below 90%. Ideally, patients with OSA should be in the line of sight of the nursing station. Supplemental oxygen should be limited to 2 L/min and the anesthesia provider and the surgeon need to be contacted if the oxygen requirement is higher than 2 L/min. Excess oxygen can suppress hypoxemic response and delay recognition of respiratory complications via pulse oximetry monitoring.[13] In patients at high risk of respiratory complications, continuous monitoring of adequate ventilation using nasal capnography is recommended as detection of airflow disruption might alter life-threatening events. Limitations of nasal capnography include poor tolerance in young children, dislodgment of nasal cannula, and inability to detect airflow in mouth breathers.[11] Postoperative use of a patient's home respiratory device (CPAP or BiPAP) for positive pressure ventilation at preoperative settings might be required during the postoperative recovery phase and during the hospital stay.

In patients with severe OSA, it is critically important to avoid the risks associated with postoperative narcotic use.[16] Codeine should be avoided, especially in children. The CYP2D6 metabolism of codeine to morphine is inconsistent, which can lead to ineffectiveness in poor metabolizers and morphine overdose and death in extensive metabolizers.[20] Use of nonopioid analgesic adjuncts and techniques is strongly recommended to reduce the risk of opioid-related respiratory complications. Discharge instructions should include educational information on OSA and follow-up with a sleep medicine consultant.

CASE STUDY: A Child With Obstructive Sleep Apnea for Adenotonsillectomy

CLINICAL SCENARIO

A 2-year-old, otherwise healthy patient presents with sleep-disordered breathing. She has snoring, breathing pauses less than 5 seconds with no gagging or gasping, restless sleep, with some tiredness during the day and with no behavior and learning issues. There is no significant history of tonsillitis with fever, pain, or dysphagia. She was full term when she was born, with normal development. Her body weight is 12 kg. She has never had anesthesia or surgery. There is no family history of problems from anesthesia or surgery. Her physical examination is unremarkable except for tonsillar hypertrophy.

SPECIAL CONSIDERATIONS

She is scheduled for a polysomnogram to evaluate her sleep-disordered breathing. The study demonstrated moderate obstructive sleep apnea associated with mild oxygen desaturation. Her oxygen nadir is 91%. The apnea–hypopnea index (AHI) was 6.8 per hour. Central sleep apnea, nonapneic hypoxemia, and alveolar hypoventilation were not observed. Due to her moderate obstructive sleep apnea, she is scheduled for adenotonsillectomy with overnight admission to the hospital instead of being discharged home as an outpatient procedure.

APPROACHES TO CARE

On the day of surgery, the anesthesia provider explains the perioperative care of the patient and obtains informed consent from the parents. Distraction methods using video and toys are used to reduce anxiety at separation and induction of anesthesia without premedication.

Inhalation induction is performed in the operating room under standard American Society of Anesthesiologists monitors with oxygen, nitrous oxide, and sevoflurane. An IV catheter is placed under anesthesia for fluid and drug administration. Propofol (2 mg/kg) and fentanyl (1 mg/kg) is given before intubation with a 4.0 oral Ring-Adair-Elwin (RAE) endotracheal tube. Anesthesia is maintained with oxygen, air, and sevoflurane, fraction of inspired oxygen (FiO2) 40%. Ondansetron (.1 mg/kg) and dexamethasone (.5 mg/kg) are given intravenously for postoperative nausea and vomiting and reduction of edema accordingly. Acetaminophen (10 mg/kg) and dexmedetomidine (.5 mcg/kg) are given as adjunctive for postoperative pain control. At the end of the procedure, the patient is extubated awake and then transported to the recovery room. The patient is observed in the recovery room to ensure adequate pain control, normal breathing, and absence of bleeding concerns before being transported to the floor.

KEY REFERENCES

Complete references for this chapter are online and available at https://connect.springerpub.com/content/book/978-0-8261-3875-0/part/part04/toc-part/ch069.

11. Patino M, Sadhasivam S, Mahmoud M. Obstructive sleep apnoea in children: perioperative considerations. *Br J Anaesth.* 2013;111 Suppl 1: i83-95. doi:10.1093/bja/aet371
14. Aurora RN, Zak RS, Karippot A, et al. . . American Academy of Sleep, M. Practice parameters for the respiratory indications for polysomnography in children. 2011;34(3):379388. doi:10.1093/sleep/34.3.379
15. Mahmoud M, Gunter J, Sadhasivam S. Cine MRI airway studies in children with sleep apnea: optimal images and anesthetic challenges. *Pediatr Radiol.* 2009;39(10):1034–1037. doi:10.1007/s00247-009-13671376
16. Arambula AM, Xie DX, Whigham AS. Respiratory events after adenotonsillectomy requiring escalated admission status in children with obstructive sleep apnea. *Int J Pediatr Otorhinolaryngol.* 2018;107:31–36. doi:10.1016/j.ijporl.2018.01.009
17. Cote CJ, Posner KL, Domino KB. Death or neurological injury after tonsillectomy in children with a focus on obstructive sleep apnea: Houston, we have a problem! *Anesth Analg.* 2014;118(6):12761283. doi:10.1213/ANE.0b013e318294fc47

Tongue Base Reduction

Hannah Kuhn

INDICATIONS/CONTRAINDICATIONS

Tongue base reduction is useful in relieving upper airway obstruction when initial medical and/or surgical treatment of obstructive sleep apnea (OSA) fails to adequately correct the condition. While first-line surgical treatment for OSA in the pediatric population is adenotonsillectomy,[1] recurrent symptoms of obstruction due to significant tongue base collapse warrant further evaluation. Tongue base reduction surgery involves inserting a narrow, needle-like probe at the base of the tongue, through which radiofrequency energy is applied. This causes contraction and shrinkage of the base of the tongue over a period of 2 months following the procedure. Frequently, surgical removal of the lingual tonsils is performed at the same time. Reducing tongue base volume proportionally increases airway size in children with significant tongue hypertrophy.

Conditions predisposing pediatric patients to tongue hypertrophy include Beckwith–Wiedemann syndrome, Down syndrome, and cerebral palsy (Box 70.1).[2] Contraindications to surgical resection of the tongue base include preexisting dysphagia, coagulopathy, unstable cardiopulmonary disease, and active infection.

SPECIAL CONSIDERATIONS AND CONCERNS

OSA is the extreme limit of the spectrum of sleep-disordered breathing. This spectrum can range from normal respiration to primary snoring, upper airway resistance syndrome, obstructive hypopnea, and OSA.[1] Obstructive events that characterize this condition include episodes of hypoxia, hypercarbia, and sleep disruption. Pediatric patients may present with a spectrum of disease affecting multiple organ systems (see Box 70.2).[1] For further information regarding care of children with sleep-disordered breathing, please see Chapter 69, "Care of Children With Sleep-Disordered Breathing."

ANESTHETIC MANAGEMENT

PREOPERATIVE EVALUATION

A thorough preoperative examination is imperative to providing a safe and effective anesthetic. Anesthesia providers should perform a detailed physical examination that includes history of treatments, both medical and surgical. Comorbidities associated with OSA should be evaluated, and the patient should be optimized prior to the surgical procedure. Upper airway endoscopy, imaging, and often a drug-induced sleep endoscopy (DISE) will have been performed prior to the day of surgery. Additional imaging and DISE provide valuable information regarding the child's upper airway anatomy and aid the surgical team in developing a comprehensive surgical treatment plan. Please see Chapter 71, "Drug-Induced Sleep Endoscopy (DISE)," for more information.

Pertinent Labs

Preoperative laboratory studies include a complete blood count including platelet count. Recent hemoglobin and hematocrit are necessary to determine allowable blood loss during the procedure. Type and screen are useful in the event a blood transfusion is required, especially if the patient has antibodies to red blood cells. Coagulation studies may be performed if there is suspicion of abnormal bleeding tendencies.

PREOPERATIVE PHARMACOLOGY

The need for preoperative medication is determined during the preanesthetic evaluation. Children with sleep-disordered breathing who require premedication should be closely monitored with pulse oximetry after administration of sedatives. Utilizing medications that have a short duration of action, those that can be antagonized, and those that have little to no effect on airway tone is advised.[1] An important factor in the determination of what premedication to utilize is patient cooperation. Oftentimes, anxiety levels hinder a child's ability to tolerate IV access placement. Medications that can be administered orally or intranasally can be beneficial in these instances. Of note, dexmedetomidine has proved to be extremely useful in cases where airway compromise needs to be avoided. Dexmedetomidine is a highly specific alpha-2-adrenergic agonist capable of producing sedation, analgesia, and anxiolysis without inducing clinically significant respiratory depression.[3]

ANESTHETIC TECHNIQUE

Intraoperative Management

Inhalation or IV techniques can be utilized for induction of general anesthesia. The choice of induction technique is largely dependent on the presence and severity of comorbidities. Endotracheal intubation should be discussed with the surgical team prior to induction of anesthesia as placement of specialized endotracheal tube (ETT) may be required. Specialized ETTs, such as an oral Ring-Adair-Elwin (RAE) ETT, nasal RAE ETT, and reinforced ETT, can allow optimal surgical exposure while decreasing the risk of inadvertent extubation during the procedure.

It is important to note that during tongue base reduction surgery, the patient is often turned 90 to 180 degrees away from the anesthesia provider. It is imperative to ensure that the ETT is secure and that there is minimal tension on the anesthesia circuit. Special precautions should also be taken to protect the patient's eyes from injury during the procedure.

Blood and secretions may be present in the oropharynx at the conclusion of surgery. These should be carefully suctioned before emergence from anesthesia, in addition to emptying the stomach with an orogastric tube. Of note, this is often performed by the surgeon under direct visualization after the completion of surgery.[1]

> **BOX 70.1 MEDICAL CONDITIONS THAT PREDISPOSE PEDIATRIC PATIENTS TO TONGUE HYPERTROPHY**
>
> - Beckwith–Wiedemann syndrome
> - Down syndrome
> - Hunter syndrome
> - Hurler syndrome
> - Pompe disease
> - Robinow syndrome
> - Maroteaux–Lamy syndrome
> - Crouzon syndrome
> - Pierre Robin sequence
> - Cerebral palsy
> - Malignancy
> - Hemangioma

> **BOX 70.2 SPECTRUM OF DISEASE AFFECTING MULTIPLE ORGAN SYSTEMS IMPACTED BY OBSTRUCTIVE SLEEP APNEA**
>
> - Failure to thrive
> - Ventricular dysfunction
>   - Depressed ventricular ejection fraction
>   - Right ventricular hypertrophy
>   - Pulmonary hypertension
> - Repeated infections of the lower respiratory tract
> - Chronic aspiration
> - Behavioral issues

Pediatric patients undergoing tongue base reduction are at a higher risk of postoperative nausea and vomiting. Anticipation of this allows the anesthesia provider to administer medications intraoperatively that can help decrease the prevalence of this complication. Total IV anesthesia (TIVA) may be an effective technique in especially high-risk populations. The avoidance of retching and vomiting can also decrease the risk of postoperative hemorrhage.

It is preferable to wait until the child is fully awake and able to clear blood and secretions from the oropharynx prior to removing the ETT. A common practice is to position the child in lateral position with the head slightly down during extubation. This position permits blood and secretions to pool in the dependent region rather than accumulate at the laryngeal inlet.[1]

Complications/Emergencies

The extent of tongue base reduction is limited by risks to the critical nerves and blood vessels to the tongue. Maintaining proper function with swallowing and speech is another factor making this surgical procedure challenging.[2] Airway edema postoperatively remains a risk and should be closely monitored.

Pediatric patients who undergo tongue base reduction are at risk of respiratory compromise postoperatively. Intact airway and pharyngeal reflexes are of utmost importance in preventing aspiration, laryngospasm, and airway obstruction.[1] As previously mentioned, it is preferable to wait until the child is fully awake prior to extubation as the use of oral airways may contribute to the risk of postoperative hemorrhage.

Postoperative hemorrhage should be addressed immediately, and the airway should be secured in a swift, efficient manner to ensure patient safety. The management of anesthesia in this situation can be challenging even in the hands of an experienced pediatric anesthesia provider.[1] In the event of acute postoperative hemorrhage, the child will present as hypovolemic, with a decrease in cardiac output secondary to ongoing blood loss. If this is not corrected immediately, lactic acidosis and a state of shock will develop. The compensatory response to acute blood loss is an outpouring of catecholamines, which causes vasoconstriction; therefore, delaying the clinical onset of hypotension in the awake child.[1] Anesthesia-induced vasodilation produces profound hypotension. Vigorous fluid resuscitation with crystalloids (20 mL/kg of balanced salt solution) and/or colloids remains the key to improvement of cardiac output and hemodynamic stability.

POSTOPERATIVE CARE

Pediatric patients who undergo this procedure should be closely monitored either in the ICU or on a complex airway unit as complications such as airway edema, hematoma, abscess formation, and permanent hypoglossal injury may occur. Narcotics should be avoided if possible or administered with great caution due to increased sensitivity to the respiratory depressant effects seen in children with OSA.[1] Continuous positive airway pressure (CPAP) may be necessary to maintain a patent airway in the immediate postoperative period.

REFERENCES

1. Coté CJ, Lerman J, Todres ID. *A Practice of Anesthesia for Infants and Children*. Saunders/Elsevier. 2009.
2. Yu JL, Afolabi-Brown O. Updates on management of pediatric obstructive sleep apnea. *Pediatr Invest*. 2019;3:228–235. doi:10.1002/ped4.12164
3. Behrle N, Birisci E, Anderson J, et al. Intranasal dexmedetomidine as a sedative for pediatric procedural sedation. *J Pediatr Pharmacol Ther*. 2017;22(1):4–8. doi:10.5863/1551-6776-22.1.4
4. Ulualp S. Outcomes of tongue base reduction and lingual tonsillectomy for residual pediatric obstructive sleep apnea after adenotonsillectomy. *Int Arch Otorhinolaryngol*. 2019;23(4):e415-e421. doi:10.1055/s-0039-1685156

CHAPTER 71

Drug-Induced Sleep Endoscopy

Yann-Fuu Kou, Mohamed A. Mahmoud, and Stacey L. Ishman

INDICATIONS/CONTRAINDICATIONS

Pediatric obstructive sleep apnea (OSA) has an estimated prevalence of 1% to 4% in the United States.[1] While first-line treatment is tonsillectomy and adenotonsillectomy (T&A), a significant percentage of children may have persistent symptoms after T&A.[2] Studies have reported rates of persistent sleep apnea to range from 20% to 75%.[3-6] Risk factors for persistent OSA include severe OSA, obesity, craniofacial abnormalities, hypotonia, and Down syndrome.[1,3,7,8] Identifying persistent OSA is important as when untreated it is associated with failure to thrive, impaired neurocognitive and neurobehavioral abnormalities, pulmonary hypertension, cor pulmonale, systemic hypertension, and metabolic syndrome.[9] Early treatment with medical or surgical intervention may reverse these complications.

Polysomnography (PSG) is the gold standard for diagnosis of OSA. Children who have concern for persistent symptoms after T&A or who are at high risk for persistent OSA should undergo a PSG after T&A.[10] However, PSG does not provide information regarding sites of obstruction, direct further therapies, or predict which children would benefit from surgical or medical interventions. As with adults, continuous positive airway pressure (CPAP) is considered for children with persistent OSA as it is an effective therapy; however, it is often poorly tolerated.[1] This was the impetus for developing further diagnostic modalities for assessing children with persistent OSA. The ideal study would closely simulate a natural sleep state while allowing the provider to visualize upper airway dynamics during obstructive episodes.

Drug-induced sleep endoscopy (DISE) is a relatively new procedure with no definite indications. The procedure itself is straightforward and similar to the manner in which flexible nasopharyngoscopy and laryngoscopy (FNL) are commonly performed on awake patients. The proper plane of anesthesia should have the child breathing spontaneously with audible snoring if possible but deep enough to not respond to the stimuli of having a scope in their nose.[11] The Ramsay sedation scale (RASS) is a commonly used measure of sedation. For this procedure, we aim to have the patients at a level 5 at which the patient would demonstrate a sluggish response to loud auditory stimulus.[12] Generally, topical decongestants and anesthetics are avoided as these can mask nasal edema and blunt upper airway reflexes.[11,13] A nasal suction catheter is passed through both nasal cavities to remove secretions and assess the patient's depth of anesthesia. A lack of patient arousal and reaction to this stimulus helps ensure an appropriate level of sedation.

The flexible fiberoptic endoscope is then passed through each nostril, and all the potential levels of airway obstruction are assessed and photo-documented. Standard sites for documentation include the nasal airway (nasal cavities and nasopharynx), palate/velum, pharyngeal airway (including lateral oropharyngeal wall and tongue base), and supraglottic larynx. A chin-lift or jaw-thrust will often be performed with the scope at different levels of the airway including when the scope is at the levels of the choana/nasopharynx, velum, and tongue base. The surgeon may ask the anesthesia provider to help with jaw thrust while assessing these sites.[11] Some providers will also advance the scope past the glottis to evaluate for tracheal and bronchial pathologies, but this is not commonly done or recommended unless there is a high index of suspicion.[11,14] If performed, a topical anesthetic is applied prior to the larynx before advancing past the glottis to avoid the risk of laryngospasm.

The American Academy of Otolaryngology-Head and Neck Surgery recently published an expert consensus statement (ECS) for pediatric DISE.[11] Persistent OSA after T&A is the most common indication as DISE allows for an assessment of different sites of obstruction to direct further surgery, and the use of DISE for this indication is supported by the ECS.[1,11,14] Similar to what is seen in adults, the majority of children have multiple levels of obstruction.[15] Commonly described sites of obstruction include the tongue base, adenoid regrowth, inferior turbinates, velum, and lateral oropharyngeal walls.[6] The ECS experts also had consensus that children with OSA and small tonsils are good candidates for DISE.[11]

Some providers will perform DISE prior to T&A, especially for children who are at high risk for persistent OSA. There is some controversy regarding its utility in these patients as removal of the tonsils and adenoids will significantly alter airway dynamics; however, some providers feel that identification of secondary surgical sites (e.g., lingual tonsillar hypertrophy) can be useful.[1] DISE has also been advocated for children with sleep-disordered breathing (SDB) or OSA who have small tonsils and adenoids.[11,16]

There are no specific contraindications for DISE outside of those for general anesthesia. It is worth noting that certain subpopulations are at high risk for cardiac comorbidities when given anesthesia, and thus, careful preoperative assessment is imperative.

ANESTHETIC MANAGEMENT

PREOPERATIVE EVALUATION

Children who have persistent OSA tend to have other comorbidities, including obesity, Down syndrome, neuromuscular diseases, or craniofacial abnormalities.[17] These factors can place also these children at higher risk for perioperative complications. This is particularly true for children with Down syndrome who have a higher rate of comorbid cardiac disease.[18]

Cincinnati Children's Hospital Medical Center (CCHMC) has developed a process for preoperative assessment of children with Down syndrome because of the high prevalence of cardiac comorbidities in this population. All these patients receive an anesthesia consult and assessment preprocedure. In addition, if there is no recent echocardiogram, patients undergo a screening ECG. In addition to preprocedure assessment, an awareness and understanding of the significant risk of neurological injury with excessive movement of the neck in these patients are extremely important. A thorough history and physical examination should also be conducted prior to anesthesia to assess for signs or symptoms suggestive of cord compression before any airway manipulation.

ANESTHETIC TECHNIQUE

Intraoperative Management

Inhalational and intravenous anesthetic agents can have independent effects and negatively impact the upper airway evaluation. The decrease in airway tone associated with inhalational and other anesthetics may lead to anatomic changes in the structures that surround the airway. These changes are more pronounced in children with OSA, who often demonstrate increased dynamic airway collapse, contributing to the clinical findings of OSA. Providing anesthesia that mimics physiological sleep prior to corrective surgery to improve OSA symptoms can be challenging but is critical for accurate interpretation of the airway evaluation (Table 71.1).

Unlike with other pediatric procedures for which midazolam is commonly used as premedication, it is recommended that midazolam be avoided because of it causes respiratory depression and can potentially increase upper airway obstruction.[19,20] In children, most studies of DISE report that sevoflurane was used for induction to allow for IV line insertion at which point sevoflurane was turned off and providers transitioned to IV sedation.[21] Sevoflurane is favored when compared to other inhalational agents because of its low incidence of breath-holding and laryngospasm.[20] While several studies of sevoflurane have shown that it has minimal effects on upper airway collapse, it is not recommended to use sevoflurane for the entire assessment as inhalational agents generally exaggerate upper airway collapse and do not appear to replicate natural sleep.[21,22]

The ideal DISE allows for assessment of the native airway free of artificial airway adjuncts. Anesthetic agents impair the ability of the upper airway muscles to overcome negative inspiratory pressures, resulting in increased upper airway resistance. Maintaining spontaneous ventilation and avoiding upper airway collapsibility associated significant oxygen desaturation in patients with OSA under anesthesia is a major challenge. Some level of oxygen desaturation must be tolerated as experts agree that supplemental oxygen can affect the study findings.[11] The PSG oxygen nadir can be used as a guide along with clinical expertise. The anesthetic technique in these patients must be tailored to improve patient safety and provide ideal study.

A 2009 survey of pediatric institutions revealed that there is significant discordance between institutions as to which medications are used.[23] The ideal anesthetic cocktail should balance a reproducible simulated sleep state without causing respiratory depression, cardiovascular effects, or exaggerating airway collapse. Multiple agents have been recommended, and many combinations are used. These medications include propofol, ketamine, remifentanil, sevoflurane, and dexmedetomidine.[9,20] The 2021 published ECS on DISE recommends propofol and dexmedetomidine as optimal forms of sedation in children.[11]

In adults, propofol is the most commonly used anesthetic and is titrated to a bispectral index (BIS) of 50 to 75.[24] Propofol is favored due to the rapid onset and ease of titration.[19] However, propofol can cause changes in sleep architecture and has dose-dependent decreases on the cross-sectional area of the upper airway.[25-27] A systematic review also showed that higher doses of propofol increased pharyngeal airway collapse in infants.[19] The effect of propofol on airway tone and sleep architecture should lead to caution in interpretation of DISE findings.

Opioids such as remifentanil are known to be associated with sedation and respiratory depression. Remifentanil is favored over other drugs in this class due to very fast onset and predictable clinical duration.[20] Opioids can also decrease upper airway reflexes, cause upper airway obstruction, and do not simulate natural sleep. Thus, they should be used cautiously for DISE.

A study at CCHMC compared a combination of dexmedetomidine/ketamine to propofol with or without sevoflurane. It was found that patients receiving dexmedetomidine/ketamine had significantly fewer desaturations, improved blood pressure stability, and a 100% successful procedure completion rate. In the propofol groups, several patients were unable to complete the procedure due to significant desaturations requiring placement of an oral airway and/or laryngospasm. Based on the results of this study, dexmedetomidine/ketamine has become the standard of care at CCHMC. One of the initial concerns with dexmedetomidine was that it replicates nonrapid eye movement (REM) sleep.[28] However, a recent study by Smith et al. reported that DISE with dexmedetomidine/ketamine can successfully identify sites of upper airway obstruction in children with REM-predominant OSA.[29]

One limitation of dexmedetomidine is the slow onset of action that necessitates a 10-minute bolus infusion prior to reaching the correct plane of anesthesia. This is why some protocols add ketamine at the time of the initial bolus to help provide sedation while the dexmedetomidine is infused. Ketamine has a fast onset of action and is a safe sedative that does not decrease respiratory drive or airway muscle tone. It is generally only used during the initiation of the

Table 71.1	Common Surgeries to Correct Obstructive Sleep Apnea			
Nasal	**Palate**	**Tongue Base**	**Larynx**	**Miscellaneous**
Inferior turbinate reduction	Uvulopalatopharyngoplasty (UPPP)	Lingual tonsillectomy	Supraglottoplasty	Tracheostomy
Septoplasty	Expansion sphincter palatoplasty (ESP)	Posterior midline glossectomy	Epiglottopexy	Hypoglossal nerve stimulator
		Tongue base suspension	Hyoid suspension	Maxillomandibular advancement
		Tongue–lip adhesion		
		Genioglossus advancement		

BOX 71.1 CINCINNATI CHILDREN'S HOSPITAL MEDICAL CENTER DRUG-INDUCED SLEEP ENDOSCOPY ANESTHESIA PROTOCOL

1. If patient not a candidate for preoperative IV, inhalational induction with sevoflurane/nitrous oxide
2. Place IV
3. Discontinue sevoflurane and nitrous oxide as soon as possible
4. Loading dose: dexmedetomidine 2 mcg/kg over 10 minutes followed by infusion 2 mcg/kg/hr[a]
5. Administer ketamine 1 mg/kg immediately after starting dexmedetomidine load
6. If uncooperative with the bolus, increase infusion rate to 3 mcg/kg/hr
7. If still uncooperative can switch to propofol
8. Oxygen can be delivered in a "blow by" fashion during titration but may need to be discontinued during parts of the examination. Alternatively, an oral airway may be used during induction but removed prior to airway evaluation[b]
9. The patient should be posited supine with the neck in neutral position (avoid shoulder rolls or pillows)
10. No topical anesthesia or nasal decongestants
11. During examination, intermittent jaw thrust may be utilized but communicate clearly with surgeon prior to performing

[a]For obese patients, use lean body weight (20% higher than ideal body weight).
[b]Children with moderate/severe OSA do not need intervention unless oxygen saturation drops below 85%. Then mask ventilate until saturation >85%.
OSA, obstructive sleep apnea.

---

dexmedetomidine infusion as it can cause increased oral and airway secretions making endoscopy difficult.[30] The current CCHMC protocol is noted in **Box 71.1**. Other institutions have used nasal dexmedetomidine in the preprocedure area to expedite the time to the DISE assessment.[23]

Traditionally, a DISE was performed in the operating room under an anesthetic separate from the MRI suite. When the procedures were combined, the child was typically assessed in the operating room and then transferred to the MRI suite for further evaluation. Recent research performed at CCHMC offers that performing both procedures in the radiology suite is safe and cost-effective.[31] In this scenario, a DISE is performed in the induction room, and after completion, the patient is taken directly to the MRI suite across the hallway. This requires close collaboration between anesthesia, otolaryngology, radiology, and nursing.

Special Techniques and Equipment

Sleep cine MRI also allows for dynamic evaluation of the upper airway.[1] Anesthetic challenges during MRI are similar to those during DISE; however, less sedation is theoretically needed due to the absence of any airway manipulation. The use of dexmedetomidine in children with OSA for sleep cine MRI provides an adequate level of anesthesia and makes it possible to successfully complete the MRI study in the majority of children without airway intervention.

The most common challenge anesthesia providers face during MRI airway dynamic studies is the inability of the child to tolerate an adequate level of sedation or anesthesia without experiencing significant oxygen desaturation without intervention. This challenge is further compounded by the need to avoid the use of airway interventions, such as oral or nasal airways, as well as other maneuvers improve airway patency, such as placement of a chin lift or shoulder roll placement. Children with severe OSA who require CPAP may be unable to complete the study without unacceptable decreases in oxygen saturation. In this situation, it may be necessary to use minimal CPAP settings or place an artificial airway to safely complete the study, recognizing that these maneuvers will compromise interpretation of the study and complicate clinical decision-making. The use of CPAP is preferable to the use of oral or nasal airways as these deform the tissue and limit the usefulness of the study unless they are removed during the time of imaging. In addition, some children can be supported with CPAP between sequences and may be able to make it through them without the CPAP turned on for the imaging itself. The decision of when to intervene with these maneuvers is another challenge and major debate among anesthesia providers.[32]

Clinical Pearls

One of the major reasons for suboptimal dynamic airway evaluation is a lack of communication between providers involved in the care of these complex children. An example of the importance of communication during DISE is the temptation to administer a nasal decongestant/anesthetic to facilitate passage and tolerance of the flexible scope. The administration of any nasal medications is discouraged, with the sole exception being intranasal dexmedotomidine prior to assessment. Vasoconstriction may decrease upstream airway resistance that will promote airway patency by affecting the starling resistor. A lack of standardized protocols during airway evaluations studies has led to wide variability in reports and the results achieved. A well-designed anesthesia protocol is essential to obtain an evaluation under anesthesia that is most likely to approximate natural sleep.

While DISE may be performed in isolation as a diagnostic procedure, there are many instances where a surgeon will bring a patient to the operating room, perform a DISE and then perform surgery as dictated by the findings of the DISE. This can theoretically involve surgery at any level of the airway from the nasal turbinates to the larynx. Due to the wide range of possibilities, it is important to discuss airway management with the surgeon including the route of intubation (oral vs. nasal).

Complications/Emergencies

A major challenge during dynamic airway evaluation in these children is significant oxygen desaturation under anesthesia, especially for those with severe OSA. There is no strict consensus among providers regarding when to intervene to improve oxygenation. Absolute lower limits of oxygen saturation below which airway intervention is required may differ from patient to patient depending on the severity of the OSA. Overnight PSG noting the severity of desaturations during natural sleep can be utilized as a guide to determine minimal acceptable arterial oxygen saturation before airway intervention. However, experts agree that oxygen supplementation can affect findings during DISE and thus should be avoided when possible.[11] A reasonable approach is to intervene in patients with mild OSA when oxygen saturation are <90%, while patients with moderate or severe OSA are allowed to oxygen saturation levels of <85% before intervention. Many of the patients experience this type of desaturation during polysomnography and natural sleep at home. An assessment of other comorbidities will also inform the decision regarding allowable desaturation as conditions such as severe cardiomyopathy may prohibit allowing significant oxygen desaturations.

POSTOPERATIVE CARE

Upon completion of the procedure, all infusions are discontinued, and the patient is awoken in the operating room to ensure a safe transition while emerging through the stages of anesthesia. In the postanesthesia care unit, key assessments should focus on the presence of airway edema, stridor, increased oxygen requirements, and the presence of respiratory distress.

KEY REFERENCES

Complete references for this chapter are online and available at https://connect.springerpub.com/content/book/978-0-8261-3875-0/part/part04/toc-part/ch071.

1. Wilcox LJ, Bergeron M, Reghunathan S, Ishman SL. An updated review of pediatric drug-induced sleep endoscopy. *Laryngoscope Investig Otolaryngol.* 2017;2(6):423–431. doi:10.1002/lio2.118
9. Kandil A, Subramanyam R, Hossain MM, et al. Comparison of the combination of dexmedetomidine and ketamine to propofol or propofol/sevoflurane for drug-induced sleep endoscopy in children. *Paediatr Anaesth.* 2016;26(7):742–751. doi:10.1111/pan.12931
11. Baldassari CMM, Lam DJM, Ishman SLMM, et al. Expert consensus statement: pediatric drug-induced sleep endoscopy. *Otolaryngol Head Neck Surg.* December 2020. doi:10.1177/0194599820985000
14. Friedman NR, Parikh SR, Ishman SL, et al. The current state of pediatric drug-induced sleep endoscopy. *Laryngoscope.* 2017;127(1):266–272. doi:10.1002/lary.26091
20. Liu KA, Liu CC, Alex G, et al. Anesthetic management of children undergoing drug-induced sleep endoscopy: a retrospective review. *Int J Pediatr Otorhinolaryngol.* 2020;139. doi:10.1016/j.ijporl.2020.110440
32. Bergeron M, Lee DR, DeMarcantonio MA, et al. Safety and cost of drug-induced sleep endoscopy outside the operating room. *Laryngoscope.* 2020;130(8):2076–2080. doi:10.1002/lary.28397

SECTION C: Ophthalmic Procedures

CHAPTER 72

Ophthalmologic Exam Under Anesthesia

Audrey Rosenblatt and Susan P. McMullan

INDICATIONS/CONTRAINDICATIONS

One of the most commonly performed pediatric ophthalmic procedures is an examination under anesthesia (EUA). The need for general anesthesia is frequently due to the inability of an infant or child to remain still and cooperative for a routine eye exam, however, may be warranted when there is a need for a motionless eye to accurately diagnose, monitor, and treat acute and chronic eye conditions.[1] In order to ensure a thorough exam, ophthalmologists may prefer an infant or child receive general anesthesia despite the short duration of the procedure.

EUA is performed on pediatric patients across the lifespan. Premature infants are evaluated and monitored for retinopathy of prematurity (ROP) and may require additional ophthalmic treatments, such as laser photocoagulation or cryotherapy, to reduce retinal proliferation and the incidence of retinal detachment. If left unchecked, retinal detachment may lead to reduced visual acuity and blindness.[2] Other common indications for EUA during infancy and childhood include assessment of the structure and function of anterior chamber of the eye (cornea, iris, and lens), including tonometry to measure intraocular pressure associated with congenital glaucoma, evaluation of congenital cataracts, and assessment of corneal issues. Should a comprehensive eye exam be needed to assess the structures of posterior chamber, including the vitreous, retina, and optic nerve, the pupil will require dilation in order for the structures to be visualized. Indications for posterior chamber exam include retinoblastoma screening and follow-up, and vitreoretinal issues. It is common that the EUA is paired with another procedure based on the initial findings.

SPECIAL CONSIDERATIONS AND CONCERNS

Should pupillary dilation be required prior to the induction of anesthesia, the anesthesia provider may consider administration of an anxiolytic as pupil-dilating drops often cause some discomfort with administration. The timing of dilating drop administration is variable, however, with some ophthalmologists preferring to wait until after the induction of general anesthesia to initiate dilation.

ANESTHETIC MANAGEMENT

PREOPERATIVE EVALUATION

A thorough preoperative evaluation, as with any preanesthetic assessment, is indicated including a review of systems, NPO status, anesthesia history, family anesthesia history, and preoperative anxiety assessment. Any constellation of symptoms indicative of a genetic syndrome should be fully vetted, including potential anesthetic implications.

PREOPERATIVE PHARMACOLOGY

As discussed in Chapter 3, "Preoperative Evaluation and Testing," it is common for pediatric patients to receive an anxiolytic to facilitate separation from their parents/caregiver. Depending on the reason for the EUA, the child may have a single EUA, such as for a screening procedure, or may be scheduled for frequent exams to assess progression of their condition, such as with retinoblastoma. Consideration should be given to the child and family who require repeat or frequent EUA requiring general anesthesia. It is important that the anesthesia provider reviews prior anesthetic records.

ANESTHETIC TECHNIQUE

Intraoperative Management

The anesthetic technique should be tailored to the specific procedure and/or planned procedures and the amount of time needed by the ophthalmologist. While an EUA may only require 5 to 10 minutes for a fundoscopic examination, the examination itself may reveal the need for additional procedure such as laser therapy. When it is known that the EUA will be the only procedure, anesthesia providers may opt to perform an inhalation induction with mask maintenance of general anesthesia, with or without placement of an IV catheter.[3] The anesthesia provider should be prepared to alter the anesthetic plan should the EUA yields information dictating another procedure be performed. In this scenario, an IV catheter should be placed if not present to allow for administration of analgesic medications, such as narcotics and nonsteroidal anti-inflammatory medications, and antiemetics such as ondansetron and dexamethasone. Depending on the subsequent procedure being performed, there may be a need for anticholinergic, medications should the oculocardiac reflex be stimulated. Additionally, placement of a laryngeal mask airway or endotracheal tube may be warranted to secure the airway and afford the ophthalmologist unimpeded access to the eyes.

Complications/Emergencies

Unless there are associated genetic syndromes with unique anesthesia considerations, complications are generally related to the surgical repair.

POSTOPERATIVE CARE

EUA does not result in significant postoperative pain, nor is it particularly stimulating during the intraoperative course. Pain relief can be accomplished with intramuscular or intravenous ketorolac, oral or rectal acetaminophen, and, less commonly, small doses of narcotic medications.

REFERENCES

1. Waldschmidt B, Gordon N. Anesthesia for pediatric ophthalmologic surgery. *J AAPOS*. 2019;23(3):127–131. doi:10.1016/j.jaapos.2018.10.017
2. Disher T, Cameron C, Souvik M, et al. Pain-relieving interventions for retinopathy of prematurity: a meta-analysis. *Pediatrics*. 2018;142(1). doi:10.1542/peds.2018-0401
3. Hung CW, Licina L, Abramson DH, Arslan-Carlon V. Anesthetic complications during general anesthesia without intravenous access in pediatric ophthalmologic clinic: assessment of 5216 cases. *Minerva Anestesiologica*. 2017;83(7):712–719. doi:10.23736/S0375-9393.17.11565-8

Strabismus Repair

Priscilla Aguirre and Veronica Y. Amos

INDICATIONS/CONTRAINDICATIONS

Strabismus occurs in 3% to 5% of the population and is defined as a disorder where the extraocular muscles are not properly aligned.[1,2] Ocular misalignment prevents binocular single vision (BSV), which can lead to discomfort, squinting, amblyopia (lazy eye), nystagmus, and diplopia.[3,4] Initial management of strabismus aims to restore alignment and/or BSV via glasses, orthoptic exercises, patching of the weaker eye, or drugs, such as echothiopate or botulinum toxin.[5] These drugs may inhibit plasma cholinesterase for up to 6 weeks.[1,5] Surgery is indicated when nonsurgical approaches have failed to adequately restore BSV.

Strabismus surgery is the most common type of ophthalmic surgery performed in the pediatric population and may be unilateral or bilateral.[6] Surgical correction can be achieved by strengthening, weakening, and/or transposition of the extraocular muscles.[4] Surgery is contraindicated in patients with fully accommodative esotropia (cross-eyed), parents or patients with unrealistic expectations, acute onset of paresis with potential for resolution, and hemodynamically unstable patients.[5]

SPECIAL CONSIDERATIONS AND CONCERNS

Overcorrection and undercorrection of strabismus is common, and reoperation may be indicated in up to 5% of pediatric patients.[2] The incidence of reoperation may be decreased by utilizing the adjustable suture technique; however, this requires patient cooperation.[4] Chronic red eye, chemosis, and suture granuloma are some minor complications that may occur.[4] Severe complications may include orbital infection, retinal detachment and, most commonly, globe perforation.[4]

ANESTHETIC MANAGEMENT

PREOPERATIVE EVALUATION

A comprehensive head-to-toe preoperative assessment is essential for any pediatric patient having surgery. The preoperative assessment should include past medical/surgical/medication history, family history related to anesthesia, and nil per os (NPO) status. Maternal history, environmental factors (such as exposure to second-hand smoke), prematurity, and postconceptual age are also valuable in guiding the anesthetic plan.[6] Although not always possible, it is recommended that all patients (healthy or with multiple comorbidities) have a completed preoperative assessment several weeks prior to surgery.[6,7] This is paramount to reducing preoperative anxiety, providing clarification, and increasing overall satisfaction while also preventing unexpected surgery cancellation.[6,7]

Key Assessment Points

Although the majority of pediatric patients having strabismus surgery are relatively healthy, anesthesia providers should be familiar with commonly associated conditions. Strabismus has been linked to several conditions, such as Down syndrome, myotonic dystrophy, and Turner's syndrome.[1] Important anesthetic implications related to these conditions include increased risk for difficult intubation, as well as cardiac and respiratory complications (Table 73.1).

Numerous studies in the past have suggested that patients diagnosed with strabismus were at risk for developing malignant hyperthermia (MH). However, a study involving more than 2,500 patients did not demonstrate a relationship between strabismus and MH.[8–10] Furthermore, the majority of pediatric patients today undergo general anesthesia using inhalational agents for strabismus surgery without MH complications.[9] It is important to note that if masseter muscle spasm or other MH symptoms occur, the MH treatment protocol should be initiated.

Pertinent Laboratories

Routine laboratory tests, consultations, and radiographic imaging are not typically required for healthy pediatric patients, and if requested or ordered, it is solely based on any existing comorbidities.[6] A pregnancy test is recommended for all pediatric patients of childbearing age.

PREOPERATIVE PHARMACOLOGY

It is estimated that up to 60% of the pediatric population experiences preoperative anxiety, which can lead to unfavorable behavioral changes, such as emergence delirium (ED), psychological trauma, and increased requirements for pain medication.[10–13] A multimodal approach is necessary and begins by utilizing nonpharmacological methods, such as play therapy, distraction/relaxation techniques (music, iPads, and games), and utilizing child life specialists if available.[10,12]

If nonpharmacological methods have failed, anxiolytics may be utilized and should only be administered if (a) the patient can be observed, (b) appropriate monitoring equipment is available, and (c) resuscitative equipment is within reach.[12] The choice of anxiolytic agents depends on the presence of multiple comorbidities, allergies, patient cooperation, and contraindications of the drug. Commonly anxiolytic medications used preoperatively include midazolam, ketamine, and dexmedetomidine.[12,14,15]

Oral midazolam can be administered to patients greater than 1 month of age. The recommended dose is 0.25 to 0.5 mg/kg with a maximum dose of 20 mg.[12] Midazolam may provide adequate amnestic effects and aid in reducing preoperative anxiety. However, higher doses of midazolam have been linked to contradictory reactions, such as agitation and ED.[12]

Ketamine, typically administered with midazolam, can be administered to patients 2 years of age and greater by mouth or IM injection. The recommended oral and IM dose for ketamine are 5 to 8 mg/kg and 4 to 5 mg/kg, respectively.[12] The sedative, anxiolytic, and analgesic properties of ketamine make it a great choice in the preoperative setting; however,

Table 73.1	Disorders Associated With Strabismus
Disorder/Syndrome	Anesthetic Implications
Apert's syndrome*	Cervical spine fusion, congenital heart disease
Cri du chat syndrome*	Micrognathia, hypotonia, hypothermia, congenital heart disease
Crouzon's disorder*	Possible elevated intracranial pressure
Down syndrome	Trisomy 21, airway obstruction, atlantoaxial instability, congenital heart disease
Goldenhar's syndrome*	Hemifacial microsoma, possible cervical spine abnormalities, possible difficult mask ventilation, hydrocephalus
Homocystinuria	Marfanoid habitus with kyphoscoliosis, sternal deformity, prone to clots and hypoglycemia
Marfan syndrome	Aortic or pulmonary artery dilation, aortic or mitral valve disease, pectus excavatum, risk for pneumothorax
Myotonic dystrophy	Prone to myotonic contractions, succinylcholine-associated contractions and hyperkalemia, cardiac conduction abnormalities, sensitive to central nervous depressants
Stickler syndrome*	Micrognathia, mitral valve prolapse, marfanoid habitus, scoliosis, kyphosis
Turner's syndrome*	Possible difficult intravenous access, congenital heart disease

*Possible difficult intubation.

Source: From "Davis P, Cladis F. Anesthesia for ophthalmic surgery. Smith's Anesthesia for Infants and Children. Elsevier, Inc; 2016. Copyright 2016 by Elsevier, Inc. Reprinted with permission.

IM administration could be very traumatic and has been linked to higher incidences of ED.[12]

Intranasal or buccal dexmedetomidine has become increasingly popular in the pediatric population and has been shown to be more effective than ketamine and midazolam in reducing anxiety.[14] Recommended doses are 1 to 4 mcg/kg with a maximum of 200 mcg and should be administered to patients older than 1 year of age.[14] Dexmedetomidine effectively decreases anxiety and provides sedation that resembles sleep without interfering with respiration. However, bradycardia and hypotension are major concerns and therefore should not be administered to patients with severe ventricular dysfunction, those with atrioventricular blocks, or patients on digoxin and/or beta-blockers.[12]

ANESTHETIC TECHNIQUES

Intraoperative Management

Limited evidence supports utilizing IV over inhalational induction or vice versa in the pediatric patient and therefore will depend on the patient.[13] The majority of patients will undergo an inhalational induction utilizing sevoflurane due to its lack of pungency. Nitrous oxide is generally avoided in these cases due to its highly emetic properties and incidence of postoperative nausea and vomiting (PONV) with eye muscle surgery, although may be considered for use briefly to facilitate an inhalational induction. A peripheral IV catheter is usually placed in the upper extremities once the patient is past the excitement stage. This may be difficult in children younger than 2 years of age, leading to cannulation of the saphenous vein, which can be easily located lateral to the medial malleolus or use of ultrasound to facilitate IV catheter placement.

A laryngeal mask airway (LMA) or endotracheal tube (ETT) can be inserted depending on the age of the patient, their comorbidities, and length of the procedure. Anesthesia providers may lean toward ETT placement due to limited airway access with an LMA.[10,15] An oral Ring-Adair-Elwyn ETT is preferred by many surgeons due to improved surgical access. Surgeons will typically administer topical or subconjunctival antibiotics; consequently, IV antibiotics are not necessary unless otherwise indicated.

Special Techniques and Equipment

Forced duction testing (FDT) is a unique consideration for patients undergoing surgery to correct strabismus. After induction, the surgeon grasps the conjunctiva via forceps and assesses the range of motion of the extraocular muscles and determines whether abnormal range of motion stems from a neurological or mechanical restriction.[16] The results of the FDT determines the surgical approach of the procedure.

Succinylcholine should not be routinely used in patients younger than age 8 years; however, if an airway emergency arises, the surgeon should not perform the FDT for at least 20 minutes after administration.[6,16] Succinylcholine could alter the FDT results as extraocular muscles have increased muscle fibers and postjunctional receptors, which account for prolonged ocular fasciculations compared with skeletal muscles.[16] If paralysis is required, nondepolarizers may be administered with no effect on FDT.[16]

Clinical Pearls

Up to 80% of pediatric patients can experience PONV due to stimulation of oculoemetic reflex.[10,15,17] Risk factors for PONV in the pediatric population include (a) age (older than 3 years), (b) duration of surgery (>30 minutes), (c) strabismus surgery, and (d) history or family history of PONV.[18] Based on the patient and their risk factors for PONV, anesthesia providers may choose to use total intravenous anesthesia (TIVA) or inhalational agents during the maintenance phase. There is robust evidence supporting the use of TIVA with propofol in pediatric patients to decrease PONV;[10,15,17] however, TIVA may accentuate the onset of the oculocardiac reflex (OCR).[19] Additionally, a systematic review comparing inhalational agents combined with prophylactic antiemetics to TIVA suggested that they are equally effective in reducing PONV.[20] Furthermore, multimodal techniques, such as hydration (20–30 mL/kg), and administration of dexamethasone (0.15 mg/kg), along with ondansetron (0.1 mg/kg), and avoidance of nitrous oxide, can further decrease the incidence of PONV.[15,21]

Complications/Emergencies

The oculoemetic, oculorespiratory, and oculocardiac reflexes are most stimulated during strabismus surgery. The onset of OCR, also known as Aschner's reflex, is one the most feared complications during eye muscle surgery.[22] OCR is defined as a 20% decrease in baseline heart rate or onset of a new arrhythmia.[10,23] The incidence of OCR is estimated to be up to 80% during strabismus surgery.[10,15,23] Stimulation of the extraocular eye muscle(s) sends signals to the afferent endings of the trigeminal nerve, which may produce a tenacious efferent vagal response, frequently leading to sinus bradycardia.[15] Other fatal arrhythmias that may occur include atrioventricular block and ventricular fibrillation, which can lead to asystole in extreme circumstances.[10,23]

Management of OCR includes (a) swiftly communicating with the surgeon to quickly release traction on the extraocular eye muscle, (b) administering atropine (0.02 mg/kg), and (c) correcting any hypoxia, hypercarbia, and acidosis as this can intensify OCR.[9,22] Anesthesia providers may choose to administer atropine prophylactically to attenuate the OCR.[10,15] Deepening the anesthetic using either sevoflurane or desflurane is also associated with a lower incidence of OCR.[20,23] Surgery should resume once hemodynamics have returned to baseline, and the surgeon should slowly reintroduce traction to prevent another event from occurring.

POSTOPERATIVE CARE

Postoperative ED may present itself as a transient state of psychomotor agitation, in which the patient is typically inconsolable and may be physically aggressive.[10,13] There are many strategies to mitigate ED; however, the literature recommends managing ED with 0.3 to 1 mcg/kg of IV dexmedetomidine, a selective alpha-2 agonist.[10,14]

Pain after strabismus surgery has been reported in up to 65% of patients and is usually treated with narcotics.[24] Respiratory depression, increased PONV, prolonged recovery, and the current global opioid epidemic, are some of the negative effects of narcotic administration in this population. Therefore, nonsteroidal anti-inflammatory drugs and intraoperative use of local anesthetics should be used to manage pain following strabismus surgery.[25] A sub-Tenon's block at the end of the procedure has shown to be superior in decreasing pain in children undergoing strabismus surgery compared with topical lidocaine.[10,24]

CASE STUDY: An Anxious 3-Year-Old Patient Undergoing Strabismus Surgery

CLINICAL SCENARIO

A healthy 3-year-old boy weighing 17 kg is scheduled for correction of unilateral strabismus. The patient has a past medical history of asthma but no surgical history. The surgeon states that the procedure will last 35 minutes.

SPECIAL CONSIDERATIONS

His mother reports that she has experienced severe postoperative nausea and vomiting (PONV) after surgery. The patient is anxious in the preoperative area and is afraid of needles. Formulate an appropriate induction plan.

APPROACHES TO CARE

Evidence-Based Approaches to Care

Nonpharmacological methods should be used prior to administration of sedative agents, such as music or games. Appropriate monitors and resuscitation equipment should be within reach if sedative agents are to be utilized. This patient can safely receive 0.25 mg/kg of midazolam or 1–4 mcg/kg of intranasal dexmedetomidine. The appropriate choice of inhalational agent is sevoflurane. Atropine (0.02 mg/kg) may be administered to prevent oculocardiac reflex (OCR) from occurring. Sevoflurane or propofol (2–3 mg/kg) can be used as the induction agent. An LMA may be beneficial for several reasons: (a) the procedure will be less than 1 hour, and (b) the patient is at risk for bronchospasm.

COMPLICATIONS

This patient's age, family history of PONV, and planned surgery place him at high risk for PONV. Preoperative anxiety may lead to emergence delirium (ED). He is also at risk for a bronchospasm or laryngospasm. Based on provider experience and the patient, a deep extubation may be warranted. Finally, because the patient is having strabismus surgery, he is at risk for onset of OCR.

RESOURCES

1. Nolan JA. Principles of paediatric anaesthesia. *Paediatric Anaesthesia* 2019;20(6):309–313. doi:10.1016/j.mpaic.2019.03.008
2. Waldschmidt B, Gordon N. Anesthesia for pediatric ophthalmologic surgery. *AAPOS*. 2019;23(3):127–131. doi:10.1016/j.jaapos.2018.10.017

KEY REFERENCES

Complete references for this chapter are online and available at https://connect.springerpub.com/content/book/978-0-8261-3875-0/part/part04/toc-part/ch073.

5. Lambert S, Lyons C. *Taylor and Hoyt's Pediatric Ophthalmology and Strabismus*. Elsevier; 2016.
6. Gropper MA, Eriksson LI, Fleischer LA, et al. *Miller's Anesthesia*. Elsevier; 2020.
10. Waldschmidt B, Gordon N. Anesthesia for pediatric ophthalmologic surgery. *J AAPOS*. 2019;23(3):127–131. doi:10.1016/j.jaapos.2018.10.017
12. Heikal S, Stuart G. Anxiolytic premedication for children. *Br J Anaesth*. 2020;20(7):220–225. doi:10.1016/j.bjae.2020.02.006
15. Smith SJ, Pettigrew TY. Anaesthesia for eye surgery in paediatrics. *Ophthalmic Anaesth*. 2019;20(12):721–724. doi:10.1016/j.mpaic.2019.10.009

CHAPTER 74

Nasolacrimal Duct Probing, Irrigation, and Dacryoplasty

Audrey Rosenblatt and Susan P. McMullan

INDICATIONS/CONTRAINDICATIONS

Nasolacrimal duct obstruction (NLDO; Figure 74.1) leads to excessive tearing and mucoid discharge that may require nasolacrimal duct probing with irrigation and/or balloon dacryoplasty to remove debris or dilate the lacrimal duct.[1] Skin irritation, crust of the lashes and rim of the eye, and infection may occur with NLDO as tears are unable to drain from the eye through the lacrimal duct into the sinus. Congenital NLDO is the most common disorder leading to epiphora, which is the abnormal overflow of tears due to excessive secretion of tears or obstruction of the lacrimal drainage passages. Congenital NLDO is caused by either a blockage or a narrowing of the lacrimal duct, often due to a persistence of an embryonic membrane at the valve of Hasner where the distal nasolacrimal duct enters the nose under the inferior turbinate.[1] The bony intrusion of the inferior turbinate can also contribute to the narrowing at this junction. NLDO in early childhood occurs in 5% to 20% of children and often does not require surgery, typically resolving with conservative treatment such as lacrimal duct massage and antibiotics.[2]

SPECIAL CONSIDERATIONS AND CONCERNS

NASOLACRIMAL DUCT PROBING

Superior and inferior puncta are dilated with a punctal dilator. A probe is passed through the canaliculus while gently retracting the upper eyelid.[3] Ductal patency can be confirmed after dilation either by using a small probe inserted through the nose and feeling the metal to metal of the lacrimal probe or by injecting a small bolus of saline colored with fluorescein and suctioning it from the nare. Probing may be performed without anesthesia in the office setting or under general anesthesia in the operating room.

BALLOON DACRYOPLASTY

Balloon dacryoplasty is used if nasolacrimal duct probing has been unsuccessful or if silicone stents have been placed without resolution of symptoms. The procedure begins as described previously followed by introduction of a balloon catheter into the duct. The balloon is then inflated for a period of 60 to 90 seconds before being deflated. This process is repeated as needed, and the position of the balloon dilator may be adjusted.

FIELD AVOIDANCE

As with many ophthalmological procedures, field avoidance is utilized to give the surgeon access to the patient's head. Depending on the layout of the surgical space, ideal positioning is with the anesthesia personnel off to the side of the patient, with the patient turned 90 degrees away from the anesthesia provider. This allows the anesthesia provider to intervene if needed during the procedure while allowing the surgeon room to operate.

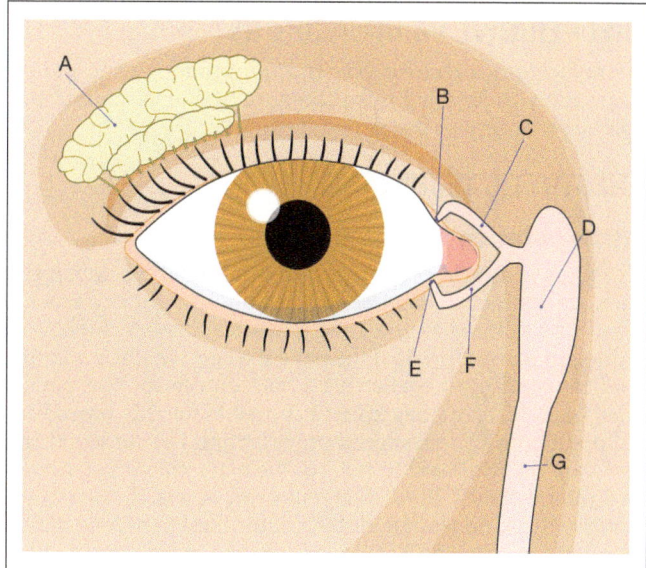

Figure 74.1: Tear system. (A) Tear/lacrimal gland. (B) Superior lacrimal punctum. (C) Superior lacrimal canal. (D) Lacrimal duct. (E) Inferior lacrimal punctum. (F) Inferior lacrimal canal. (G) Nasolacrimal canal.

Source: From Melnyk J, Zeno R, Teall AM. Evidence-based assessment of the eye. In: Gawlik KS, Melnyk BM, Teall AM, eds. *Evidence-Based Physical Examination: Best Practices for Health and Well-Being Assessment.* Springer Publishing Company. 2021;327, Fig. 12.38.

EMERGENCE DELIRIUM

Emergence delirium is a risk for this patient population given the average patient age, short duration of the procedure, and use of inhalation anesthetic agents.[4] Informed anesthesia consent for these patients should include the risk for emergence delirium and information for the parents on what postoperative behavior they might experience when they join their child in the recovery room. Using elbow restraints in immediate postanesthesia recovery may be used to protect the eye from aggressive rubbing as the patient emerges from anesthesia but should be removed as soon as the patient has emerged from anesthesia.

ANESTHESIA MANAGEMENT

PREOPERATIVE EVALUATION

NLDO occurs in otherwise healthy children, as well as in children with facial dysmorphic syndromes.[1] Unless the child has other indicators of syndromic or genetic abnormalities, the presence of nasal lacrimal duct obstruction would not indicate concern in this regard. There is no increased incidence of malignant hyperthermia in this patient population, beyond the general increased risk in pediatrics. A thorough preoperative evaluation, as with any preanesthetic assessment, is indicated including a review of systems, NPO status, anesthesia history, family anesthesia history, and preoperative anxiety assessment. This procedure is not emergent, and proper preoperative optimization is indicated.

PREOPERATIVE PHARMACOLOGY

Premedication for anxiolysis is appropriate for the patient population undergoing this procedure in the presence of preoperative anxiety or per parental request.

ANESTHETIC TECHNIQUE

Intraoperative Management

NLDO is a quick procedure with minimal postoperative pain. Anesthesia management is usually straightforward and should be tailored to the child's medical history. Inhalation induction is appropriate if the patient's age, weight, and other medical conditions make this a safe choice for the patient otherwise. Mask management is possible for this procedure, although both the anesthesia provider and the surgeon must be aware that the need to remove the mask from the patient's face intermittently to facilitate surgeon access to the patient may result in inadequate depth of anesthesia, laryngospasm, or patient movement. For this reason, the placement of either a laryngeal mask airway or endotracheal tube for the duration of the procedure is ideal as it allows the ophthalmologist unimpeded access to the patient's face to perform the procedure in addition to ensuring a consistent and appropriate anesthetic depth is provided.

Securing IV access is at the anesthesia provider's discretion. This is a procedure in which IV placement may be safely avoided; however, anesthesia providers must remain vigilant given the risk for laryngospasm.[5] After dilation of the lacrimal duct, fluorescein is instilled into the lacrimal duct and subsequently suctioned from the nares to ensure patency of the lacrimal duct and success of the procedure. Careful observation of the volume of injected fluid is warranted as increased fluid or secretions in the nasopharynx or oropharynx may increase the risk of laryngospasm, which is especially problematic if the patient does not have an IV. As with any procedure where an IV is not placed, the management of intraoperative complications is more challenging until IV access is secured.

Complications/Emergencies

Potential complications associated with nasolacrimal duct probing, irrigation, and dacryoplasty include creation of a false passage and injury to the nasolacrimal duct, canaliculi and puncta, bleeding, laryngospasm, or aspiration.

POSTOPERATIVE CARE

Nasolacrimal duct probing and balloon dacryoplasty do not result in significant postoperative pain, nor are they particularly stimulating during the intraoperative course. Pain relief can be accomplished with intramuscular or intravenous ketorolac, oral or rectal acetaminophen, and less commonly small doses of narcotic medications. Bradycardia due to stimulation of the oculocardiac reflex is rare during this procedure as the muscles of the eye are not retracted.[6]

REFERENCES

1. Petris C, Liu, D. Probing for congenital nasolacrimal duct obstruction. *Cochrane Database Syst. Rev.* 2017;7(7):CD011109. doi:10.1002/14651858.CD011109.pub2
2. Durrani J. Crigler massage for congenital blockade of nasolacrimal duct. *J Coll Physicians Surg Pak JCPSP*. 2017;27(3):145–148.
3. Valcheva KP, Murgova SV, Krivoshiiska EK. Success rate of probing for congenital nasolacrimal duct obstruction in children. *Folia Med*. 2019;61(1):97–103. doi:10.2478/folmed-2018-0054
4. Mehrotra S. Postoperative anaesthetic concerns in children: postoperative pain, emergence delirium and postoperative nausea and vomiting. *Indian J. Anaesth*. 2019;63(9):763–770. doi:10.4103/ija.IJA_391_19
5. Hung CW, Licina L, Abramson DH, Arslan-Carlon V. Anesthetic complications during general anesthesia without intravenous access in pediatric ophthalmologic clinic: assessment of 5216 cases. *Minerva Anestesiol*. 2017;83(7):712–719. doi:10.23736/S0375-9393.17.11565-8
6. Ducloyer JB, Couret C, Magne C, et al. Prospective evaluation of anesthetic protocols during pediatric ophthalmic surgery. *Eur. J. Ophthalmol*. 2019;29(6):606–614. doi:10.1177/1120672118804798

CHAPTER 75

Retinal Surgery

Suzanne M. Wright

INDICATIONS/CONTRAINDICATIONS

Pediatric patients present for a wide variety of ophthalmic surgeries in large part for conditions related to congenital defects, injury, and infection. It is imperative that anesthesia providers have a sound understanding of the disease processes and surgical techniques related to retinal surgery as this special patient population poses unique challenges. This chapter discusses the indications for pediatric retinal surgery, as well as the anesthetic management in this special patient population including preoperative evaluation, pharmacology, anesthetic technique, and postoperative care.

The retina is a mutiple-layer structure that contains the sensory receptors of the eye. Also called photoreceptors, these sensory receptors include the rods, which detect dim light and are mainly responsible for black and white and night vision, and the cones, which are responsible for color vision. After light passes through the ocular lens, it passes through various layers of the retina before stimulating the rods and cones, thereby sending impulses that travel through successive layers of neurons in the retina, the optic nerves, and, finally, the cerebral (visual) cortex in the brain (Figure 75.1). The macular area lies in the center of the retina. The fovea is a small area located in the center of the macula and plays a significant role in acute and detailed vision largely due to the action of the central foveola, an area even smaller than the fovea, which is composed of a high concentration of specialized cones.[1]

The central retinal artery and the choroidal circulation supply oxygen and nutrients to the retina. The central retinal artery provides blood supply to the inner portion of the retina and the choroid, by way of the posterior ciliary arteries, provides oxygen and nutrients to the outer areas of the retina. Both the central retinal artery and the choroid arise from the ophthalmic artery, the first branch of the internal carotid artery, which passes through the optic canal near the optic nerve.[1]

It is essential that the retina and retinal structures are healthy and functioning properly in order for vision to be optimal. Most retinal disorders involve disruption in the transmission of impulses from the lens to the sensory receptors. The treatment of retinal disorders varies widely depending on the type of disease but can include laser treatment, eye drops or other medications, observation and monitoring, or surgery.

Of all eye surgeries, retinal surgery in particular is less common in the pediatric population than in the adult population. Indications for retinal surgery in the newborn, for example, may include congenital conditions and tractional retinal detachments (RDs) related to retinopathy of prematurity (ROP), persistent fetal vasculature, or familial exudative vitreoretinopathy (FEVR). As a child advances in age, trauma becomes another significant etiologic factor.[2]

RETINAL DETACHMENT

Retinal surgery is usually indicated as a result of detachment of the retina (Figure 75.2). When the retina becomes detached

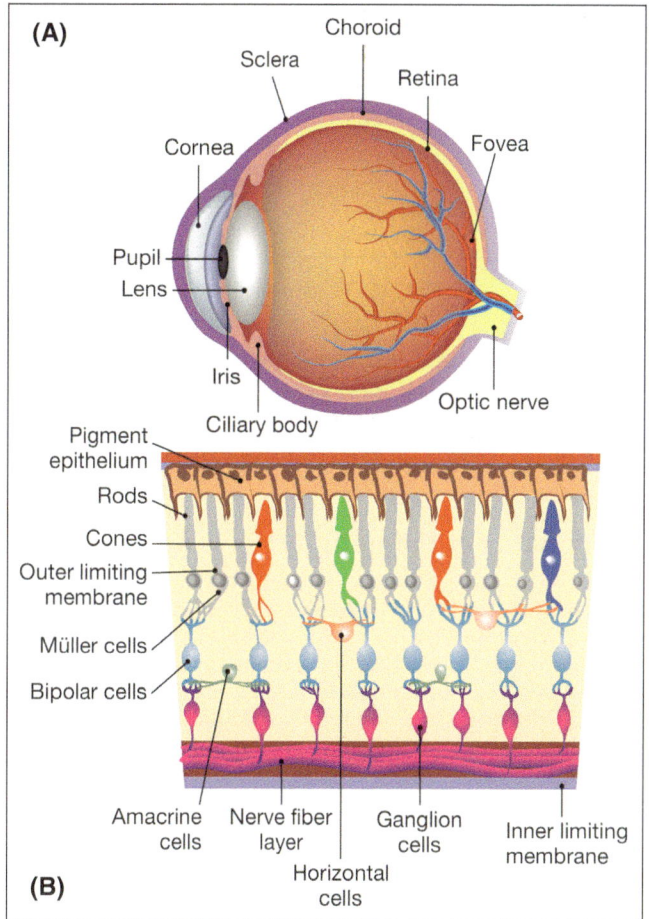

Figure 75.1: Anatomy of the retina. (A) Location within the eye. (B) Specialized pigmented and neural layers.

Source: From Melnyk J, Zeno R, Teall AM. Evidence-Based Assessment of the Eye. In KS Gawlik, BM Melnyk, AM Teall, eds. *Evidence-Based Physical Examination: Best Practices for Health and Well-Being Assessment.* Springer; 2021:311, Fig. 12.10.

or lifts away from the back of the eye, it cannot function properly resulting in the perception of flashing lights, cobweb-like floaters, or shadows. A detached retina should be treated as a medical emergency, and timely attention from an ophthalmologist is necessary to avoid the loss of sight in the eye. Early diagnosis and treatment have been reported to be more difficult in infants and children, in many cases, but are necessary to halt the progression of retinal diseases.

Retinal detachment (RD) is less common in the pediatric population with an annual incidence of 0.38 to 0.69/100,000 and mean and median ages for children of 9 and 13 years, respectively.[3] Procedures requiring anesthesia may be necessary to repair recurring RDs or incomplete repairs. In the case of a subsequent retinal tear, it is important for the surgeon to distinguish a dialysis, a retinal tear with specific

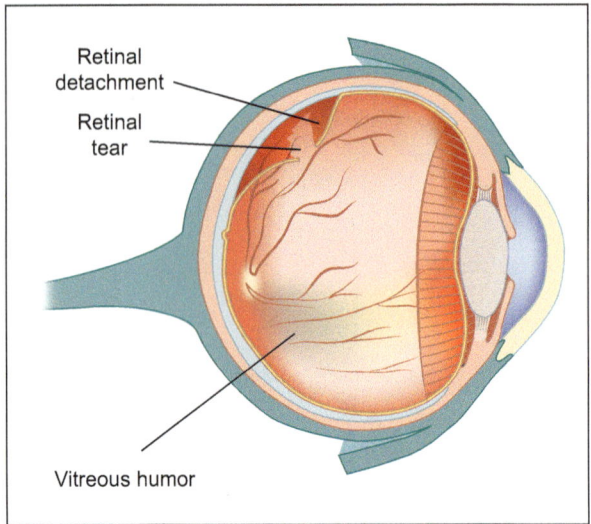

Figure 75.2: Retinal detachment.

characteristics, from a larger tear, to determine which type of retinal surgery is indicated. Ocular trauma, especially blunt trauma with blood in the anterior chamber of the eye and posterior chamber involvement, can lead to later RD or glaucoma. Lifelong follow-up is important to assess for complications.

Retinopathy of Prematurity

ROP is a disorder of the developing retinal blood vessels in preterm infants who are low birth weight and is a leading cause of childhood blindness. These abnormal blood vessels are fragile and can leak thereby scarring the retina and pulling it out of position, resulting in RD. Most full-term infants have fully developed retinas and retinal vasculature; under normal gestational terms, conditions do not support the development of ROP. In preterm infants, however the development of the retina is incomplete, and the degree of immaturity of the retina is largely related to the extent of prematurity at birth.[4] Any delay in the diagnosis or treatment of ROP can result in permanent blindness. Therefore, it is important that at-risk infants are identified and screened as early as possible. It is important to remember that not all infants with the disease will necessarily require surgical treatment.

Rhegmatogenous Retinal Detachment

Rhegmatogenous retinal detachment (RRD) is a common form of RD that occurs in approximately 12.4 persons per 100,000 population and results from a tear or break in the retina. As vitreous gel accumulates under the retina due to the tear, the retina pulls away from the nourishing layer beneath it. In children younger than 18 years of age, RDD accounts for 3.2% to 5.6% of all cases of RD. It is ideal to avoid surgically entering pediatric eyes whenever possible; typically, the repair of pediatric RRD is with scleral buckling, which is discussed later in this chapter.[5]

X-linked retinoschisis (XLRS) is a juvenile onset retinal degenerative condition seen mostly in males with a prevalence of 1 in 25,000 to 1 in 5,000.[6] XLRS is the result of a genetic mutation that miscodes for retinoschisin, a protein that helps in cellular adhesion as well as in cell-to-cell interaction. It typically manifests in the first decade of life with poor of vision resulting from splitting of the retinal layers and involves the fovea. Complications including rhegmatogenous and/or tractional RD, vitreous hemorrhage (VH), progressive disease involving the macula, and hemorrhage can occur suddenly, which may require surgical intervention. RRD is seen in 10% to 22% of cases with XLRS.[7]

Trauma-Related Retinal Detachment

Another cause of RD in the pediatric population is ocular trauma in which a penetrating injury occurs from a foreign object that has become embedded in the eye. Managing pediatric patients with retinal trauma requires an individualized approach. No two trauma cases are alike, and there is insufficient scientific evidence to recommend one particular surgical or medical approach to management or treatment over another.[8] If surgery is indicated, it can be staged to allow for stabilizing the patient if other injuries exist. The prompt removal of intraocular foreign bodies (IOFBs) and closure of the globe in open globe injuries are the top priorities, followed by vitrectomy to prevent or repair RD. Other surgical treatments may be necessary to optimize vision outcomes depending on the extent and individual characteristics of the trauma.[8]

Imaging studies may be necessary in the management of pediatric patients with retinal trauma. Preoperative B-scan ultrasonography can be used to assess choroidal or RDs or IOFBs in self-sealing wounds but might better be avoided in open-globe injuries or injuries that include a protruding IOFB. A B-scan, short for brightness scan, offers a two-dimensional cross-sectional view of the eye as well as its orbit. A B-scan is used on the outside of the closed eyelid to view the structures beneath. If it confirmed an IOFB does not contain metal, magnetic resonance imaging (MRI) scanning should be considered because it reduces radiation exposure when compared with a CT scan. If there is any chance the IOFB contains metal, MRI scanning is contraindicated, and a computed tomography (CT) scan can be performed.[8]

Surgery for pediatric retinal trauma is often performed at a pediatric hospital so that pediatric anesthesia providers and other pediatric experts are available to provide care in the event there are other extensive injuries. The proper equipment and an operating room (OR) team with expertise in treating pediatric retinal trauma emergencies are critical. Special knowledge related to the operative setup, equipment, and surgical processes as well as the ability to troubleshoot problems and anticipate operative needs are essential.

Pediatric retinal trauma often also involves other areas of the eye, and providers with specialized knowledge of the anterior segment of the eye, oculoplastics, glaucoma, and pediatric ophthalmology may be called on. In infants and young children, media opacity from corneal scars, vitreous hemorrhage, and cataracts can cause amblyopia, or lazy eye, so it is important that a pediatric ophthalmologist develops a plan to minimize this adverse condition through postoperative visual rehabilitation.

Exudative Retinal Detachment

Exudative RD, which involves a collection of fluid in the subretinal space, is rare and may be caused secondary to ocular syndromes such as Coats disease. Coats disease is a congenital nonhereditary sporadic retinal vascular disease characterized by telangiectasia, subretinal and intraretinal exudation, and exudative RD.[9] The disease may be complicated by vitreous hemorrhage, neovascular glaucoma, or phthisis bulbi, a shrunken, nonfunctioning eye. Coats disease occurs most commonly in young males and is classified into five stages. The medical management and prognosis depend largely on the stage of disease at presentation. The aim of treatment is to preserve the vision and the globe.[10] If diagnosed early, a laser can be used to constrict the abnormal blood vessels and stop the leakage of fluid. In more advanced stages where partial or complete detachment of the retina has occurred, surgery will likely be necessary.

FEVR is a genetic condition that affects the blood vessels that support the retina. Patients with FEVR may be asymptomatic, but the disease can cause a wide variety of eye issues, including bleeding and RD. In the case of FEVR, treatment with laser or surgery may be performed.

Tractional Retinal Detachment

Another rare form of RD is tractional RD and in the pediatric population is usually caused by vasoproliferative diseases, such as ROP, FEVR, incontinentia pigmenti (IP), and developmental diseases such as persistent fetal vasculature (PFV) and trauma (as discussed earlier).[11]

SPECIAL CONSIDERATIONS AND CONCERNS

See Box 75.1 for a summary of special considerations and concerns in the anesthetic management of retinal surgery.

ANESTHETIC MANAGEMENT

There are special anesthetic considerations related to the preoperative, intraoperative, and postoperative phases for the pediatric patient presenting for retinal surgery. A systematic approach that considers these phases can contribute to the development of an individualized plan of care that thoughtfully incorporates all patient and surgical factors as well as ways in which these factors may influence outcomes.

PREOPERATIVE EVALUATION

Generally speaking, anesthesia providers should perform and document or verify documentation of a preanesthesia evaluation that includes an assessment of the patient's general health, allergies, medication history, preexisting conditions, anesthesia history, and any relevant diagnostic tests.[13] The comprehensive medical history, history of current illness, and physical examination should be performed with goals to (a) identify and minimize risks related to the patient and surgery, (b) establish an individualized plan of care, and (c) optimize surgical outcomes and safety.

The preoperative evaluation should uncover acute and chronic medical problems and the extent to which they are adequately managed, as well as screen for any family history or history of complications related to anesthesia, including malignant hyperthermia (MH). It is not unusual for children who present for retinal surgery to have other systemic physical conditions, of which the anesthesia provider should be mindful. These conditions may be related to, for example, retinoblastoma, Coats disease, Aicardi syndrome, a rare genetic disorder that interferes with the formation of the corpus callosum, or Stickler syndrome, a group of hereditary conditions characterized by facial deformities, eye abnormalities, hearing loss, and joint problems.[14]

Gathering information about previous eye conditions and eye surgeries and verifying the correct eye for the current surgery are important to avoid unnecessary complications. For example, the use of nitrous oxide should be avoided after recent retinal surgery that involved the placement of an expandable gas bubble. Also, surgery times may be longer than expected in patients who have had multiple eye surgeries. The correct surgical site should always be verified and reverified. Laterality misjudgments in ophthalmic surgeries are rarely mentioned in the medical literature, but the results can be devastating.[15] The American Academy of Ophthalmology updated a universal protocol in 2014 to prevent confusions of side in eye surgeries. The protocol recommends implementation of a consistent approach before surgeries, such as preoperative verification, site marking, and time-out procedures.[16]

Although surgical procedures on the eye in adults are frequently performed using local anesthesia, children undergoing retinal surgery will nearly always require general anesthesia with or without orbital regional anesthesia.[17] General anesthesia necessitates IV catheter placement and the use of a laryngeal mask airway or endotracheal tube if neuromuscular blocking medications are used, due to the length of the procedure and the need to move the head of the stretcher away from the anesthesia provider. A meticulous airway assessment and adequate preparation for the management of a difficult airway are invaluable for adept management of the airway.

Retinal surgery can be elective, urgent, or emergent; therefore, special attention to the patient's NPO status is necessary to avoid complications related to pulmonary aspiration. Infants and children with a full stomach who present for retinal surgery should be identified as a pulmonary aspiration risk and treated accordingly with rapid sequence induction while avoiding unnecessary increases in intraocular pressure (IOP). Sudden increases in IOP in patients with an open globe injury can lead to vitreous loss and blindness. It is important

---

BOX 75.1 SPECIAL CONSIDERATIONS AND CONCERNS: RETINAL DETACHMENT

- Pediatric patients have smaller eyes with anatomical and surgical landmarks that differ from adults. Surgeons must appreciate and anesthesia providers must be aware of such anatomical differences when retinal surgeries are performed in this population.[12]
- The pediatric eye has a shorter axial length and a larger lens relative to the size of the globe. There are more adherent vitreoretinal attachments, and the eye may be affected by congenital anatomic abnormalities.[2]
- It can be challenging to obtain an accurate understanding of patient symptoms or history of trauma from a pediatric patient because they are often unable to describe what happened, and if the trauma was not witnessed or is associated with abuse, accurate details may not be obtained from adults.
- Imaging studies may be necessary in the management of pediatric patients with retinal trauma to detect choroidal or RDs or the orientation of intraocular foreign bodies. Anesthesia services may be requested and necessary for preoperative imaging.
- Subsequent procedures may be needed to repair RD. Pediatric patients may present with unusual levels of fear and anxiety if they are required to return for multiple surgeries on the eye.

to try to avoid situations that may increase IOP and therefore risk further eye damage including straining related to crying, coughing, and vomiting, an improperly placed anesthesia face mask, and succinylcholine.

Anticipating the needs of the surgeon and surgery in the preoperative period can facilitate a successful surgical outcome and contribute to a swift intraoperative course. Because retinal pathologies vary greatly from patient to patient and the surgical approach to treating retinal disorders varies from surgeon to surgeon, communication with the surgeon about disease characteristics, surgical approach, positioning of the patient, and critical points of the surgery allows the anesthesia provider to make the best practice decisions and to be prepared to respond quickly to the patient's changing condition. For example, most cases of RD result in decreased IOP as a result of increased outflow by active pumping of fluid through the exposed retinal pigment epithelium. Conversely, in the case of Schwartz-Matsuo syndrome, there is elevated IOP associated with RRD.[19] In this instance, efforts to avoid medications and interventions that increase IOP should be weighed against their benefit. A brief but focused discussion about each case is helpful in establishing an appropriate anesthetic plan of care.

ANESTHETIC MANAGEMENT

Intraoperative Management

Surgical procedures that address retinal pathologies in the pediatric population are usually those designed to treat retinal detachment and are most likely to include vitrectomy, scleral band or buckle (Figure 75.3), and pneumatic retinopexy (tamponade). The choice of surgical procedure depends on clinical and anatomical features and patient characteristics with goals to improve visual acuity through sustained retinal attachment.[21.] Table 75.1 describes various surgical approaches to retinal surgery.

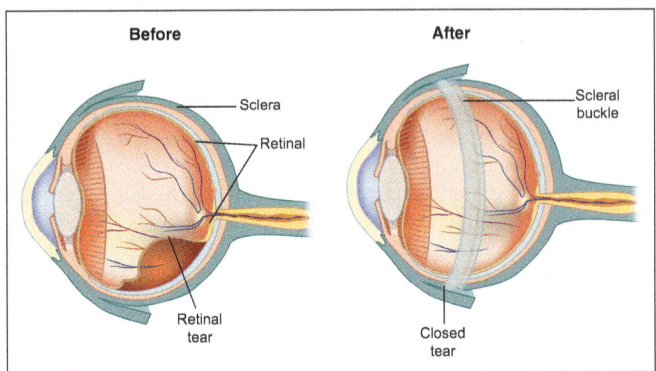

Figure 75.3: Scleral band or buckle in treatment of retinal detachment.

Patients lie supine for retinal surgery, and standard monitoring that assesses the patient's oxygenation, ventilation, circulation, neuromuscular status, level of consciousness and temperature should be utilized for continuous evaluation of the patient's physiologic condition. In certain circumstances of higher American Society of Anesthesiologists (ASA) classification, advanced monitoring may be considered. Depending on the patient's age and comorbidities, an appropriately sized IV catheter is placed either preoperatively or following induction of general anesthesia.

The anesthesia work environment can be challenging during retinal surgical cases. The procedure or operating room can be extremely dark due to the retinal specialist's use of a light pipe to illuminate the posterior segment of the eye in order to optimize the surgical field. It can be difficult for the anesthesia provider to visualize the patient, medication

Table 75.1	Retinal Surgeries in the Pediatric Population
Type of Surgery	**Description**
Pars plana vitrectomy (PPV)	• PPV involves the removal of vitreous humor, the gel-like substance that fills the posterior segment (vitreous chamber) of the eye, to facilitate the attachment of the retina to the back of the eye. The posterior segment is accessed through the pars plana, commonly identified as the anatomical safe zone through which microsurgical tools, lenses, illuminating devices, and lasers can be introduced into the eye to avoid damage to the retina and lens. The pars plana may not be developed in eyes less than 7 years old, so a different approach to vitrectomy may be used.[22]
Scleral band or buckle	• Scleral buckle surgery or scleral banding involves the surgical placement of a silicone band from one side of the eye, across the back of the eye, to the other side of the eye to bring the eye closer to the retina that has torn away from its foundation. The band provides support to allow for healing that will sustain the surgical retinal attachment.
Pneumatic retinopexy (PR)	• PR is the least invasive method to reattach the retina and involves the injection of an expandable gas or silicone oil along with retinal cryotherapy or laser photocoagulation to seal retinal breaks. PR works best for small superior retinal breaks.[23] The use of silicone oil as a retinal tamponade is preferred over expandable gas in some children because of difficulties with postoperative positioning and IOP monitoring. Silicone oil also allows for earlier visual rehabilitation, which is especially important in the younger population who are at risk for amblyopia.[22]
	• If expandable gas is used for PR, it is imperative to avoid the use of nitrous oxide. Nitrous oxide will rapidly diffuse into the gas bubble and alter its size, resulting in rapid expansion of the bubble and an acute rise in pressure within the globe causing irreversible ischemic damage to the retina and optic nerve. These gases may remain in the eye for several weeks, and patients and their caregivers should be given very clear instructions about communicating this information to anesthesia providers in the event other surgery is necessary during this time.

labels, syringes, markings on the anesthesia machine, and other equipment such as flow meters. Unlike laparoscopic surgeries that require the room lights to be dimmed but allow for a reasonable degree of light during the case, retinal surgical cases demand nearly complete room darkness.

In some retinal surgeries, laser photocoagulation may be performed to seal a retinal tear to stop the progression to complete RD, a potentially blinding condition. Retinal laser photocoagulation can also be used to seal or destroy leaking blood vessels to prevent further retinal damage and preserve sight. Laser photocoagulation creates scar tissue to stop a tear from growing larger and can repair leaking blood vessels and slow neovascularization in the eye.[10,22] In rooms where the laser is being utilized, all providers must wear protective eyewear, which further compromises the ability to see.

Additionally, the anesthesia provider can expect that the head of the bed, and therefore, the patient's airway will be turned away from the anesthetizing area, where the anesthesia cart and anesthesia machine are located. As in most ophthalmic cases, it is critical to avoid patient movement or movement of the stretcher or anything attached to it during retinal surgeries.

Many children requiring retinal surgery will be taking or may be administered medications in the perioperative period. A basic knowledge of commonly used preparations of eye drops and their potential effects is especially useful. There is a risk that these medications could be absorbed through the pharyngeal mucosa via the nasolacrimal ducts, resulting in adverse systemic effects.

Newborns and infants are especially subject to the systemic side effects of eye drop medications. The eye of a newborn is approximately two thirds of its adult size and does not fully develop until around the age of 3 or 4 years. The ocular membranes of newborns and infants are much thinner than those in adults allowing for more rapid drug absorption. Lower tear volume in this same group can lead to a higher concentration of topically applied medications.[26] Therefore, it is estimated that, as a guide, a newborn may require only one-half of the adult dosage of eye drops to obtain an equivalent ocular concentration. Similarly, about two thirds of the adult dosage is required at the age of 3 years, while it reaches 90% at the age of 6 years.[27] Ocular dosing is not weight-adjusted, and, therefore, pediatric patients are particularly vulnerable to dosing as drug metabolism is reduced in the young and an immature blood–brain barrier may be present.

It is important to understand the concentration and be mindful of dosing of all medications, including those delivered as "eye drops" to avoid unintentional adverse effects. Table 75.2 lists commonly used ocular medications with indications and potential side effects.

POSTOPERATIVE CARE

The postoperative care of children presenting for retinal surgery mirrors postoperative care of the pediatric patient after other eye surgeries and includes monitoring for early recognition of issues related to general anesthesia and surgery. Inadequate oxygenation, cardiovascular instability, pain, postoperative nausea and vomiting, and emergence delirium should be anticipated and a plan to address these swiftly and effectively should be in place.[24]

More specific to retinal surgery, postoperative discomfort has been described as achy, itchy, and scratchy, much like sand or an eyelash in the eye. The presence of an eye patch to prevent accidental injury, reduce pain that may be caused by light exposure, or limit swelling can further aggravate infants and children as they are in recovery. Care should be given to

Table 75.2	Commonly Used Eye Preparations With Indications and Potential Systemic Effects	
Eye Preparation	**Indication**	**Systemic Side Effect**
Beta-blockers: Timolol maleate Betaxolol hydrochloride	Glaucoma	Bradycardia refractory to atropine Bronchospasm in asthmatics
Carbonic anhydrase inhibitors: Acetazolamide (Diamox)	Glaucoma	Metabolic acidosis Electrolyte abnormalities Allergies (*avoid in those allergic to sulfonamide*) Stevens–Johnson syndrome
Antimuscarinic agents: Cylopentolate Atropine	Pupil dilation	Dry mucous membranes Nausea, vomiting Tachycardia
Alpha-adrenergic sympathomimetic agents: Phenylephrine 2.5%	Pupil dilation	Hypertension Tachycardia
NSAIDs: Diclofenac sodium Ketorolac trometamol 0.5%	Analgesia	Worsen acute asthma
Local anesthetic agents: Amethocaine (Tetracaine) Oxybuprocaine Proxymetacaine	Analgesia	Local anesthetic toxicity (*especially in preterm infants*)
Steroids: Dexamethasone Prednisolone	Treat inflammation (redness, swelling, itching)	None Headache, itching, and dysgeusia

NSAIDs, non-steroidal anti-inflammatory drugs.

be sure the eyelid is closed and that the cornea is protected beneath the eye patch. It is not uncommon to see blood-tinged tears or fluid drainage, and caution should be given to the administration of aspirin or nonsteroidal analgesics due to their association with an increased risk of bleeding.

Special attention will be given during the postoperative phase to infection prevention through universal precautions (e.g., strict handwashing and antibiotic eye drops). Other eye drop medications ordered in the postoperative phase may include cycloplegics, a class of medications that paralyze the ciliary muscle and lower the risk of adhesions and pain, and steroids, which reduce the risk of inflammation thereby reducing pain, photophobia, and the formation of adhesions.[25]

KEY REFERENCES

Complete references for this chapter are online and available at https://connect.springerpub.com/content/book/978-0-8261-3875-0/part/part04/toc-part/ch075.

2. Baumal CR, Berrocal AM. Pearls for pediatric retinal surgery. *Retina Today*. July/August 2018:32–34.
8. Hartnett ME. Pediatric trauma requires an individual approach. *Retina Today*. July/August 2018:35–40.
9. Amer R, Hilal N, Yalcindag N. Exudative retinal detachment. *Surv Ophthal*. 2017;62(6):723–769. doi:10.1016/j.survophthal.2017.05.001
10. Nuzzi R, Lavia C, Spinetta R. Paediatric retinal detachment: a review. *Int J Ophthalmol*. 2017;10(10). doi:10.18240/ijo.2017.10.18
11. Balakrishnan D. Pediatric retinal detachment: an overview. *Kerala J Ophthalmol*. 2018;30:87–93. doi:10.4103/kjo.kjo_32_18
12. Gan NY, Lam W. Special considerations for pediatric vitreoretinal surgery. *Taiwan J Ophthalmol*. 2018;8(4):237–242. doi:10.4103/tjo.tjo_83_18
17. Sekhara C, Rajiva I. Balanced anaesthesia for paediatric ophthalmic procedures. J *Anest & Inten Care Med*. 2017;2(3):555–590. doi: 10.19080/JAICM.2017.01.555590
21. Read SP, Aziz HA, Kuriyan A, et al. Retinal detachment surgery in a pediatric population: visual and anatomic outcomes. *Retina*. 2018;38(7):1393–1402. doi:10.1097/IAE.0000000000001725
22. Torrado LA, Fivgas GD. *Surgical Treatment in Pediatric Retinal Detachment* American Academy of Ophthalmology. 2020. https://www.aao.org/disease-review/surgical-treatment-in-pediatric-retinal-detachment
24. Mehrotra S. Postoperative anaesthetic concerns in children: postoperative pain, emergence delirium and postoperative nausea and vomiting. *Indian J Anaesth*. 2019; 63(9):763–770. doi:10.4103/ija.IJA_391_19

CHAPTER 76

Ptosis Repair

Audrey Rosenblatt and Susan P. McMullan

INDICATIONS/CONTRAINDICATIONS

Congenital blepharoptosis (ptosis) is characterized by a drooping eyelid appearance that can obscure visual field and thus visual development via deprivational amblyopia (**Figure 76.1**).[1] Ptosis can be either unilateral (more common and usually the left eye) or bilateral.[2] Its origin is either neurological, mediated by cranial nerve III, or neuromuscular, involving the levator palpebral superioris muscle and the superior rectus muscle.[3] Ptosis may be hereditary, presenting in the absence of a genetic syndrome, or may occur in association with a wider spectrum of birth defects and ocular conditions.[4] If eyelid closure is complete, this surgery may be performed during infancy. Otherwise, surgical correction of congenital blepharoptosis is generally performed in later childhood.

SPECIAL CONSIDERATIONS AND CONCERNS

SURGICAL INTERVENTIONS

Surgical correction of congenital blepharoptosis can be accomplished by a variety of surgical interventions including frontalis sling, levator resection, Muller's muscle resection, Whitnall ligament sling, and the Fasanella–Servat procedure.[3] The goal of each of these procedures is eliminating the obstruction in the field of vision secondary to the drooping eyelid. None of these procedures is intraocular, with all involving incisions in either the eyelid and/or the brow. The anesthesia requirements for the varying surgical interventions are not significantly different. The sole exception is when an autologous fascia lata is harvested from the lateral thigh for a frontalis sling, in which case surgical positioning changes as does postoperative pain relief management.[3]

POSTOPERATIVE EYELID IMMOBILIZATION

Anesthesia providers should be aware of the methods used to prevent surgical disruption of the eyelid following surgical intervention. The surgeon can employ a variety of protection measures, such as the application of a "frost" silk suture stitch, which holds the lower and upper lids together by anchoring them to the brow; use of skin closure strips; an eye pad; transparent adhesive dressing; and/or an eye shield. With young children, elbow immobilizers may be applied

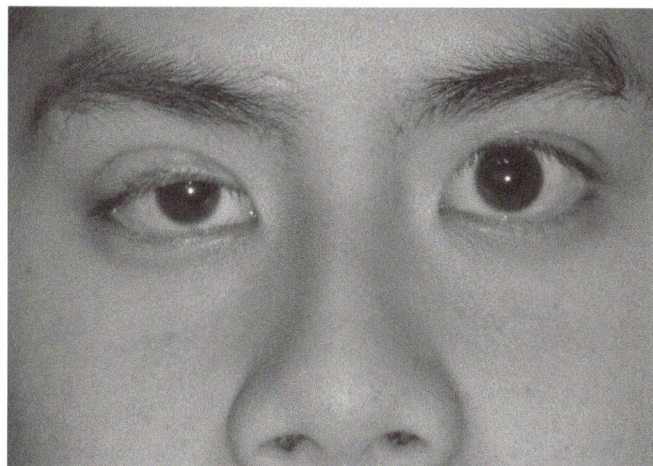

Figure 76.1: Ptosis of the right upper eyelid.
Source: Chiocca EM. *Advanced Pediatric Assessment*, 3rd ed. Springer. 2019;326. Fig. 15.7.

prior to emergence from anesthesia to prevent rubbing of the eye or face and subsequent injury to the surgical site. Eyelid immobilization or closure may result in significant distress for the child during the postanesthesia recovery period. Age-appropriate psychological preparation is important, and medications to facilitate a smooth emergence from anesthesia, such as dexmedetomidine, narcotics, and benzodiazepines, are often indicated.

ANESTHETIC MANAGEMENT

PREOPERATIVE EVALUATION

Congenital blepharoptosis may be associated with genetic syndromes that have anesthetic implications beyond those associated with the ptosis surgery alone. A thorough preoperative evaluation should include a review of systems, with careful assessment of any constellation of symptoms indicative of a genetic syndrome.[1] For children presenting with a diagnosed genetic syndrome, a thorough review of the associated anesthesia considerations for that syndrome must be completed by the anesthesia provider prior to the start of the procedure.

PREOPERATIVE PHARMACOLOGY

Premedication with an anxiolytic is appropriate as indicated and may help smooth emergence through synergistic interaction with intraoperative narcotics and alpha-2 adrenergic agonists.[5] If available, child life specialists can bolster preoperative preparation by providing age-appropriate information regarding eyelid immobilization in the postoperative period.

ANESTHETIC TECHNIQUE

Intraoperative Management

Congenital blepharoptosis repair varies in length depending on the degree of surgical correction required and surgical technique utilized.[3] General anesthesia is indicated, and intraoperative anesthesia management should be adaptable to variations in length of surgical procedure. An inhalation induction is appropriate providing there are no patient factors precluding this from being a safe choice. Placement of a single peripheral IV catheter is indicated for this procedure. Neuromuscular blocking drugs are not contraindicated, so muscle paralysis prior to intubation is acceptable although generally not required. Airway management can be accomplished with either a laryngeal mask airway (LMA) or an endotracheal tube. The decision regarding airway management should be guided by the anticipated length of the procedure; need for a secure airway without the necessity to intervene during the surgical procedure; likelihood of the need for positive pressure ventilation; and risk of fire when using electrocautery around the face. Accordingly, these authors preferentially use an oral Ring–Adair–Elwyn (RAE) endotracheal tube for this procedure for the aforementioned reasons.

Surgical positioning is supine, with the exception of when a fascia lata harvest from the lateral thigh is indicated for a frontalis sling. In this scenario, the patient is placed supine with the leg bent at the knee and flexed medially across the body, thereby shifting the hips and exposing the lateral thigh.[4] The patient is secured in this position with tape, so it is imperative that the tape does not create pressure on a bony prominence and careful padding is used to prevent peripheral nerve damage. Surgical positioning should be done in collaboration with surgery and nursing.

Complications/Emergencies

Unless there are associated genetic syndromes with unique anesthesia considerations, complications are generally related to the surgical repair and include undercorrection, overcorrection, corneal staining, ectropion, entropion, and a loss of lashes. Undercorrection is a complication encountered more frequently in surgery for congenital ptosis.

POSTOPERATIVE CARE

Postoperative pain, nausea and vomiting, and emergence agitation and delirium are the main postoperative morbidities that the anesthesia care plan should address. A less common complication is cardiac arrhythmia, especially the risk for bradycardia and nodal dysrhythmias triggered by the oculocardiac reflex.[3] Although this occurs less frequently than during eye muscle surgery for strabismus or esotropia, it may occur and is more likely in patients who have Marcus Gunn (jaw-winking) syndrome.[6] If bradycardia occurs, the first step is to request the surgeon cease surgical manipulation and release any applied tension, possibly followed by the administration of IV atropine should the bradycardia not resolve. Postoperative pain can be managed with narcotic pain medication and nonnarcotic adjuncts, such as ketorolac and acetaminophen. The addition of a lateral femoral cutaneous peripheral nerve block for fascia lata harvest provides optimal pain relief and is a welcome addition to a general anesthetic for postoperative pain control of this surgical site. Postoperative nausea and vomiting (PONV) can be addressed with IV dexamethasone, ondansetron, and crystalloid fluids for optimum hydration.[7] As narcotics are a contributor to PONV, a reduction in narcotic use can improve PONV. Strategies to limit narcotics include increasing the use of nonnarcotic adjuncts, as well as utilization of dexmedetomidine and benzodiazepines for treatment of emergence delirium.

CASE STUDY: 2-Year-Old Presenting for Left-Sided Frontalis Sling and Autologous Fascia Lata Harvest

CLINICAL SCENARIO

A 13-kg, 2-year-old male presents for left-sided frontalis sling and autologous fascia lata harvest. The patient was born full term after an uncomplicated pregnancy. He has never had surgery or anesthesia before, and there is no family history of complications with anesthesia. He takes no medications and has no diagnosed comorbidities. His review of systems is negative, and he is appropriately NPO. In the preoperative area, the patient is fearful and refuses a trial separation, preferring to sit on his mom's lap and watch a movie.

APPROACHES TO CARE

The parents are consented for general anesthesia and a lateral femoral cutaneous nerve block. Based on the patient's anxiety and concern for combative behavior during parental separation, a premedication of midazolam 0.5 mg/kg of PO is administered along with acetaminophen 15 mg/kg PO. After 15 minutes the patient is appropriately sedated, he easily separates from his parents and is taken to the operating room.

General anesthesia is induced via an inhalation induction technique with 4 L nitrous oxide, 4 L oxygen, and 8% sevoflurane. After the patient loses consciousness, the nitrous is discontinued. A 22-gauge IV is placed in his hand, and rocuronium 1 mg/kg IV and fentanyl 1 mcg/kg IV are administered. Following intubation with a 4.0 oral RAE endotracheal tube, bilateral breath sounds are confirmed with an air leak at 20 cm H_2O, the endotracheal tube is secured, and sevoflurane is administered at 1 MAC. An ultrasound-guided lateral femoral cutaneous nerve block is performed utilizing 2 mL of 0.2% ropivacaine. Prior to surgical incision dexamethasone 0.1 mg/kg IV is administered.

Anesthesia is maintained with sevoflurane titrated to effect, air, and oxygen. Fentanyl 1 mcg/kg IV is administered as needed for surgical stimulation. Atropine is immediately available in case of cardiac arrhythmia.

Prior to emergence from anesthesia, dexmedetomidine 0.5 mcg/kg IV and ondansetron 0.1 mg/kg IV and ketorolac 0.5 mg/kg IV are administered. Neuromuscular blockade is reversed with a combination of IV neostigmine and glycopyrrolate or sugammadex if available. The patient is emerged from anesthesia in the operating room, and the trachea is extubated. After insuring adequate spontaneous ventilation, the patient is assessed for agitation. Given the careful titration of narcotic and use of adjuncts, the patient is breathing well and returns to sleeping comfortably. The patient is administered oxygen via blow by face mask and taken to the postanesthesia recovery room. Morphine 100 mcg/kg IV times three doses are ordered for postoperative pain, as well as telemetry monitoring until the patient meets requirements for phase 2 recovery.

REFERENCES

1. Finsterer J. Ptosis: causes, presentation, and management. *Aesthetic Plast Surg.* 2003;27(3):193–204. doi:10.1007/s00266-003-0127-5
2. Griepentrog GJ, Diehl NN, Mohney BG. Incidence and demographics of childhood ptosis. *Ophthalmology.* 2011;118(6):1180–1183. doi:10.1016/j.ophtha.2010.10.026
3. Marenco M, Macchi I, Macchi I, et al. Clinical presentation and management of congenital ptosis. *Clin Ophthalmol.* 2017;11:453–463. doi:10.2147/OPTH.S111118
4. Jubbal KT, Kania K, Braun TL, et al. Pediatric Blepharoptosis. *Semin Plast Surg.* 2017;31(1):58–64. doi:10.1055/s-0037-1598631
5. Song IA, Seo KS, Oh AY, et al. Dexmedetomidine injection during strabismus surgery reduces emergence agitation without increasing the oculocardiac reflex in children: a randomized controlled trial. *PloS one.* 2016;11(9):e0162785. doi:10.1371/journal.pone.0162785
6. Pandey M, Baduni N, Jain A, et al. Abnormal oculocardiac reflex in two patients with Marcus Gunn syndrome. *J Anaesthesiol Clin Pharmacol.* 2011;27(3):398–399. doi:10.4103/0970-9185.83693
7. Shaikh SI, Nagarekha D, Hegade G, Marutheesh M. Postoperative nausea and vomiting: a simple yet complex problem. *Anesthesia, essays and researches.* 2016;10(3):388–396. doi:10.4103/0259-1162.179310

CHAPTER 77

Enucleation

Suzanne M. Wright

INDICATIONS/CONTRAINDICATIONS

Surgical removal of the eye is performed in the pediatric population for conditions that cannot be treated by other means. The surgical goals of eye removal surgery include clearance of the damaged tissue, a reduction of pain, the replacement of the volume originally taken up by the globe, and the restoration of appearance.[1] The thought of having an eye removed is understandably unimaginable and one often wrought with fear and uncertainty. It is important for patients and families to know that surgeries performed to remove an eye as a treatment for significant pathology are not entirely uncommon and have significant potential to, in the end, enhance the patient's quality of life.[2]

From a psychological standpoint, the removal of an eye can be devastatingly traumatic for any patient. In addition to a specialized surgical team, a psychologist familiar with the psychological trauma related to the loss of an eye may be able to provide support before the procedure and may be helpful in securing informed consent. It can be extraordinarily difficult to come to terms with such an irreversible loss and one that will have a drastic impact on facial aesthetics until a prosthesis is properly placed. An ocularist, a specialist with expertise in creating ocular prostheses, will likely play a critical role in the patient's postoperative recovery and physical and psychological rehabilitation.

Pediatric patients present for enucleation for a multitude of reasons, including congenital cosmetic defects such as microphthalmia and anophthalmia, severe trauma, and intraocular malignancy and, most commonly, retinoblastoma (Table 77.1).

ANOPHTHALMIA AND MICROPHTHALMIA

Anophthalmia and microphthalmia are congenital anomalies of the fetal eye that may be bilateral or unilateral. Anophthalmia refers to the absence of an eye and is a condition rarely compatible with life due to associated cerebral defects. Most cases diagnosed as anophthalmia are most often found to be severe microphthalmia.[4] Microphthalmia is a condition in which the eye is unusually small, often determined by axial length and corneal diameter.[5] Bilateral microphthalmia is often associated with intellectual disability and the extent of visual impairment depends on the extent to which the retina develops.

When caring for pediatric patients with these congenital anomalies, it is important to consider all related pathological conditions that may be secondary to genetic defects, such as triploidy and mosaic trisomies 9 and 13. Triploidy, also known as hypertelorism, is associated with anomalies of the heart, brain, and face. Trisomy 13 is associated with midline facial and brain defects, cardiac anomalies, and polydactyly, a condition involving extra fingers and toes. Features of trisomy 9 include abnormalities of the heart, face, and skull and most often results in early pregnancy loss.[4] Microphthalmia may also result from various environmental factors, including maternal exposure to radiation, maternal vitamin A deficiency, or intrauterine infection.[6]

While mild to moderate microphthalmia can be managed with clear, plastic conformers to encourage adequate growth of the eye socket, severe cases may require surgical intervention.

TRAUMA

Pediatric patients suffer injury to the eyes from penetrating objects, chemical burns, corneal abrasions, eyelid lacerations, and orbital fractures, many associated with sports and other recreational activities, as well as accidents. In a study to determine diagnoses related to enucleation in the pediatric population, Huang et al.[3] found acute trauma, as well as complications from trauma, to be the second-most common circumstances for referral for pediatric enucleation after retinoblastoma. The study also revealed promising evidence that pediatric enucleation procedures resulting from trauma decreased nearly fivefold from the 1960s to the 2000s due to better microsurgical techniques for treating wounds, the use of antibiotics for eye injury, and increased compliance with eye protection guidelines. Pediatric eye injuries are treated according to severity and with a goal of minimizing long-lasting visual deficits. Treatment may include a wide range of interventions from placement of an ice pack and rest for soft tissue damage or a black eye to enucleation for unsalvageable penetrating trauma to the globe.

RETINOBLASTOMA

Retinoblastoma is a rare childhood cancer of the eye with about 9,000 cases diagnosed yearly worldwide. Retinoblastoma is the most common primary intraocular malignancy of childhood with an incidence of about 11 new cases per million individuals under 5 years old or 1 case in every 15,000 to 20,000 live births.[7] Retinoblastoma is a disease of infants and toddlers, with 95% of cases occurring before the age of 5 years. Seventy-five percent of patients with retinoblastoma will present with unilateral disease, with a median age peak of 2 to 3 years. Pediatric patients can present with bilateral retinoblastoma, but it is far less common and usually occurs in infants.[7] The management of bilateral retinoblastoma has improved significantly over the past several decades and includes earlier diagnosis and the use of nonsurgical treatment methods, such as

Table 77.1	Frequency of Primary Diagnoses for Pediatric Enucleations From 1960 to 2008		
Diagnosis		**Number of Patients**	**%**
Retinoblastoma		330	45.3
Trauma		233	32.0
• Post-traumatic complication		• 165	
• Acute trauma		• 88	
Congenital anomalies		44	6.0
• Multiple (>5) congenital anomalies		• 7	
• Microphthalmos		• 5	

Source: From Huang S, Crawford JB, Porco T, Rutar T. Clinicopathologic review of pediatric enucleations during the last 50 years. *J AAPOS.* 2010;14(4):328–333. doi:10.1016/j.jaapos.2010.05.006.

plaque brachytherapy, stereotactic and proton beam radiotherapy, cryotherapy, chemoreduction, and chemothermotherapy.[3]

If diagnosed early, the eye and vision may be preserved with non- or minimally invasive therapy. Enucleation is necessary when all other options, in which the eyeball is left intact with the hope of retaining vision, do not offer the best chance of managing the pathological condition.

An enucleation is contraindicated in cases of intraocular malignancy with evidence of orbital metastasis as these patients generally require the more extensive exenteration. Patients with sympathetic ophthalmia, a rare bilateral granulomatous inflammation that results from a physical insult to the uvea of one eye, can be poor candidates for enucleation because the sympathizing eye can have better vision, and longitudinal studies have not found a significant advantage of enucleation over evisceration for the prevention of sympathetic ophthalmia.[8] Finally, enucleation can be relatively contraindicated in patients who will experience significant psychological trauma due to the loss of the eye.[9]

ENUCLEATION, EVISCERATION, AND EXENTERATION

There are three major surgical procedures designed to remove the eye: enucleation, evisceration, and exenteration. While this section focuses on enucleation, a discussion on evisceration and exenteration is included for educational purposes. It is important to remember that the anesthetic management of pediatric patients undergoing any of the eye removal surgeries is largely the same. Caring for pediatric patients and their families during this profoundly emotional time necessitates effective communication among all members of the healthcare team, including anesthesia providers, in order to promote patient and family well-being, facilitate their coping capabilities, enhance understanding, and foster hope for and trust in the future.[10]

ENUCLEATION

The eye, sometimes referred to as the globe, is a complex sensory organ that is secured in the orbital fossa by way of multiple attachments including extraocular muscles and the optic nerve (Figure 77.1). The orbital fossa houses the eye, extraocular muscles, nerves, blood vessels, fat, and anatomical structures related to lacrimation. Each orbit is pear-shaped, and its margins are formed by the frontal, zygomatic, and maxillary bones (Figure 77.2). The orbital fossa holds about 30 mL of total content, with the globe consuming 7 to 9 mL of that volume.

Enucleation is a surgical procedure that involves removal of the globe in its entirety once it is separated from the extraocular muscles and the optic nerve.[11] Enucleation preserves the eyebrows and eyelids and four of the extraocular muscles that remain attached to their origin, the annulus of Zinn (a dense, fibrous ring of connective tissue located at the apex of the orbit).[12] Enucleation aims to remove diseased tissue, improve patient comfort, provide a good functional and cosmetic result, and replace orbital volume. Replacing any volume removed is important for normal growth of the orbit but can be particularly challenging in the pediatric population because the eye has not reached its full size.[11] At 2 years of age,

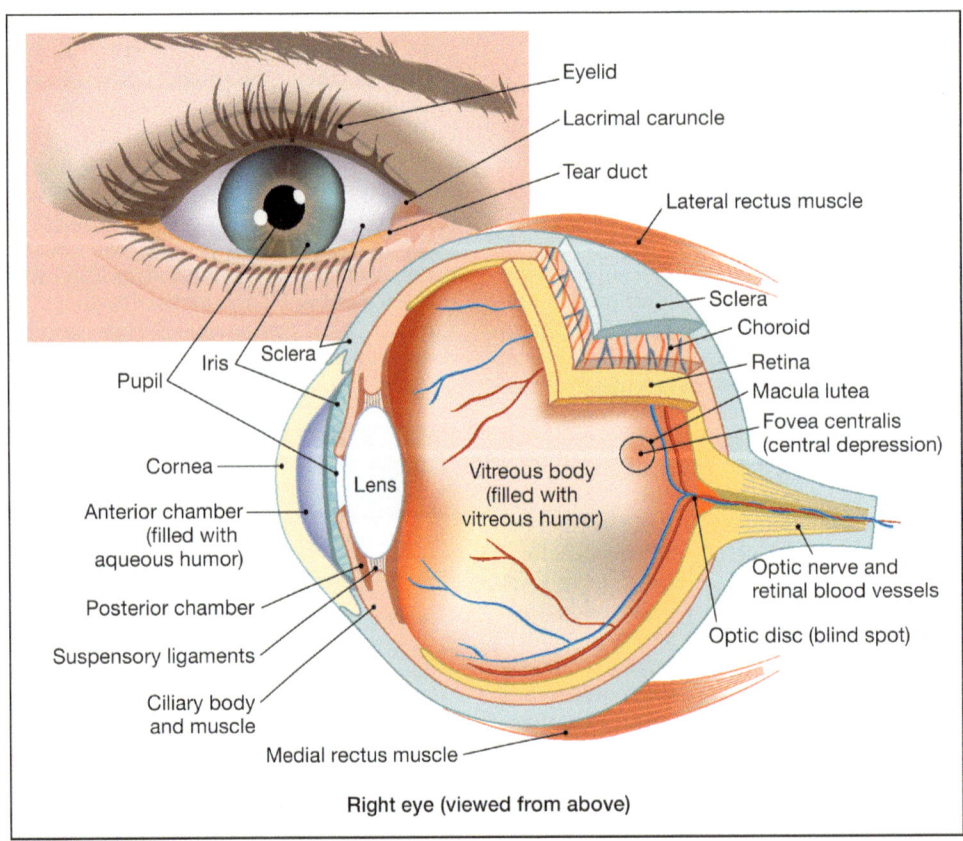

Figure 77.1: Anatomy of the eye.
Source: Melnyk J, Zeno R, Teall AM. Evidence-based assessment of the eye. In: Gawlik KS, Melnyk BM, Teall AM, eds. *Evidence-Based Physical Examination: Best Practices for Health and Well-Being Assessment.* Springer; 2021:311, Fig. 12.1.

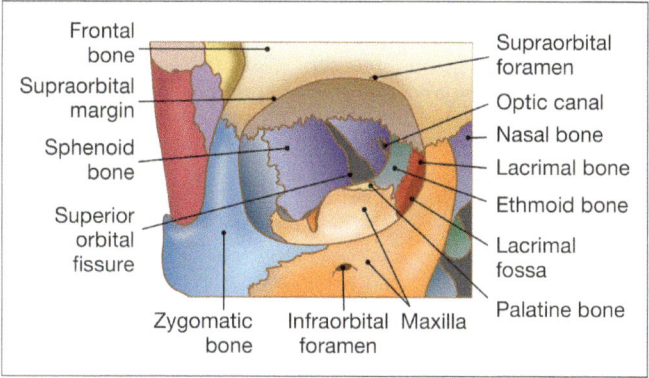

Figure 77.2: Bones of the orbit.
Source: Melnyk J, Zeno R, Teall AM. Evidence-based assessment of the eye. In: Gawlik KS, Melnyk BM, Teall AM, eds. *Evidence-Based Physical Examination: Best Practices for Health and Well-Being Assessment.* Springer; 2021:311, Fig. 12.2.

for example, the pediatric eye has an axial length, defined as the distance from the anterior corneal surface to the retinal epithelium, of about 85% of that of an adult and continues to grow about 1% per year until adulthood.[11]

Pediatric patients who undergo enucleation may require an implant, or prosthesis, exchange as they grow or, alternatively, a larger implant may be placed at the time of enucleation to make the need for secondary procedures less likely.[11] A good surgical outcome after enucleation is dependent on a number of factors including adequate volume replacement, an appropriately sized ocular prosthesis, and functional eyelids. Surgical caution must be exercised to prevent damage to the lacrimal system that produces and drains the lubricating tears or the patient may suffer a dry socket resulting in significant difficulty retaining the prosthesis.

After surgical enucleation, patients should be able to blink, produce tears, and maintain motor control of the eye and brow area. The operation usually takes less than an hour, and pediatric patients can go home the same day once pain has been controlled and postoperative instructions and care have been explained. A follow-up office visit is scheduled for the next day.[2]

EXENTERATION

Exenteration refers to the surgical removal of the globe and the surrounding tissues, which can include the eyelids, ocular muscles, nerves and fatty tissue that surrounds the globe. An orbital exenteration is a major operation that is usually performed to address a malignant tumor that involves the eyelid or structures surrounding the eye such as in the case of orbital recurrence following enucleation for retinoblastoma. An orbital exenteration usually takes around an hour or more and is performed under general anesthesia in the pediatric population. Following exenteration and when indicated, the eye socket may be reconstructed with a skin graft. Once postoperative pain is adequately managed and there is no evidence of surgical complications, most patients are able to go home the following day.[13]

EVISCERATION

Orbital evisceration is performed to remove the iris, cornea, and the intraocular contents while preserving the remaining white fibrous sclera, extraocular muscle attachments, and surrounding orbital tissues. An evisceration in the pediatric patient is rare because the pathology does not usually lend itself to this type of sparing procedure, and the salvaged scleral shell would likely be too small to eventually accommodate an adult-sized prosthesis or adequate volume replacement for optimal growth of the orbital.[14]

While appreciating the differences in surgical technique, patients undergoing enucleation and evisceration will have the same external appearance postoperatively[2]; those undergoing exenteration will have a more striking physical outcome (**Figure 77.3**).

Special considerations and concerns are noted in **Box 77.1**.

ANESTHESTIC MANAGEMENT

There are special anesthetic considerations related to the preoperative, intraoperative, and postoperative phases for the pediatric patient presenting for enucleation. A systematic approach that considers these phases can contribute to the development of an individualized plan of care that thoughtfully incorporates all patient and surgical factors as well as ways in which these factors may influence outcomes.

PREOPERATIVE EVALUATION

Pediatric patients presenting for enucleation are usually fairly healthy otherwise. They may have an associated infection or comorbidities related to a traumatic event. A thorough preoperative assessment that examines associated conditions as well as the ill effects of systemic treatments such as chemotherapy will uncover potential risks that need to be communicated to the patient and/or family. The patient's history and physical should guide decisions about preoperative laboratory testing or imaging. It is important to remember that the surgical loss of an eye is extraordinarily overwhelming for patients and families and that sufficient time should be allowed to help the family come to grips with the fact that the next time they see their child, they will look quite different. Anesthesia providers may consider preoperative anxiolysis to facilitate a smooth induction.

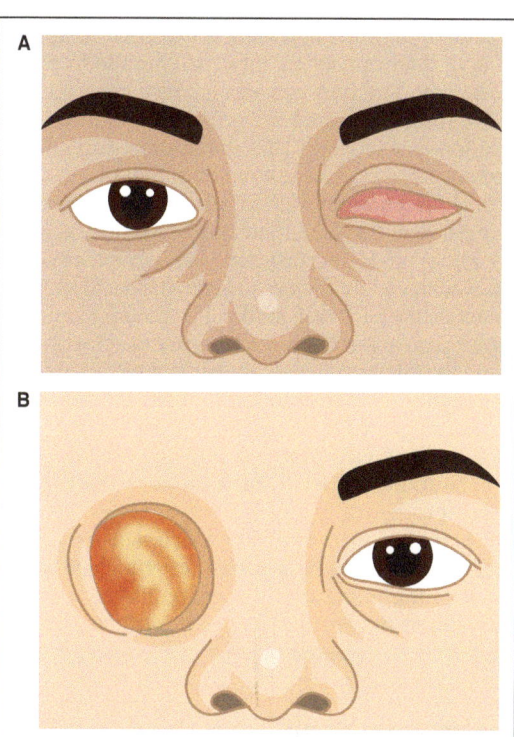

Figure 77.3: Differences in postoperative result between enucleation or evisceration (A) and exenteration (B).

> **BOX 77.1 SPECIAL CONSIDERATIONS AND CONCERNS: RETINOBLASTOMA**
>
> - Pediatric patients diagnosed with retinoblastoma may be treated nonsurgically with ophthalmic artery chemotherapy, radiation, laser, or cryotherapy.
> - Enucleation can cure retinoblastoma but is a poor choice in the case of bilateral disease.
> - When patients present with retinoblastoma that has metastasized to surrounding tissues, an exenteration will likely be required.

ANESTHETIC TECHNIQUE

Intraoperative Management

Enucleation is performed under general anesthesia in the pediatric population. Once the patient is anesthetized, an oral Ring–Adair–Elwyn (RAE) tube may be considered to enhance surgical exposure. Anesthesia is usually maintained with anesthetic gas. Muscle relaxation is rarely necessary, but patient coughing or other movements should be prevented to avoid damage to surrounding structures. The surgical table is usually turned 90 to 180 degrees from the provider; therefore, special attention should be given to ensure the patient is properly positioned, the endotracheal tube is secured, the nonoperative eye is properly protected, the IV catheter is working optimally, and the anesthesia provider has adequate access to administer medications through it. The patient's head is usually positioned on a gel doughnut, and attention should be given to keep the patient warm. Expected blood loss is minimal, but rarely, excessive bleeding can occur. An age appropriate sized IV catheter can be used; a pain level of 3 to 4 out of 10 can be anticipated and can be dependent on the extent to which local anesthesia is used intraoperatively by the surgeon.[15]

From a surgical standpoint, the enucleation procedure begins with retraction of the eyelids and a circumferential periotomy at the limbic margin of the eye. Care is exercised to keep the conjunctiva and Tenon's capsule intact so that the implant can be placed securely. The four extraocular recti muscles are identified, and a suture is placed in each, which is then clamped to the drape for easy retrieval later in the procedure. Each muscle is then removed from the eye anterior to the suture, and the two oblique muscles are usually left to fall back into the orbital fossa.[16] The optic nerve is then clamped and transected, and the eye is free to be removed. Hemostasis can take a couple to several minutes and is achieved by the use of local anesthetic with epinephrine-soaked gauze pads and/or bipolar cautery. Communication with the surgeon about their intended use of epinephrine is critical to avoid the mis- or overuse, as well as the ill effects that would ensue. The eye is sent to pathology for further examination.[16]

The next stage of the surgery involves securing the properly sized conformer or implant into the orbital fossa with a goal to encourage proper development of the socket and to achieve an anesthetically desirable result. Once the conformer or the implant are placed, a Tenon's capsule is sutured over the implant, and the recti muscles are attached to allow for movement of the implanted device. Antibiotic ointment will be administered intraocularly once the conjunctiva is closed over the device. A pressure patch is placed over the operative eye before the patient is transferred to the recovery area.[15,16,17]

POSTOPERATIVE CARE

Anesthetic management in the postoperative phase is similar to the postoperative phase of other pediatric eye surgeries following enucleation with special attention to monitor for adequate ventilation, pain management, postoperative nausea and vomiting, and bleeding. The patient will continue antibiotic therapy and will be watched closely over the next several weeks by their provider. Once the inflammation in the eye socket has resolved, the patient and family will meet with an ocularist for their permanent ocular prosthesis.

REFERENCES

1. Koylu MT, Gokce G, Uysal Y, Ceylan O, Dorukcan A, Gunal A. Indications for eye removal surgeries: a 15-year experience at a tertiary military hospital. *Saudi Med J.* 2015; 36(10):1205–1209. doi:10.15537/smj.2015.10.12031
2. Yom KH, Ricca AM, Shriver EM, Ko AC. Enucleation and evisceration: what to expect. EyeRounds.org. posted September 27, 2017. http://EyeRounds.org/cases/279-anophthalmic-socket.htm
3. Huang S, Crawford JB, Porco T, Rutar T. Clinicopathologic review of pediatric enucleations during the last 50 years. *J AAPOS.* 2010;14(4):328–333. doi:10.1016/j.jaapos.2010.05.006
4. Benacerraf BR, Bromley B, Jelin AC. Anophthalmia and microphthalmia. *Am J Obstet Gynecol.* 2019;221(5):B20–B21. doi:10.1016/j.ajog.2019.08.054
5. Skalicky S, White AJ, Grigg, JR, et al. Microphthalmia, anophthalmia, and coloboma and associated ocular and systemic features: understanding the spectrum. *JAMA Ophthalmol.* 2013;131(12):1517–1524. doi:10.1001/jamaophthalmol.2013.5305
6. Ludwig PE, Lopez MJ, Czyz CN. *Embryology and Eye Malformations.* StatPearls. 2020. https://www.ncbi.nlm.nih.gov/books/NBK482496/
7. Ortiz MV, Dunkel IJ. Retinoblastoma. *J Child Neurol.* 2016;31(2):227–36. doi:10.1177/0883073815587943
8. Chu X, Chan C. Sympathetic ophthalmia: to the twenty-first century and beyond. *J Ophthalmic Inflamm Infect.* 2013;3:49. doi:10.1186/1869-5760-3-49
9. Tan XL, Seen S, Dutta Majumder P, et al. Analysis of 130 cases of sympathetic ophthalmia - a retrospective multicenter case series. *Ocul Immunol Inflamm.* 2019;27(8):1259–1266. doi:10.1080/09273948.2018.1517894
10. Dobrozsi S, Trowbridge A, Mack JW, Rosenberg AR. Effective communication for newly diagnosed pediatric patients with cancer: Considerations for the patients, family members, providers, and multidisciplinary team. *Am. Soc. Clin. Oncol. educ. Book.* 2019;39:573–581. doi:10.1200/EDBK_238181
11. Fu L, Patel BC. Enucleation. In: *StatPearls.* StatPearls Publishing; 2020. https://www.ncbi.nlm.nih.gov/books/NBK562144/
12. Khan K, Almarzouqi SJ, Morgan ML, Lee AG. Annulus of Zinn. In: Schmidt-Erfurth U, Kohnen T, eds. *Encyclopedia of Ophthalmology.* Springer; 2018. doi:10.1007/978-3-540-69000-9_1160
13. Honavar SG, Rao R. Enucleation and exenteration. In: S Chaugule, S Honavar, P Finger, eds. *Surgical Ophthalmic Oncology.* Springer; 2019:131–139
14. Kherani F, Mehta S, Katowitz J. Pediatric enucleation, evisceration, and exenteration techniques. In: *Pediatric Oculoplastic Surgery.* Springer; 2018:921.
15. Callaway NF, Moshfeghi DM, Jaffe RA. Chapter 2: Ophthalmic surgert. In: Jaffe RA, Schmiesing CA, Golianu B, eds. *Anesthesiologist's Manual of Surgical Procedures.* 5th ed. Lippincott-Williams; 2014:168–171.
16. Jovanovic N, Carniciu A, Russell W, et al. Reconstruction of the orbit and anophthalmic socket using the dermis fat graft: a major review. *Ophthal Plast Reconstr Surg.* 2020;36(6):529–539. doi:10.1097/IOP.0000000000001610
17. Davis SA, Slonim CB. Enucleation. In: El Toukhy E, ed. *Oculoplastic Surgery.* Springer; 2020. doi:10.1007/978-3-030-36934-7_44

SECTION D: Oral, Maxillofacial, and Dental Procedures

CHAPTER 78

Dental Rehabilitation

Corey Southworth and Shannon Zhang

INDICATIONS/CONTRAINDICATIONS

Early childhood caries (ECCs) have frequently been reported as one of the most common childhood health concerns despite readily available treatment options and preventative habits. ECC is defined by the American Academy of Pediatric Dentistry (AAPD) as the presence of one or more decayed tooth, a missing tooth from caries, or a filled tooth surface of any primary tooth in children younger than 6 years of age.[1] When left untreated, EEC can lead to pain as well as structural damage of the teeth and infection. In addition, it can have a profound negative impact on a patient's overall quality of life as a result of the difficulties with speech; disturbances in eating, sleeping, and growth patterns; and social disruptions at home and school that can ensue. While there is no single best plan of care for restorative treatment, a variety of nonpharmacological and pharmacological treatment options can be employed to optimize a patient's dental health. Over the last decade, dental rehabilitation under general anesthesia has become more common for pediatric patients as this approach facilitates high-quality, preventive, and restorative dental treatment in as few visits as possible.[2]

The AAPD Best Practices for Use of Anesthesia Providers in the Administration of Office-Based Deep Sedation/General Anesthesia to the Pediatric Dental Patient offers that some children may require deep sedation or general anesthesia to receive dental treatment in a safe and humane fashion. This includes, but is not limited to, those with special care needs, acute situational anxiety, immature cognitive functioning, and certain medical conditions or those who are uncooperative with care.[3] When patients are noncommunicable, display behavior disruptions uncontrolled by other nonpharmacological or pharmacological techniques or are in need of protection from potential negative psyche development related to extreme anxiety and fear, general anesthesia allows children to receive oral healthcare they may not otherwise be able to receive. Likewise, poor oral health causing airway obstruction may be deemed an emergency requiring general anesthesia. General anesthesia may also be warranted if the patient has an allergy to local anesthetics or when use of local anesthetics may be ineffective due to an acute localized infection or anatomic variation (Box 78.1). Finally, general anesthesia should be considered when there is an anticipation of multiple appointments due to the severity of the oral disease, a need for complex restorative or surgical care, or extremely limited access to dental care.[4]

Contraindications to pediatric dental rehabilitation under general anesthesia are few, although the child's comorbidities or ongoing disease process should be considered to ensure the delivery of safe, effective anesthetic care.[4] It should be noted that if a child is able to tolerate mild or moderate sedation for treatment or when the presenting history and radiographic images indicate a lack of inflammation of carious teeth, efforts should be made to avoid general anesthesia. Even if dental rehabilitation under general anesthesia is the preference of the patient and/or guardian, general anesthesia should be reserved for those patients in whom other techniques to complete care have failed.

SPECIAL CONSIDERATIONS AND CONCERNS

Frequently, children with special needs have trouble maintaining adequate oral health due to physical limitations or a lack of cooperation. Patient present with a continuum of medical needs that preclude routine dental care. Anesthesia providers should make every effort to facilitate coordination of care, which often requires of clearance from specialties such as cardiology, endocrinology, or hematology; care of this patient population often presents challenges for all providers during the perioperative period.[5]

ANESTHETIC MANAGEMENT

PREOPERATIVE EVALUATION

Like any pediatric patient, a detailed preoperative evaluation is needed to ensure delivery of safe, effective anesthetic care and to determine if general anesthesia is warranted. This includes a thorough history and physical exam, including determining the presence of allergies to local anesthetics, latex, inhaled anesthetics, or paralytics (Box 78.2). It is important to determine if a family history of anesthetic exists, including a history of malignant hyperthermia (MH) or pseudocholinesterase deficiencies. A clean technique will be required for patients with a history or family history of MH and should be greatly considered for patients who are diagnosed with congenital myopathies. Refer to Chapter 126, "Malignant Hypothermia" for

---

BOX 78.1 INDICATIONS FOR PEDIATRIC DENTAL REHABILITATION UNDER GENERAL ANESTHESIA

1. Special care needs with extensive oral healthcare needs
2. Acute situational anxiety
3. Uncooperative or disruptive age-appropriate behavior
4. Immature cognitive functioning
5. Certain disabilities or medical conditions
6. Allergy to local anesthesia
7. Acute local infection or anatomic variation rendering local anesthesia ineffective
8. Noncommunicable patients
9. Potential for negative psyche development
10. Dental concerns creating life-threatening obstruction or occlusion of the airway
11. Anticipation of need for multiple appointments
12. Planned complex restorative or surgical care
13. Limited access to dental care

> **BOX 78.2 KEY ASSESSMENT POINTS**
>
> 1. History and physical
> 2. Allergies
> 3. NPO status
> 4. History of prematurity
> 5. History of neurological developmental delays or anomalies
> 6. Detailed airway assessment and history
> 7. History of genetic or dysmorphic syndromes
> 8. History of malignant hypothermia (MH) or family history of MH
> 9. History or family history of pseudocholinesterase deficiency
> 10. History of cardiac problems
> 11. History of acute or chronic respiratory ailments
> 12. History of obstructive sleep apnea (OSA)

additional information on the management of the patient presenting with MH.

A child who presents with any genetic or dysmorphic syndrome should be further evaluated by the patient's pediatrician or specialist as this can often be secondary to craniofacial abnormalities influencing the plan of care. Patients with cardiac histories can be higher risk for perioperative morbidity and may also need antibiotic prophylaxis. Evaluation by cardiology preoperatively is needed in order to determine the appropriate level of care. Patients presenting with active or recent respiratory infections, a history of asthma, or obstructive sleep apnea are at a greater risk of perioperative complications. Thus, it is important to elicit this information as with any procedures. Referral to specialists for further evaluation prior to undergoing general anesthesia may be warranted based on the patient's medical history and presenting symptoms.[6]

Pertinent Labs

Children who are otherwise healthy presenting for dental rehabilitation generally do not require preoperative lab work. Should there be a concern of significant blood loss, a complete blood count and a type and screen may be obtained preoperatively. Although bleeding time, prothrombin time, and partial thromboplastin time are not shown to be reliable in predicting bleeding risk, anesthesia providers may consider ordering these labs preoperatively if there is a patient or family history of bleeding disorder.[6]

PREOPERATIVE PHARMACOLOGY

Many pediatric patients presenting for dental rehabilitation under general anesthesia are anxious and may benefit from an anxiolytic. Not only will administration of an anxiolytic aid with parental separation but also can decrease the ensuing physiological response to stress and total anesthetic requirements. Administering an anxiolytic preoperatively may also help with placement of an IV catheter if required prior to induction of general anesthesia. Midazolam, clonidine, dexmedetomidine, ketamine, and fentanyl are all potential options.[7] Please refer to Chapter 3, "Preoperative Evaluation and Testing" and Chapter 131, "Pediatric Pain Management" for further information regarding the pharmacological management of preoperative anxiety. When giving any of these medications, however, appropriate monitoring for respiratory depression is required in accordance with institutional policies.

Anesthesia providers should also be aware that patients presenting with certain cardiac conditions may require antibiotic prophylaxis prior to dental procedures due to an increased risk for bacteremia.[6] Please refer to **Chapter 93** in this text for information regarding the care of children with heart disease undergoing noncardiac surgery.

ANESTHETIC TECHNIQUE

Intraoperative Management

Dental procedures under general anesthesia may be relatively brief or may require several hours depending on the amount of preventative and/or restorative work needed. Dental restorations in pediatric patients typically require more surgical time than dental extractions alone. Prior to arrival in the operating room, a conversation among the dental, anesthesia, nursing, and surgical teams should occur to review the case in detail. A more comprehensive restorative plan, including extractions or stainless steel crowns as opposed to amalgam or composite restorations and pulp treatments, may minimize the need for dental rehabilitation under general anesthesia in the future. Stainless steel crowns are often more durable and functional for patients, but if there is a doubt about the success of the restorative therapy, tooth extraction should be considered.[8]

As children may have many fears about the procedure, including the fear of needles or injections, inhalation inductions with inhaled volatile anesthetics are used frequently. Sevoflurane, often in conjunction with a mixture of oxygen and nitrous oxide, is commonly the induction inhalation agent of choice because of its more pleasant odor, fast onset, and minimal respiratory irritability.[8] Depending on institutional protocol, parents may be permitted to be present during the induction process to help reduce the patient's anxiety.[6] Once general anesthesia is induced, IV access should be established. The maintenance of anesthesia can be achieved with continued delivery of inhaled volatile anesthetics or via total intravenous anesthetic (TIVA) infusions.[8]

Airway management can vary, with placement of an oral endotracheal tube (ETT), nasal ETT, or laryngeal mask airway (LMA) all having been reported previously in the literature. The placement of a nasal ETT, however, is most common for intraoral procedures as this gives the dentist or oral and maxillofacial surgeon full access to the mouth. Anesthesia providers should be aware that placement of a nasal ETT may lead to epistaxis both during placement of the nasal ETT and following removal. Suctioning of excess blood and secretions may be necessary to avoid untoward airway complications. For further information regarding nasal intubation, please refer to Chapter 6 in this text. Depending on the anesthesia provider's and dental teams' comfort, an LMA may be used for pediatric dental rehabilitation. The use of an LMA has been reported as not only being safe, it has been associated reduced postoperative pain, a reduced incidence of ED, and higher parental satisfaction.[9]

A multimodal approach to pain management is encouraged to decrease the reliance on opioid administration and incidence of opioid-induced sequelae. This may include the administration of acetaminophen, nonsteroidal anti-inflammatory drugs, glucocorticoids, and local anesthetics. Specific practice for the administration of local anesthetics by dentists in the intraoperative period is varied during dental rehabilitation. Local anesthetics may improve hemostasis, decrease postoperative pain, and decrease anesthesia requirements. Teeth extraction is the most common procedure for which local anesthetics are administered by dentists.[8] The use of local anesthetics is not universally agreed on, however. It has been offered that the use of local anesthetics increases the risk of inadvertent lip and cheek biting in children.

Clinical Pearls

Emergence delirium (ED) is common after general anesthesia in pediatric patients. While there is no definitive way to prevent ED from occurring, there are a number of techniques that may help decrease the incidence of ED.[10] Administering dexmedetomidine, a potent alpha adrenergic receptor agonist, has been found to decrease the likelihood of ED and improve postoperative pain scores, especially when compared with the administration of midazolam.[11] Dexmedetomidine, however, may increase the total time required for emergence and time to meet discharge criteria.[12]

Administration of 1 mg/kg of propofol prior to extubation may decrease ED and lower Pediatric Anesthesia Emergence Delirium (PAED) scores in pediatric patients presenting for dental rehabilitation.[13] A meta-analysis of propofol administered at the end of an inhaled volatile agent-based anesthetic reported there was a small decrease in the severity of ED, a significant decrease in the incidence of ED, a significant increase in the emergence time but not a significant increase in the total recovery time. Potential complications with this technique include laryngospasm, apnea, desaturation, and hypotension.[14] Similarly, transitioning to TIVA after the placement of an IV catheter and securing the airway can lower ED, lower pain scores, such as a Face, Legs, Activity, Cry, Consolability (FLACC) score,

and increase parental satisfaction without delaying extubation and recovery times.[10]

Complications/Emergencies

While complications under general anesthesia have decreased due to the improved knowledge of pathophysiology, a safe profile of anesthetic drugs, and advances in monitoring equipment, general anesthesia should not be considered a benign process. Fortunately, most pediatric patients presenting for dental rehabilitation under general anesthesia are older than 1 year of age, the age group with the overall highest incidence of reported fatalities under general anesthesia.

Thankfully, the complications that commonly occur are considered mild and not severe. These include pain, sleepiness, and inability to consume food/drink due to bleeding, sore throat, vomiting, coughing, or fever.[3] Injury to teeth, lips, and soft tissues may occur from laryngoscopy and the use of forced mouth retractors. Cardiac arrhythmias, dislodged or obstructed ETTs, IV catheter infiltration, and edema of lips or tongue have also been described.[8]

POSTOPERATIVE CARE

In the postanesthesia care unit (PACU), the emphasis of focus is most often on pain control.[15] Anesthesia providers should be aware that the patient's pain will likely peak 2 hours postoperatively and then slowly decrease over the course of the next several days. Adequate pain management perioperatively will aid in transitioning to an effective regimen postdischarge, including the use of oral analgesic medications when necessary. Parents should be encouraged to provide around the clock oral pain medications for 2 days rather than dosing pain medication "as needed."[16] Postoperatively, eating difficulties, nasal bleeding, hoarseness, sleep disturbances, weakness, drowsiness, dehydration, fever, nausea or vomiting, diarrhea, and constipation may also be experienced. The success of dental rehabilitation under general anesthesia relies on follow-up care. Parents and guardians must be educated and encouraged to comply with postoperative visits and regular oral hygiene to prevent relapse and obtain the best outcomes.[3]

CASE STUDY: Dental Rehabilitation

CLINICAL SCENARIO

A 9-year-old girl with a history of dental caries and situational anxiety presents for full dental restoration under general anesthesia. Per the patient's parents, she has a history of high anxiety and fear secondary to previous negative experiences with dental appointments. Other relevant history includes birth at 36 weeks of gestation by uncomplicated vaginal delivery. The patient has short stature and is in the 18th percentile for height. She is otherwise healthy, and her airway exam is unremarkable.

SPECIAL CONSIDERATIONS

Preoperatively she was offered oral midazolam, but the parents declined it. Acetaminophen 15 mg/kg orally was administered. Special attention was given to the patient to establish some trust prior to entering the operating room. This included giving the patient the opportunity to ask her own questions and state her own fears. She was also reassured that a parent could be present with her as she went off to sleep under general anesthesia.

An inhalation induction with a mixture of oxygen, nitrous oxide, and sevoflurane was performed with her parents present. A 22-gauge peripheral IV catheter was placed, and the patient was nasally intubated with a 5.5 nasal Ring-Adair-Elwin (RAE) endotracheal tube (ETT) per the dentist's request. For pain

(continued)

CASE STUDY: Dental Rehabilitation (continued)

control associated with planned dental extractions, the patient received fentanyl and ketorolac intravenously, in addition to 1 mL of 1% lidocaine with 1:100K epinephrine via local infiltration by the dentist.

This patient had a smooth emergence from general anesthesia and was extubated and transferred to the postanesthesia care unit (PACU), where no complications were noted.

APPROACHES TO CARE

Evidence-Based Approaches to Care

Based on the literature we reviewed, some dentists believe it is not necessary to inject local anesthetics for dental procedures. However, we believe proactive pain control for dental procedures is very important and thus routinely have given acetaminophen PO in the preop holding area and a small dose of fentanyl and ketorolac intraoperatively and encourage dentists to give local anesthetics.

The pediatric dentist we worked with for this patient preferred intubation with a nasal RAE ETT. We have observed very minimal complications from this practice.

KEY REFERENCES

Complete references for this chapter are online and available at https://connect.springerpub.com/content/book/978-0-8261-3875-0/part/part04/toc-part/ch078.

1. Policy on Early Childhood Caries (ECC): classifications, consequences, and preventive strategies. *Pediatr Dent.* 2016;38(6):52–54.
2. Oubenyahya H, Bouhabba N. General anesthesia in the management of early childhood caries: an overview. *J Dent Anesth Pain Med.* 2019;19(6):313. doi:10.17245/jdapm.2019.19.6.313
4. Andreeva R. Indications for dental treatment under general anesthesia. *Scripta Scientifica Medica.* 2018;50(3):26. doi:10.14748/ssm.v50i3.5327
6. Basel A, Bajic D. Preoperative evaluation of the pediatric patient. *Anesthesiol Clin.* 2018;36(4):689–700. doi:10.1016/j.anclin.2018.07.016
7. Dave N. Premedication and induction of anaesthesia in paediatric patients. *Indian J Anaesth.* 2019;63(9):713. doi:10.4103/ija.ija_491_19
8. Ramazani N. Different aspects of general anesthesia in pediatric dentistry: a review. *Iran J Pediatr.* In press. 2016. doi:10.5812/ijp.2613
10. Kocaturk O, Keles S. Recovery characteristics of total intravenous anesthesia with propofol versus sevoflurane anesthesia: a prospective randomized clinical trial. *J Pain Res.* 2018;11:1289–1295. doi:10.2147/jpr.s164106
15. Hu Y, Tsai A, Ou-Yang L, et al. Postoperative dental morbidity in children following dental treatment under general anesthesia. *BMC Oral Health.* 2018;18(1). doi:10.1186/s12903-018-0545-z
16. Wong M, Copp PE, Haas DA. Postoperative pain in children after dentistry under general anesthesia. *Anesth Prog.* 2015;62(4):140–152. doi:10.2344/14-27.1

CHAPTER 79

Mandibular Distraction

Heather J. Rankin, Edgar Soto, and René P. Myers

INDICATIONS/CONTRAINDICATIONS

Mandibular distraction osteogenesis (MDO) is a surgical technique commonly used to correct or improve upper airway obstructions in neonates and infants with micrognathia and resulting glossoptosis. MDO was first introduced in 1992 by McCarthy and has been increasingly prevalent over the last two decades by surgeons worldwide.[1]

Potential surgical candidates include pediatric patients with hemifacial microsomia, including patients with Pierre–Robin sequence, Treacher-Collins syndrome, Goldenhar syndrome, and other syndromic micrognathia. Indications for MDO include obstructive sleep apnea as evidenced by a polysomnography (PSG) test measuring the degree of obstruction, the apnea–hypopnea index (AHI), and oxygen desaturations.

A number of more conservative methods may be tried first to alleviate the tongue-based obstruction, including prone positioning (Figure 79.1), supplemental oxygen, continuous positive airway pressure, nasopharyngeal airway, or nasal noninvasive ventilation.[1] If the more conservative methods are not successful, or if the obstruction is severe at baseline, MDO may be considered.

The success of MDO is due to the movement of the mandible and tongue base anteriorly, thereby functionally relieving the previous airway obstruction. In a systematic review, MDO was reported to prevent tracheostomy placement in 95% of cases presenting for the relief of obstruction. MDO is also a potential consideration for patients who had tracheostomies placed prior to MDO yet has been found to be less effective.[1] As MDO provides an anatomic solution, if the patient is a candidate, this will be the preferred definitive treatment. MDO has been shown to significantly improve obstructive sleep apnea as evidenced by comparison of preoperative and postoperative PSGs[2] and as evidenced by combined comparison of preoperative and postoperative PSGs and flexible fiberoptic (FO) imaging.[3]

Contraindications for MDO include unilateral dysplasia, mandibular infection, or a lack of glossoptosis seen on flexible FO inspection, which involves a nasal flexible endoscopic exam by otolaryngology, where the tongue is manually displaced anteriorly to examine obstruction.[4] Severe cases of obstruction or moderate or higher amounts of central sleep apnea are an indication for tracheostomy.[5] While a tracheostomy does provide a definitive airway for the infant, it does not resolve the problem of obstruction from the tongue causing the difficulty breathing and has a significant degree of risk.

SPECIAL CONSIDERATIONS AND CONCERNS

Patients presenting with hemifacial microsomia can present many special considerations and concerns, particularly relating to anesthesia and intubation of the trachea. The degree of obstruction can be severe enough to necessitate an immediate emergency surgical airway tracheostomy to be performed if the airway is unable to be otherwise secured, and otolaryngology should be available for elective procedures should this scenario occur.

ANESTHETIC MANAGEMENT

PREOPERATIVE EVALUATION

Preoperative evaluation considerations are noted in Box 79.1.

ANESTHETIC TECHNIQUE

Intraoperative Management

After preoperative considerations noted in Box 79.1 have been evaluated and anesthesia consent is obtained, the patient will be brought to the operating room; standard monitors will be applied; and vital signs will be obtained. Specialized pediatric anesthesia equipment should be available for induction and intubation. In addition, all equipment available necessary for rigid bronchoscopy should be readily available should otolaryngology need to assist with securing the airway. Examples of the recommended equipment can be found in Box 79.2.

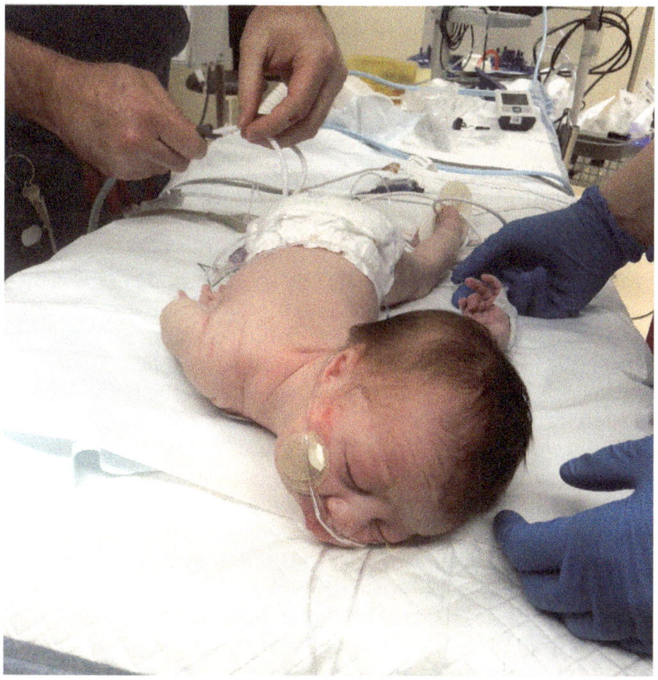

Figure 79.1: Patient with Pierre-Robin sequence prior to mandibular distraction osteogenesis in prone position due to moderate-to-severe obstruction when supine.

Source: Courtesy of René P. Myers, MD.

BOX 79.1   PREOPERATIVE EVALUATION CONSIDERATIONS

- Physical exam including degree of visual micrognathia present
- Measured maxillomandibular discrepancy
- Oxygen requirements
- Oxygen nadir on PSG
- Supplemental respiratory devices present such as nasopharyngeal airway or use of continuous positive airway pressure
- Degree of severity of obstruction or respiratory distress present when positioned supine
- Results from flexible fiberoptic evaluation including other airway diagnoses such as laryngomalacia or tracheomalacia
- Results from rigid bronchoscopy if performed
- Comorbidities present
- PSG results
- Pertinent labwork including blood gas readings
- Computed tomography or ultrasound airway studies if available
- Family history of anesthesia complications

PSG, polysomnography.

> **BOX 79.2** **SPECIALIZED PEDIATRIC ANESTHESIA EQUIPMENT AVAILABLE FOR INDUCTION AND INTUBATION**
>
> - Appropriately sized mask
> - Multiple sizes endotracheal tubes
> - Variety of laryngoscope blades
> - Laryngoscope handle
> - Appropriately sized laryngeal mask airways
> - Stylet
> - Bougie
> - Video laryngoscope
> - Fiberoptic scope
> - Appropriately sized oral airways
> - Appropriately sized nasopharyngeal airway
> - ENT specialist available with set-up for rigid bronchoscopy

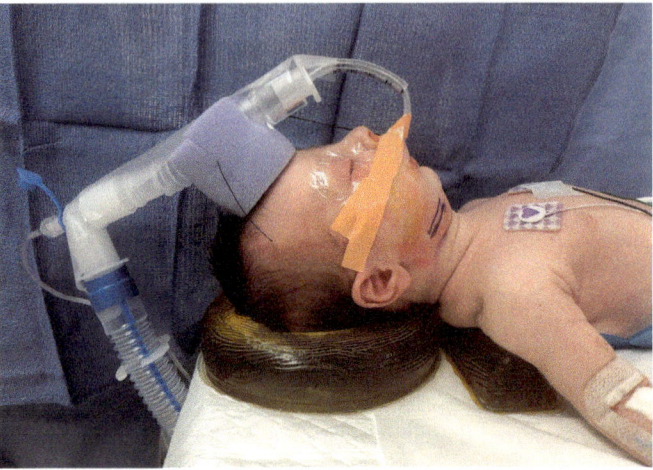

Figure 79.2: Patient intubated and ready for mandibular distraction osteogenesis surgery to begin.
Source: Courtesy of René P. Myers, MD.

Several methods to induce general anesthesia may be used, whether it be an inhalation induction, IV induction, or a combination of both. Inhalation induction with sevoflurane may be preferred to keep the patient spontaneously breathing and to decrease episodes of obstruction and hypoxia. Depending on the presentation of the patient, those with severe obstruction may require induction in the prone or lateral position.[6] IV adjuncts of propofol, ketamine, and dexmedetomidine may be used to deepen anesthesia for the bronchoscopy if one is performed or for tracheal intubation if an inhalation induction is preferred. Conversely, an IV induction may provide better intubation conditions. Anesthesia providers should proceed with an IV induction with caution, however, as they may be presented with a cannot-ventilate, cannot-intubate situation if spontaneous ventilation is obliterated with IV agents. As sugammadex can swiftly reverse aminosteroidal neuromuscular blocking agents in the event of a cannot-ventilate, cannot-intubate situation, administration of a neuromuscular blocking agent should be considered as it may improve intubating conditions. Furthermore, sugammadex has been used safely in pediatric patients.[7,8]

If severe hypoxia occurs during attempted induction or intubation, FO intubation via a laryngeal mask airway (LMA) with the patient awake should be considered.[9] A multistage approach to intubation in this scenario has been described, beginning with placement of LMA in an awake neonate followed by an inhalation induction with sevoflurane and finally administration of a neuromuscular blocking agent.[6] An intubating LMA can then be placed, followed by FO intubation through the LMA. The use of a neuromuscular blocking agent has been reported to facilitate intubation and considered a superior technique due to the decreased likelihood of laryngospasm.[6]

Traditional difficult airway algorithms can be followed when securing the airway prior to MDO, including LMA, FO, and video laryngoscope (VL) use. VL use is relatively new in the pediatric arena but has become more common and gaining favor with some anesthesia providers.[10–15] Clear communication among anesthesia, otolaryngology, and plastic surgery is essential to ensure patient safety.

Following successful intubation and preparation of the patient, mandibular distraction can be performed. See Figure 79.2 for an example of a patient intubated, prepped, and ready for the procedure. The osteotomy phase of the surgical procedure is performed via an extraoral approach to the mandibular area in which the distraction device is internally placed across the bony segment. The distraction device is a 20-mm semi-buried uniplane with a ratcheting mechanism that is placed to the lower border of each side of the mandible. Once the device is secured to the mandible using high-profile screws, the device is activated for several millimeters to verify that there is no opposition. After the distraction device is used to confirm complete mandibular osteotomy, the incision is closed in layers. Prior to exiting the operating room, a feeding tube is placed and an x-ray is taken to confirm both feeding tube and endotracheal tube placement.

POSTOPERATIVE CARE

Postoperatively, patients are typically transported to the NICU or pediatric intensive care (PICU), intubated, sedated, and paralyzed after the surgery is completed. Collaboration among anesthesia, NICU or PICU staff, respiratory therapy, and plastic surgery is key to ensure safe transport and care of the critical airway while the patient remains intubated. An appropriately sized LMA and emergency intubation equipment should be available at the patient's bedside in case an inadvertent extubation occurs. Many facilities have a sign on the patient's door designating a critical airway patient is in the room.

A latency phase follows, with varying time frames dependent on patient age to allow for the healing process to initiate and for callus formation. The device is activated during the distraction phase to create tension at a set rate per day dependent on the device to the maximum length of the distraction device (20 mm). Bone formation begins within the callus, as the segments are distracted. During the initial phase postoperatively, all patients are intubated and undergo weaning of sedation medications used; the choice of sedation is facility dependent but may include midazolam, fentanyl, dexmedetomidine, or a combination of the three. Patients are often brought to the operating room for airway evaluation prior to extubation, with most patients extubated within a week of the initial distraction hardware surgery. Patients are discharged once airway stabilization has occurred, assuming there are no other comorbidities to keep the patient hospitalized.

After the distraction phase, the consolidation phase follows in order to allow the distracted bone segments to become stabile and regenerate. The consolidation phase lasts roughly 8 weeks. There is no activation during this phase in order to allow for complete maturation. The patient then returns to the operating room for a second operation with the devices removed after the 8-week time frame after cohesion of the bone has been assessed.

Management following post–MDO involves follow-up by a multidisciplinary team including a plastic surgeon and pulmonologist to monitor the development of the mandible and the reemergence of obstructive breathing patterns and feeding difficulties. A sleep study analysis is performed within 3 months of the operation to identify and quantify the presence of residual airway obstruction.

CASE STUDY: Full-Term Neonate With Pierre-Robin Sequence and Feeding Difficulty

CLINICAL SCENARIO

The patient presented at 17 days as a former 39-week, 2-day infant via the NICU transferred from an adjacent state for Pierre-Robin sequence. Of note, there was a family history of Pierre-Robin sequence, with her father also having this diagnosis. High-flow nasal cannula oxygen was needed to maintain saturations, and craniofacial plastic surgery was consulted. The patient tired quickly with feeding and was eventually switched to nasogastric feeds only secondary to a swallow study that showed penetration to the vocal cords. Her mother reported several episodes of the patient "turning blue" when feeding prior to presenting to our institution.

Of note, a sleep study and computed tomography (CT) scan were requested, but the patient required intubation for the CT (Figure 79.3). A recommendation from plastic surgery was for the patient to remain intubated following the CT for the distraction process to follow the next day. Unfortunately, the patient self-extubated on the morning of the operation.

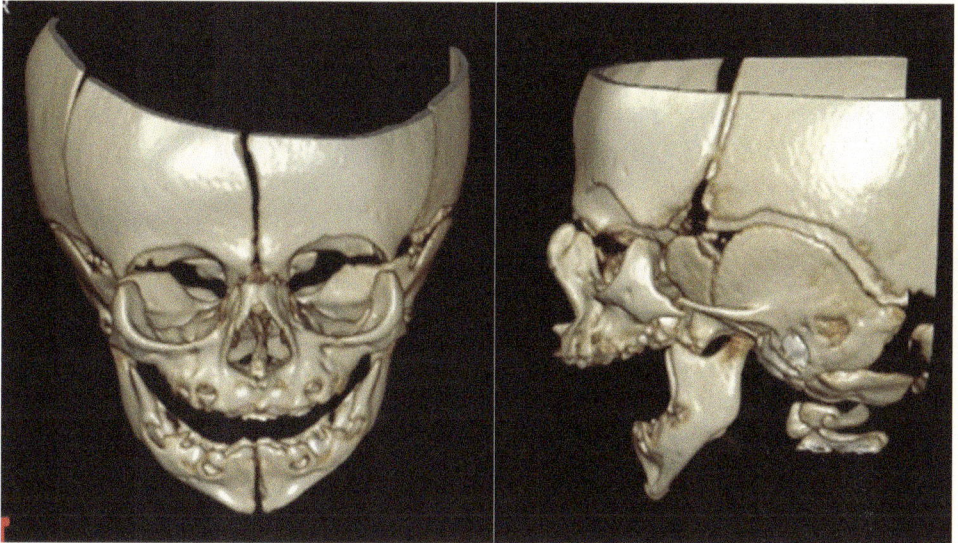

Figure 79.3: Computed tomography of the patient.
Source: Courtesy of René P. Myers, MD.

APPROACHES TO CARE

Evidence-Based Approaches to Care

Otolaryngology was consulted to perform a nasal and rigid endoscopy after an uneventful induction of anesthesia in the operating room and noted a Grade 3 view on scope and laryngomalacia. Forward advancement of the tongue relieved the upper airway obstruction, and as a team, the decision was made to move forward with distraction, given the extent of her micrognathia. The patient was intubated and prepped for surgery (Figure 79.2).

The plastic surgery team proceeded with bilateral inverted-L osteotomies and internal distraction per our standard. A nasogastric feeding tube was reinserted and intraoperative views off the ETT were obtained via x-ray prior to having the respiratory therapist from the NICU resecure the ETT. She thereafter underwent uneventful distraction osteogenesis of the mandible with a cadence of three turns twice daily for a total of 1.8 mm/day of distraction. She was sedated and intubated throughout

(continued)

CASE STUDY: Full-Term Neonate With Pierre-Robin Sequence and Feeding Difficulty (*continued*)

the initial distraction, and then repeat flexible nasoendoscopy was performed on postoperative day 9. She was subsequently discharged and did well with subsequent visits to the cleft and craniofacial center, as well as cardiology, for her atrial septal defect and ventricle septal defect.

Following a consolidation phase, her distraction devices were removed around 2 months later. After-distraction sleep study was performed a month after device removal and showed an AHI of 4.7 and a rapid eye movement (REM) sleep apnea-hypopnea index (AHI) of 14.1. She had 22 central apneas, two mixed apneas, and no obstructive apneas. Her mean oxygen saturation was 97%. Repeat sleep study at the age of 8 months showed improvement with three central apneas, no mixed apneas, no obstructive apneas, and no hypopneas. Her AHI was 0.5 and had an REM AHI of 0. She underwent uncomplicated palatoplasty with a Furlow technique and most recently saw us at the age of 2 years, 7 months (Figures 79.4 and 79.5). There was some relapse despite the overcorrection performed with the distraction but there had been no other problems. She continues in speech therapy and will continue to be followed up.

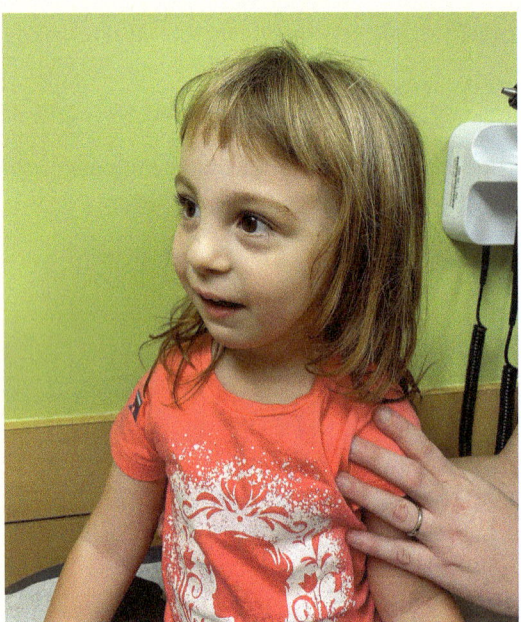 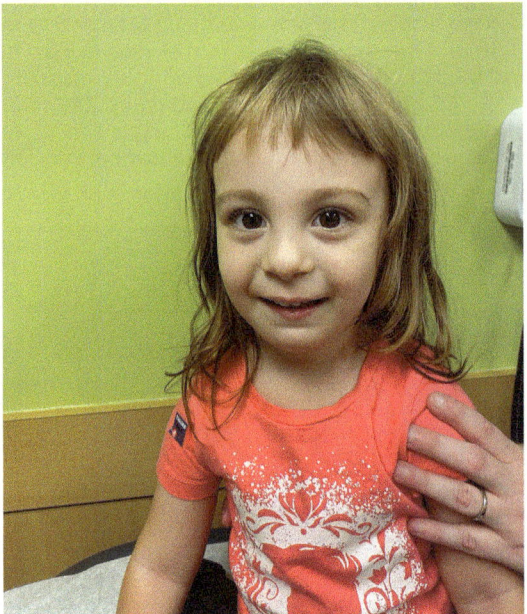

Figure 79.4: Follow-up visit for patient at 2 years, 7 months, following mandibular distraction osteogenesis.
Source: Courtesy of René P. Myers, MD.

KEY REFERENCES

Complete references for this chapter are online and available at https://connect.springerpub.com/content/book/978-0-8261-3875-0/part/part04/toc-part/ch079.

3. da Costa AL, Manica D, Schweiger C, et al. The effect of mandibular distraction osteogenesis on airway obstruction and polysomnographic parameters in children with Robin sequence. *J Craniomaxillofac Surg.* 2018;46:1343–1347. doi:10.1016/j.jcms.2018.05.030

6. Templeton TW, Goenaga-Diaz EJ, Runyan CM, et al. A generalized multistage approach to oral and nasal intubation in infants with Pierre Robin sequence: a retrospective review. *Paediatr Anaesth.* 2018;28:1029–1034. doi:10.1111/pan.13499

8. Liu G, Wang R, Yan Y, et al. The efficacy and safetly of sugammadex for reversing postoperative residual neuromuscular blockade in pediatric patients: a systematic review. *Sci Rep.* 2017;7(1):5724. doi:10.1038/s41598-017-06159-2

11. Raimann FJ, Cuca CE, Kern D, et al. Evaluation of the C-MAC Miller video laryngoscope sizes 0 and 1 during tracheal intubation of infants less than 10 kg. *Pediatr Emerg Care.* 2020;36(7):312–316. doi:10.1097/PEC.0000000000001296

15. Suzuki K, Kusunoki S, Tanigawa K, Shime N. Comparison of three video laryngoscopes and direct laryngoscopy for emergency endotracheal intubation: a retrospective cohort study. *BMJ Open.* 2019;9:1–7. doi:10.1136/bmjopen-2018-024927

CHAPTER 80

LeFort Osteotomy

Terri M. Cahoon and Kris Redden

INDICATIONS/CONTRAINDICATIONS

LeFort fractures can be classified according to the specific plane of injury and subsequently divided into three distinct classifications. With a LeFort type I fracture, the plane of injury is horizontal generally traverses the alveolar ridge, the lateral nose, and the inferior part of the maxillary sinus, typically separating the teeth from the upper face. Patients presenting with a LeFort type II fracture will have a distinct pyramidal-shaped appearance, with the upper teeth forming the base of the pyramid and the nasofrontal suture being apex of the pyramidal fracture. The plane of injury occurs through the alveolar ridge, maxillary sinuses, and orbital rim, often extending through the nasal bones. With a LeFort type III fracture, the plane of injury is transverse or horizontal beginning at the nasofrontal area and extending across the orbital walls, zygomatic arch, and pterygoid plates. A type III LeFort fracture is the most extensive of the three classifications of LeFort fracture as it can result in complete dislocation of the midface from the base of the skull, known as a craniofacial dislocation (Figure 80.1).

LeFort osteotomy is an orthognathic procedure that uses the anatomic patterns associated with a LeFort fracture to correct a broad spectrum of midfacial skeletal abnormalities whether congenital, developmental, or acquired in origin (Figure 80.2). A LeFort I osteotomy, often combined with sagittal split osteotomies, is indicated for dentofacial deformities and maxillary deficiencies with the intent to alter facial appearance and improve function related to malocclusion of the jaw. The surgical bone fracture extends from the nasal septum along the tooth apices and through the pterygomaxillary junction to allow adjustment of the lower portion of the maxilla, including both teeth and the bony palate. A LeFort I osteotomy is also indicated for midface hypoplasia, maxillary excess, obstructive sleep apnea (OSA), and cleft lip and palate repair.[1,2] In addition, the patient population presenting for LeFort I osteotomy often includes older teens and young adults who have mature growth of maxillary and mandibular bones. Coordination of the procedure with orthodontic preparation optimizes correction of various malocclusions. LeFort II and III osteotomies are indicated for severe midface hypoplasia, maxillary hypoplasia, syndromic craniosynostosis, and class 3 malocclusion.[3,4]

SPECIAL CONSIDERATIONS AND CONCERNS

Anesthesia providers should be aware that patients presenting for LeFort osteotomy are often considered difficult intubations.[5,6] In addition, nasal intubation is often requested to allow the surgeon the ability to verify surgical improvement of malocclusion during the procedure. While nasal intubation was traditionally contraindicated in LeFort II or III fractures due to the possible disruption of the cribriform plate and the risk of cranial intubation or meningitis, multiple reports have described the successful placement of a nasotracheal tube over a fiberoptic bronchoscope without cranial intubation or other complications.

Positioning of patients presenting for LeFort osteotomy may also present challenges as the surgical team may prefer turning the operating table 90° or 180°. Conversely, if the operating table is left in the standard position, the anesthesia provider is charged with sharing access to the patent and will have limited access to the patient from the cephalad approach.

ANESTHETIC MANAGEMENT

PREOPERATIVE EVALUATION

A thorough preoperative evaluation should vet the presence of comorbidities impacting the cardiovascular, respiratory, gastrointestinal, renal, and endocrine systems. Special attention should be given to the airway examination to determine extent of mouth opening and neck mobility, as well as the presence of fractures and/or bony alterations that may negatively impact the ability to successfully intubate the patient. Preoperative airway assessment includes typical Mallampati class, thyromental distance, and oral opening, as well as evaluations related to nasal patency, previous nasal or sinus surgery (Box 80.1). Anesthesia providers must examine for signs of difficult airway such as micrognathia, maxillary or midface hypoplasia, or cleft palate as patients presenting for oral or maxillofacial surgery frequently (40%) include risk factors for a difficult airway.[7] In addition, it is important to inquire about a history of signs and symptoms of OSA, such as drowsiness during the day, snoring, mouth breathing, or pauses in breathing pattern.

As with all cases, patient preparation and education play a large role in achieving optimal patient outcomes. It should be discussed at length with the patient preoperatively that they will awaken with rubber bands or wires on their teeth, as well as a tight cold compression around their chin and head, which

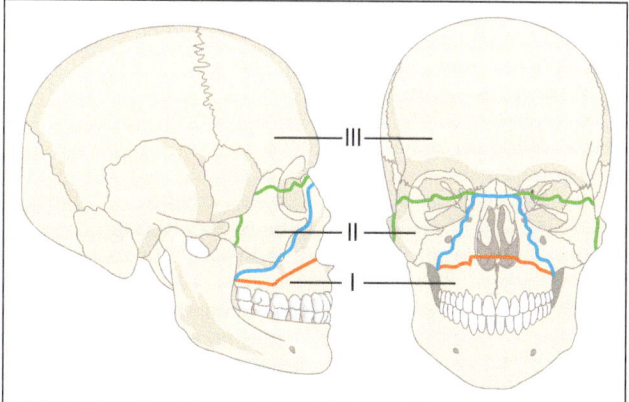

Figure 80.1: LeFort fractures.

I, Type I, horizontal, alveolar ridge; II, Type II, pyramidal, nasofrontal suture; III, Type III, horizontal, craniofacial dislocation.

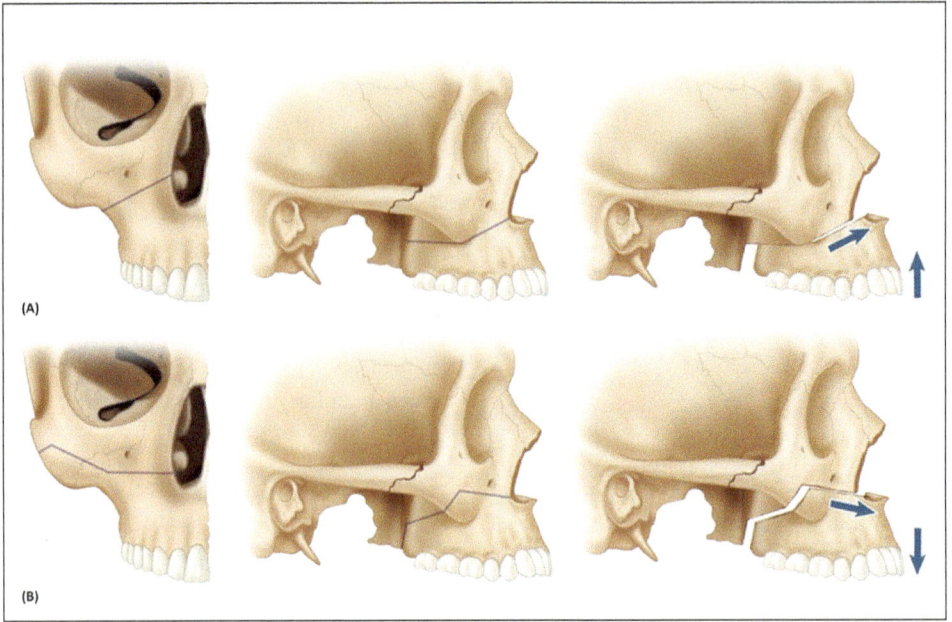

Figure 80.2: Maxillary osteotomies. (A) Type I, (B) Type II.

Source: From Patel PK. Maxillary osteotomies. In: P Taub, P Patel, S Buchman, M Cohen, eds. *Ferraro's Fundamentals of Maxillofacial Surgery*. Springer; 2015.

BOX 80.1	KEY ASSESSMENT POINTS

- Mallampati class
- Thyromental distance
- Mouth opening
- Neck mobility
- Micrognathia
- Maxillary or midface hypoplasia, or cleft palate
- Nasal patency, previous nasal or sinus surgery
- Signs and symptoms of obstructive sleep apnea

postoperatively. Reassurance and setting appropriate expectations are key to mitigating anxiety and complications in the postoperative period.

Pertinent Labs

Based on patient history, gender, age and risk for blood loss, the pertinent labs may include a hemoglobin and hematocrit and a urine chorionic gonadotrophin (UCG).

PREOPERATIVE PHARMACOLOGY

Prior to surgery, premedication includes administration of an anxiolytic if indicated, surgical infection and postoperative nausea and vomiting (PONV) prophylaxis, and potential initiation of controlled hypotensive regimen if indicated. Midazolam, either oral or IV, is commonly administered to decrease preoperative anxiety.[6] Dexmedetomidine, an alpha-2 adrenergic agonist, has both anxiolytic and opioid-sparing analgesic properties that may contribute to controlled hypotension as well.[8,9] Prophylactic antibiotics, often consisting of a first-generation cephalosporin, such as cefazolin, should be administered prior to surgical incision.[10–12] A scopolamine patch should be considered for PONV prophylaxis in patients aged 12 years and older.

ANESTHETIC TECHNIQUE

Intraoperative Management

Mask ventilation can often prove to be very difficult in patients presenting for LeFort osteotomy due to the associated midface hypoplasia (Box 80.2). Therefore, an IV induction using propofol and nondepolarizing neuromuscular blockade (NMB) is advisable. Prior to intubation, oxymetazoline should be administered to both nares to induce mucosal vasoconstriction and to minimize epistaxis secondary to nasal intubation. Additionally, oxymetazoline will induce decongestion that will facilitate nasal breathing postoperatively. Intubation with a nasal Ring–Adair–Elwin (RAE) endotracheal tube (ETT) allows securing the ETT for stability and avoiding interference with surgeon access. To provide a foundation on which to secure the breathing circuit to the forehead, the patient's head is securely wrapped with a nonsterile towel. The breathing circuit should be directed cephalad with a straight connector and secured to avoid pressure on nasal alar rim or forehead.[6]

Choice of volatile anesthetic agent should be guided by the importance of a smooth, rapid awakening with minimization of bleeding related to localized vasodilation. Sevoflurane may reduce airway irritability compared to desflurane yet offers low solubility for quick emergence. Total IV anesthesia with a propofol infusion, guided by the level of consciousness monitoring, may decrease PONV and speed emergence.[12] Balanced anesthesia including NMB may be used, although the use of sugammadex should be considered to avoid nausea secondary to neostigmine administration.

The analgesia component of the balanced anesthetic may be achieved by multiple methods. Traditional administration of fentanyl (2–3 mcg/kg) is effective; however, short-acting opioids may decrease the risk of postoperative respiratory depression. While remifentanil provides potent intraoperative analgesia, which can be titrated to variations in surgical stimulus and has rapid offset, it has been associated with postoperative hyperalgesia.[8] Multimodal analgesia might include the use of small

> **BOX 80.2 AIRWAY MANAGEMENT FOR LEFORT OSTEOTOMY**
>
> - In preparation for nasal intubation, an alternative or addition to mucosal vasoconstriction is inserting a warmed, lubricated nasal airway for mechanical dilation prior to inserting the ETT.
> - Warm (soften) cuffed end of nasal RAE ETT in a bottle of warm sterile water; lubricate just prior to insertion; and have Magill forceps available if needed to guide the ETT to the glottic opening.
> - Unless contraindicated, insert the ETT via the right naris to angle the bevel away from turbinates and minimize visual interference for direct laryngoscopy.
> - With the surgeon manipulating the patient's head, it may be necessary to use a larger size nasal RAE ETT to provide the sufficient length from the naris opening to the cuff below the glottic opening.
> - With nasal intubation, video laryngoscopy may not be helpful if Magill forceps are needed due to decreased space. The patient's orthodontic appliances may also contribute to difficulty.
> - If the ETT tip becomes lodged on the arytenoid cartilages during insertion, pull the ETT back slightly, rotate it 90° to 180°, and reattempt to insert before resorting to Magill forceps.
> - Stabilize the breathing circuit to the patient's padded forehead and top of head to avoid surgical field interference but allow surgeon ability to reposition the head.
> - Develop a fail-safe method to ensure throat pack removal at the end of the procedure. Place an obvious indicator in a conspicuous place on insertion and remove the indicator with removal of throat pack. Do not rely on the sponge count!
>
> ETT, endotracheal tube; RAE, Ring–Adair–Elwin.

> **BOX 80.3 TECHNIQUES TO MINIMIZE BLOOD LOSS**
>
> - Controlled hypotension: monitoring with invasive arterial line or a continuous noninvasive system with a finger cuff, appropriate pharmacologic agent(s) and administration equipment; avoiding reflex tachycardia
> - Tranexamic acid, administered IV or topically, may reduce intraoperative blood loss
> - Positioning in reverse Trendelenburg
> - Local anesthetic agent with epinephrine injected per surgeon into surgical field

dose ketamine, acetaminophen, ibuprofen, or ketorolac.[12] The potential negative effect of nonsteroidal anti-inflammatories on bleeding must be weighed against potential benefits and should be discussed with the surgical team prior to administration. The surgeon will inject local anesthetic (e.g., lidocaine 1% with 1:100,000 epinephrine or lidocaine 0.25% with 1:400,000 epinephrine) in the surgical field to aid in analgesia and vasoconstriction.

Controlled hypotension may be requested and can be achieved a variety of ways. Intraoperative management involves minimizing intraoperative bleeding with the use of controlled hypotension, especially during the down fracture of the maxilla and until the splint is secured (Box 80.3). Deliberate hypotension decreases blood loss, improves surgical field quality, decreases need for transfusion, and decreases length of stay postoperatively.[13] Different techniques may be employed to induce hypotension: remifentanil, propofol, volatile anesthetics, atenolol, enalapril, dexmedetomidine, labetalol, sodium nitroprusside, and nitroglycerine.[13–15] The use of remifentanil (0.05–0.5 mcg/kg/min) as opposed to a propofol infusion (50 mcg/kg/min) to induce controlled hypotension is recommended as remifentanil alters perfusion in the mandibular bone marrow, which may offset local vasodilation effects of volatile agents.[16,17] A continuous infusion of remifentanil may therefore yield reductions in blood loss and improved management of blood pressure. Compared to remifentanil, dexmedetomidine has better opioid-sparing effects postoperatively in addition to providing hypotensive benefits and should be considered.[8] In addition, controlled hypotension regimens may be achieved via administration of antihypertensive medications, although this is rarely required for the pediatric patient. Tranexamic acid, administered IV or topically, may also reduce intraoperative blood loss.[18,19] Regardless of the technique employed, the benefits of hypotension should be accurately controlled and closely monitored to ensure the balance of appropriate tissue perfusion with decreased blood loss.

Perioperative fluid management needs to meet the deficit and maintenance needs of the patient without contributing to excessive edema. With young, healthy patients who will be reluctant to take oral fluids postoperatively, the volume deficit can be minimized by encouraging clear fluids up to 2 hours before surgery. Fluids should be administered according to the needs of the patient to achieve euvolemia.[12] Dexamethasone is administered early in the operative period to reduce both postoperative edema and PONV.[20–22] Ondansetron should be administered prior to the completion of surgery for additional PONV prophylaxis. Administrating lidocaine or dexmedetomidine may facilitate a smooth emergence with minimal sympathetic stimulation and minimize coughing and respiratory depression.[23]

At the end of the procedure, it is recommended that the surgeon suction the oropharynx with a flexible catheter under direct visualization after the throat pack is removed and prior to attaching rubber bands of maxillomandibular fixation (MMF). Additional suctioning should be limited as it has potential to cause trauma to the suture line of the vestibular intraoral incision; it is difficult to thread the catheter between the rubber bands. During emergence, the optimal position is with the patient's head elevated in a reverse Trendelenburg's position and semi-Fowler's position to minimize bleeding and swelling. Fixation of the maxilla and mandible presents potential extubation challenges. It can be difficult to avoid having patients clench their jaw during emergence; however, this should be tempered if possible as clenching has the potential to break the miniplates used for internal fixation. While deep extubation is an alternative, it is not advisable as it may lead to laryngospasm and require manipulation of the jaw to open the airway. Small hardware might also be damaged with aggressive chin lift or jaw thrust. Once extubated and airway stability is confirmed, a cooling apparatus may be applied before transferring the patient to the postanesthesia care unit (PACU).

Complications/Emergencies

Potential complications and emergencies are summarized in Box 80.4.

BOX 80.4 COMPLICATIONS/EMERGENCIES

- Respiratory compromise: laryngospasm, respiratory depression, airway affected by edema or hematoma
- Bleeding: continued bleeding, the most common complication in maxillary surgery, may allow secretions to induce laryngospasm or gastric accumulation[24]
- Postoperative nausea and vomiting: concerns for aspiration, if patient vomits with maxillomandibular fixation, and hypovolemia
- Surgery related: cranial nerve injury or sensory symptoms, temporomandibular joint disorders, auditory changes[24]

POSTOPERATIVE CARE

Airway and respiratory stability require vigilance in the early period after surgery. PACU monitoring should include capnography, if possible, to provide greater sensitivity for detection of airway compromise.[23] Continued bleeding, edema, and residual anesthetic respiratory depression may cause airway obstruction. The preparation for emergency airway management includes the proximity of band or wire cutters and suction setup. Airway compromise may necessitate emergency induction and reintubation using a rapid sequence and oral intubation for initial stabilization.

During the remainder of the postoperative period, the emphasis is on minimizing the possible effects on respiratory compromise. With MMF, patients may perceive a feeling of inability to breathe sufficiently or suffocation. Calming reminders to breathe nasally and reassurance may reduce exacerbating anxiety. Nasal decongestants, saline solution spray, and topical corticosteroids may facilitate nasal breathing.[12] A multimodal approach to both PONV prophylaxis and postoperative pain may reduce the incidence and risks of respiratory depression. Decreased desire to take oral fluids and swallowing blood may contribute to nausea. A cooling system or ice wrap, positioning of head elevation greater than 30°, and dexamethasone are used to minimize swelling.[12]

CASE STUDY: 17-Year-Old Female With Dentofacial Anomaly Presenting for LeFort I Osteotomy, Bilateral Sagittal Split Osteotomy, and Genioplasty

CLINICAL SCENARIO

A female, 17-year-old, with dentofacial anomaly presents for a LeFort I, bilateral sagittal split osteotomy, and genioplasty. She has no significant medical history and denies smoking, illicit drug use, or alcohol consumption. She has orthodontic appliances in place.

SPECIAL CONSIDERATIONS

The anesthesia provider reinforces instructions and expectations for the early postoperative period. A thorough airway assessment is completed; it is remarkable for slight micrognathia. The patient denies OSA and notes that the airflow through the right naris is better. She self-administers oxymetazoline spray in bilateral nares. She has a scopolamine patch behind her left ear, which she applied as instructed prior to arriving. After confirmation of a negative urine pregnancy test (UCG), she receives midazolam 2 mg IV to relieve her anxiety. Once in the operating room with monitors applied, she self-administers additional oxymetazoline spray in bilateral nares and starts breathing oxygen at 8 L/min flow via a face mask. General anesthesia is induced with fentanyl 100 mcg, propofol 160 mg, and rocuronium 40 mg IV. After onset of relaxation, a pliable, lubricated 6.5-mm nasal RAE ETT is inserted via her right naris, and direct laryngoscopy is performed to visualize the proper placement of the ETT using Magill forceps.

Mechanical ventilation and sevoflurane administration are initiated, dexamethasone 6 mg is given, and infusions of dexmedetomidine 0.7 mcg/kg/hour and propofol 25 mcg/kg/minute are started. Cefazolin 1 g is administered after a test dose. Prior to incision, the surgeon infiltrates the surgical site with 1% lidocaine with 1:100,000 epinephrine. The surgeon places a throat pack to protect the airway.

After the procedure is completed, the surgeon removes the throat pack, which is confirmed by all in the room with the magnet removal. He passes a flexible suction catheter through the oropharynx for orogastric suctioning. The rubber bands are placed on the orthodontic appliances to main the alignment of the maxilla and mandible. With sevoflurane, dexmedetomidine and propofol weaned off, the patient spontaneously ventilates with appropriate tidal volumes and responds to quiet encouragement to take deep breaths. After extubation and the oxygen mask is gently applied, the patient is calmly reminded to breathe through her nose and that she has rubber bands on her teeth restricting mouth opening. A cooling wrap is secured around the patient's head; the head of the stretcher is in semi-Fowler's position; and humidified oxygen is applied on arrival to the PACU. The patient has no respiratory distress, is easily arousable, responds to commands appropriately, and denies PONV or pain. She will remain in the hospital for observation overnight. An emergency airway kit with band cutters remains with the patient in the PACU and through discharge to home.

(continued)

CASE STUDY: 17-Year-Old Female With Dentofacial Anomaly Presenting for LeFort I Osteotomy, Bilateral Sagittal Split Osteotomy, and Genioplasty (*continued*)

APPROACHES TO CARE

Evidence-Based Approaches to Care

LeFort I osteotomy is combined with bilateral sagittal split osteotomy to improve function related to jaw malocclusion and to alter facial appearance related to dentofacial deformities. Evidence shows that appropriate nasal mucosal vasoconstriction, softening of the nasal ETT in warm water, and lubrication reduce the risk for epistaxis.[6] Bleeding is a known intraoperative complication, especially during the down fracture of the maxilla.[24] Blood loss is reduced, and quality of the surgical field is improved with the use of controlled hypotension and the injection of local anesthetic with epinephrine.[15,25] Controlled hypotension is possible using a variety of agents, including volatile agents, opioids, dexmedetomidine, and propofol.[14–16] Multimodal analgesia is us to reduce the respiratory depressant effect of opioids in the postoperative period.[6,9,12] Multimodal PONV prophylaxis is essential as PONV incidence (46.1%) after orthognathic surgery is high. Postoperative MMF is an additional factor with an increased Apfel score.[26,27] Respiratory distress postoperatively is a key concern. Swelling, bleeding, laryngospasm, and anxiety related to the MMF may contribute to decreased ventilation.[6] Opioid-sparing agents, such as dexamethasone, dexmedetomidine, and acetaminophen, us in addition to the local anesthetic infiltration by the surgeon intraoperatively can minimize the need for opioids postoperatively.[12]

COMPLICATIONS

The patient remained in the hospital overnight for observation and continued prophylaxis of PONV. She received ondansetron 4 mg IV every 6 hours and acetaminophen liquid 500 mg PO every 4 hours. Oral intake was encouraged. A cooling system was used to the patient's head with the bed in semi-Fowler's position to minimize swelling and patient discomfort. Saline nasal spray and lip lubrication was encouraged. The patient was discharged home the following morning.

KEY REFERENCES

Complete references for this chapter are online and available at https://connect.springerpub.com/content/book/978-0-8261-3875-0/part/part04/toc-part/ch080.

6. Stein KM, Titler S. Maxillomandibular fixation and anesthesia management. *AANA J.* 2017;85(6):469–477.
10. Brignardello-Petersen R, Carrasco-Labra A, Araya I, et al. Antibiotic prophylaxis for preventing infectious complications in orthognathic surgery. *Cochrane Database Syst Rev.* 2015;5(1):CD010266. doi:10.1002/14651858.CD010266.pub2.
12. Otero JJ, Detriche O, Mommaerts MY. Fast-track orthognathic surgery: an evidence-based review. *Ann Maxillofac Surg.* 2017;7(2):166–175. doi:10.4103/ams.ams_106_17
19. Olsen JJ, Skov J, Ingersley J, et al. Prevention of bleeding in orthognathic surgery—a systematic review and meta-analysis of randomized controlled trials. *J Oral Maxillofac Surg.* 2016;74(1):139–150. doi:10.1016/j.joms.2015.05.031
20. Jean S. Perioperative systemic corticosteroids in orthognathic surgery: a systematic review and meta-analysis. *J Oral Maxillofac Surg.* 2017;75(12):2638–2649. doi:10.1016/j.joms.2017.06.014
23. Joyce JA. The other side of the difficult airway: a disciplined, evidence-based approach to emergence and extubation. *AANA J.* 2017;85(1):61–71.
24. Jedrzejewski M, Smektala T, Sporniak-Tutak K, Olszewski R. Preoperative, intraoperative, and postoperative complications in orthognathic surgery: a systematic review. *Clin Oral Investig.* 2015;19(5):969–977. doi:10.1007/s00784-015-1452-1

SECTION E: Plastics Procedures

CHAPTER 81

Cleft Lip and Cleft Palate Repair

Joshua Lea, Eleanor Mullen, and Julianne Ryan

INDICATIONS/CONTRAINDICATIONS

Oral clefts are a split or opening in the upper lip and/or palate and are the most common craniofacial abnormalities among newborns. The three main types of oral clefts are (a) cleft lip (CL), (b) cleft palate (CP), and (c) a combination of both cleft lip and palate (CLP). Oral clefts can be further classified by laterality, completeness, and primary or secondary palate (Box 81.1). In the United States, the incidence of oral clefts is approximately 1 in 690 births, with CP being the most prevalent of the oral clefts.[1] Depending on the specific oral cleft, the relationship among race, sex and prevalence can vary (Table 81.1). Oral clefts develop in vitro, between the 3rd and 12th week of gestation, and their contributing risk factors may be syndromic or nonsyndromic. Common syndromes associated with oral clefts include Pierre Robin, Treacher-Collins, Van der Woude, Apert, and Crouzon. Nonsyndromic risk factors include maternal age, cigarette smoking, folate deficiency, antiseizure medications, and genetic factors. Considering the prevalence and risk factors for oral clefts, it is paramount for the pediatric anesthesia providers to be familiar with the anesthetic management of these craniofacial anomalies.

The repair of CLs and/or CPs usually occurs during the first year of an infant's life.[2] The timing of surgery balances the need for early repair to allow for a functional velum during sound and speech development, against the need to avoid impairment of facial growth associated with early surgery. Therefore, CL repair is usually performed within the first 6 months after delivery to ensure proper sucking; CP repair should be performed within the first 2 years after delivery but usually occurs within 6 to 12 months, to ensure proper speech development and to limit interference with growth.[3]

While there are no absolute contraindications for CL and/or palate repairs, patients may have various comorbidities with which the use of general anesthesia may be a relative contraindication. The child should be medically optimized, with some surgeons still abiding by the "rule of 10s," meaning the surgery would only be performed once the child is older than 10 weeks, weighs greater than 10 pounds, and has a hemoglobin level greater than 10 g/dL.[4] Furthermore, the surgery should be conducted at an appropriate time in the child's development based on the aforementioned current guidelines.

BOX 81.1 CLASSIFICATION FOR CLEFT LIP AND PALATE

- Bilateral versus unilateral (left or right)
- Complete versus incomplete (left or right)
- Primary palate or secondary palate
- Combination of all

Source: Data from Zhang JX, Arneja JS. Evidence-based medicine: the bilateral cleft lip repair. *Plast Reconstr Surg.* 2017;140(1):152e–165e. doi:10.1097/PRS.0000000000003474

Table 81.1 Oral Clefts Malformations

Oral Clefts	Prevalence (per 10,000 live births)	Male-to-Female Ratio	Race/Ethnicity
Cleft lip	3.1	Constant between sexes	Highest among American Indians and Alaska Natives, lowest among African Americans
Cleft lip and palate	5.6	2:1	
Cleft palate	5.9	1:2	Constant between race and ethnicities

Source: Data from Mai CT, Cassell CH, Meyer RE, et al. Birth defects data from population-based birth defects surveillance programs in the United States, 2007 to 2011: highlighting orofacial clefts. *Birth Defects Res A Clin Mol Teratol.* 2014;100(11):895–904. https://doi-org.treadwell.idm.oclc.org/10.1002/bdra.23329

SPECIAL CONSIDERATIONS AND CONCERNS

Communication among members of the operating room (OR) team (e.g., anesthesia provider, surgeon, and circulating nurse) is essential to patient safety. Incorporating time into the perioperative workflow dedicated to sharing information, concerns, and solutions has been shown to decrease the incidence of errors and near misses while promoting multidisciplinary relationships.[5]

Regarding the huddle for oral cleft surgery, the surgical safety checklist should include the patient's name, procedure and laterality, allergies, antibiotics, procedure length, equipment needed, expected blood loss, airway concerns, throat packs, and recovery. While the details of these components can vary depending on the institution, patient, and OR team members, Table 81.2 includes a list of key elements commonly incorporated.

Table 81.2 Components of the Preoperative Huddle for Oral Cleft Surgery

Time	Anticipated Estimated Blood Loss (EBL)	Position	Special Considerations
1.5 to 2.5 hr	50 to 150 mL	Supine, table turned 90° to 180°, roll under neck/shoulders	Monitor throat pack in/throat pack out

ANESTHETIC MANAGEMENT

PREOPERATIVE EVALUATION

The preoperative evaluation of the pediatric patient with an oral cleft should include a thorough respiratory and airway assessment. When considering the respiratory system, upper respiratory infections (URIs) are common in this population, with a higher incidence in CPs than CLs. In fact, acute URI symptoms (e.g., fever, cough, and runny nose) are one of the most common causes of postponing surgery because of the increased risk of laryngospasm and bronchospasm. Chronic otitis and aspiration are also common among pediatric patients with oral clefts. Therefore, the anesthesia providers should collect a thorough respiratory history from the patient's guardian(s), and consider the patient's pulse oximeter reading, temperature, and breath sounds on auscultation.

With regard to the airway assessment of the patient with an oral cleft, obstructive sleep apnea, retrognathia, bilateral clefts and subglottic stenosis can be suggestive of difficulty with ventilation and/or intubation. Based on these findings, the anesthesia professional may consider using an advanced airway technique during intubation, such as glidescope or fiberoptic intubation. In the case of severe airway anomalies, an elective tracheostomy might be warranted. When planning for recovery, admission to the pediatric intensive care unit (PICU) should be considered for patients with a complicated medical history, especially those with severe obstructive sleep apnea and/or extensive palatal surgery.

An advanced assessment of different systems might be needed in pediatric patients with oral clefts related to syndromes (e.g., Apert, Klipel–Feil, Pierre–Robin, or Treacher-Collins syndromes). These considerations are listed in Table 81.3.

PREOPERATIVE PHARMACOLOGY

In general, patients less than 9 months rarely require premedication for anxiolysis. Conversely, patients older than 1 year of age may benefit from a preoperative anxiolytic (midazolam .5 mg/kg PO) or, alternatively, an anesthetic agent (ketamine 5 mg/kg PO).

Table 81.3 Key Assessment Points

	Associated Disorders/Illnesses	Assessment/Consults	Perioperative Planning
Cardiac	Congenital heart disease	ECG Chest x-ray Hct baseline O_2 saturation Consider cardiac consult	Optimize cardiac condition
Respiratory	Chronic otitis (Eustachian tube dysfunction) URI	Auscultation of breath sounds	Consider antibiotics for otitis prior to procedure Consider postponing due to URI if there are copious secretions and fever

Airway	Apert syndrome
	Goldenhar
	Kipel–Feil
	Pierre Robin
	Treacher-Collins
		• Airway examination
		  • Mallampati score
		  • B/l cleft
		  • Retrognathia
		• ICU bed should be available for patients with OSA
			Prepare for difficult intubations
			• Consider FOI or glidescope intubation
			• Consider elective tracheostomy placement for severe airway abnormalities or severe subglottic stenosis

Nutritional	NPO status Baseline malnutrition related to ineffective sucking		NPO • Liquids >3 hr • Breast milk >6 hr • Formula and solid food >8 hr
Neurological	Delayed speech Hearing impairment Developmental delays associated with other syndromes	Consult child life specialist	Ensure patient is fully prepared for experience prior to surgery to minimize communication problems
Hematological	Iron deficiency anemia	Hematocrit Type and screen	Consider setting up 1 unit of packed red blood cells
Psychological		Consult child life specialist	Multiple procedures for these patients mean increased anxiety • Consider premedication

B/l, bilateral; FOI, fiberoptic intubation; Hct, hematocrit; OSA, obstructive sleep apnea; URI, upper respiratory infection.

ANESTHETIC TECHNIQUE

Intraoperative Management

For most patients presenting for CL and CP repair, general anesthesia can be induced via an inhalational mask induction. For those patients who are suspected of having a difficult airway or for those who have a peripheral IV catheter in place, an IV induction may be considered (see Box 81.2). Anesthesia providers should anticipate challenges with mask ventilation and endotracheal intubation in patients presenting with craniofacial anomalies. In this scenario, it is recommended to have advanced airway management equipment readily available in the OR prior to induction of anesthesia. This may include either a video laryngoscope, fiberoptic bronchoscope, or both. It is also advisable to keep the patient breathing spontaneously until the airway has been secured. Intubation with an oral Ring–Adair–Elwin (RAE) endotracheal tube (ETT) is recommended to optimize the surgeon's access to the lesion being repaired. Care should be taken when securing the ETT, as tape securing the ETT may become loose secondary to surgical prep solution, secretions, or blood (see Box 81.3).

Anesthesia can be maintained via inhalation of volatile anesthetic agent or use of a total IV anesthesia (TIVA) technique; however, it is important to recognize that anesthetic techniques differ based on the patient, surgical team, institutions, and available resources. Standard monitors should be employed, including ECG, blood pressuring monitoring, pulse oximetry, and temperature monitoring. A single peripheral IV catheter is often sufficient, as anticipated blood loss is minimal.

A multimodal analgesic strategy should be employed to reduce the incidence of negative opioid-related sequelae, with the primary goal being avoidance of respiratory depression in the postoperative period. Acetaminophen (10–15 mg/kg IV or PR = rectal), fentanyl (1 mcg/kg IV), morphine (.05–.1 mg/kg IV), and dexmedetomidine (.5–1 mcg/kg IV) are routinely incorporated to achieve adequate pain management postoperatively. Bilateral infraorbital nerve blocks have been proven to provide excellent analgesia as well.

Complications and/or Emergencies

Bleeding, airway complications (especially airway obstruction), and postoperative nausea and vomiting (PONV) are the most common postoperative complications of CLs/CPs. Blood loss is greater in CP repairs than CL repairs.[3] Airway complications occur more commonly with a combined CLP repair and CPs alone.[6] Airway obstruction is one of the most common airway complications that occur but can be prevented by the surgeon placing a tongue stitch. When obstruction occurs, the stitch can be pulled to retract the tongue and relieve the obstruction. Anesthesia providers must execute caution upon extubation so as not to rip the stitch. Other airway complications include difficult intubations, ETT disconnection or compression, airway edema, bronchospasm, and laryngospasm.[6]

> **BOX 81.2   SPECIAL EQUIPMENT**
> - Oral airway
> - Video laryngoscope and/or fiberoptic bronchoscope
> - Oral right angle endotracheal tube

> **BOX 81.3   CLINICAL PEARLS**
> - Risk of endotracheal tube migration with movement of head/neck
>   - Neck extension and rotation → extubation
>   - Neck flexion → endobronchial intubation
> - Table is rotated 45°, 90°, or 180°
>   - Ensure ample circuit and IV tubing
> - Throat pack may be used
>   - Monitor peak inspiratory pressure (PIP) before and after placement to assess for endotracheal tube or inadvertent extubation
> - Epinephrine may be infiltrated to decrease blood loss
>   - Monitor for dysrhythmias

PONV is a common occurrence. To prevent PONV, anesthesia providers should ensure that the patient receives all antiemetics prior to extubation and may consider use of a TIVA technique, as well as placing an orogastric tube to suction prior to extubation.

POSTOPERATIVE CARE

Complications can transcend into the postoperative period as well, with a postoperative complication rate of 13%.[7] Complications specific to the postoperative period include edema of the tongue and oropharynx, airway obstruction, bronchospasm, pain, bleeding, wound dehiscence, and nausea and vomiting.[7] Tongue swelling may occur from the use of retractors during CP repairs; a nasopharyngeal airway may be placed at the completion of surgery to minimize airway obstruction due to such swelling.[8] Adequate pain control and the prevention of emergence agitation are vital, as sequelae from these complications include wound dehiscence and alterations in ventilation.[7] Dexmedetomidine administration prior to emergence and extubation has been shown to be a useful adjunct in preventing emergence agitation, although it may increase respiratory recovery time.[7] Arm restraints are frequently applied postoperatively to prevent the child from accessing the surgical site.[8]

Prior to hospital discharge, the patient should not have edema of the tongue and oropharynx and must have adequate nutritional intake and pain control.[8] Many patients will require secondary procedures for revisions.[8]

CASE STUDY: Airway Management During Induction in a Pediatric Patient Undergoing Cleft Lip and Palate Repair

CLINICAL SCENARIO

A 10-month American Indian female patient with a history of a left-sided, complete CLP presents for a CLP repair. According to the electronic medical record, the infant's height and weight are 7 kg and 65 cm today. No known drug allergies are reported. She has a medical history significant for obstructive sleep apnea, micrognathia, and malnutrition related to difficulty sucking, with no surgical history. The patient's electrolytes are within normal limits, and she does not take any medications.

(continued)

> **CASE STUDY: Airway Management During Induction in a Pediatric Patient Undergoing Cleft Lip and Palate Repair (*continued*)**
>
> ## SPECIAL CONSIDERATIONS
>
> During the preoperative interview, the parents of the infant report a history of recurrent respiratory infections but deny symptoms within the past 2 weeks. The infant was last fed 5 ounces of Pedialyte over 3 hours ago. On physical assessment, the patient's heart rate is regular, and her lungs are clear to auscultation. She is being held by her parent, who wish to be present for the induction of anesthesia.
>
> ## APPROACHES TO CARE
>
> ### Evidence-Based Approaches to Care
>
> Upon entering the warmed OR, accompanied by the child life specialist, the parent holding the infant sits on the OR table. The anesthesia provider places the pulse oximeter on the infant's large toe as she begins to cry and squirm. At this point, the infant's oxygen mask is placed over her nose and mouth; the anesthesia professional administers oxygen at 8 L/min and sevoflurane at 5%, which is titrated to 8% after a few minutes. Once loss of consciousness is demonstrated, the parent is reassured and escorted out of the room with the child life specialist.
>
> A 24 g IV is placed in the right saphenous vein and the patient is noted to be partially obstructing. An oral airway is placed with improvement of ventilation. Propofol 10 mg IV and rocuronium 4.2 mg IV are administered.
>
> ## COMPLICATIONS
>
> A 3.5 uncuffed ETT is placed using a Miller 1 with a Grade 3 view; however, there is an absence of chest rise and end-tidal carbon dioxide waveform on the anesthesia machine. Gurgling is reported to be auscultated over the epigastrium by another anesthesia professional. Meanwhile, the infant's pulse oximetry has dropped to 72%.
>
> Fortunately, the anesthesia provider was well prepared and a video laryngoscope was in the room and ready to use. With the aid of the video laryngoscope, the patient was atraumatically intubated, with the oxygen saturations quickly returning to baseline.

KEY REFERENCES

Complete references for this chapter are online and available at https://connect.springerpub.com/content/book/978-0-8261-3875-0/part/part04/toc-part/ch003.

4. Zhang JX, Arneja JS. Evidence-based medicine: the bilateral cleft lip repair. *Plast Reconstr Surg.* 2017;140(1):152e–165e. doi:10.1097/PRS.0000000000003474
5. Urdaneta F. A time-out for anesthesia professionals. *APSF Newsletter.* 2019;34(2):36. https://doi.org/10.1213/01.ane.0000270266.32684.12
8. Chang J. *Global Reconstructive Surgery.* Elsevier; 2019.
9. Huang AS, Hajduk J, Rim C, et al. Focused review on management of the difficult pediatric airway. *Indian J. Anaesth.* 2019;63(6):428–436. doi:10.4103/ija.IJA_250_19
11. Nagelhout JJ, Elisha S. *Nurse Anesthesia.* 6th ed. Elsevier. 2018.

CHAPTER 82

Venous Malformations

Nicole K. Damico and Rajanya S. Petersson

INDICATIONS/CONTRAINDICATIONS

Venous malformations (VMs) are the most common type of vascular anomalies found in the body, comprising approximately two-thirds of all congenital vascular malformations.[1]

According to one commonly used classification system,[2] the two major groups of vascular anomalies are tumors and malformations. Different vascular malformations are distinguished by nomenclature based on presentation, such as lesions of one type only (simple), of two or more types (combined), of major named vessels, or occurring in association with other anomalies. Vascular malformations can further be subdivided as low-flow or high-flow lesions. Venous and lymphatic malformations are low-flow lesions, whereas arteriovenous malformations are high-flow lesions. The distinction between low-flow and high-flow lesions is of relevance when making treatment decisions. Venous malformations are composed of a network of serpiginous interconnected veins with ectatic venous channels that lack vascular smooth muscle in the vessel wall.[3] Venous malformations can occur anywhere in the body, although most are found in the extremities or the head and neck, with the oral cavity, airway, or muscles of mastication most commonly involved in the latter subgroup.[1,4]

VMs can be challenging to diagnose as there is no characteristic pattern or presentation for patients with VM and are often confused with hemangioma in terminology as well as with imaging. As a congenital condition, VMs are always present at birth, occurring in isolation or as part of a syndrome, but may not be evident until the child reaches preschool or school age.[5,6] VMs increase in size with normal growth and development and will not regress without intervention.[7] Significant lesion progression is common during adolescence due to normal hormonal fluctuations during puberty.[8]

VMs are associated with a host of sequelae. Unlike nearly all other vascular anomalies, VMs are frequently painful, especially when engorged. A dependent position, Valsalva maneuver, or thrombi development within the lesion all have the potential to further accentuate the associated pain. Chronic thrombosis can trigger localized intravascular coagulopathy (LIC), a dreaded and potentially very serious complication marked by elevated D-dimer, decreased plasma fibrinogen and ultimately, disseminated intravascular coagulation (DIC).[9] Mass effect from VMs of the head and neck can cause a myriad of significant functional impairments of speech, mastication, swallowing, or airway patency. Cosmetic defects associated with venous malformations vary with the size and specific location of the lesion. Superficial lesions are associated with dynamic soft tissue swelling, often with an irregular contour, and blue or purple skin discoloration.

Treatment of VMs is generally indicated for management of symptoms, avoidance of complications, and/or cosmesis, versus cure. Lesion size and complexity are key factors in treatment decision-making. A single treatment modality may be appropriate for small, well-localized lesions, while multimodal and/or sequential interventions are typically indicated for large or infiltrative lesions. Simple, noninvasive interventions, such as sleeping with the head of bed elevated for head and neck lesions or wearing compression garments for lesions of the extremities, are generally helpful in preventing venous stasis and associated sequelae.[4] Medical management with low-dose aspirin or low-molecular-weight heparin can help prevent thrombosis. Nonsteroidal anti-inflammatory drugs (NSAIDs) and warm compresses are recommended for treatment of mild to moderate pain, while referral to a chronic pain specialist may be necessary for patients with very painful lesions.[10,11]

Several invasive treatments for VMs are commonly used for patients of all ages. Primary surgical excision may be an option for lesions that are small, discrete, and in easily accessible locations. Sclerotherapy, or injection of a sclerosing agent directly into the VM under fluoroscopy or ultrasound guidance, is a mainstay of treatment for a wide variety of lesion types and locations, alone or in combination with other approaches.[10] Due to the risk of swelling and hemorrhage, sclerotherapy of VMs in or near the airway carries a high risk of compromised airway protection[5,10] and may be ill advised, especially in children. Light amplification by the stimulated emission of radiation (laser) phototherapy is a viable alternative or adjunct to other invasive treatments for superficial VMs of the face, oral cavity, and the aerodigestive tract. Given its particular utility in the treatment of head and neck VMs in pediatric patients, laser treatment will be the focus of the remaining portion of this chapter.

Contraindications to laser are few and nearly entirely related to consideration of lesion characteristics. VM that are infiltrative, large, deeper than about 7 to 8 mm, very near to nerves or other vital structures, or in an area that is very challenging to access are unlikely to be amenable to laser treatment as a stand-alone modality and usually require multimodality therapy.

LASER TREATMENT

Several types of lasers can be used to treat VMs, with the determination based on a multitude of factors, such as the lesion size, location, depth, wall thickness, and flow characteristics. While many types of laser have been described for treatment of VMs in the literature, the most common types of laser used for head and neck VMs in children are carbon dioxide (CO_2) and neodymium-doped yttrium aluminum garnet (Nd:YAG). A CO_2 laser emits far-infrared, long-wavelength (10,600 nm) light, while a Nd:YAG emits near-infrared light at a relatively shorter wavelength (1064 nm). These properties highlight the most fundamental distinction among laser types: depth of penetration. Carbon dioxide lasers penetrate relatively shallow depths, up to approximately .25 mm, while Nd:YAG can achieve depths of 4 to 7 mm.[12] The chromophore for Nd:YAG laser is deoxyhemoglobin, whereas it is water for the CO_2 laser. While the CO_2 laser vaporizes the surface of tissue in the area being treated, the Nd:YAG laser penetrates below the treated surface and is absorbed by pigment-carrying bodies as well as proteins carried in small, to medium-sized veins, making it a superior choice for superficial and deep mucosal VM.[13] The type of laser used in a given case has little direct impact on anesthetic decision-making and is a vital factor to consider when determining appropriate safety precautions to be used intraoperatively.

SPECIAL CONSIDERATIONS AND CONCERNS

Unique intraoperative risks associated with procedures involving lasers include fire, patient or healthcare personnel injury, and exposure to smoke plume.[14] Recommendations for fire prevention during laser surgery of the head and neck are summarized in Box 82.1. Facilities at which lasers are used must have a comprehensive laser safety program per the *Standard for Safe Use of Lasers in Healthcare*.[15] The anesthesia team is generally most directly charged with ensuring compliance with appropriate eye protection guidelines for the type of laser used, such as covering the patient's eyes with saline-soaked gauze pads. Evidence-based guidelines to reduce risks of smoke exposure do not currently exist.

ANESTHETIC MANAGEMENT

PREOPERATIVE EVALUATION

Preoperative evaluation must be tailored to the patient's biological and developmental age. In addition to routine anesthetic history and physical, in-depth airway evaluation is critical. Vascular malformations are space-occupying lesions with characteristic slow, monophasic inflow. They are compressible and variable in size in association with positional changes, fluctuating hormonal conditions, and trauma.[1] The dynamic nature of VMs highlights the importance of attention to positional and hemodynamic conditions during preoperative physical assessment and the peri-induction period. Comprehensive ultrasonography with or without Doppler and duplex imaging is frequently performed as part of the initial workup for suspected vascular anomalies, and MRI is the gold standard for definitive diagnosis and procedural planning.[1,4] Review of imaging reports is likely to yield pertinent information key to anesthetic management and decision-making.

> **KEY TAKEAWAY**
>
> - Thorough airway assessment is vital for procedures of the head and neck. Evaluation in the upright and supine positions may help anticipate the conditions likely to be encountered during airway management.

Pertinent Labs

Patients with VMs are at risk of local and systemic coagulopathic complications. LIC is characterized by elevated D-dimer and low fibrinogen levels due to chronic activation of fibrinolytic pathways and, if present, increased risk of perioperative hemorrhage and development of DIC.[17] It is generally recommended that invasive interventions are delayed in patients with preoperative evidence of LIC to facilitate patient optimization and possible initiation of prophylactic low–molecular-weight (LMW) heparin therapy.[9] Candidates for laser treatments for VMs of the head and neck, by virtue of the nature of their lesions as relatively simple, discrete, and superficially located, may be less likely to manifest LIC preoperatively, given the observed positive correlation between D-dimer levels and lesion characteristics such as large lesion surface area (10 cm^2), truncal location, and deeper tissue involvement.[17]

Preoperative laboratory analysis is the best method to detect LIC, as patients with VMs are characteristically otherwise asymptomatic for the condition. It is important to note that isolated elevated D-dimer (>500 ng/mL, normal reference <500 ng/mL) is common in patients with VMs[18] but is not diagnostic for LIC. The presence of phleboliths and the combination of markedly elevated D-dimer (>1000 ng/mL) and low fibrinogen levels are associated with LIC.[17]

PREOPERATIVE PHARMACOLOGY

Several considerations related to preoperative medications are important for pediatric patients scheduled for laser photocoagulation of head or neck VMs. Preprocedural administration of sedatives and/or analgesics may be indicated for control of anxiety and pain or to prevent vigorous crying and straining preoperatively. Crying and straining have the potential to raise intrathoracic pressure and cause engorgement of the VM, thereby decreasing functional airway diameter and increasing the risk of difficult airway management. However, commonly used sedatives and analgesics, such as midazolam and short-acting opioids, are associated with respiratory depression and potential airway compromise, especially if given in combination. Selection and titration of preoperative sedative and/or analgesic medications should aim to carefully balance these risks and benefits. Patients on LMW heparin or aspirin may continue these medications perioperatively.

BOX 82.1   RECOMMENDED FIRE PREVENTION MEASURES DURING LASER SURGERY OF THE HEAD AND NECK

- Preassign specific fire management tasks to team members prior to the case.
- Display the fire management protocol in the operating room.
- Consider a sealed airway device if moderate or deep sedation is needed or the patient is likely to be oxygen dependent.
- Use a cuffed endotracheal tube instead of an uncuffed tube for procedures inside the airway.
- Use a laser-resistant tube whenever possible and fill the cuff with saline colored with indicator dye.
- Prior to activating the laser,
  - the surgeon should alert the anesthesia team;
  - reduce oxygen delivery to the lowest concentration needed to avoid hypoxia;
  - stop nitrous oxide flow, if applicable; and
  - pause until the reduction in oxygen concentration has had time to take effect.
- Consider application of suction scavenging to reduce oxidizer concentration near the surgical field.

Source: From American Society of Anesthesiologists (ASA) Committee on Standards and Practice Parameters: Apfelbaum JL, Chicago, Illinois.

ANESTHETIC TECHNIQUE

Anesthetic planning is fundamentally based on the location and extent of the VM to be treated. Laser treatments must be precisely applied in order to be effective and avoid damage to adjacent normal tissues. While relatively short procedures, small, superficial VMs on the face or the anterior oral cavity may be treated on an outpatient basis under local anesthesia or IV sedation, although general anesthesia is very often necessary to achieve adequate lesion exposure and an absolutely still surgical field.[19,20] The airway management plan further dictates options for achieving general anesthesia. The anesthetic plan should be discussed with the perioperative team in advance to ensure all relevant factors are considered prior to patient arrival in the operating room.

Intraoperative Management

Mask inhalational induction with nitrous oxide and sevoflurane is preferred in younger children without established IV access. If possible, it may be helpful to elevate the head of bed, even slightly, to optimize airway patency in patients with lesions in or very near to the airway. Maintaining spontaneous respirations until after placement of IV access is ideal. In patients with lesions in the oropharynx, oral airways should be placed only in the event of intractable peri-induction upper airway obstruction and, even then, with great care to avoid trauma to the VM.

The selection of the most appropriate airway management plan must incorporate the surgeon's requests and preferences. Very short procedures can be done under IV general anesthesia with spontaneous ventilation and no artificial airway. Following inhalational induction and placement of IV access, an appropriate depth of general anesthesia is established with IV agents, such as propofol or dexmedetomidine and titrated doses of short– or ultra–short-acting opioids. Mask ventilation can be maintained until the operating room table and patient are positioned. Supplemental oxygen can be administered intermittently via blow-by or periods of facemask-assisted ventilation, although periods of administration of room air are likely needed, especially during application of laser, which may not be tolerated by some patients.

Suspension laryngoscopy may be necessary for procedures on the periglottic area or trachea and placement of an endotracheal tube in such cases could conceivably obscure the surgical field. Due to the depth of general anesthesia needed, maintaining sufficient spontaneous respiratory effort may be challenging. When supplemental ventilatory assistance is needed in such circumstances, jet ventilation may be helpful, though anesthesia providers must be cognizant of the potential for barotrauma. Following establishment of an appropriate depth of general anesthesia with IV agents and placement of the suspension laryngoscope, the jet ventilator cannula is inserted through a dedicated side port on the laryngoscope and advanced until it reaches the desired supra- or subglottic position. Ventilation can be delivered with a manual system (low frequency) or a commercial ventilator (high frequency). Regardless of technique, it is recommended that inspiratory driving pressure not exceed 15 to 30 pounds per square inch (PSI). It is critical to ensure adequate gas egress to avoid complications such as hemodynamic instability or tension pneumothorax, especially when using subglottic catheter placement.[21]

Due to the well-documented risk of fire, placement of a sealed airway device is preferred when moderate or deep anesthesia is needed during laser procedures on the head and neck.[16] If the lesion is external, or outside the aerodigestive tract, placing a cuffed supraglottic airway may be an option. When treating a lesion in the oral cavity or anywhere else in the aerodigestive tract, endotracheal intubation is likely need for surgical exposure. Using a laser-resistant endotracheal tube (ETT) is recommended if the patient's size permits. Unfortunately, due to the wall thickness of laser-resistant ETTs, very few options are available for pediatric patients in general, and no currently marketed devices are suitable for children under the age of approximately 4 to 5 years. The minimum outside diameter of available laser-resistant ETTs is 5.8 mm for cuffed tubes (Sheridan LTS microlaryngeal ETT; Teleflex Medical, Morrisville, NC), and 5.2 mm for uncuffed tubes (Shiley laser oral tracheal tube; Medtronic ENT, Minneapolis, MN). Both products are marketed for use during procedures involving CO_2 and potassium titanyl phosphate (KTP), but not Nd:YAG, lasers. Standard ETTs are the best and only option for many children.

There are additional benefits to having a secure airway during laser procedures of the head and neck. Unlike when spontaneous or manual jet ventilation is used, continuous capnography monitoring can be employed. In addition, a far wider variety of pharmacological options for maintenance of general anesthesia are possible. Nitrous oxide should be discontinued, and the fraction of inspired oxygen reduced to less than 30% prior to commencing laser treatment. Volatile inhalational agents, alone or in combination with IV infusion of hypnotics such as propofol or dexmedetomidine, and titrated doses of short– or ultra–short-acting opioids are commonly used techniques. Neuromuscular blockade and controlled mechanical ventilation can facilitate surgical access and ensure maintenance of a still surgical field.

Several anesthetic adjuncts are recommended regardless of the specific techniques of anesthesia used. IV dexamethasone .15 to .5 mg/kg may help prevent postoperative nausea and vomiting (PONV) and airway swelling. When volatile agents are used, procedure time is greater than 30 minutes and/or the pediatric patient is older than 3 years, additional PONV prophylaxis with a 5-hydroxytryptamine 3 ($5\text{-}HT_3$) antagonist, such as ondansetron, is recommended, especially if other patient risk factors are present.[22] Other intraoperative interventions such as liberal fluid replacement (up to 30 mL/kg), opioid-sparing, acetaminophen (15 mg/kg), and lidocaine infusion (1.5 mg/kg bolus, 2 mg/kg/hr infusion) may further reduce PONV risk in patients with many risk factors.[22] Lidocaine would offer the added benefit of blunting protective reflexes during stimulation of the airway. Perioperative cefazolin may be given per the surgeon's discretion, although the indication varies based on the location of the VM and the extent of intervention.

Special Equipment

Equipment and supply needs are significant for laser procedures on the head and neck area. Recommended eye protection includes saline-soaked gauze pads for the patient and specialized glasses or goggles suitable for the laser wavelength to be used for all personnel in the room, as shown in **Box 82.1**. Whether intubation is planned or will be used as a rescue technique, several appropriately sized, cuffed ETTs should be readily available. A bottle of sterile saline should be kept handy at all times to flood the surgical field to rapidly extinguish a fire and cool the tissues should this unfortunate situation occur.

Clinical Pearls

While laser procedures on the head, neck, and tissues of the aerodigestive tract and/or techniques to achieve surgical exposure in these areas (e.g., suspension laryngoscopy) are intensely stimulating while in progress, little residual pain is anticipated once the procedure is completed. Accordingly, highly titratable, short-acting hypnotic and analgesic agents are strongly preferred as part of all anesthetic plans.

Complications/Emergencies

Intraoperative complications during laser procedures can be severe and include fire, bleeding, aspiration, and airway loss. Recommendations for prevention and management of fire were previously described in Box 82.1. Significant intraoperative bleeding is very rare, especially during procedures on relatively small lesions. Risks may be higher in patients taking aspirin or LMWH, or with abnormal preoperative coagulation studies (elevated D-dimer and low fibrinogen). While risk of aspiration during laser procedures has not been described in the literature, this dreaded complication is clearly a possible during any periods when a secure airway in not in place. Acute airway obstruction or complete loss of airway patency, which, again, has not previously been described in the literature, could conceivably occur due to a number of factors, including, among others, bleeding, swelling, ineffective patient position, mechanical obstruction by equipment, and ETT kinking. Excessively deep anesthesia during cases without an ETT in place may result in periods of apnea and may necessitate temporary halting of the procedure to facilitate effective assisted or controlled ventilation. Using standard monitors, such as capnography (whenever feasible), pulse oximetry, and the precordial stethoscope can aid in rapid detection and intervention in the event of acute airway compromise.

POSTOPERATIVE CARE

Patient disposition and details of postoperative care are dependent upon the extent of the procedure performed and patient tolerance. Significant swelling or bleeding after laser procedures is uncommon.[23] Accordingly, patients may often be discharged to home once recovered from anesthesia and they meet the facility's discharge criteria. Mild swelling and lesion ulceration may occur during normal healing and may result in mild to moderate scarring or other cosmetic changes over time.[24] When treating areas such as the lips, patients are instructed to liberally apply petroleum-based products to keep the tissue from drying out, which can lead to bleeding. Paresthesias are an uncommon and often self-limited postoperative complication.[25] However, if significant swelling is encountered during treatment of laryngeal, periglottic, tongue-base, or other upper airway lesions, the surgeon may elect to keep the patient intubated overnight to protect the airway while edema resolves, especially in pediatric patients with smaller airways. When treating large upper airway lesions, the surgeon may elect to place a temporary tracheostomy for the duration of the treatment period, which can allow for serial outpatient procedures.

KEY REFERENCES

Complete references for this chapter are online and available at https://connect.springerpub.com/content/book/978-0-8261-3875-0/part/part04/toc-part/ch082.

4. Fowell C, Verea Linares C, Jones R, et al. Venous malformations of the head and neck: current concepts in management. *Br J Oral Maxillofac Surg*. 2017;55(1):3–9. doi:10.1016/j.bjoms.2016.10.023
9. Zhuo KY, Russell S, Wargon O, Adams S. Localised intravascular coagulation complicating venous malformations in children: associations and therapeutic options. *J Paediatr Child Health*. 2017;53(8):737–741. doi:10.1111/jpc.13461
10. Gallant SC, Chewning RH, Orbach DB, et al. Contemporary management of vascular anomalies of the head and neck—part 1: vascular malformations: a review. *JAMA Otolaryngol Head Neck Surg*. 2020;1, 1–10. doi:10.1001/jamaoto.2020.4353
16. Caplan RA, Barker SJ, Connis RT, et al. Practice advisory for the prevention and management of operating room fires: an updated report by the American Society of Anesthesiologists Task Force on Operating Room Fires. *Anesthesiology*. 2013;118(2):271–290. doi:10.1097/ALN.0b013e31827773d2
20. Stevic M, Ristic N, Budic I, et al. Comparison of ketamine and ketofol for deep sedation and analgesia in children undergoing laser procedure. *Lasers Med Sci*. 2017;32(7):1525–1533. doi:10.1007/s10103-017-2275-x
23. Ridgway R, Dumbarton T, Brown Z. Update on ENT anaesthesia in children. *Anaesth Intensive Care Med*. 2019;20(1):56–60. doi:10.1016/j.mpaic.2018.11.003

CHAPTER 83

Pharyngoplasty

D. Julie Soelberg and Tomas Lazo

INDICATIONS/CONTRAINDICATIONS

Pharyngoplasties are performed to treat velopharyngeal dysfunction (VPD), a generic term comprising disorders that disrupt the velopharyngeal closing pattern.[1,2] The velopharyngeal space is a complex and dynamic structure that serves to separate the oropharynx and nasopharynx during speech and swallowing.[1] Adequate closure of the velopharynx is required for normal phonation and swallowing (Figure 83.1). Failure of the velopharyngeal mechanism to close completely can result in nasal air emission, hypernasal speech, and nasopharyngeal regurgitation.[1,3,4]

Multiple etiologies are responsible for VPD in children. The spectrum of disorders comprising VPD include velopharyngeal insufficiency (VPI), incompetence, and mislearning. These disorders may result from surgery on the velopharynx, as part of a craniofacial syndrome, due to neuromuscular impairment or from functional articulation errors[1,3] (Box 83.1). VPI refers to a structural abnormality resulting in incomplete closure of the velopharyngeal space and is most commonly seen in children with a history of cleft palate repair. After cleft palate repair, VPI and subsequent hypernasal speech are noted in 20% to 30% of children.[2,5] Pharyngoplasties are often performed as secondary speech procedures following palatoplasty, with the primary goal of normalizing speech and phonation.[3] Children generally present for speech-correcting procedures at 4 to 6 years of age.[6]

Several surgical approaches are described for the management of VPI, including superior-based pharyngeal flaps, sphincter palatoplasty, Furlow double-opposing Z-palatoplasty, or a combination of these procedures.[7,8,9,10] All are preformed via the transoral route. Surgical treatment aims to close the velopharyngeal defect by creating a functional seal between the oropharyngeal and nasopharyngeal space during speech.[4,11] Pharyngoplasty augmentation procedures are a less invasive option and include injection of a tissue filler or grafts into the palate to increase palatal bulk and to facilitate closure, which may be effective in some patients with VPI.[4,12] No absolute contraindications to pharyngoplasty exist, although it should be noted that pharyngoplasty is a speech-correcting, elective procedure.

SPECIAL CONSIDERATIONS AND CONCERNS

See Box 83.2 for special considerations and concerns.

ANESTHETIC MANAGEMENT

PREOPERATIVE EVALUATION

Appropriate preoperative assessment should occur prior to induction of general anesthesia. This should include a history with a thorough review of systems, as well as a physical examination. Special attention should be taken to evaluate for existing craniofacial abnormalities, congenital syndromes, and the possibility of difficult mask ventilation and/or intubation.[13] Patients should be screened for any recent or existing signs of respiratory illnesses since this may increase their likelihood for perioperative pulmonary complications.[14]

As patients often have a surgical palatoplasty performed before undergoing a pharyngoplasty, a thorough review of prior anesthetic records is highly recommended. The ability to

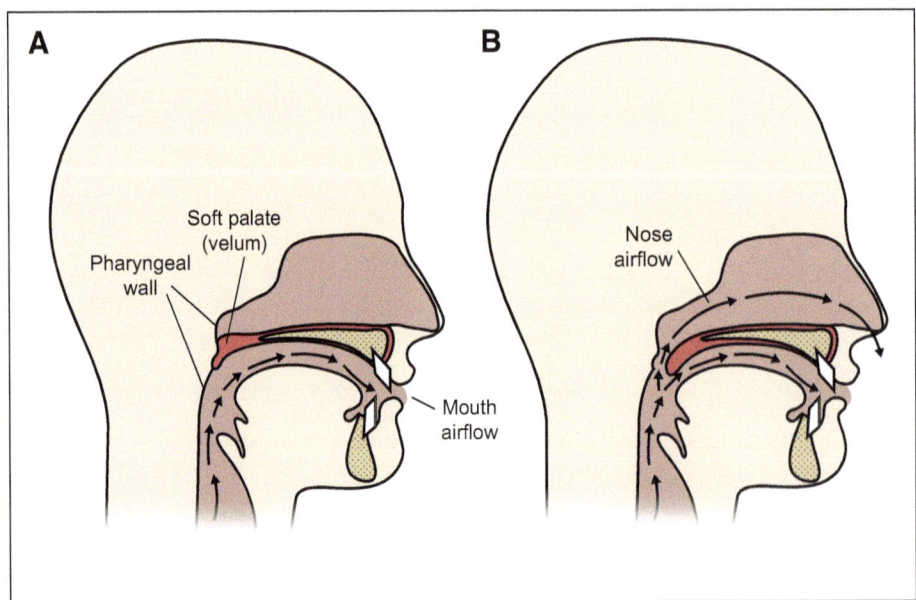

Figure 83.1: Velopharyngeal dysfunction (VPD). (A) During normal speech, the velum closes the velopharynx. (B) In VPD, the velum is too short to adequately close the velopharynx.

> **BOX 83.1 ETIOLOGIES OF VELOPHARYNGEAL DYSFUNCTION (VPD)**
>
> **Velopharyngeal Insufficiency**
> - Congenital: cleft palate, submucosal cleft, velopharyngeal disproportion in 22q11.2 deletion syndrome
> - Mechanical: enlarged tonsils, mass, trauma, velopharyngeal surgery
>
> **Velopharyngeal Incompetence**
> - Neurological: cerebrovascular accident
> - Neuromuscular: myasthenia gravis, global hypotonia, cerebral palsy, muscular or myotonic dystrophy, demyelinating diseases
>
> **Velopharyngeal Mislearning**
> - Functional, without evidence of anatomic or physiological cause

> **BOX 83.3 CLINICAL PEARLS FOR THE ANESTHETIC MANAGEMENT OF PHARYNGOPLASTY**
>
> Perform a thorough preop assessment evaluating for
> - upper respiratory infection symptoms.
> - congenital syndromes with associated abnormalities, and
> - likelihood of a difficult mask ventilation or intubation.
>
> Review prior anesthetic records.
>
> Prepare difficult intubation equipment.
>
> Provide multimodal analgesia.
>
> Be wary of postoperative nasal or oropharyngeal obstruction.
>
> Extubate patients awake.

> **BOX 83.2 SPECIAL CONSIDERATIONS WITH VELOPHARYNGEAL INSUFFICIENCY (VPI) AND PHARYNGOPLASTY**
>
> - VPI may be present in syndromic or nonsyndromic children.
> - Children with VPI will have reduced intelligibility of speech, ranging from mild to severe nasality.
> - Retropharyngeal course of carotid arteries may increase surgical risks and/or alter surgical planning.
> - Speech therapy and prosthesis are alternatives to surgical treatment for mild VPI.

review prior airway management notes is not always a luxury afforded to anesthesia providers and should be taken advantage of when possible. This may reveal prior difficulty with mask ventilation and/or intubation, which may aid in the preparation for airway management for the pharyngoplasty procedure. Additionally, prior records may offer information about the success of previously employed premedication strategies. As these patients may have some degree of developmental delay, assessing the need for premedication and which administration route would be most effective is warranted.[15]

ANESTHETIC TECHNIQUE

Intraoperative Management

Refer to **Box 83.3**. In the intraoperative setting, most patients can be treated similarly to those undergoing primary palate repair. Thus, the principles of beginning with an inhalational induction, obtaining IV access, intubating with an oral Ring–Adair–Elwyn (RAE) tube, using IV steroids to mitigate airway swelling, and providing multimodal analgesia would all apply to pharyngoplasty patients.[16] Caveats to this approach may include patients with a history of difficult mask ventilation due to micrognathia or retrognathia, or prior known difficult mask ventilation, where additional airway management techniques may be employed. Additionally, if a patient has had a previous palatoplasty procedure, nasal intubation should be avoided, if possible, to prevent damage to prior surgical repairs.[17]

Complications

Complications in the intraoperative and postoperative periods are also similar to those of palatoplasties. The potential for postoperative airway obstruction from local tissue edema and tongue swelling due to the operative retractor is important to consider.[17] Of note, one study demonstrated a longer term effect of increased incidence of apnea/hypopnea in patients undergoing multiple procedures for VPI, notably the dynamic sphincter pharyngoplasty.[18] This may be further worsened by the effects of residual anesthetics or neuromuscular blockers, in addition to the respiratory depressing effects of benzodiazepines and opioids.[17,19] To maintain patent airways, surgeons will often place a conduit, such as a nasopharyngeal airway device, into one or both nares. These are often sutured in and are left in for hours to days after surgery to ensure appropriate ventilation.[15] Since obstruction, apnea, and hypopnea are reasonable considerations, most anesthesia providers recommend extubating these patients when fully awake.

POSTOPERATIVE CARE

While bleeding following a palatoplasty may be common, postoperative bleeding requiring reexploration seems to be a fairly rare complication in pharyngoplasty patients.[20] Other more common postoperative complications include emergence delirium, pain, and nausea. Emergence delirium can be lessened by appropriate use of multimodal analgesia, potentially including the use of palatal nerve blocks.[21] The increased popularity of dexmedetomidine has also shown benefit in reducing the likelihood of emergence delirium and postoperative pain in the pediatric otolaryngology population.[22] The use of liposomal bupivacaine has also demonstrated improvement in postoperative pain relief, less opioid use, and earlier time to feeding.[23] Prior to discharge, it is important to convey to the parents that the roof of the mouth may be without feeling for several weeks. Parents must take extra care to avoid injury to the surgical site secondary to the lack of feeling at the surgical site.

KEY REFERENCES

Complete references for this chapter are online and available at https://connect.springerpub.com/content/book/978-0-8261-3875-0/part/part04/toc-part/ch083.

1. Raol N, Hartnick CJ. Anatomy and physiology of velopharyngeal closure and insufficiency. *Adv. Oto-Rhino-Laryngol.* 2015a;76:1–6. doi:10.1159/000368003

16. Coté CJ, Anderson BJ, Lerman J. *Cote and Lerman's A Practice of Anesthesia for Infants and Children.* 6th ed. Elsevier/Saunders.

17. Kang JYJ. Anesthetic implications of common congenital anomalies. *Anesthesiol Clin.* 2020;38(3):621–642. doi:10.1016/j.anclin.2020.06.002

CHAPTER 84

Alveolar Cleft Repair

Michele Baker

INDICATIONS/CONTRAINDICATIONS

Cleft lip and palate deformities are noted to be one of the most common congenital craniofacial birth defects, with an incidence of 1 in 800 live births.[1] A multitude of factors have been shown to cause cleft palate development in utero, although cleft lip and palate deformities are typically repaired within the first of year of life (see Chapter 81, "Cleft Lip and Cleft Palate Repair"). Quite often, repair of the palate deformity results in an alveolar cleft which subsequently requires surgical correction. Alveolar clefts (Figure 84.1) may also occur in response alterations in normal frontonasal prominence growth, contact, and fusion.[2] The goal of alveolar cleft repair is stabilization and provision of bone continuity to the maxillary arch. Alveolar cleft repair should ultimately facilitate normal eruption of teeth, eliminate oronasal fistulas, and improve facial symmetry and growth. Patients undergoing alveolar cleft repair should witness improvements in speech. Additionally, alveolar graft repair should eliminate oronasal communication and prevent the retention of food particles, thereby improving oral hygiene and preventing inflammation.

Alveolar cleft closure is typically performed around 8 to 12 years of age, during the mixed dentition period (between 6 and 11 years of age). During this period, the root of the permanent canine teeth has typically formed and undergoes accelerated periods of growth leading to active eruption. Performing alveolar cleft repair at this time allows the permanent teeth to erupt through the bone graft placed during the surgical repair, thereby promoting facial symmetry and providing a stable dental arch. It should be noted that most children will also require orthodontic planning, along with surgical intervention to correct the congenital deformity.[3] While alveolar cleft repair with bone graft is typically the last procedure performed in a series of repairs for cleft lip and palate deformities, it can yield significant improvements in the quality of life for these patients.

SPECIAL CONSIDERATIONS AND CONCERNS

Many patients with a history of cleft lip and palate deformity have coexisting syndromes, with the most common being Pierre–Robin sequence. The impact of any coexisting syndromes should be considering when developing the anesthetic plan. Syndromes commonly associated with cleft lip and palate deformity are presented in Box 84.1.

ANESTHETIC MANAGEMENT

PREOPERATIVE EVALUATION

It is imperative anesthesia providers explore the presence of coexisting syndromes that may have a deleterious impact on the anesthetic plan (Box 84.2). A focused exam should include identification of heart defects, as well as a thorough airway exam. The results of all diagnostic testing performed preoperatively should be reviewed, including electrocardiograms, echocardiograms, and polysomnography if available.

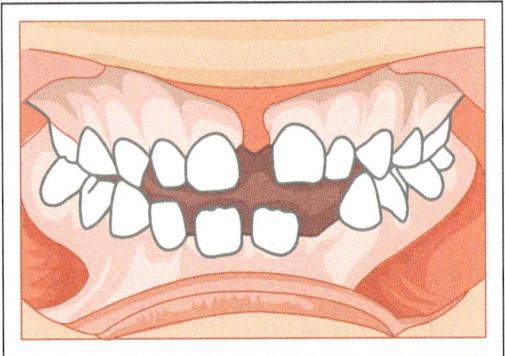

Figure 84.1: Alveolar cleft seen between upper incisors.

> **BOX 84.1 SYNDROMES COMMONLY ASSOCIATED WITH CLEFT LIP AND PALATE**
>
> Pierre–Robin sequence
> Down's syndrome
> Klippel–Feil syndrome
> Treacher–Collins syndrome
> Velocardiofacial syndrome
> Fetal alcohol syndrome
> Nager syndrome
> Goldenhar syndrome
>
> Source: From Cote CJ, Lerman J, Andersen, B. *A Practice of Anesthesia for Infants and Children*. 5th ed. Saunders; 2013.

> **BOX 84.2 KEY ASSESSMENT POINTS**
>
> Extensive airway evaluation
> Cardiac testing if indicated
> Recent illness including upper respiratory infection
> Review of previous anesthetic records
> Syndrome-specific concerns if present

Many of these patients may be considered to have a difficult airway secondary to anatomic variations associated with their coexisting syndrome. Unfortunately, they may not be cooperative enough to allow for an extensive airway evaluation, making it difficult to discern the extent of potential airway concerns. A review of previous anesthetic records may provide useful information relating to airway management. There are no preoperative labs specifically needed for this procedure.

PREOPERATIVE PHARMACOLOGY

Significant anxiety may be a concern in patients presenting for alveolar cleft repair. Typically, these patients have undergone multiple surgical procedures and physician visits prior to presenting for alveolar cleft repair. Adequate premedication should be considered, with midazolam and dexmedetomidine both providing adequate anxiolysis in the preoperative period.

ANESTHETIC TECHNIQUE

Intraoperative Management

Anesthetic management for alveolar cleft repair is straightforward. Depending on institutional protocol, patients will receive either a mask or IV induction. A single IV catheter is usually sufficient for this procedure, with invasive lines and blood products not typically required. The airway should be secured with an oral Ring–Adair–Elwyn (RAE) endotracheal tube as the patient is often positioned with the head of the bed away from the anesthesia provider to allow the surgeon access to the bone graft site. Given this patient population often has a history of having a difficult intubation, alternate airway equipment should be present in the room prior to the induction of anesthesia. The typical duration of the surgical procedure ranges from 2 to 6 hours, depending on the severity of the defect. Hence, appropriate measures to maintain the patient's temperature should be taken.

Special Techniques and/or Equipment

A number of sources have been used to provide bone graft material for the surgical repair. While both cortical and cancellous bones can be used for a bone graft, cancellous bone is the preferred technique because of the cell transfer and revascularization in osteoinduction and osteoconduction.[2] Potential harvest sites include the iliac crest, cranium, tibia, and mandibular symphysis. Of these, the iliac crest is the most commonly employed as it can provide a large amount of cancellous bone. Harvesting from the cranium yields a graft survival rate similar to that of iliac crest harvested bone; however, this donor site is associated with the potential for serious complications including hematoma, seroma, dural tear, and cerebrospinal fluid leakage.[5] While harvesting from the tibia is associated with less pain and bleeding and required operative time, it may be necessary to harvest from bilateral lower extremities to yield enough bone graft. Although graft harvested from the mandibular symphysis produces bone graft that revascularizes relatively fast, harvesting bone graft from site has the potential to damage the teeth or elicit nerve root injury. In addition to autologous bone graft, a variety of allogeneic and xenogeneic bone materials, along with growth factors, have been used for alveolar cleft repair.

Complications/Emergencies

Airway edema and postoperative airway obstruction are concerns after any surgery involving the oral cavity. This is especially important to monitor for in patients with known difficult airway anatomy. Infection of the incision is also a potential complication, with both the bone graft donor site and the surgical site having the potential for infection. It is important to monitor for infection postoperatively as it can decrease the integrity of the surgical correction. Should the surgical site become infected, normal tooth eruption and development will be inhibited.[6]

POSTOPERATIVE CARE

Postoperative pain management can be challenging, with many patients reporting the donor bone graft harvest site is more painful than the oral surgical site. While IV opioid administration has been the standard approach to pain management following alveolar cleft repair, the reliance on opioids alone is undesirable, given the many undesired side effects associated with this approach. Dexmedetomidine has been proven to be a useful adjunct to pain management. Not only does it shorten the overall time to discharge readiness and decrease opioid requirements but also dexmedetomidine promotes maintenance of natural airway tone as opposed to other sedatives and analgesics. Furthermore, the addition of dexmedetomidine has replaced the need for patient controlled anesthesia in some institutions.[7]

Novel approaches to pain management have been reported, with the transversalis facial plane block having emerged as an alternative to local wound infiltration for iliac crest bone graft harvesting.[8] This can be performed as either a single injection or a catheter can be placed for continuous infusion of local anesthetic over several days postoperatively to provide extended analgesia. The extended analgesia may facilitate earlier ambulation postoperatively and expedite the transition to the use of acetaminophen and ibuprofen as the primary analgesics following discharge.

REFERENCES

1. Steward D. Anesthesia for patients with cleft lip and palate. *Seminars in Anesthesia, Perioperative Medicine and Pain.* 2007;26(3):126–132. doi:10.1053/j.sane.2007.06.004
2. Kang NH. Current methods for treatment of alveolar cleft. *Arch Plast Surg.* 2017;44(3):188–193. doi:10.5999/aps.2017.44.3.188
3. Miller L, Kauffmann D, St. John D, et al. Retrospective review of 99 patients with secondary alveolar cleft repair. *J Oral Maxillofac Surg.* 2010;68(6):1283–1289. doi:10.1016/j.joms.2009.09.106
4. Cote CJ, Lerman J, Andersen, B. *A Practice of Anesthesia for Infants and Children.* 5th ed. Saunders; 2013.
5. Cohen M, Figueroa AA, Haviv Y, et al. Iliac versus cranial bone for secondary grafting of residual alveolar clefts. *Plast Reconstr Surg.* 1991;87(3):423–427.
6. Lilja J. Alveolar bone grafting. *Indian J Plast Surg.* 2009;42:110–115. doi:10.4103/0970-0358.57200
7. Lopez M, Zech D, Linton J, Blackwell S. Dexmedetomidine decreases postoperative pain and narcotic use in children undergoing alveolar bone graft surgery. *Cleft Palate-Craniofacial J.* 2018;55(5):688–691. doi:10.1177/1055665618754949
8. Sequera-Ramos L, Ruby JM, Jackson OA, et al. Continuous transversalis fascia plane catheter infusion in a pediatric patient undergoing alveolar cleft repair with iliac crest bone graft: a case report. *A&A Pract.* 2019;13(5):162–165. doi:10.1213/XAA.0000000000001013

CHAPTER 85

Breast Reduction

Nicole K. Damico and Gregory Lynam

INDICATIONS/CONTRAINDICATIONS

Breast reduction, or reduction mammaplasty, is a commonly performed cosmetic surgery procedure in the United States.[1] Although patients younger than the age of 18 years represent a small proportion of the overall population of patients who have this procedure,[2] the number of breast reductions done annually in adolescents has risen significantly over the past decade.[3] Recent evidence suggests particularly positive long-term outcomes and patient satisfaction following breast reduction in this patient subset,[4] which may support a future trend toward increasing numbers of procedures in young patients.

Indications for breast reduction include the desire for aesthetic enhancement and symptomatic breast hypertrophy (hyperplasia). Treating physical and psychosocial consequences of breast hypertrophy is the more common indication of the two, especially in younger adult and adolescent patients.[5] Breast hypertrophy is associated with lower healthcare quality of life, self-esteem issues, breast issues, and disordered eating patterns in adolescent females.[6] Breast reduction has been shown to significantly improve pain and quality of life when using a validated, condition-specific patient-reported outcome instrument such as the Breast-Q reduction module.[7] The benefits of breast reduction are generally sustained long term.[4]

There are no specific, absolute contraindications to breast reduction. General contraindications include those common to other elective surgeries, such as coagulopathy, active infection or other acute conditions, and poorly controlled chronic medical conditions. Although there is no set minimum age for elective breast reduction, it is often recommended that the procedure is delayed until breast growth has stabilized, with at least 3 years after the onset of puberty being the earliest the procedure may be performed at some centers.[8] Some insurance carriers require a minimum patient age of 16–18 years or evidence of physical maturity, yet this requirement is not supported by the American Society of Plastic Surgeons.[9] Smoking is associated with an increased risk of wound-related complications,[10] and accordingly, many surgeons advocate that elective plastic surgery is delayed until following a period of smoking abstinence of at least 2–4 weeks.[11]

SPECIAL CONSIDERATIONS AND CONCERNS

Pediatric patients who present for breast reduction inherently have multiple risk factors for postoperative nausea and vomiting (PONV). According to a recent systematic review, risk factors for PONV in children include age ≥3 years, female gender/postpuberty, and surgery duration of ≥60 minutes, meaning essentially that all patients scheduled for breast reduction have an elevated baseline risk of PONV.[12] Additional nonmodifiable factors include personal history of PONV or motion sickness and family history of PONV, which, if present, suggest an anticipated incidence of PONV in this patient group of 55% in the absence of intervention.[13]

Breast reduction may carry an increased risk of acute pain relative to other, similar plastic surgery procedures. Patients who have a breast reduction are routinely prescribed hydrocodone or oxycodone with acetaminophen postoperatively.[14] While this may be attributable to increased pain and a greater need for opioids in association with breast reduction versus other outpatient plastic surgery procedures,[15] some researchers have suggested that, counterintuitively, opioid prescribing patterns could be a contributing factor to increased opioid use in this patient group.[16] Few published studies of pain after breast surgery have noted the inclusion of patients under the age of 18 years, and further research is needed to determine the relative risk of acute postoperative pain in this patient population.

Patients who have a breast reduction may also be at risk of the development of chronic postsurgical pain. Breast surgeries in general have been associated with development of postbreast surgery pain syndrome (PBSPS).[17] While the incidence of PBSPS is highest after cancer and reconstructive breast surgeries, aesthetic procedures such as breast reduction have also been implicated.[18] In surveys of women who have had breast reduction surgery 1 to 10 years previously, the incidence of chronic pain has been found to be ≥20%.[19] Risk factors for chronic pain after breast reduction in adults include younger age, body mass index greater than 26 kg/m^2, and psychosocial characteristics such as elevated baseline depression, anxiety, and catastrophizing scores.[18]

ANESTHETIC MANAGEMENT

PREOPERATIVE EVALUATION

The majority of pediatric patients who have breast reduction are generally healthy, with no comorbidities,[5] despite often being overweight or obese.[20] Preoperative diagnostic testing is generally not needed prior to breast reduction. Determining the need for preoperative laboratory or other diagnostic assessments is therefore based on patient history and presence of any comorbidities. Questions about the date of the last period and potential for pregnancy are indicated in female patients beyond the age of menarche. Preoperative urine pregnancy testing is generally required per local, institutional guidelines.

The preoperative interview focuses on gathering relevant patient history, discussion of anesthetic options, education about immediate postoperative care, and developing rapport. If the patient is a minor, the parent or legal guardian must be included in preoperative discussions and the informed consent process. Compliance with recommended fasting guidelines of 2 hours for clear liquids, 6 hours for light meals, and 8 hours for fatty solid foods should be verified.[21] Due to the elevated risk of PONV in pediatric patients having breast reduction, further inquiry about additional patient risk factors for PONV during the preoperative assessment, such as personal or family history of PONV or motion sickness, may inform selection of appropriate perioperative strategies to mitigate this risk. Patients with breast hypertrophy commonly have mild anxiety prior to surgical intervention, especially those who are younger.[22] The preoperative interview is an opportunity to assess the patient's level of anxiety on the day of surgery and to determine if pharmacologic intervention is indicated.

PREOPERATIVE PHARMACOLOGY

Goals of premedication in the pediatric patient scheduled for breast reduction are to reduce the risk of PONV, initiate multimodal analgesia, and treat patient anxiety, if present. While most prophylactic antiemetic agents are administered during the intraoperative period, two notable exceptions may be considered in this patient group. Transdermal scopolamine, a systemic anticholinergic commonly recommended for PONV prophylaxis in adults, may be considered for patients older than age 12. The scopolamine patch is ideally placed the evening before or as soon as possible on the day of surgery, as the onset of therapeutic drug effect can take as long as 4 hours.[23] Preoperative oral gabapentin may also help prevent PONV.[12]

Preoperative administration of multimodal analgesic therapies may be considered, especially in older adolescents. When given in conjunction with intraoperative local anesthetics, a preoperative combination of oral acetaminophen, gabapentin, and celecoxib has been shown to decrease opioid use and pain scores in the immediate postoperative period in adult patients having outpatient breast surgery.[24] Consensus guidelines support the use of oral gabapentin or pregabalin, and celecoxib preoperatively as part of a multimodal analgesia regimen in adults;[25] however, similar guidelines for pediatric patients do not exist. As stand-alone agents, preoperative acetaminophen and dextromethorphan (1 mg/kg) have been shown to reduce perioperative opioid requirements in pediatric patients, but there is insufficient evidence of such benefits in association with gabapentin, pregabalin, or celecoxib.[26] Ideally, oral preoperative medications are given 1–2 hours before surgery to allow time for drug absorption and gastric emptying.

Placement of an IV line preoperatively is routine in this patient age group and, if indicated, preoperative anxiolytic medications, such as midazolam, may be given parenterally. Of note, many surgeons routinely perform final baseline measurements and mark the planned surgical incisions preoperatively with the patient in the standing position. IV midazolam should be withheld until after these procedures are completed to reduce the risk of patient fall. A dose of IV prophylactic antibiotic prior to surgical incision is frequently ordered, unless contraindicated, in accordance with the recommendation of the American Board of Plastic Surgery Patient Safety Task Force,[2] which may be initiated during the preoperative period at the provider's discretion.

ANESTHETIC TECHNIQUE

Intraoperative Management

Selection of specific anesthetic management techniques during breast reduction surgery is largely on the basis of surgical factors, patient factors, and planned postoperative patient disposition. Likely due to the location and extent of surgical incisions made during breast reduction, general anesthesia is the most commonly employed primary anesthetic technique.[2] IV induction is preferred over inhalational induction in adolescents, although from a procedural standpoint, there are no contraindications to the use of an inhalational induction technique. Propofol is the IV induction agent of choice to reduce the risk of PONV.[12] If general anesthesia is used, either a supraglottic airway or endotracheal tube is acceptable for airway management. Maintaining muscle paralysis following airway management is unnecessary since neither the surgical resection nor field exposure involves skeletal muscle. Maintaining anesthesia with propofol infusion, minimal doses of opioids, and avoidance of volatile anesthetics and nitrous oxide may reduce the risk of PONV.[12] Single intraoperative doses of antiemetic drugs such as ondansetron and/or dexamethasone may further reduce the risk of PONV, if not contraindicated. Most breast reductions are performed on an outpatient basis, whether in a hospital or an ambulatory surgery center,[2] and accordingly, short-acting agents are preferred.

Intraoperative fluid replacement can serve the dual purposes of restoring homeostasis and mitigating the risk of PONV. Estimated blood loss during breast reductions using modern surgical techniques is modest, 100–200 mL,[27] which represents a downward trend over time. As recently as the 1990s, breast reduction was commonly associated with intraoperative blood loss sufficient to warrant blood transfusion perioperatively.[28] Over the past 20 years, infiltration of epinephrine in the surgical field has consistently been found to significantly reduce blood loss and the rate of transfusion during breast reductions,[29] and this practice has become increasingly more common.[2] Another commonly used intervention, tumescent technique of epinephrine injection, which involves injection of relatively large volumes of a dilute solution (epinephrine 1:200,000 to 1:1,000,000) into SC tissue, has also been found to reduce intraoperative blood loss and the need for blood transfusion.[30] Isotonic crystalloid solutions can effectively replace evaporative, third-space, and estimated blood losses intraoperatively. Liberal fluid replacement volume of 10–30 mL/kg should additionally be considered to reduce the risk of PONV.[12]

A wide variety of strategies of analgesia can be used in conjunction with general anesthesia during breast reduction. The simplest intraoperative technique is to administer analgesic medications by the IV route. One option, arguably still the most widely used technique, is an opioid-based approach featuring short-acting opioids such as fentanyl, with or without supplementation with hydromorphone as needed. In light of the opioid crisis, there is a growing emphasis on use of opioid-sparing and opioid-free techniques.[31] The aforementioned risk of chronic pain following breast surgery and high incidence of preoperative anxiety in this patient population, plus the recognized risk of new, persistent opioid use following surgery,[32] are factors that weigh in favor of selection of nonopioid analgesic drugs for pediatric breast reduction.

Due to the relatively little research that has been done to evaluate comprehensive nonopioid intraoperative strategies during plastic surgery in pediatric patients, strong recommendations in favor of one approach over others cannot be made. Several nonopioid IV analgesic options are worthy of consideration as adjuncts to general anesthesia. Acetaminophen 30 mg/kg (up to a maximum dose of 1 g) can provide pain relief for up to 4 hours postoperatively.[33] Dexamethasone ≥.1 mg/kg can reduce postoperative pain scores and opioid requirements.[34] Intraoperative administration of ketorolac is controversial, given its association with increased risk of hematoma formation following breast reduction in adults.[35] In a single-center prospective study of adolescents and young adults having breast reductions, ketorolac 30 mg was found to decrease intraoperative requirements for short-acting opioids with no increase in the risk of hematoma formation.[36]

Across numerous trials in pediatric patients, including many in ambulatory surgery settings, ketamine has been found to reduce pain scores whether given as a single bolus (.25–1 mg/kg), an infusion (.25–1 mg/kg/hr), or a combination of the two.[26] Dexmedetomidine has been found to decrease postoperative pain scores and opioid consumption in the setting of a wide variety of outpatient surgeries. The range of dexmedetomidine doses used in prior students has been quite variable, with bolus doses ranging from .15 to 4 µg/kg and infusions doses between .2 and 2 µg/kg/hr reported in the studies included in two published meta-analyses.[26] According to one study, the optimal analgesic dose of dexmedetomidine in pediatric patients is a bolus of ≥.5 µg/kg, with or without infusion.[37]

Intraoperative administration of lidocaine, via any one of several possible routes, may be of limited use during breast reduction in pediatric patients. IV lidocaine has been found to decrease intraoperative anesthetic and opioid requirements and postoperative pain scores in adults.[38] These benefits are likely dependent upon the procedure performed, however, and the benefits in breast surgeries have been found to be limited.[39] Furthermore, there are currently insufficient data to support widespread use in pediatric patients.[26] Lidocaine is frequently added to epinephrine solutions used with tumescent techniques in the hope of providing analgesia, yet little evidence to date supports this claim in patients having breast reductions, particularly beyond the immediate postoperative period.[40]

Novel interfacial regional anesthetic techniques, such as the pectoral nerve block (PECS II), thoracic paravertebral block, and erector spinae block, can be employed as part of a multimodal pain management strategy. The PECS II block is an interfacial block that consists of two injections of local anesthetic: the first injection between the pectoralis minor muscle and pectoralis major muscle and the second injection between the pectoralis major muscle and serratus muscle. While this block provides reliable anesthesia for the breast and axilla region, it may fail to cover the parasternal branches of the intercostal nerves leaving areas unaffected. The thoracic paravertebral block (TPVB) provides postoperative analgesia by injection of local anesthetics near the thoracic spinal nerves at the point, where they exit the intervertebral foramina. This results in ipsilateral somatic and sympathetic nerve blocks without dense motor block. Ultimately, a segmental blockade can be achieved in the consecutive dermatomes of the thoracic and breast surgical areas. The erector spinae plane block (ESPB) has been proven to be a useful adjunct in the management of acute pain as an injection at the level of T5 can sufficiently anesthetize unilateral multidermatomal sensation from T1 to L3. When compared with the commonly used TPVB, the ESPB has been reported to offer similar pain relief results with fewer adverse effects.

Consideration of other procedural details may further facilitate individualization of the anesthetic management plan. Average case duration for a breast reduction is between 2 and 3 hours.[3,41] The preferred patient position is supine, possibly with the head of the bed elevated slightly. The arms may be abducted on arm boards or tucked per the surgeon's preference. Resected breast tissue volume is routinely measured and recorded by the surgeon during the case. Regardless of patient age, surgical specimens are typically sent for pathologic examination; however, specimen analysis does not impact intraoperative decision-making. In patients younger than age 40, the likelihood of abnormal findings is expected to be very low.[42] Compression stockings and sequential compression devices are frequently used for deep vein thrombosis prophylaxis.

Box 85.1 summarizes special techniques and Box 85.2 highlights clinical pearls related to safe airway removal.

Complications/Emergencies

Reported complications of breast reduction range from relatively minor to severe or even fatal. Minor complications

> **BOX 85.1 SPECIAL TECHNIQUES AND EQUIPMENT**
>
> - Hypothermia, defined as body temperature less than or equal to 36°C, commonly occurs during plastic surgery procedures, including breast reduction.[43]
> - Due to the potential for hypothermia, intraoperative temperature monitoring is indicated.
> - Active body-surface warming devices can reduce the risk of hypothermia-related complications and postoperative shivering.[44]
> - The area of exposure for an isolated breast reduction is the anterior torso, which facilitates placement of standard blankets or forced-air warming blankets on much of the lower body.
> - Other interventions such as increasing the ambient temperature, wrapping the patient's head, and IV fluid warming may also be helpful.

> **BOX 85.2 CLINICAL PEARLS**
>
> - Removal of the artificial airway while the patient is still "deep" should be considered following breast reduction, provided there are no patient factors that contraindicate this technique.
> - The location of the surgical field, patient's supine position, and operating room table routinely left in the neutral position allow ready access to the patient's airway and the area around the head of the bed.
> - Muscle relaxants are not necessary during surgical closure, which often requires a relatively lengthy period due to the length of the incisions involved.
> - Extended period of low surgical stimulation facilitates reversal of neuromuscular blockade (if indicated), return of spontaneous breathing, and assessment of the return of respiratory function to a level sufficient to support safe airway removal.

include seroma, superficial skin infection, wound-healing issues, altered nipple sensation, and postoperative breast regrowth; major complications include bleeding/hematoma, fat tissue necrosis, nipple necrosis, deep vein thrombosis, and pulmonary embolism.[20,45,46] While complications following breast reductions occur frequently in adults, overall risk of complications is substantially lower in patients under the age of 18 years, ranging from under 5%[3,5] to 31%,[20] likely owing to a lower prevalence of comorbidities in this patient subset.

Patient and surgical factors may increase the risk of complications following breast reductions. Obesity increases the risk of some surgical complications, such as fat necrosis, in adult patients.[47] In adolescent patients, obesity (body mass index [BMI] >30 kg/m²) has been associated with a threefold higher chance of experiencing an adverse event following breast reduction.[3] Smoking has been found to significantly increase the risk of postoperative complications following plastic surgery, with a specific association with increased rates of infection, skin necrosis, delayed wound healing, and reoperation after breast reduction.[48] The period of smoking abstinence needed to reduce the risk of complications is currently unknown. The volume of breast tissue has also been found to directly correlate with the rate of certain postoperative complications, such as wound healing issues and fat tissue necrosis.[46]

POSTOPERATIVE CARE

Pediatric breast reductions can be done on an inpatient or outpatient basis. The majority of pediatric patients admitted to the hospital following breast reduction stay only 1 day, with higher lengths of stay generally associated with performance of additional concurrent procedures or the occurrence of early postoperative complications such as hematoma.[5] There are no published evidence-based guidelines for patient disposition following breast reduction, largely because of the scarcity of high-quality prior studies,[49] and the decision is generally on the basis of the surgeon's judgment. Although a substantial body of evidence suggests there is little to no benefit derived from postoperative drains, the majority of plastic surgeons continue to place them during breast reductions.[2] Roughly half of plastic surgeons order prophylactic antibiotics postoperatively following breast reduction,[2] although it is unlikely that continued dosing beyond 24 hours reduces the risk of surgical site infection.[50]

CASE STUDY: Anesthetic Management of an Adolescent Female Undergoing Bilateral Breast Reduction

CLINICAL SCENARIO

A 16-year-old female presented for a bilateral breast reduction at a free-standing ambulatory surgery center. Her preoperative diagnosis was macromastia, with approximately G-cup-sized breasts at baseline, associated with significant chronic back and shoulder pain and self-esteem issues. The patient had no significant medical history, no known drug allergies, no prior surgeries, and no family history of nausea and took no medications on a daily basis. The patient was obese, with a BMI of 31 kg/m². Her baseline vital signs revealed a slightly elevated systolic blood pressure of 144/74 and a normal heart rate of 74 bpm. The planned surgical approach was an "inverted T," or Wise technique,[51] and the patient's skin was marked accordingly in the preoperative holding area. After skin markings were complete, sequential compression device sleeves were placed, and the patient was given IV doses of midazolam 2 mg and cefazolin 2 g.

(continued)

CASE STUDY: Anesthetic Management of an Adolescent Female Undergoing Bilateral Breast Reduction (*continued*)

SPECIAL CONSIDERATIONS

Several key patient factors impacted surgical and anesthetic decision-making in this case. The anticipated breast resection volumes were quite high, above the weight-based criterion for gigantomastia of >1.5 kg/breast, although at less than 3% of the patient's total body weight, not within the range associated with this clinical diagnosis.[52] Due to the size of the patient's breasts, which would accommodate fluid injection without derangement of the surgical field, and the overall large length of the planned incisions, which increased potential for significant intraoperative blood loss, the surgeon opted to inject tumescent solution prior to making the initial incision. A total of 870 mL of tumescent solution, created by reconstituting 30 mL of lidocaine 1% and 1 mL of epinephrine 1:1,000 in 1 L of normal saline, was injected bilaterally throughout the planned incision and resection areas. Care was taken by the surgeon not to inject the base of the inferior pedicle, in an effort to preserve blood flow to the nipple areola complex[51] and thereby to decrease the risk of one of most devastating major complications of breast reduction, namely, nipple necrosis.

The selected anesthetic technique for this procedure was a balanced IV and inhalational technique, given there was no patient or family history of PONV weighing in favor of alternate techniques such as total IV anesthesia. The anesthetic plan determination was further impacted by the fact that the surgeon's routine practice does not include administration of preoperative multimodal analgesics. The time from patient arrival in the facility to the scheduled procedure was approximately 30 minutes, arguably far too little time to initiate such therapies in the absence of an existing protocol.

APPROACHES TO CARE

The relatively "traditional" anesthetic approach, with reliance on a combination of short- and long-acting opioids, was associated with exceptional short-term outcomes and patient satisfaction. General anesthesia was induced via IV induction with lidocaine 60 mg, propofol 250 mg, and fentanyl 50 mcg. A size 4 laryngeal mask airway was placed without difficulty, and sevoflurane was initiated at approximately 2.5 vol%, titrated to effect during the remainder of the procedure. Prior to the initial incision, IV dexamethasone 10 mg was given for nausea prophylaxis. Once spontaneous respirations resumed, additional fentanyl was titrated IV to a total dose of 100 mcg over approximately 10 minutes during the surgical field prep. The patient was intermittently reactive to surgical stimulation, largely in the form of elevated heart rate and blood pressure, and accordingly received bolus doses of propofol 20–50 mg (total dose 70 mg) and hydromorphone .5 mg (total dose 2 mg) as needed during the case to facilitate control of hemodynamic responses while maintaining the targeted sevoflurane concentration of 1 MAC or less. Her vital signs ranged from a blood pressure of 89 to 117/34 to 44 mm Hg, heart rate of 75 to 119 bpm, respiratory rate of 10–23 bpm, and oxygen saturation of 98%. Zofran 4 mg was given intravenously during final incision closure. Upon arrival in the postanesthesia care unit, the patient reported very mild incisional discomfort and denied nausea. She was discharged from the facility to the care of her mother by 60 minutes postoperatively.

KEY REFERENCES

Complete references for this chapter are online and available at https://connect.springerpub.com/content/book/978-0-8261-3875-0/part/part04/toc-part/ch085.

2. Greco R, Noone B. Evidence-based medicine: Reduction mammaplasty. *Plast Reconstr Surg*. 2017;139(1):230e–239e. doi:10.1097/PRS.0000000000002856
3. Fairchild B, Wei S, Bartz-Kurycki M, et al. The influence of obesity on outcomes after pediatric reduction mammaplasty: a retrospective analysis of the pediatric national surgical quality improvement program–pediatric database. *Ann Plast Surg*. 2020;85(6):608–611. doi:10.1097/sap.0000000000002311
4. Krucoff KB, Carlson AR, Shammas RL, et al. Breast-related quality of life in young reduction mammaplasty patients: a long-term follow-up using the BREAST-Q. *Plast Reconstr Surg*. 2019;144(5):743E–750E. doi:10.1097/PRS.0000000000006117
12. Gan TJ, Belani KG, Bergese S, et al. Fourth consensus guidelines for the management of postoperative nausea and vomiting. *Anesth Analg*. 2020;131(2):411–448. doi:10.1213/ANE.0000000000004833
15. Rose KR, Christie BM, Block LM, et al. Opioid prescribing and consumption patterns following outpatient plastic surgery procedures. *Plast Reconstr Surg*. 2019;143(3):929–938. doi:10.1097/PRS.0000000000005351
16. Merola D, Calotta NA, Lu ZA, et al. Initial opioid prescriptions predict continued narcotic use: analysis of 24,594 reduction mammaplasty patients. *Plast Reconstr Surg*. 2020;145(1):20–30. doi:10.1097/PRS.0000000000006318
17. Kokosis G, Chopra K, Darrach H, et al. Re-visiting post-breast surgery pain syndrome: risk factors, peripheral nerve associations and clinical implications. *Gland Surg*. 2019;8(4):407–415. doi.org/10.21037/gs.2019.07.05
20. Nuzzi LC, Firriolo JM, Pike CM, et al. Complications and quality of life following reduction mammaplasty in adolescents and young women. *Plast Reconstr Surg*. 2019;144(3):572–581. doi:10.1097/PRS.0000000000005907
26. Zhu A, Benzon HA, Anderson TA. Evidence for the efficacy of systemic opioid sparing analgesics in pediatric surgical populations: a systematic review. *Anesth Analg*. 2017;125(5):1569–1587. doi:10.1213/ANE.0000000000002434
34. Moore, S. G. (2018). Intravenous dexamethasone as an analgesic: a literature review. *AANA journal*, 86(6), 488-493.

CHAPTER 86

Microtia Repair

Kristen Deveras and Pacifico Tuason

INDICATIONS/CONTRAINDICATIONS

Microtia, small or malformed ear, is a congenital deformity of the pinna that may be isolated or occurring in conjunction with a spectrum of other abnormalities. Seventy-five percent of microtia cases are associated with aural atresia, involving an underdeveloped auditory canal and malformed middle ear ossicles. The incidence of micortia occurs in approximately 1–20 per 10,000 births worldwide, affecting almost 50% more males than females and a higher prevalence among Native Americans, Asians, and Hispanics.[1] Risk factors include low birth weight and acute maternal illness, as well as in utero exposure to teratogens, such as thalidomide and retinoids. In vitro, the external ear starts to form at 6 weeks from tissue derived from first and second branchial arches; by 13 weeks, the tympanic membrane is formed, and at 18 weeks, the meatus and all parts of the external ear are formed.[2] Microtia can occur in isolation and often unilaterally; however, the microtia phenotype is associated with a spectrum of disorders, which most commonly include craniofacial microsomia, Goldenhar's syndrome, and Treacher–Collins' syndrome. The following syndromes and genetic causes have been associated with microtia in less than 50% of cases: auriculocondylar, Bixler, Bosley–Salih–Alorainy, branchio-oculofacial, branchio-otorenal/branchio-otic, CHARGE, Fraser, Kabuki, Kilppel–Feil, labyrinthine aplasia, Meier–Gorlin, Miller, Nager, oculoauricular, Pallister–Hall, Townes-Brocks, and Treacher–Collins.[2]

Microtia is diagnosed at birth, and global assessment of both structural and functional abnormalities is warranted.[1] Diagnostic investigation of microtia includes clinical examination, audiological testing, genetic analysis and in higher grade malformations, computed tomography (CT) or cone beam CT is needed for the planning of surgery and rehabilitation, including the implantation of hearing aids.[3]

Multiple classification systems are used to delineate the degree of microtia. Marx and Rogers describes four classes of microtia as such: Grade I, the ear is small or abnormal, but all landmarks are discernible; Grade II, some of the landmarks are identifiable; Grade III has very small external auricle components, often only a skin tag; and Grade IV is anotia. OMENS, a classification system for hemifacial microsomia, examines orbital, mandibular ear, neural, and soft tissue phenotypes. This system was useful in showing that approximately 67% of patients with hemifacial macrosomia also presented with extracraniofacial anomalies and 26% with cardiac anomalies. HEAR MAPS is a classification method that describes the physical and radiological findings in patients with congenital aural atresia and microtia that incorporates multiple staging systems and thus may be useful to improve interdisciplinary communication among providers (Table 86.1).[2]

While the primary goals for microtia repair are cosmesis and acoustic functionality, indications for microtia repair depend on the severity of the deformity as well as any associated anomalies. For example, patients with high-grade microtia, Jahrsdoerfer score less than 5, and abnormal cochlear function, with no apparent middle ear space, may not be considered good surgical candidates, as these would unlikely

Table 86.1	HEAR MAPS Classification Method
Hear	Airbone gap
Ear	Microtia Grades 1–4
Atresia	Jahrsdoerfer CT scale 1–10
Remnant earlobe	Grade 1–4
Mandible asymmetry	Grade 1–4
Asymmetry soft tissue	Grade 1–4
Paresis of facial nerve	House-Brackmann scale 1–6
Syndrome	Yes/no

Source: From Bly RA, Bhyrany AD, Sie KC. Microtia reconstruction. *Facial Plast Surg Clin North Am.* 2016;24(4):577–591. doi:10.1016/j.fsc.2016.06.011.

benefit hearing.[1] Thus, indications for microtia repair should be based on a thorough interdisciplinary discussion with the patient and the patient's family to generate a cohesive plan on management of the ear and hearing.[2]

Optimal timing for microtia repair is dependent on the maturity of the external ear and the adequacy of donor rib cartilage. The external ear grows to reach approximately 85% of its maximal size by the age of 5 years, while the donor rib is not adequate in volume and stability until the ages of 5–6 years. Thus, 6–7 years is typically of optimal age for auricular reconstruction and atresiaplasty.[1]

While several options for microtia reconstruction exists, the primary three options include autologous reconstruction with autologous rib, composite reconstruction using alloplastic framework, and prosthetic reconstruction (Table 86.2).[1]

ANESTHETIC MANAGEMENT

PREOPERATIVE EVALUATION

Interdisciplinary communication is essential for the child undergoing microtia repair see Table 86.3. Considering microtia is associated with a spectrum of conditions, a thorough preoperative evaluation is vital. The child should be medically optimized and cleared for surgery as indicated. The severity of symptoms of children with upper respiratory infections or reactive airway diseases should be evaluated as they are predisposed to laryngospasm and/or bronchospasm during induction and emergence. Wheezing, fever, and cough are signs of lower respiratory infection and are associated with increased risk of perioperative airway complication and may warrant postponing surgery.[4]

Bilateral (not unilateral) microtia has been associated with difficulty in visualizing the laryngeal inlet (Grade 3 or 4 view) in up to 42% of cases as opposed to only 2.5% in children with unilateral microtia. It is believed that microtia may represent a mild form of hemifacial microsomia and its associated mandibular hypoplasia. The advantage of such an association is that ear deformity is easily recognized clinically than mandibular hypoplasia.[5]

Table 86.2 Microtia Management Options

Type	Details	Advantages	Disadvantages
Autologous cartilage reconstruction	Stage 1: done under general anesthesia, may require two surgical teams to harvest cartilage and prepare recipient site, involves rib harvest and framework carving Stage 2: usually done outpatient	• Autologous tissue • Minimal maintenance • Atresia repair	• Multiple surgeries • Donor sites • Appearance
Alloplastic reconstruction	Temporoparietal fascial flap: done as a single stage under general anesthesia	• Less donor site morbidity • Less variability in carving • Appearance • Single surgery	• Foreign body • More challenging to do atresia repair
Prosthesis		• Appearance	• Ongoing prosthetic care • Maintenance • Use restrictions

Source: From Bly RA, Bhyrany AD, Sie KC. Microtia reconstruction. *Facial Plast Surg Clin North Am.* 2016;24(4):577–591. doi:10.1016/j.fsc.2016.06.011.

Table 86.3 Key Assessment Points

	Assessment	Perioperative Planning
Respiratory	Upper respiratory infection Reactive airway diseases	Consider severity of symptoms; may warrant postponing surgery
Airway	Associated syndromes/disorders	Airway examination: Mallampati score Microsomia Cranio- and extracraniofacial anomalies Consider video laryngoscopy or fiberoptic intubation
Cardiovascular	Congenital heart disease	Cardiac clearance/cardiac consult Optimize cardiac conditions Obtain baseline ECG, chest x-ray, and ECHO as indicated
Neurological	Development delays associated with syndromes Hearing deficits	Consult child life and/or parental participation with induction Examination of the ears, diagnostic audiological assessment, and radiographic imaging
Hematological	Anemia	Baseline hemoglobin and hematocrit
Nutritional	NPO status	Fasting guidelines: Clear fluids >2 hr Breast milk >4 hr Nonhuman milk >6 hr Solid food >8 hr
Psychological	Pre-existing depression and anxiety	Consult child life and/or parental participation with induction

When airway is presumed difficult, it is necessary to communicate with the operative team, as well have backup measures in place such as video laryngoscopy or fiberoptic intubation. Patients with cardiac anomalies may require preoperative ECG, echocardiogram, chest x-ray, and/or cardiac clearance. It is important to determine the child's baseline neurological status, hearing deficits, and psychosocial status and involve family and child life therapy as indicated. Clear communication with the surgical team is vital and the surgical safety checklist should include but should not be limited to patient identifiers, procedure, laterality, allergies, antibiotics, length of procedure, equipment needed, airway concerns, and recovery.[6]

PREOPERATIVE PHARMACOLOGY

Older children may be able to proceed without sedation preoperatively; however, anesthesia providers may want to consider the administration of oral midazolam (0.5 mg/kg) or intranasal dexmedetomidine (0.5–2 mcg/kg) to facilitate parental separation, decrease anxiety, or improve mask acceptance if an inhalation mask induction is planned.

ANESTHETIC TECHNIQUE

Intraoperative Management

Essential intraoperative management requirements for microtia repair include airway management, assurance of satisfactory intraoperative and postoperative analgesia, patient immobility, quiet surgical field, and smooth emergence from anesthesia. Thus, general endotracheal anesthesia is most widely employed.[6]

Inhalational mask induction is most commonly employed in younger children who are otherwise healthy and have no airway concerns. For older children, a peripheral IV catheter may be placed in the preoperative setting to facilitate an IV induction with propofol in the operating room. Neuromuscular blockade can be achieved with rocuronium (0.6–1.2 mg/kg IV) or cistatracurium, (0.15–0.2 mg/kg IV) to facilitate endotracheal intubation. Anesthesia providers must consider an alternate course for patients who are known to have or are presumed to have a difficult airway. In this scenario, it may be prudent to keep the patient breathing spontaneously and to consider using succinylcholine (1–2 mg/kg IV). Atropine (0.2 mg/kg IV) or glycopyrrolate (0.01 mg/kg IV) may be given prior to administration of succinylcholine to prevent profound bradycardia.

Once the airway has been secure, anesthesia can be maintained with a volatile anesthetic agent or via a total IV anesthetic. Should maintenance with a volatile anesthetic agent be selected, sevoflurane is the agent of choice given this is the least irritation to the airway. Standard monitors include ECG, blood pressure, pulse oximetry, and temperature monitoring. Estimated blood loss is anticipated to be minimal, and a single peripheral IV catheter most often proves sufficient.

Intraoperative fluid management should entail administration of 4 mL/kg/hr for the first 10 kg of body weight, 2 mL/kg/hr for the second 10 kg, adding 1 mL/kg/hr for over 20 kg. The usual solution for replacement of fluid deficit and ongoing losses in healthy child is lactated Ringer's solution.

Pain management should be multimodal in nature. While fentanyl (0.5–1 mcg/kg every 1–2 hours) or hydromorphone (0.02 mg/kg every 2–4 hours) can be administered to provide intra- and postoperative analgesia, the administration of nonopioid adjuncts may limit the incidence of negative opioid-related sequelae, such as respiratory depression, pruritis, and nausea and vomiting. Acetaminophen (10–15 mg/kg PO or IV), ketorolac (0.5 mg/kg IV), and dexmedetomidine (0.5–1 mcg/kg IV) are commonly employed to foster a multimodal approach to pain management. Likewise, infiltration of the local anesthetic may be beneficial when a rib harvest is involved.

In most cases, tracheal extubation occurs after emergence of anesthesia as the child demonstrates purposeful activity. Alternatively, extubation may occur when the child is in a deep plane of anesthesia and spontaneously ventilating; however, this should be avoided for children who are difficult to intubate or at risk of full stomach. Emergence delirium is known to be associated with a host of factors, many of which are present in patients presenting for microtia repair. This includes patient 1–5 years of age, those undergoing ENT/ophthalmic procedures, patients with preoperative anxiety, a rapid emergence from anesthesia, or heightened pain postoperatively. Anesthesia providers should consider the administration of fentanyl (1 mcg/kg), propofol (1 mg/kg), or dexmedetomidine (0.5 mcg/kg) to temper emergence delirium should it occur (see Boxes 86.1–86.3).

POSTOPERATIVE CARE

Microtia repair is generally well tolerated. General anesthesia warrants recovery in a postanesthesia care unit. Children with preexisting disorders may require overnight stay. Discharge often follow the Aldrete Scoring System as well as pain control. The goal is for the child to return to preprocedural parameters before discharge.[7]

BOX 86.1 SPECIAL TECHNIQUES AND/OR EQUIPMENT

Airway: Consider video laryngoscopy or fiberoptic bronchoscope for presumed difficult airway.

BOX 86.2 COMPLICATIONS

- **Postoperative nausea and vomiting:** Consider multimodal prophylaxis or total intravenous anesthesia (TIVA) technique.
- **Pneumothorax:** Valsalva maneuvers with wound irrigation may be warranted to assess for air leak when rib harvest is involved.
- **Infection:** Administer prophylactic antibiotics.

BOX 86.3 CLINICAL PEARLS

- **Position**
  - Supine
  - Table may be rotated 90°, or 180°, ensure adequate circuit tubing and secured endotracheal tube (ETT)
  - Movement of head and neck during procedure, ensure well secured ETT
- **Incision**
  - Posterior/anterior ear, stage dependent, chest wall
- **Local Anesthetic**
  - Epinephrine may be infiltrated, monitor for arrhythmias
- **Closing Considerations**
  - Consider dressing ear/head dressing
  - Consider drainage system in first stage microtia repair fixed to head dressing
- **Smooth Emergence**

REFERENCES

1. Ali K, Mohan K, Liu Y. Otologic and audiology concerns of microtia repair. *Semin Plast Surg.* 2017;31(3):127–133. doi:10.1055/s-0037-1603957
2. Bly RA, Bhyrany AD, Sie KC. Microtia reconstruction. *Facial Plast Surg Clin North Am.* 2016;24(4):577–591. doi:10.1016/j.fsc.2016.06.011
3. Bartel-Friedrich S. Congenital auricular malformations: description of anomalies and syndromes. *Facial Plast Surg.* 2015;31(6):567–580. doi:10.1055/s-0035-1568139
4. Pino RM. *Clinical Anesthesia Procedures of the Massachusetts General Hospital.* 9th ed. Lippincott Williams & Wilkins; 2016.
5. Cote C, Lerman J, Todres D. *A Practice of Anesthesia for Infants and Children.* 4th ed. Saunders Elsevier; 2009:247–248.
6. Jaffe RA, Schmiesing CA, Golianu B. *Anesthesiologist's Manual of Surgical Procedures.* Lippincott Williams & Wilkins; 2014.
7. Nagelhout JJ, Elisha S. *Nurse Anesthesia.* 6th ed. Elsevier; 2018.

CHAPTER 87

Burns

Alison Henry and Lisa Wahlers

INDICATIONS/CONTRAINDICATIONS

The prevalence of traumatic injuries in children is significant. In the United States, burns are the fifth leading cause of unintentional injury in children, and the third most common cause of preventable death.[1] Swift effective care is essential for optimal outcomes. Children with airway compromise or edema, or those who present with respiratory distress, should be intubated immediately. The primary survey of a burn patient should include two key priorities: establishing the extent of the burn wound or total body surface area (TBSA) and the depth of the wound.[2]

The TBSA of the injury is commonly calculated using the Lund–Browder diagram (**Figure 87.1**). However, the depth of the wound determines need for surgical excision and grafting, which is generally recommended for all deep partial or full thickness burns that would take more than 2 to 3 weeks to heal. In addition to wound depth or thickness, other predictors of surgery (for children with 20% TBSA or greater) are infection and blood loss. The only contraindication that would detour surgery for a burn patient would be a condition that would normally prevent the induction of general anesthesia.[3]

SPECIAL CONSIDERATIONS AND CONCERNS

It is important to consider not only the TBSA of a burn injury but also the mechanism (i.e., thermal, electrical, or chemical) and how the injury occurred. If the patient was in a motor vehicle accident or other traumatic event, identifying concomitant injuries, such as organ damage, traumatic brain injury, or spinal injury, is imperative. The TBSA is an important determinant of physiological changes that occur and help guide the resuscitation process. Cell destruction occurs in thermal injuries and increases cellular permeability and capillary leakage, which can lead to significant fluid loss. Initial goals revolve around repletion of intravascular volumes to protect tissue perfusion and reduce ischemic and inflammatory responses. Before noticeable reductions of plasma volume, cardiac output depression occurs, and continues for 24 to 36 hours (**Figure 87.2**). The hypermetabolic and hyperdynamic phase begins 48 to 72 hours after injury (**Figure 87.3**); increases in oxygen consumption, carbon dioxide production, and protein wasting are prevalent during this time.[4] Electrical injuries allow heat generation by current conduction (greater in high water-content tissues: blood vessels, nerves, and muscles) and can lead to compartment syndrome. The nervous system is especially susceptible to damage because of the low resistance of neurons; this can lead to paresthesias. Surgical excision and grafting help promote healing time and can decrease pain. There are different types of grafts that can be used, such as an allograft, xenograft, or synthetic graft.[1] Anesthesia providers should realize that if an allograft is being used, wherein the patient's own tissue is excised, there will be increased pain at the donor site.

ANESTHETIC MANAGEMENT

PREOPERATIVE EVALUATION

Airway assessment in relation to the burn injury is important. If an inhalation injury has occurred, morbidity and mortality increase significantly.[4] The mechanism of inhalational injury is multifactorial but can be devastating to oxygen transport and utilization (**Figure 87.4**). Additionally, patients with burns to the head or neck may require fiberoptic intubation or a surgical

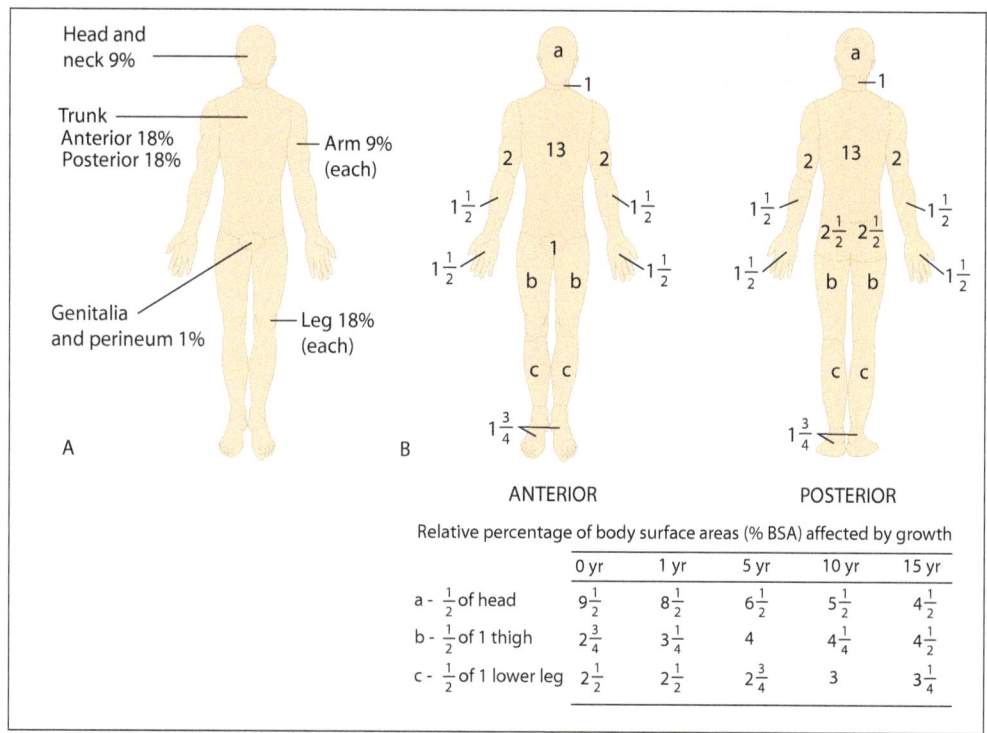

Figure 87.1: Lund–Browder diagram. Estimating percentage of total body surface area in children affected by burns. (A) Rule of "nines"; (B) Lund–Browder diagram for estimating extent of burns.

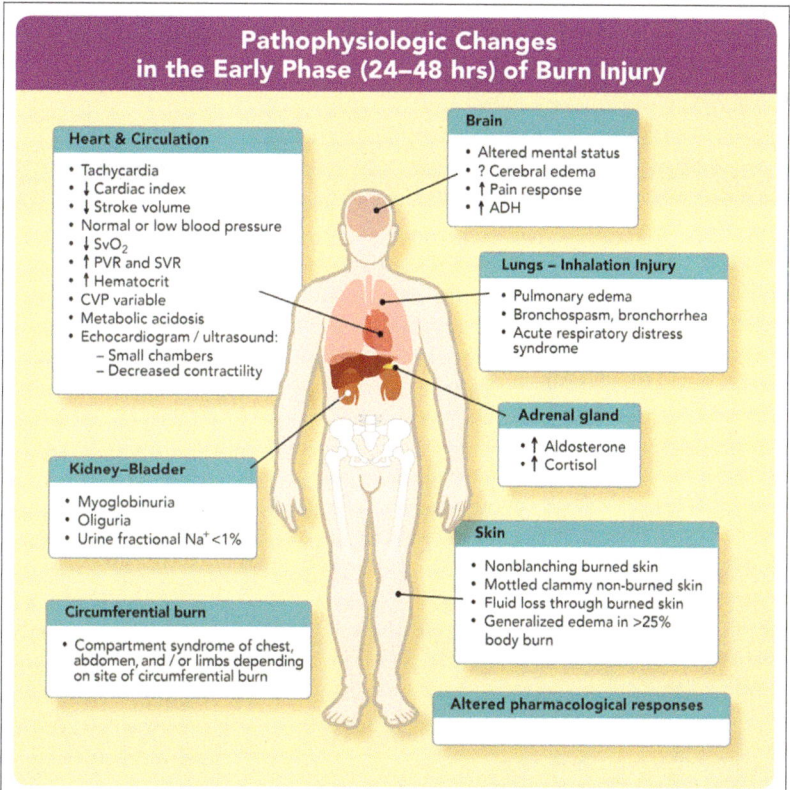

Figure 87.2: Early pathophysiological changes following burn injury (24–48 hours).

ADH, antidiuretic hormone; CVP, central venous pressure; PVR, pulmonary vascular resistance; SvO_2, mixed venous oxygen saturation; SVR, systemic vascular resistance.

Source: From Bittner EA, Shank E, Woodson L, et al. Acute and perioperative care of the burn-injured patient. *Anesthesiology.* 2015;122(2):448–464. doi:10.1097/ALN.0000000000000559.

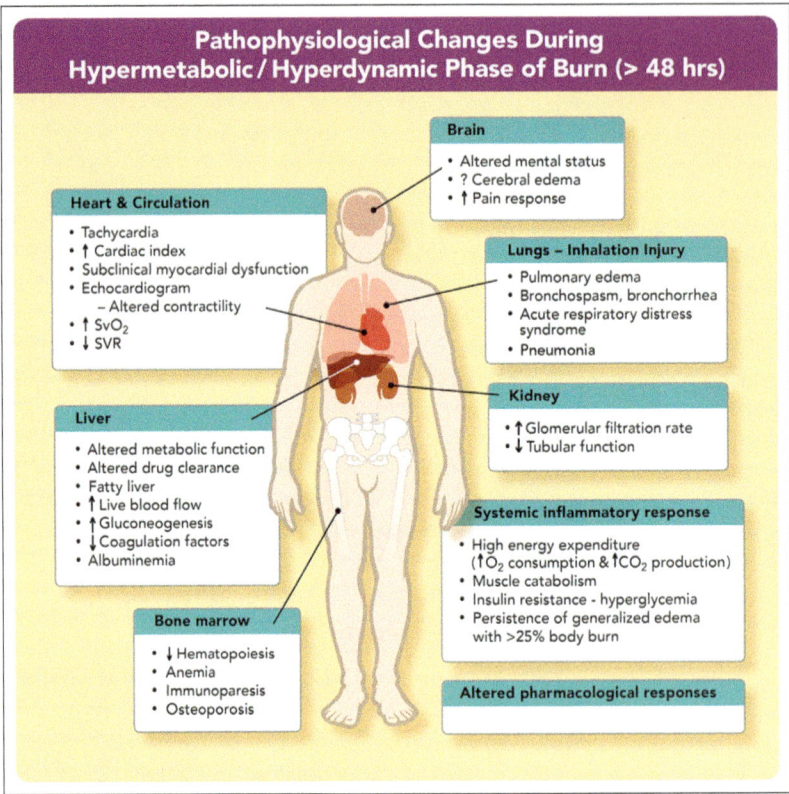

Figure 87.3: Pathophysiological changes 48 hours following burn injury.

SvO$_2$, mixed venous oxygen saturation; SVR, systemic vascular resistance.

Source: From Bittner EA, Shank E, Woodson L, et al. Acute and perioperative care of the burn-injured patient. *Anesthesiology.* 2015;122(2):448–464. doi:10.1097/ALN.0000000000000559.

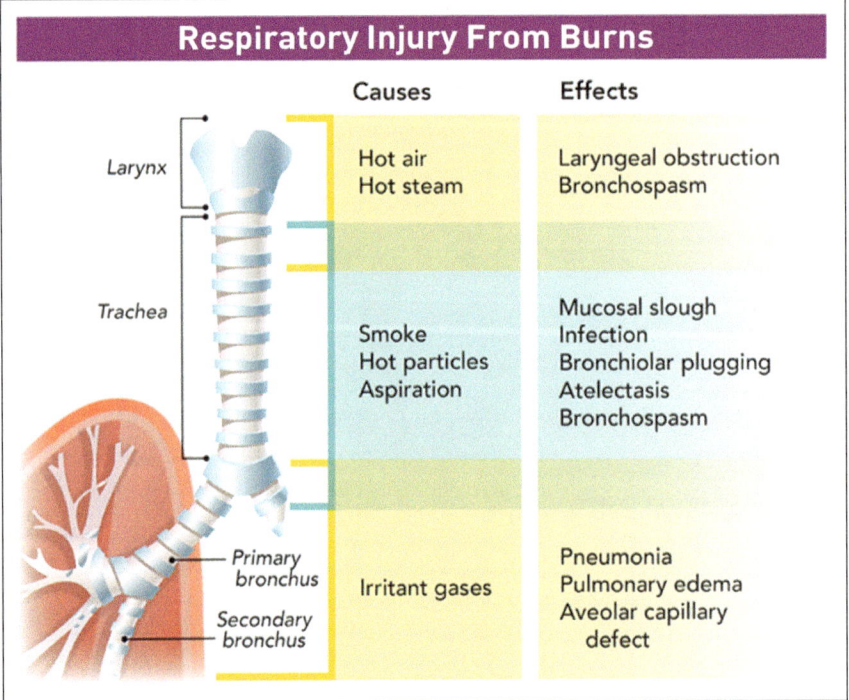

Figure 87.4: Effects of inhalational burn injury.

Source: From Bittner EA, Shank E, Woodson L, et al. Acute and perioperative care of the burn-injured patient. *Anesthesiology.* 2015;122(2):448–464. doi:10.1097/ALN.0000000000000559.

airway.[5] Mandibular mobility may reveal tightness, and mouth opening can be limited due to edema or contractures that can make laryngoscopy challenging. Anesthesia providers should thoroughly assess the patient's anxiety level and consider premedication with an anxiolytic, such as a benzodiazepine, dexmedetomidine, or ketamine. Evaluate current fluid resuscitative state. Patients with <10% TBSA typically do not require formal resuscitation; however, those with >30% TBSA develop systemic physiological changes and may require increased fluid administration during surgery.[6] For the pediatric patient, the Lund–Browder chart provides an age-based algorithm that considers the child anatomy of a large head and small limbs and may be more accurate for estimating burns in children.[7] A minor burn in a child is <5% TBSA, a moderate burn is 5% to 10% TBSA, and a major burn is >10% TBSA.[5]

PERTINENT LABS

Important laboratory values to consider for the burn patient are a complete blood count, coagulation studies, type and screen/cross, electrolytes, blood urea nitrogen, serum protein, and creatinine clearance. Special emphasis should be placed on correcting any acid–base disturbances.[6]

PREOPERATIVE PHARMACOLOGY

After a thermal injury, there are differences in organ flow, plasma protein levels and binding, body water distribution, and end-organ receptor population and affinity. The most important drug to avoid 24 hours post burn injury is succinylcholine. Its use produces a potentially fatal hyperkalemic response due to potassium efflux from muscle.[8] Non-depolarizing agents may require up to five times the usual dose for effect with shorter duration of action.[8] This is due to altered protein binding and increased number of extrajunctional acetylcholine receptors that bind nondepolarizing drugs without causing a neuromuscular effect.[9]

Pain secondary to burns is an underrated problem in children, due to acute exacerbation and repeated procedures. Burn patients typically require larger doses of opioid medications. Opioids have a greatly reduced distribution and elimination half-lives (as little as 20% of usual values) and tolerance develops rapidly.[8] Options to consider for non-narcotic pain management include acetaminophen, opioids, gabapentin, dexmedetomidine, or ketamine. Nonsteroidal anti-inflammatory drug use in burn patients is limited by concerns for potential side effects, such as bleeding risk, gastrointestinal side effects, and renal toxicity.[10] It is important to consider the use of multimodal agents to decrease opioid use that could lead to tolerance and addiction.

ANESTHETIC TECHNIQUE

INTRAOPERATIVE MANAGEMENT

Routine monitoring is affected in severely burned patients. Noninvasive blood pressure monitoring may be contraindicated over burned extremities, necessitating placement of arterial lines, sutured in place. Adhesive ECG leads, and pulse oximeters may similarly be contraindicated. Needle ECG electrodes and nonadhesive pulse oximeters (under tongue, across nasal septum or lip, or on the penis) may be needed.[8]

Inhalation induction is acceptable for the child that does not have an IV catheter. If inhalation injury has occurred, bronchodilators and mucolytic agents have proven useful for stabilization before intubation.[7] Cuffed endotracheal tubes are preferable compared to uncuffed in order to match the high-minute volume and positive-end expiratory pressure requirements of burn patients.[7] Laryngeal mask airways are also acceptable in appropriate patients. Maintenance is achieved with potent inhalation agents, a nitrous-narcotic technique or a total IV agent depending on the physiological needs of the patient.[6]

Fluid management can be accomplished using a calculated fluid plan per the patient's weight. Keep in mind that younger patients have limited glycogen storage, and dextrose-containing solutions are recommended in addition to the standard isotonic solutions.[11] Anesthesia providers should be aware of the potential for fluid overload and potential cardiac side effects (e.g., tachycardia or dysrhythmias) from systemic absorption of tumescent solutions containing vasoconstrictors being used in the surgical field.[6] Urine output is an important indicator of fluid resuscitation, and 0.5 to 1 mL/kg/hr has been suggested as reasonable output.[11] Heat loss through denuded skin is a serious problem in the burn patient; warming blankets, increased operating room temperature, humidified inspired gases, and warmed IV fluids should be used.[9] Increased ambient temperature prevents the untoward effects of hypothermia, such as altered effects of IV and inhalation anesthetics, prolonged neuromuscular blockade, increased bleeding, and impaired wound healing. Regional anesthesia using ultrasound-guided, catheter-delivered, or single-injection local anesthetic techniques has recently provided superior pain control and should be considered (Table 87.1 and Box 87.1).

COMPLICATIONS/EMERGENCIES

Perioperative complications include fluid overload, arrhythmias, and cardiac arrest from inadvertent succinylcholine

TABLE 87.1	Special Techniques and Equipment in Surgical Treatment of Burn Injury
Airway management	- If there is concern for upper airway patency/mobility and fiberoptic intubation is needed, consider ketamine because it induces sedation but maintains pharyngeal muscle tone. - A tie harness that goes circumferentially around the head or wire securement for patients with facial burns so the ETT can stay safely fixed in place.

Ventilation	- Ventilation rates (due to increased carbon dioxide production), PEEP, and inspiratory pressure may need to be higher during the hypermetabolic state.
	- Use lower tidal volumes in the OR (~6 mL/kg ideal body weight).
	- Depending on burn severity/location, patients may have
	  ○ FRC or lung/chest wall compliance.
	  ○ a gradient carboxyhemoglobinemia and methemoglobinemia.

(continued)

TABLE 87.1	Special Techniques and Equipment in Surgical Treatment of Burn Injury (*continued*)
Maintenance anesthetic	• Inhalational agents are preferred during the acute phase of injury due to increased volume of distribution (need for higher dosing), changes in protein binding, and decreased hepatic blood flow. However, if patients come to the OR on sedation or narcotic infusions, these should not be stopped.
Neuromuscular monitoring	• Neuromuscular function monitoring is useful when patients are receiving paralytics because their dose requirements will often be altered. • Avoid succinylcholine administration 48 hrs after the burn injury to avoid a significant hyperkalemic response and possible cardiac arrest. • 3–7 days after a burn injury, the dose of NDMRs increases to achieve paralysis. For maximal effect, an induction dose of 1.5 mg/kg takes ~90 sec; 1.2 mg/kg ~105 sec; 0.9 mg/kg ~150 sec.
Temperature management	• The body's inflammatory response to large burns can cause the core temperature set point to increase. Hypothermia increases oxygen consumption and exacerbates the catabolic response to injuries; it can also increase blood loss during surgery. • Increasing the OR temperature (typically 80 °F–100 °F), warming blankets, radiant warmers, blood/fluid warmers (all fluids should be warmed), wrapping the head or nonsurgical extremities with insulation, and minimizing skin exposure can all be effective ways in maintaining body temperature.
Pain control	• If the patient is receiving opioid infusions, these can be titrated to effect. Patients often become tolerant to narcotics; a multimodal approach of clonidine, dexmedetomidine, ketamine, and methadone is an effective pain treatment.
Regional anesthesia	• Central neuraxial techniques, such as spinals or epidurals, can have good pain attenuation both intraoperatively and postoperatively. • Other peripheral or truncal blocks have also provided adequate analgesia, especially a lateral femoral cutaneous block because it is exclusively a sensory nerve and covers the lateral thigh, which is often chosen for split-thickness skin grafts.

ETT, endotracheal tube; FRC, functional residual capacity; NDMRs, nondepolarizing muscle relaxants; OR, operating room; PEEP, positive end-expiratory pressure.

BOX 87.1 CLINICAL PEARLS

Parenteral nutrition
- Keep parenteral nutrition running to prevent hypoglycemia.

Premedication
- Midazolam is acceptable for these patients at the anesthesia providers, discretion; also consider additional pain medicine before transport or moving the patient to the OR table as these patients are often on high-dose narcotics.

Airway
- For long surgeries or large injury sites, an ETT is recommended due to possible large amount of blood loss and need for fluid resuscitation, airway edema can occur.

Antibiotics
- Cefazolin (unless allergy or otherwise indicated by surgical team)

Positioning
- The positioning will be based on surgical need but note that burn patients are particularly susceptible to facial, laryngeal, and upper airway edema in the prone position.
- Caution should be used before extubation.

Fluid management
- Avoid giving too much fluid intraoperatively to prevent edema, follow normal perioperative fluid replacement guidelines and consider colloid instead of crystalloid.
- There may be SC infiltration of fluid or fluid containing epinephrine solution.

Blood loss
- For large excision and grafting surgeries, blood loss can be massive.
- Make sure blood is available and in the room; be vigilant in watching for blood loss, as it often does not get collected by suction.
- Surgeons may use epinephrine-soaked sponges to decrease blood loss, watch for systemic absorption of this and subsequent tachycardia and dysrhythmias.

ETT, endotracheal tube.

administration and postoperative reintubation secondary to airway edema. Anesthesia providers can play a role in preventing many of these complications. Fluid overload and arrhythmia can occur from the absorption of epinephrine-containing solutions used to obtain hemostasis of the burned area. Fluid management should be administered as per the patient's calculated needs. Succinylcholine should be avoided 24 hours after thermal injury and up to 1 year thereafter to prevent the hyperkalemic response that may lead to cardiac arrest. Assessing for extubation criteria, keeping in mind any lung injury from the burn, could prevent reintubation from occurring.

POSTOPERATIVE CARE

The decision to extubate in the operating room depends on standard criteria with specific concerns for burn patients including assessment of airway patency, metabolic status, potential for ongoing bleeding, and when the patient will return for surgery.[4] The mechanism of injury and lack of an endotracheal cuff air leak are key prognostic indicators of extubation failure.[7] Anesthesia providers should consider administering longer acting opioids or non-narcotics medications, such as acetaminophen, dexmedetomidine, or ketamine. Inadequate control of pain or anxiety can adversely affect wound healing and psychological status.[4]

CASE STUDY: Excision and Grafting in a 6-Year-Old Female With Scald Burn

CLINICAL SCENARIO

A 6-year-old female with scald burn covering 10% TBSA to chest/trunk and upper right arm presents for excision and grafting of these locations. She presented 3 days ago with a scald burn from pulling a small pot of boiling water off of the stove. Her burn TBSA has been determined to be 10% with differing depths ranging from superficial to deep partial thickness. She has been on crystalloid maintenance fluid and adequately resuscitated by the managing team. She is on morphine (PRN) and dexmedetomidine infusion at 0.4 mcg/kg/hr for pain control. She has been NPO for over 12 hours. Her vital signs are as follows: core temperature 36.8, blood pressure 88/55, heart rate 122 beats per minute, and respiration rate 26. She has two IV sites, a 22 g in her left hand and a 20 g in her left antecubital space.

SPECIAL CONSIDERATIONS

Make sure to check the patient's record to see what medications she has been receiving and when (i.e., pain medications and antibiotics if any). Make sure the operating room temperature is greatly increased, use an underbody radiant warmer and fluid to ensure her temperature is maintained especially because she will be fairly exposed. Have midazolam and narcotic ready for premedication (moving her may be painful). Check her labs and make sure her type and screen is up to date, have 1 unit of blood available in the room, and albumin to refrain from giving too much crystalloid.

APPROACHES TO CARE

Evidence-Based Approaches to Care

Once in the operating room, standard monitoring should be applied, and the patient should be induced in a normal fashion through her IV and an endotracheal tube placed. Considering that she is 3 days postburn, nondepolarizing muscle relaxant dosing will need to be increased to achieve adequate muscle relaxation. Continue her dexmedetomidine infusion and consider use of morphine since she has been receiving it already. Ketamine boluses of 0.5 mg/kg can be used for additional non-narcotic pain control. Monitor blood loss vigilantly and recognize that it is generally not retrieved by suction. Judicious fluid management with the use of colloid fluids is appropriate to avoid unnecessary edema.[4] At the conclusion of the procedure, if the patient is hemodynamically stable and does not exhibit any signs of airway edema, the patient can be extubated before proceeding to the postanesthesia care unit (PACU).

COMPLICATIONS

The patient had an uneventful perioperative course; she was safely extubated and taken to PACU. She did receive additional pain medication and one dose of 0.5 mg Haldol for nausea but otherwise did well and returned to her inpatient room without issue.

ETT, endotracheal tube; OR, operating room.

REFERENCES

1. Bosques G, Singh M. *Pediatric Burns*. 2019. https://now.aapmr.org/pediatric-burns
2. Leon-Villapalos J, Dziewulski P. *Overview of Surgical Procedures Used in the Management of Burn Injuries*. 2020. https://www.uptodate.com/contents/overview-of-surgical-procedures-used-in-the-management-of-burn-injuries
3. Fabia R. *Surgical Treatment of Burns in Children Treatment & Management*. 2020. https://reference.medscape.com/article/934173-treatment#d10
4. Bittner EA, Shank E, Woodson L, Martyn JA. Acute and perioperative care of the burn-injured patient. *Anesthesiology*. 2015;122(2):448–464. doi:10.1097/ALN.0000000000000559
5. Singh-Radcliff N. *The 5-Minute Anesthesia Consult*. Lippincott Williams & Wilkins; 2013.
6. Fuzaylov G, Fidkowski C. Anesthetic considerations for the major burn injury in pediatric patients. *Paediatr Anaesth*. 2009;19(3):202–211. doi:10.1111/j.1460-9592.2009.02924.x
7. Preston D, Ambardekar A. The pediatric burn: current trends and future directions. *Anesthesiol Clin*. 2020;38(3):517–530. doi:10.1016/j.anclin.2020.05.0038
8. Holzman R, Mancuso T, Polaner D. *A Practical Approach to Pediatric Anesthesia*. 2nd ed. Lippincott Williams & Wilkins; 2016.
9. Butterworth J, Mackey D. *Morgan & Mikhail's Clinical Anesthesiology*. McGraw Hill McGraw-Hill Education; 2013.
10. Pardesi O, Fuzaylov G. Pain management in pediatric burn patients: review of recent literature and future directions. *J Burn Care Res*. 2017;38(6):335–347. doi:10.1097/BCR.0000000000000470
11. Sofia J, Ambardekar A. Pediatric burn resuscitation, management, and recovery for the pediatric anesthesiologist. *Curr Opin Anaesthesiol*. 2020;33(3):360–367. doi:10.1097/ACO.0000000000000859

SECTION F: Endocrine Procedures

CHAPTER 88

Thyroidectomy and Parathyroidectomy

Tracy Beckham

INDICATIONS/CONTRAINDICATIONS

Although thyroid and parathyroid surgeries are not common in the pediatric population, it is imperative that anesthesia providers have a sound understanding of the surgical procedure and potential complications that may ensue as these procedures are associated with higher rates of complication when compared to their adult counterparts. Moreover, the surgical procedures can vary greatly, ranging from relatively simple to very complicated. Despite the complexity of the procedure, however, all are associated with potential complications and risks.

Not only must anesthesia providers manage a shared airway throughout the surgical procedure, but they must also remain ever ready to manage a host of known perioperative complications. Thorough preparation best prepares anesthesia providers to deliver safe, effective care when caring for pediatric patients undergoing thyroidectomy and/or parathyroidectomy.

THYROIDECTOMY

The thyroid gland is a butterfly-shaped gland located directly in front of the larynx. The principle thyroid hormones produced are thyroxine (T_4) and triiodothyronine (T_3). T_4 is the primary circulating thyroid hormone and T_3, which is converted from T_4, is the major physiologically active thyroid hormone. The serum T_3 and T_4 concentrations are both regulated by thyroid-stimulating hormone (TSH), which is secreted by the anterior pituitary. As thyroid hormones affect all metabolically active cells, dysfunction must be treated and managed swiftly and effectively to stave off negative sequelae. Thyroid cancer comprises 0.5% to 3% of all pediatric malignancies, but generally has a good prognosis. While some types of thyroid disease can be treated conservatively, others will require surgical intervention.[1,2]

A thyroidectomy may be either total or partial in nature, depending on the type and extent of disease. A total thyroidectomy aims to remove the entire thyroid gland and may be necessary for patients with Grave's disease or thyroid cancer. Removing the target tissue for the TSH receptor antibody will necessitate lifelong T_4 replacement therapy. A partial, or subtotal, thyroidectomy describes one of two procedures. It may consist of a lobectomy that removes only one side of the thyroid gland, or it can be a bilateral subtotal thyroidectomy, which leaves behind bilateral thyroid remnants. A subtotal thyroidectomy is indicated when the removal of thyroid nodules is necessary or as part of the conservative treatment of Grave's disease and leaves a portion of the functioning gland intact (Box 88.1).[2,3]

Historically, pediatric patients presenting with thyroid nodules and cancers were treated using the same management guidelines as adults. Trends in management have shifted, however, as it is now recognized that pediatric patients, including adolescents up to the age of 21, exhibit differences in pathophysiology, clinical presentation, and long-term outcomes (Figure 88.1).[4] While children are at a lower risk of death, they remain at a higher risk of developing long-term negative sequelae secondary to overly aggressive treatment. Subsequently, the American Thyroid Association (ATA) has developed recommendations unique to the pediatric population. Optimal care for children presenting with thyroid nodules and cancers now follows guidelines specific to the pediatric population.[4]

PARATHYROIDECTOMY

There are four parathyroid glands, all of which are located in close proximity to the posterior four corners of the thyroid gland. These glands function to maintain calcium homeostasis by secreting parathyroid hormone (PTH) in response to a decrease in serum ionized calcium. PTH acts directly on the kidneys and on the bones, resulting in an increase of serum calcium while decreasing serum phosphate levels. As osteoclasts are stimulated to release calcium and phosphate into the extracellular fluid, increased phosphate excretion and calcium reabsorption occurs in the kidneys.[2] The elevated circulating calcium levels associated with hypercalcemia lead to fatigue, as well as symptoms stemming from alterations in bone, abdominal, urological, and even mental function (Box 88.2).

Hyperparathyroidism can be primary or secondary in nature. Primary hyperparathyroidism is often secondary to a noncancerous growth, such as a parathyroid adenoma, but can also be secondary to hyperplasia of two or more parathyroid glands or a cancerous tumor. Parathyroid adenoma is the most common reason for parathyroidectomy, with cancerous tumors being very rare. Secondary hyperparathyroidism is the result of another condition that lowers calcium levels, such as severe calcium deficiency, severe vitamin D deficiency, or chronic renal disease and/or failure.

Intraoperatively, hyperparathyroidism is associated with a higher incidence of cardiovascular deaths and glucose intolerance.[3] One of the most frequent complications of thyroid surgery is hypoparathyroidism, which occurs in approximately a third of patients. Parathyroid glands are very small and have similar tissue, causing them to be accidentally

---

BOX 88.1 INDICATIONS FOR THYROIDECTOMY IN PEDIATRIC PATIENTS

- Adenoma
- Grave's disease/hyperthyroidism
- Hashimoto's disease
- MEN type 2, a hereditary thyroid syndrome associated with certain thyroid cancers
- Thyroid cancer (female:male ratio 2:1)
- Thyroid nodules, which may be either malignant or benign in nature

MEN, multiple endocrine neoplasia.

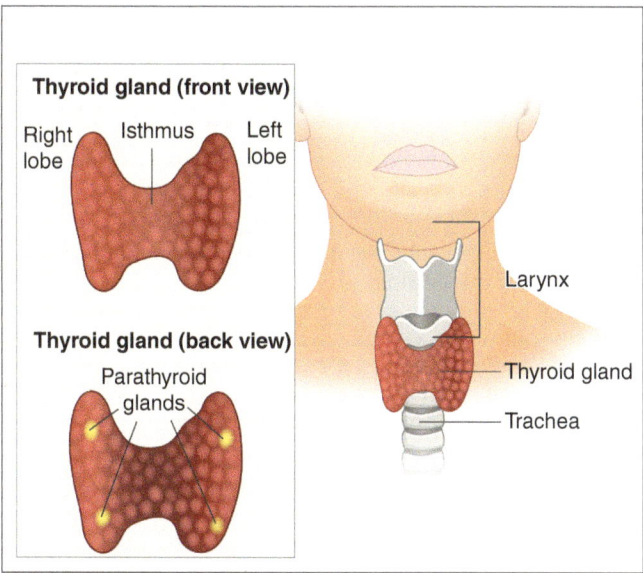

Figure 88.1: Pediatric thyroid and parathyroid.

excised or damaged frequently.[5] During a parathyroidectomy, overactive glands are identified based on the hypertrophied appearance or by special techniques, such as Sestambi scanning. Often only one gland is enlarged and is removed. If all the glands are enlarged, they will all be removed, with the exception of approximately half of one gland with hope of preventing hypoparathyroidism and hypocalcemia by leaving a portion of function tissue. Confirmation is done by tissue biopsy and frozen section. Additionally, indocyanine green dye can be injected to allow imaging of the parathyroid glands by autofluorescence intraoperatively, which allows for location and preservation of the glands intraoperatively.[5]

SPECIAL CONSIDERATIONS AND CONCERNS

Given the rarity with which thyroidectomy and parathyroidectomy surgeries are performed in the pediatric population, it has been suggested that optimal outcomes are achieved when surgery is performed at a high-volume pediatric surgical center. Referral to a high-volume center provides patients access to surgeons with expertise in performing these surgeries, which can decrease the incidence of serious postoperative complications.[2, 6] Regardless of the location surgery is performed, clear, concise communication between the multidisciplinary team caring for the patient is essential to ensure optimal outcomes. It is recommended that all patients be medically optimized prior to surgery. While patients with complicated medical histories or those requiring inpatient procedures would not be candidates, the majority of pediatric thyroidectomies can be safely and effectively managed on an outpatient basis.[7]

> **BOX 88.2 INDICATIONS FOR PARATHYROIDECTOMY IN PEDIATRIC PATIENTS**
>
> - Hyperparathyroidism (neonatal or primary)
> - Parathyroid hyperplasia
> - Familial hypocalciuric hypercalcemia (benign)
> - Parathyroid cancer (rare)

ANESTHETIC MANAGEMENT

PREOPERATIVE EVALUATION

Prior to surgery, a thorough history and physical assessment is paramount. In addition to a careful airway assessment including assignment of a Mallampati score, examining mandibular protrusion and performing Patil's test are highly recommended. Goiters and infiltrating carcinomas may hinder neck movement, obscure cord visualization, and thus, cause difficult intubation.[3] In addition to assessing the patient's neck for the presence, the size and consistency of a goiter should be noted. A large goiter has the potential to cause tracheal deviation or compression, thus, it is imperative that anesthesia providers assess for airway compromise preoperatively. Any history of positional dyspnea or difficulty swallowing should be noted. A hard goiter generally suggests malignancy.

Patients presenting for thyroidectomy should be clinically and pharmacologically euthyroid prior to surgery. Vital signs should be within normal limits; therefore, tachycardia, palpitations, goiter, dyspnea, fatigue, tremor, muscle weakness, hyperreflexia, insomnia, heat intolerance, nervousness, and weight loss are all concerning findings preoperatively and should alert the anesthesia provider that the patient may not be euthyroid the day of surgery. Patients with known hyperthyroidism especially need to be euthyroid before surgery to avoid precipitation of thyroid storm. They should no longer have tachycardia and have a pulse pressure and resting pulse within normal limits. If cardiovascular parameters are not within normal ranges, surgery should be postponed until the thyroid hormone levels are normalized or controlled with beta-adrenergic blockers. Patients with hyperthyroidism presenting emergently for surgery will need careful preparation with antithyroid drugs, beta-blockers, iodine, and corticosteroids to prevent further thyroid release. Children with a diagnosis of Grave's disease may have ocular involvement characterized by inflammation and edema of retro-orbital tissues and extraocular muscles causing proptosis and impaired function of the eye muscles.

It is also important to inquire about prior surgeries, head and neck radiation, or radioiodine therapy as it may impact the patient's neck range of motion. Interestingly, undocumented hypothyroid is associated with the majority of complications, so it is important to ask about all potential thyroid-related symptoms. Patients with a diagnosis of Down syndrome, diabetes mellitus, celiac disease, or other genetic disorders are at an increased risk and should be screened for hypothyroidism.[2,3]

Patients presenting for parathyroidectomy may have tumors secondary to hypercalcemia, although this is an uncommon finding in children. They may present with nonspecific symptoms, such as nausea and vomiting, failure to thrive, irritability, polyuria, constipation, and fatigue. Children who may have persistent hypocalcemia, resulting from hypoparathyroidism, may present with symptoms, such as poor feeding, laryngospasm, tetany, seizures, myocardial dysfunction, and myopathy. Calcium and vitamin D levels should be normalized before surgery.[2,3]

Pertinent Labs

Recommended preoperative laboratory work includes a complete blood count, electrolytes, thyroid function tests including T_3, T_4, and TSH levels, and a serum calcium level. Assessment of phosphate, magnesium, alkaline phosphatase, 25-hydroxyvitamin D, and creatinine is indicated with hypocalcemia and hypercalcemia.[2]

A chest x-ray may be indicated to assess for tracheal deviation and narrowing based on the patient's presenting history. In complex or suspicious cases, a lateral chest x-ray with thoracic inlet views may be indicated to better detect tracheal compression in the anteroposterior plane. CT scans may be needed for patients who have a history of airway involvement or positional dyspnea. A CT scan is helpful when there is suspicion of malignancy that could encroach onto the trachea. Any narrowing of the trachea seen on chest x-ray should be looked at more closely with a CT scan to accurately pinpoint the site that is compromised and the degree of narrowing to plan for intubating the trachea.

PREOPERATIVE PHARMACOLOGY

Prior to surgery, it is recommended that children be euthyroid. Antithyroid medications, such as methimazole, are the first line of conservative treatment and are frequently used to treat Grave's disease, which is the most common cause of hyperthyroidism. Approximately 25% to 40% of children will go into remission with antithyroid medications. Propylthiouracil is no longer used to treat Grave's disease in children due to the risk of hepatotoxicity and liver failure.[1,2] Radioactive iodine therapy may be indicated for pediatric patients who fail to respond to antithyroid medication regimens or have a reaction to them.

In emergent situations that preclude treatment with the aforementioned medications, the child can be given antithyroid drugs followed by oral iodine (Lugol solution or saturated potassium iodine solution) to block the thyroid gland from further releasing thyroid hormone.

Beta-adrenergic blockers, such as esmolol and propranolol, can be used preoperatively and intraoperatively to control cardiovascular responses. Corticosteroids can also be given to limit T_4 to T_3 conversion and increase vasomotor stability. If the patient presents with hypothyroidism and urgent surgery is needed, IV levothyroxine (LT4) can be administered. Additionally, anesthesia providers should anticipate the patient being sensitive to opioid and benzodiazepine administrations.[2,3]

ANESTHETIC TECHNIQUE

Intraoperative Management

See clinical pearls in **Box 88.3**. Most thyroid and parathyroid surgeries in the pediatric population are performed under general anesthesia. The patient should be considered to be a possible difficult airway with the potential of tracheal deviation. Therefore, it is recommended advanced airway devices are in the room prior to induction and are readily available. Prior to induction, the patient should be adequately preoxygenated. In cases of known compromised airway, the bed may be placed in semi-supine position. While either an inhalational mask induction or IV induction is acceptable, it is advisable to keep the patient breathing spontaneously until it is determined that the patient can be easily mask ventilated and there is no obstructive pathology. Once it has been established that the patient can be easily mask ventilated, a neuromuscular blocking agent can be given to facilitate tracheal intubation.

Fiberoptic intubation may be required if the airway is displaced or narrowed. If the airway is severely compromised, the surgeon may elect to do a tracheostomy under local anesthesia to secure the airway. A rigid bronchoscope can also be used to secure ventilation if attempts to intubate with an endotracheal tube fail due to obstruction. A reinforced endotracheal tube is commonly used and should be taped into position away from the surgical site. Regardless of which technique is used, the surgeon should be immediately available in the operating room at the time of induction to manage any emergency airway situation.

Intraoperatively, anesthesia providers must share the patient's airway with the surgical team. Endotracheal tube placement and connections must be closely monitored. The patient must have full American Society of Anesthesiologists monitoring and is generally positioned supine with their head slightly elevated and extended to optimize surgical exposure and prevent venous engorgement (**Figure 88.2**). This position can be stabilized using a gel head ring and a shoulder roll or gel pad between the shoulder blades to extend the neck. The eyes should be carefully taped and padded, and possibly covered with goggles, especially if exophthalmos is present. Most thyroid and parathyroid surgeries are done through a standard collar-type transverse surgical incision. As the thyroid lobe is dissected, the thyroid vessels are ligated and the superior laryngeal nerve is identified. The parathyroid glands are then identified and preserved or, in the case of hyperparathyroidism, excised. The patient's arms are generally tucked to provide access to the surgical site.

Anesthesia can be maintained with inhalation agents or with total intravenous anesthesia (TIVA). If preoperative stridor is present, sevoflurane in heliox may be used if available. Anesthesia providers should be aware that hypothyroidism increases sensitivity to anesthetics and neuromuscular blocking agents. Remifentanil may be used to provide analgesia, blunt the laryngeal reflexes, reduce the need for further neuromuscular blocking agents, and help maintain stable hemodynamics, which decreases bleeding. Depending on the

---

BOX 88.3 CLINICAL PEARLS

- Eucapnia should be maintained by continuous end-tidal CO_2 monitoring to avoid causing alterations in ionized calcium levels.
- Local anesthetic infiltration is commonly done by the surgeon at the end of the case and improves pain control and decreases opioid needs.
- The surgeon may send tissue for frozen section and wait for the pathology, which can delay closure. This is to identify the presence of cancer and to verify thyroid tissue versus parathyroid tissue, making sure the parathyroid glands were not inadvertently removed or, in the case of hyperparathyroidism that the correct amount of tissue was taken.
- The surgeon may request a Valsalva maneuver, maintaining the positive pressure for 10–20 sec, possibly with the patient in head down position, to ensure homeostasis before wound closure.
- The cords may be examined under direct vision and the cuff of the endotracheal tube should be deflated and a "leak test" performed immediately before extubation.
- The patient should be fully awake and spontaneously breathing before extubation. The anesthesia provider may inspect the cords post-extubation but may have difficulty visualizing. A fiberoptic scope can also be passed through a laryngeal mask airway if better visualization is needed.
- Recurrent and superior laryngeal nerve function should be checked perioperatively.

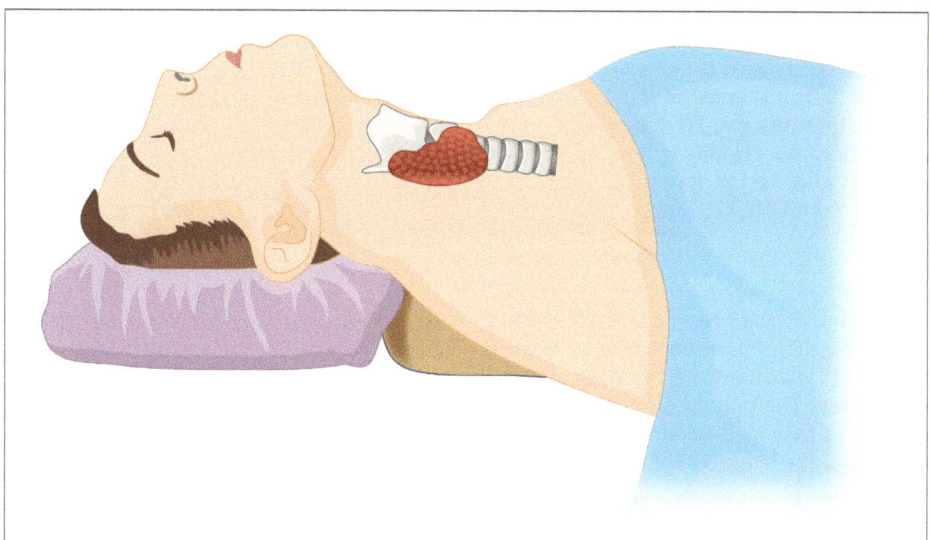

Figure 88.2: Positioning for thyroid and parathyroid surgeries. The patient must have full ASA monitoring and is generally positioned supine with their head slightly elevated and extended to optimize surgical exposure and prevent venous engorgement.

ASA, American Society of Anesthesiologists.

location and type of the procedure, regional anesthesia may be utilized, using superficial and deep cervical plexus blocks to provide intra- and postoperative analgesia. Sedation can also be given, but this technique still requires full cooperation by the patient, so it is not as commonly used with children.[1,3] Dexamethasone may be administered to decrease postoperative edema and airway swelling. Dexamethasone also contributes to decreased postoperative nausea and vomiting.

Blood loss is usually minimal, less than 100 mL; however there is the potential for major hemorrhage due to the glands being extremely close to large blood vessels.[1–3]

Special Techniques
One of the most common injuries following both pediatric thyroidectomy and parathyroidectomy is recurrent laryngeal nerve (RLN) damage. Intraoperative monitoring of the RLN during these surgeries has become the standard of care for adults and is strongly recommended in the pediatric population. Monitoring of the RLN should be done with a double-needle electrode inserted through the cricothyroid ligament. This is connected to a specialized nerve integrity monitor (NIM) endotracheal tube. The placement of a NIM endotracheal tube should be with the middle of the exposed electrodes well in contact with the true vocal cords under direct laryngoscopy (Figure 88.3). This method has been shown to be reliable and is not associated with any known complications at any age. However, there are instances where the child may need a smaller size endotracheal tube than what was available with the smallest monitoring tube.[8]

The role of intraoperative nerve monitoring during parathyroidectomy is unclear in preventing injury to the RLN and can add cost and setup time to the procedure. Visual identification remains the gold standard in preventing RLN damage.[9]

Complications/Emergencies
Thyroidectomy and parathyroidectomy are both associated with complications that have the potential to have profound effects on the quality of life of the children involved. Fortunately, the incidence of complications is relatively low, especially when surgery is performed at high-volume centers.[6]

Thyroid Storm
Thyroid storm is a rare but very serious event. It is usually witnessed following a precipitating event, such as surgery, infection, trauma, or diabetic ketoacidosis. It can mimic acute malignant hyperthermia, but usually develops 6 to 18 hours

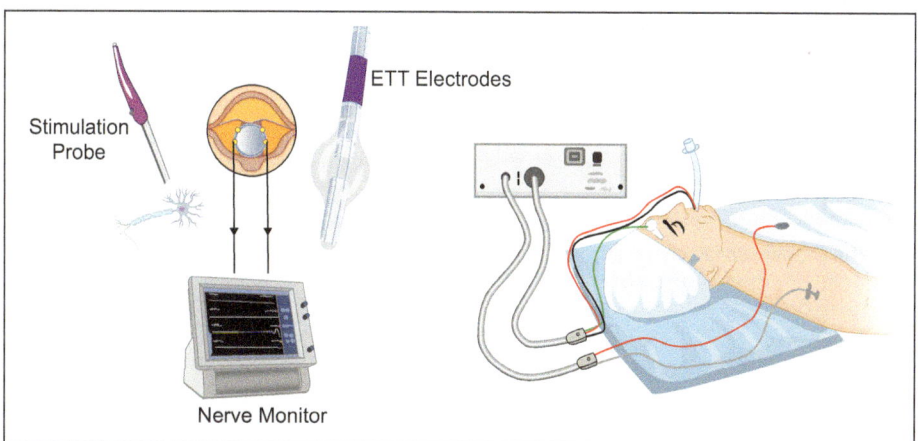

Figure 88.3: Positioning of a nerve integrity monitor (NIM) endotracheal tube.
ETT, endotracheal tube.

after surgery, although it can occur precipitously during surgery as well. If unable to differentiate between malignant hyperthermia and thyroid storm based on labs or symptoms, dantrolene should still be administered as it will treat the hypermetabolic states of either process. Treatment of thyroid storm includes antithyroid drugs, oral iodine, beta-adrenergic blocking agents, such as esmolol and propranolol, corticosteroids, and supportive treatment with IV fluids.[2]

Postoperative Hematoma
Postoperative hematoma is an emergent complication that typically requires reoperation in the presence of respiratory difficulties. Scissors or surgical clip removers should be kept at the bedside to emergently evacuate the hematoma if the patient is in extreme distress. The patient should be reintubated as early as possible as they will need to return to the operating room for control of the hemorrhage.

Tracheomalacia or Laryngeal Edema
Tracheomalacia may be present following goiter or tumor excision, and in rare instances may cause airway collapse and obstruction due to erosion of the tracheal rings. Laryngeal edema may be secondary to a traumatic intubation or prolonged surgery. Treatment with corticosteroids and humidified oxygen may be adequate, although immediate reintubation may be required.

RLN Damage
RLN damage may occur either unilaterally or bilaterally. RLN damage can be caused by ischemia or contusion from prolonged retraction, exposure to air, or accidental transection. With unilateral damage or partial cord paralysis, the patient may only complain of hoarseness or have difficulty with phonation, specifically the long "E" sound. Bilateral RLN damage often presents with more severe respiratory difficulty or stridor and may require reintubation.[2,3] Electrophysiological monitoring of the RLNs during surgery and careful dissection and identification of the RLNs have proven to be the most reliable way to avoid injury (Figure 88.4).[8]

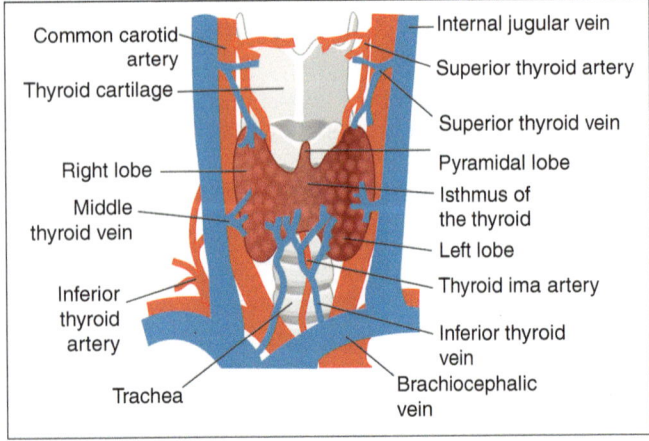

Figure 88.4: Relevant vessel and nerve anatomic locations.

Hypocalcemia
Temporary hypocalcemia is common following both thyroidectomy and parathyroidectomy but is rarely permanent. The incidence of postoperative hypocalcemia and hypoparathyroidism among children undergoing total thyroidectomy, however, is considerable. The inability to preserve the parathyroid glands during surgery seemingly plays a role, making it key to preserve the parathyroid glands if possible to ensure optimal outcomes.[10]

The presenting symptoms of hypocalcemia include perioral and fingertip tingling or twitching. Laryngeal stridor may also be present. If untreated, hypocalcemia can progress to tetany, seizures, or ventricular arrhythmias. Prolonged QT intervals may be noted on an ECG. Additional clinical signs include carpopedal spasm with cuff inflation (Trousseau's sign) or facial muscle spasm with tapping over the facial nerve at the parotid gland (Chvostek's sign).

Oral calcium may be given if the serum calcium is >2 mmol / L; if calcium levels drop below this, IV calcium gluconate or calcium chloride should be given immediately. A 4-hour PTH level <10 pg/mL has been shown to be a good predictor of symptomatic hypocalcemia and the need for supplemental calcium.[1-3,11]

POSTOPERATIVE CARE

Postoperatively, the patient should be recovered with the head of the bed up to avoid venous congestion and edema. The airway needs to be monitored carefully and reassessed before discharge, as the status can quickly change with the onset of complications, such as edema, hypocalcemia, or hematoma.

In most instances, the surgeon infiltrates the surgical area with local anesthetic and epinephrine, but a superficial cervical plexus block can be considered to reduce the need for opioids. However, postoperative pain in most pediatric patients is adequately controlled with acetaminophen and nonsteroidal anti-inflammatory drugs. Calcium levels will need to be monitored carefully postoperatively, with calcium supplementation administered as indicated.

KEY REFERENCES

Complete references for this chapter are online and available at https://connect.springerpub.com/content/book/978-0-8261-3875-0/part/part04/toc-part/ch088.

1. Holzman RS, Mancuso TJ, Polaner DM. *A Practical Approach to Pediatric Anesthesia.* 2nd ed. Lippincott Williams & Wilkins, Wolters Kluwer; 2015.
2. Coté C, Lerman J, Anderson B. *A Practice of Anesthesia for Infants and Children.* 6th ed. Elsevier; 2019:644–650.
3. Davis P, Cladis F. *Smith's Anesthesia for Infants and Children.* 9th ed. Elsevier; 2017:1109–1112.
7. Dream S, Rongzi W, Lovell K, et al. Outpatient thyroidectomy in the pediatric population. *Am J Surg.* 2020;219(6):890–893. doi:10.1016/j.amjsurg.2020.03.025

SECTION G Cardiovascular Procedures

CHAPTER 89

Cardiac Surgery: On-Pump

Jamie W. Sinton and Zhe Amy Fang

INDICATIONS/CONTRAINDICATIONS

Each year in the United States, about 40,000 children are born with congenital heart disease (CHD), with one quarter of them undergoing cardiac surgery during infancy.[1] Most will remain into adulthood and will have required a cardiac surgical procedure. The care of children undergoing cardiac surgery with cardiopulmonary bypass (CPB) has many similarities to that of adults; however, it is the salient features and differences that are discussed in this chapter.

Heart disease exists along a spectrum, though many heart diseases, regardless of severity, will be repaired in predetermined age windows. Timing of cardiac surgery on CPB is largely dependent on the type of lesion and medical optimization. Neonatal operations are offered to those with ductal-dependent lesions, such as critical aortic stenosis, hypoplastic left heart syndrome (HLHS), and other single-ventricle lesions, d-transposition of great arteries (d-TGA), truncus arteriosus, and obstructed totally anomalous pulmonary venous return (TAPVR). Operations are offered in infancy (depending on spectrum of disease) for those with atrioventricular (AV) or ventricular septal defects (VSDs) and tetralogy of Fallot (TOF).

SPECIAL CONSIDERATIONS AND CONCERNS

Children with CHD present unique anesthetic challenges to anesthesia providers, specifically increased incidence of difficult airway,[2] syndromic status and its implications, and anesthetic considerations of the cardiac lesion itself. There may be additional extracardiac abnormalities that must be addressed prior to congenital heart surgery (CHS), such as tracheoesophageal fistula or intestinal atresia. In addition to complex medical issues, ethical challenges become poignant in the context of offering extremely resource-intensive operations to infants with expected poor duration or quality of life.[3] Multidisciplinary discussion and input should be sought for patients with complex malformations, and extracorporeal membrane oxygenation (ECMO) candidacy should be discussed prior to intervention.

CYANOSIS

Many cardiac lesions involve mixing of oxygenated and deoxygenated blood resulting in cyanosis. Cyanosis may lead to increased blood viscosity and derangements in coagulation. Bleeding tendency is attributed to inappropriate platelet activation and fibrinogen dysfunction.[4] Complications of chronic cyanosis include hyperviscosity, stroke, and brain abscess. The body's physiological alterations in response to cyanosis are listed in **Box 89.1**.

SOCIETY OF THORACIC SURGEONS-EUROPEAN ASSOCIATION FOR CARDIO-THORACIC SURGERY MORTALITY RISK CATEGORY AND OUTCOMES

Estimating and managing mortality risk during CHS are most commonly classified using the Society of Thoracic Surgeons-European Association for Cardio-Thoracic Surgery (STAT) categories.[6,7] STAT scores are categorized into five categories, with category five having the highest mortality. The STAT score serves as a benchmark for comparing outcomes across institutions. Perioperative death is defined as death within 30 days of the congenital heart operation.

BOX 89.1 PHYSIOLOGICAL ADAPTATIONS TO CHRONIC CYANOSIS

Postnatal fetal hemoglobin production[4]
Lack of physiological anemia of infancy[5]
Right shift of the Hb–O_2 dissociation curve
Increased erythropoietin production

Hb, hemoglobin.

Source: From Rudolph A, Nasas A, Borges W. Hematologic adjustments to cyanotic congenital heart disease. *Pediatrics.* 1953;11(5):454–65; Zabala. Cyanotic congenital heart disease (CCHD): focus on hypoxemia, secondary erythrocytosis, and coagulation alterations. *Pediatr Anesth.* 2015;25(10):981–989. doi:10.1111/pan.12705.

ANESTHETIC MANAGEMENT

PREOPERATIVE EVALUATION

As with any patient presenting for anesthesia, performance of a careful history and physical examination is imperative in the care of children with CHD presenting for cardiac surgery. History should include birth history, previous interventions, medications, and exercise tolerance. Exercise tolerance is assessed based on weight gain and feeding in infants. If the infant is able to breastfeed or drink a bottle in under 20 minutes without cyanotic episodes, diaphoresis, or tachycardia (as noticed by the parent), then exercise tolerance is normal. Mothers of infants who are breastfeeding should be offered a clean space to express milk while the infant is in surgery as they will miss several feeds.

Physical examination begins with notation of vital signs and attention to baseline oxygen saturation. Particular attention should be paid to the infant's color, respiratory pattern, and cardiac auscultation. Auscultation of heart sounds for S3, S4, and (unexpected) murmurs offers clues to the presence of heart failure or decompensation. Laboratory and imaging studies should be reviewed and compared to the expected values for healthy children and those with similar lesions. The echocardiogram and cardiac catheterization laboratory data should be reviewed for systemic ventricular end-diastolic pressure (for determination of adequate coronary perfusion pressure) and hemodynamic significance of each cardiac lesion. In the presence of an active upper respiratory infection, anesthesia providers should exercise caution and postpone elective cardiac surgeries when possible.

Preoperative admission the evening prior to CHS is rare. However, in a shunt-dependent infant, dehydration may lead to life-threatening shunt thrombosis. In this scenario, preoperative admission ensuring IV hydration is prudent.

PREOPERATIVE PHARMACOLOGY

It is not unusual for children with CHD to require frequent visits to the hospital and repeated procedures. These children often develop fear of healthcare providers and have exaggerated separation anxiety. The anesthesia provider should develop a rapport with these patients and their parents, and sedative premedication should be strongly considered. Medications, such as oral midazolam, oral ketamine, and dexmedetomidine, are commonly employed preoperatively to safely temper anxiety in children with CHD.

ANESTHETIC TECHNIQUE

Intraoperative Management

Pediatric patients with CHD have a higher incidence of difficult airway.[2] Route of intubation should also be considered when planning for the case. Nasal intubation is associated with a lower incidence of inadvertent extubation when transesophageal echocardiography (TEE) is employed during pediatric cardiac surgery with CPB.[8]

Cardiac monitoring is most commonly achieved with a 5-lead ECG. Lead II should be monitored for detection of arrhythmias and ischemia, while lead V1 can be monitored for ischemia. As the epicardial courses of the coronary arteries are usually not known with certainty, ischemia should be monitored in all leads. Defibrillator pads are placed laterally on the chest of the children in case of redo sternotomies as unintended entry into the right ventricle may lead to catastrophic bleeding, ischemia, ventricular fibrillation, and others. Defibrillator pads should also be placed for primary sternotomy in a patient with reasonable likelihood of arrest on induction of anesthesia, such as the infant with Williams syndrome.

Use of TEE is routine for most on-pump cardiac surgeries as it confers cost-savings to the hospital by reducing reoperations.[9] The American Society of Echocardiography has published TEE guidelines for children and those with CHD.[10] During insertion of the TEE probe, ventilation should be monitored and adjusted as needed. Endotracheal tube cuff pressure is also affected with insertion of the TEE probe, albeit only transiently.[11] Contraindications are similar to those of adults. The cardiac contraindication or notable exception is children with TAPVR in which case TEE probe insertion may cause additional pulmonary vein obstruction making the procedure not tolerable. A history of tracheoesophageal fistula is also a contraindication to the use of TEE that is not frequently encountered in the adult population. VACTERL associations indicate an increased incidence of tracheoesophageal fistula in children with CHD.

Intraoperatively, near-infrared spectroscopy is often used to noninvasively detect oxygen content in the brain. In significantly cyanotic patients, this monitor may not function until hemodilution or CPB has been initiated.[12] For any infant surgery that involves aortic arch reconstruction, transcranial Doppler can be used to prevent excessive flow during antegrade cerebral perfusion.[13]

Standard temperature monitoring includes at least two locations: core (nasal) and peripheral (rectal). Temperature measurement at these sites (and often the foot or toe) facilitates maintenance of even cooling and rewarming following surgery. Temperature monitoring should continue into the postoperative period.

Considerations for Specific Cardiac Lesions

Septal Defects

Septal defects can be atrial, ventricular, or AV in nature. During the initial stages of life, left-to-right shunting across the defect is expected. The natural history of unrepaired septal defects, especially atrioventricular and ventricular septal defects, can result in overcirculation which can result in reversal of shunt flow, and right-to-left shunting (i.e., Eisenmenger syndrome). It should be noted that if Eisenmenger syndrome has developed, intracardiac repair may not be feasible.

ATRIAL SEPTAL DEFECTS There are several types of atrial septal defects (ASDs) including ostium secundum (most common), ostium primum, coronary sinus, and sinus venosus (either superior or inferior). The magnitude of shunt depends on the difference in compliance between the two ventricles, the location and size of the defect, and the blood viscosity (determined by hematocrit). The right ventricle typically has a higher compliance compared to the left ventricle (LV) in normal hearts, hence the direction of the shunt is normally left to right.

Repair of an ASD is indicated if right heart dilation is present on echocardiogram. Preschool age is a common time for repair of a secundum ASD. Patients undergoing isolated ASD repair may be minimally symptomatic; however, repair is still indicated in childhood period. ASD repairs may be catheter-based or open surgical repairs. These patients are generally at low risk of postoperative bleeding.

VENTRICULAR SEPTAL DEFECTS For ventricular and great vessel level shunts, the magnitude of shunting depends on pressure gradient between the chambers, the ratio of pulmonary to systemic vascular resistance (SVR), and the size of the defect. Qualitatively, VSD size is compared to the aortic valve annulus size of that patient. For VSDs that are larger in diameter than the aorta, no pressure gradient is expected and significant pulmonary overcirculation is present (Qp/Qs >> 1). Patients present with tachypnea and poor weight gain and are often on diuretic/anticongestive therapy. Because the pulmonary vasculature is exposed to both pressure and volume load, Eisenmenger syndrome will develop much earlier in patients with VSD compared with ASD.

Prebypass, the anesthesia provider should be careful not to exacerbate pulmonary overcirculation with high FiO_2 and hyperventilation. Following sternotomy, a piece of autologous pericardium is harvested and preserved. On CPB, a cross-clamp is applied and cardioplegia is administered to achieve diastolic and asystolic arrest. For a perimembranous VSD, surgical exposure is achieved via a right atriotomy with or without detachment of the septal leaflet of the tricuspid valve. The previously harvested pericardial patch is sewn in place very close to the AV node and other conduction tissue. Separation from bypass is often well tolerated as long as sinus rhythm is present. Myocardial edema may lead to temporary AV node dysfunction; therefore, epicardial pacing wires are often placed for maintenance of AV synchrony.

ATRIOVENTRICULAR SEPTAL DEFECTS An atrioventricular septal defect (AVSD) or atrioventricular canal (AVC) defect is an endocardial cushion defect. The AVC forms from endocardial cushion and the AV septum separates the tricuspid from the mitral valve. A partial AVSD includes an ostium primum defect, with a cleft mitral valve, with no ventricular level shunting. A transitional AVSD includes an ostium primum defect, a common AV orifice, and a restrictive VSD. In a complete AVSD, there is an ostium primum defect, an unrestrictive VSD, and a common AV valve. Left-to-right shunting in this defect is often torrential, and operative repair is undertaken in early infancy. As in the case of VSD, it is imperative that the anesthesia provider does not exacerbate pulmonary over circulation in the prebypass period with excessive FiO_2 and hyperventilation.

Repair of AVC lesions never results in completely normal AV valves.[14] Post-bypass, there may be some degree of left-sided AV valve regurgitation. Furthermore, due to the location of the patch, heart block may also occur as in VSDs, necessitating epicardial pacing wires. If a chromosomal anomaly is present, it is often trisomy 21 and anesthetic considerations for Down syndrome apply.

Tetralogy of Fallot

TOF is the most common cyanotic CHD (CCHD). The four lesions classically involved are pulmonic stenosis, a VSD, overriding aorta, and right ventricular (RV) hypertrophy. TOF may occur in an otherwise healthy baby, or it may occur with extracardiac malformations, such as VACTERL association, CHARGE association, Alagille syndrome, and 22q11 deletion syndrome. TOF is classified into three different types: the classic TOF with RV outflow tract obstruction, TOF with pulmonary atresia (PA) and major aortopulmonary collateral arteries (MAPCAs), and TOF with absent pulmonary valve (also called absent pulmonary valve syndrome). Depending on the pulmonary artery anatomy, TOF with PA/MAPCAs may be a prostaglandin (PGE)-dependent lesion requiring supplemental PGE administration to maintain ductal patency and promote pulmonary blood flow. TOF with absent pulmonary valve syndrome has a physiology that is different compared to the classic TOF in that the bidirectional flow across the RV outflow tract (RVOT) during fetal life massively dilates the pulmonary artery, which leads to surrounding airway malacia and respiratory distress at birth. Repair of absent pulmonary valve syndrome may be urgent or emergent.

The clinical course of newborns with TOF is related to the severity of their obstruction RVOT. During agitation, paroxysms of RV infundibular muscle spasm trigger increased RVOT obstruction and reduced Qp, leading to what is commonly known as a hypercyanotic or "tet" spell. Treatment aims to reduce infundibular muscle spasm and to promote pulmonary blood flow. Common interventions include oxygen administration, fluid volume loading, sedation, agents to increase afterload, and beta-blockade. Sedation and beta-blockade reduce inotropy and therefore infundibular muscle spasm. Volume and agents that increase afterload will increase SVR and increase the left-to-right shunt across the VSD to improve pulmonary blood flow.

Standard aortic and bicaval cannulation will usually suffice. The type of repair needed depends on the anatomy of the pulmonary artery. A transatrial transpulmonary approach is common and involves a right atriotomy, with RVOT muscle resection performed as needed and VSD closure. At this point, the cross-clamp may be released. The transannular patch of the main pulmonary artery may be performed either with the heart stopped or beating, depending on surgeon preference. If the native pulmonary artery is inadequate, an RV-to-PA conduit may be placed instead of a transannular patch.

On release of the aortic cross-clamp, the ECG should return promptly to sinus rhythm with a right bundle branch block expected. Heart block may occur due to edema of the conduction system. Junctional ectopic tachycardia (JET) is a rhythm traditionally associated with postoperative TOF repairs. JET is a rhythm that is junctional in nature with high ventricular rates, often ranging from 140 to 160 beats/min and is catecholamine-sensitive. JET worsens cardiac output as the RV, whose diastolic function is already poor, now has minimal filling time during diastole. Treatment is aimed at reducing catecholamines, with interventions often including discontinuation of epinephrine infusions, cooling, sedation, and neuromuscular blockade (Figure 89.1). Overdrive pacing also has utility in maintaining ventricular synchrony, which is useful in the setting of diastolic dysfunction.

Despite surgical palliation, TOF is a lifelong disease. Some residual RVOT obstruction may be present with the intention of limiting the size of the transannular patch and ultimately the amount of pulmonary insufficiency. If a transannular patch is placed, pulmonary regurgitation is common due to pulmonary insufficiency and/or RV dilation. Additionally, RV-to-PA conduits become stenotic and regurgitant over time. Indications for pulmonary valve replacement (PVR) include signs or symptoms of heart failure, syncope related to arrhythmia, sustained tachyarrhythmias in the presence of RV volume load, and exercise intolerance not explained by extracardiac causes. Cardiac MRI is often used to evaluate RV end-diastolic volume as an indication for PVR.

d-Transposition of Great Arteries

d-TGA is a cyanotic heart disease that may be diagnosed pre- or postnatally. In TGA, the pulmonary artery is connected to the LV and the aorta is connected to the right ventricle. TGA is occasionally associated with a VSD. The coronary anatomy varies widely among patients with TGA. Those with intramural coronaries are at higher surgical risk of ischemia postoperatively. Oxygenated blood returning from the pulmonary veins enters the left atrium and LV but is pumped to the pulmonary artery for further oxygenation. Meanwhile, systemic venous return does not pass through the lungs for oxygenation; therefore, newborns with TGA exhibit reverse differential cyanosis. They can be quite sick, and a source of mixing of oxygenated and deoxygenated blood is essential for survival. The best site for mixing is at the atrial level as the pressure gradient between the two atria is low, whereas mixing at the level of the ventricular septum (VSD) is less efficacious. Shortly after birth, many newborns with TGA undergo balloon atrial septostomy if the ASD is restrictive.

In the neonatal period, patients with TGA undergo definitive repair with the arterial switch operation (ASO, also called the Jatene operation). Cannulation for bypass includes a more distal aortic cannula in order to accommodate the aortic cross-clamp distal to the future aortic anastomosis. Surgery includes great vessel suture lines and coronary reimplantation. A left atrial (LA) line may be placed to monitor the pressure in the left side of the heart. LA distension should be avoided with careful fluid administration. LA distension may indicate the LV overload, which can be an early sign of LV dysfunction. Also, LA distension may lead to PA distension, which may lead to coronary ischemia. Anesthesia providers should attempt to maintain LA pressures in the single digits (e.g., <4 mm Hg). LA distension may be corrected by aspirating blood from the central line. Due to the presence of high-pressure suture lines, bleeding may be a risk in the post-bypass period. In the long term, these children do well.[15]

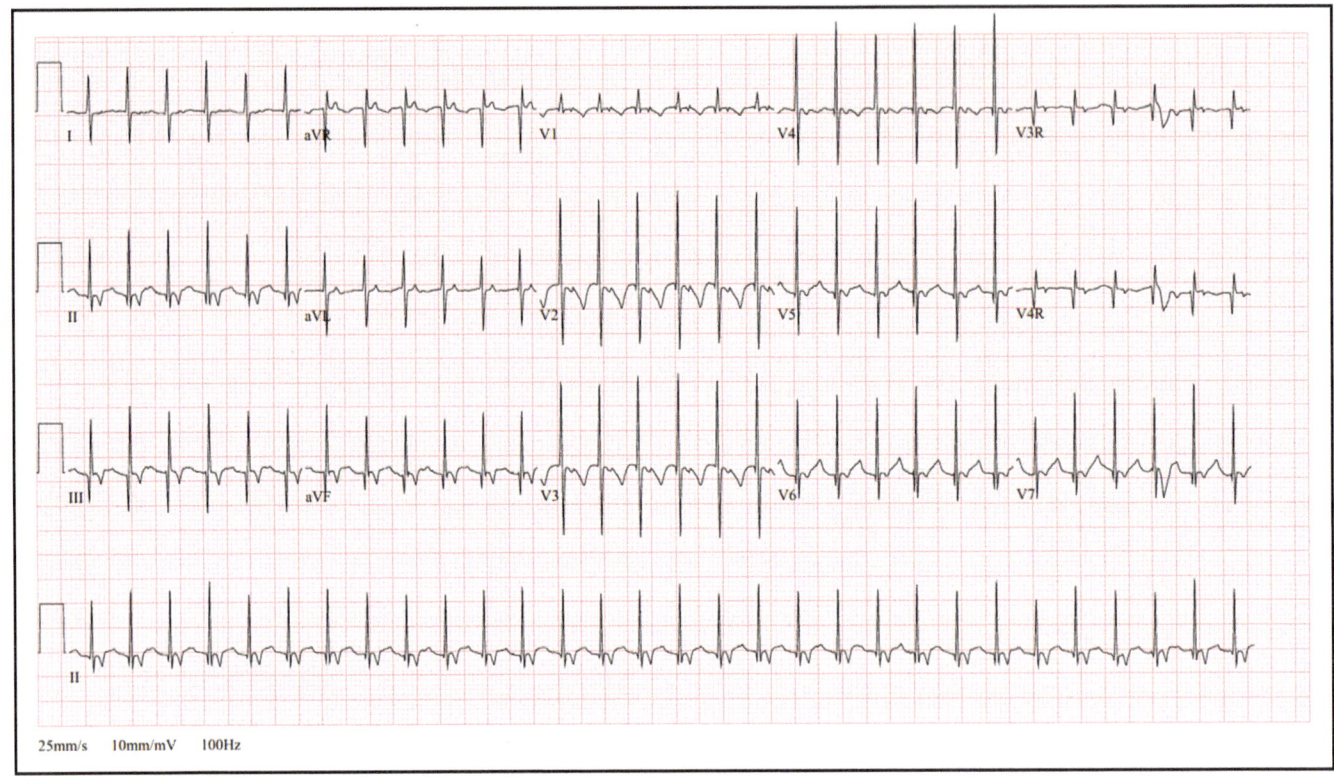

Figure 89.1: ECG of an infant in junctional ectopic tachycardia (JET) following complete repair of tetralogy of Fallot.

Truncus Arteriosus

Truncus arteriosus is a cyanotic cardiac lesion with a single great vessel arising from both ventricles, along with an obligate VSD. As blood is ejected from both ventricles, desaturated and oxygenated blood mix at the level of the single great vessel supply both the aorta and pulmonary arteries in parallel. The truncal valve is abnormal and valve repair is often required. Repair of truncus arteriosus is undertaken in the neonatal period due to the risk of early pulmonary hypertension given that the pulmonary vasculature is exposed to both volume and pressure overload. The natural history of unrepaired truncus arteriosus is one of pulmonary hypertension and pulmonary vascular occlusive diseases leading to mortality in infancy. Additionally, in the first few weeks of life, pulmonary artery pressure falls creating coronary steal and myocardial ischemia. Truncus arteriosus is associated with velocardiofacial syndrome and DiGeorge syndrome. It is classified by the relationship of the pulmonary arteries in relation to the truncus.

In the prebypass period, the anesthesia provider must take care not to exacerbate pulmonary overcirculation. In certain circumstances, the surgeon may place a temporary pulmonary artery band to help alleviate pulmonary overcirculation and improve coronary perfusion. Separation from CPB may be complicated by high RV pressures (if PVR had risen preoperatively) and truncal valve insufficiency. In this case, an ASD may be created to maintain cardiac output (at the expense of saturation). Long-term, truncal valve insufficiency is the predominant concern. Due to the manipulation in the area of the AV node, transient or permanent heart block may also occur.

Single-Ventricle Palliation

There are many anatomic variations of single-ventricle physiology, including HLHS, tricuspid atresia, double inlet LV, unbalanced AVC, pulmonary atresia with intact VSD with RV-dependent coronary arteries and others. Single-ventricle physiology is a condition in which the pulmonary and systemic circulations mix and are supplied in parallel. With parallel circulation, increases in blood flow to one circulatory system produce reductions in flow to the other.

HLHS PALLIATION STAGE 1 HLHS is the prototypical single-ventricle CHD. There is typically mitral stenosis or atresia in combination with aortic stenosis or atresia, and a hypoplastic LV. In the neonatal period prior to repair, systemic venous blood enters the right atrium, and pulmonary venous return enters the left atrium. There is mixing of both systemic and pulmonary venous blood at the atrial level across the ASD. Blood flow is obstructed at the mitral (and aortic) valve so it crosses the ASD and ejects into the PA, where it may cross the patent ductus arteriosus (PDA) to perfuse the body or reenter the lungs. Coronary perfusion is retrograde from the PDA. An ASD and a PDA are required for survival and are maintained by balloon atrial septostomy if needed and PGE, respectively. Within the first few weeks or so of life, patients undergo stage 1 palliation with a Norwood or Hybrid operation. The purpose of stage 1 palliation is to construct an unobstructed aortic arch and provide a stable source of pulmonary blood flow.

The Norwood operation refers to the aortic arch reconstruction while the source of pulmonary blood flow is variable.[16] Either a Blalock-Taussig shunt (BTS), Sano, or Braun shunt may be used. A 3.5-mm BTS diverts blood from the (usually right) subclavian artery to the pulmonary artery. A Sano shunt directs blood from the single ventricle directly to the pulmonary artery. The Norwood operation is performed with CPB under regional low-flow perfusion (also called antegrade cerebral perfusion) and/or with deep hypothermic circulatory arrest. The choice between a BTS versus a Sano shunt was addressed in the Single Ventricle Reconstruction Trial.[17] Within the first year, Sano shunts had improved transplant-free survival but required more interventions.

HLHS Palliation Stage 2 Around age 3 to 6 months, infants undergo superior cavopulmonary anastomosis (Glenn) in which the superior vena cava (SVC) is anastomosed to the pulmonary artery (PA). The purpose of this stage is to (partially) volume unload the single ventricle. Six-month old infants receive approximately 50% of their venous return from their upper body and 50% from their lower body. As children grow, an increasing portion of venous return is from the lower body. Consequently, the resting oxygen saturation of a patient with Glenn physiology does fall over time as more desaturated blood is ejected into the systemic circulation.

The anesthesia provider should thoughtfully place and interpret monitors; for example, avoid placing an arterial line on the side of a modified BTS or on the side of an aberrant subclavian artery if a TEE is to be used. For those with HLHS, volume expansion with packed red blood cells (pRBCs) and fresh frozen plasma (FFP) is reasonable to ensure adequate hemoglobin and response to heparin. Ventilation with room air also maintains PVR and prevents overcirculation; however, the Sano or the BTS is usually restrictive and pulmonary overcirculation is not as problematic as in the neonatal period. In addition to standard and invasive monitors, give volume slowly and observe for cardiac enlargement on the surgical field. Post-bypass, ventilation favors mild hypercarbia as it increases pulmonary blood and improved oxygenation.[18] When troubleshooting desaturation, consider inadequate pulmonary blood flow due to increased PVR, venous drainage obstruction, collateral vessels, and cerebral vasoconstriction. Treatment should be instituted according to etiology. Clinically significant bleeding may be related to hemostatic defects associated with cyanosis or surgical bleeding.

Of the three stages of single-ventricle palliation, the Glenn stage is considered the most hemodynamically stable. In cases of increased PVR and decreased pulmonary blood flow, systemic preload is maintained because of inferior vena cava (IVC) blood return. For single-ventricle patients who require nonurgent noncardiac surgery, such as G-tubes, the Glenn stage is the favored time to complete such operations.

HLHS Palliation Stage 3 Children with Glenn physiology who present for Fontan completion are typically around 3 years of age. The Fontan operation, usually the final stage in palliation for single-ventricle heart disease, occurs after the child learns to ambulate. The ability to ambulate is key, with contraction of calf muscles necessary to propel blood through an extracardiac conduit and directly to the lungs as there is no subpulmonary pumping chamber. Liver disease is characterized by centrilobular fibrosis. Hepatic injury may occur even before the Fontan operation.[19]

In the modern Fontan operation, total cavopulmonary anastomosis is accomplished with an extracardiac conduit, where the IVC is anastomosed to a tube that connects it to the PA. Cyanosis is relieved, ventricular volume overload decreases, and pulmonary blood flow is passive. The surgeon may create a fenestration in the Fontan pathway, creating it right to left to maintain systemic preload in cases of increased PVR in the perioperative period. Separation from bypass requires generous volume administration. However, excessive volume administration leads to lymphatic failure and chylothorax and pleural effusions. Oxygen saturation may be normal or slightly cyanotic if there is shunting across the fenestration, and the function of the single ventricle is often mildly depressed. Preload and cardiac output depend on low PVR and adequate intravascular volume. The transpulmonary gradient (TPG) drives blood to the lungs. TPG is the difference between the mean (PA) pressure and the mean LA pressure or mean pulmonary capillary wedge pressure. Optimal hemodynamics incorporate sinus rhythm, low PVR, spontaneous ventilation, zero aortic arch obstruction, and minimal AV valve regurgitation. Postoperatively, spontaneous ventilation pulls blood into the thorax and enhances pulmonary blood flow and therefore preload. It is therefore desirable for extubation in the operating room.

Total Anomalous Pulmonary Venous Return Obstruction in the vertical vein may occur and this group of patients often presents in extremis with pulmonary edema and poor systemic perfusion as evidenced by elevated lactate. Obstructed TAPVR is a true neonatal emergency (**Box 89.2**).

Prebypass management is dictated by physiology. Those with obstruction will be very sick, and the goal is to go on to CPB while minimizing oxygen consumption. Nitric oxide is often indicated for separation from CPB for TAPVR repair as pulmonary vasculature is abnormal, and these patients are prone to pulmonary hypertension. Furthermore, the left-sided structures are often small in TAPVR, and volume overload of the LV is best avoided. Post-bypass bleeding is likely for types 1 and 3 TAPVR as very low temperatures are needed to facilitate surgical repair. Given the location of the suture lines, it may be difficult to control the bleeding. Exposure may require significant manipulations of the heart

---

BOX 89.2 TAPVR CLASSIFICATION

- TAPVR occurs where the pulmonary venous return connects to a place other than the left atrium.
- Classified into four different types based on the location of the pulmonary venous drainage
  - **Supracardiac TAPVR (Type 1):** The pulmonary veins drain highly oxygenated blood into a vertical vein that connects the pulmonary vein confluence with the innominate vein or the SVC, above the heart.
  - **Cardiac TAPVR (Type 2):** Systemic venous blood flows from pulmonary veins to the coronary sinus. Less frequently obstructed. It may be repaired via right atriotomy, unroofing of the coronary sinus and baffling such that pulmonary venous blood is directed to the left atrium.
  - **Infracardiac TAPVR Veins (Type 3):** The pulmonary veins may drain oxygenated blood into any vein below the diaphragm, such as the portal vein, IVC, or hepatic vein. More commonly obstructed due to the longer course the vertical vein traverses.
  - **Mixed TAPVR (Type 4):** a combination of any of types 1 through 3

IVC, inferior vena cava; SVC, superior vena cava; TAPVR, totally anomalous pulmonary venous return.

to get to the sutures, which invariably decreases preload and causes hemodynamic instability. Direct measurement of LA pressure via a surgically placed LA line aids in transfusion clotting factors without overwhelming the small left-sided structures. Outcomes are suboptimal in the first year of life, however, children who survive beyond 1 year of age have excellent long-term survival.[20] Long term, the veins must be monitored for development of stenosis and need for reintervention.

OTHER DEFECTS There are a multitude of other congenital heart defects, such as aortopulmonary window, double outlet right ventricle, congenitally corrected transposition, interrupted aortic arch, anomalous origin of the left coronary artery from the pulmonary artery (ALCAPA), and Ebstein's anomaly. The details of these lesions are beyond the scope of this book.

CARDIOPULMONARY BYPASS

Coagulation

Fibrinolysis

CPB induces fibrinolysis, and antifibrinolytic agents have been used to reduce transfusion in cardiac surgery. Tranexamic acid and e-aminocaproic acid are two commonly used antifibrinolytic agents. There is evidence for the use of both agents in congenital cardiac surgery and the choice is often institution-dependent.[21-23] One concern with the use of high-dose tranexamic acid is that while it may reduce blood loss after cardiac surgery, it has been associated with seizures.[24]

Prebypass

Sternotomy, especially during reoperation, may lead to significant bleeding; therefore, allogeneic packed red blood cells and plasma (thawed or fresh frozen) should be in the operating room and checked prior to incision. During prebypass dissection, care must be taken to maintain hemodynamic stability and react in the face of trespass and retraction of the heart and great vessels. PGE must be continued until initiation of CPB. Acid–base status and hemoglobin should be continually optimized with care to avoid excessive crystalloid administration and hemodilution prebypass.

Anticoagulation

Adequate anticoagulation must be achieved prior to CPB. Heparin is the most commonly used anticoagulants for CPB in children with CHD. Heparin dosing is often higher (400 units/kg) in infants than children, adolescents, and adults (350 units/kg). Neonates often have physiologically low levels of antithrombin, which may lead to apparent heparin resistance. Administering plasma and additional heparin aids in achieving adequate activated clotting time (ACT). If the ACT remains inadequate, then antithrombin concentrates should be considered. Bivalirudin may be used for those with contraindications to heparin, such as those with heparin-induced thrombocytopenia (antibodies form against the heparin-platelet factor 4 complex) or other heparin contraindications. Bivalirudin is not approved for use in children; however, it has been used for CPB and in the cardiac catheterization lab.[25]

Cannulation

As in adults undergoing CPB, arterial cannulation precedes venous cannulation. Purse string sutures are placed around candidate cannulation vessel sites. At this time, heparin administration is often discussed with the surgeon. The placement of the cannulae are often in the ascending aorta and SVC and IVC, respectively. Particular anatomic considerations for cannulation are unique to each type of lesion.

Circuits and Prime Volume

CPB circuit and prime volume are institution-dependent. Figure 89.2 shows a CPB circuit with adult and pediatric considerations. Preoperative discussion with the perfusionist can be useful not only in determining cannula size and anticipated fluid dynamics but also for understanding the prime volume, electrolytes, and hematocrit needed to optimize oxygen delivery during CPB. Gerrah et al. provide an interesting resource on this topic.[26]

A variety of strategies have been used to prime the CPB pump and this varies according to institution. For larger patients, patient blood volume-to-pump prime volume ratio may allow for clear prime. For neonates and infants, this strategy often leads to unacceptable hemodilution. Some institutions prime the CPB circuit with fresh whole blood, but this is not available in most places. Many programs prime the CPB circuit with reconstituted whole blood using pRBCs and FFP at varying ratios. For toddlers and children, the decision to add pRBC depends on the pump prime volume needed to prime the circuit, the desired bypass hematocrit, the patient's blood volume and the patient's hematocrit, and the hematocrit of the pump prime.

Initiation of CPB

Adequate ACT must be achieved prior to CPB initiation. The definition of an adequate ACT varies by institution but is generally 400 to 480 seconds. Should the anticipated physiological changes associated with the initiation of CPB not occur, troubleshooting should begin immediately. Adequacy of oxygenation and perfusion should be routinely checked. A venous blood gas with a partial pressure of oxygen (PO_2) greater than 40 indicates adequate oxygenation. An arterial lactate less than 1 mEq/dL indicates adequate perfusion and removal of metabolic waste. Physical examination of the patient should reveal a flat fontanelle and absence of plethora or facial edema. Once on full-flow CPB, ventilation is accomplished by the CPB pump and mechanical ventilation of the lungs ceases in order to provide the surgeon an akinetic surgical field.

Flow While on CPB

Upon initiation of CPB, the heart should empty and non-pulsatile flow should commence. The arterial line tracing will flatten to read only mean arterial pressure (MAP). Optimal flow on CPB balances the need for visceral perfusion with the risk of excess blood in the surgical field. Maintenance of MAP on CPB provides optimal brain perfusion. Cerebral autoregulation is impaired in a time-varying manner in infants with CHD.[27,28] Further, the MAP that represents the lower limit of autoregulation during CPB should guide execution of optimal MAP for that period.

Physiological Impact of CPB

CPB in children often necessitates more physiological trespass than needed for adult patients witness for several reasons, such as children having a smaller blood volume in relation to the CPB circuit, and an aortic arch repair is often conducted requiring exposure to a greater degree of hypothermia and antegrade cerebral perfusion if not circulatory arrest (Box 89.4).

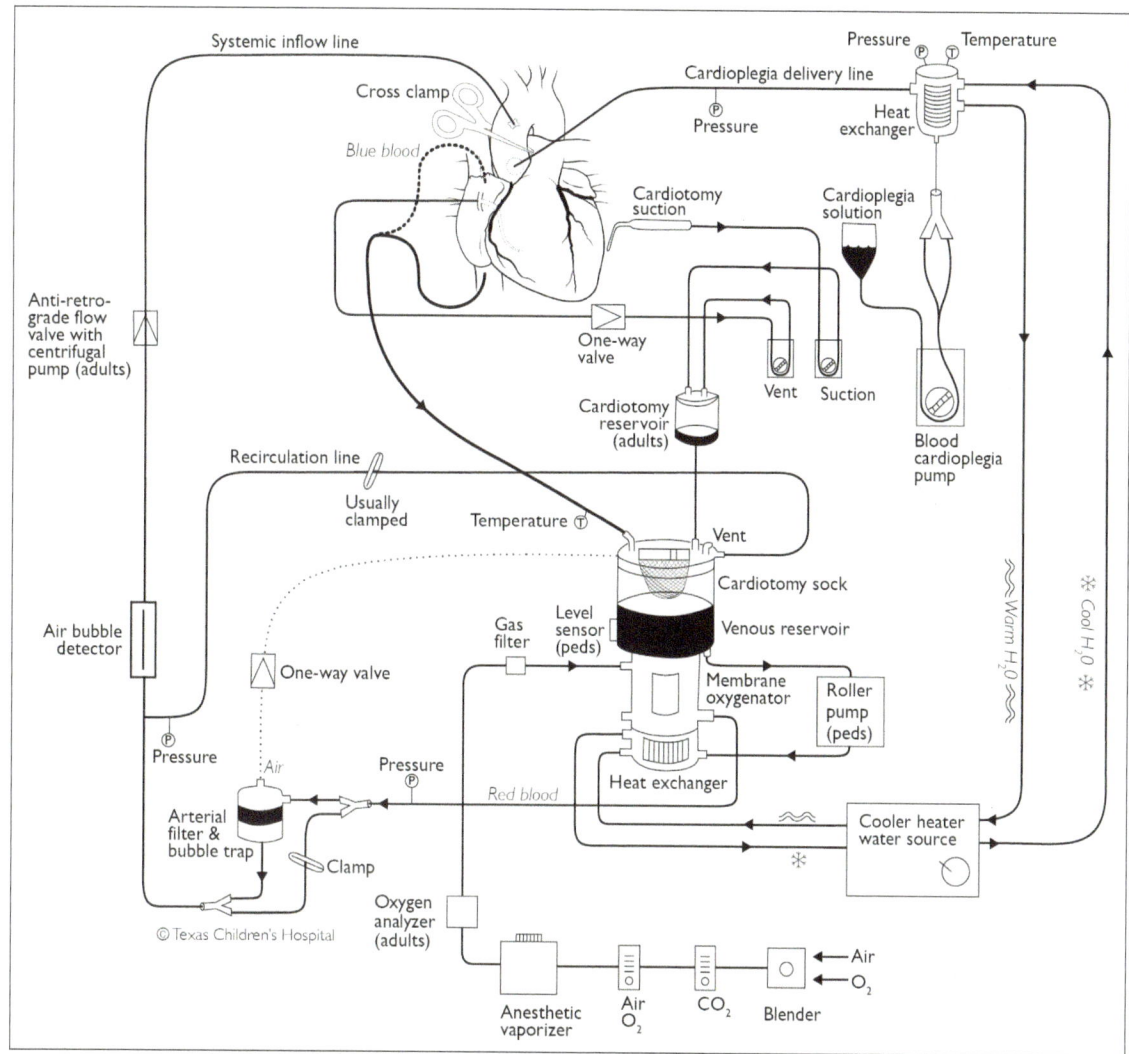

Figure 89.2: The cardiopulmonary bypass circuit with designation for components available in pediatric and adult circuits. Dotted lines represent tubes through which air is evacuated from the system.

Source: From Texas Children's Hospital.

Hypothermia

Hypothermia is often employed to facilitate lower flows and decrease oxygen consumption (organ protection). Hypothermia is classified as mild (30 °F–36 °F), moderate (22 °F–30 °F) or deep (16 °F–22 °F). Lower CPB temperatures predispose the patient to cerebral vasoconstriction that limits cerebral blood flow. This can be overcome with the addition of carbon dioxide to the CPB circuit. Notably, neonates and infants have a remarkable ability to maintain sinus rhythm at low temperatures and heart rates in contrast to their adult peers who may fibrillate during mild or moderate hypothermia.

Acid–Base Management

Changes in temperature affect the dissociation of water (into hydrogen and hydroxyl ions) and the solubility of carbon dioxide (CO_2). Lower temperatures increase the solubility of CO_2 while total CO_2 content is unchanged. Acid–base management at cooler temperatures is important for cerebral protection and therefore neurological outcome following surgery with CPB.

Pediatric patients are managed with pH-stat acid–base management,[29] meaning that the patient's pH is kept constant regardless of temperature. In this way, carbon dioxide levels are high (or even added to the circuit) to maintain cerebral vasodilation (and therefore even cooling), luxury perfusion, and even cooling during cold temperatures. Ratios of intra- and extracellular proton and hydroxide ions are altered. Addition of carbon dioxide also reduces the left shift of the hemoglobin–oxygen dissociation curve during cooling so that more oxygen is available to the tissues. It is associated with less metabolic acidosis after surgery and a trend toward improved neurological outcomes.[30]

In contrast, the idea behind alpha-stat management is to maintain stable intra- and extracellular ion gradients (electrochemical neutrality) as well as enzyme function with a constant ratio of hydroxyl to hydrogen ions. The "alpha" refers to the ratio of unprotonated to protons on the imidazole ring of histidine. The appealing advantage is to maintain cerebral autoregulation with mild or moderate hypothermia, reduce cerebral blood flow, and therefore reduce cerebral edema and formation of microemboli to the brain. In adult cardiac surgery, the use of alpha-stat management shows better neurological outcomes, but in pediatrics, pH-stat management may confer superior outcomes.[31,32]

Hemodilution and Blood Conservation

The optimal hemoglobin concentration for children following CPB is unknown, though the use of a conservative transfusion strategy appears to be safe.[33] Based on previous research, neurodevelopmental outcomes are improved with a hematocrit up to 23.5%, after which there is a plateau effect.[34–36] Blood conservation beyond scavenging from the surgical field is of great importance in terms of reducing transfusions and its inherent risks. Facilitating this aim in small patients means miniaturizing circuit tubing, and therefore, the prime volume utilized,[37] among other strategies (Box 89.3).[38]

Oxygen and Hyperoxia

On initiation of CPB, extreme hyperoxia is possible and is advocated by some in order to afford a degree of protection should there be a catastrophic bypass-related event. However, a cyanotic infant, whose PO_2 is below 40 mm Hg preoperatively, could instantaneously become 500 mm Hg. The balance of the safety margin of additional oxygen and the dangers of hyperoxia are presently controversial.[39] It has been offered that there is less myocardial damage when oxygen levels are controlled on initiation of CPB.[40] Additionally, myocardial reoxygenation injury may occur with hyperoxic CPB in cyanotic children.[41]

Stress and Inflammation

CPB induces a significant stress response in children undergoing CHS. This stress response is likely injurious hence a variety of strategies have been offered to try and mitigate the deleterious impact including administration of high-dose steroids and the use of ultrafiltration. One of the difficulties with studying stress and inflammatory response is that while trials may show a decrease in inflammatory mediators, they do not always correlate with clinical outcomes. Steroids in adult cardiac surgery have not been shown to improve mortality and may potentially increase morbidity.[42,43] In children, the evidence on whether steroids improve outcomes in neonates and infants is limited due to small sizes. To better define best practice, the STRESS trial (STeroids to REduce Systemic Inflammation After Infant Heart Surgery), a multicenter steroid study, is under way. Ultrafiltration strategy is institution-dependent, with continuous (CUF) or modified (MUF) often employed. Ultrafiltration during CPB removes excess volume and inflammatory mediators while aiding in hemoconcentration.[44] Most institutions utilize some form of ultrafiltration or MUF.

Renal Function and Metabolism

Acute kidney injury following bypass may be secondary to inflammatory mechanisms as the body reacts via an immune response to the CPB circuit. It can be predicted in children at least 2 years of age by interleukin-8 and tumor necrosis factor-alpha levels. In this group, higher postoperative levels are associated with longer periods of postoperative mechanical ventilation and overall hospital stay.[45] Even years after cardiac surgery, chronic kidney disease and hypertension are common. Renal tissue oxygenation monitoring via near-infrared spectroscopy may prove to be a viable mechanism for monitoring and protecting renal function.[46]

Weaning From CPB

Expected physiological change following anatomic repair should be used to guide pharmacological support on weaning from CPB. Neonates and young infants have a poorly developed sarcoplasmic reticulum and subsequently are inefficient at managing calcium. As such, calcium should be replaced prior to separation from CPB. Furthermore, the patient's lungs should be suctioned and ventilated, the heart de-aired, and hemoglobin, electrolytes, acid–base balance, temperature, and rhythm optimized.

Temporary epicardial pacing leads are often placed on the right atrium and ventricle during rewarming, though this is dependent on the specific surgery performed. Once placed, the leads are passed by the surgeon over the drapes and connected to a temporary pacemaker. Postsurgical edema of the conduction system may lead to transient heart block and necessitate pacing to maintain cardiac output. Anesthesia providers should remain cognizant that post-bypass the myocardium is in a state of recent ischemia, especially in operations necessitating a cross-clamp. In infants, an ischemic myocardium is poorly compliant with diastolic dysfunction commonly present. As cardiac output depends largely on heart rate, temporary pacing may optimize heart rate perioperatively.

Complications/Emergencies

Inability to wean from CPB on the first attempt is associated with poorer outcomes.[47] If weaning attempts are unsuccessful, transition to mechanical support, either ECMO or a temporary ventricular support device, should be considered.

Despite anticoagulation, CPB leads to thrombin generation and consumption of coagulation factors. In addition, blood contact with the circuit leads to platelet activation and dysfunction. Platelets and fibrinogen concentrate or cryoprecipitate are frequently required for neonates undergoing CHS. There is significant interest in using evidence to guide transfusion management post bypass. Point-of-care viscoelastic testing has shown some evidence in guiding post-bypass transfusion in the pediatric cardiac population, but currently no high-grade evidence exists for its use.[48]

POSTOPERATIVE CARE

The need for postoperative mechanical ventilation depends largely on the specific surgery performed. In 2016, a collaborative learning initiative was undertaken to increase rates of early extubation (defined as extubation on the operating room table or within 6 hours of arrival in the intensive care unit [ICU]). This quality improvement project did result in significantly increased rates of early extubation for the patient populations studied: isolated coarctation repairs and TOF repairs. However, length of ICU stay was unaffected. Following surgery, the patient is transferred to the ICU for continued hemodynamic status monitoring, respiratory support, and pain management. If the anesthesia team extubates the patient in the operating room, pain control can be facilitated by initiating patient-controlled analgesia prior to arrival in the ICU. If the patient remains intubated postoperatively, in most instances they are able to be extubated within the first 24 hours postoperatively.

Traditional IV opioid analgesia has prevailed for decades as the primary approach to providing postoperative sternotomy analgesia with few challenges, although there have been intermittent attempts to incorporate regional anesthesia. Opioid

---

BOX 89.3 EQUATION TO CALCULATE PRBCS NEEDED TO PRIME CPB PUMP

Blood prime required (mL) = [(PBV + circuit vol)(desired CPB Hct) − PBV*Pt Hct]/Hct of blood prime

CPB, cardiopulmonary bypass; Hct, hematocrit; PBV, patient blood volume; pRBCs, packed red blood cells; Pt, patient; vol, volume.

> **BOX 89.4 EXPECTED PHYSIOLOGICAL CHANGES WITH INITIATION OF CPB**
>
> Relief of cyanosis (if present preoperatively)
> Significant decrease in end-tidal carbon dioxide
> Loss of arterial line pulsatility
> Increase in NIRS
> Central venous pressure near zero
>
> CPB, cardiopulmonary bypass; NIRS, near-infrared spectroscopy.

administration not only offers analgesic benefits but is also associated with reductions in systemic inflammation, provides hemodynamic stability, and may prevent tachycardia at high doses. The use of regional anesthesia to temper sternotomy-related pain has historically been with caudal analgesia (non-site specific) or thoracic epidural analgesia. While use of these techniques is theoretically safe, concerns related to the potential for, and management of, a spinal cord hematoma following full anticoagulation for CPB have largely precluded the use of regional anesthesia with this population. The American Society of Regional Anesthesia has guidelines on systemic heparinization and CPB that should be followed if caudal or epidural anesthesia is planned. Novel approaches, such as the erector spinae block, have been recently reported to provide reliable, effective postoperative analgesic following pediatric cardiac surgeries utilizing a midline sternotomy.[49]

Complications

Common complications encountered in the perioperative period after TOF repair include rhythm disturbances, RV dysfunction, and bleeding. JET and heart block are the common rhythm disturbances. JET can be confirmed with an atrial wire study in the ICU. Treatment of JET includes sedation, cooling, overdrive atrial pacing, and amiodarone.

The RV hypertrophy leads to diastolic dysfunction and potential difficulty with cardioprotection during cross-clamp resulting in systolic dysfunction. Separation from CPB frequently requires some inotropic support. Care should be taken to avoid tachycardia and increases in PVR. The transannular patch causes pulmonary insufficiency further placing a strain on a stiff RV.

In the long term, pulmonary insufficiency leads to RV dilation and patients present for either catheter-based pulmonary valve replacement or open pulmonary valve replacement. Eventually, the aortic root dilates in older patients with a history of TOF repair, and these patients may present in adulthood for aortic root replacement.[50]

CASE STUDY: Repair of Tetralogy of Fallot

CLINICAL SCENARIO

A 4-month-old male presents for TOF repair. The child was diagnosed with TOF at birth following auscultation of a cardiac murmur. The anatomy on echocardiography was noted to be TOF with valvar pulmonary stenosis. The child was sent home after 1 week of observation in the NICU. He has been growing and gaining weight well, though he has experienced occasional hypercyanotic spells. Accordingly, preventive therapy with propranolol was initiated.

SPECIAL CONSIDERATIONS

This is an infant with an unrepaired TOF that has hypercyanotic spells on propranolol. NPO time should be limited as hypovolemia can exacerbate tet spells particularly on induction of anesthesia. Emergency medications should be immediately available to treat tet spells and propranolol should be continued the morning of the operation.

APPROACHES TO CARE

After applying standard monitors, the infant is given a mask induction with sevoflurane. Induction of anesthesia may lead to cyanotic spells due to the increased sympathetic stimulation; thus, it may be prudent to have a second anesthesia provider available to help with IV access as this may be difficult in infants of this age.

During induction, the patient begins to turn blue and oxygen saturation drops to 75%. IV access is immediately obtained, and the patient is treated with an IV fluid bolus, 100% oxygen, and phenylephrine. The saturation improves with the previously mentioned maneuvers. The patient is then given fentanyl and rocuronium to facilitate nasal endotracheal intubation. Next, radial artery and central vein cannulation are performed.

Incision and dissection are uneventful. After successful aortic and venous cannulation, CPB is initiated. The VSD is closed then a transannular patch repair of the RV outflow tract is performed. With the release of the aortic cross-clamp, the rhythm is noted to be sinus. Pacing wires are placed and the patient successfully separates from CPB with milrinone and low-dose epinephrine infusions. Post-CPB TEE showed no residual VSD, normal biventricular systolic dysfunction, and no residual RVOT obstruction.

While hemostasis was being achieved, the patient's heart rate increases to 155 beats per minute, with A–V dissociation. JET is suspected. Dexmedetomidine bolus is followed by an infusion, the epinephrine infusion is terminated and the forced air warmer was turned to ambient to cool the patient to 35.5 °C. The patient remains intubated for transport to the ICU. On arrival to the ICU, an atrial wire study is completed, and the diagnosis of JET is confirmed.

KEY REFERENCES

Complete references for this chapter are online and available at https://connect.springerpub.com/content/book/978-0-8261-3875-0/part/part04/toc-part/ch089.

3. Wingate JR, Adachi I, Fenton K, et al. Case 14--2014: Tetralogy of Fallot with severe cyanosis in an infant with trisomy 18: ethical dilemmas in the perioperative period. *J Cardiothorac Vasc Anesth*. 2014;28(6):1677–1685. doi:10.1053/j.jvca.2014.04.004
10. Puchalski MD, Lui GK, Miller-Hance WC, et al. Guidelines for performing a comprehensive transesophageal echocardiographic: examination in children and all patients with congenital heart disease: recommendations from the american society of echocardiography. *J Am Soc Echocardiogr*. 2019;32(2):173–215. doi:10.1016/j.echo.2018.08.016
15. Lee J, Abdullah Shahbah D, El-Said H, et al. Pulmonary artery interventions after the arterial switch operation: unique and significant risks. *Congenit Heart Dis*. 2019;14:288–296. doi:10.1111/chd.12726
21. Faraoni D, Rahe C, Cybulski KA. Use of antifibrinolytics in pediatric cardiac surgery: where are we now? *Paediatr Anaesth*. 2019;29(5):435–440. doi:10.1111/pan.13533
26. Gerrah R, Haller SJ. Computational fluid dynamics: a primer for congenital heart disease clinicians. *Asian Cardiovasc Thorac Ann*. 2020;28(8):520–532. doi:10.1177/0218492320957163
37. Wang L, Chen Q, Qiu YQ, et al. Effects of cardiopulmonary bypass with low-priming volume on clinical outcomes in children undergoing congenital heart disease surgery. *J Cardiothorac Surg*. 2020;15(1):118. doi:10.1186/s13019-020-01151-w
38. Boettcher W, Dehmel F, Redlin M, et al. Cardiopulmonary bypass strategy to facilitate transfusion-free congenital heart surgery in neonates and infants. *Thorac Cardiovasc Surg*. 2020;68(1):2–14. doi:10.1055/s-0039-1700529
46. Harer MW, Chock VY. Renal tissue oxygenation monitoring an opportunity to improve kidney outcomes in the vulnerable neonatal population. *Front Pediatr*. 2020;8:241. doi:10.3389/fped.2020.00241
47. Gellings JA, Johnson WK, Ghanayem NS, et al. Norwood procedure-difficulty in weaning from cardiopulmonary bypass and implications for outcomes. *Semin Thorac Cardiovasc Surg*. 2020;32(1):119–125. doi:10.1053/j.semtcvs.2019.08.005
49. Kaushal B, Chauhan S, Magoon R, et al. Efficacy of bilateral erector spinae plane block in management of acute postoperative surgical pain after pediatric cardiac surgeries through a midline sternotomy. *J Cardiothorac Vasc Anesth*. 2020;34(4):981–986. doi:10.1053/j.jvca.2019.08.009

CHAPTER 90

Cardiac Surgery: Off-Pump

Jamie W. Sinton and Zhe Amy Fang

INDICATIONS/CONTRAINDICATIONS

Cardiac surgery off a cardiopulmonary bypass (CPB) often addresses major vascular disease. The etiology of major vascular disease habitually occurs in the embryonic period as pathology in the primitive paired dorsal aortic arches (namely, 4 and 6). The term *vascular ring* includes several malformations, such as double aortic arch, right aortic arch with left-sided ligamentum, and pulmonary artery (PA) sling. The following operations are considered and discussed in this chapter: end-to-end repair of coarctation of the aorta, vascular ring division, pulmonary artery banding (PAB), modified Blalock–Taussig shunt (BTS), patent ductus arteriosus (PDA) ligation, and pacemaker generator placement or change.

SPECIAL CONSIDERATIONS AND CONCERNS

COARCTATION OF THE AORTA

Coarctation of the aorta is a relatively common type of congenital heart disease (CHD) accounting for approximately 5% to 8% of all CHDs and is due to the presence of extra ductal tissue in the aortic arch extending into the adjacent aorta. When the ductus arteriosus constricts shortly after birth, so does ductal tissue in the aortic arch, thereby creating the coarctation. The presentation of coarctation of the aorta depends on the location of the coarctation, namely, preductal, (juxta) ductal, and postductal.

Preductal Coarctation

Preductal coarctation obstructs aortic flow distal to the coarctation and systemic perfusion depends on the PDA. Blood shunting right to left across the PDA results in differential cyanosis; the head and right upper extremity are fully saturated while the lower extremities, which are supplied by the PA, are desaturated.

Ductal Coarctation

Ductal coarctations are normally not detected until the second week of life when the PDA closes. Prenatal diagnosis or suspicion for coarctation depends on fetal echocardiographic findings of ventricular asymmetry, arterial disproportion, and hypoplasia of the aortic arch or isthmus.[1] For neonates with known risk of this physiology, prostaglandin E1 (PGE1) can be infused following birth to maintain ductal (and therefore arch) patency. Next, coarctation is formally diagnosed when PGE1 is discontinued, and serial measurements are taken of the neonate's aortic arch and lactate. This process is called an "arch watch." Infants whose coarctation is unsuspected prior to birth present in extremis with elevated lactate levels following natural PDA closure. In this case, there is minimal systemic perfusion distal to the PDA, anaerobic metabolism leads to lactate accumulation and metabolic acidosis.

Postductal Coarctation

Postductal coarctation occurs in older children and adults. Patients present with upper extremity hypertension and heart failure. The classic chest roentgenogram finding is rib notching due to collateral circulation. Common comorbid cardiac conditions include PDA, decreased left ventricular function, and mitral valve disease.

VASCULAR RING DIVISION

Congenital anomalies of the aortic arch result from anomalies during embryonic development of paired dorsal aortic arches 3, 4, and 6. Recall from embryology that the paired dorsal aortae form and connect to the aortic sac. In this way, all embryos begin their development with multiple vascular rings. Timed asymmetric resorption of some aortic arches comprises the final great vessel anatomy.

Clinical presentation of a vascular ring is related to compression of the trachea and esophagus. Rings may be complete, incomplete, or involve the PA. The anatomically complete ring is a double aortic arch as shown in Figure 90.1. Embryologically, failure of the fourth right aortic arch to obliterate leads to a double aortic arch.

The incomplete ring is right aortic arch with a left ligamentum arteriosum. A right aortic arch may accompany other CHDs. Finally, a pulmonary sling occurs when the left pulmonary artery (LPA) arises from the right pulmonary artery (RPA) and crosses to the left side between the trachea and esophagus. Major vascular disease often presents as respiratory pathology or dysphagia. The vascular ring may comprise a right-sided aortic arch that gives off in order: left common carotid artery, right subclavian, and left subclavian. The left subclavian artery is forced to come off so far distally that it may course posterior to the esophagus (Figure 90.2).

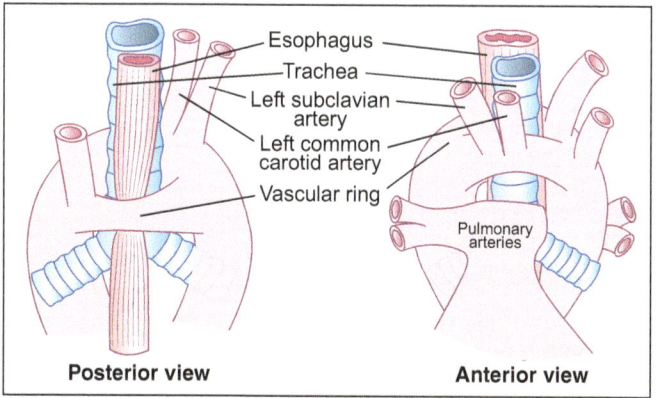

Figure 90.1: Double aortic arch. A double aortic arch is an anatomically complete vascular ring. Failure of the fourth right aortic arch to obliterate leads to a double aortic arch.

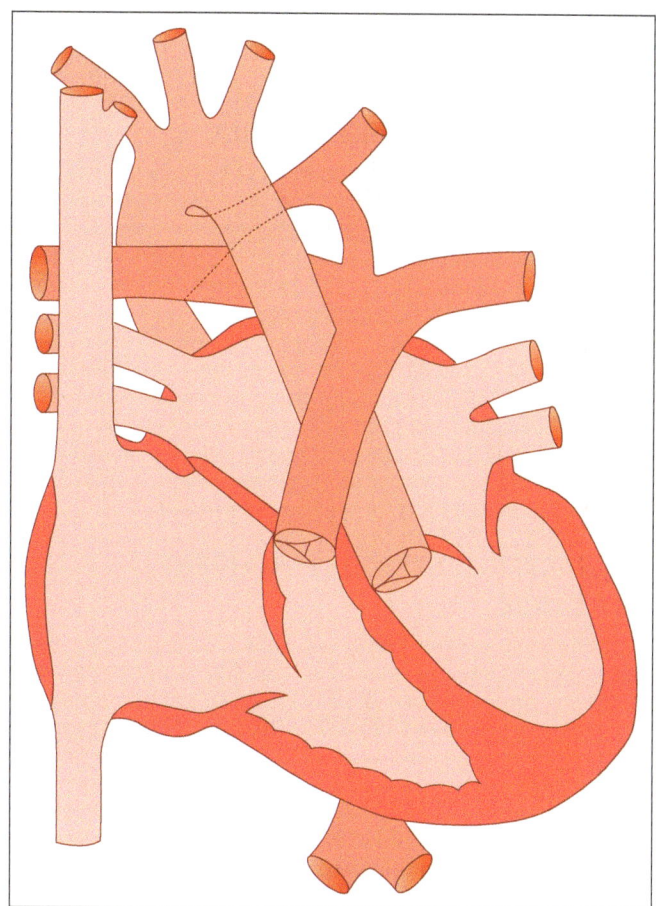

Figure 90.2: Vascular ring. The left subclavian artery is forced to come off so far distally that it may course posterior to the esophagus.

PA BANDING

PAB placement is a palliative procedure employed to restrict pulmonary blood flow and prevent pulmonary overcirculation. PAB is considered when infants are too small to undergo definitive corrective surgical procedures, as a temporizing measure. For example, an infant with multiple muscular ventricular septal defects (VSDs) may undergo PAB placement to prevent overcirculation while waiting for the defects to close spontaneously. Bilateral PABs are placed in the case of the hybrid stage 1 single-ventricle palliation.

BLALOCK–TAUSSIG SHUNT

The infant with a ductal-dependent cardiac lesion (PDA supplying either pulmonary or systemic circulation) may present for a BTS. The most common reason for this is Tetralogy of Fallot (TOF). Other lesions may include tricuspid atresia with a restrictive VSD, and pulmonary atresia with intact ventricular septum. Commonly, the PDA may be stented in the cardiac catheterization laboratory as a less invasive alternative source of pulmonary blood flow. However, the modified BTS is discussed here as it is used when ductal anatomy is not amenable to stenting or as part of a larger operation, such as a Norwood procedure. For historical purposes, the classic BTS is worth mentioning. The classic BTS involves using a subclavian artery flap to anastomose to the PA. It may still be used in an infant with chronic infection, for example, urogenital malformation that predisposes to repeated infection. In this case, foreign material as required for a modified BTS is likely to become infected so a subclavian flap is preferable.

LIGATION AND DIVISION OF A PDA

The first description of division of a PDA occurred in 1938 by Dr. Robert Gross.[2] Increasingly and with favorable anatomy, PDA disease can be addressed in the cardiac catheterization laboratory even in premature infants weighing 1 kg or less.[3] It is mentioned here, though, that institutional experience and ductal anatomy may favor a thoracoscopic or open surgical approach.

Indications for PDA ligation are left heart dilation, respiratory compromise (e.g., requiring persistent mechanical support), heart failure, hemodynamic compromise such as reversal of flow in the descending aorta during diastole, oliguria or rising serum creatinine concentration, hypotension, necrotizing enterocolitis, or wide pulse pressure.[4]

PACEMAKER GENERATOR PLACEMENT OR CHANGE

Pacemakers pace the heart and may sense intrinsic heart beats. Indications for placement include sinus node dysfunction, congenital heart block, symptomatic bradycardia, and acquired heart block 7 to 10 days following cardiac surgery. Pacing systems may be transvenous or epicardial. Transvenous systems are generally preferred for older children and adults due to decreased complication burden. Epicardial systems may be placed in children smaller than 15 to 25 kg or with single-ventricle cardiac disease in which the subclavian vein does not connect to the right ventricle. Epicardial systems do not touch the endocardium and therefore do not present the risk of endocarditis nor require endocarditis prophylaxis. Any patient (adult or pediatric) with a cardiac rhythm management device should be approached with the following issues listed in **Box 90.1**.

Systems may have unipolar or bipolar electrode design. Bipolar systems offer the advantage of smaller inter-electrode (cathode and anode) distance. Unipolar systems require more energy and are more susceptible to electromagnetic interference (EMI). The three main reasons for pacemaker failure are failure to capture, lead failure (fracture, over-, or undersensing), and generator failure.

BOX 90.1 CONSIDERATIONS FOR PATIENTS WITH CARDIAC RHYTHM MANAGEMENT DEVICES

- Coexisting CHD
- Dependency (i.e., underlying rhythm)
- Function of impulse generator, battery life
- Indication for implantation
- Lead integrity (i.e., not fractured on CXR)
- Location (e.g., transvenous or epicardial)
- Manufacturer
- Mode
- Other intraoperative sources of EMI
- Type of leads (i.e., unipolar vs. bipolar)

CHD, congenital heart disease; CXR, chest x-ray; EMI, electromagnetic interference.

Pediatric patients with dual-chamber (DDD) pacing who develop sinus tachycardia may reach their Wenckebach or 2:1 block point, so it is helpful to know what these are for each patient and try to avoid extreme sinus tachycardia. Implantable cardioverter defibrillator (ICD) systems may be implanted to treat life-threatening arrhythmias and also contain pacing functions. ICDs are indicated for primary and secondary prevention for increased risk of sudden cardiac death and sustained ventricular arrhythmias. Cardiac resynchronization therapy improves mechanical efficacy in hearts with dysynchrony and may be placed in children with left bundle branch block morphology on ECG.

ANESTHETIC MANAGEMENT

PREOPERATIVE EVALUATION

The preoperative history and physical examination should focus on symptoms referable to the cardiovascular system, such as angina, syncope, and congestive heart failure. Congestive heart failure may be right or left sided and manifest as edema or dyspnea, respectively. Congestive heart failure in an infant is associated with poor weight gain and diaphoresis and tachypnea with feeding. Recent weight gain related to edema fluid should be noted. A usual cardiovascular examination for pulses and perfusion is appropriate. Medications taken on the day of surgery may impact perioperative beta-blockade guidelines or risk of hypotension with administration of angiotensin-converting enzyme inhibitors (ACEIs). For patients presenting for pacemaker generator insertion or change, the indications for the pacemaker should be sought and the patient's baseline rhythm and pacemaker dependence should be determined.

Pertinent Labs

In addition to preoperative chest roentgenogram and ECG, echocardiogram and interrogation report or Holter monitor should be reviewed as indicated. Baseline chemistry levels, hemoglobin, and hematocrit should be reviewed prior to induction of anesthesia, as well as coagulation studies as indicated. A type and screen should be sent for cross-matching blood. All cardiac rhythm management devices should be interrogated if in place.

PREOPERATIVE PHARMACOLOGY

No special considerations, however, when choosing to advise a patient regarding home medications on the day of surgery, the risk–benefit analysis of each may be considered. For patients with cardiac rhythm management devices in situ, hyperkalemia, metabolic acidosis (more than alkalosis), hypothermia, and hyperglycemia all significantly increase the pacing threshold.

ANESTHETIC TECHNIQUE

Intraoperative Management

End-to-End Repair of Coarctation of the Aorta
Coarctations are often repaired end to end with aortic cross-clamp and division of the descending thoracic aorta. Another approach is a subclavian flap, which is rarely seen in modern times. To reduce oxygen consumption in the (nonperfused) lower body, the patient's temperature is allowed to fall following prep and drape.

Invasive and noninvasive monitors apply as in on-pump cardiac surgery. General considerations for anesthetic management include monitors as described in the chapter on cardiac surgery except for transesophageal echocardiography (TEE). TEE is used less frequently in children undergoing nonpump cardiac surgery. Monitoring should include right radial arterial cannulation and a lower extremity blood pressure. Femoral arterial cannulation may be challenging due to delayed or absent pulse in the lower extremities, even with ultrasound guidance. However, non-invasive blood pressure (NIBP) measured at the femur correlates strongly with femoral arterial pressures.[5]

Special attention should be paid to anatomic considerations for location of invasive arterial lines. The location of the arterial line should be based on the patient's anatomy and planned surgical procedure. For example, the aortic cross-clamp for a coarctation repair might render blood pressure unmeasurable in any limb other than the right upper extremity.

Airway management requires equally thoughtful planning. Lung isolation is helpful in children undergoing thoracoscopy or thoracotomy as it produces better exposure than surgical packing or retraction. Physiology of lateral positioning, infant age, and thoracic anesthesia are relevant but beyond the scope of this chapter. Briefly, infants have a flatter diaphragm that is less loaded while supine or lateral, more elastic chest wall, and a smaller hydrostatic pressure gradient from the dependent lung to the operative lung in lateral position. For these reasons, oxygenation of the infant in lateral position with a diseased lung is best when the infant is lying on the diseased lung.[6] Of course, this rarely happens as the diseased lung is often the operative lung if the child has lung pathology.

Vascular Ring Division

Surgical approach is via thoracotomy. If reimplantation of the left subclavian is considered, lung isolation with a bronchial blocker or Fogarty catheter should be considered to aid surgical exposure. When the esophagus is instrumented as with a esophagogastroduodenoscopy (EGD) or TEE probe, it may be compressed and not read a blood pressure. This may be alarming for circulatory arrest especially if directly proceeded by compromised ventilation and secretions secondary to flexible bronchoscopy (with lavage) and rigid bronchoscopy. Postoperative pain control is similar to PDA ligation and coarctation repair. Long term, vascular ring patients do well.

Vascular rings are often associated with a diverticulum of Kommerell, which is a large diverticulum from the proximal descending thoracic aorta. Luciano et al. suggest control of the diverticulum of Kommerell at the time of vascular ring division to prevent aneurysm formation, dissection, or medial necrosis.[7]

PA Banding

Standard and invasive monitoring is used, and the surgical approach is a sternotomy. TEE is very useful in this case in order to optimize restriction to PA blood flow, that is, tightness of the PA band. For infants who are too small to accept a TEE probe or when systemic perfusion depends on the PDA and bilateral branch PABs must be placed, this procedure may occur in the cardiac catheterization laboratory. There are no set criteria for how to determine the correct band tightness and there are variations across institutions. Ideally, the patients should be saturating in the mid to high 80s on room air if single-ventricle physiology is present. A common target for flow acceleration across the PAB is 4 meters per second. Alternatively, tightening of the PAB occurs until right ventricular pressure is so high that the tricuspid valve becomes incompetent, then it is loosened to restrict flow to the lungs but maintain function of the tricuspid valve. After the PABs are in place, it is common to complete an oxygen saturation run, which includes saturations from the aorta, superior vena cava (SVC), PA, and left atrium to determine the ratio of pulmonary blood flow to systemic blood flow (Qp/Qs ratio).

Blalock–Taussig Shunt

Surgical approach to the modified BTS may be sternotomy or thoracotomy. An advantage of sternotomy is little risk of damage to the right recurrent laryngeal nerve (ansa cervicalis). The azygos vein may be retracted and paratracheal lymph nodes may be removed to sit posteriorly enough to maintain its geometry while it is in use. For infants about 2.5 to 3.5 kg, a 3.5-mm graft is chosen. During the neonatal period, a 3.5-mm BTS will generally cause overcirculation, oxygen must be carefully titrated to maintain pulmonary vascular resistance. As the infant grows, the shunt does not, this will lead to decreasing pulmonary blood flow and therefore oxygen saturation with time. Hence, it is commonly referred to that the neonate grows into their shunt.

During the operation, following sternotomy (or thoracotomy) and opening of the pericardium, dissecting the relevant structures could contact the PDA and cause it to spasm creating low Qp, hypoxia, and low cardiac output. The procedure begins at the subclavian artery. Heparin, usually 100 units/kg (institution and surgeon-dependent), is given to facilitate vascular surgery. A c-shaped clamp is placed at the takeoff of the subclavian artery (and some of the innominate artery). The graft is sewn circumferentially at the subclavian. Next, the RPA then receives the c-clamp and the distal anastomosis.

Upon opening the shunt, hemodynamic instability can be expected. During a right-modified BTS, a right subclavian artery cross-clamp may be required, which may severely dampen a right radial arterial line. Also, after the BTS is in place, a right radial artery blood pressure may not be accurate due to runoff from the shunt. Certainly, oxygenation should be maintained; however, the immediate concern with providing supplemental oxygen is its dramatic effect on reducing pulmonary vascular resistance. Hypotension is common owing to diastolic runoff into the pulmonary arteries. Increasing systemic vascular resistance is usually required realizing that increased systemic pressure promotes additional pulmonary circulation. Immediately postclamp release, the infant will be appropriately or overcirculated, and coronary ischemia is a major concern. As the infant grows and the shunt does not, undercirculation develops. However, caution is advised whenever desaturation out of proportion is noted as other causes of desaturation should be sought as shunt occlusion may be life-threatening.

Ligation and Division of a PDA

Intraoperatively, standard and invasive monitors are placed, although TEE is not used. Blood pressure should be measured in the right upper extremity and lower extremity to compare the two before and after ligation. A right thoracotomy may be used to expose the PDA. Careful dissection is conducted, and the target vessel is temporarily clamped. If diastolic blood pressure rises with unchanged ventilation (expected), the vessel is ligated proximally and distally and then divided. Surgical misadventure could lead to inadvertent ligation of the right bronchus or aorta. Therefore, it is important to monitor ventilation and lower extremity blood pressure, respectively.

Pacemaker Generator Placement or Change

Changes of these generators will usually be performed in the cardiac operating room with a cardiac surgeon although transvenous systems may be exchanged in the cardiac catheterization laboratory. External defibrillator pads are placed prior to induction of anesthesia along with standard monitors. Arterial access is obtained. If the patient is completely pacemaker dependent with no reasonable escape rhythm, then considerations should be made for alternative pacing strategies. Central venous access may be obtained with an introducer that can accommodate a temporary transvenous pacing system in the event the leads are damaged during surgical dissection. However, if the patient has a Fontan circulation, central venous access does not directly connect to the right ventricle. Surgical dissection will often interfere with pacing function. Following placement or replacement of the device or leads, pacing and sensing thresholds will be measured by a representative of the device company.

Adult congenital heart disease (ACHD) patients often had multiple sternotomies making entry into the chest challenging, with the potential for catastrophic bleeding. Hence, reliable IV access is imperative. Furthermore, for ACHD patients, scarring of the myocardium may make placing pacemaker leads with appropriate thresholds very difficult. Subxiphoid incisions may not be adequate, and a sternotomy may be required. This increases the risk of potential bleeding, and the need for CPB being readily available.

In general, placement of an ICD (but not a plain pacemaker) requires fibrillation of the heart to test the new device. The device company representative can provide electrical energy directly for an R on T shock that ought to initiate ventricular fibrillation. On rare occasions, this is (repeatedly) unsuccessful. If the patient does not fibrillate with this intervention, then a fibrillator may be used. A fibrillator delivers direct current to the heart until fibrillation occurs. Following fibrillation, the patient's new device should defibrillate appropriately (or else CPR begins).

While sources of EMI will be carefully planned for pacemaker generator changes, children undergoing other procedures are exposed to EMI as well. Sources of EMI include cautery, large tidal volumes, Cavitron (ultrasonic dental cleaning device), nerve stimulators, shivering, fasciculation, extracorporeal shockwave lithotripsy (ESWL), and MRI. EMI can cause either inappropriate triggering or inhibition of paced output as well as reversion to an asynchronous (noise suppression) mode.[8]

If defibrillator and pacemaker generators will likely receive interference with surgical electrocautery, disabling of the anti-tachycardia function is reasonable. However, it should be noted that bipolar cautery is preferred. The dispersion pad should not be placed in the path of the generator and cautery should be at least 15 centimeters from the generator.

Complications/Emergencies

Complications during any thoracic surgery are many and can be classified into neurologic, airway, hemodynamic, and metabolic. Paraplegia is the foremost concern due to spinal cord ischemia beyond the cross-clamp. Neuraxial analgesia with a local anesthetic-containing solution should be deferred as it may delay a diagnosis of spinal cord ischemia or injury post coarctation repair.

During lung isolation whether by surgical packing or one lung ventilation, ventilation–perfusion mismatch, intrapulmonary shunt, and obstruction to the endotracheal tube (ETT) occur. Surgical manipulation of the lung may result in disruption of the visceral pleura and pulmonary hemorrhage as well.

Hemodynamic complications are expected during aortic cross-clamping and unclamping. Preparing these events minimizes physiologic trespass. Metabolic derangements result from acidosis and lower body hypoperfusion. These derangements are not definitively corrected until surgery. Entry into the operating room, especially in emergent cases, promises metabolic acidosis and elevated lactate. The aortic cross-clamp time required to repair the coarctation is enough to contribute further to metabolic derangements.

Notably absent in patients presenting with coarctation of the aorta is an impact on autonomic function given surgical disruption of the aortic arch.[9] The aortic arch is rich with baroreceptors. Increased blood pressure increases stimulation of baroreceptors, which synapse in the nucleus tractus solitarius. Here, vagal outflow results in increased inhibition of the tonically active sympathetic flow. The result is vasodilation and decreased peripheral vascular resistance.

The most feared complication of coarctation repair is paraplegia due to inadequate perfusion to the lower body during aortic cross-clamp. Many patients have what is judged to be adequate collateral flow to tolerate aortic cross-clamping, however, if not, partial CPB may be used.[10] Late complications are common and include hypertension and recoarctation. Smaller aortic arch was a stronger predictor of recoarctation than age and weight at surgery.[11] Anatomically, important autonomic nervous system structures underlie the great vessels, such as baroreceptors. Notably, autonomic nervous system effect is not measurably different in those with history of coarctation compared to controls.[9] Finally, coarctation repair may have long-term impacts on left atrial function.[12]

While CPB is not required for BTS placement, if the infant is very unstable or does not tolerate lung retraction, then bypass is initiated. In the case of PA/intact ventricular septum (IVS), avoidance of bypass is especially important if the coronary circulation depends on high pressure in the right ventricle (RVDCC). In this case, the venous cannula can decompress the right ventricle and ischemia may result.

Complications of pacemaker or ICD generator changes include bleeding and arrhythmias. Bleeding is likely to occur and may be catastrophic if the patient has had sternotomies in the past and surgical dissection disrupts the integrity of the inferior vena cava or right ventricle. An indication for central venous access would be back-up transvenous pacing during the procedure; however, if the patient has a Fontan circulation, central venous access does not directly connect to the right ventricle.

Arrhythmias may occur as mentioned during dissection or during fibrillation to test the device.

POSTOPERATIVE CARE

Many off-pump cardiac surgeries in children occur via thoracotomy. Immediately postoperatively and long term, pain is a significant consideration.[13] Multimodal analgesia is the standard of care. In addition to IV medication, regional analgesia via peripheral nerve blockade can be employed. It reduces the stress response in children undergoing surgery[14] and may have similar benefits in neonates.[15] Peripheral nerve blockade provides analgesia with less severe complications compared to neuraxial blocks and does not require American Society of Regional Anesthesia (ASRA) anticoagulation for neuraxial block guidelines to be followed.[16] Popular intermuscular plane blocks, such as the serratus anterior plane and erector spinae plane blocks, require substantial volumes of local anesthetics. The concentration, volume, and milligram dose of local anesthetic drug must be chosen carefully to avoid local anesthetic systemic toxicity.

Routine postoperative care for BTS includes prevention of thrombosis of the shunt. Commonly, if hemostasis is achieved within 6 hours of the operation, aspirin is initiated. By the time the infant is 3 to 6 months old (or so) and presents for TOF repair, Glenn, and so on, the shunt will be more restrictive, and oxygen can be given with much less concern for coronary ischemia due to hypoperfusion (inadequate coronary perfusion pressure).

Analgesia following pacemaker generator change is amenable to regional analgesia as well. For transvenous devices with the generator in the chest, pectoralis I and II blocks unilaterally show promise. In adults, it has been described as providing adequate anesthesia;[17] however, for children, general anesthesia will likely be necessary with regional techniques primarily for postoperative analgesia. Nomenclature of these relatively new blocks is evolving as well.[18] For epicardial pacing and defibrillation systems, a truncal block can be chosen for the insertion site of the generator. Again, plane blocks are commonly used, such as erector spinae, quadratus lumborum, or transversus abdominis plane block. Anticoagulation must be considered if paravertebral analgesia is planned.

CASE STUDY: 8-Day-Old With Coarctation of the Aorta

CLINICAL SCENARIO

A neonate was discharged home after an uneventful delivery. She returns to the hospital on day of life 8 in extremis with tachypnea, respiratory distress, and elevated serum lactate. She is intubated and initiated on PGE1 at 0.05 mcg/kg/min. Her echocardiogram reveals coarctation of the aorta, a structurally normal heart, and moderately depressed left ventricular (LV) function. Dopamine supports her cardiac function, and she presents to the operating room for coarctation repair.

APPROACHES TO CARE

Following application of standard monitors, the patient undergoes IV induction with midazolam, fentanyl and rocuronium. Her oral ETT is exchanged for a nasal ETT. A right radial arterial line is placed for monitoring. A lower extremity noninvasive blood pressure cuff is placed around her femur for comparison of upper and lower extremity blood pressure. She has an in situ femoral peripherally inserted central catheter (PICC) line; however, it is in the infrahepatic IVC. PGE continues through this line; however, an additional central line is placed for vasoactive infusions.

An oroesophageal (OE) tube is placed to aid in surgical dissection by providing rigidity to the esophagus. She is positioned in right lateral decubitus position. Following skin preparation and draping, the forced-air warmer is discontinued in order to allow passive cooling and therefore reduction in oxygen consumption. Lung isolation is not attempted; surgical packing is used to retract the left lung.

Intraoperative management initially prioritizes the reopening of the PDA with PGE1. If the patient stabilizes with PGE1, surgery is urgent (but not emergent). Supplemental oxygen is necessary during (effectively) one lung ventilation; however, oxygen dilates pulmonary vessels, increases blood flow through the PDA, and reduces diastolic blood pressure and therefore coronary perfusion pressure. Heparin 100 units/kg is given prior to cross-clamping of the aorta. The aorta is cross-clamped during which time the left arm and lower body are not receiving perfusion from the aorta. Inhalational agents are used to control hypertension; however, if the coarctation is very tight, application of the cross-clamp will add little afterload. During the cross-clamp, which often lasts 20 minutes, she receives 100% oxygen. Upon release of the cross-clamp, she becomes hypotensive due to the expected acidosis resulting from lack of lower extremity perfusion. She stabilized with sodium bicarbonate (after controlling ventilation), calcium, epinephrine (1 mcg/kg) and volume. Right radial and lower extremity blood pressures are compared and found to be similar. The patient's LV function recovers fairly rapidly with relief of the aortic obstruction (coarctation). Consequently, she becomes hypertensive. Nitroprusside is initiated to prevent hypertension given the fresh aortic suture lines. She remains intubated and is transferred to the intensive care unit in stable condition.

Evidence-Based Approaches to Care

Evidence for spinal cord protection during coarctation repair is sparse. Reduction in oxygen consumption via temperature drift is performed with passive cooling. It cannot ethically be studied by maintaining warmth in some subjects and risking paralysis or other complications. In older children and adults, hypothermic circulatory arrest or partial CPB has been suggested for complex coarctations involving the proximal aortic arch.[19] Steroids and mannitol have been proposed, albeit without great evidence of efficacy and safety.

(continued)

CASE STUDY: 8-Day-Old With Coarctation of the Aorta (continued)

Postoperative pain control may be underprioritized in a neonate in extremis. Additionally, immaturity of the neonate's liver with albumin bound to bilirubin from neonatal jaundice may limit safe local anesthetic dosing. However, in infants aged 4 to 12 months, analgesia from thoracotomy for coarctation with paravertebral nerve blockade is improved when supplemented with dexamethasone 0.1 mg/kg.[20] The analgesic effect of paravertebral blockade results from absorption of local anesthetic from the paravertebral space into the spinal nerves. In this way, cerebral cortical response to thoracic stimulation is blunted.

KEY REFERENCES

References for this chapter are online and available at https://connect.springerpub.com/content/book/978-0-8261-3875-0/part/part04/toc-part/ch090.

1. Vigneswaran TV, Bellsham-Revell HR, Chubb H, Simpson JM. Early postnatal echocardiography in neonates with a prenatal suspicion of coarctation of the aorta. *Pediatr Cardiol.* 2020;41(4):772–780. doi:10.1007/s00246-020-02310-5
3. Hubbard R, Edmonds K, Rydalch E, et al. Anesthetic management of catheter-based patent ductus arteriosus closure in neonates weighing <3 kg: a retrospective observational study. *Paediatr Anaesth.* 2020;30(4):506–510. doi:10.1111/pan.13838
9. Nederend I, de Geus EJC, Kroft LJM, et al. Cardiac autonomic nervous system activity and cardiac function in children after coarctation repair. *Ann Thorac Surg.* 2018;105(6):1803–1808. doi:10.1016/j.athoracsur.2018.01.084
11. Dias MQ, Barros A, Leite-Moreira A, Miranda JO. Risk factors for recoarctation and mortality in infants submitted to aortic coarctation repair: a systematic review. *Pediatr Cardiol.* 2020;41(3):561–575. doi:10.1007/s00246-020-02319-w
20. Saleh AH, Hassan PF, Elayashy M, et al. Role of dexamethasone in the para-vertebral block for pediatric patients undergoing aortic coarctation repair. Randomized, double-blinded controlled study. *BMC Anesthesiol.* 2018;18(1):178. doi:10.1186/s12871-018-0637-y

CHAPTER 91

Cardiac Catheterization Laboratory

Joanna Rosing Paquin

INTRODUCTION

The role of the pediatric and congenital cardiac catheterization laboratory (PCCCL) has advanced considerably over time. In recent years, the PCCCL has transitioned from primarily a diagnostic tool to a therapeutic procedural suite offering nonsurgical options, with novel primary treatment and palliation strategies for congenital heart disease (CHD) continually emerging.[1,2]

INDICATIONS/CONTRAINDICATIONS

Cardiac catheterization procedures can be both diagnostic and therapeutic in nature. A diagnostic cardiac catheterization procedure is often performed to gather information about the cardiac morphology and physiology of a patient. Frequently, this involves either a right heart catheterization (RHC), a left heart catheterization (LHC), or a combination of both procedures. Therapeutic cardiac catheterization procedures involve correction of a defect or lesion in the heart.

DIAGNOSTIC CARDIAC CATHETERIZATION

Right Heart Catheterization

During an RHC, a fluid-filled catheter is passed through a large vein into the central venous system under fluoroscopic guidance. While the femoral vein is typically accessed, variations in anatomy, vessel thrombosis, or stenosis may necessitate additional or alternative access. Alternate points of access include the internal jugular vein, the subclavian vein, or the hepatic vein utilizing a percutaneous transhepatic approach. In neonates, the umbilical vein may also serve as an alternative during the first few days of life.[3] Once placed, the catheter can measure the intravascular pressures and cardiac output (CO), as well as be used to obtain blood samples for analysis. An RHC offers direct hemodynamic feedback, providing information that can be used to determine CO or evaluate intracardiac shunts and valvular dysfunction. The addition of angiography furthers the diagnostic profile of an RHC by better defining the patient's anatomy and physiology.

LEFT HEART CATHETERIZATION

An LHC measures systolic, diastolic, and mean arterial blood pressures by passing a catheter retrograde through a femoral, brachial, or axillary artery. In doing so, pressures in the aorta, left ventricle, and left atrium can be directly measured. The left heart may also be accessed via the right atrium should the patient have a patent foramen ovale (PFO), allowing the atrial septum to be crossed or through an atrial septal defect (ASD).[3] A diagnostic LHC is indicated to measure arterial blood pressures, define complex anatomy, such as left-sided cardiac lesions, and evaluate the coronary arteries.

Hemodynamic Measurements Obtained During Cardiac Catheterization

The data gathered during a diagnostic cardiac catheterization are applied to a variety of equations to calculate CO, pulmonary vascular resistance (PVR), systemic vascular resistance (SVR), oxygen consumption (VO_2), and shunt fractions. Shunt fractions, or the percentage of blood ejected by the heart that is not completely oxygenated, can be used to monitor the effectiveness of pulmonary oxygenation. In addition, the presence of an intracardiac shunt can be localized and quantified by directly measuring mixed venous oxygen saturations.

CO can be measured through a process called thermodilution. With thermodilution, a known volume of iced water or saline solution is injected into the right atrium followed by measurement of the temperature at the catheter tip in the pulmonary artery (PA). CO is then calculated using a modified Stewart–Hamilton equation. PA thermodilution is not the only approach, however, with transpulmonary thermodilution (TPTD) gaining popularity in the pediatric population due to its limited invasive nature. TPTD involves an ice-cold saline injection via a central venous line, with the change in temperature assessed distally via an arterial line catheter equipped with a thermistor. It should be noted that TPTD measurements are prone to error given the longer distance the indicator (injectate) has to travel. Pulse contour analysis (PCA), a minimally invasive and continuous measurement of CO, has emerged as another method for measurement of CO. Hemodynamic parameters can also be measured using a combination of TPTD and PCA techniques via a specific thermodilution arterial catheter (pulse contour cardiac output monitoring, PiCCO) that measures temperature changes following the injection of the bolus through a central vein catheter.

The Fick principle, which is based on the body's VO_2 and arterial to venous oxygen content difference, can also be used to calculate CO, cardiac index (CI), and stroke volume (see Table 91.1). VO_2 can be extrapolated from the LaFarge tables for use in the Fick equation; however, this has been shown in multiple studies to overestimate VO_2 relative to measured values, particularly in neonates and infants. The LaFarge tables relate VO_2 to body surface area or to a patient's heart rate and age. Unfortunately, the accuracy of the LaFarge tables is diminished in children younger than 3 years of age and those with complex CHD. Therefore, in these populations, it is recommended that VO_2 be directly measured.[4] Real-time measurement of VO_2 can be achieved by measuring samples proximally from the endotracheal tube during inspiration and expiration to calculate VO_2. In children younger than 3 years old with a structurally normal heart, real-time VO_2 generates highly accurate determinations of Fick CI as compared with thermodilution.[5]

The Fick principle can also be used to measure both systemic blood flow (Qs) and pulmonary blood flow (Qp). Comparison of the pulmonary-to-systemic blood flow, commonly referred to as Qp:Qs, is an accurate means of identifying and quantifying intracardiac shunts.[3] Poiseuille's equation approximates the volume flow rate of blood through the blood vessels of our body. It can be used to measure intravascular resistance and contributes valuable information about the systemic and pulmonary vasculature.[6]

TABLE 91.1 Hemodynamic Calculations and Normal Values		
	Equation	**Normal**
Flows		
Pulmonary	$Qp = VO_2/(S_{PV}O_2 - S_{PA}O_2) \times Hgb \times 1.34 \times 10$	3.5–5 L × min^{-1} × m^{-2}
Systemic	$Qs = VO_2/(S_{AO}O_2 - S_{MV}O_2) \times Hgb \times 1.34 \times 10$	3.5–5 L × min^{-1} × m^{-2}
Resistance (Wood Unit)		
Pulmonary	$Rp = PAP - LAP/Q_p$	Newborns: 8–10 Older children: 1–3
Systemic	$Rs = AOP - RAP/Q_s$	Newborns: 10–15 Older children: 15–30
Shunts		
Pulmonary to systemic	$Qp/Qs = (S_{AO}O_2 - S_{MV}O_2)/(S_{PV}O_2 - S_{PA}O_2)$	1:1
VO$_2$		
	$VO_2 = (CO \times CaO_2) - (CO \times CvO_2)$	LaFarge equations below
LaFarge equation for VO$_2$	Boys $VO_2 = 138.1 - [11.49 \times \log_e \text{(age in yrs)}] + 0.378 \text{(heart rate)}$ Girls $VO_2 = 138.1 - [17.04 \times \log_e \text{(age in yrs)}] + 0.378 \text{(heart rate)}$	

AO, aorta; AOP, aortic pressure; CaO$_2$, arterial oxygen content; CO, cardiac output; CvO$_2$, venous oxygen content; LAP, left atrial pressure; MV, mixed venous; PA, pulmonary artery; PAP, pulmonary artery pressure; PV, pulmonary vein; Qp, pulmonary flow; Qs, systemic flow; RAP, right atrial pressure; Rp, pulmonary vascular resistance; Rs, systemic vascular resistance; S, saturation; VO$_2$, oxygen consumption.

ADDITIONAL INDICATIONS FOR DIAGNOSTIC CARDIAC CATHETERIZATION

Additional indications for cardiac catheterization include angiography, myocardial function evaluation, and endocardial biopsy sampling.[7] Coronary anatomy may also be evaluated with angiography. While a diagnostic cardiac catheterization is able to identify vascular anatomy and congenital anomalies through angiography, other less invasive imaging modalities, such as computerized tomography (CT) and MRI, have replaced cardiac catheterization for diagnostic imaging as they can provide similar data regarding patient anatomy in a less invasive fashion.[8] Patients with varying degrees of cardiomyopathy or pulmonary hypertension may benefit from a cardiac catheterization to optimize therapy and medical planning through evaluation of myocardial function and hemodynamic response to drugs or interventions performed. Finally, endocardial biopsies provide additional information, specifically orthotopic heart transplant surveillance, cardiomyopathy, or myocarditis diagnoses. Overall, a diagnostic cardiac catheterization procedure provides insight into a patient's anatomy and physiology so that the appropriate treatment strategies are implemented.

THERAPEUTIC CARDIAC CATHETERIZATION

Therapeutic interventions via a cardiac catheterization procedure focus on the treatment of a specific diagnosis. Although very few procedures and/or specific devices are approved for use in pediatric and congenital heart lesions in the United States by the Food and Drug Administration (FDA), therapeutic catheterization procedures now represent the primary indication for performing cardiac catheterizations in congenital heart patients. These advanced therapeutic options allow the risks and complications associated with cardiopulmonary bypass (CPB) to be delayed or avoided. Interventions, such as balloon valvotomies, radiofrequency catheter ablations, endovascular stenting, percutaneous valve placement, closure of vascular shunts, and combined catheter and surgical interventions, are being performed with increased frequency due to continued advances in cardiac catheterization techniques.[1]

During therapeutic procedures, a catheter is placed into the vasculature and components of a diagnostic cardiac catheterization procedure are performed. Following an initial diagnostic, evaluation wires, balloons, and/or devices are introduced for the desired intervention. It is imperative that anesthesia providers understand the intervention being performed so they can develop the anesthetic plan accordingly. In addition, a sound understanding of the procedure being performed allows the anesthesia provider to better anticipate procedure-related complications. For example, during balloon dilation of a ventricular outflow tract (right or left), balloon inflation can completely obstruct blood flow impairing CO. In this scenario, the anesthesia provider must be prepared to mitigate derangements in CO. While short and repetitive inflations are ideal to improve patient tolerability of the procedure, rapid ventricular pacing may be required to maintain CO during balloon inflation.[9]

The percutaneous closure of shunts is another therapeutic cardiac catheterization procedure associated with a wide array of medical challenges. Helical wire coils or particle embolization can be used to close unwanted vascular shunts, such as veno-venous or aortopulmonary collateral blood vessels.[10] Persistent ASDs, patent ductus arteriosus, and ventricular septal defects require the use of more complex devices to achieve closure of the defect. Each of these techniques is associated with a host of device-related complications, such as malposition or emboli of the device, vascular occlusion, myocardial perforation, hemolysis, and vascular trauma.[8]

Unfortunately, as the complexity of interventions increases, so does the incidence of serious adverse events, especially among the neonatal population. The lack of availability of emergency surgical services and circulatory support, such as CPB or extracorporeal membrane oxygenation (ECMO), may be a contraindication for certain interventions. For patients at highest risk during cardiac catheterization, elective use of ECMO should be considered as it has been proven safe and preferable as a rescue therapy.[11]

SPECIAL CONSIDERATIONS AND CONCERNS

WORK ENVIRONMENT CHALLENGES

The PCCCL presents unique environmental challenges. Large immobile radiological equipment, necessary for appropriate imaging, obstructs and limits access to a patient. The lateral and anteroposterior fluoroscopy cameras, monitors, and anesthesia machine also limit the functional space in a cardiac catheterization laboratory. It is recommended that all IV tubing and ventilation circuit tubing be secured, positioned, and of sufficient length to accommodate for anticipated movement of the fluoroscopy cameras and the patient table. Communication between medical staff in the PCCCL can be challenging due to these physical environmental constraints. Since communication is imperative between all members of the team, it is recommended that headsets be used to facilitate communication and care coordination.

Further confounding work environment-related issues is that the physical location of the PCCCL is typically remote from the main operating suite and additional emergency resources. Establishing clear emergency response protocols can facilitate management of emergencies in the PCCCL. Challenges often arise from accommodating additional patient equipment for mechanical circulatory support and surgical intervention, such as CPB or ECMO. Due to the special considerations of the PCCCL, it is favorable that anesthesia providers have the skill set necessary to anticipate, prevent, and treat complex patients with CHD in this challenging environment.[2]

RADIATION EXPOSURE

Both patients and staff alike are at risk of radiation exposure due to the use of fluoroscopy. Cine fluoroscopy, in particular, delivers extremely high doses of radiation potentially putting the patient at increased risk of harm from radiation exposure.[12] Chromosomal damage secondary to radiation exposure in the PCCCL is not unheard of, with cumulative radiation exposure in patients with CHD being significant. In fact, children are three to four times more likely than adults to develop malignancies from radiation exposure.[13] As survival in CHD continues to improve, monitoring and strategizing radiation exposure will be imperative to minimize the cumulative risks of radiation exposure in this high-risk population.[13]

The concern for radiation exposure is not reserved for just the patients. The maximum recommended exposure for healthcare professionals is less than 5 rem/year; however, it is recommended that exposure is ideally maintained to less than 0.12 rem/year. Minimizing the time of exposure, maintaining the maximal allowable distance from a radiation source, and the use of protective barriers, such as a lead apron, thyroid shield, eyeglasses, and a lead screen all reduce cumulative radiation exposure.[14] To safeguard anesthesia providers' health, monitoring of radiation exposure with dosimeter badges is advised.

ANESTHETIC MANAGEMENT

PREOPERATIVE EVALUATION

Children with CHD are at an increased risk of perioperative morbidity and mortality, thereby demanding a thorough preoperative evaluation.[15] Preoperative evaluation of a child presenting to the PCCCL includes an assessment of baseline functional status, identification of congenital cardiac disease, prior surgical interventions, residual lesions from prior surgeries, and baseline oxygen saturation. Alarming symptoms of cardiac disease include fatigue, shortness of breath, diaphoresis, tachypnea, decreased feeding, and worsening cyanosis. Recent respiratory illnesses are also important to identify as they pose an increased risk of adverse events under general anesthesia. More specifically, a recent respiratory illness can increase PVR, which is unlikely to be tolerated in the patient with CHD.

On physical examination, anesthesia providers should be sure to take note of cardiac-specific findings. Concerning signs of cardiac disease include clubbing, cyanosis, mottled skin, delayed capillary refill, lethargy, failure to thrive, murmurs, hepatomegaly, tachypnea, pre- and post-ductal oxygen saturation discrepancies, and diminished pulses. All available imaging studies should be reviewed, including chest radiographs, ECG, echocardiograms, MRI scans, and prior cardiac catheterization procedures.

IV access may be difficult to obtain in patients with CHD. This may be the result of scarring from multiple access points during prior procedures or hospitalization, clotted or stenotic blood vessels from prior central lines, and/or abnormal vasculature. Ultrasound guidance may facilitate peripheral IV catheter placement. Radiographs to confirm the location of indwelling lines, such as peripherally inserted central catheters (PICCs) and umbilical catheters should be reviewed.

The Congenital Cardiac Interventional Study Consortium developed and validated a preprocedural scoring system to predict the risk of serious adverse events for pediatric patients undergoing cardiac catheterization procedures.[16] The 20-point scoring system assesses 10 patient variables and is referred to as the CRISP score (Catheterization Risk Score for Pediatrics). When developing the criteria for the CRISP score, the frequency of significant adverse events was evaluated in over 18,000 procedures. It was determined that the complexity of the procedure, underlying diagnosis, and patient's physiological status all contribute to the frequency of serious adverse events.[16] Children less than 1 year of age with at least two abnormal hemodynamic values who are scheduled to undergo a high-risk procedure are at the highest risk of experiencing a serious adverse event.[4,16] It is essential that anesthesia providers incorporate the CRISP score into their preoperative evaluation and planning routine (Box 91.1).

Pertinent Labs

Preprocedural blood sampling may be indicated for certain patients and procedures. A baseline hematocrit and blood product type and screen are reasonable to obtain prior to an intervention and/or high-risk procedures. In procedures with contrast administration, close evaluation of the patient's renal function is also recommended.

> **BOX 91.1 CRISP SCORING VARIABLES**
>
> - Patient status/timing (elective, emergent/urgent, postoperative)
> - Age (>1 yr, 30 days–1 yr, <30 days)
> - Weight (>10 kg, 2.5–10 kg, <2.5 kg)
> - Inotropic support (none, yes; stable, yes; unstable or ECMO)
> - Respiratory status (natural airway, stable on ventilator, respiratory failure on mechanical ventilation)
> - Systemic illness/failure (none, medically controlled, uncontrolled or >1 organ system failure)
> - ASA score (1 or 2, 3, 4 or 5)
> - Physiological category (1, 2, or 3)
> - Precatheterization diagnosis (1, 2, or 3)
> - Procedure risk category (1, 2, or 3)
>
> ASA, American Society of Anesthesiology; CRISP, Catheterization Risk Score for Pediatrics ECMO, extracorporeal membrane oxygenation.

PREOPERATIVE PHARMACOLOGY

It is beneficial to minimize preprocedural stress in patients with CHD. The most common premedication used is midazolam (oral, IV, or intranasal). Midazolam is safe and effective in CHD. Intranasal dexmedetomidine has also proven helpful for anxiolysis. However, caution is advised in patients presenting with atrioventricular (AV) nodal heart block, significant uncontrolled pulmonary hypertension, or those taking AV nodal blocking agents (e.g., digoxin) when administrating dexmedetomidine, as resulting bradycardia could be detrimental.[17,18]

ANESTHESIA TECHNIQUE

When determining the optimal anesthesia technique for a procedure in the PCCCL, anesthesia providers must carefully consider the patient's overall health, the demands of procedure, and the associated risks. The choice between general anesthesia and sedation requires a sound understanding of the advantages and disadvantages each technique affords. Likewise, thoughtful consideration should also be given to airway management for the procedure, as an advanced airway may or may not be preferred to maintaining spontaneous ventilation.

Although cardiac catheterization procedures typically involve little noxious stimuli, both the procedures and the patients can be complex, frequently involving a broad range of hemodynamic stability and comorbidities. Complex high-risk procedures, such as aortic valvotomy, dilation of severe pulmonary stenosis, percutaneous device placement, and hybrid surgical catheterization procedures, warrant consideration for general anesthesia with an advanced airway to ensure patient safety throughout the procedure.[8,19] General anesthesia will blunt reflexes, ensure immobility and a secure airway, and allow control of the $PaCO_2$. Smaller patients, such as neonates and infants and those with additional noncardiac comorbidities or low mixed venous oxygen saturations, are more likely to fail procedural sedation for cardiac catheterization procedures and should also be considered candidates for general anesthesia with an advanced airway.[19]

Intraoperative Management

Patient monitoring should include all standard American Society of Anesthesiology (ASA) monitors. The PCCCL is susceptible to low ambient temperature; therefore, patient temperature should be closely monitored. Warming devices, such as convective warming blankets, do not inhibit imaging. These devices should be used to regulate temperature. Additional invasive monitors, such as an arterial and/or venous pressure lines, may be indicated by a patient's disease state and the procedure being performed. During an LHC the arterial catheter can be transduced to closely monitor the arterial blood pressure.

Careful positioning and padding to avoid pressure injuries are recommended. A patient's arms are typically required to be placed above the head to optimize imaging. It is recommended that a patient be positioned with their arms up with elbow flexion less than a 90-degree angle to avoid stretch and injury to the brachial plexus. Additionally, a proceduralist may request a bump under the hips to facilitate femoral vascular access. This position may compromise ventilation in neonates and small infants.

Ideally, hemodynamic data should be acquired on room air when dissolved oxygen is negligible and contributions to resistance and flow equations are not significant. If supplemental oxygen is needed, it is imperative to communicate with the proceduralist so that data obtained can be appropriately interpreted. Common equations used for hemodynamic calculations in a diagnostic cardiac catheterization procedure and associated normal values can be referenced in **Table 91.1**.

Antibiotic administration may be indicated if a therapeutic catheterization procedure involves deployment of a device. Typically, blood loss during a cardiac catheterization procedure is minimal; however, neonates and infants with CHD may not tolerate the smallest decrease in blood volume as they may rely on a higher hematocrit for oxygen-carrying capacity. This is especially true in patients with cyanotic CHD. Volume overload and hemodilution could also result, even with judicious catheter flushing. Close monitoring of blood levels including electrolytes and heparin concentration through an activated clotting time (ACT) is imperative.

Unfractionated heparin use during a cardiac catheterization is beneficial in reducing arterial thrombosis in pediatric patients.[20] Unfortunately, the ideal dose of heparin in children remains unclear. Current guidelines recommend 100 units/kg to be administered for arterial or venous entry.[21] The concentration of heparin can be followed by monitoring the ACT, with subsequent doses of heparin administered throughout the procedure per institutional protocol. Although heparin has a short half-life, it may need to be emergently reversed at times. Therefore, is it important to have protamine readily available.[20]

Special Techniques
General Anesthesia
Cardiac catheterization, whether diagnostic or therapeutic, is invasive and for the majority of children, general anesthesia is necessary. Induction of anesthesia will vary with the individual patient's cardiac defect and functional status. Considerations should be made for the presence of shunts, myocardial contractility, ventricular dilation or hypertrophy, outflow tract obstructions, dysrhythmias, and pulmonary hypertension when formulating an anesthetic plan.

Some patients may be appropriate for an inhalational induction. The most common inhalational agent used is sevoflurane, which can reduce myocardial contractility and decrease SVR by vasodilation. Nevertheless, because heart rate increases with sevoflurane, the CO is generally not affected. It has been shown to result in less hypotension and less negative inotropy when compared to halothane.

Nitrous oxide, often used during induction of anesthesia for its second gas effect, allows for use of less sevoflurane, thereby ameliorating the decrease in SVR and hypotension during induction. Nitrous oxide is also known to expand an air embolism, which is a significant risk in patients with CHD. While nitrous oxide has a utility in inhalational induction of anesthesia, the risk of air embolism makes it a poor choice for maintenance of anesthesia.

Varying agents are available for use in an IV induction of anesthesia, including fentanyl, propofol, ketamine, and etomidate. A multimodal, slowly titrated, patient-specific IV induction is recommended to maintain cardiac function and hemodynamic balance during induction of anesthesia.

General anesthesia can be maintained with a variety of anesthetic techniques. Inhalational anesthetics, in conjunction with neuromuscular blockade and IV narcotics, are most commonly used. While a primary narcotic anesthesia may be beneficial in some instances, cardiac catheterization procedures are typically not painful. Therefore, an abundance of narcotics may hinder a planned extubation.

The disadvantages of general anesthesia are that it alters a patient's hemodynamics resulting in vasodilation, decreased SVR, and myocardial depression. In addition, it is important to be mindful of the impact of mechanical ventilation. Positive pressure ventilation decreases VO2, alters cardiac preload, and impedes shunt flow and flow across the cardiac valves. The addition of a respiratory VO_2 monitor to the endotracheal tube may alter measured tidal volumes in the smallest patients and should be taken into consideration to avoid barotrauma to the lungs.

Sedation
In a cooperative patient, sedation is a valid approach.[22,23] Sedation affords cardiovascular stability, as it most reflects a patient's natural hemodynamics. However, oversedation can result in hypoventilation and impair hemodynamic measurements with resulting increased $PaCO_2$ and PVR.[4] Careful selection of anesthetic agents can reduce the effects of oversedation; however, these effects are not fully eliminated. Understanding of these variables and the effects of the anesthetics used will allow appropriate data interpretation within the context of the patient's current state.

Complications/Emergencies
Adverse events in the PCCCL are likely to be sudden and unexpected, despite occurring in up to 10% of all catheterization procedures.[2] The Pediatric Perioperative Cardiac Arrest (POCA) registry documented that one third of all perioperative cardiac arrests occur in children with CHD, with 17% of these arrests occurring in the PCCCL.[15] This reinforces the importance of understanding the physiology and pathophysiology of each patient, the challenges and risks accompanied with each procedure, and the potential impact of a chosen anesthetic technique.

The most common adverse events associated with cardiac catheterization are vascular injuries and arrhythmias, which account for approximately 34% and 23% of complications, respectively.[2,4] Minor events are transient and typically self-limiting. Major adverse events are described as those requiring significant intervention with potential permanent and detrimental effects. Examples of major events include bleeding, hypotension, perforation, cardiac arrest, stroke, and death. Despite the potential for major adverse events, the mortality in the cardiac catheterization laboratory remains low with death rates reported at 0.2% to 0.29%.[4,24]

POSTOPERATIVE CARE

Following the procedure, catheters are removed and pressure is held at the catheter access site to achieve hemostasis. A calm emergence facilitates hemostasis and allows for a smooth transition to the postoperative phase. Standard protocols advise a postprocedural "flat time" following femoral vascular access to avoid bleeding and hematoma formation.[25] During this time, it is recommended that a patient remain supine for typically a 2- to 6-hour period depending on the access obtained and the size of the catheters placed during the procedure.

In addition to maintaining flat time, appropriate postprocedure care includes standard postanesthesia concerns, such as managing nausea and vomiting, emergence delirium, hypoxemia, and apnea. During this time, additional procedures, such as echocardiograms or ECGs may be required. This can be facilitated with additional sedation if a patient is unlikely to be cooperative.

Overall, the care of patients in the pediatric congenital cardiac catheterization laboratory requires a comprehensive understanding of the procedure being performed and the specific cardiac lesion being addressed, thorough preoperative evaluation, and thoughtful planning. It is essential the anesthesia provider be in constant communication with the proceduralists throughout the entirety of the perioperative period to ensure optimal patient outcomes.

CASE STUDY: Cardiac Catheterization for New-Onset Pulmonary Hypertension

CLINICAL SCENARIO

An 8-year-old female is seen by her pediatrician for new onset of dyspnea and fatigue. Following a thorough evaluation, a transthoracic echocardiogram was obtained. The imaging demonstrated supra-systemic right ventricular pressures, a leftward bowing of the interventricular septum, and mild right ventricular dysfunction. These findings are concerning for idiopathic pulmonary hypertension. The patient now presents for a diagnostic cardiac catheterization procedure and PICC line placement. She has no prior medical diagnosis. Her family history is significant only for a maternal uncle with idiopathic pulmonary hypertension.

SPECIAL CONSIDERATIONS

Children with pulmonary hypertension have a 20-fold higher risk of perioperative cardiac arrest when compared to children without pulmonary hypertension.[28] Cardiac catheterization is the gold standard for the diagnosis of pulmonary hypertension as it is necessary to assess disease severity and plan appropriate treatment. In these patients, a full diagnostic cardiac catheterization procedure is performed in addition to acute vasoreactivity testing. Acute vasoreactivity testing assesses the hemodynamic response to therapies, such as pulmonary vasodilators (inhaled nitric oxide [iNO] and oxygen). The data obtained during the procedure will guide medical management.

APPROACHES TO CARE

Prior to inducing anesthesia, it is imperative that these patients receive a multidisciplinary team approach to formulate a safe plan, including emergency rescue support in the event of cardiac collapse. In addition to peripheral access, consider arterial access prior to induction as it will facilitate close blood pressure monitoring during induction of anesthesia. The goals of induction of anesthesia in patients with severe pulmonary hypertension are to maintain preload and SVR while avoiding increases in PVR. Generally, an inhalational induction should be avoided or undertaken with extreme caution in patients with severe pulmonary hypertension. Rather, slow titration of a combination of IV medications at lower doses is recommended.

Resuscitation medications, such as epinephrine, vasopressin, and/or phenylephrine, should be immediately available. For higher risk patients, inotropic and vasopressor infusions should be prepared with iNO readily available. Consider running a vasopressin or phenylephrine infusion during induction to maintain SVR and balance the decreased preload and vasodilation result of inducing general anesthesia. In these high-risk patients, ensuring that a team is available to place the patient on ECMO if decompensation occurs is advised.

Overall, from induction to emergence from anesthesia, the hemodynamic goals in patients with severe pulmonary hypertension continue—maintain preload, SVR, and minimize hypercarbia and hypoxia to avoid increases in PVR. These patients require extreme vigilance.

RESOURCES

Abman SH, Hansmann G, Archer SL. Pediatric pulmonary hypertension: guidelines from the American heart association and American thoracic society. *Circulation*. 2015;132(21):2037–2099. doi:10.1161/CIR.0000000000000329

Latham GJ, Yung D. Current understanding and perioperative management of pediatric pulmonary hypertension. *Pediatr Anesth*. 2019;29:441-456. DOI:10.1111/pan.13542

Rosenzweig E, Abman S, Adatia I, et al. Paediatric pulmonary arterial hypertension: updates on definition, classification, diagnostics and management. *Eur Respir J*. 2019;53(1):1801916. doi:10.1183/13993003.01916-2018

KEY REFERENCES

Complete references for this chapter are online and available at https://connect.springerpub.com/content/book/978-0-8261-3875-0/part/part04/toc-part/ch091.

1. Daaboul DG, DiNardo JA, Nasr VG. Anesthesia for high-risk procedures in the catheterization laboratory. *Pediatr Anesth*. 2019;29:491–498. doi:10.1111/pan.13571
2. Odegard KC, Vincent R, Baijal R, et al. SCAI/CCAS/SPA expert consensus statement for anesthesia and sedation practice: recommendations for patients undergoing diagnostic and therapeutic procedures in the pediatric and congenital cardiac catheterization laboratory. *Catheter Cardiovasc Interv*. 2016;88:912–922. doi:10.1002/ccd.26692
4. Lam JE, Lin EP, Alexy R, Aronson LA. Anesthesia and the pediatric cardiac catheterization suite: a review. *Pediatr Anesth*. 2015;25:127–134. doi:10.1111/pan.12551
7. Feltes TF, Bacha E, Beekman RH, et al. Indications for cardiac catheterization and intervention in pediatric cardiac disease: a scientific statement from the American Heart Association. *Circulation* 2011;123:2607–2652. doi:10.1161/CIR.0b013e31821b1f10
13. Lloyd DFA, Goreczny S, Austin C, et al. Catheter, MRI and CT imaging in newborns with pulmonary atresia with ventricular septal defect and aortopulmonary collaterals: quantifying the risks of radiation dose and anaesthetic time. *Pediatr Cardiol*. 2018;39:1308–1314. doi:10.1007/s00246-018-1895-7
19. Lin CH, Desai S, Nicolas R, et al. Sedation and anesthesia and congenital cardiac catheterization: a prospective multicenter experience. *Pediatric Cardiology*. 2015;36:1363–1375. doi:10.1007/s00246-015-1167-8
23. O'Byrne ML, Millenson ME, Steven JM, et al. Operator-directed procedural sedation in the congenital cardiac catheterization laboratory. *JACC Cardiovasc Interv*. 2019;12(9):835–843. doi:10.1016/j.jcin.2019.01.224

CHAPTER 92

Cardiac Electrophysiology Laboratory Procedures

Whitney S. Roberts, M. Leona A. Sayson, and Anne M. Peeke

INDICATIONS/CONTRAINDICATIONS

Electrophysiology studies (EPS) and radiofrequency catheter ablation (RFCA) have become a common intervention for cardiac arrhythmias largely due to the high success rates, low complication rates, and inefficacy of many antiarrhythmic medications. During the last two decades, the development of successful ablative strategies and better understanding of different arrhythmia mechanisms have resulted in RFCA being applied to increasingly complex substrates. Although RFCA has been associated with significant success rates, the natural history of cardiac arrhythmias and its potential life-threatening complications, and the effects of antiarrhythmic agents should all be considered against the risks associated with RFCA in young children.[1]

According to the American College of Cardiology and the American Heart Association Guidelines for Clinical Intracardiac Electrophysiological and Catheter Ablations, the performance and interpretation of intracardiac electrophysiological studies in children are generally similar to general indications in adults. The patient's age can influence indications for an electrophysiological study and dictate technical decisions, as can the presence of associated congenital heart lesions.[2] According to these guidelines, electrophysiological studies are performed to evaluate electrophysiological properties, such as automaticity, conduction, and refractoriness. Studies are also performed to initiate and terminate tachycardias, map activation sequences, evaluate patients' various forms of therapy, and judge response to therapy. These guidelines also acknowledge that each patient needs to be considered on a case-by-case basis, an electrophysiology procedure may not be the best treatment plan for all patients, some may have other treatments before, such as medical management, and all risks and benefits must be reviewed.[2]

Indications for ablation in the pediatric patient continue to develop as technology advances. While some patients require surgical intervention, others are medically managed. For example, ectopic atrial tachycardia (EAT) treatment depends on the patient's age and ventricular contractility. Patients with depressed function can benefit from slowing the ventricular rate. Agents including digoxin, beta-blockers, amiodarone, sotalol, and flecainide have all been used, but an empirical trial is necessary for each agent.[3] When EAT is persistent despite drug therapy or patients have displayed a tachycardia-induced myopathy, catheter ablation is an accepted therapy.[3]

Atrial flutter (AF) is an unusual rhythm for pediatric patients, and it is often associated with a history of congenital heart disease (CHD).[3] As previously mentioned, it is important to treat these patients on a case-by-case basis. Decisions need to take into account hemodynamic status, other possible arrhythmias, and the condition of the sinoatrial/atrioventricular (SA/AV) nodes. An AV blocking agent can be considered after conversion, but if the flutter becomes a recurrent issue, consulting an electrophysiologist is advised. Therapy for atrial fibrillation is similar to that of AF. If arrhythmia duration is uncertain, risk for atrial thrombi may alter treatment decisions.[3]

AV nodal reentrant tachycardia (AVNRT) can occasionally be managed conservatively with vagal maneuvers if symptoms are minimal. If tachycardia is prolonged, the decision between medication and ablation is dependent on the age of the patient and the family's preference. Ventricular tachycardia (VT) in children can have multiple causes, and there is no single condition sufficiently common in children to permit treatment recommendations. Some sites rely on electrophysiological studies to help guide therapy along a middle course for these patients.[3]

Wolff–Parkinson-White (WPW) syndrome has multiple presentations. It is important to assess patient age, presenting symptom severity, accessory pathway (AP) location, and anterograde conduction properties.[3] Pharmacology options are recommended in the first year of life, with propranolol most frequently used. If the orthodromic reciprocating tachycardia (ORT) symptoms are persistent, flecainide, sotalol, and amiodarone have been used. Ablation becomes an attractive treatment option for older children.[3]

ETIOLOGY OF CARDIAC ARRHYTHMIAS

The etiology of cardiac arrhythmias can be classified by (a) disorders related to impulse formation (automaticity or triggered activity), (b) disorders regarding impulse conduction (reentry or block), or (c) a combination of these two disorders. As classically known, the rapid spontaneous depolarization of the SA node makes it the natural pacemaker of the heart. Therefore, premature beats and tachycardias may be initiated before the SA node activity causing the disorders of either reentry or automaticity.[3,4]

Reentry

The most common mechanism for tachycardia is referred to as reentry. Reentry describes the single stimulus wave that can return and reactivate the same tissues from which it came from (Figure 92.1). The stimulus cannot simply walk backwards in its old pathway because cardiac cells require a refractory period after the initial depolarization; therefore, there must be a second pathway in the circuit (refer to limb B of Figure 92.1). The reentry pathway will cease promptly if one of the conduction limbs is adequately modified or interrupted using techniques like overriding pacing, pharmacological intervention, electrical cardioversion, or catheter ablation.[3]

The classic example of reentry pathway occurs in WPW. This pathway utilizes the AV node and an AP (like limb B in Figure 92.1) as the two limbs of the circuit. Reentry is also considered to be the operative mechanism for AF, atrial fibrillation, AV node reentry, and probably most forms of VT.

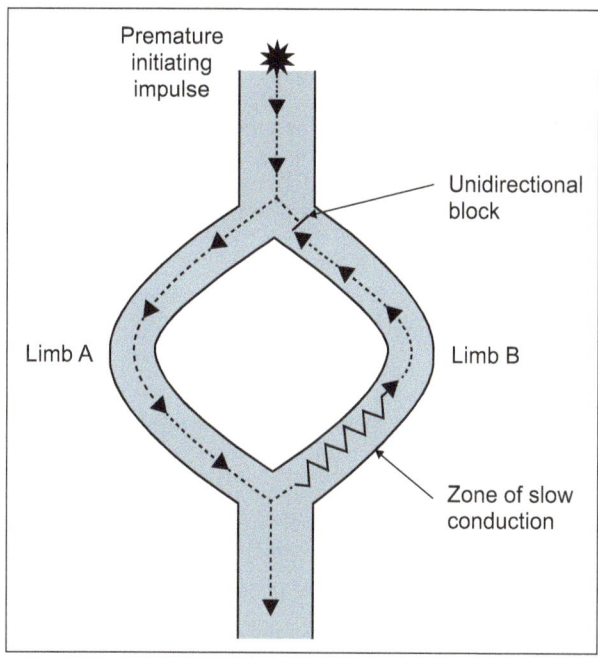

Figure 92.1: Reentry tachycardia.

Source: From Keane JF, Fyler DC, Lock JE, Teele S. *Nadas' Pediatric Cardiology Cardiac Arrhythmias.* 2nd ed. Elsevier; 2006: Chapter 29.

Reentry mechanisms more commonly attribute to narrow QRS tachycardia. AF is a single atrial entry circuit, which is a type of reentry mechanism within atrial muscle. Atrial fibrillation is another type of reentry mechanism except with multiple small reentry circuits.[3]

Abnormal Automaticity

Another mechanism of clinical tachycardia is enhanced automaticity with a focus outside the SA node, which promotes early achievement of threshold for the action potential. One abnormal activation can generate an isolated ectopic beat versus repetitive activation, which can generate a sustained tachycardia. This type of mechanism has been attributed to the possible mechanism of a few arrhythmias seen in children, such as EAT, multifocal atrial tachycardia (FAT), and junctional ectopic tachycardia (JET).[3]

Triggered Automaticity

The third mechanism is triggered automaticity. With this mechanism, the electrical triggers are small oscillations, which occur during the phase 3 or phase 4 of an action potential. These oscillations can trigger the action potential and generate one or more premature beats. It can be difficult to define the clinical features of triggered tachycardias in structurally normal hearts as there are often coinciding characteristics of both reentry and abnormal automaticity.[3]

TERMINOLOGY AND CLASSIFICATION OF TACHYCARDIA MECHANISM

When considering the effective management of tachycardia, an accurate identification of the mechanism of arrhythmia is essential. It is important anesthesia providers understand the site of origin and whether it is a reentrant or automatic type of tachycardia. It should be noted that the terms *supraventricular tachycardia* (SVT) and VT are extremely vague in describing the mechanism. The term SVT refers to any rapid rhythm from the atrium, the AV junction, or an AP. The term VT refers to any disordered rhythm, which originates from below the bifurcation of the bundle of His.[3] The vague nature of this nomenclature provides no guidance for a therapeutic management. A more effective classification scheme is offered in Table 92.1, one that can be more useful when determining the best approach to therapy.[3] Furthermore, ECG can help in providing diagnostic clues, such as timing, atrial depolarization ratio, and wide or narrow QRS width (Figure 92.2).[3]

The most common SVT seen in children with structurally normal hearts are AV reentry tachycardia (AVRT) facilitated by an AP, an AVNRT, and a FAT.[1] The occurrence of AVRT is most common in the neonatal and infant groups. Most of these patients will be free from symptomatic arrhythmia by the end of the first year of life, although it is well recognized that recurrence may be seen later in childhood or adolescence. It is also worth noting that spontaneous remission for those children older than 5 years of age at presentation is less common. AVNRT is rare in early childhood, although it becomes more frequent with increasing age.[1] Catheter ablation is an effective therapy for AVNRT in pediatric patients. There is a 78% to 100% nonrecurrence of AVNRT after ablation in children after follow-up time of 1 to 3 years. Most AVNRT

Table 92.1	Mechanisms for Clinical Tachycardia		
Sinoatrial Node		**Sinus Tachycardia**	
Atrium	Flutter	Ectopic at tachycardia	Some ectopic tachycardia?
	Fibrillation	Multifocal at tachycardia	
AV junction	AV node reentry	Junctional ectopic tachycardia	
Ventricle	Monomorphic VT	Focal VT	Torsades de pointes?
	Polymorphic VT		Some focal VT?
Accessory pathways	ORT (WPW)		
	ORT (URAP)		
	ORT (PJRT)		
	ART (WPW)		
	ART (Mahaim)		
	Preexcited atrial fibrillation		

ART, antidomic reciprocating tachycardia; AV, atrioventricular; ORT, orthodromic reciprocating tachycardia; PJRT, permanent junctional reciprocating tachycardia; URAP, unidirectional retrograde anomalous pathway. VT, ventricular tachycardia; WPW, Wolff–Parkinson–White syndrome.

Source: From Keane, JF, Fyler DC, Lock JE, Teele S. *Nadas' Pediatric Cardiology Cardiac Arrhythmias.* 2nd ed. Elsevier; 2006: Chapter 29.

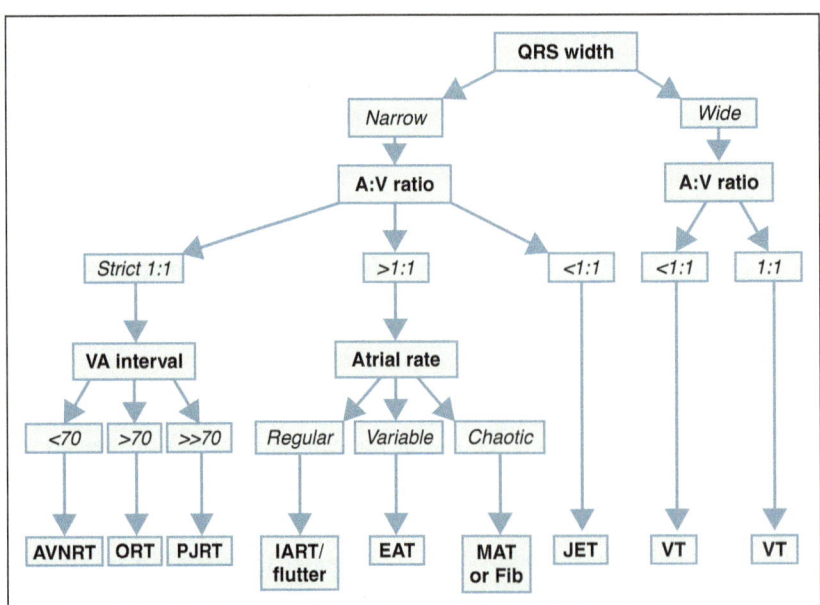

Figure 92.2: Differential diagnosis of tachycardia. Practical scheme for determining the most likely mechanism for a clinical tachycardia based on ECG features.

AVNRT, atrioventricular nodal reentry tachycardia; EAT, ectopic atrial tachycardia; IART, intra-atrial reentrant tachycardia; JET, junctional ectopic tachycardia; MAT, multifocal atrial tachycardia; PJRT, permanent junctional reciprocating tachycardia; ORT, orthodromic reciprocating tachycardia; VA, ventriculoatrial; VT, ventricular tachycardia.

Source: From Keane, JF, Fyler DC, Lock JE, Teele S. *Nadas' Pediatric Cardiology Cardiac Arrhythmias.* 2nd ed. Elsevier; 2006: Chapter 29.

recurrences were noted within the first year after ablation. The long-term follow-up study performed by Backhoff et al. demonstrated a substantial portion of AVNRT recurrences occurred well after ablation, sometimes even 5 years after.[5] Other less common mechanisms include JET, and permanent junctional reciprocating tachycardia (PJRT).

CATHETER ABLATION

Catheter ablation is performed by applying energy to the cardiac tissue using an ablation catheter. The applied energy creates a transmural lesion in the myocardial wall to interrupt the disordered pathway. There are various types of energy which can be applied, but radiofrequency energy is the most utilized because it is effective and simple to use. The ablation catheter is used to apply the radiofrequency to heat the cardiac tissue through direct resistive heating. This results in irreversible coagulation necrosis, which evolves into a scar.[4]

Cryoablation is an alternative energy source used for catheter ablation. Cryoablation delivers liquid nitrous oxide under pressure through the catheter tip or within the balloon (if balloon-based catheter is used) where it turns to gaseous state. This results in freezing the cardiac tissues and disrupts the cell membranes, leading to cell death.[4]

Catheter ablation has become the choice for treating pediatric patients with tachyarrhythmias for several reasons. Catheter ablation avoids the prolonged exposure to antiarrhythmic agents, which may have unideal side effects. Secondly, ablation targets specific areas, such as APs, which are congenital disorders that may often produce its most debilitating effects in the earlier years of life and therefore, require definitive treatment before the patient reaches adulthood. Furthermore, there is an increasing number of young patients who undergo surgical repair of CHD who develop scar-related atrial and ventricular arrhythmias. These tachyarrhythmias have been known to be particularly resistant to pharmacological interventions.[6] The recent evolution of techniques for high-density mapping of postoperative atrial tachycardia has resulted in improved ability to determine specific activation pathways and target these specific sites for ablation.[7] These are some of the reasons for which catheter ablation has been widely accepted as a cornerstone of treating tachyarrhythmias in pediatric patients. Table 92.2 offers a summary of the indications for RFCA procedures in pediatric patients as reported by a recent expert consensus conference.[1] However, as technology advances and new clinical outcome data become available, indications for catheter ablation in children will evolve. The final decision to recommend catheter ablation will require case-by-case considerations.

SPECIAL CONSIDERATIONS AND CONCERNS

CATHETER ABLATION IN INFANTS (<1 YEAR OF AGE)

RFCA in infants less than 15 kg has traditionally been associated with increased complications. Typically, RFCA is deferred because of the known predominant tachycardia mechanism related to this age group unless a refractory or life-threatening arrhythmia with associated ventricular dysfunction is known.[1] A retrospective analysis concluded that RFCA performed by experienced operators is an advantage to the management of life-threatening arrhythmia in this age group. Additionally, there is no difference in success rates in all tachycardia mechanisms or incidence of major complications.[8]

ISSUES RELATED TO CONGENITAL HEART DISEASE

Children and young adults with CHD pose unique challenges during ablation procedures. The distorted anatomy makes it difficult to identify fluoroscopic landmarks that are conventional to catheter manipulation in an anatomically normal heart. Therefore, it is paramount to understand the underlying cardiac anatomy and surgical interventions to safely anticipate chamber malposition, surgical patches, or redirected vasculature. This is especially true with patients who have intra-atrial baffles placed, such as those used for Mustard, Senning, and Fontan operations.[6]

Among older children and young adults who have undergone these operations, a large number of them encounter late-onset postoperative tachyarrhythmias; most common of which is intra-atrial reentrant tachycardia (IART). This tachyarrhythmia continues to be a source of high morbidity in this patient population.[6] VT can occur in late postoperative period in a subset of these patients who undergo ventriculotomy or ventricular patch during their cardiac surgery. This is most concerning following surgical repair of tetralogy of Fallot, as VT and sudden cardiac death occur in 4.2% and 2.0% of patients, respectively, postoperatively.[9] Because VT can result in sudden cardiac death and catheter ablation is less-than-certain intervention at present, there is hesitation to rely solely on ablative therapy. Although ablation maintains an important role in therapy, implantable cardioverter defibrillator (ICD) is the preferred therapy for VT in patients with CHD.[6]

WPW can cause sudden death in otherwise healthy children. This occurrence is rare but potentially preventable. The sudden death is usually due to atrial fibrillation with rapid conduction over an AP, which causes ventricular fibrillation

Table 92.2	Key Assessment Points
Key Points	**Notes**
Medical/surgical history	A thorough review of all systems, particular attention to the cardiovascular portion, past surgeries/cardiac interventions, functional status
Medications	Current antiarrhythmic agents, diuretics, heart failure medications, etc.
Diagnostic imaging	ECG, echocardiogram, chest x-ray, CT/MRI
Laboratory tests	Patient specific, electrolytes, complete blood count, coagulation panel
Physical examination	Overall appearance, signs of heart failure, current vital signs (compared to previous vital signs?)

Source: From Deng, Y., Naeini PS, Razavi, M., Collard CD, Tolpin DA, Anton JM. Anesthetic management in radiofrequency catheter ablation of ventricular tachycardia. *Tex Heart Inst J.* 2016;43(6):496–502.

(VF). Therefore, it is important to consider EPS as a preventative strategy against this life-threatening event (LTE). EPS that can identify inducible AVRT or pathway capable of rapid anterograde conduction is considered a predictor of malignant arrhythmia. This finding may render catheter ablation and cure WPW syndrome and eliminate the risk of LTE.[10]

Congenital cardiac defects are often associated with the presence of APs. Although these APs can occur in a variety of malformations, it is most associated with Ebstein's malformation. Patients with this malformation often undergo catheter ablation before surgical correction because catheter access may be rendered difficult following repair. In addition, recurrent SVT can be problematic and associated with morbidity postoperatively.[6]

Overall, catheter ablation in patients with CHD is a challenging task, even with advances in preoperative anatomical mapping. Lower acute success rates reported at 80% to 85% and the recurrence risk reported as high as 15% to 20%.[6]

ANESTHETIC MANAGEMENT

PREOPERATIVE EVALUATION

There are a wide range of patients who come to the electrophysiology laboratory for a variety of procedures and disease processes. This requires anesthesia providers to be flexible in the preprocedural planning; they need to be familiar with the pathophysiology while anticipating hemodynamic changes and possible complications from the procedure. A comprehensive pre-procedure evaluation is crucial to the safety and success of the procedure (see Table 92.2). The preoperative assessment is guided by the patient's medical history, with particular attention to the cardiovascular review. A thorough assessment includes exploration of their previous cardiac interventions, ECG, echocardiogram, and chest radiography. Laboratory data should include, but not limited to, complete blood cell count and chemistry and coagulation panel. Current and/or recent changes to their medications or functional status are essential.[11] Patients with arrhythmias can be sensitive to metabolic derangements, and preoperative laboratory analysis is important.[4,12] Some arrhythmias, such as long QT syndrome (LQTS), can have a genetic component, so a thorough family history is warranted.[12] On the day of the procedure, or preoperative clinic if available, a thorough physical examination is important, along with reviewing vital signs and if this patient remains at their baseline hemodynamics. Many of these patients have had multiple blood draws and procedures in the past. As such, obtaining IV access may be difficult, and anesthesia providers should consider having ultrasound readily available.[13]

PREOPERATIVE PHARMACOLOGY

The preoperative period can be a time of significant anxiety for pediatric patients undergoing any procedure conducted in the electrophysiology laboratory. Anxiety, fear of the unknown, and ultimately the separation from parents all contribute to inducing a significant stress response. Abating this response as well as the profound sympathetic surge that accompanies it may be an important consideration. Commonly used medications for anxiolysis in the pediatric population include midazolam, ketamine, and dexmedetomidine.[12]

Midazolam, a benzodiazepine, is one of the most used sedatives in the electrophysiology laboratory. Its sedative, anxiolytic, and amnestic properties are valuable in most types of anesthetics. It has a relatively short half-life, minimal effect on hemodynamics, and causes very few effects on the cardiac conduction system.

Ketamine, an N-methyl-D-aspartate (NMDA) receptor antagonist, exhibits unique qualities in relation to its effect on cardiac electrophysiology while also having sedative and pain-relieving properties. Ketamine stimulates the sympathetic nervous system, increases heart rate and blood pressure, and may facilitate the induction of arrhythmias.[14] These stimulatory effects may be useful in patients with preexisting hemodynamic instability.[4] However, these same effects may be detrimental in some syndromes, such as LQTC, and should be avoided if possible.[12]

The use of dexmedetomidine, an alpha-2 receptor agonist, has been increasing in frequency for both premedication and sedation in the pediatric population.[12] Its ability to sedate and relieve pain without depressing the respiratory system makes it an ideal choice for many procedures. However, data regarding the use of dexmedetomidine during an EPS are conflicting. Several studies have shown it to cause decreased central sympathetic outflow with subsequent bradycardia and hypotension, potentially making it a poor choice for ablations of tachyarrhythmias.[4,14,15] In contrast, it has been reported that the use of dexmedetomidine does not interfere with EPS for SVT ablation; however, the greater use of isoproterenol was required for success.[16] So, while the use of dexmedetomidine may be discussed with the electrophysiologist preoperatively as a safe option for some pediatric patients, more studies are needed to clarify its use in the electrophysiology laboratory.[14]

ANESTHETIC MANAGEMENT

Intraoperative Management

There is a wide range of patients who present for EPS, ranging from young, otherwise healthy patients with intermittent SVT to more complex patients with congenital abnormalities and multiple comorbidities. When choosing the best choice of anesthetic for patients presenting to the electrophysiology laboratory, anesthesia providers must consider a multitude of factors. Anesthesia providers should appreciate that EPS and related procedures can cause significant discomfort and anxiety for many patients due to the placement of multiple IV and arterial catheters, the long duration of some procedures, and the uncomfortable symptoms arrhythmias can induce.[14] In addition, the procedure being performed, whether inducibility is required, and what the pediatric patient will be able to tolerate must all be considered.

EPS and RFCA have been successfully done with sedation, monitored anesthesia care (MAC), and general anesthesia (GA). The choice of anesthetic agent and adjuncts must also be carefully considered, as many of the medications used by anesthesia providers may contribute to hemodynamic instability or have direct effects on the arrhythmia being diagnosed and/or treated.

Although some procedures can be done under sedation provided by a trained registered nurse,[14] several patient factors may require the need for anesthesia's involvement. These include nonreassuring airway examination, obesity, pulmonary disease, hemodynamic instability, chronic pain, and previous failed sedation.[17] In some cases, the type of anesthetic required may be subject to change during the procedure and conversion from sedation to GA may be necessary.[14] Anxiety, as well as the patient's inability to lie still for a significant period, may ultimately deem sedation inappropriate and unsafe.

When choosing between MAC and GA, anesthesia providers must consider that many of the anesthetic agents commonly used can affect cardiac electrophysiology and conduction, altering the ability to induce the abnormal rhythm and having a negative impact on mapping and ablation treatment.[14] For certain arrhythmias, inducibility is vital for diagnostics, potentially making MAC a better choice.[15] In some instances, diagnostics and mapping may be completed under light sedation, and once complete, the conversion to GA for the ablation portion of the procedures is indicated. The ideal anesthetic would provide patient comfort, adequate airway and ventilation, minimal patient motion, and optimal catheter stability.[14] The flexibility of anesthesia providers is essential when considering anesthetic options, and adequate communication with the cardiology interventionalists is required.

The induction agent of anesthesia in the pediatric population is always chosen on a case-by-case basis. While IV catheter placement is often the safer option, doing so with an awake child may have deleterious effects, both psychologically and hemodynamically, depending on the patient's medical history.[12] Premedication may be helpful, but even this can be challenging with an uncooperative child. In these cases, an inhalation induction may be the best option.

Volatile anesthetic agents are known to slow the rate of SA conduction node discharge as well as prolong AV conduction time.[14] In addition, they can prolong action potential duration, delay atrial and ventricular repolarization, and decrease the inducibility of tachyarrhythmias in vitro.[15] However, modern inhaled anesthetics, such as isoflurane, sevoflurane, and desflurane, have been used successfully in children undergoing procedures in the electrophysiology laboratory.[14] This is particularly true in patients presenting for prolonged and complex procedures when catheter stability and control of ventilation are required.[15,17] Some evidence suggests a higher success rate and shorter procedural and fluoroscopy times with GA; however, it is not necessarily attributed to the anesthetic agent.[14,17] Nitrous oxide has been used safely, although should be used with caution as it possesses sympathomimetic properties, which may be undesirable in some arrhythmogenic syndromes.[12]

Propofol is a widely used sedation, induction, and maintenance anesthetic agent due to its rapid onset and recovery. In the electrophysiology laboratory, propofol is often used as it has little or no clinically significant effect on the electrophysiological expression of the AP and refractoriness of the normal AV conduction system and has no direct effect on SA node activity or intra-atrial conduction.[4,18] Propofol's disadvantages include its depressive effects on hemodynamics. In addition, propofol infusions may decrease the inducibility of tachyarrhythmias in the pediatric population.[14]

Fentanyl is commonly used for sedation and GA given its relatively short half-life, stable hemodynamic profile, and a lack of significant effect on arrhythmia inducibility.[12,14,17] Fentanyl is useful for achieving adequate depth of anesthesia, as light anesthesia during laryngoscopy may produce sympathetic stimulation resulting in cardiac events in certain patients.[12] Fentanyl can increase vagal tone and prolong sinus node recovery, so minimal usage for certain VT ablation procedures is sometimes advised, as inducibility of these arrhythmias may be extremely sensitive to sedation.[14,15]

Remifentanil infusions should be used with caution due to the inhibition of the sinus and AV node function and subsequent bradycardia. While some studies report success with remifentanil for EPS, its use remains controversial and sometimes contraindicated in the electrophysiology laboratory because of its cardiac depressant effects.[4,12,14]

Neuromuscular blocking agents are often employed, and certain procedures require control of ventilation, deeming muscle relaxation necessary.[15] When extensive mapping is required, the use of neuromuscular blocking agents may be the only way to ensure immobility of the pediatric population and avoid prolongation of the procedure and possible injury to the patient.[4,17,19] When choosing a muscle relaxant, there are several key considerations. Succinylcholine can precipitate both brady- and tachyarrhythmias, as well as prolong the QT interval and abruptly shift potassium levels.[4,12] For these reasons, succinylcholine is often avoided. Pancuronium has vagolytic properties and may increase the heart rate and is associated with histamine release, making it a less desirable option in the electrophysiology laboratory. While vecuronium and rocuronium have little association with histamine release, vecuronium has been associated with bradycardia. There are some studies that show no significant change in heart rate associated with rocuronium.[4] As the use of sugammadex for reversal becomes more widely available, rocuronium has the added advantage of easy reversibility without the hemodynamic effects and QT prolongation of traditional reversal agents, such as neostigmine and glycopyrrolate.[12] In some instances, muscle relaxation should be avoided in the electrophysiology laboratory, such as in cases where the phrenic nerve requires monitoring. But when indicated, rocuronium may be the agent of choice.

As with any procedure requiring anesthesia, EPS and ablation are performed with standard monitors as recommended by the American Society of Anesthesiologists.[15] The need for invasive arterial monitoring may be indicated if the patient is hemodynamically unstable or has comorbidities that warrant more close monitoring.[15,19] In some cases, surgically placed femoral arterial access can be shared with the anesthesia provider; however, separate radial artery access may be preferred if continuous monitoring is preferred or continuous monitoring postoperatively is required.[4] Similarly, femoral central venous access obtained for the procedure can be shared, but if separate central monitoring is needed or peripheral access is inadequate, jugular or subclavian access should be considered.[4] Generally, two peripheral IV catheters are adequate, although this should be decided on an individual basis. Esophageal temperature monitoring is useful for preventing intraprocedural hypothermia as well as esophageal injury during certain ablation techniques.[15,19] Defibrillator pads should be positioned prior to initiating the procedure if cardioversion, defibrillation, or external pacing is required.[4,19] Foley catheter insertion may be necessary for longer procedures and when careful monitoring of fluid balance is indicated. In addition to monitoring the fluids administered by the anesthesia provider, fluid administered by the electrophysiology team must also be accounted for.[4,19] For longer duration procedures, anesthesia providers must consider the risk of pressure ulcers. Careful positioning and padding of pressure points are imperative.

Emergence from anesthesia is a dynamic time with potential for sympathetic stimulation. In addition to coughing associated with extubation, the potential for rebleeding is increased during this time. Deep extubation may be considered to avoid the effects of emergence with an airway in place.[12] Some form of sedation is often employed, and a calm quiet environment must be established to assist the child in lying flat for this extended period.

Special Techniques and/or Equipment

Systemic anticoagulation is often required for electrophysiology procedures after insertion of the femoral sheaths to prevent thrombus formation. Typically, a bolus of heparin is administered, sometimes followed by an infusion, to a targeted activated clotting time (ACT) 300 to 400 seconds.[4,15,19] At the end of the procedure, depending on the ACT, protamine may be used to reverse the effect of heparin prior to removing vascular sheaths.[4,15] Protamine should be administered slowly as it has several detrimental side effects and can cause severe hypotension.

Vasoactive agents may be necessary for inducing arrhythmias and cardiac mapping.[4,15] Isoproterenol is a beta-adrenergic drug used to increase the heart rate and facilitate the induction of SVT and VT. It is also used to test the results of ablation. Isoproterenol is typically administered by infusion in incremental doses between 0.01 and 0.1 mcg/kg/min.[4] Hemodynamic instability can occur during arrhythmias and mapping and may require the use of inotropic/vasopressor agents. The use of these agents should be communicated to the cardiologist to achieve successful mapping while maintaining patient safety.[19]

An adenosine challenge has been widely used for decades as a tool for the evaluation and diagnosis of AV preexcitation. Its safety for use has been demonstrated at length in the adult population and there are data to suggest that it is also safe to use in pediatrics even in the presence of complex CHD.[20] It is typically administered by the cardiologist starting at 0.1 mg/kg and can be doubled if subsequent doses are necessary. Anesthesia providers should be aware that bronchospasm has occurred in patients with reactive airway disease and the patient's respiratory status should be monitored regardless of anesthetic technique being employed.

The risk of postoperative nausea and vomiting (PONV) should be considered, especially in high-risk patients. Ondansetron is an effective antiemetic but has been shown to interact with cardiac ion channels and prolong the QT interval. Current recommendation is to administer with caution with appropriate cardiac monitoring.[12] Dexamethasone can also be effective for PONV prophylaxis but is often undesired by the electrophysiology team after ablation procedures due to the many side effects including hyperglycemia, poor wound healing, and potential for inadequate scar formation at the ablation sites.[21] Low-dose propofol infusions at sub-hypnotic doses (15–25 mcg/kg/min) have demonstrated the ability to reduce postoperative vomiting[21] and should be considered in high-risk patients.

Clinical Pearls

The electrophysiology laboratory itself poses unique challenges for the anesthetist as they are often designed according to the preference of the cardiologist performing the procedures.[4] Careful management and organization of anesthesia equipment are necessary. Frequently, anesthesia providers must work around electrophysiology equipment, such as fluoroscopes, that are required for many of the procedures. This may present an added challenge when accessing the patient or manipulating the airway, particularly once the procedure has begun and space is limited. Anesthesia circuits, IV and arterial lines, and monitoring cables often require extensions to overcome the field avoidance and increased distance between the anesthesia equipment and the patient.[4,11] It is imperative that anesthesia providers understand and feel comfortable with their surroundings in this off-site anesthetizing location.

Radiation exposure is another aspect of the electrophysiology laboratory that needs to be considered for both anesthesia providers and the patients. The use of minimally invasive techniques has increased steadily over the past several years, making the use of fluoroscopy even more common. In many institutions, women of childbearing age are screened for pregnancy before the procedure is performed.[22] Anesthesia providers in these locations are also at a higher risk of radiation exposure, and effort should be made to limit exposure. This can be done by decreasing time exposed to radiation as much as possible and increasing personal distance from the source of radiation.[23] Anesthesia providers should don appropriate personal safety equipment as well, including front and back lead with a thyroid shield and lead glasses. Many institutions require providers who are frequently in the electrophysiology laboratory to wear a personal dosimeter.[23] Stationary and rolling lead shields are often available and should be used whenever long periods of radiation exposure are unavoidable.[4]

Complications/Emergencies

Complications related to EPS include cardiac tamponade, pulmonary vein stenosis, thromboembolism, embolic stroke, and atrioesophageal fistula formation. Pulmonary edema and heart failure can occur in cases of fluid overload resulting from fluid administered via ablation catheters unaccounted for by the anesthetist.[4,15] Catheter-induced heart block (CIHB) has been reported in the pediatric electrophysiology laboratory, although the incidence is low (2.2%) and the majority regain conduction within a week.

CASE STUDY: Electrophysiology Study and Ablation for Wolff–Parkinson–White

CLINICAL SCENARIO

A 7-year-old female 28.3 kg, 126 cm, with no known drug allergies presents with WPW for EPS and ablation. Diagnosed after ECG obtained for abnormal heart sound auscultated by primary care physician (PCP). Complains of self-terminating palpitations two to three times per month for several months. Denies syncope, shortness of breath, or other symptoms during episodes. Another medical history includes attention-deficit/hyperactivity disorder without medical intervention.

Preoperative Testing

- **ECG**: sinus rhythm with shortened PR interval (due to conduction over the faster AP) and slurred upstroke of QRS complex "delta wave" (due to fusion of impulses that pass through AV node and those that pass via the AP)
- **Echo**: structurally and functionally normal heart

(continued)

CASE STUDY: Electrophysiology Study and Ablation for Wolff–Parkinson–White (*continued*)

- **Labs:** hemoglobin 13.9; hematocrit 38.2; white blood cell count 5.61; platelets 233; type and screen
- **Vital Signs:** temperature 36.7 °C; heart rate 83; respiratory rate 20; blood pressure 110/58 (68); SaO_2 99%

Physical Examination

Well-appearing cooperative child. Breath sounds clear to auscultation bilaterally, heart sounds S1, S2 with 2/6 vibratory murmur best heard at lower left sternal border. Skin warm, capillary refill less than 2 seconds. Adequate mouth opening, Mallampati score 1, thyromental distance >2 finger breadths, full neck range of motion.

SPECIAL CONSIDERATIONS

- Use caution to avoid increases in sympathetic tone as this may induce tachycardias.
- Reduce anxiety, pain, and hypovolemia.
- Patients with WPW who develop atrial arrhythmia intraoperatively should not be given nodal blockers or carotid massage.
- Cardioversion and/or sodium channel blockers (e.g., procainamide) are the first-line therapy for atrial fibrillation/flutter in patients with WPW.
- Treatment of narrow complex arrhythmias (AVRT) is similar to that of SVT.

Drugs to Avoid in WPW	
Sympathomimetics Desflurane, atropine, glycopyrrolate, ketamine	Sympathomimetics can increase AV nodal conduction time, which may result in greater conduction via AP
Neostigmine	Slows AV nodal conduction and facilitates AP conduction
Nodal blockers (for Afib, Aflutter) Adenosine, calcium channel blocker, beta-blockers, digoxin	Slow AV nodal conduction and allow for greater conduction through the faster conducting AP
Note: Nodal blockers can be administered for **narrow complex** arrhythmias to slow the rate.	

APPROACHES TO CARE

Preoperative
- PO midazolam 0.5 to 0.75 mg/kg max 20 mg

Intraoperative
- Standard American Society of Anesthesiologists monitors
- Defibrillator pads applied
- Antiarrhythmics available
- Inhalation induction with N_2O/O_2/Sevo
- Peripheral intravenous catheter (PIV) × 2
- After PIV established, administer fentanyl (0.5–1 mcg/kg) and rocuronium (0.6–1.2 mg/kg)
- GETA with cuffed endotracheal tube 5.0 mm. Placement verified with fluoroscopy
- Careful positioning with pressure points padded and checked (procedure time several hours)
- Maintained with inhalation agent (isoflurane used in this case)
- Muscle relaxation for cardiac mapping maintained with rocuronium
- Adequate hydration based on weight and NPO time (4–2–1 rule)
- Vascular access for EPS and ablation: right femoral vein, left femoral vein
- Heparin administered for clot prophylaxis
- Isoproterenol administered per cardiologist order for arrhythmia induction
- Adenosine administered after ablation to evaluate for latent AV preexcitation
- At conclusion of procedure, pressure held on groin until hemostasis achieved
- Muscle relaxant reversal with sugammadex (2 mg/kg), patient with >2/4 twitches on train-of-four monitor
- Pain control: fentanyl, Tylenol, local injected by cardiologist at vascular access sites
- PONV prophylaxis with Zofran (0.1 mg/kg)
- Patient lies flat for 4 hours post-hematosis; care taken to avoid rebleeding as vascular access sites. May require sedative (dexmedetomidine 0.5 mcg/kg titrated to effect). Dim and quiet recovery room

However, a small number of patients may require pacemaker placement.[24]

POSTOPERATIVE CARE

Once the procedure is complete, removing vascular sheaths requires several minutes of direct pressure to achieve hemostasis. For venous sheaths, this is typically 10 to 15 minutes while arterial sheaths require 15 to 20 minutes or more. Percutaneous closure devices may be considered for patients who were not able to receive protamine or may not tolerate lying flat for extended periods.[4] Hemodynamics, fluid balance, and patient neurological status should be monitored closely in the postoperative period. The likelihood of complications associated with electrophysiology procedures should also be considered when postoperative disposition is decided.

Patients are required to lie flat for 4 to 6 hours postoperatively, maintaining this during that time; however, this can often be a challenge. Patients are also discouraged from lifting their heads without assistance due to the risk of rebleeding at the femoral site.[4,15] Hence, additional sedation may be required to facilitate patient compliance with remaining immobile. If rebleeding does occur, direct pressure will have to be applied again and the patient must lie flat for an additional 4 hours after hemostasis is achieved.[4]

KEY REFERENCES

Complete references for this chapter are online and available at https://connect.springerpub.com/content/book/978-0-8261-3875-0/part/part04/toc-part/ch092.

10. Etheridge S, Escudero C, Blaufox A, et al. Life-threatening event risk in children with Wolff-Parkinson-White Syndrome. *Clin Electrophysiol.* 2018;4:433–444. doi:10.1016/j.jacep.2017.10.009
12. Staudt G, Watkins S. Anesthetic considerations for pediatric patients with congenital long QT syndrome. *J Cardiothorac Vasc Anesth.* 2019;33:2030–2038. doi:10.1053/j.jvca.2018.11.005
14. Vladinov G, Fermin L, Longini R, et al. Choosing the anesthetic and sedative drugs for supraventricular tachycardia ablations: a focused review. *Pacing Clin Electrophysiol.* 2018;41:1555–1563. doi:10.1111/pace.13511
20. Follansbee CW, Beerman LB, Wu L, et al. Utility and safety of adenosine challenge for subtle ventricular pre-excitation in the pediatric population. *J Cardiovasc Electrophysiol.* 2019;30:1036–1041. doi:10.1111/jce.13935
21. Lee Y, Banooni A, Yuki K, et al. Incidence and predictors of postoperative nausea and vomiting in children undergoing electrophysiology ablation procedures. *Paediatr Anaesth.* 2019;30(2):147–152. doi:10.1111/pan.13797
23. Fujii S, Zhou JR, Dhir A. Anesthesia for cardiac ablation. *J Cardiothorac Vasc Anesth.* 2018;32. doi:10.1053/j.jvca.2017.12.039

CHAPTER 93

Care of Children With Heart Disease Undergoing Noncardiac Surgery

Jamie W. Sinton, Brian J. Gronert, Peace C. Madueme, and Karen S. Bender

INDICATIONS/CONTRAINDICATIONS

The incidence of congenital heart disease (CHD) has been estimated to be 6 out of every 1,000 live births.[1] CHD can be broadly classified into acyanotic, cyanotic, major vascular disease, and pulmonary hypertension (PH). This classification, in addition to single-ventricle lesions and adult CHD, is used to organize the anesthetic management for remainder of the chapter.

Noncardiac surgery is often needed in children and adults with CHD and carries substantial risk.[2] While the indications and contraindications are procedure specific, perioperative risks can be impacted by the type of surgery,[3] stage of heart defect palliation[4] and case volume at a given center.[5] The overall mortality in children with CHD undergoing noncardiac (CNC) surgery is 2.8% compared to 1.2% in patients without CHD.[6] Those at the highest risk of complications are patients with single-ventricle heart disease, PH, cardiomyopathies, and ventricular assist devices in place.[7-9]

At the time of the writing of this text, a multicenter study titled "Outcomes and Healthcare Resource Utilization in Patients With Congenital Heart Disease Undergoing Noncardiac Procedures" is planned to better discern more granular details for risk stratification, resource utilization, and management of this group of patients.

COMMON PRESENTING CARDIAC CONDITIONS

Please refer to Chapter 17, "Cardiovascular Conditions" for more information regarding cardiac conditions pediatric patients may present with.

Acyanotic Defects

Acyanotic defects include left-to-right shunting lesions as well as cardiomyopathy, obstructive and valvular lesions. See Figure 93.1 for further classification of acyanotic lesions by magnitude of pulmonary blood flow.

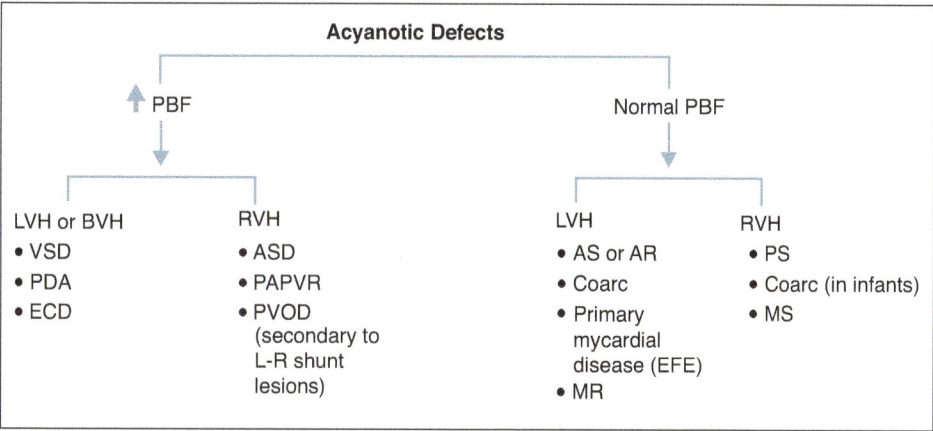

Figure 93.1: Acyanotic defects.

AS, aortic stenosis; ASD, atrial septal defect; BVH, biventricular hypertrophy; LVH, left ventricular hypertrophy; PAPVR, partial anomalous pulmonary venous return; PBF, pulmonary blood flow; PDA, patent ductus arteriosus; PS, pulmonic stenosis; PVOD, pulmonary veno-occlusive disease; RVH, right ventricular hypertrophy; VSD, ventricular septal defect.

Septal Defects

Left-to-right shunts are often due to septal defects. Magnitude of shunt depends on the size of the defect and the blood viscosity (determined by hematocrit). See **Figure 93.2** for details. For atrial level shunts, magnitude of shunt is also determined by relative ventricular compliance. In normal hearts, the right ventricle is much more elastic than the thicker left ventricle. Therefore, blood flows left to right across the atrial septum. Repair of an atrial septal defect (ASD) is indicated if right heart dilation is present. Preschool age is a common time for repair of a secundum ASD. ASD repairs may be catheter-based or open surgical repairs. **Figure 93.3A** shows types of ASDs.

For ventricular and great vessel level shunts, magnitude of shunting depends on pressure gradient between the chambers and the ratio of pulmonary to systemic vascular resistance. Qualitatively, ventricular septal defect (VSD) size is compared to the aortic valve annulus size of that patient. Indications for repair of VSDs include aortic valve insufficiency and left-sided heart dilation. See **Figure 93.3B** for types of VSDs.

An atrioventricular septal defect (AVSD) or atrioventricular canal (AVC) defect is due to absence of the AV septum and is an endocardial cushion defect. The AVSD forms from endocardial cushion and the AV septum separates the tricuspid from the mitral valve. With a complete atrioventricular canal (CAVC) defect, the AV septum is absent, and the AV valves share an annulus. Left-to-right shunting in this defect is often torrential and operative repair is undertaken in infancy. Davey et al. explain that repair of AVSD lesions never results in completely normal AV valves.[10]

Obstructive Lesions

Acyanotic lesions with normal pulmonary blood flow are obstructive lesions, such as aortic stenosis and Williams syndrome. Left ventricular outflow tract obstruction (LVOTO) promotes development of left ventricular hypertrophy (LVH), increasing its myocardial oxygen consumption and reducing ability to increase coronary perfusion pressure. Critical neonatal aortic stenosis occurs when a minimal amount of blood is ejected across the native aortic valve such that systemic and coronary perfusion must be retrograde via the patent ductus arteriosus (PDA). Neonates are prostaglandin-dependent. If they have adequately sized left-sided structures, they undergo dilation of the aortic valve. Post-dilation, infants are often left with residual obstruction and iatrogenic aortic insufficiency. If there is significantly turbulent flow across the diseased valve, endocarditis prophylaxis may be recommended by the cardiologist.

Deletion of the elastin gene on chromosome 7 produces Williams syndrome. A decreased amount and function of elastin collectively lead to thickening and reduced compliance of arterial media. Supravalvar aortic stenosis, pulmonic stenosis, and hooded coronary ostia result. The aorta is poorly distensible during systole and has poor diastolic recoil leading to limited coronary perfusion (Windkessel effect). Children with Williams syndrome are at exceedingly high risk of arrest under anesthesia.[11] Classically, children with Williams syndrome have elfin facies and a cocktail personality. Other manifestations include prolonged QT interval, generalized anxiety disorder (or other psychiatric condition), endocrine problems such as hypercalcemia, abdominal pain, subclinical hypothyroidism, and glucose intolerance. Surgical treatment of supravalvar aortic stenosis occurs prior to the onset of severe LVH. Any infant undergoing noncardiac surgery should have immediate access to extracorporeal support. If a child has not required intracardiac repair by preschool age, anesthetic risk is decreased and noncardiac surgery could be considered without immediate availability of extracorporeal support. Goals of anesthetic induction for a patient with Williams syndrome include maintaining preload, afterload, and coronary perfusion pressure (CPP). Adequate CPP is a diastolic blood pressure that is 20 mm Hg above left ventricular end-diastolic pressure (LVEDP). LVEDP can be found in previous cardiac catheterization laboratory data (if available).

Valvular Lesions

Valvular lesions are uncommon in children beyond endocarditis-related damage and repaired AVC patients. Previous endocarditis usually leads to valve insufficiency. Valve replacements are tricky in children due to a lack of growth of the new valve, anticoagulation if mechanical, and so on. Therefore, children with valvular lesions are often allowed to grow until the valve begins to cause intolerable effects. Patients with previous endocarditis may receive endocarditis prophylaxis depending on the surgical procedure.

Children with repaired CAVC, as previously discussed, usually have some element of AV valve insufficiency and less likely stenosis. While the valvular insufficiency is acceptable in infancy, as the child grows, hemodynamics due to the valve worsen over

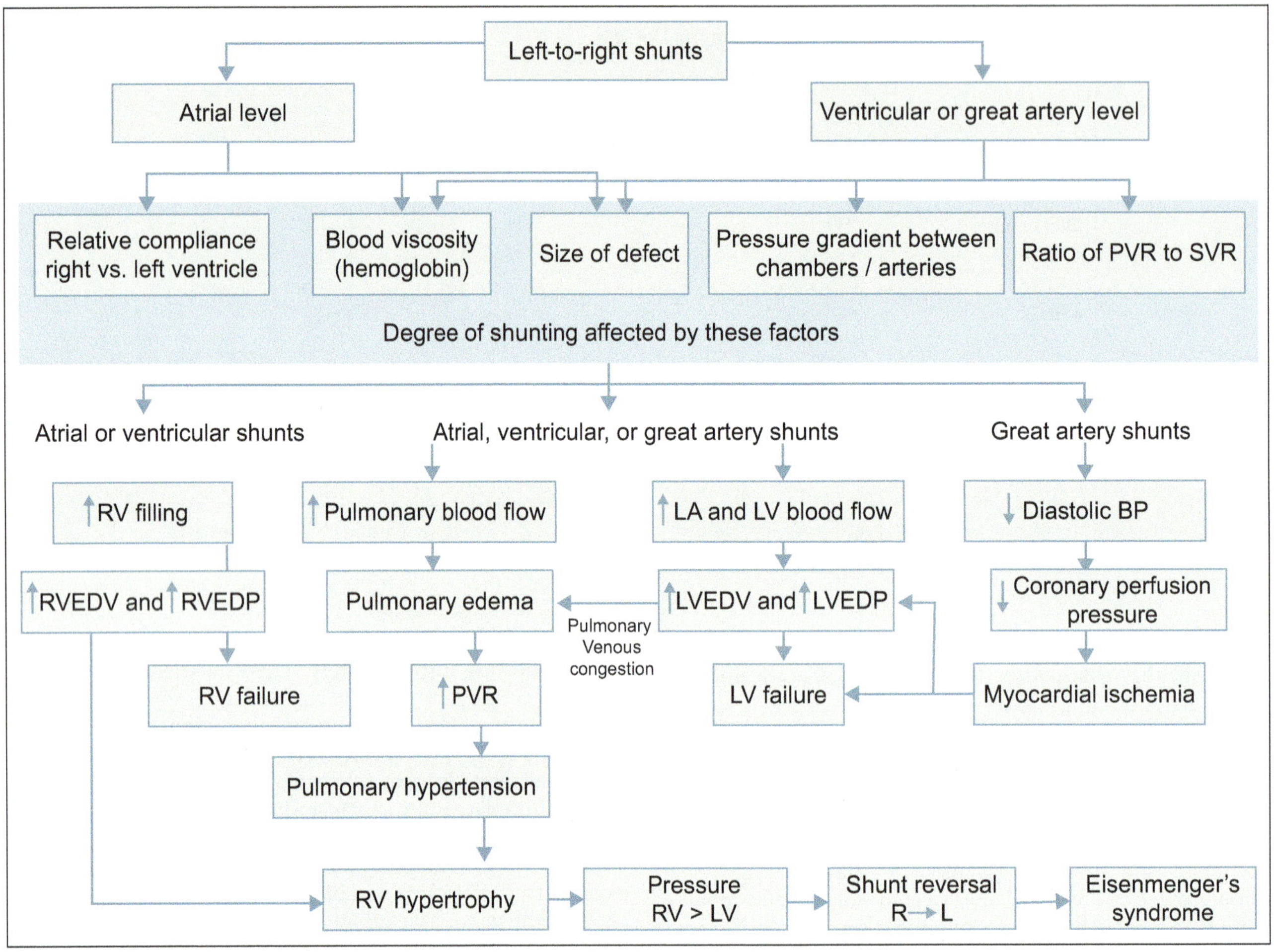

Figure 93.2: Determinants of left-to-right shunts.

BP, blood pressure; LA, left atrium; LV, left ventricle; LVEDP, left ventricular end-diastolic pressure; LVEDV, left ventricular end-diastolic volume; PVR, pulmonary vascular resistance; RV, right ventricle; RVEDP, right ventricular end-diastolic pressure; RVEDV, right ventricular end-diastolic volume; SVR, systemic vascular resistance.

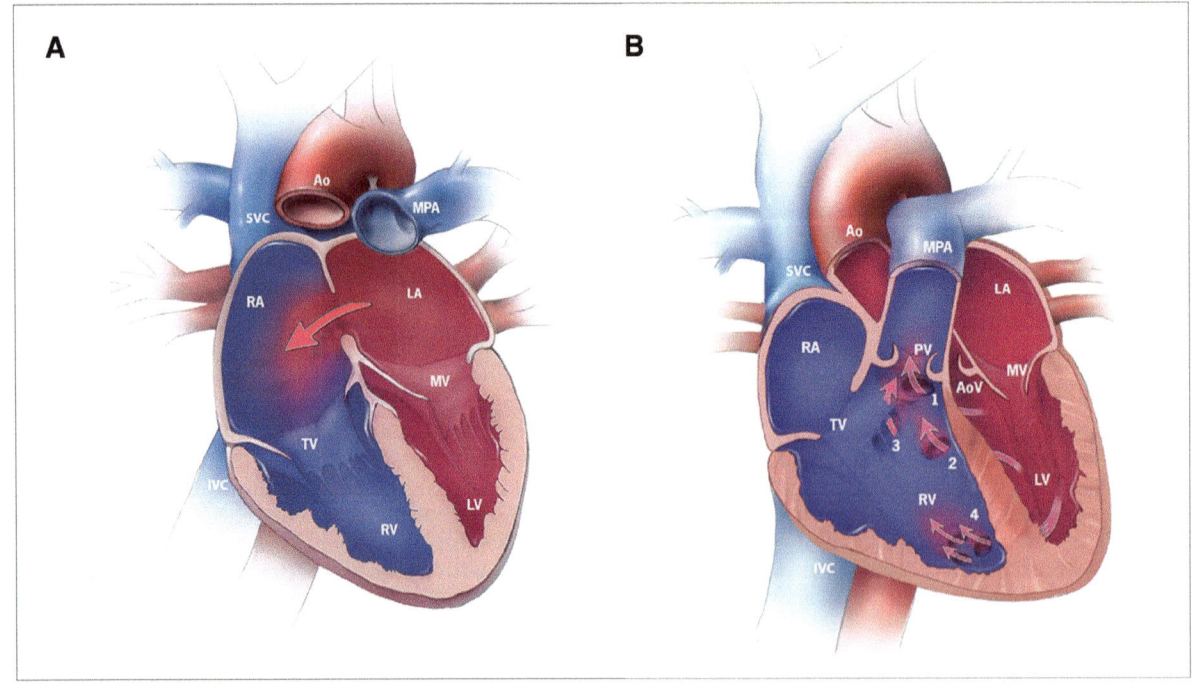

Figure 93.3: (A) Atrial septal defect. (B) Ventricular septal defects.

time. If the left AV valve is insufficient, left atrial dilation is common leading to potential for atrial arrhythmias. If severe enough, flow reversal into the pulmonary veins occurs and eventual postcapillary PH is a concern. However, in mild or moderate cases, vasodilation from low-dose inhaled anesthetics promotes forward flow and is tolerated. If pulmonary congestion is present, so is potential for failure to thrive. If the right AV valve is insufficient, anesthesia providers should be cautious with hydration. Pulmonary vasodilation promotes forward flow and is easily achieved with some supplemental oxygen. Right AV valve disease is well tolerated compared to left AV valve disease.

Coarctation of the Aorta

Coarctation of the aorta can be classified in relation to the ductus arteriosus: preductal, ductal, and postductal. Preductal coarctation obstructs aortic flow distal to the coarctation and systemic perfusion depends on the PDA. Ductal coarctations are normally not detected until around 2 weeks of life when the PDA closes. Infants present in extremis with elevated lactate levels as systemic perfusion distal to the PDA is compromised. Postductal coarctations occur in older children and adults. Patients present with upper extremity hypertension. The classic chest roentgenogram finding is rib notching due to collateral circulation.

Vascular Rings

Congenital anomalies of the aortic arch complex can result in compression of the trachea and esophagus. Rings may be complete, incomplete, or involve the pulmonary artery. The anatomically complete ring is a double aortic arch. The incomplete ring is right aortic arch with a left ligamentum arteriosum. A right aortic arch may accompany CHD. Finally, a pulmonary sling occurs when the left pulmonary artery (LPA) arises from the right pulmonary artery (RPA), and crosses to the left side between the trachea and esophagus.

Cyanotic Defects

Cyanotic defects represent a wide range of pathology. Figure 93.4 classifies cyanotic congenital heart disease (CCHD) based on pulmonary blood flow. Many lesions listed in Figure 93.4 are also single-ventricle lesions.

CCHD accounts for 1,300 per million live births with CHD.[1] This section begins with an explanation of systemic adaptations and complications to chronic cyanosis. The two lesions considered here are Tetralogy of Fallot (TOF) and Ebstein's anomaly.

Other biventricular cyanotic lesions, such as truncus arteriosus and transposition of great arteries (TGA), are repaired in the neonatal period. Newborns with these cardiac pathologies usually do not receive noncardiac surgery prior to repair.

Hypoxemia is a PaO_2 below the normal 80 to 100 mm Hg. Cyanosis is the appearance of blue skin and mucus membranes due to at least 5 grams of desaturated hemoglobin. The presence of anemia decreases the clinical appearance of cyanosis. During long-standing cyanosis, physiological adaptations occur to preserve oxygen delivery. See Figure 93.1 for details.

The three side effects of cyanosis are increased blood viscosity, coagulopathy, and urate metabolism. Bleeding tendency is attributed to inappropriate platelet activation and decreased plasma volume, which leads to hypofibrinogenemia. Complications of chronic cyanosis include hyperviscosity and stroke, brain abscess, hypervolemia, gout, and microcytic anemia.

TOF With Pulmonary Stenosis

TOF is the most common CCHD. Its four classic lesions are pulmonic stenosis, VSD, overriding aorta, and right ventricular hypertrophy. Newborns with TOF have a clinical course related to the severity of their right ventricular outflow tract obstruction (RVOTO). During agitation, paroxysms of RV infundibular muscle spasm trigger increased RVOTO and reduced Qp, hypotension, and ischemia: a hypercyanotic or "Tet" spell. Treatment includes oxygen, volume, afterload, and beta-blockade.

Transposition of Great Arteries

Newborns with d-TGA can be quite sick and may require balloon atrial septostomy early in life, followed by an arterial switch operation (ASO) as a neonate. The surgery includes great vessel suture lines and coronary reimplantation. However, long term, these children do well.[12]

Major Vascular Disease

The etiology of major vascular disease often occurs in the embryonic period as the primitive paired dorsal aortic arches. Pathology in aortic arches 4 and 6 are common sources of major vascular diseases, such as coarctation of the aorta and vascular rings. The term *vascular ring* includes malformations, such as double aortic arch, right aortic arch with ligamentum,

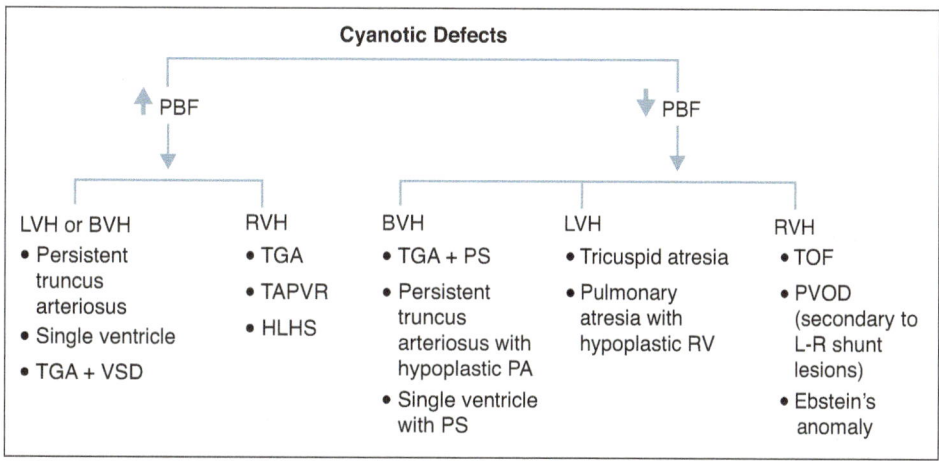

Figure 93.4: Cyanotic defects.

BVH, biventricular hypertrophy; HLHS, hypoplastic left heart syndrome; LVH, left ventricular hypertrophy; PA, pulmonary artery; PBF, pulmonary blood flow; PS, pulmonic stenosis; PVOD, pulmonary veno-occlusive disease; RV, right ventricle; RVH, right ventricular hypertrophy; TAPVR, total anomalous pulmonary venous return; TGA, transposition of the great arteries; TOF, tetralogy of Fallot; VSD, ventricular septal defect.

pulmonary artery sling, and left aortic arch with aberrant right subclavian artery.

Cardiomyopathy

Cardiomyopathy may be hypertrophic, dilated, or restrictive. It may also be anthracycline induced, endocardial fibroelastosis, noncompaction, catecholamine induced, arrhythmogenic right ventricular cardiomyopathy, or metabolic. The spectrum of pathophysiology and severity dictates the anesthetic considerations. Noncardiac elective surgery is rarely performed; however, to follow disease progression, serial MRI scans may be performed. In young children, sedation is required. If myocardial function (systolic or diastolic) is poor, additional support, such as a milrinone infusion or automated implantable cardiac defibrillator, may be in place.

Pulmonary Hypertension

PH is defined by a mean pulmonary artery pressure (mPAP) of at least 25 mm Hg at rest or 30 during exercise regardless of age. Also, it is present if pulmonary vascular resistance is greater than or equal to 3 Woods units/m^2.[13] The mPAP is equal to the systolic PAP times 0.61 plus 2 mm Hg.[14,15] PH is classified into five groups by the World Health Organization (WHO): (1) pulmonary arterial hypertension, (2) PH due to left heart disease, (3) PH due to lung disease and or hypoxia, (4) chronic thromboembolic PH, and (5) PH with unclear multifactorial mechanisms. The Panama Classification of PH is widely used in pediatrics because it includes more granular etiologies of PH.

PH due to lung disease is commonly related to bronchopulmonary dysplasia (and prematurity). The outcome of PH in this group is directly related to respiratory robustness. Notably, children with Down syndrome have a high incidence of PH even with a structurally normal heart;[16] PH in this population is of heterogeneous origin but usually falls into WHO groups 1 and 3.

Arrhythmias and Epicardial Pacemaker Systems

CHDs or their treatments can result in arrhythmia burden. Scar-related reentrant atrial tachycardia and atrial flutter are the most common.[17] Fontan patients would have epicardial-implanted electrical systems. Epicardial systems do not obviate subacute bacterial endocarditis (SBE) prophylaxis and are more prone to complications than transvenous systems.

Chronic Disease

Congestive heart failure (CHF) encompasses cardiac dysfunction and its neurohormonal effects. It is due to pressure overload in a single ventricle or volume overload (e.g., Ebstein's anomaly). Noncardiac contributors include hypertension and obstructive sleep apnea (OSA). Late complications, such as pulmonary arterial hypertension, are not compatible with passive pulmonary blood flow as in the Fontan. Cancer risk is elevated due to radiation exposure. Long-term cyanosis can lead to brain abscess and stroke.

Adult CHD

By adulthood, most patients with CHD will have undergone some type of cardiac repair. Many will have a complication, increased risk of sudden death, and eventually transition to adult care.

SPECIAL CONSIDERATIONS AND CONCERNS

When caring for children and adults with heart disease presenting for CNC surgery, it is imperative that there is a strong emphasis on medical optimization. Anesthesia providers must ensure the patient is in otherwise good health, and medications have been taken or withheld appropriately. Ideally, patients presenting for elective CNC surgery have no pending cardiac procedures planned. This is often not the case, however, as CNC surgery may be a prerequisite to intracardiac repair or heart transplantation. For example, children with heart disease frequently require dental clearance (and often anesthesia) prior to cardiac operations or interventions to reduce endocarditis risk.

In contrast to children with heart disease undergoing cardiac surgery, those presenting for CNC surgery may not have preoperative data such as a recent echocardiogram (ECHO), ECG, chest roentgenogram, or complete blood count as the surgeon would not order them for the average child undergoing noncardiac surgery, such as dental rehabilitation or central line placement. Additionally, patients presenting for CNC surgery often have noncardiac pathology as the reason to present for surgery, which must be considered. Evaluation of exercise tolerance in infants relates to feeding tolerance. If the infant is able to breastfeed or drink from a bottle an entire feed in under 20 minutes without cyanotic episodes, diaphoresis, or tachycardia (as noticed by the parent), then exercise tolerance is near normal.

Universal anesthetic considerations for children with CHD undergoing CNC surgery are listed in **Box 93.1**.

CRISIS RESOURCE MANAGEMENT

Importantly, outside of the cardiac operating room (OR), providers from all fields are less comfortable with caring for a child with heart disease. To that end, crisis resource management and giving anticipatory guidance to the surgeons, nurses, and scrub technicians are essential.

BOX 93.1 UNIVERSAL ANESTHETIC CONSIDERATIONS FOR CHILDREN WITH CHD UNDERGOING NONCARDIAC SURGERY

- Question any deviation from expected clinical trajectory
- Preoperative laboratory evaluation and cardiologist follow-up
- Evaluation of exercise tolerance
- Careful airway evaluation as difficult airway is more common in children with CHD[18]
- Discuss limits of care and ECMO candidacy
- Surgical operating suite with the appropriate resources
- *Nil per os* time
- Medications to be taken the day of surgery
- Preoperative anxiolysis with hemodynamic goals
- Availability of outside consultants for cardiac rhythm device and electromagnetic interference
- Availability of vasoactive substances and defibrillator
- Endocarditis prophylaxis
- Adjust ventilation to optimize hemodynamics for that patient's lesion

ECMO, extracorporeal membrane oxygenation.

UPPER RESPIRATORY INFECTION

Elective surgery is often postponed for 4 to 8 weeks following an upper respiratory infection (URI) to allow airway reactivity and therefore anesthetic risk to decrease. In children with CHD, also consider the effects of treatment of laryngospasm or bronchospasm. While Larson's maneuver (upward pressure on the mastoid process) is benign, other treatments can cause circulatory instability. Positive pressure ventilation reduces venous return; and in a Fontan patient, cardiac output falls quickly. Succinylcholine could be used in a small dose with rapid return of spontaneous ventilation and negative intrathoracic pressure. Propofol given to reinduce anesthesia for laryngospasm has profound venodilation (and vasodilation) effects reducing preload. This is perilous for those with poor systolic function, single-ventricle physiology and LVOTO. Bronchospasm treatment with albuterol or IV epinephrine causes tachycardia and worsens the physiology of those with obstructive cardiac lesions. Although the aforementioned considerations would imply a conservative approach to the child with CHD and a URI, data from children undergoing catheterization laboratory procedures suggested no long-term harm from perioperative consequences of URI despite the need for acute resuscitation.[19]

TIMING OF SURGERY

The child's heart disease may influence the timing of surgery. For example, scoliosis surgery in Duchenne muscular dystrophy should occur prior to the onset of significant cardiac disease. On preoperative examination, if the patient's clinical status or objective data vary substantially from what is expected, further workup prior to surgery is reasonable.

ANESTHETIC MANAGEMENT

PREOPERATIVE EVALUATION

The preanesthetic evaluation of a pediatric patient with congenital or acquired heart disease is an essential clinical assessment used to optimize a patient prior to an anesthetic and to develop the safest anesthetic plan. This plan includes premedication, IV versus mask induction, use of invasive monitoring, the appropriate location for the procedure and optimal time of day, best-suited anesthesia team to quickly recognize and respond to adverse physiological changes, post-procedure pain management, admission versus discharge, and need for intensive care. It also includes consultation with the primary cardiologist and other specialists involved in the patient's management to reveal the extent of residual disease and allow for risk stratification.[20]

The process begins with a thorough history of the current condition that led to the planned diagnostic or therapeutic procedure. An in-depth understanding of the procedure is an essential component for anesthesia planning, and discussion with the proceduralist may be necessary. Review the medical history including previous hospitalizations, surgeries, transcatheter interventions, information about prior anesthetics and anesthesia-related complications, allergies, current prescription and over-the-counter medications, recent laboratory tests, chest x-ray (CXR), ECG, ECHO, cardiac MRI (CMR), CT angiography (CTA), cardiac catheterization data, and recent notes from the primary cardiologist. Pulmonary pressure greater than half-systemic blood pressure may require additional considerations for anesthetic care.

A detailed review of systems may reveal associated congenital anomalies and comorbidities. During the cardiac review, determine the functional severity of the cardiovascular disorder. Limitations on age-appropriate daily activities reflect reduced cardiac function and limited cardiac reserve. Are there concerns about too much pulmonary blood flow? Ask parents of infants if their child has difficulty feeding (frequent stops, becomes diaphoretic, breathes rapidly, or appears cyanotic). Parents/guardians of nonverbal or young children may notice their child tires easily and cannot keep up with their siblings or peers. Ask older children about palpitations, chest discomfort, dizziness, syncope, fatigue, and dyspnea at rest or on exertion. Review any exercise testing. If cyanotic, does the child seem bluer? Children may limit their physical activity instinctively and the caretaker may not be aware of the extent of their limitations. For example, a parent/guardian may not realize that their teenager who used to like to play a sport is now exclusively playing video games because of increasing exercise intolerance.

Before proceeding with the physical examination, review the recorded weight and vital signs. Heart rate, blood pressure, and respiratory rate vary with age (Tables 93.1–93.3).

Table 93.1	Vital Signs in Children: Heart Rate	
Age	Awake Rate (beats/min)	Sleeping Rate (beats/min)
Newborn–3 mos	85–205	80–160
3 mo–2 yrs	100–190	75–160
2–10 yrs	60–140	60–90
>10 yrs	60–100	50–90

Source: From https://chemm.nlm.nih.gov/pals.htm.

Table 93.2	Vital Signs in Children: Respiratory Rate
Age	Rate (breaths/min)
Infant	30–60
Toddler	24–40
Preschooler	22–34
School-age child	18–30
Adolescent	12–16

Source: From https://chemm.nlm.nih.gov/pals.htm.

Table 93.3	Vital Signs in Children: Definition of Hypotension by Systolic Blood Pressure and Age
Age	Systolic Blood Pressure
Term neonates (0–28 days)	<60 mm Hg
Infants (1–12 mos)	<70 mm Hg
Children 1–10 yrs (5th BP percentile)	<70 mm Hg + (age in years × 2) mm Hg
Children >10 yrs	<90 mm Hg

Source: From https://chemm.nlm.nih.gov/pals.htm.

Oxygen saturation measurement by pulse oximetry is an important part of the preanesthetic assessment. If the patient has a history of cyanosis, compare the current reading with previous recorded measurements. A decreasing oxygen saturation may indicate the need for cardiac reevaluation prior to an elective procedure. Occasionally, a team member unfamiliar with the patient's baseline records a saturation that is not reflective of the patient's usual oxygenation status, a low reading is considered erroneous, and a momentary higher saturation recorded. Visible cyanosis occurs when the level of deoxygenated hemoglobin is around 5 g/dL. A greater degree of hypoxia is present when anemic patients appear cyanotic. Jaundice and darker pigmentation also affect detection of cyanosis. The best areas to assess for cyanosis have a thin outer layer of skin (cheeks, nose, ears, lips, and oral mucosa).

Is the patient's weight appropriate for age? Children with limited cardiac reserve and CHF gain weight slowly. Look at the growth chart. Examine the airway; patients with syndrome-associated CHD may have an abnormal airway (e.g., trisomy 21). Careful planning will avoid harm. When listening to breath sounds, observe the patient for signs of increased work of breathing (head bobbing, nasal flaring, retractions, or tachypnea). Rales, rhonchi, stridor, and wheezing require further investigation. Examination of the heart includes not only listening for murmurs, gallops, and clicks but feeling for thrills and heaves. A brief abdominal examination is important to check for hepatomegaly. An examination of the extremities will reveal cyanosis, clubbing, poor peripheral perfusion, and the most appropriate sites for IV lines and invasive monitoring placement.

Angiotensin-converting-enzyme (ACE) inhibitors are often held on the day of the planned anesthetic to avoid exaggerated hypotension at induction. It should be noted that ACE inhibitors do not appear to produce post-induction hypotension in the pediatric patient as frequently as they do in adults, however, the only study that described this lack of phenomenon was in children undergoing cardiac surgery.[21] Consider holding diuretics to lessen difficulty with IV access. Pulmonary vasodilators should be continued. Patients may be taking anticoagulants. Well in advance of an elective procedure, a discussion between the cardiologist and proceduralist needs to take place to discuss whether to hold anticoagulants and if a heparin bridge is indicated.

In general, NPO time should be minimized to avoid the added negative effect of hypovolemia in patients with diminished cardiovascular reserve. Schedule outpatients early in the day and order IV hydration for inpatients. Children with long-standing cyanotic heart disease may demonstrate significant polycythemia (hematocrit >65) and need an exchange transfusion to reduce the risk of a cerebral vascular accident from hyperviscosity.[22] Electrolyte disturbances (hypokalemia, hypocalcemia, and hypomagnesemia) may be secondary to diuretic use and require treatment.

Key Assessment Points

See Box 93.2 for history and physical examination considerations for children with left-to-right shunting lesions. If children have had prior experience with volume overload during an anesthetic, the parent may be able to share whether it manifested as pulmonary edema and tachypnea or body wall, periorbital edema. In this case, severity of left versus right heart disease can be postulated. If an indication for cardiac surgery is present, elective noncardiac surgery should be deferred.

When major vascular disease is suspected, cardiac CT or three-dimensional printed models are employed to define anatomy. Additionally, children with heart disease have a higher-than-average incidence of difficult airway. Many children have had extensive hospital stays and venous access may be challenging.

Pertinent Labs

Many patients with CHD presenting for CNC surgery have undergone extensive preoperative planning for cardiac surgery including basic labs, CXR, ECHO, and perhaps even cardiac catheterization (Box 93.3). A recent cardiac workup, however, is often unavailable as routine labs are generally not indicated for elective CNC surgery. This adds emphasis to the history and physical examination.

Ordering of coagulation tests may be complicated by severe polycythemia. Plasma volume is reduced and therefore less citrate is needed per blood collection tube. Communicate with the laboratory to determine if citrate adjustment is required for your patient.

Perioperative Transthoracic Echocardiography

Monitoring of various cardiac concerns can be addressed by performing focused assessed transthoracic echocardiogram

---

BOX 93.2 CONCERNING FINDINGS IN CHILDREN WITH ACYANOTIC LESIONS

Presence of an indication for cardiac surgery disqualifies a patient from elective surgery (unless it is a prerequisite to cardiac repair)

- ASD with right-sided heart enlargement
- VSD with left-sided heart enlargement or aortic valve insufficiency
- PDA with left-sided heart enlargement

Congestive symptoms, such as tachypnea, failure to thrive, and diuretic use

---

BOX 93.3 ECHO INTERPRETATION OF LEFT-TO-RIGHT SHUNTING LESIONS

- For ASDs, recall the atria contract during (ventricular) diastole. Therefore, flow through an ASD may be in diastole. Relative ventricular compliance determines the direction of shunt.

- VSDs are sized based on the size of the patient's aortic valve because during systole, blood is ejected via the path of least resistance. Therefore, if the VSD is larger than the aortic valve, it is termed large, and blood will preferentially flow through it (rather than the aorta).

- A large amount of flow across a VSD results in a large amount of flow across the pulmonary valve. This may create turbulence and result in an ECHO interpretation of pulmonic stenosis. If pulmonic valve morphology is normal, concern for an obstructive lesion (pulmonic stenosis) is low.

- VSDs are often repaired with a piece of pericardial patch. This patch does not contract, so an ECHO interpretation of paradoxical ventricular septal motion requires clinical correlation rather than immediate concern.

> **BOX 93.4 ECHO INTERPRETATION IN SINGLE-VENTRICLE DEFECTS**
>
> - BTS in older infants (e.g., 3 months old) may have flow acceleration across them in the absence of BTS pathology. The infant may just be outgrowing their source of pulmonary blood flow.
> - Glenn anastomoses should be widely patent (but are sometimes difficult to visualize).
> - Systolic ventricular function is usually at least mildly depressed (i.e., do not expect normal function even in a healthy single-ventricle patient).
> - Extracardiac Fontans may be fenestrated, however the patency of the fenestration is not guaranteed (they do spontaneously close). The direction of shunt through the fenestration is right to left.

(FATE) perioperatively. A phased array ultrasound probe (pediatric and neonatal versions available) should be used for excellent depth of penetration and resolution. Transthoracic echocardiography for the interested provider is attainable by enrolling in a course and completing an online module prior to in-person certification (Box 93.4). The FATE program promotes placing the probe in four positions to obtain cardiac and pulmonary ultrasound images. The extended FATE examination includes additional images obtained from positions 2 and 3. More information is available at usabcd.org.

During an intraoperative emergency, use crisis resource management. Use directed, closed-loop communication, and following 6 minutes of cardiopulmonary resuscitation in pediatric advanced life support, activate extracorporeal membrane oxygenation (ECMO) support if available. Details vary based on candidacy, and feasibility of cannulation sites according to cardiac anatomy and somatic size.

PREOPERATIVE PHARMACOLOGY

Psychological preparation is important. Families of patients and patients with CHD suffer significant anxiety related to multiple times of hospitalization and the use of pharmacological and nonpharmacological means of stress reduction warranted. Preoperative anxiolysis is often administered even to young infants to prevent physiological perturbations on induction of anesthesia rather than for specifically separation anxiety. For example, crying may have a more dramatic impact on pulmonary vascular resistance and cardiac output than mild hypoventilation as a side effect of oral midazolam. In healthy cyanotic children, oral midazolam premedication is well tolerated and may be indicated to prevent excessive stress and crying. Anesthesia providers should defer premedication for those in extremis who are relying on sympathetic tone for survival preoperatively.

Part of the planning for each patient includes deciding the need for antibiotics to prevent endocarditis. Follow the most recent American Heart Association (AHA) guidelines.[23] Infective endocarditis is associated with a 6-month mortality of 20%.[24] The AHA guidelines include a list of the cardiac conditions requiring prophylaxis (Box 93.5), high-risk procedures for which antibiotics are recommended (Box 93.6), and the antibiotic regimens (Table 93.4).

> **BOX 93.5 CARDIAC CONDITIONS ASSOCIATED WITH THE HIGHEST RISK OF ENDOCARDITIS REQUIRING PROPHYLAXIS**
>
> Prophylaxis
>
> - Prosthetic cardiac valve including transcatheter-implanted prostheses and homografts
> - Prosthetic material used for cardiac valve repair, such as annuloplasty rings, chords, or clips
> - Previous IE
> - CHD*
>   - Unrepaired cyanotic CHD, including palliative shunts and conduits
>   - Completely repaired congenital heart defect with prosthetic material or device, whether placed by surgery or by catheter intervention, during the first 6 months after the procedure†
>   - Repaired CHD with residual shunts or valvular regurgitation at the site or adjacent to the site of a prosthetic patch or prosthetic device (which inhibit endothelialization)
> - Cardiac transplantation recipients who develop cardiac valvulopathy
>
> CHD, congenital heart disease; IE, infective endocarditis.
> *Except for the conditions listed above, antibiotic prophylaxis is no longer recommended for any other form of CHD.
> †Prophylaxis is reasonable because endothelialization of prosthetic material occurs within 6 months after the procedure.
>
> Source: From Otto CM, Nishimura RA, Bonow RO, et al. 2020 ACC/AHA guideline for the management of patients with valvular heart disease. *J Am Coll Cardiol.* 2021;77(4):e25-e197. doi:10.1016/j.jacc.2020.11.018.

> **BOX 93.6 PROCEDURES FOR WHICH ANTIBIOTIC PROPHYLAXIS IS RECOMMENDED**
>
> - All dental procedures involving manipulation of gingival tissue or periapical region of teeth or perforation of oral mucosa
> - Respiratory tract procedures that involve incision or biopsy of respiratory mucosa
> - Tonsillectomy and adenoidectomy
> - Patients only with an established GI or GU infection
> - Surgical procedures that involve infected skin or musculoskeletal tissue
>
> GI, gastrointestinal; GU, genitourinary.
>
> Source: From Wilson W, Taubert KA., Gewitz M, et al. Prevention of infective endocarditis: guidelines from the American Heart Association: A Guideline From the American Heart Association Rheumatic Fever, Endocarditis, and Kawasaki Disease Committee, Council on Cardiovascular Disease in the Young, and the Council on Clinical Cardiology, Council on Cardiovascular Surgery and Anesthesia, and the Quality of Care and Outcomes Research Interdisciplinary Working Group. *Circulation.* 2007;116(15):1736–1754.

Table 93.4	American Heart Association Guidelines for Prevention of Infective Endocarditis: Antibiotic Regimens	
Situation	**Agent**	**Regimen (dose 30–60 min before procedure)**
Oral	Amoxicillin	50 mg/kg (maximum 2 g)
Unable to take oral medication	Ampicillin OR Cefazolin or ceftriaxone	50 mg/kg IM or IV (maximum 2 g) 50 mg/kg IM or IV (maximum 1 g)
Allergic to penicillins or ampicillin—oral	Cephalexin*† OR Clindamycin OR Azithromycin or clarithromycin	50 mg/kg (maximum 2 g) 20 mg/kg (maximum 600 mg) 15 mg/kg (maximum 500 mg)
Allergic to penicillins or ampicillin and unable to take oral medication	Cefazolin or ceftriaxone+ OR Clindamycin	50 mg/kg IM or IV (maximum 1 g) 20 mg/kg IM or IV (maximum 600 mg)

*Or other first- or second-generation oral cephalosporin in equivalent adult or pediatric dosage.
†Cephalosporins should not be used in an individual with a history of anaphylaxis, angioedema, or urticarial with penicillins or ampicillin.

Source: From Wilson W, Taubert KA, Gewitz M, et al. Prevention of infective endocarditis: guidelines from the American Heart Association: A Guideline From the American Heart Association Rheumatic Fever, Endocarditis, and Kawasaki Disease Committee, Council on Cardiovascular Disease in the Young, and the Council on Clinical Cardiology, Council on Cardiovascular Surgery and Anesthesia, and the Quality of Care and Outcomes Research Interdisciplinary Working Group. Circulation. 2007;116(15):1736–1754.

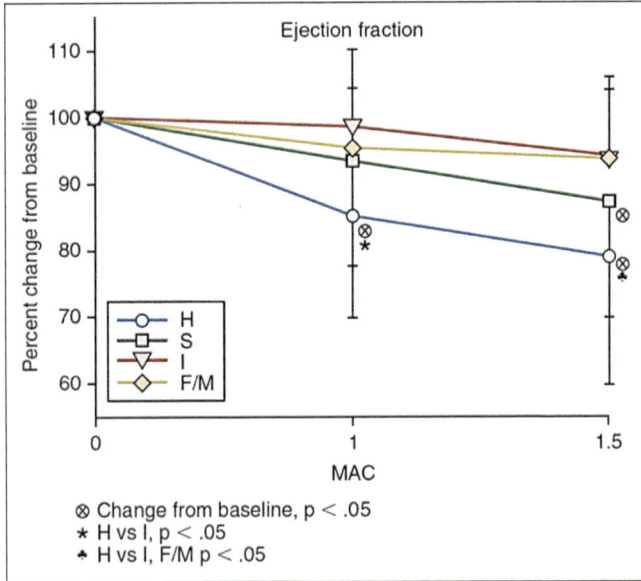

Figure 93.5: Effects of different maintenance anesthetics on cardiac index.

F/M, fentanyl/midazolam; H, halothane; I, isoflurane; S, sevoflurane.

Source: From Rivenes SM. Cardiovascular effects of sevoflurane, isoflurane, halothane, and fentanyl-midazolam in children with congenital heart disease: an echocardiographic study of myocardial contractility and hemodynamics. Anesthesiology. 2001;94(2):223–229.

ANESTHETIC TECHNIQUE

Intraoperative Management

The anesthetic management of congenital and acquired heart disease is as varied as the types of defects and pathophysiological states. The neonatal myocardium has disorganized, reduced density of muscle fibers. The neonatal myocardium also has rapid myocardial uptake of inhalation anesthetics. Due to a high ratio of minute ventilation to functional residual capacity, insoluble inhalation agents undergo faster equilibration. Consequently, infants have a higher incidence of cardiac arrest during induction.[25] In children, sevoflurane depresses myocardial function less than halothane.

Depending on the perceived risk of induction of anesthesia, the surgical team and perfusionist may be in attendance in case of emergent need for mechanical circulatory support. The classic example of this is an infant with Williams syndrome in whom coronary insufficiency and myocardial ischemia accompany induction. For healthy patients with CHD, the same inhalational and IV anesthetics used for healthy patients can be used as long as hemodynamic effects are considered. Children with extensive history of anesthetics and intensive care unit (ICU) stays may have developed significant physical dependence and tachyphylaxis to IV agents.

Inhalation anesthetics distribute in the body according to tissue partial pressure and solubility (partition coefficient)[26] and in the case of patients with CHD, pulmonary blood flow. In children with left-to-right intracardiac shunts, pulmonary blood flow is excessive, and anesthetic uptake is rapid, speeding induction. Induction of anesthesia for patients with cyanosis should proceed with the head of bed up to allow gravity to aid venous drainage to the lungs and preload. Due to a paucity of pulmonary blood flow, inhalation induction is prolonged. Slowly up-titrated sevoflurane mask induction takes a long time and predisposes to minutes of agitation. Another approach, increasing brain tissue concentration of sevoflurane quickly, is to allow three breaths of sevoflurane at 8% and then immediately reduce the concentration. In this way, induction is expedited without a prolonged exposure to high concentrations of sevoflurane.

Nitrous oxide should be used with caution in patients with CHD due to potential impact on pulmonary vascular resistance (PVR). In infants, there is no increase in PVR when nitrous oxide is used.[27] At the same time, inhalation induction with potent (and more pungent) agent, such as sevoflurane, may precipitate crying and significant increases in PVR. In this case, the choice of use of nitrous oxide is multifactorial.

However, in adults, nitrous oxide does increase PVR. Low cardiac output states predispose patients to overdose with soluble agents, as the rate of rise in alveolar concentrations will be markedly increased.

Induction and maintenance of anesthesia should preserve cardiac index. Rivenes et al. found that in children with CHD, cardiac index was preserved at 1 MAC and at 1.5 MAC (or equivalent) with various anesthetics.[28] See **Figure 93.5** for a graphical representation of the effects of different maintenance anesthetics on cardiac index. Laparoscopic surgical technique tends to decrease systolic function on transesophageal echocardiography and reduced preload due to pneumoperitoneum; however, children with single-ventricle physiology tend to tolerate it.[29]

Consider the physiological effects of high concentrations of oxygen prior to providing it. The closure of a necessary PDA, pulmonary overcirculation, and coronary steal are possible consequences when more than momentary supplemental oxygen is provided. Depending on the lesion, ventilation with room air may help maintain PVR and prevent overcirculation. Provision of oxygen is tenuous in the infant with a Blalock–Taussig shunt (BTS) as increasing inspired oxygen leads to decreased PVR and pulmonary overcirculation. This steals blood from the systemic circulation, specifically the coronaries, whose perfusion is already retrograde.

For patients with TOF, maintain systemic vascular resistance (SVR) to maintain coronary perfusion and pulmonary blood flow even before a hypercyanotic spell occurs. Some would advocate for initiation of low-dose vasopressin as soon as the central line is in place. For those with hypoplastic left heart syndrome (HLHS), volume expansion with packed red blood cells and fresh frozen plasma is reasonable to ensure adequate hemoglobin and response to heparin.

A five-lead ECG should be monitored on CNC as the epicardial course of their coronary arteries and conduction system may be aberrant and unpredictable.[30] Monitoring of pulse oximetry and cerebral saturation via near-infrared spectroscopy may be inaccurate or inadequate respectively if hematocrit is high.[31,32] An upper extremity peripheral intravenous catheter (PIV) aids in provision of preload with some protection against systemic air emboli.

When a cardiac rhythm management device is in place, sources of electromagnetic interference (EMI) should be sought. Sources of EMI include cautery, cavitron, nerve stimulators, shivering, fasciculation, extracorporeal shockwave lithotripsy (ESWL), and MRI. EMI can cause either inappropriate triggering or inhibition of paced output as well as reversion to an asynchronous (noise suppression) mode.[33] If disabling anti-tachycardia function, place defibrillator pads in the anterior and posterior positions or any way such that current from one to the other does not intersect the generator. Hyperkalemia, metabolic acidosis and alkalosis, hypothermia, and hyperglycemia all significantly increase the pacing threshold.

SBE prophylaxis is often necessary as many adults have implanted prosthetic conduits or valves. Note that SBE prophylaxis in patients with cardiac rhythm management devices only applies to transvenous systems. Epicardial systems do not touch the endocardium and therefore do not present additional risk of endocarditis.

Defibrillator and pacemaker generators may be subxiphoid and interfere with surgical electrocautery. In this case, disabling of the anti-tachycardia function is indicated. Bipolar cautery is preferred. The dispersion pad should not be placed in the path of the generator and cautery should be at least 15 centimeters from the generator. EMI can inhibit the necessary pacing function of the device or inappropriately trigger the device.[33] Other sources of electrical interference in the OR include ultrasonic scaler used by a dentist (cavitron), nerve stimulators, shivering, fasciculation, extracorporeal shock wave lithotripsy, and MRI.

Special Techniques and/or Equipment

When caring for children with PH, additional resuscitation equipment should be available, including inhaled nitric oxide, iloprost and a mesh nebulizer to deliver it, and vasoactive medications. Norepinephrine is endorsed by the Congenital Cardiac Anesthesia Society in the management of the patient with PH undergoing anesthesia. Other options include phenylephrine or vasopressin in order to maintain SVR. Pressors serve two purposes: to maintain SVR and coronary perfusion pressure. RV hypertrophy may prevent coronary perfusion around the cardiac cycle. Then, as with the left ventricle, the at-risk right ventricle is also now only receiving perfusion during diastole. The second purpose is maintenance of ventricular geometry. The interventricular septum normally thickens and bows slightly into the RV cavity during systole. In PH patients, RV pressure may be so high that the septum may flatten or even exhibit paradoxical motion during systole. If this occurs, the LV stroke volume will be compromised and thus so will cardiac output and coronary perfusion pressure, which begets itself in a dangerous spiral. Calcium should be used with caution as bolus doses elevate pulmonary artery pressures. A failing right ventricle should be supported early with inotropes over volume. Ketamine may be used safely as long as ventilation is controlled.[34]

Clinical Pearls

All IV lines need to be carefully de-aired. Poor venous access is common in patients with congenital or acquired heart disease related to past procedures and long intensive care stays. A handheld infrared light (vein finder) and ultrasound system are often needed. Palpate pulses, a diminished pulse in one wrist, will exclude that site as the best location for an arterial line. Reasons for one wrist to have a weaker pulse include a prior cutdown, sacrifice of the subclavian artery for surgical repair, or more commonly, a Gore-Tex shunt directly blood from the innominate artery to the pulmonary artery (modified BTS) that reduces flow to the arm. Frequent cardiac catheterizations can lead to a diminished or absent femoral pulse due to thrombosis and scarring. Central venous access may also be difficult. If the child has a single ventricle, weigh the pros and cons of central venous access. A thrombosis of the superior or inferior vena cava is a serious complication in this population and may prevent further palliative heart surgery, leaving transplant as the only option.

Patients with Glenn physiology will have high upper extremity venous pressure. This is relevant for peripheral IV or central line placement. Trendelenburg position may not be as helpful and may impede pulmonary blood flow and cardiac output by decreasing preload. During arterial line placement, expect dark, slightly sluggish blood return (the opposite of a healthy patient with anemia).

Complications/Emergencies

When troubleshooting desaturation, consider inadequate pulmonary blood flow and a fluid bolus. Clinically significant bleeding may be related to hemostatic defects associated with cyanosis or surgical bleeding. In this case, consider point-of-care coagulation testing (e.g., rotational thromboelastometry (ROTEM) or thromboelastography (TEG)). Expect low levels of fibrinogen or, if the patient is taking aspirin, poor platelet function.

Pulmonary hypertensive crisis is a worrisome complication. It can occur unexpectedly at any time during a general anesthetic. Tachycardia may be the presenting symptom as the right ventricle struggles to maintain cardiac output in the face of acutely elevated PVR. The right heart will dilate acutely and fail. End-tidal carbon dioxide falls lower with each breath indicating reduction in cardiac output. At this point, the interventricular septum is likely bowing into the left ventricle and reducing stroke volume and therefore CPP. Hypotension leads to poor CPP, which leads to poorer ventricular function, which leads to more hypotension. This is an emergency. Treatment revolves around reducing PVR and supporting the failing right ventricle. To reduce PVR, hyperventilate with 100% oxygen and normalize plasma pH with sodium bicarbonate (assuming ventilation is adequate). To aid the failing right ventricle, minimize fluid administration, support CPP by increasing SVR (e.g., phenylephrine or vasopressin), and increase intropy with norepinephrine (or epinephrine if it is more quickly available).

Adults with CHD are also at risk of cardiovascular disease, such as systemic hypertension, thromboembolism, aortic dilation heart failure, arrhythmias, and atherosclerotic coronary disease. The risk varies by lesion and Bigras et al. review this topic extensively.[35] The risk of hypertension is elevated in coarctation and Ebstein's anomaly. The risk of coronary disease is elevated in coarctation and transposition patients (who are status post-ASO). The risk of aortic dilation is common to many lesions. The risk of thromboembolism is greatest in those with pulmonary atresia and VSD. Heart failure risk is elevated in those with Eisenmenger's, pulmonary atresia with VSD, congenitally corrected TGA (cc-TGA), TOF, and Ebstein's anomaly. Finally, arrhythmias predominate in lesions such as Eisenmenger's, pulmonary atresia with VSD, Fontan circulation, cc-TGA, TOF, and Ebstein's anomaly. These risks are for the lifetime of the patient and not necessarily while under general anesthesia.

POSTOPERATIVE CARE

If postoperative mechanical ventilation is required, the patient is transported to the ICU often with manual ventilation. Ventilation en route to the ICU is exceedingly important especially for those who are status post-Norwood with modified BTS. Hyperventilation during this short transport will result in decreased PVR (avoid supplemental oxygen), and coronary steal potentially with myocardial ischemia. Neonatal myocardium that has just undergone significant ischemic time on bypass will not tolerate it. Conversely, hypoventilation will worsen blood pH in the setting of (nearly certain) metabolic acidosis and impair myocardial function. Postoperative stroke and subclinical seizure are gaining attention. These events will be difficult to attribute to a cannulation/bypass misadventure versus long-standing erythrocytosis.

Fluid resuscitation in the OR may necessitate postoperative diuresis to minimize pulmonary congestion especially if the mitral or left AV valve is involved, such as in AV valve disease. Postoperatively, fluid shifts present a significant source of morbidity. Even appropriate intraoperative fluid administration may lead to pulmonary edema and dyspnea, dependent edema, and lymphatic failure with chylous pleural effusions in single-ventricle patients.

For outpatient procedures, attention should be given to the return of activities of daily living without dyspnea or hypoxia. In practice, this may include asking the patient to walk while monitoring oxygen saturation and work of breathing prior to discharge from the postanesthesia care unit (PACU). If there is a cardiac rhythm management device in place, device interrogation should occur prior to discharge from the PACU.

KEY REFERENCES

Complete references for this chapter are online and available at https://connect.springerpub.com/content/book/978-0-8261-3875-0/part/part04/toc-part/ch0093.

2. Taylor D, Habre W. Risk associated with anesthesia for noncardiac surgery in children with congenital heart disease. *Paediatr Anaesth*. 2019;29(5):426–434.

7. Brown MLM, James M, DiNardo A. Anesthesia in pediatric patients with congenital heart disease undergoing noncardiac surgery: defining the risk. *J Cardiothorac Vasc Anesth*. 2020;34:470–478.

35. Bigras JL. Cardiovascular risk factors in patients with congenital heart disease. *Can J Cardiol*. 2020;36(9):1458–1466.

SECTION H: General Surgery Procedures

CHAPTER 94

Appendectomy

Tamra Nicole Kelly

INDICATIONS/CONTRAINDICATIONS

Acute appendicitis (AA) is one of the most common surgical emergencies worldwide. Between 1% and 8% of children who present to the ED with abdominal pain are diagnosed with AA and require open or laparoscopic surgical intervention.[1] The patient may be diagnosed with complicated or uncomplicated appendicitis (Figure 94.1). *Complicated appendicitis* is defined as the presence of perforation, rupture, necrosis, or inflammatory mass.[2] *Uncomplicated appendicitis* is usually early appendicitis and is acutely inflamed without perforation.[3]

The World Society of Emergency Surgery (WSES) updated its guidelines for diagnoses and treatment in 2020. For pediatric patients with suspected AA, laboratory work and imaging together are recommended to confirm a diagnosis. White blood cell count greater than 16,000 per milliliter and a C reactive protein greater than 10 mg/L have been found to be strong predictors of AA in pediatric patients presenting to the ED with right iliac fossa pain.[4] Ultrasound is the recommended first-line imaging to diagnose AA, with CT recommended if ultrasound is inconclusive.[4] Once the diagnosis is made, uncomplicated AA should have surgical intervention within 24 hours and complicated AA within 8 hours.[4]

SPECIAL CONSIDERATIONS AND CONCERNS

Laparoscopic appendectomy has become the standard treatment for complicated and uncomplicated AA.[5] Laparoscopic appendectomy is associated with lower incidence of surgical site infections, lower postoperative pain due to fewer adhesions and smaller incisions, minimal scarring, shorter hospital stays, and facilitates visualization of the full abdomen[5,6] (Figure 94.2). The WSES recommends laparoscopic over open appendectomies in children when there is appropriate equipment, expertise, and no contraindication to abdominal insufflation.[4] There are many physiologic factors related to the pneumoperitoneum that can make the anesthetic management of the laparoscopic approach more complicated than the open approach.

ANESTHETIC MANAGEMENT

PREOPERATIVE EVALUATION

Children presenting for appendectomy should have a thorough history and physical as they may present with nausea, vomiting, dehydration, ileus, peritonitis, or sepsis. Their level of dehydration and pain should also be assessed. Anesthesia providers

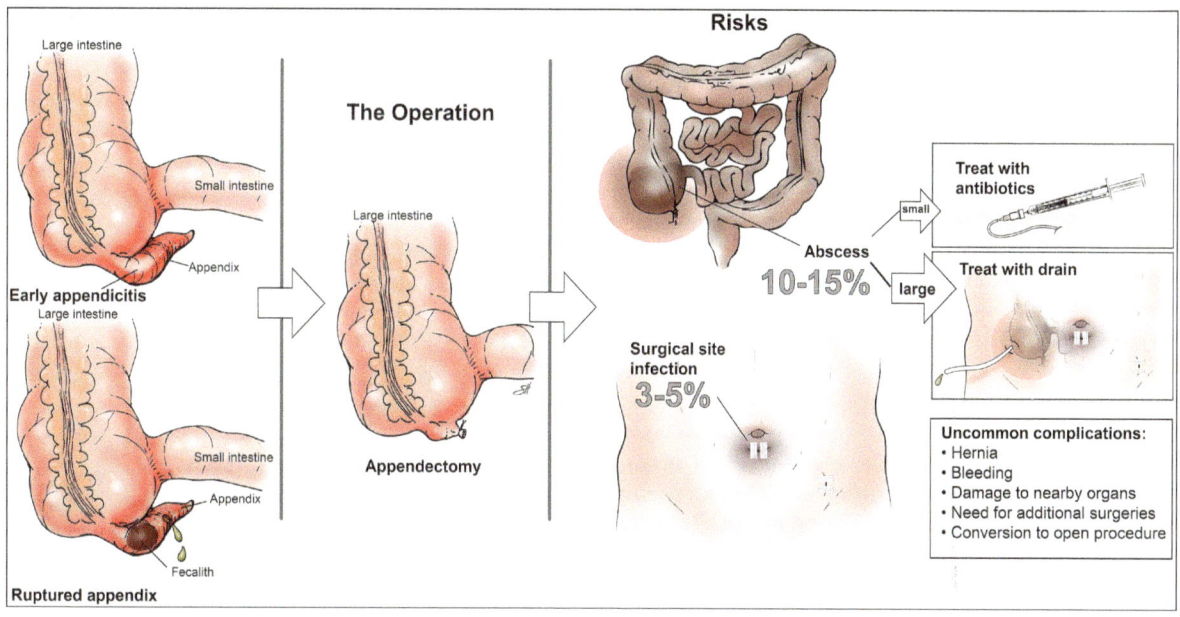

Figure 94.1: Appendicitis classification, operation, and risks.

Source: From Rosenfeld EH, Lopez ME, Yu YR, et al. Use of standardized visual aids improves informed consent for appendectomy in children: a randomized control trial. *Am J Surg.* ;216(4):730–735. doi:10.1016/j.amjsurg.2018.07.032; Copyright Baylor College of Medicine.

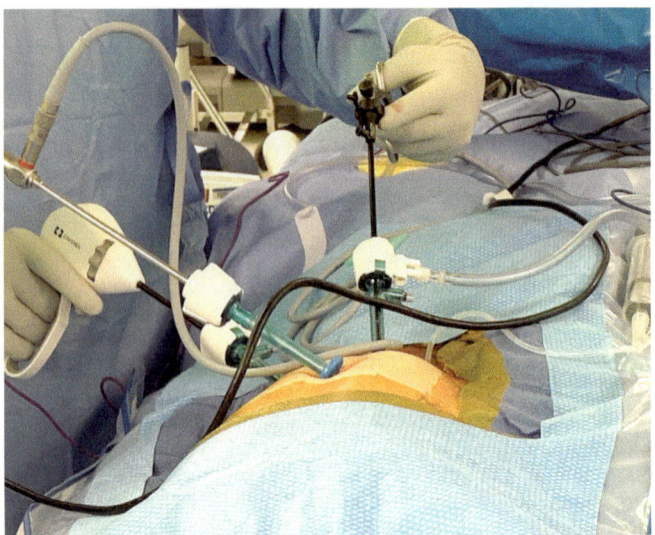

Figure 94.2: Laparoscopic surgery utilizing three trocar sites.
Source: From Texas Children's Hospital.

should note when the last dose of antibiotics was administered, as well as the amount of IV fluid already given for resuscitation.[7] NPO status is not applicable to these patients as they should be considered with full stomach. Prior to surgery, patients presenting with AA should have sent to laboratories for evaluation of complete blood count and electrolyte status.

PREOPERATIVE PHARMACOLOGY

It is not uncommon for children presenting for appendectomy to be anxious preoperatively. Anesthesia providers should assess the patient's level of anxiety to determine if pharmacologic anxiolysis is needed. While some institutions favor parental presence during induction, other institutions more commonly utilize anxiolytics. The use of an induction room, however, is precluded should a rapid sequence induction be planned. IV midazolam is the most common medication used to help ease anxiety and parental separation prior to surgery. Other medications that should be considered prior to surgery include antacids, H2 antagonists, antisialagogues, opioids, and ketamine.[7] If the patient has not been adequately rehydrated, anesthesia providers should consider administering a 20 mL/kg bolus of isotonic crystalloid to minimize hemodynamic changes associated with pneumoperitoneum.[5]

ANESTHETIC TECHNIQUE

Intraoperative Management

Patients with AA require a rapid sequence IV induction (RSI) with cricoid pressure until the endotracheal tube is secured to reduce the risk of aspiration of gastric contents.[7] A cuffed endotracheal tube is preferred due to Trendelenburg positioning and increases intra-abdominal pressure (IAP) from the pneumoperitoneum.[6] An upper extremity peripheral IV line is needed in case IAP obstructs the inferior vena cava (IVC).[7] Standard monitors including end-tidal CO_2 and temperature should be utilized. Following induction, the stomach should be decompressed using an orogastric tube. This will improve surgical visualization of structures and reduce the risk of accidently perforating the stomach during trocar placement.[7]

The choice of anesthetic is based on preexisting conditions, but a combination of inhaled anesthetics, such a sevoflurane, IV opioids, nondepolarizing neuromuscular blockers, and nonsteroidal anti-inflammatory drugs (NSAIDs), is typically used.[6,7] Nitrous oxide should be avoided intraoperatively due to the small risk of venous CO_2 air embolism with pneumoperitoneum. Avoidance of nitrous oxide also helps decrease the risk of bowel distention.[6,7] Anesthetic management for open versus laparoscopic appendectomy is directly related to the changes induced by pneumoperitoneum and Trendelenburg positioning associated with the laparoscopic approach (Box 94.1).

BOX 94.1 POSITIONING CONCERNS IN APPENDECTOMY

During laparoscopy, CO_2 gas is used to create a pneumoperitoneum, which elevates the IAP. This, combined with the Trendelenburg position for visualization, results in several important physiologic changes:

- Increased $ETCO_2$. Increase the rate to bring $ETCO_2$ back to baseline.
- Decreased FRC, increased PIP, preferential ventilation to the nondependent areas of the lung causing a VQ mismatch. Use PEEP.
- Increased CO_2 causes increased heart rate, contractility, BP, and risk of dysrhythmias.
- If the IAP is <15 mm Hg, the patient will have increased CO and BP due to increased venous return from the splanchnic bed.
- If the IAP is >15 mm Hg, the patient will have decreased CO and BP from IVC compression.
- An IAP of 6 mm Hg does not change the CO and is recommended for cardiac patients.
- Children have high resting vagal tone, which could cause bradycardia on insufflation. If this occurs, have the surgeon desufflate and then slowly reinsufflate.
- Increased ICP, but maintain cerebral oxygenation if the patient remains well hydrated.

BP, blood pressure; CO, cardiac output; $ETCO_2$, end-tidal carbon dioxide; FRC, functional residual capacity; IAP, intra-abdominal pressure; ICP, increased intracranial pressure; IVC, inferior vena cava; PEEP, positive end-expiration pressure; PIP, peak inspiratory pressure; VQ, pulmonary ventilation/perfusion.

Sources: From Pennant J. Anesthesia for laparoscopy in the pediatric patient. *Anesthesiol Clin North Am.* 2001;19(1):69–88. doi:10.1016/S0889-8537(05)70212-1; Oztan MO, Aydin G, Cigsar EB, Bozkurt PS, Koyluoglu G. Effects of carbon dioxide insufflation and trendelenburg position on brain oxygenation during laparoscopy in children. *Surg Laparosc Endosc Percutan Tech.* 2019;29(2):90–94. doi:10.1097/SLE.0000000000000593.

Appendectomy is typically a short surgical procedure. Although the peritoneum is deflated at the end of the surgery, a small amount of CO_2 gas will remain trapped in the peritoneum. This gas can cause referred right shoulder pain due to irritation of the diaphragm and can increase the incidence of postoperative nausea and vomiting.[7] Ondansetron should be given prior to extubation. Postoperative pain can be managed with administration of IV NSAIDs, such as ketorolac, IV acetaminophen, and IV opioids. In addition, the surgeon should inject local anesthetic at the incision site to help alleviate postoperative pain.[6,8]

BOX 94.2	COMPLICATIONS AND EMERGENCIES DURING APPENDECTOMY

- CO_2 air embolism
- Pneumopericardium
- Hemorrhage
- Gastrointestinal injury
- Genitourinary injury

Complications/Emergencies

Potential complications and emergencies include CO_2 air embolism, pneumopericardium, hemorrhage, gastrointestinal injury, and genitourinary injury (Box 94.2).

POSTOPERATIVE CARE

Postoperatively, pain typically lasts approximately 5 days for an open appendectomy and 2 days for a laparoscopic appendectomy.[9] The pain peaks for both open and laparoscopic on postoperative day 1.[9] Regional anesthesia has been trialed to help diminish postoperative pain. A meta-analysis found paravertebral blocks reduced pain scores at 4 hours postoperatively, but there was no difference at 24 hours postoperatively.[10] Transversus abdominis plane block has been found effective in reducing pain in open appendectomies at 4 and 18 hours postoperatively.[11] Studies have found a patient-controlled analgesia (PCA) is beneficial in complicated appendicitis but not useful in uncomplicated appendicitis.[8,12] One study found that patients with uncomplicated appendicitis could be managed postoperatively on oral analgesia alone if they were given intraoperative NSAIDs.[2]

CASE STUDY: A 13-Year-Old Male With Acute Appendicitis

CLINICAL SCENARIO

A 13-year-old male (156 cm, 64 kg) presents with acute appendicitis (AA) by CT showing a possible microperforation. His heart rate is in the 130s, respiratory rate in the 40s, blood pressure 128/79, febrile, and with 2+ pulses. He is complaining of pain and has mild confusion when given PRN morphine. He has had 2 days of nausea and vomiting.

SPECIAL CONSIDERATIONS

Given the vitals, the patient is in compensated shock. Fluid status needs to be assessed. He was given 1 L normal saline (NS) bolus and started on a second liter. He was given one dose of antibiotics, one dose of ondansetron, and 4 mg of morphine prior to arrival to the holding area.

APPROACHES TO CARE

Evidence-Based Approaches to Care

IV midazolam was given in the holding area. Standard monitors were applied prior to induction. The patient required a rapid sequence IV induction with fentanyl, lidocaine, propofol, and rocuronium. A cuffed endotracheal tube was placed. He was given dexamethasone, ondansetron, morphine, and 1 L of lactated Ringer's solution (LR). On insufflation, there was a slight increase in heart rate (HR) and blood pressure. He was fully reversed with neostigmine and glycopyrrolate and was extubated awake. A patient-controlled analgesia was ordered for postoperative pain.

COMPLICATIONS

The patient had complicated AA due to perforation. He developed an abscess on postoperative day 6 that required a drain in interventional radiology. He was hospitalized for a total of 16 days and was discharged home on oral antibiotics.

KEY REFERENCES

Complete references for this chapter are online and available at https://connect.springerpub.com/content/book/978-0-8261-3875-0/part/part04/toc-part/ch094.

2. Ousley R, Burgoyne L, Crowley N, et al. An audit of patient-controlled analgesia after appendicectomy in children. *Paediatr Anaesth*. 2016;26(10):1002–1009. doi:10.1111/pan.12964
4. Di Saverio S, Birindelli A, Kelly M, et al. WSES Jerusalem guidelines for diagnosis and treatment of acute appendicitis. *World J Emerg Surg*. 2016;11(1):34–34. doi:10.1186/s13017-016-0090-5
5. Oztan MO, Aydin G, Cigsar EB, et al. Effects of carbon dioxide insufflation and Trendelenburg position on brain oxygenation during laparoscopy in children. *Surg Laparosc Endosc Percutan Tech*. 2019;29(2):90–94. doi:10.1097/SLE.0000000000000593
6. Muñoz C, Nguyen H, Houck C. Robotic surgery and anesthesia for pediatric urologic procedures. *Curr Opin Anaesthesiol*. 2016;29(3):337–344. doi:10.1097/ACO.0000000000000333
7. Pennant J. Anesthesia for laparoscopy in the pediatric patient. *Anesthesiol Clin North Am*. 2001;19(1):69–88. doi:10.1016/S0889-8537(05)70212-1

CHAPTER 95

Tracheoesophageal Fistula Repair

Judith M. Lewis and Ashley J. Austin

INDICATIONS/CONTRAINDICATIONS

Tracheoesophageal fistula (TEF) is a relatively rare congenital anomaly with an incidence of approximately 1 in 3,000 live births.[1] TEF is an abnormal communication between the posterior wall of the trachea and the anterior wall of the esophagus and is the most common type of airway fistula.[2,3] TEF is often associated with esophageal atresia (EA), which, with or without TEF, is the most frequent congenital anomaly of the upper digestive tract with an occurrence ranging from 1 in 2,500 to 4,000 live births.[4]

TEF is classified into five subtypes according to the Gross classification[5] (Figure 95.1). The most common subtype of TEF/EA is Gross classification type C (85%), in which the upper segment of the esophagus terminates in a blind pouch and the lower segment is connected to the trachea via a fistula.[5,6]

The clinical presentation of TEF depends on the presence or absence of EA. EA should be suspected when a stomach bubble is absent on prenatal ultrasound.[7] A diagnosis of EA prenatally should be considered if maternal polyhydramnios, or excessive amniotic fluid, is seen on prenatal ultrasound as well. When undiagnosed prenatally, TEF/EA is readily identified early after birth during physical examination of the newborn. The presence of excessive salivation, choking with oral feeds, coughing, cyanosis and respiratory distress, abdominal distention, pneumonia, and failure to thrive should all raise suspicion of TEF/EA.[2] Inability to pass a 10-French gastric tube on an anterior–posterior chest radiograph is considered the gold standard for diagnosis of EA, while air in the stomach and distal bowel confirms the presence of a distal TEF.[6,8] Infants with type H fistula are more difficult to diagnose and may be asymptomatic in the newborn period presenting with mild respiratory distress or recurrent pneumonia, with 90% being diagnosed during their first year of life.[8]

Preoperative medical management of a neonate with suspected TEF/EA starts shortly after birth and should begin prior to transport to the NICU or within the NICU itself. Once TEF/EA has been diagnosed, the neonate is given nothing by mouth and remains NPO and is administered IV fluids to maintain normoglycemia and euvolemia. A Replogle tube can be placed for continuous suction of secretions, or regular intermittent oropharyngeal suction should be performed. To further prevent aspiration of gastric fluid, the head of the bed (HOB) is elevated 30 to 40 degrees to help prevent gastric reflux from the lower portion of the esophagus through the fistula and into the trachea and lungs in types C, D, and E. Placing the infant prone may also help minimize the risk of pulmonary aspiration.[6,9] Antibiotic administration is indicated if there is a suspicion of aspiration or if infective perinatal risk factors are present.[9]

Healthy neonates without pulmonary sequelae are usually repaired within the first few days of life. Infants with low birth weight, pneumonia, or other major congenital anomalies have delayed repair.[7] Depending on the extent and type of TEF/EA, primary repair reconstruction can be from the native esophagus or from parts of the stomach or intestines, but keeping the native esophagus reduces the risk of recurrent aspiration and chronic respiratory issues.[10] Staged repair may be necessary if primary anastomosis is not possible with the esophageal segment. A long-gap EA, defined as a gap length of three or more vertebral bodies, requires esophageal elongation procedures on the esophageal segment.[6,8] Although several surgical techniques have been attempted, the recommended treatment for long-gap EA remains controversial. The most common technique currently used is to allow the infant to grow 2 to 3 months with a Replogle tube in the proximal pouch and a gastrostomy for feeds.[6,11]

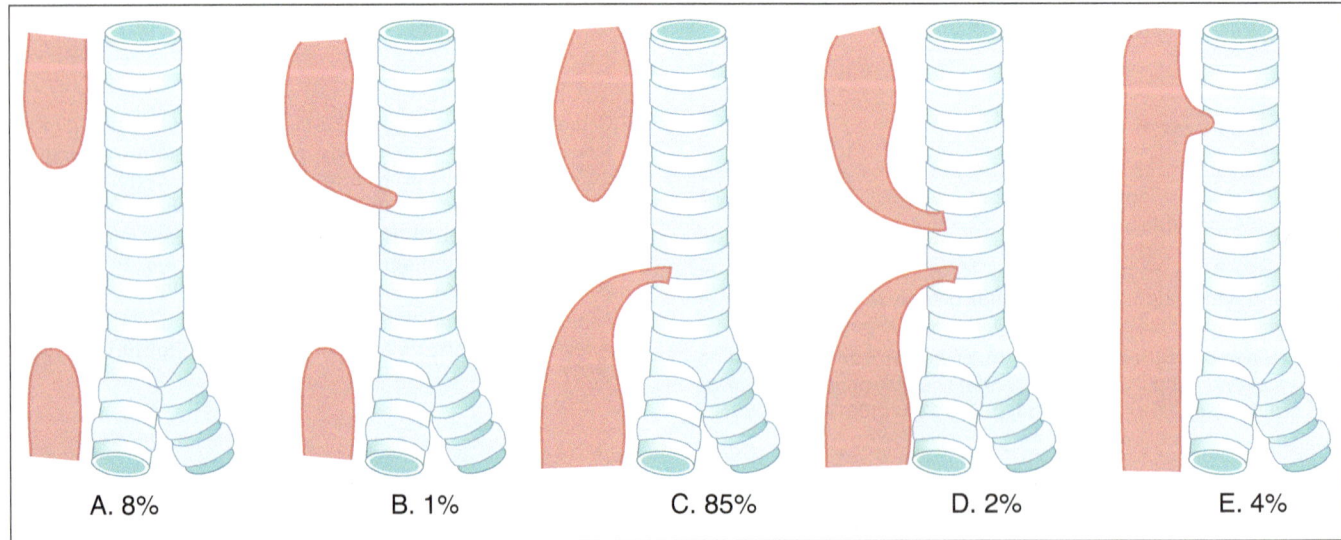

Figure 95.1: Gross classification of tracheoesophageal fistula, types A through E.

SPECIAL CONSIDERATIONS AND CONCERNS

TEF/EA can occur as the sole congenital anomaly; however, it is estimated between 40% and 60% of cases are associated with one or more additional major anatomical birth defects.[6,12,13] The most common linked anomalies are those within the VACTERL spectrum (V, vertebral anomalies; A, anorectal atresia; C, congenital heart defects; TE, tracheoesophageal defects; and L, anomalies), with congenital heart defects the most common comorbidity (13%–34%).[13] There are also some genetic syndromes associated with TEF/EA, including CHARGE syndrome (C, coloboma; H, heart defects; A, choanal atresia; R, retardation of growth and/or development; G, genital and/or urinary defects; E, ear anomalies), as well as trisomies 18 and 21 and DiGeorge syndrome.[8,13] Refer to Chapter 28, "CHARGE Syndrome"; Chapter 31, "Down Syndrome"; and Chapter 47, "VACTERL Association," for more information regarding the anesthetic management of children with these syndromes.

Survival rates of healthy neonates with TEF/EA can approach 100%, but when associated with other anomalies or in neonates who are not healthy enough for early repair, reported survival decreases to 85% to 95%, with a greater impact on quality of life noted.[6,7] Accordingly, associated anomalies are more indicative in predicting neonatal outcomes when compared with weight alone. Term neonates typically tolerate primary repair. In contrast, extremely low-birth-weight (ELBW) or very low-birth-weight (VLBW) neonates may be too frail, with prematurity and birth weight recognized as primary indicators of neonatal survival.[6]

ANESTHETIC MANAGEMENT

PREOPERATIVE EVALUATION

Preoperative physical examination, evaluation, and preparation are similar to surgical repair by either thoracotomy or thoracoscopy. A complete airway examination is recommended to locate the site of the TEF. The gold standard for identifying the location of the TEF is direct visualization with a bronchoscopy and esophagoscopy.[2] An airway examination can also identify frequent secondary airway anomalies, such as a fistula at an unusual site, concurrent tracheomalacia, laryngeal cleft, vocal fold paresis or immobility, and subglottic stenosis.[4]

With coexisting congenital anomalies occurring between 40% and 60% in infants with TEF/EA, evaluation for other congenital anomalies is imperative.[1,6,12] The overall morbidity and mortality of newborns do not only depend on the TEF/EA subtype but also on the type, severity, and number of coexisting anomalies.[5] Diagnostic workup should include all organ systems, including a renal ultrasound, genetic testing, and an echocardiogram to evaluate for any clinically pertinent structural cardiac defects and determine the position of the aortic arch. A right-sided aortic arch is present in approximately 2.5% of cases and is important with regard to the surgical approach taken for repair if an open thoracotomy is planned by the surgical team.[1,9]

Pertinent Laboratories

Routine preoperative blood test should include a complete blood count, coagulation studies, baseline chemistry, and blood type and crossmatching. Although the need for a blood transfusion is rare during or after repair, requiring a transfusion may delay the opportunity for genetic testing. Therefore, genetic testing should also be drawn preoperatively.[9]

PREOPERATIVE PHARMACOLOGY

Antibiotics are started preoperatively in the presence of aspiration or suspected aspiration. Other medications, such as vasopressors, may be indicated to support stabilization of neonates presenting with unstable cardiorespiratory status.[6,10]

ANESTHETIC TECHNIQUE

Intraoperative Management

Surgical repair and management of the airway and ventilation during a TEF/EA repair can be challenging and complex. Several factors need to be considered in planning the airway and ventilation, with both the surgical and anesthesia teams working in close partnership. Several techniques and management options should be available. The location and size of the fistula are typically unknown prior to intubation; therefore, preoperative prediction of which intubation technique will work best may prove difficult.[14]

Management of the airway and ventilation strategies are accomplished after taking into consideration the size, exact location, and orientation of the TEF. Fiberoscopy is needed to determine the TEF location and size and the tracheobronchial tree anatomy and to verify the endotracheal tube (ETT) placement, along with possibly assisting the surgeon during the actual fistula ligation.[14] The classic approach is placing the ETT below the level of the fistula and proximal to the carina to prevent gastric distention and reflux of gastric contents into the lungs.[7,14] When the fistula is close to the carina, it can be extremely difficult to position the tip of the ETT between the fistula and the carina with the tip migrating into the right mainstem or upward toward the fistula with very little movement of the ETT. Inadvertent intubation of the actual fistula or right mainstem bronchus can then occur when trying to correct for the slight migration of the ETT tip.[14] Turning the bevel of the ETT to face backward (anterior) after it passes through the larynx can help avoid inadvertent intubation of the fistula. This also increases the possibility of blocking the fistula, and using a cuffed ETT further increases the chance of blocking the fistula.[14]

Another option for intubation is placing the tip of the ETT proximal to the fistula. This causes the distal end of the trachea to dilate and contract with ventilation, but with the risk of air going into the stomach. Airway pressure needs are limited with this technique and can be troublesome for neonates with an already poor respiratory status or distended abdomen.[14] Placing the ETT tip into the left mainstem bronchus is another choice, with the fistula being blocked in most cases. Reducing ventilation to the right lung may help with surgical access. In this approach, the ETT bevel should be directed to the right without the need for fiberoptic placement. Alternating between one- and two-lung ventilation throughout the surgical procedure may be necessary and less complicated without fiberoptic navigation.[14] Fogarty balloon-type blockers can also be used and can be placed by either the surgeon or the anesthesia provider. This technique places the balloon of the catheter through the TEF until the balloon disappears under fiberoptic visualization. This technique allows for the ETT to be placed mid-trachea and for positive pressure ventilation with less risk. With this technique, the Fogarty balloon-type blocker does not need to be removed prior to TEF ligation.[14]

Surgical repair of TEF/EA can be performed via either a thoracoscopic approach or a traditional open approach. The thoracoscopic approach is preferred by many due to better visualization of the surgical field, less surgical damage, reduced pain, and better long-term outcomes, such as reduced musculoskeletal deformities, including scoliosis.[15,16] In a thoracoscopic approach, the patient is placed in a modified prone position with the right side elevated at 30 degrees. If a right-sided aortic arch has been identified during a preoperative echocardiogram, the approach may be from the left side. This position is to provide exposure to the fistula by allowing the lung to fall away from the posterior mediastinum.[1] When the surgeon is ready to work on the thoracic outlet, anesthesia may be asked to put pressure on the nasogastric tube to help the surgeon find the upper pouch.

This approach has few contraindications except when there is severe hemodynamic instability, in addition to the relative contraindications of prematurity, small size (<1500 g), significant congenital heart anomalies, and abdominal distention.[1] An advantage of a thoracoscopic approach is the avoidance of complications from a thoracotomy, although an open approach can be beneficial in identifying anastomotic leaks.[1] A right posterolateral thoracotomy is used when a thoracotomy approach is preferred by the surgeon.[1] A right thoracotomy is also a viable approach if the defect is below T3.[2] Anesthesia providers should be aware, however, that when spreading the ribs for a posterolateral thoracotomy, damage to thoracic nerves can occur, leading to respiratory complications and chest wall morbidity.

Special Techniques and/or Equipment

Spontaneous respirations, even with poor lung compliance, have very little risk of gastric insufflation. To prevent the complications associated with mechanical ventilation, mechanical ventilation is avoided preoperatively, if possible. Neonates experiencing respiratory distress requiring intubation should be ventilated gently with low peak pressures. Whether intubated prior to arriving at the operating room or after the induction of general anesthesia, it is imperative that the end of the ETT be placed below the fistula, if possible, to avoid gastric distention.[6,9]

Neonates with distal TEF have a smaller risk of gastric distention and ventilatory compromise involving impingement on the diaphragm or pneumoperitoneum from gastric rupture.[9] Ventilation with positive end-expiratory pressure on lungs with poor compliance can cause air to be trapped in the stomach, with potential leakage through the distal fistula, as in types C and D.[6,9] Gastric distention leads to worsening respiratory distress and impaired diaphragmatic movement, along with an increased risk of gastric perforation.

Emergency ligation of the distal TEF is performed with possible gastrostomy tube placement to decompress the stomach if gastric perforation is to be prevented.[6] Broemling and Campbell[17] (as cited in Hunt et al.[9]) state that the purpose of the gastrostomy is to eliminate life-threatening gastric rupture. However, placement may actually worsen the already ineffective ventilation by creating a low-pressure leak via a bronchocutaneous fistula. It is therefore retained in cases of impending or actual gastric perforation.[9] An additional indication for emergency repair is a premature infant with worsening respiratory distress syndrome (RDS), in which the ventilation preferentially goes to the stomach via the TEF and contributes to a significant decline in respiratory status.[15]

Clinical Pearls

Clinical pearls for TEF repair are summarized in **Box 95.1**.

Complications

Once the ETT is in position, it should be carefully secured and every precaution must be taken to avoid the need for adjustment of the ETT during the resection of the fistula. Evidence of inadequate ventilation (declining O_2 saturation and end-tidal CO_2) may be from migration of the ETT, but could also be attributable to blockage of ETT from secretions or blood, hemodynamic instability, or surgical retraction causing pressure on the bronchus or the trachea.[14] Other complications revolve around periods of one-lung ventilation with problems of oxygenation and elimination of CO_2. Neonates having surgical repair for TEF/EA often develop intraoperative acidosis and hypercapnia regardless of the surgical technique but is typically more severe during thoracoscopic repair.[18] Therefore, it is important anesthesia providers routinely assess arterial blood gases intraoperatively and maintain arterial oxygenation to prevent the potential for any long-term sequelae for which further study is needed.

Upper airway pathology can make postoperative extubation a challenge. It has been found that vocal cord dysfunction occurs at a higher rate than previously reported and a higher rate of cord dysfunction is present in infants having long-gap EA repairs.[10] The higher rate of vocal cord dysfunction is attributed to injury of the recurrent laryngeal and vagus nerves when performing a thoracoscopic dissection of the

---

BOX 95.1 CLINICAL PEARLS: TRACHEO-ESOPHAGEAL FISTULA REPAIR

Anesthetic Management

- Standard ASA monitoring
- Upper and lower (preductal and postductal) pulse oximetry
- Arterial line access
- IV lines × 2
- Place Replogle for continuous suction
- Underbody forced-air warmer
- Induction with sevoflurane and/or propofol
- Maintain spontaneous ventilation
- Obtain additional IV access if needed
- Obtain arterial access if not in situ
- Topicalize vocal cords with lidocaine if preoperative bronchoscopy is being performed
- Consider glycopyrrolate for vagal stimulation and to reduce secretions
- Intubate with bevel anteriorly and place as indicated by location of the fistula and consider cuffed ETT
- Neuromuscular blockade after placement of ETT
- Position left lateral or semiprone 30 degrees by surgeon preference
- Fentanyl for analgesia
- Regional anesthesia if indicated
- Low peak pressure ventilation

Postoperative Care

- Transfer to ICU
- Postoperative ventilation (avoid hyperextension of the neck)
- Multimodal analgesia for postoperative pain (±paralytic)

ASA, American Society of Anesthesiologists; ETT, endotracheal tube.

esophagus high in the thoracic inlet.[19] In addition to long-gap EA repairs, vocal cord paresis can be attributed to anastomotic leakage and longer periods of mechanical ventilation[20] (as cited in Hunt et al.[9]). Unilateral cord paralysis can be manageable, but bilateral paralysis may require a tracheostomy.[9]

Lung contusions can occur on the side of the thoracotomy where lung retraction has occurred during surgical repair. It can be seen on chest x-ray as an opacity and may require an increase in oxygen and ventilatory pressure for 12 to 24 hours postoperatively.[9]

Postoperative complications should be anticipated as most patients will have at least one complication.[10] Early surgical complications occurring postoperatively include anastomotic leak, anastomotic stricture, and recurrent TEF. Anastomotic leaks commonly occur within 48 hours postsurgical repair and can be treated medically with antibiotics to prevent mediastinitis from salivary leakage, parenteral nutrition, and drainage.[1,6,9] Larger leaks may require emergency chest tube placement following acute decompensation from a tension pneumothorax or sepsis; however, minor leaks are more common.[15] Anastomotic strictures are the most common type of complication and require dilatation with a balloon or bougie.[6,9] Acid suppression is an important treatment to reduce the risk of stricture formation.[9] Recurrent TEF is the least common of the postoperative complications with infants presenting with recurrent chest infections or feeding difficulties.[1,6,15] Operative treatment, however, should occur promptly after diagnosis.[1]

POSTOPERATIVE CARE

Determination for postoperative tracheal extubation relies on several factors. Most infants return to the ICU intubated with potential paralysis to prevent shearing or distraction of the esophageal anastomosis.[6] Careful attention to avoid hyperextension of the neck prevents accidental extubation and trauma to the surgical site.[6] Early tracheal extubation may be possible in infants who preoperatively had good lung function and whose anastomosis is not under significant tension, with the caveat that laryngoscopy puts stress on the anastomosis, and weaning infants over several days with paralysis may be more beneficial to allow for surgical healing.[14] In infants who required intubation preoperatively due to acute respiratory failure or poor lung compliance, delayed extubation should be considered to prevent the need for emergency reintubation.[14] Prolonged mechanical ventilation has the added risk of pneumonia, atelectasis, and other morbidities. Keeping all factors in mind, earlier extubation is recommended if possible.[21]

Infants are kept NPO for 1 to 2 days postoperatively and are started on enteral feeds through a transanastomotic feeding tube placed during surgery.[6,9] Care is taken during extubation of the ETT so that the feeding tube is left in the proper location through the anastomosis. An x-ray of the chest and abdomen can confirm correct placement. If enteral feed cannot be started, then the infant can be started on total parenteral nutrition.[6]

Postoperative pain management in neonates following TEF/EA repair can be achieved in a number of ways, including IV opioid infusion, epidural catheter, subcutaneous wound catheter, and local infiltration. Surgeons may request postoperative muscle relaxation to prevent damage to the anastomotic site, making pain assessment difficult and reliant on vital signs alone.[9] Managing postoperative pain with opioids and benzodiazepines alone may cause respiratory depression. Therefore, it is recommended that once the surgeon's concern for tension on the surgical anastomotic site has diminished, analgesia is lightened and the neonate can then be placed on an assist mode in preparation for extubation at the earliest and safest time.[9]

KEY REFERENCES

Complete references for this chapter are online and available at https://connect.springerpub.com/content/book/978-0-8261-3875-0/part/part04/toc-part/ch095.

1. Slater BJ, Rothenberg SS. Tracheoesophageal fistula. *Semin Pediatr Surg.* 2016;25:176–178. doi:10.1053/j.sempedsurg.2016.02.010
6. Lee S. Basic knowledge of tracheoesophageal fistula and esophageal atresia. *Adv Neonatal Care.* 2018;18(1):14–21. doi:10.1097/ANC.0000000000000464
9. Hunt RW, Perkins EJ, King S. Peri-operative management of neonates with oesophageal atresia and trachea-oesophageal fistula. *Paediatr Respir Rev.* 2016;19:3–9. doi:10.1016/j.prrv.2016.01.002
10. Lal DR, Gadepalli SK, Downard CD, et al. Perioperative management and outcomes of esophageal atresia and tracheoesophageal fistula. *J Pediatr Surg.* 2017;52:1245–1251. doi:10.1016/j.jpedsurg.2016.11.046
14. Ho AM, Dion JM, Wong JCP. Airway and ventilator management options in congenital tracheoesophageal fistula repair. *Journal of Semin Cardiothorac Vasc Anesth.* 2016;30(2):515–520. doi:10.1053/j.jvca.2015.04.005
15. Teague WJ, Karpelowsky J. Surgical management of oesophageal atresia. *Paediatr Respir Rev.* 2016;19:10–15. doi:10.1016/j.prrv.2016.04.003

CHAPTER 96

Hernia Repair

Tomas Lazo and Courtney Miller

INDICATIONS/CONTRAINDICATIONS

Hernias are one of the most common conditions of infancy and childhood and are a common reason for pediatric patients to present to their primary care provider and ultimately to see either a pediatric surgeon or a pediatric urologist.[1-3] Hernias are defined as the protrusion of part of a tissue or organ through the wall containing it, normally a weakened portion of the abdominal wall. They occur in both adult and pediatric populations and can present at various stages of life, from the intrauterine stage into adulthood. The most common types of pediatric hernias in order of prevalence are inguinal hernia, umbilical hernia, and incisional hernias.[2-4] Other types include spigelian hernias, epigastric hernias, femoral hernias, and lumbar hernias, although these are not as common.[1] Congenital diaphragmatic hernias, as well as other major abdominal wall defects, such as gastroschisis and omphalocele, are discussed in Chapter 127, "Neonatal Emergencies."

Inguinal hernias are associated with incomplete closure of the processus vaginalis during fetal development. This process involves the descent of the gonads (in males and females) from below the diaphragm to the lower abdominal cavity between 8 and 15 weeks' gestation. Ultimately the gonads, particularly the testes in males, descend through the inguinal canal and into the scrotum between 25 and 35 weeks' gestation. In normal fetal development, the processus vaginalis closes after descent of the testes, with the left processus vaginalis closing earlier than the right side, resulting in higher incidence of right-sided inguinal hernias.[3]

It is estimated that up to 5% of mature infants and up to 30% of premature babies will develop an inguinal hernia.[1,5,6] Parents are often the first to notice an inguinal hernia, commonly during bathing, which appears as an abnormal bulge that may or may not cause distress to the child, with a higher male versus female predominance. Notably, inguinal hernias occur three to five times more frequently in males than in females, with approximately 80% of inguinal hernia repairs (IHR) being performed in male babies.[1,3] Furthermore, the incidence of inguinal hernias is inversely correlated with gestational age and birth weight.[3] This trend is attributed to an increased likelihood of a patent processus vaginalis in preterm infants at birth. Interestingly, bilateral inguinal hernias are found more commonly in this population, with a higher female predominance, compared with infants born at term and older children.[1,3]

Prematurity and clinical presentation are two important factors to consider when planning surgical intervention of inguinal hernias. Some surgeons advocate for early repair (prior to discharge from the NICU in preterm infants), while others prefer delayed surgical intervention, assuming the patient is asymptomatic.[3] A notable advantage of an early repair includes preventing incarceration, which would warrant readmission and urgent surgery. Conversely, the benefit of delayed intervention includes overall reduction in hernia recurrence that accompanies early intervention, thereby minimizing exposure to additional anesthetics.[3] However, delaying surgery may put the child at risk of multiple episodes of herniation that cannot be reduced, thereby compromising blood flow, eventually leading to testicular atrophy. Delayed management also risks the need for emergent surgery in infants and children who have signs of strangulation with ischemic bowel and who may have comorbid conditions that have yet to be fully optimized.[2,3] Early versus late surgical intervention is an ongoing debate and requires careful identification of risks and benefits.[2,5]

Surgical repair of inguinal hernias is one of the most common pediatric procedures and involves ligation of the patent processus vaginalis at the level of the internal ring.[4,6] This can be achieved through open hernia repair (OHR), considered the gold standard, or laparoscopic hernia repair (LHR). OHR has the advantage of reduced incisional pain in comparison with traditional three-port laparoscopy; for cosmetic purposes, the incision can be concealed by the groin crease.[6] Newer laparoscopic techniques have comparable recovery times when compared with traditional laparoscopy and only require a small umbilical incision and a 1-mm stab incision at the site of the hernia.[2] In addition, visualization of the contralateral inguinal canal is easy and efficient when using laparoscopy, reducing handling, and thus injury, of delicate structures passing through the inguinal canal (i.e., vas deferens, spermatic vessels) without an additional incision, as well as decreased operative time as proficiency is gained.[2,4,6] Examination of the contralateral side for inguinal hernia is often done automatically in children under 2 years of age as patency of the contralateral processus vaginalis is common in infants and children younger than 2 years of age, 44% and 34%, respectively.[3] Intraoperative examination for bilateral inguinal hernias and repair of the contralateral processus vaginalis decrease the likelihood of hernia development and the possibility of exposure to a second anesthetic, although some find this practice controversial.[3-5] Meta-analyses show similar outcomes for LHR and IHR, with recurrence rates of less than 4%.[4] Despite these findings, LHR continues to be utilized less than OHR.[3,7]

SPECIAL CONSIDERATIONS AND CONCERNS

Asymptomatic hernias have the potential to become symptomatic and develop signs of hernia strangulation or incarceration. Strangulation occurs when a tissue, such as the bowel, testis, or ovary, protrudes through the patent processus vaginalis and incurs compromised blood flow. The narrow canal in this circumstance has the potential to obstruct venous return, leading to edema and ultimately increasing hernial sac pressure that causes decreased arterial blood flow, which can lead to ischemia and necrosis.[3] Initial presentation of strangulation is pain, and signs of ongoing intra-abdominal process, such as abdominal distension, and signs of tissue ischemia or necrosis, such as increasing lactate levels, although this is rare outside of diaphragmatic hernias.[8] In the event of strangulation, immediate attempt to reduce the hernia should be performed. Notably, 80% to 90% of cases are easily reduced, allowing for a 24- to 48-hour delay in surgical intervention.[3] On the other hand, if manual reduction is unsuccessful, then an urgent repair is warranted. Herniation is a less concerning sign and represents extrusion of tissue into the canal without compromise to blood supply or lymphatic drainage. Once the condition of the infant or the child is determined to be elective, urgent, or emergent, the anesthetic technique requires consideration.

ANESTHETIC MANAGEMENT

PREOPERATIVE EVALUATION

Anesthetic considerations include preoperative evaluation of the patient, obtaining relevant histories, examining pertinent laboratory findings, communicating with the surgical team (and the neonatologist if applicable), and determining the anesthetic technique.[3] A careful history and physical examination should be conducted preoperatively. A birth history, particularly in infants, should be obtained. Evaluating comorbidities and the family is vital to not only identify risk factors for inguinal hernia occurrence but also to identify conditions that may not be adequately optimized and may increase the likelihood of perioperative complications, such as existing respiratory symptoms.[9]

Often infants and children with disease processes resulting from increased abdominal pressure, such as chronic respiratory distress, mechanical ventilation, or constipation, are at risk of iatrogenic inguinal hernias.[3] Instances of increased intra-abdominal pressure from ventriculoperitoneal shunts placed for hydrocephalus (VPS) have also been reported.[3] In addition, familial history of congenital inguinal hernia and connective tissue disorders such as Ehlers–Danlos syndrome have been associated with occurrence inguinal hernias.[3] Lastly, medical conditions resulting in poor nutritional status (such as necrotizing enterocolitis) may predispose patients to inguinal hernias secondary to inadequate muscle and connective tissue development.[3] These hernia risk factors may have anesthetic implications and a thorough history should be obtained to proper perioperative management.

ANESTHETIC TECHNIQUE

Intraoperative Management

Decades ago, nearly all these procedures were performed under general anesthesia (GA). However, there has been an increasing amount of evidence for concern over neuronal apoptosis in the developing brain when exposed to GA.[10] However, within the past 15 years, more evidence has emerged disputing these claims, noting a favorable safety profile in most young patients undergoing GA at a young age, particularly for anesthetic exposures of 1 hour or less.[10] These findings are particularly reassuring as most children present for short elective surgeries with anesthetic exposure less than 1 hour.[3,10]

With the continued spotlight on neurotoxicity in young infants and children receiving GA, a common decision for anesthesia providers to make is whether to perform a GA or choose an alternative such as a regional anesthetic (RA) or sedation with infiltration of local anesthetic at the surgical site. Selecting anesthetic technique requires careful consideration of patient history and comorbidities, location and complexity of the hernia, length of case, surgical technique, as well as surgeon preference. GA with an endotracheal tube (ETT) or a laryngeal mask airway (LMA) is often preferred in cases requiring extensive repair of bilateral, complex, or large hernias with a long case duration.[3,6] In addition, the use of laparoscopic technique and the need for neuromuscular blockade are indications for GA with a secure airway.[3]

RA techniques for IHR include neuraxial anesthetics such as spinal or caudal epidural, as well as local anesthetic, nerve blocks around the ilioinguinal and iliohypogastric nerves.[3] While caudal epidurals or local anesthetics can be used as the sole anesthetic for surgery, they are often combined with inhalation or intravascular (IV) anesthetics. Per recent reports, this approach has a similar postoperative complication profile to a spinal anesthetic alone.[3]

Neuraxial anesthetics have gained traction as cost-effective, opioid-sparing alternatives to GA for IHR. Some studies found fewer complications, notably with postoperative apnea, bradycardia, and hypoxemia, among patients undergoing neuraxial anesthesia.[3] More recent findings indicate RA approaches have reduced the incidence of postoperative apnea within 30 minutes after the procedure has finished. However, the incidence was the same as patients receiving GA when compared at the 12-hour postoperative period, when the majority of these episodes were related to prematurity.[3] Comparatively, neuraxial and local anesthetics may not offer appropriate anesthetic duration for longer and more complex hernia repairs. Spinal anesthesia, for instance, tends to have shorter action in infants due to increased cerebrospinal fluid (CSF) circulation and blood flow.[3] Thus, multiple factors, including gestational age, likelihood of postoperative apnea, duration and complexity of surgery, and additional comorbidities, should be considered when deciding to proceed with a regional versus a general anesthetic.

POSTOPERATIVE CARE

From a surgical perspective, patients usually do quite well. Hernia recurrence is always a possibility, with a higher incidence noted in premature infants and earlier repairs.[1,3] Other complications include wound infection and injury to adjacent structures. For males in particular, patients may incur inadvertent cryptorchidism or testicular atrophy.[3]

In terms of anesthesia, the largest concern surrounds the likelihood of postoperative apnea events. Ex-preemies and infants who are less than 45 to 50 weeks postconceptional age, including those born at term, are at increased risk of postoperative apnea.[11] For this reason, the recommendation for patients under 50 weeks, gestational age is to undergo a 12- to 24-hour observation period after a GA.[3] While this is the most common reason for postoperative apnea, other factors, including presence of pulmonary disease (such as bronchopulmonary dysplasia), residual neuromuscular blockade, and oversedation, may also increase this risk.[11] If patients do not fall under these higher risk categories, such as older children, they may be managed under traditional postoperative and day-patient standards. A summary of anesthetic management strategies for inguinal hernia surgery can be found in **Box 96.1**.

BOX 96.1 CLINICAL PEARLS FOR ANESTHETIC MANAGEMENT OF INGUINAL HERNIA PATIENTS

- Perform a thorough preoperative assessment: calculate postgestational age and evaluate for upper respiratory infection symptoms and congenital syndromes with associated abnormalities.
- Be wary of postoperative apnea.
- Consider regional anesthesia approaches for patients at high risk of postoperative apnea.
- Extubate patients awake if using general anesthesia.

REFERENCES

1. Abdulhai SA, Glenn IC, Ponsky TA. Incarcerated pediatric hernias. *Surg Clin North Am.* 2017;97(1):129–145. doi:10.1016/j.suc.2016.08.010
2. Chan YY, Durbin-Johnson B, Kurzrock EA. Pediatric inguinal and scrotal surgery — practice patterns in U.S. academic centers. *J Pediatr Surg.* 2016;51(11):1786–1790. doi:10.1016/j.jpedsurg.2016.07.019
3. Ramachandran V, Edwards CF, Bichianu DC. Inguinal hernia in premature infants. *NeoReviews.* 2020;21(6):e392–e403. doi:10.1542/neo.21-6-e392
4. Thomas DT, Göcmen KB, Tulgar S, Boga I. Percutaneous internal rivvvvng suturing is a safe and effective method for the minimal invasive treatment of pediatric inguinal hernia: experience with 250 cases. *J Pediatr Surg.* 2016;51(8):1330–1335. doi:10.1016/j.jpedsurg.2015.11.024
5. Maillet OP, Garnier S, Dadure C, et al. Inguinal hernia in premature boys: should we systematically explore the contralateral side? *J Pediatr Surg.* 2014;49(9):1419–1423. doi:10.1016/j.jpedsurg.2014.01.055
6. Timberlake MD, Herbst KW, Rasmussen S, Corbett ST. Laparoscopic percutaneous inguinal hernia repair in children: review of technique and comparison with open surgery. *J Pediatr Urol.* 2015;11(5):262.e261–262.e266. doi:10.1016/j.jpurol.2015.04.008
7. Chong AJ, Fevrier HB, Herrinton LJ. Long-term follow-up of pediatric open and laparoscopic inguinal hernia repair. *J Pediatr Surg.* 2019;54(10):2138–2144. doi:10.1016/j.jpedsurg.2019.01.064
8. Fox C, Stewart M, King SK, Patel N. Acute gastrointestinal compromise in neonates with congenital diaphragmatic hernia prior to repair. *J Pediatr Surg.* 2016;51(12):1917–1920. doi:10.1016/j.jpedsurg.2016.09.012
9. Mamie C, Habre W, Delhumeau C, et al. Incidence and risk factors of perioperative respiratory adverse events in children undergoing elective surgery. *Paediatr Anaesth.* 2004;14(3):218–224. doi:10.1111/j.1460-9592.2004.01169.x
10. Vutskits L, Culley DJ. GAS, PANDA, and MASK. *Anesthesiology.* 2019;131(4):762–764. doi:10.1097/aln.0000000000002863
11. Lamoshi A, Lerman J, Dughayli J, et al. Association of anesthesia type with prolonged postoperative intubation in neonates undergoing inguinal hernia repair. *Am J Perinatol.* 2020. doi:10.1038/s41372-020-0703-4

CHAPTER 97

Pectus Excavatum Repair

Nicholas Detchon

INDICATIONS/CONTRAINDICATIONS

Pectus excavatum (PE) is a congenital abnormality of the sternum, ribs, and costal cartilages (Figure 97.1). PE is cited as the most common chest wall deformity in children and adolescents, occurring in 1 in every 1,000 live births.[1] While some children are born with PE or have a genetic predisposition, such as Marfan's syndrome, most do not develop the deformity until their prepubescent and early teenage years.[2] The role of surgery in correcting PE is multifactorial and supported by findings that postbar removal there is an increase in cardiopulmonary function, chest wall mechanics, subjective clinical improvement in exercise tolerance, and self-image.[3]

Classic operative repair involves extrapleural excision of the sternocostal cartilage and mobilization of the sternum and ribs, known as the Ravitch procedure. The majority of patients now undergo the more minimally invasive Nuss procedure, in which the costal cartilages are preserved and the sternum is elevated with bars to correct the deformity. Through the direct vision of a thoracoscope (Figure 97.2), a transmedial tunnel is created and a prebent bar(s) is passed behind the sternum with the convex side down. Once in place, the bar is rotated 180 degrees to elevate the sternum and is then fixed to the ribs on both sides (Figure 97.3). The bars are left in place temporarily, typically being removed after a 2- to 4-year period as an outpatient procedure.[3]

Despite the minimally invasive approach of the Nuss procedure, which utilizes smaller incisions, entails no cartilage resection and requires less operative time, the stretch and pressure on the chest wall following repair yield a more painful postoperative course when compared with the Ravitch.[4] The significant and lengthy postoperative pain can last for weeks, causing distress to patients, families, and clinicians. The ability to adequately control postoperative pain is the primary determinant of hospital stay following the Nuss procedure, as insufficient pain control often necessitates prolonged hospitalization.[5]

SPECIAL CONSIDERATIONS AND CONCERNS

The Haller index (HI) is the most common measure of PE defect and severity using CT scans for accurate measurement. CT is used to demonstrate the abnormal ratio between the patient's transverse diameter and their anterior–posterior diameter at the deepest part of the deformity. An index of 2 to 3 is considered normal, while an HI greater than 3.25 is considered a moderately severe defect possibly requiring surgical repair. Since the HI does not account for asymmetry of the defect, an asymmetry index is often utilized in combination with the HI to more accurately characterize the degree of asymmetry of PE.[6]

ANESTHETIC MANAGEMENT

PREOPERATIVE EVALUATION

Preoperative evaluation of patients with PE focuses on exercise tolerance and signs of cardiopulmonary compromise. Clinically, symptoms of dyspnea, anterior chest wall pain,

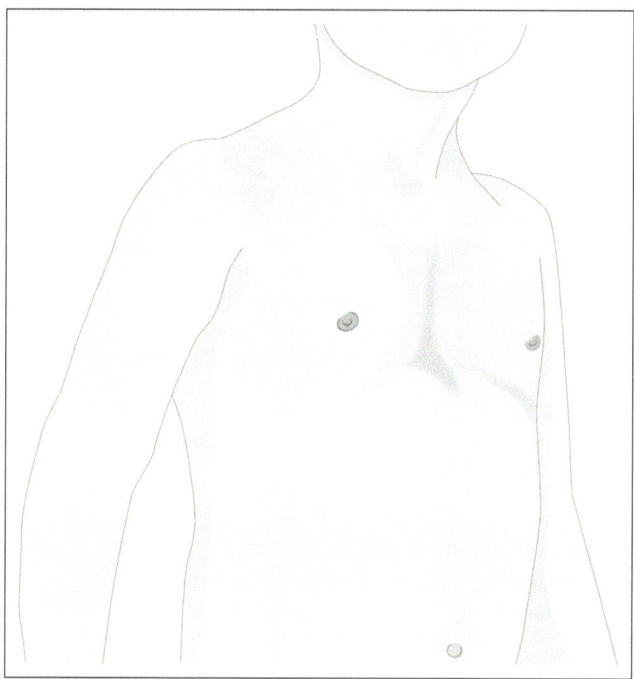

Figure 97.1: Pectus excavatum.
Source: Chiocca EM. Chapter 17: Assessment of the thorax, lungs, and regional lymphatics assessment of the thorax, lungs, and regional lymphatics in the pediatric patient. In *Advanced Pediatric Assessment*. 3rd ed. Springer; 2019:Fig. 17.6.

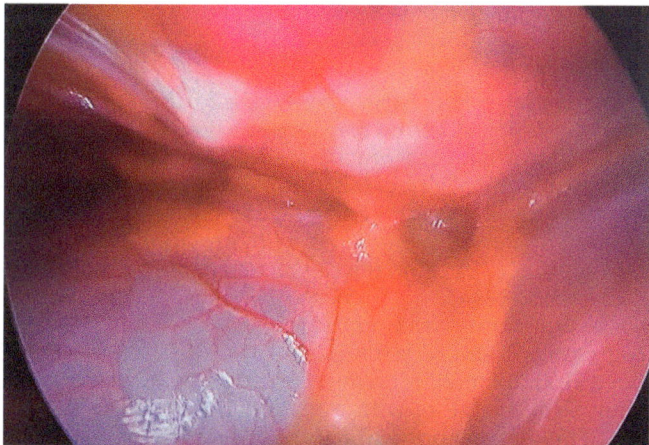

Figure 97.2: Thoracoscopic view across the chest during dissection.
Source: Courtesy of Dr. Victor Garcia.

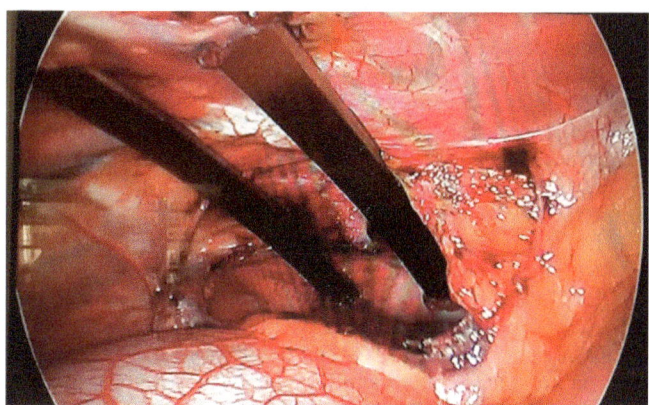

Figure 97.3: Thoracoscopic view across the chest after bar placement.
Source: Courtesy of Dr. Victor Garcia.

easy fatiguability, palpitations, and recurrent lower respiratory tract infections may be present, but most patients are healthy and asymptomatic.[3] The preoperative evaluation for PE repair should include review of a CT scan of the chest to evaluate and document the severity of the deformity, the degree of cardiac compression and displacement, as well as the degree of lung compression and any other unexpected problems. Other preoperative tests may include an echocardiogram to further investigate compression of the right atrium and ventricle, an ECG, and pulmonary function test (PFT). Most patients with significant PE have low normal or below normal PFT results. Both static and exercise PFTs are useful in eliciting a physiologic effect of the PE defect. Also, in patients with known cardiac issues, a cardiac MRI is often indicated.[7]

Preoperative education days or weeks prior to surgery is vital to managing pain expectations and helps temper anxiety prior to PE repair for both patients and families. The various methods of postoperative pain management need to be thoroughly reviewed in the preoperative education, which can occur via a class, participation in a virtual meeting, or by having the patient view a video. On the day of the procedure, the patient and their family will be met by a member of the acute pain service who will be charged with managing the pain regimen perioperatively. At this time, the patient and their family will be reeducated on the pain management methods available and realistic pain expectations will again be discussed. An analgesia plan will be agreed on by the patient, their family, and the acute pain service, and proper informed consent for the agreed-on pain procedures will be obtained.

PREOPERATIVE PHARMACOLOGY

In older teenagers and young adults, a peripheral IV catheter is placed preoperatively, a scopolamine patch is ordered, and oral pregabalin is administered. In many cases, an anxiolytic, such as midazolam, is indicated and administered prior to transferring the patient to the operating room (OR). In younger patients, oral midazolam can be administered 20 minutes prior to going to the OR, and an IV catheter can be placed following an inhalation mask induction or sedation with nitrous oxide once in the OR.

ANESTHETIC TECHNIQUE

Intraoperative Management

Once in the OR, standard monitors will be applied and the patient will be positioned in a manner that facilitates performance of regional anesthesia. A Salter nasal cannula is placed on the patient and midazolam and fentanyl can be titrated for patient comfort. A variety of regional anesthetic techniques can be employed to provide perioperative analgesia. Should a thoracic epidural (TE) be the analgesic plan, the patient is typically positioned sitting on the side of the OR table, leaning forward onto a small table with the aid of a nurse for TE placement.

Thoracic paravertebral and erector spinae plane blocks are also viable techniques that have proved to provide effective analgesia. While both blocks are typically performed with the patient in the upright, sitting position, they can also be performed in the prone or lateral position. In some instances, general anesthesia may be induced and the patient intubated on the stretcher and then positioned prone or lateral on the OR table sto facilitate placement of ultrasound-guided thoracic paravertebral or erector spinae plane block catheters depending on institutional protocol. After placement is complete, the catheters are secured, and the patient is turned supine back onto the stretcher and then moved onto the OR table for surgical positioning.

An IV induction is most commonly performed, although inhalation mask inductions may be warranted in younger patients. IV inductions typically consist of propofol 1 to 2 mg/kg, fentanyl 1 mcg/kg, and a nondepolarizing paralytic, such as vecuronium or rocuronium. Following induction of anesthesia and endotracheal intubation, another IV catheter is placed. One of the infusing IV catheters should be connected to a fluid warmer with blood tubing in anticipation of the need for blood transfusion. Intraoperative mortality from exsanguination secondary to cardiac or vascular injury has been described but is rare. Nonetheless, it is imperative the anesthesia provider ensures the availability of packed red blood cells, with adequate vascular access that can accommodate rapid resuscitation prior to surgical incision. Arterial catheters are typically not indicated unless there is a history of significant cardiac or pulmonary compromise.

The patient is positioned supine with gel rolls placed longitudinally under their back for the procedure. The arms are tucked to the side in anatomic position, with thoracic elevation provided by the gel rolls affording the surgeon access to the lateral chest walls. A rectal temperature probe is preferred and a lower body forced-air warmer should be placed on the patient prior to placing the surgical drapes. It is advisable to have a phenylephrine infusion in-line, connected at a port close to the patient prior to draping. The infusion can be titrated as needed to maintain adequate mean arterial blood pressure (MAP) during the surgical procedure. Pain management is multimodal in nature. After incision, the epidural, thoracic paravertebral, or erector spinae plane block infusions are started and IV methadone .1 mg/kg up to 5 mg should be administered. A ketamine bolus of .25 to .5 mg/kg should be considered in patients with a history of chronic pain. Additionally, IV acetaminophen 15 mg/kg and ketorolac .5 mg/kg (max 15 mg) should be administered along with antiemetics.

After the incisions and thoracoscopy, a clamp is placed around the sternum, which is then elevated to facilitate careful dissection around the lungs, mediastinum, and pericardium, followed by thoracoscopic placement of the bar(s) by the surgeon. Anesthesia providers should be aware that arrhythmias can occur during advancement of the bar(s) and ongoing communication with the surgical team is vital during this phase of the procedure. Accordingly, the pulse oximetry volume should be increased to alert the anesthesia provider of cardiac arrhythmias, and the ECG tracing should be monitored closely during bar advancement.

Once the bars are in place, managing bilateral pneumothoraces is important. The surgeon may ask the anesthesia provider to perform the Valsalva maneuver several times while suction is simultaneously applied to the pleural spaces. A chest x-ray is often used to evaluate lung expansion either intraoperatively or while in the recovery area. If the patient is easy to ventilate and intubate, a deep extubation is preferred to avoid coughing, thereby decreasing the likelihood of developing subcutaneous emphysema.

Following extubation IV diazepam .05 mg/kg is administered to prevent muscle spasms and to reduce postoperative anxiety. Dexmedetomidine .5 mg/kg up to 20 mg can also be given at this time if the patient is extremely anxious preoperatively. Supplemental doses of hydromorphone may be given in small weight-based increments if the patient reports pain once awake.

Special Techniques and/or Equipment

There is no standardized optimal pain management following this procedure; however, TE analgesia and patient-controlled analgesia (PCA) remain the two most commonly used techniques employed, whether it be together or independently. The placement of a TE consists of infiltration of a local anesthetic subcutaneously, then inserting an 18-g Tuohy needle between the spinous processes of T5 to T6, or T6 to T7. The epidural space is noted by loss of resistance to air or preservative free saline and a catheter is advanced 3 to 4 cm and secured in place. A test dose is then administered, and once confirmed negative the catheter is secured and a sterile dressing is placed. The TE is then usually loaded with ropivacaine .15% to .2% with or without clonidine .5 to 1 mcg/mL at .5 mL per level, which is typically 6 to 10 mL, depending on height and catheter position. The infusion pump can then be programmed with a basal rate of .2 to .3 mL/kg/hr.[4]

TE analgesia has been shown to be more effective than PCA alone in the early postoperative period, and although considered safe it carries risks including nerve damage, infection, one-sided block, upper extremity weakness or tingling, respiratory depression, and in rare instances epidural hematoma or epidural abscess. Epidural anesthesia is typically limited to the first 2 or 3 postoperative days (POD), then transitioned to oral regimens.[7] A meta-analysis of six studies confirmed that a TE is associated with lower pain scores through to 48 hours after surgery, without significant differences in secondary outcomes, compared with IV opioids alone.[1]

Continuous thoracic paravertebral nerve blocks are nonneuraxial nerve blocks being used as an alternative to TE to help manage pain postoperatively following PE repair. Thoracic paravertebral nerve blocks involve placing peripheral bilateral spinal nerve catheters into the paravertebral space, inserting at T2 and reaching T5 using ultrasound guidance. After negative aspiration for blood and cerebral spinal fluid (CSF), .15 mL/kg of 0.2% or .25% ropivacaine with dexmedetomidine .25 mcg/kg is injected on each side. An infusion is initiated at .2 mg/kg/hr with or without a clonidine max of .1 mcg/kg/hr to the catheter on each side after surgical incision.

Several studies and meta-analysis of randomized trials comparing thoracic paravertebral nerve blocks with TE have found thoracic paravertebral nerve blocks to have equivalent analgesia with a better side effect profile than TE.[8] The more peripheral nature of thoracic paravertebral nerve blocks makes them an attractive alternative to TE in cases of mild anticoagulation or if there are other concerns for placing a TE.[9]

Erector spinae plane blocks are a novel technique being employed with more regularity in pediatric practice. While the exact mechanism is not fully understood, it is thought that following injection of local anesthetic deep to the erector spinae muscles and superficial to the transverse process the local anesthetic diffuses anteriorly into the paravertebral space. There is likely interfascial spread toward the posterior rami of the spinal nerves as well, which may account for the primary mechanism of action. As the use of this technique is employed more frequently in pediatric practice, there is a need for a better understanding of the efficacy of management of postoperative pain following PE repair.

Intraoperative cryoanalgesia is a newer pain control strategy in which the surgeon freezes the nerve axon directly perpendicular to the intercostal nerves via application of a cryoprobe. Freezing prevents transmission of electrical signal along the axon, thereby negating pain signaling and providing analgesia. The fibrous neural structures remain intact, as do the intercostal vessels facilitating axonal regeneration, which has been found to be complete in animal studies in 4 to 6 weeks.

Single-lung ventilation may be needed to improve visualization during probe application, which was best achieved with a double-lumen endotracheal tube in a study by Graves et al. The benefits of cryoanalgesia include analgesia effects that can last at least 2 months as compared with less than 23 hours in injectable regional blocks and the gradual return of sensation as opposed to short-acting blocks, which can cause a difficult transition period requiring "catch-up" with oral regimens.[5] The utility of cryoanalgesia in pediatrics is still being explored.

Complications/Emergencies

Major anesthetic complications can occur during bar placement or when the patient returns for removal, which include myocardial perforation, diaphragmatic perforation, pneumothorax, and flail chest. Fortunately, these complications are rare. Common complications associated with the Nuss procedure include atelectasis, subcutaneous emphysema, and pericardial and pleural effusions. Blood loss is usually minimal though and patients often leave the OR with a chest tube in place.

Metal allergies pose another potential complication, as the bars were historically made of stainless steel which contains various metals such as iron, chromium, and nickel. These metals are not antigens themselves but can become ionized in the body and bind with natural proteins, leading to allergic reactions. Titanium, a biocompatible metal that rarely becomes ionized and thus provokes few allergic reactions, is now more widely used for pectus bars.[10]

POSTOPERATIVE CARE

Postoperative pain management can be challenging despite the procedure being minimally invasive; the pain is intense and generally lasts days to weeks (Box 97.1). Pain can be attributed to the surgical retraction and dissection of intercostal muscles, as well as the conformational change of the rib cage. Pain management can be especially challenging in

---

BOX 97.1 COMMON PECTUS SURGERY PAIN MANAGEMENT PROTOCOL

Preoperative Preparation
- Pectus surgery education, set expectations, and create pain plan.
- Consent for agreed-on regional anesthesia.

Day of Surgery (POD 0)
- PO pregabalin (Lyrica): in In patients <50 kg, 25 mg; >50 kg, 50–75 mg, and place scopolamine patch.
- Epidural placement (T5–T7) or PVNB catheter placement by anesthesia/pain team.
- Epidural analgesia with ropivacaine .15%–.2% with clonidine .5–1 mcg/mL (or no clonidine).
- PVNB initial bolus: 20 mL (.15 mL/kg) .2% or .25% ropivacaine with dexmedetomidine .25 mcg/kg each side; maintenance: ropivacaine infusion to bilateral catheters at .2 mg/kg/hr to each catheter on pump with/without clonidine max .1 mcg/kg/hr each side.
- IV methadone .1 mg/kg, up to 5 mg × 1 dose (before incision or during surgery); second dose at 9 p.m.
- Intraoperative bolus .25–.5 mg/kg in patients with chronic pain issues only.
- IV acetaminophen (Ofirmev) 15 mg/kg q6h for 2 days.
- IV ketorolac (Toradol) 0.5 mg/kg (max 30 mg) q6h from 8 p.m. of day of surgery.
- IV methocarbamol (Robaxin) 15 mg/kg IV q8h ATC, convert to PO after 48 hr for muscle spasms.
- IV diazepam (Valium) .05 mg/kg IV every 4–6 PRN for pain and chest tightness.
- IV ondansetron (Zofran) .1 mg/kg (max 8 mg) q8h ATC for 2 days followed by PRN (confirm no prolonged QTc); first dose to be given 8 hr after last intraoperative/PACU dose.

POD 1
- Continue epidural analgesia or PVNB catheter infusions, IV acetaminophen, IV methocarbamol, and IV diazepam PRN.
- Start oxycodone q4h ATC (start when the patient is tolerating solid diet and adjust dose and frequency based on weight and effect).
- Continue pregabalin (Lyrica) q12h.
- Continue scheduled IV ondansetron (Zofran) q8h ATC.
- Place order on the electronic record to stop epidural infusion on POD 2 at 6 a.m.
- IV hydromorphone or morphine for breakthrough pain on POD 1 and 2.
- Remove Foley catheter prior to first physical therapy session.
- Bowel regimen per surgery.
- If PVNB catheters in place, transition all medications to PO by end of day if possible

> **BOX 97.1 COMMON PECTUS SURGERY PAIN MANAGEMENT PROTOCOL** (*cont.*)
>
> **POD 2**
>
> - Stop epidural infusion at 6 a.m. and remove catheter.
> - Once epidural is out, continue/transition to PO oxycodone q4h ATC or PRN for moderate and severe pain. Transition to PO methocarbamol ATC and PO diazepam q4h ATC or PRN if sedated. Continue PO pregabalin (Lyrica) q12h and stop after 2 days of use. Transition to PO acetaminophen q6h (max 75 mg/kg/d). Start scheduled PO ibuprofen (10 mg/kg/dose, give q6h).
> - Transition from IV ondansetron to oral ondansetron (4 mg; max 8 mg q8h PRN) after 48 hr.
> - For patients with PVNB catheters, connect On-Q pumps
>
> **POD 3 Until the Day of Discharge**
>
> - Continue PO pain medications started on POD 2. Go over all the recommendations and instructions for pain management at home and educate the patient and the family about On-Q pump care and how to remove catheters on POD 5.
> - Follow up until hospital discharge and daily home calls until POD 6.
>
> Postdischarge follow-up should already be scheduled (especially for patients >12 years of age). Please encourage pain clinic follow-up if a patient continues to require opioid medications beyond 2 weeks after surgery or has other pain issues.
>
> ATC, around the clock; PACU, post-anesthesia care unit; POD, postoperative day; PVNB, paravertebral nerve block.

older patients with more rigid and ossified rib cages. There are numerous protocols established and utilized by various institutions to help manage postoperative pain control. Strategies commonly employed incorporate the use of systemic opioids, TEs, thoracic paravertebral blocks, erector spinae plane blocks, and more recently cryoanalgesia. Multiple studies have shown similar recovery characteristics following the use of TE and thoracic paravertebral blocks, although more systemic opioids are required on POD 0 and 1 by those receiving thoracic paravertebral blocks, with no difference in pain scores after POD 0 and a shorter length of stay in the hospital.[4]

Whichever method of postoperative pain control is employed, the regimen will require a multimodal approach, including a combination of diazepam, methocarbamol, ketorolac, and acetaminophen. As the patient begins to increase oral intake postoperatively, medication regimens can be transitioned to oral route and doses adjusted as needed. Pain medications are continued for 2 weeks postoperatively, and patients older than 17 years may require longer coverage. Patients with excessive pain issues after discharge may need to be followed by a chronic pain service until transitioned off medications.[6]

REFERENCES

1. Frawley G, Frawley J, Crameri J. A review of anesthetic techniques and outcomes following minimally invasive repair of pectus excavatum (Nuss procedure). *Paediatr anaesth*. 2016;26(11):1082–1090. doi:10.1111/pan.12988
2. Obermeyer RJ, Cohen NS, Jaroszewski DE. The physiologic impact of pectus excavatum repair. *Semin pediatr surg*. 2018;27(3):127–132. doi:10.1053/j.sempedsurg.2018.05.005
3. Siddiqui A, Tse A, Paul JE, et al. Postoperative epidural analgesia for patients undergoing pectus excavatum corrective surgery: a 10-year retrospective analysis. *Local Reg Anesth*. 2016;9:25–33. doi:10.2147/LRA.S80710
4. Muhly WT, Beltran RJ, Bielsky A, et al. Perioperative management and in-hospital outcomes after minimally invasive repair of pectus excavatum: A multicenter registry report from the society for pediatric anesthesia improvement network. *Anesth analg*. 2019;128(2):315–327. doi:10.1213/ANE.0000000000003829
5. Graves C, Idowu O, Lee S, et al. Intraoperative cryoanalgesia for managing pain after the Nuss procedure. *J pediatr surg*. 2017;52(6):920–924. doi:10.1016/j.jpedsurg.2017.03.006
6. Sesia SB, Heitzelmann M, Schaedelin S, et al. Standardized haller and asymmetry index combined for a more accurate assessment of pectus excavatum. *Ann Thorac Surg*. 2019;107(1):271–276. doi:10.1016/j.athoracsur.2018.07.086
7. Mavi J, Moore DL. Anesthesia and analgesia for pectus excavatum surgery. *Anesthesiol Clin*. 2014;32(1):175–184. doi:10.1016/j.anclin.2013.10.006
8. Hall Burton DM, Boretsky KR. A comparison of paravertebral nerve block catheters and thoracic epidural catheters for postoperative analgesia following the Nuss procedure for pectus excavatum repair. *Paediatr anaesth*. 2014;24(5):516–520. doi:10.1111/pan.12369
9. Beltran R, Veneziano G, Bhalla T, et al. Postoperative pain management in patients undergoing thoracoscopic repair of pectus excavatum: a retrospective analysis of opioid consumption and adverse effects in adolescents. *Saudi J Anaesth*. 2017;11(4):427–431. doi:10.4103/sja.SJA_339_17
10. Sakamoto K, Ando K, Noma D. Metal allergy to titanium bars after the Nuss procedure for pectus excavatum. *Ann Thorac Surg*. 2014;98(2):708–710. doi:10.1016/j.athoracsur.2013.10.089

CHAPTER 98

Bowel Resection and Gastrojejunal Tube Placement

Caren Bergdahl and Jingjing Sparrow

BOWEL RESECTION

Bowel resection is the surgical removal of a portion of the bowel, including the small intestine, large intestine, or rectum, followed by primary anastomosis of the proximal and distal ends or creation of an ostomy. Successful management of pediatric patients undergoing bowel resection surgery depends on a thorough understanding of indication for surgery, existing treatments the patient is receiving, and the patient's comorbidities. It requires communication and collaboration within the multidisciplinary team.

INDICATIONS/CONTRAINDICATIONS

Indications for neonatal bowel resections often include congenital anomalies involving the intestinal tracts, such as duodenal or intestinal atresia, Hirschsprung disease, anorectal malformation, and occasionally, intestinal malrotation and meconium ileus when necrotic bowel is involved. Some of these conditions are associated with other congenital anomalies. For example, anorectal malformation can be part of the vertebral defects, anal atresia, cardiac defects, tracheoesophageal fistula, renal anomalies, and limb abnormalities (VACTERL) association. Similarly, malrotation has an increased incidence in heterotaxy.[1] Necrotizing enterocolitis (NEC) is another important indication for neonatal bowel resection. NEC is intestinal inflammation that could progress into tissue necrosis and shock. Resection of the necrotic bowel and ostomy formation are indicated if medical management fails.[2] Other indications for bowel resection in the pediatric population include strangulated inguinal hernia, abdominal trauma, neoplasm, and inflammatory bowel disease (IBD). The most common forms of IBD are Crohn's disease (CD) and ulcerative colitis (UC). Surgical intervention is required during childhood in approximately 25% of children diagnosed with CD and 10% of children diagnosed with UC.[3]

With advances in medical technology and equipment, laparoscopy has replaced laparotomy in many abdominal surgical cases. However, there are some situations that preclude using the laparoscopic technique for bowel resection surgery. Laparoscopy involves insertion of trocars into the abdomen and insufflation of the peritoneal cavity with carbon dioxide (CO_2). The small size of neonates can make this technique difficult. A history of prior abdominal surgery that causes extensive adhesions and scarring can make dissection extremely challenging in laparoscopic surgery. In addition, CO_2 insufflation of the peritoneal cavity causes many physiological changes that are ill tolerated by patients with marginal cardiovascular status (Table 98.1). Occasionally, in emergent cases, such as in abdominal trauma, laparotomy is required for rapid access and exposure.

Table 98.1	Special Considerations for Laparoscopic Surgery
Respiratory	↓ FRC, lung compliance, and VC from cephalad shift of the diaphragm Small airway collapse, atelectasis, and hypoxemia ↑ Airway resistance, V/Q mismatch, shunting, physiological dead space, and PIP ↑ CO_2 absorption across peritoneum
Cardiovascular	↑ SVR, MAP, and CVP <15 mm Hg: ↑ venous return = ↑ CO >15 mm Hg: ↓ venous return = ↓ CO and hypotension Bradyarrhythmias: significant bradycardia, AV dissociation, asystole—most occur with initial insufflation
Intracerebral	↑ ICP, ↓ CPP from hypercapnia, ↑ SVR, and head-down position
Renal	↑ Renovascular resistance: ↓ flow through renal veins ↑ ADH: activation of renin–angiotensin system ↓ UO (oliguria): during procedure and lasting several hours postoperatively
Endocrine	Stress response activation: ↑ insulin, cortisol, prolactin, and epinephrine
Immunological	↓ Local immunity from suppression of monocyte and macrophage function Preserved systemic immunity because ↓ tissue trauma with smaller incisions

ADH, antidiuretic hormone; AV, atrioventricular; CO, cardiac output; CO_2, carbon dioxide; CPP, cerebral perfusion pressure; CVP, central venous pressure; FRC, functional residual capacity; ICP, intracranial pressure; MAP, mean arterial pressure; PIP, peak inspiratory pressure; SVR, systemic vascular resistance; UO, urine output; VC, vital capacity; V/Q, ventilation/perfusion.

Source: From Muñoz CJ, Nguyen HT, Houck CS. Robotic surgery and anesthesia for pediatric urological procedures. *Current Opinion in Anaesthesiology*. 2016;29(3):337–344. doi:10.1097/aco.0000000000000333 and Pennant JH. Anesthesia for laparoscopy in the pediatric patient. *Anesthesiol Clin North Am*. 2001;19(1):69–88. doi:10.1016/s0889-8537(05)70212-1.

SPECIAL CONSIDERATIONS AND CONCERNS

Patients undergoing urgent bowel resection frequently present with vomiting and abdominal distension. These patients are at high risk of aspiration and must be considered as having a "full stomach." Vomiting and nasogastric suction causes dehydration, electrolyte imbalances, and deranged acid–base status. It is important to optimize the patient's fluid and electrolyte status preoperatively. Many patients are NPO prior to surgery due to an ongoing feeding intolerance and subsequently are receiving glucose-containing IV fluids or total parenteral nutrition (TPN). It is imperative anesthesia providers do not stop these solutions abruptly as doing so would place the patient at an increased risk of hypoglycemia. Preoperative antibiotic therapy should be continued through the perioperative period, with the need for supplemental prophylactic antibiotics a possibility. Critically ill patients may present in a state of shock, requiring interventions such as intubation and inotropic and/or vasopressor support.

Patients with certain congenital anomalies of the gastrointestinal tract have associated cardiac and other body system abnormalities, which must be taken into consideration while developing the anesthesia plan. Patients with IBD and neoplasm may undergo elective bowel resections when medical therapy fails or as an adjunct therapy. These patients are likely malnourished from long-standing disease states. Their preoperative medical therapy usually includes steroids, immunomodulators, and chemotherapy agents. It is important to consider the anesthesia implications of these medications. Additionally, if laparoscopic surgery is planned, the anesthesia provider must anticipate and be able to treat associated hemodynamic instability and complications associated with abdominal insufflation.

ANESTHETIC MANAGEMENT

Preoperative Evaluation

A complete history and physical exam should be performed with special attention paid to several aspects, such as the patient's current vital signs and fluid status as these directly relate to the patient's hemodynamic stability during surgery. Tachycardia with hypotension, delayed capillary refill (>3 seconds), sunken fontanelle, poor skin turgor, and decreased urine output are all signs of dehydration. Fluid resuscitation with a balanced salt solution should be initiated if not already infusing. The presence of vomiting and abdominal distension places the patient at higher risk of aspiration during induction, making rapid sequence induction (RSI) indicated. In the context of RSI, a careful airway assessment is even more important. If difficult airway is anticipated, appropriately sized video laryngoscope or fiberoptic bronchoscope should be used to facilitate successful tracheal intubation. In intubated patients, attention should be paid to ventilator settings as abdominal distension can make ventilation difficult. Higher inspiratory pressures may be needed to adequately ventilate these patients, but care must be taken to avoid barotrauma.

Anomalies of the gastrointestinal tract can be associated with cardiac and other body system anomalies. If cardiac defects are present, nonurgent surgeries should be postponed until after the cardiac repair. In the case of emergency surgery, ECG and echocardiography must be obtained and reviewed. Computed tomography (CT) angiography and cardiac catheterization reports, if available, should also be reviewed. Other diagnostic studies, chest x-ray, abdominal ultrasound and radiograph, gastrointestinal contrast study, CT and MRI are useful for assessing disease severity. The patient's home- and facility-administered medications should also be reviewed. These medications may include antibiotics, fluid and electrolyte replacements, TPN, vasoactive infusions, and long-term treatment medications such as steroid, immunomodulators, biologics, and chemotherapeutic agents. For patients with IBD undergoing bowel resection, preoperative steroid administration should be minimized to reduce the risk of complications such as infection, sepsis, and venous thromboembolism, whereas data are lacking on the influence of preoperative administration of thiopurine immunomodulatory and biological agents.[3] However, biological agents, including infliximab, adalimumab, and vedolizumab, have been reported as safe to use in the preoperative period and are associated with a shorter postoperative length of stay (LOS).[4] Due to the lack of definitive evidence on preoperative administration of these medications, discussion with the involved specialty services should be undertaken to decide on their preoperative use.

Pertinent Labs

Laboratory tests offer invaluable information on patient status and the development of treatment plan. Complete blood count (CBC) with differential should be ordered for all patients undergoing bowel resection surgery. An elevated hematocrit may indicate dehydration or inadequate fluid replacement, while a high or low white blood cell count is associated with infectious process. An abnormal platelet count should prompt further coagulation studies, and transfusion of platelets may be indicated prior to the surgery to minimize bleeding. Along with the patient's cardiovascular status, CBC and coagulation studies will help the anesthesia provider plan for types and quantities of blood products needed for the surgery. Chemistry and blood gases provide important information on the patient's fluid and electrolyte status, renal function, and acid–base balance, thus providing guidance on ventilation management and fluid and electrolyte replacement therapy.

ANESTHETIC TECHNIQUE

Intraoperative Management

Patients undergoing urgent bowel resection should have an IV placed preoperatively. The vascular access team (VAT) should be consulted if difficult IV placement is anticipated. Short-acting IV anxiolytic medications, such as midazolam, should be considered preoperatively, especially for those infants and children who are inconsolable. For patients undergoing elective bowel resection, an oral anxiolytic can be administered if the patient is a candidate for inhaled induction and cannot tolerate having an IV placed while awake.

If a nasogastric tube (NGT) is present, it should be connected to suction prior to induction to ensure that the stomach is decompressed. Preoxygenation with 100% oxygen is performed to stave off desaturation during apneic periods associated with intubation. It is especially important in RSI as bag–mask ventilation does not occur. Typically, a hypnotic and a rapid-acting muscle relaxant, such as propofol and rocuronium, are administered, and the endotracheal tube (ETT) is placed while cricoid pressure is being held. In hemodynamically unstable patients, alternative induction agents, such as etomidate or ketamine, should be considered. Once the airway is secured, additional vascular access

> **BOX 98.1 ERAS PROTOCOL FOR ELECTIVE BOWEL SURGERY**
>
> - Preoperative education.
> - Avoid mechanical bowel preparation
> - Avoid prolonged fasting: allow clear liquids to 2 hours prior to surgery.
> - Multimodal analgesia: non-opioid, neuraxial, and regional blocks
> - Preincision antibiotic prophylaxis
> - Goal-directed fluid therapy
> - Minimize the use of nasogastric tubes (NGTs) and drains.
> - Early mobilization
>
> ERAS, enhanced recovery after surgery; NGT, nasogastric tube.
>
> Sources: Phillips M, Adamson W, McLean S, et al. Implementation of a pediatric enhanced recovery pathway decreases opioid utilization and shortens time to full feeding. J Pediatr Surg. 2020;55(1):101–105. doi:10.1016/j.jpedsurg.2019.09.065; Short H, Heiss K, Burch K, et al. Implementation of an enhanced recovery protocol in pediatric colorectal surgery. J Pediatr Surg. 2018;53(4):688–692. doi:10.1016/j.jpedsurg.2017.05.004.

lines can be placed if warranted based on the patient status and surgery complexity. In surgeries with anticipated large blood loss, additional IVs, an arterial line, and central venous access should be obtained to facilitate invasive pressure monitoring, blood gas assessment, administration of fluids and blood products, and vasoactive medication infusion. A Foley catheter is used as urine output is an important indicator of the patient's fluid status. Muscle relaxation is needed to help improve operative conditions for the surgery team. However, muscle relaxation should be monitored and fully reversed if extubation is planned at the end of the procedure.

Fluid management is fundamental in the anesthetic management of bowel resections. Historically, fluid administration was based on combining maintenance fluid according to the 4–2–1 rule, NPO deficit, and insensible loss. This method can lead to large volumes of fluid being administered. In recent years, there has been a shift to fluid management that is based on the patient's hemodynamic response. Goal-directed fluid management, including use of colloid solution, blood products, and vasopressors when necessary, is associated with better postoperative recovery. High-volume fluid administration is associated with longer hospital LOS, increased time to first meal, and supplemental oxygen use greater than 24 hours in pediatric patients undergoing colectomy at a tertiary pediatric hospital.[5] It has been strongly recommended to employ goal-directed fluid therapy (GDFT) in high-risk patients and for patients undergoing gastrointestinal surgery when a large intravascular fluid loss is anticipated.[6] GDFT has also been incorporated into the enhanced recovery after surgery (ERAS) protocol for colorectal surgery in some pediatric centers (Box 98.1).[7,8] Additional intraoperative considerations include maintenance of normothermia, adequate pain control, and prevention of postoperative nausea and vomiting (PONV). Many children presenting for bowel resection experience nausea and vomiting at baseline. In addition, dehydration, laparoscopic surgery, and general anesthesia with volatile anesthetics and opioids increase their risks of PONV.[9] These patients should receive a combination of antiemetics with different mechanisms of action. Opioid-sparing multimodal analgesic techniques should also be used when possible.[10]

Complications

Hemorrhage is an inherit risk of bowel resection surgeries regardless of the operative technique. Blood products should be available, especially for high-risk patients and extensive surgeries. Ventilation may be challenging due to abdominal distension and/or insufflation. Abdominal insufflation may also cause CO_2 embolism, bradycardia, or asystole. The surgery team should be alerted, insufflation stopped, and meaures to support cardiopulmonary function implemented.

POSTOPERATIVE CARE

Avoidance of postoperative ileus is important for patient recovery because it allows for early return of bowel function and tolerance of feeding. Pulmonary toileting and early mobilization are also beneficial for recovery. These efforts partly rely on adequate pain control. Epidural analgesia can be used as an adjunct to general anesthesia in major abdominal surgeries to decrease the amount of opioids required.[11] Caudal blockade and multimodal analgesia, such as paracetamol, ketorolac, and ketamine infusion, and local anesthetic infiltration, are superior to the reliance on morphine when comparing the time to first analgesic requirement and total requirement postoperatively.[12] Regional blocks such as rectus sheath,[13] transversus abdominis,[14] erector spinae plane,[15,16] and quadratus lumborum[15] are all effective options to help reduce intra- and postoperative pain. There is no single superior anesthesia technique for pediatric patients undergoing bowel resection surgery. The anesthesia provider should base the decision on patient characteristics, operative technique, and location of the surgery.

GASTRIC AND GASTROJEJUNAL TUBE PLACEMENT

Gastric (G) tubes are percutaneously inserted in patients with inadequate oral intake. The most common method for G tube placement is percutaneous endoscopic gastrostomy (PEG).[17] If the patient is unable to tolerate gastric feeding following placement of a G tube, a postpyloric gastrojejunal (GJ) tube is placed via existing gastrostomy or creation of a jejunostomy. The prevalence of enteral feeding requirements is growing due to the increased survival rate of children with severe chronic illnesses and/or neurological disabilities, with approximately 40% to 70% of them having feeding issues.[17]

INDICATIONS/CONTRAINDICATIONS

Placement of enteral feeding access is one of the most common procedures done by pediatric surgeons.[18] Indications for G- or GJ-tube placement include chronic or medication-resistant gastroesophageal reflux disease (GERD), poor swallow coordination or aspiration risk, developmental delays, intestinal dysmotility/gastroparesis, and conditions with high metabolic demands.[19,17] Contraindications for G- or GJ-tube placement include family and/or patient refusal, uncorrected coagulopathy, peritonitis, and sepsis.

SPECIAL CONSIDERATIONS AND CONCERNS

The approach to G-tube placement can be open (Stamm) laparotomy, laparoscopic, endoscopic, fluoroscopic, or ultrasound guided.[20] Laparotomy is usually reserved for patients weighing less than 6 kg or if an emergency occurs during a laparoscopic procedure, such as hemorrhage,

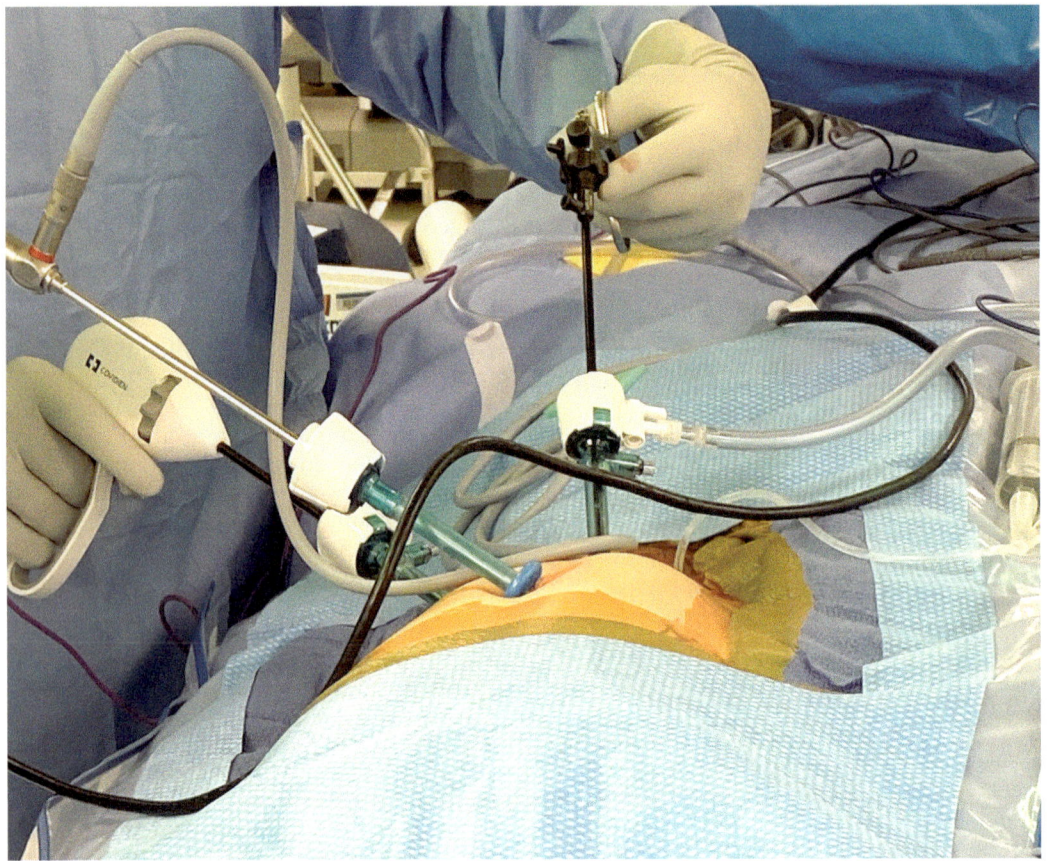

Figure 98.1: Trocars in the abdomen during laparoscopic surgery.

Source: From Texas Children's Hospital.

requiring conversion to open laparotomy.[17,21] Laparoscopic G-tube placement requires placement of trocars, as seen in Figure 98.1, into the abdomen with creation of pneumoperitoneum. Due to the increased intracranial pressure (ICP) from the pneumoperitoneum, the laparoscopic approach for G- and GJ-tube placement is discouraged in patients with decreased intracranial compliance and premature infants because of risk of intraventricular hemorrhage.[21] Endoscopic placement involves use of a fiberoptic scope inserted through the mouth into the stomach, and then a trocar is placed directly into the stomach via endoscopic visualization.[17] Placement using fluoroscopy or ultrasound guidance is not as common.

ANESTHETIC MANAGEMENT

PREOPERATIVE EVALUATION

A thorough history and physical and chart review should be performed before placing a child under anesthesia.[22] Patients requiring G- or GJ-tube placement usually have poor oral intake and weight gain.[23] Local and regional anesthesias for G-tube placement are generally not tolerated by the pediatric population; hence, general anesthesia is usually performed.

Key Assessment Points

Hydration status of the patient should be addressed as these patients may be NPO for an extended amount of time with or without IV fluids, depending on their clinical status. If the patient is dehydrated, IV placement may require ultrasound guidance. If the patient is on maintenance fluids or TPN prior to surgery, they should be continued. Patients requiring G- or GJ-tube placement often present with additional comorbidities, such as complex cardiac disease, prematurity, respiratory disease, and neurological disorders.[24] Patients with cardiovascular disease, anemia or hypovolemia have a higher risk for decompensation from the hemodynamic changes associated with pneumoperitoneum, seen in Table 98.1.[21]

Pertinent Labs

Healthy children who require surgical enteral feeding tube placement usually do not require specific preoperative labs or testing. If the child has a complex medical history, then chest x-ray, ECG, and preoperative blood tests (CBC with differential, chemistry panel, and coagulation studies) may be appropriate to obtain.[22]

PREOPERATIVE PHARMACOLOGY

Most institutions support the use of premedication for anxiolysis, with some combining or substituting this with parental presence during induction. Anxiolytics may be administered via the oral, IV, IM, intranasal, rectal or transmucosal route depending on clinical situation. Patients presenting for G-tube placement may also require antacids, H_2 antagonists, gastrokinetic agents (e.g., metoclopramide), opioids, or antisialogogues.[22] Some anesthesia providers may choose to premedicate with an anticholinergic to prevent vasovagal reflexes associated with laparoscopy.[22]

ANESTHETIC TECHNIQUE

INTRAOPERATIVE MANAGEMENT

Standard anesthesia monitors are often adequate for G- or GJ-tube placement in healthy patients, although patients with severe cardiovascular, respiratory, or renal compromise may benefit from arterial line placement (Box 98.2).[21] An inhaled induction is usually tolerated by most patients, unless significant GERD or other indications exist that require RSI with preoperative IV placement.[21] Muscle relaxation should be used to facilitate ventilation and avoid patient movement, especially in the beginning of a laparoscopic procedure during placement of the trocars and insufflation.[21] Muscle relaxation should be reversed based on the patient's train-of-four prior to extubation in the operating room. Anesthesia providers must closely monitor and adjust ventilation and fluid status during laparoscopic cases, given the influence of a pneumoperitoneum. A urinary catheter should be inserted to monitor urine output during the procedure and to prevent accidental injury to the genitourinary system if laparoscopy is performed.

Intra-abdominal pressures in pediatric patients should be kept less than 12 mm Hg to limit alterations in splanchnic perfusion and to prevent organ damage.[21] Should bradyarrhythmias occur, they are most likely secondary to vagal stimulation from initial needle placement and peritoneal stretch from the pneumoperitoneum.[21] It is important anesthesia providers are cognizant that children have a high resting vagal tone, which is more likely to lead to bradycardia or asystole with insufflation.[22]

Special equipment for laparoscopy is summarized in Box 98.3.

Complications/Emergencies

The most common minor complication following G or GJ tube placement is peristomal leakage, with other minor complications including peristomal infection, granulation tissue, occlusion, and tube migration with associated reflux. The most common major complication is gastrocolocutaneous fistula. Other major complications include intussusception, small bowel obstruction, peritonitis, and perforation.[17,23,24]

The laparoscopic approach has specific complications including pneumothorax and pneumopericardium, which are more likely to occur with higher intra-abdominal pressures.[22] SC emphysema can also occur during laparoscopic placement but usually resolves spontaneously without treatment. During laparoscopy, serious and fatal complications can result from accidental placement of the trocar into any major vessel (e.g., aorta, iliac vessels, inferior vena cava).[21]

CO_2 embolism is an intraoperative emergency during laparoscopy resulting from placement of the needle intravascularly. Signs and symptoms of CO_2 embolism include sudden rise in end-tidal carbon dioxide ($ETCO_2$), acute hypotension, hypoxemia, dysrhythmias, pulmonary edema, cyanosis of the head and neck, and "mill-wheel" murmur. If a CO_2 embolism is suspected, treatment includes informing the surgeon to stop and deflate pneumoperitoneum, calling for help, hyperventilating with 100% O_2, placing the patient in left lateral decubitus position in the Trendelenburg position, placing a central line to aspirate CO_2, performing cardiopulmonary resuscitation if indicated, and initiating cardiopulmonary bypass if there is hemodynamic collapse.[21]

POSTOPERATIVE CARE

Postoperative care will differ based upon the surgical approach for G- or GJ-tube placement. Pain is generally well controlled after laparoscopic placement with nonsteroidal anti-inflammatory drugs (NSAIDs); however, open laparotomy may require use of IV opioids or patient-controlled analgesia (PCA). Antiemetics should be administered to prevent PONV. Pneumoperitoneum can lead to shoulder pain in the postoperative period thought to be caused by irritation and desiccation of the peritoneal surface of the diaphragm

---

BOX 98.2 CLINICAL PEARLS FOR G- OR GJ-TUBE PLACEMENT

- Obtain IV access above the diaphragm: avoid IVC compression during pneumoperitoneum.
- Avoid nitrous oxide: ↑ risk of nausea/vomiting, ↑ bowel distention.
- Cuffed endotracheal tube ± RSI for severe GERD
- Use PCV with PEEP: goal tidal volume 6–8 mL/kg, $ETCO_2$ <50 mm Hg, PIP <20 cm H_2O
- Calculate and replace fluid deficit prior to insufflation for laparoscopic placement.
- Medications to treat bradyarrhythmias: glycopyrrolate, atropine, and epinephrine.
- Monitor for endobronchial intubation during pneumoperitoneum.
- Bair hugger: increased risk of hypothermia with cold, nonhumidified CO_2
- Prophylactic antiemetic: 5-HT3 antagonist, dexamethasone, and so forth.
- Local anesthetic infiltration by surgeon at trocar insertion site with systemic pain medications

$ETCO_2$, end-tidal carbon dioxide; G, gastric; GERD, gastroesophageal reflux disease; GJ, gastrojejunal; IVC, inferior vena cava; PCV, pressure-controlled ventilation; PEEP, positive end-expiratory pressure; PIP, peak inspiratory pressure

Sources: Muñoz CJ, Nguyen HT, Houck CS. Robotic surgery and anesthesia for pediatric urologic procedures. *Curr Opin Anaesthesiol.* 2016;29(3):337–344. doi:10.1097/aco.0000000000000333; Pennant JH. Anesthesia for laparoscopy in the pediatric patient. *Anesthesiol Clin North Am.* 2001;19(1):69–88. doi:10.1016/s0889-8537(05)70212-1.

BOX 98.3 SPECIAL EQUIPMENT FOR LAPAROSCOPIC G- AND GJ-TUBE PLACEMENT

- OG tube sized appropriately for patient
- 60 mL piston irrigation syringe
- Large stainless steel hemostat clamp
- Technique: Place OG tube to aspirate gastric contents; then provide gastric insufflation during laparoscopy by instilling air via the irrigation syringe and maintaining with the hemostat clamp.

G, gastric; GJ, gastrojejunal; OG, orogastric.

Source: Muñoz CJ, Nguyen HT, Houck CS. Robotic surgery and anesthesia for pediatric urologic procedures. *Curr Opin Anaesthesiol.* 2016;29(3):337–344. doi:10.1097/aco.0000000000000333 and Pennant JH. Anesthesia for laparoscopy in the pediatric patient. *Anesthesiol Clin North Am.* 2001;19(1):69–88. doi:10.1016/s0889-8537(05)70212-1.

from insufflation, although this is less common in pediatric patients.[21,22]

Feeds are usually initiated 4 hours up to 24 hours postoperatively.[17] Patients will usually have a low-profile "button" G tube that is flush with the skin or a continuous G tube with a long external portion (Figure 98.2). Some patients may experience worsening of GERD after G-tube placement and may require exchange for a GJ tube.[23] If a GJ tube was placed, the G port is placed to suction, and the jejunal (J) port is used for feeding.

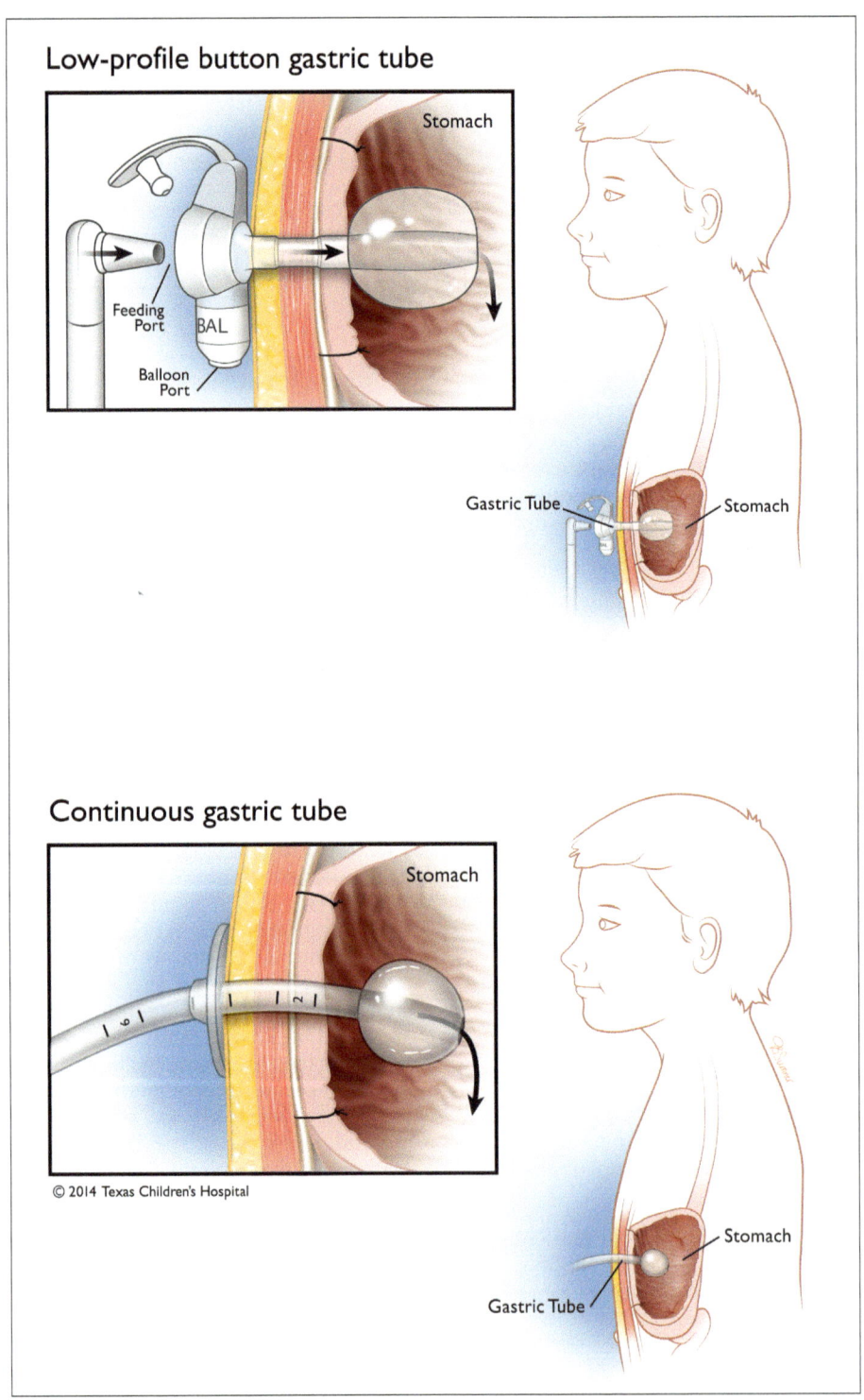

Figure 98.2: Examples of gastric tubes.

Source: From Texas Children's Hospital.

CASE STUDY: A 10-Month-Old Male Status Post–Heart Transplant Requiring Long-Term Enteral Feeding

CLINICAL SCENARIO

The patient is a 10-month-old 10.4-kg male with medical history of severe hypertrophic cardiomyopathy with pulmonary vein stenosis s/p heart transplant at 9 months of age, pulmonary hypertension, left vocal cord paralysis, respiratory distress syndrome (with multiple intubations), failure to thrive, oral aversion, GERD, aspiration pneumonia, and chronic renal failure. The patient requires enteral feeding via nasojejunal (NJ) tube (goal 75 mL/kg/d) and was scheduled for laparoscopic gastrostomy and G-tube placement. He is currently requiring 8 liters per minute (LPM) 80% O_2 high-flow nasal cannula (HFNC) in the ICU with infusions of dexmedetomidine (2 mcg/kg/hr), dextrose 5% (22 mL/hr), and hydromorphone (80 mcg/kg/hr).

SPECIAL CONSIDERATIONS

The patient was critically ill in the ICU and had multiple tests completed prior to placement of laparoscopic G tube. His most recent echocardiogram showed mild to moderately dilated right ventricle with mild right ventricular hypertrophy and low normal systolic function, and normal left ventricular systolic function. His chest x-ray showed stable postoperative changes, slightly increased right upper lobe atelectasis, and persistent left-sided retrocardiac opacities and pleural effusion. Preoperative laboratory testing showed hemoglobin 11.9, hematocrit 38.6, white blood cell 15, platelets 635, blood urea nitrogen 14, creatine 0.16, and electrolytes within normal limits.

APPROACHES TO CARE

Evidence-Based Approaches to Care

The patient was premedicated with 1 mg IV midazolam via femoral central line before being transported to the operating room. Once in the operating room and attached to the monitors, the patient was induced intravenously with 10 mcg fentanyl, 15 mg ketamine, and 10 mg rocuronium. He was successfully intubated with a 3.5 cuffed ETT and placed on pressure-controlled ventilation (PCV) for the duration of the procedure. After securing the airway, a 22-g IV was placed in the right forearm via ultrasound guidance. The patient remained on the infusions of dexmedetomidine, dextrose 5% and hydromorphone during the procedure. Prior to incision, his NJ tube was removed; stomach contents were aspirated with a 14 Fr orogastric (OG) tube, and 300 mg IV cefazolin was given. The patient tolerated abdominal insufflation with no significant change in heart rate, and upon surgeon request, the stomach was insufflated via the OG tube for better visualization. Upon completion of the G-tube placement, the patient remained intubated on his current infusions and was given 15 mg IV ketamine before returning to the ICU.

COMPLICATIONS

There were no complications during the procedure or postoperative period. The patient was safely extubated in the ICU and placed back on 8 LPM 80% O_2 HFNC. He was started on gastric feeds approximately 8 hours after returning to the ICU and he tolerated them well with full advancement to the goal rate.

KEY REFERENCES

Complete references for this chapter are online and available at https://connect.springerpub.com/content/book/978-0-8261-3875-0/part/part04/toc-part/ch098.

3. Kelay A, Tullie L, Stanton M. Surgery and paediatric inflammatory bowel disease. *Transl Pediatr*. 2019;8(5):436–448. doi:10.21037/tp.2019.09.01
15. Aksu C, Şen M, Akay M, et al. Erector spinae plane block vs quadratus lumborum block for pediatric lower abdominal surgery: A double blinded, prospective, and randomized trial. *J Clin Anesth*. 2019; 57;24–28. doi:10.1016/j.jclinane.2019.03.006
17. Burdall OC, Howarth LJ, Sharrard A, Lee ACH. Paediatric enteral tube feeding. *Paediatr Child Health*. 2017;27(8):371–377. doi:10.1016/j.paed.2017.05.001
21. Muñoz CJ, Nguyen HT, Houck CS. Robotic surgery and anesthesia for pediatric urologic procedures. *Current Opinion in Anaesthesiology*, 2016;29(3):337–344. doi:10.1097/aco.0000000000000333
22. Pennant JH. Anesthesia for Laparoscopy in the Pediatric Patient. *Anesthesiology Clinics of North America*. 2001;19(1):69–88. doi:10.1016/s0889-8537(05)70212-1
23. Mahant S, Cohen E, Nelson KE, Rosenbaum P. Decision-making around gastrostomy tube feeding in children with neurological impairment: engaging effectively with families. *Paediatr Child Health*. 2018;23(3):209–213. doi:10.1093/pch/pxx193

CHAPTER 99

Sleeve Gastrectomy

Lisa A. Durako

INDICATIONS/CONTRAINDICATIONS

Sleeve gastrectomy has become the most common metabolic and bariatric surgery (MBS) among the adolescent population, comprising 80% of all elective procedures performed for the treatment of severe obesity in this age group.[1] The gold standard indications for all MBS, including the sleeve gastrectomy, were published in the 1991 National Institutes of Health (NIH)[2] Consensus Development Conference Statement on Gastrointestinal Surgery for Severe Obesity. Over time, as the frequency of MBS has increased, the indications and contraindications have evolved. Additionally, the American Society for Metabolic and Bariatric Surgery (ASMBS) has since established evidence-based guidelines specific to the pediatric population. These updated guidelines published in 2018 address comorbidities specific to the pediatric population and use the modern definitions of Class II and III obesity set forth by the Centers for Disease Control and Prevention.

According to the ASMBS guidelines, sleeve gastrectomy is indicated for adolescents whose body mass index (BMI) is ≥ 35 kg/m^2 or 120% of the 95th percentile (Class II obesity) and associated with significant comorbidities such as obstructive sleep apnea (OSA), type 2 diabetes (T2D), idiopathic intracranial hypertension (IIH), nonalcoholic steatohepatitis (NASH), Blount's disease, slipped capital femoral epiphysis (SCFE), gastroesophageal reflux (GERD), or hypertension (HTN). In addition, those adolescents who have a BMI of ≥ 40 kg/m^2 or are 140% of the 95th percentile (Class III obesity) should also be considered candidates for sleeve gastrectomy. Contraindications to the sleeve gastrectomy include a medically correctable cause of the patient's obesity—although exceptions may be made in some syndromic obesities; an ongoing or recent (within 1 year) history of substance abuse—and medical, psychiatric, psychosocial, or cognitive conditions that prevent compliance with dietary and medication regimens; and current or planned pregnancy within 18 months of the procedure (Box 99.1).[3]

SPECIAL CONSIDERATIONS AND CONCERNS

Prior to undergoing a sleeve gastrectomy, proper consent must be obtained from the parent and/or legal guardian, in addition to obtaining assent from the patient.[4] It is essential all parties involved have a thorough understanding of both the surgery and postoperative regimen associated with the sleeve gastrectomy as this is an elective procedure which requires significant long-term commitment, including behavior and lifestyle changes, adhering to dietary and supplement protocols, strict medication regimens, and continued medical follow-up with the potential need for future surgical procedures. Understanding and assenting to this commitment are complicated by the fact that the adolescent is still undergoing cognitive, personal, emotional, and social development. For this reason, it is recommended that an adolescent-trained counselor, psychologist, or psychiatrist be part of the perioperative multidisciplinary team caring for the patient.[3,4]

BOX 99.1 INDICATIONS AND CONTRAINDICATIONS TO SLEEVE GASTRECTOMY IN ADOLESCENT PATIENTS

Indications
- BMI > 35 kg/m^2 or 120% of 95th percentile with at least one of the following:
  - obstructive sleep apnea,
  - type 2 diabetes,
  - idiopathic intracranial HTN,
  - Blount's disease,
  - nonalcoholic steatohepatitis,
  - slipped capital femoral epiphysis,
  - gastroesophageal reflux disorder, and
  - HTN

or
- BMI > 40 kg/m^2 or 140% of the 95th percentile

Contraindications
- Substance abuse within past year
- Medically correctable cause of obesity (with some exceptions)
- Current or planned pregnancy within next 18 months
- Medical, psychiatric, psychosocial, or cognitive condition that prevents compliance with dietary and medication regimens

BMI, body mass index.

ANESTHETIC MANAGEMENT

PREOPERATIVE EVALUATION

Prior to surgery, all patients will undergo extensive medical and surgical evaluation from a variety of medical specialties involved with the perioperative management of the patient, including anesthesia. When performing a preoperative anesthetic evaluation of an adolescent undergoing a sleeve gastrectomy, it is important anesthesia providers thoroughly assess for the presence of all comorbidities known to be associated with obesity.[5] Specifically, anesthesia providers inquire about the presence of cardiac, pulmonary, and endocrine disease. As part of the cardiac evaluation, all patients should at the minimum receive a chest x-ray and ECG; for those with higher risks of changes in cardiac function and morphology, an echocardiogram and stress test (either pharmacological or traditional) should be performed.[5,6]

Airway management, including mask ventilation, direct laryngoscopy, and tracheal intubation, has been proved to be more difficult in both obese adults and children when compared to their normal weight counterparts.[5,7] Therefore, a thorough airway assessment, including neck range of motion, degree of mouth opening, thyromental distance, and Mallampati score, should be performed preoperatively to identify potential difficulties with airway management.

OSA is reported to be present in nearly 50% of severely obese children, although it is important to be cognizant that is often undiagnosed in this population.[6] For this reason, it is recommended that OSA screening be performed on all patients, with those identified as being "at risk" having a sleep study performed prior to surgery as well. If the patient has been previously diagnosed with OSA, any requirement of continuous positive airway pressure (CPAP) or bilevel positive airway pressure (BiPAP) devices should be assessed.[5,6] In addition to OSA, a number of other respiratory comorbidities exist in the obese adolescent, including an increased prevalence of asthma and atelectasis and decreased lung volumes, diffusion capacity, and pulmonary compliance.[7] Pulmonary function tests (PFTs) may also be useful tool in predicting pulmonary complications in both the intraoperative and postoperative periods.[6]

With this population of patients being at an increased risk of T2D, an endocrinology consult is warranted and may include a glucose tolerance test.[5] For those with a preexisting T2D diagnosis, endocrinology should be consulted for recommendations regarding perioperative glucose management. Thyroid function may also be evaluated and medically controlled, if warranted, by the endocrinology team (Box 99.2).

Pertinent Labs

Patients presenting for sleeve gastrectomy undergo extensive evaluation leading up to their sleeve gastrectomy. During this time, numerous labs will be assessed by the multidisciplinary team caring for the patient. Relevant labs that anesthesia providers review include a complete blood count (CBC), type and screen, and blood glucose.

PREOPERATIVE PHARMACOLOGY

Postoperative nausea and vomiting (PONV) is the most common anesthesia-related complication that occurs in patients undergoing a sleeve gastrectomy.[8] Prophylaxis for PONV should start in the preoperative period and often includes placement of a scopolamine patch.[9]

Obesity is a risk factor for perioperative venous thromboembolism (VTE), with the risk of developing a blood clot increasing as the BMI increases.[10] Therefore, administration of low-molecular-weight heparin (LMWH), such as enoxaparin, should be considered and started preoperatively with 40 mg, given subcutaneously to patients with BMIs of 40 to 49 and 60 mg given to patients with a BMI of >50.

Preoperative sedation with benzodiazepines and/or opioids should be used judiciously in this patient population due to the increased incidence of OSA, as even a small dose has the potential to result in pronounced respiratory obstruction and depression. If an anxious patient requires sedation preoperatively, consider giving a decreased dose and closely monitor their respiratory status.[7]

ANESTHETIC TECHNIQUE

Intraoperative Management

Sleeve gastrectomy is usually performed laparoscopically under general endotracheal anesthesia (GETA) (Box 99.3). When preparing the operative suite for these patients, ensure that appropriately sized monitors and equipment are available, including large or extra-large blood pressure cuffs, sequential compression devices, an operating table rated for your patient's weight, and any airway equipment anticipated to be needed.[5] As previously mentioned, airway management, including bag-mask ventilation, direct laryngoscopy, and tracheal intubation can be difficult in these patients.

BOX 99.2 KEY ASSESSMENT POINTS

- **Cardiac**
  - Chest x-ray
  - ECG
  - Consider echocardiogram.
  - Consider stress test.
- **Pulmonary**
  - Obstructive sleep apnea screening
  - Consider sleep study
  - Consider pulmonary function tests (PFTs).
- **Endocrine**
  - Glucose tolerance test
  - Consult endocrinology for perioperative glucose control plan.
- **Airway**
  - Assess
    - neck range of motion,
    - degree of mouth opening,
    - Mallampati score, and
    - thyromental distance.
  - Plan for potential difficult mask ventilation and tracheal intubation.

BOX 99.3 CLINICAL PEARLS

- Plan for a difficult airway.
  - Consider positioning techniques, such as "ramping" and reverse Trendelenburg.
- Combat both PONV and respiratory complications by decreasing opioid use.
  - Consider IV acetaminophen, ketorolac, and dexmedetomidine as adjuncts.
- Prophylactically treat PONV multimodally.
  - Consider scopolamine patch, ondansetron, and dexamethasone.
- Discuss use and placement of the surgeon's preferred calibration device.
  - Nothing besides this device should reside in the esophagus and/or stomach.

PONV, postoperative nausea and vomiting

Anesthesia providers should prepare accordingly. In addition to having the appropriate equipment, the patient should be positioned in a manner that facilitates intubation. It is recommended the patient start in an augmented sniffing position with their upper body and head "ramped" up on blankets and/or pillows such that the occiput is raised to the point where the external acoustic meatus is horizontally aligned with the sternal notch. This position improves the anesthesia provider's visibility of the vocal cords during direct laryngoscopy.[1,5,7] Placing the operative table in a reverse Trendelenburg position will help to increase the patient's lung volumes, including functional residual capacity (FRC), and assist with preoxygenation, which is especially important in this population, given the combination of OSA and increased BMI is associated with a higher risk of laryngospasm.[7]

Maintenance of anesthesia can be accomplished with either volatile anesthetic agents or via total IV anesthesia (TIVA). If the procedure will last greater than 2 hours in length and use of a volatile anesthetic agent is planned, the use of desflurane should be considered as desflurane's fat:blood solubility is almost half that of sevoflurane's, resulting in a more rapid emergence. The use of TIVA during a sleeve gastrectomy may be beneficial in controlling PONV; however, dosing of medications can prove difficult in obese adolescents. The use of intraoperative EEG during a TIVA may provide guidance regarding dosing and adjusting medications in an effort to prevent a delayed emergence.[5,7]

Prevention of PONV should start preoperatively and then be continued intraoperatively. Antiemetic agents, such as ondansetron and dexamethasone, should be given as prophylaxis and reduction of opioids should be considered.[1,9] Reducing the use of opioids not only is an effective strategy in reducing the incidence of PONV, but it may also decrease the occurrence of adverse respiratory events in patients with OSA. Patients with OSA, particularly those with nadir oxygen saturations while asleep less than 85%, have an increased sensitivity to opioids and are more likely to experience complications such as upper airway obstruction and apnea from standard doses.[7,11] IV acetaminophen and ketorolac are often included as nonopioid analgesics in an anesthetic plan for an adolescent undergoing a sleeve gastrectomy.[9] The selective alpha-2 agonist dexmedetomidine has also been reported to provide promising opioid-sparing effects in obese adolescents.[11]

Special Techniques and/or Equipment

During a sleeve gastrectomy, anesthesia providers may be charged with placing a gastric sleeve calibrator during the procedure. Typically, this entails placement of an orogastric device which allows the surgeon to measure and maintain the size and shape of the gastric sleeve accurately and consistently. There are a number of different devices that could be used for this purpose, including bougie dilators and inflatable calibrators.[12,13] Communication with the surgeon regarding placement of the device and any special instructions specific to the device is of utmost importance. It is imperative that there is nothing else in the esophagus and/or stomach during these procedures, including temperature probes and orogastric or nasogastric suctioning tubes.

Complications/Emergencies

Intraoperative bleeding is a possible complication during a sleeve gastrectomy, though the risk is relatively low. If bleeding were to occur, it tends to be during the gastric stapling or the division of vessels in the greater curvature of the stomach.[14,15] Should this occur, the anesthesia provider should assess and support the patient's blood volumetric needs.

As discussed previously, a bougie or other calibration device is often placed intraoperatively by the anesthesia provider. During placement and adjustment of such device, the anesthesia provider should be aware that mechanical injuries could occur to the oral cavity, pharynx, epiglottis, and esophagus.[12] As such, care should be taken during insertion, adjustment, and removal.

It is important to note that nothing besides the calibration device reside in the stomach during gastric stapling to avoid retention of such objects in the staple line.

POSTOPERATIVE CARE

Airway management, PONV, and pain control are the main anesthetic concerns in the immediate postoperative period. The use of opioid-sparing adjuncts and use of a multimodal analgesic approach, along with PONV prophylaxis, optimize postoperative outcomes. Nonetheless, additional medications and patient care may be required in the immediate postoperative period. Pain should be addressed, and if necessary, opioids administered in a judicious manner as to not contribute to PONV and respiratory depression.[1] If PONV is an issue, additional ondansetron may be administered and an additional class of antiemetic, such as an antihistamine, should be considered.[8,9] Anesthesia providers should consider any possible sedative effects prior to administration.

If a patient with OSA uses CPAP or BiPAP at home, this may be considered in the immediate postoperative period to assist with airway obstruction; however, this remains controversial and is not recommended by some bariatric surgeons

---

CASE STUDY: 17-Year-Old Male With BMI of 54 Undergoing Sleeve Gastrectomy

CLINICAL SCENARIO

A 17-year-old male with Class III obesity (BMI of 54) who carried medical diagnoses of OSA and prediabetes presented to the general surgery team as a consult for bariatric surgery. According to the ASMBS pediatric metabolic and bariatric surgery guidelines published in 2018, the patient was deemed a candidate to be worked up for a sleeve gastrectomy. A comprehensive medical and social evaluation was performed over the course of several months by a multidisciplinary team, which included specialists in psychology, nutrition, cardiology, gastroenterology, sleep medicine, and endocrinology as suggested in the aforementioned guidelines and additional publications.[3,4,7] Parental consent and patient assent were obtained for the procedure and the anesthesia team was consulted preoperatively.

(continued)

CASE STUDY: 17-Year-Old Male With BMI of 54 Undergoing Sleeve Gastrectomy (*continued*)

SPECIAL CONSIDERATIONS

A standard preanesthetic evaluation was performed and focused on the patient's comorbidities related to his obesity, including OSA and prediabetes. The patient's OSA was diagnosed as moderate, and the patient reported to be compliant with CPAP while asleep. For this reason, the patient was advised to bring their CPAP machine on the day of the procedure. The patient's prediabetic state had been evaluated by endocrinology, and there were no specific regimens ordered for the perioperative period. There were no additional diagnoses or concerns brought forth by any of the multidisciplinary teams involved in the preoperative evaluation. Assessment of the airway proved benign, with a Mallampati score of II, neck range of motion within normal limits, as well as adequate mouth opening and thyromental distance.

APPROACHES TO CARE

Evidence-Based Approaches to Care

On the day of surgery, a final anesthesia evaluation was performed, and a peripheral IV (PIV) catheter was placed under ultrasound guidance. A CBC and type and screen was drawn at the time of PIV placement. PONV was discussed with the patient and a scopolamine patch was placed behind their ear. The patient was taken to the operating room suite and positioned on the surgical table in a "ramped" reverse trendelenberg position to assist with pre-oxygenation and direct laryngoscopy.[1,5,7] Appropriately sized monitoring equipment was utilized, and the patient underwent a standard IV induction consisting of fentanyl, dosed on lean body weight (LBW), propofol, also dosed on LBW, and a nondepolarizing muscle relaxant, dosed on ideal body weight (IBW).[1,5] Once the endotracheal tube was placed, GETA was maintained with the volatile anesthetic agent desflurane, which was chosen related to its low fat:blood coefficient.[5,7] Dexamethasone and ondansetron were administered as antiemetic prophylaxis.[9] In an attempt to limit opioid use for purposes of decreasing PONV and adverse respiratory events, nonopioid analgesics were administered, including IV acetaminophen and ketorolac.[7,9] A dexmedetomidine infusion was also used throughout the procedure for its opioid-sparing effects.[11] The procedure was completed without complication; the patient emerged from anesthesia; and the muscle relaxant reversed with sugammadex. During emergence, the patient received two small doses of hydromorphone totaling 0.4 mg. The patient was then extubated and transferred to recovery while receiving oxygen via a simple face mask. While the patient's CPAP mask remained available, its use was deemed unnecessary.

COMPLICATIONS

The lone complication in this case occurred in the postanesthesia care unit. Upon arrival to recovery, the patient reported nausea and received one dose of diphenhydramine. Following this rescue antiemetic, the patient was able to rest comfortably and maintain his own airway without CPAP support.

due to the perceived potential of disruption of staple lines in the stomach secondary to positive pressure ventilation.[11] Although the immediate postoperative period may be difficult to manage regarding airway management and PONV, a thoughtful plan that is initiated preoperatively and continued intraoperatively will contribute to a positive outcome.

KEY REFERENCES

Complete references for this chapter are online and available at https://connect.springerpub.com/content/book/978-0-8261-3875-0/part/part04/toc-part/ch099.

1. Lemmens HJM, Morton JM, Ku CM, Jones SB. Anesthetic considerations. In NT. Nguyen, SA. Brethauer, JM. Morton, J. Ponce, RJ. Rosenthal, eds. *The ASMBS Textbook of Bariatric Surgery*. 2nd ed. 2020;89–101. doi:10.1007/978-3-030-27021-6
3. Pratt JSA, Roque SS, Valera R, et al. Preoperative considerations for the pediatric patient undergoing metabolic and bariatric surgery. *Semin Pediatr Surg*. 2020;29(1):150890. doi:10.1016/j.sempedsurg.2020.150890
8. Mulier JP, Reis Falcao LF. Intraoperative anesthesia management. In M. Gagner, AR. Cardoso, M. Palermo, P. Noel, D. Nocca, eds. *The Perfect Sleeve Gastrectomy*. 2020;153–166. doi:10.1007/978-3-030-28936-2
9. Derderian SC. Rove KO. Enhance recovery after surgery among adolescents undergoing bariatric surgery. *Semin Pediatr Surg*. 2020;29(1):150885. doi:10.1016/j.sempedsurg.2020.150885
12. Almustafa M, Obeidat F, Mismar A, et al. Role of preoperative dexamethasone nebulization in reducing bougie complications encountered after sleeve gastrectomy: a prospective double-blind control interventional study. *Obes Surg*. 2020;30:501–506. doi:10.1007/s11695-019-04202-x
13. Ingram MC, Wulkan ML, Lin E. Technical review: vertical sleeve gastrectomy in adolescents. *Semin Pediatr Surg*. 2020;29(1):150886. doi:10.1016/j.sempedsurg.2020.150886
15. Lamoshi A, Chernoguz A, Harmon CM, Helmrath M. Complications of bariatric surgery in adolescents. *Semin Pediatr Surg*. 2020;29(1):150888. http://doi.org/10.1016/j.sempedsurg.2020.150888

CHAPTER 100

Nissen Fundoplication

Mary J. Scott-Herring and Aileen Mendez

INDICATIONS/CONTRAINDICATIONS

Gastroesophageal reflux disease (GERD) is common in the pediatric population. It is estimated that approximately 60% of infants have GERD due to immaturity of the lower esophageal sphincter (LES) and consumption of a liquid diet. By approximately 1 year of age, the incidence of GERD will decrease to approximately 5% when solid foods are introduced into the diet. By 2 years of age, most pediatric patients experience resolution of their symptoms with no intervention.[1] Patients who continue to have symptoms beyond the age of 2 years are likely to present with complications secondary to GERD, such as failure to thrive (FTT), respiratory disease, apnea, apparent life-threatening events (ALTEs), or esophageal stricture.[1] Infants most often present with regurgitation, vomiting, and irritability, while older children complain of dysphagia, hoarseness, chronic cough, epigastric pain, and asthma.[1]

While medical management is attempted initially in all cases, patients may continue suffer from FTT, severe vomiting, aspirational pneumonia, apneas, bradycardias, ALTE, esophageal strictures, or esophagitis, requireing surgery to abate all symptoms (see **Box 100.1**).[2] This is particularly true in children who are at high risk due to coexisting neurological conditions or in those that have had prior surgeries for tracheal esophageal fistulas or diaphragmatic hernias. In these patients, incompetence of the LES often allows gastric contents to reflux into the lower esophagus, resulting in the presenting symptoms.

There are two types of fundoplication procedures, one of which involves a complete (360-degree) wrap of the fundus of the stomach around the lower esophagus to support the LES with the other only partially wrapping the fundus around the lower esophagus.[1,3,4]

SPECIAL CONSIDERATIONS AND CONCERNS

It is important to be aware that many pediatric patients who require a Nissen fundoplication often have severe neurological compromise or a history of seizures (see **Box 100.2**). Concurrent respiratory compromise is also frequently

BOX 100.1 INDICATIONS FOR NISSEN FUNDOPLICATION

- Aspiration pneumonia
- Apneas
- Bradycardias
- Apparent life-threatening events
- Severe vomiting
- Failure to thrive
- Esophageal strictures
- Esophagitis

BOX 100.2 COMMON COMORBIDITIES WITNESSED IN PATIENTS PRESENTING FOR NISSEN FUNDOPLICATION

- Neurological compromise
- Cerebral palsy
- Seizure history
- Aspiration
- Bronchospasm
- Asthma

seen due to aspiration, bronchospasm, and asthma.[3] A careful history and physical should explore these issues and plans should be made prior to surgery for a monitored bed postoperatively as appropriate.

During the procedure, anesthesia providers must be aware of physiological changes that may occur, especially during insufflation. For instance, cardiovascular collapse may occur due to gas emboli which is believed to be caused by intravascular carbon dioxide (CO_2), although it may be nitrogen or air. This can occur when the insufflation pressure is greater than the venous pressure as it may force bubbles into venous circulation. This can be especially problematic in infants and children with patent foramen ovale (PFO) as they are more susceptible to gas emboli. Essentially, as insufflation pressure increases, a rise in adverse respiratory events is often seen. Meanwhile, decreases in pulmonary and thoracic compliance occur, which leads to decreases in vital capacity (VC), functional residual capacity (FRC) and closing volumes. A resultant ventilation/perfusion (VQ) mismatch is created, and hypoxemia can result. The decrease in pulmonary compliance leads to increased peak inspiratory pressures (PIPs) and overall decreased compliance. For this reason, a cuffed endotracheal tube (ETT) is preferred over uncuffed to obtain optimal alveolar ventilation. It is important to monitor for high intra-abdominal pressure (IAP) as that can cause pneumomediastinum or pneumothorax. In addition, high IAP can decrease cardiac output (CO), venous return, myocardial contractility, and left ventricular systolic function (see **Table 100.1**).[4] For additional information regarding the anesthetic management of children undergoing laparoscopic surgery, please refer to Chapter 102, "Laparoscopic Surgery."

Increased IAP along with increased systemic vascular resistance (SVR), increased $PaCO_2$, and Trendelenburg positioning may increase intracranial pressure (ICP) to unsafe levels. It is important to assess and evaluate the patient's neurological status prior to surgery and to evaluate ventricular peritoneal (VP) shunt function prior to proceeding. An increased IAP may also decrease renal blood flow, renal function, and creatinine clearance. Special care should be taken to avoid fluid overload, as it is with all patients.[4]

Specific to Nissen fundoplication, a bougie is positioned in the esophagus to help the surgeon determine how tight to tie the muscles around the esophagus. Care should be

Table 100.1 Physiological Changes Anticipated During Laparoscopic Nissen Fundoplication

Physiological Changes	Increase	Decrease
Cardiovascular	Systemic vascular resistance (SVR)	Cardiac output Venous return Contractility Left ventricular systolic function
Respiratory	Peak inspiratory pressures (PIPs) $PaCO_2$	Compliance Vital capacity (VC) Functional residual capacity (FRC) Closing volume
Neurological	Intracranial pressure (ICP)	
Renal	Intra-abdominal pressure (IAP)	Renal blood flow Renal function Creatinine clearance

taken to gently advance the bougie without forcing it to pass. Anesthesia providers must also be careful to not extubate the patient during bougie manipulation or push the bougie forcefully as trauma can occur in the oropharynx. At the end of the procedure, anesthesia providers may be asked to "bolus" 50 to 60 mL of air into the patient's stomach via a syringe to test the anastomosis for leakage. Overall, postoperative pain is usually easily managed.[4]

ANESTHETIC MANAGEMENT

PREOPERATIVE EVALUATION

As with all patients, it is important to optimize a child's condition preoperatively, especially any cardiac issues or any chronic lung disease due to chronic aspiration.[5]

Pertinent Labs
If the patient has experienced excessive vomiting, laboratory values should be normalized prior to proceeding.

PREOPERATIVE PHARMACOLOGY

Premedication with benzodiazepines is controversial.[5] Any antiseizure medications or any bronchodilators should be continued as scheduled.[3]

ANESTHETIC TECHNIQUE

Intraoperative Management
Anesthetic management for Nissen procedures entails general anesthesia with an ETT.[4] Preoperative IV access should be obtained due to the risk of aspiration and the need to secure the airway quickly. If the patient has on an orogastric or nasogastric tube in place, it should be connected to suction to decompress the stomach prior to induction. Any gastric tube will need to be removed during the case when the Maloney type bougie/dilator is being used.

Intraoperative management includes the use of standard monitors, such as ECG, noninvasive blood pressure monitoring, pulse oximetry, and temperature monitoring. Rapid sequence intubation should be performed if the patient exhibits excessive vomiting.[5] Standard induction medications include propofol and a muscle relaxant, with additional medications to include antiemetics, opioids for pain, and acetaminophen and/or nonsteroidal analgesics for further management. Local infiltration by the surgeon is helpful in decreasing postoperative pain, while epidural analgesia is helpful in pain management for open procedures.[3] Regional anesthesia may or may not be beneficial in treating pain postoperatively and results are mixed. Patients who received a surgeon-performed abdominal wall nerve block have demonstrated a shorter hospital stay when compared to local wound infiltration and ultrasound-guided nerve blocks.[6] However, in matched groups, there was no significant difference in patient pain scores in the first 8 hours.[6]

Decompress the patient's stomach with a nasogastric tube (NGT) or orogastric tube (OGT), and after induction, a urinary catheter should be placed to empty the bladder. A foley catheter is not always placed, but surgeons may use the Credé maneuver on the bladder to decompress it when the patient is asleep. Generally, there is minimal fluid and blood loss.

Surgeons should try to keep pneumoperitoneum pressure as low as the risk of cardiovascular and respiratory compromise—and even potentially fatal emboli—have been directly correlated to peak pneumoperitoneal pressure. Generally used are pressures of 6 to 8 mm Hg in infants, 10 to 12 mm Hg in children, and not more than 15 mm Hg in any case. High pressures may cause cardiac and respiratory depression, hypothermia, pneumothorax, SQ emphysema, endobronchial intubation.[4] The CO_2 used to insufflate the abdomen is rapidly absorbed and the peak end-tidal carbon dioxide ($ETCO_2$) measurement is greater in infants than in children. There is an inverse relationship between age and the rate of CO_2 absorption that is attributed to a thinner peritoneum and fat deposits in babies compared to older children; the longer the surgery, the higher the $ETCO_2$. This requires increasing the minute ventilation by up to 50% to 100% in order to maintain physiological pH.[4]

Most patients are able to be extubated at the end of the procedure. Those with preexisting neurological or respiratory compromise may need to stay intubated or go to an ICU or monitored bed.[3]

Special Techniques and/or Equipment
A Maloney-type bougie/dilator is placed in esophagus during the case so surgeons can use it as a guide to wrap the fundus around the esophagus. It is important to ensure that the dilator is mobile, that it has not been sutured into, and that the wrap itself is not too tight. When it is time to remove the dilator, if there is resistance, the anesthesia provider must not pull too hard. They should let the surgeon know there is difficulty in removing the dilator so they can release suture. Occasionally, the surgeon may request that a nasogastric tube be placed for postoperative management. If so, care should be taken when passing it through the distal esophagus and undue force should not be exerted.

Complications/Emergencies
With a Nissen repair, it is desirable to avoid retching and gas bloat.[2] These can be avoided by adequately decompressing the stomach and by administration of adequate opioid analgesics and antiemetics. Additional complications include dysphagia, atelectasis, pneumonia, wound infection, dehiscence, small bowel obstruction due to adhesions, delayed gastric emptying, wrap failure, slipped wrap, herniation of wrap into the chest, and excessively tight wrap.[7]

The highest risk is for aspiration on induction, so make sure suction is immediately available and be able to perform bronchial lavage if needed in the event that aspiration does occur. There have been some studies suggesting that the use of cricoid pressure for rapid sequence intubation is not supported and may in fact make visualization more challenging.[5]

POSTOPERATIVE CARE

Most commonly, patients experience pain arising from the incision sites, gas in the abdomen, shoulder pain referred from the diaphragm, or position stretch in their back and shoulder. It is most common for surgeons to inject local anesthetics along the incision sites and to incorporate multimodal analgesics such as acetaminophen, non-steroidal anti-inflammatory drugs (NSAIDs), and opioids.[4]

REFERENCES

1. Jackson HT, Kane TD. Surgical management of pediatric gastroesophageal reflux disease. Gastroenterology research and practice. *Gastroenterol Res Pract*. 2013;2013:863527. doi:10.1155/2013/86527
2. Dekonenko C, Holcomb GW. Laparoscopic fundoplication for the surgical management of gastroesophageal reflux disease in children. *Eur J Pediatr Surg*. 2020;30:150–155. doi:10.1055/s-0040-1702139
3. Davis PJ, Cladis FP. *Smith's Anesthesia for Infants and Children*. 9th ed. Elsevier; 2017.
4. Cote CJ, Lerman J, Anderson BJ. *A Practice of Anesthesia for Infants and Children*. 6th ed. Elsevier; 2019.
5. Houck PJ, Hache M, Sun LS. *Handbook of Pediatric Anesthesia*. McGraw Hill; 2015.
6. Landmann A, Visoiu M, Malek MM. Laparoscopic-guided abdominal wall nerve blocks in the pediatric population: a novel technique with comparison to ultrasound-guided blocks and local wound infiltration alone. *Surgery*. 2018;163(3):622–626.
7. Jaksic T. Pediatric Gastroesophageal Reflux Surgery. *Medscape*. 2020. https://emedicine.medscape.com/article/936596-treatment. Accessed 9/1/20201

CHAPTER 101

Intussusception

Lisa Herbinger and Karen Knight

INDICATIONS/CONTRAINDICATIONS

Intussusception is a condition in which an intestinal segment slides into the lumen of a more distal intestinal segment. The portion of bowel that slides into the other portion is known as the intussusceptum; the outer, more distal segment around the intussusceptum is known as the intussuscipiens. When this telescoping of the bowel occurs, material passing through the intestine becomes blocked, and blood flow to the affected portions of the intestine becomes compromised. As a result, the patient is at risk of bowel necrosis, perforation, and sepsis. For this reason, intussusception is considered an emergent finding requiring immediate treatment.

The area of affected bowel segments can vary. However, 85% of intussusceptions are ileocolic, as the distal ileum invaginates into the cecum and ascending colon (see **Figures 101.1 and 101.2**). The intussusceptum can progress through the transverse colon and into the descending or even sigmoid colon.[1] Other possible intussusception sites include ileoileal, ileo-ileocolic, and colocolic.[2]

The etiology of intussusception is unknown; however, researchers have observed an increased risk after a gastrointestinal (GI) infection.[3] While fighting the infection, local lymphatic tissue swells, creating pressure that can pull a segment of bowel into another segment. In fact, diagnosis is often delayed because early symptoms of intussusception can mimic those of the GI infection. Pain can be intermittent for hours or days before the diagnosis is made.[4] Spontaneous reduction with no treatment occurs in approximately 20% of intussusception events.[2]

Intussusception is the most common cause of intestinal obstruction in children between 3 months and 6 years of age. Males are four times more likely to have an intussusception event than females.[5] Although rare, there are documented cases of in utero and neonatal intussusception. Intussusception is categorized as either idiopathic or secondary to a pathological lead point. Approximately 90% of intussusception events are idiopathic, meaning there is no obvious cause other than swollen or hyperplasic lymphatic tissue known as Peyer's patches.[6] This lymphatic hyperplasia is most often caused by adenovirus; however, rotavirus, norovirus, enterovirus, herpesvirus 6, cytomegalovirus, Epstein–Barr virus, and bacterial infections have been implicated.[7]

Of the nonidiopathic cases, multiple types of lead points can project into the lumen of the bowel, predisposing the child to intussusception. Documented lead points include Meckel's diverticula, the appendix, intestinal polyps, duplication cysts, neoplastic tumors, foreign bodies (including feeding tubes), thick or hardened feces (commonly seen with cystic fibrosis) and hematomas (commonly seen in celiac disease[2]).

Historically, concerns have been raised related to an association between the rotavirus vaccine and intussusception. The vaccine was first licensed in the United States in 1998 but was withdrawn from the market in 1999. Researchers found a link between vaccination and intussusception, especially during the first week postvaccination. The vaccine was reintroduced in 2006, and clinical trials since that time have not included evidence of an associated increase in the incidence of intussusception.[8] The Centers for Disease Control and Prevention (CDC) does, however, state that there is a small risk of intussusception after rotavirus vaccination, usually during the first week after the first or second dose.[9] The CDC list of contraindications to the rotavirus vaccine includes a history of intussusception.

The symptoms associated with intussusception can be vague and variable. Only about 20% have the classic triad of intussusception, which includes colicky abdominal pain, presence of an abdominal mass, and red currant–jelly stool. It has been suggested that more useful clinical signs include abdominal pain, vomiting, pallor and lethargy. If the diagnosis is missed or treatment is delayed, dehydration and sepsis will be evident. **Box 101.1** summarizes the differential diagnoses associated with intussusception.[10]

Although several tools have historically been used for diagnosis, abdominal ultrasonography (US) is now considered the gold standard with greater than 90% sensitivity and specificity.[2,10] Computed tomography can detect an intussusception but is generally avoided in children due to the high level of radiology exposure. Conventional radiology is less reliable and lacks the advantages that come with US. Direct visualization of the defect is possible during US. When color Doppler is used, areas of decreased blood flow with associated higher risks of perforation can be identified so that the decision to proceed with pneumatic or hydrostatic reduction is more safely made. A contrast enema with dilute barium, a water-soluble contrast, or air is considered diagnostic and therapeutic.[1] Approximately 75% of ileocolic intussusceptions are reduced during a contrast enema procedure,[11] which negates the need for surgical intervention.

Nonoperative reduction should proceed immediately after the diagnosis of intussusception is made and the child's hydration status has been normalized. Before proceeding, a bolus of 20 mL/kg of isotonic crystalloid should be administered to prevent or treat dehydration. A nasogastric (NG) tube should be inserted to decompress the stomach and to minimize the risk of vomiting. Occasionally, these children will present with hypovolemic shock symptoms requiring advanced pediatric life support measures, such as intubation, aggressive fluid resuscitation and observation in a critical care unit. A broad-spectrum antibiotic should be administered intravenously before nonoperative or operative interventions. Cautious use of opioids or sedatives with monitoring may be considered.[2]

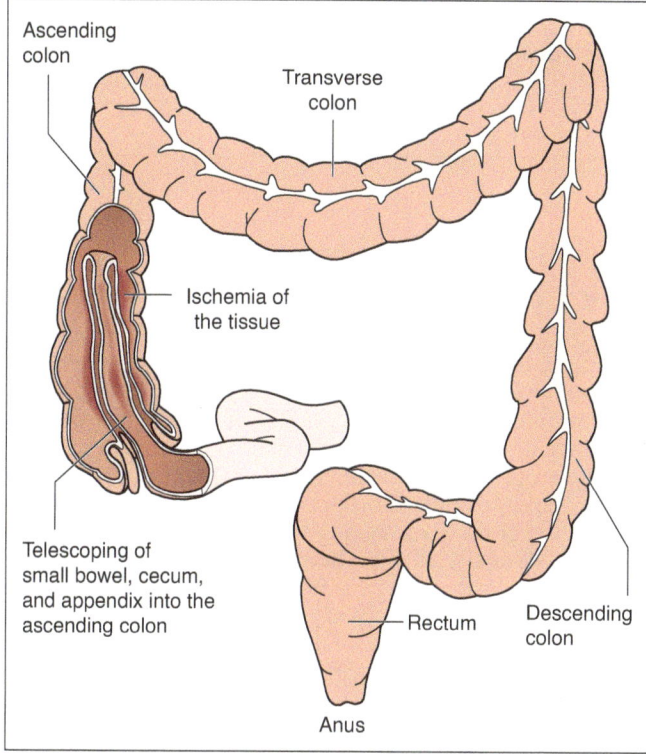

Figure 101.1: Ileocolic intussusception.

Source: From Small A. Advanced health assessment of the abdomen, rectum, and anus. In: Myrick KM, Karosas LM, eds. *Advanced Health Assessment and Differential Diagnosis.* Springer; 2019:Fig. 8.39.

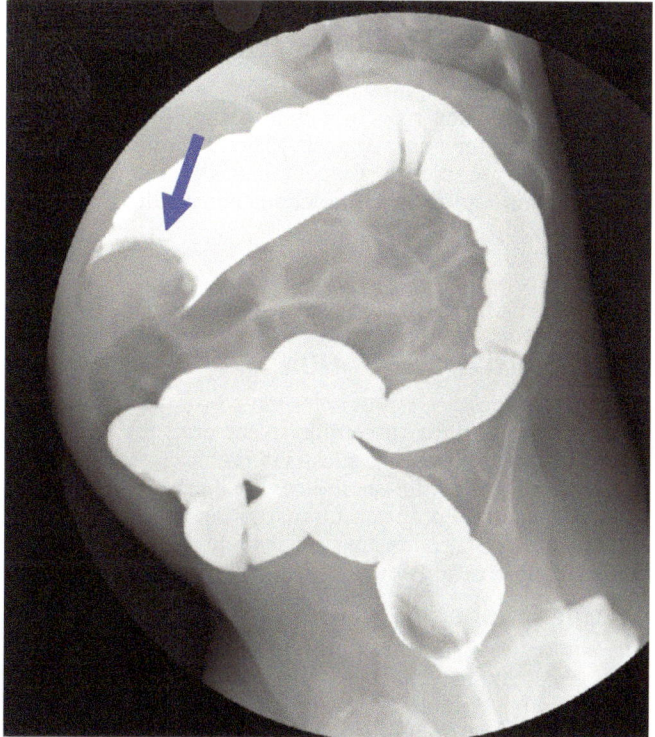

Figure 101.2: Radiograph of crescent sign with ileocolic intussusception.

BOX 101.1 DIFFERENTIAL DIAGNOSES ASSOCIATED WITH INTUSSUSCEPTION

- Gastroenteritis
- Sepsis related to another condition
- Strangulated hernia
- Urinary tract infection
- Acute appendicitis
- Hirschsprung disease

> **BOX 101.2 EXEMPLAR PROTOCOL FOR NON-OPERATIVE PNEUMATIC REDUCTION OF INTUSSUSCEPTION**
>
> - Preprocedure
>   - Obtain informed consent from parent/legal guardian
>   - Prepare equipment (pressurized air delivery system or sphygmomanometer, and emergent air aspiration)
>   - Warm the radiology suite
>   - Ensure availability of necessary staff
>   - Apply pulse oximetry and ECG leads
>   - Consider sedation and/or analgesia
> - Procedure
>   - Insert 24-Fr catheter into the rectum
>   - Hold/tape buttocks to create a seal
>   - Insufflate to 60 to 80 mm Hg; increase to 120 mm Hg
>   - Limit to 3 minutes per attempt; repeat up to three times
>   - Assess with fluoroscopy
>   - Air moving into bowel loops signals successful reduction
>   - If unsuccessful, repeat 2 to 6 hours later
> - Postprocedure
>   - Monitor respiratory status if sedation and/or analgesia has been given
>   - Consider repeat ultrasound
>   - Observe for 24 hours for signs of recurrence

> **BOX 101.3 INDICATIONS FOR SURGICAL INTERVENTION OF INTUSSUSCEPTION**
>
> - Bowel perforation
> - Peritonitis
> - Hemodynamic instability
> - Known pathological lead point
> - Failed nonoperative reductions
> - Prematurity

Bradshaw and Johnson[2] describe a typical sequence of events for a nonoperative enema reduction procedure. **Box 101.2** illustrates this sequence. Pneumatic (air) reduction with radiology guidance reduces the risk of peritoneal contamination should a perforation occur during insufflation. However, hydrostatic reduction with ultrasound guidance is also used in some facilities. Normal saline, Ringer's solution, Hartmann's solution, and tap water have been successfully used. The advantage to this technique in that ionizing radiation can be avoided. Although there is historical widespread use of barium for hydrostatic reduction, it is no longer used due to the risk of life-threatening peritonitis should a perforation occur.[12] Little difference exists in success rates of pneumatic versus hydrostatic reductions, and the decision of which technique to use is based on institutional or practitioner preference.[10]

Although many intussusceptions are reduced without surgical intervention, evidence-based criteria exist for deciding when a child should proceed to the operating room (OR).[2,13] **Box 101.3** includes a summary of these findings. Intussusception in the neonatal population is rare but can occur prenatally or postnatally. Pneumatic or hydrostatic enema reduction is contraindicated in preterm infants due to immature and frail intestinal tissue with an accompanying high risk of perforation.[13] Another absolute contraindication to attempting a nonoperative enema reduction is evidence or strong clinical suspicion of full-thickness bowel necrosis, which significantly increases the risk of pressure-induced perforation.[10]

SPECIAL CONSIDERATIONS AND CONCERNS

A perforation during pneumatic reduction can progress to a tension pneumoperitoneum. If a perforation is suspected, a needle aspiration of the air with a large bore catheter (18 ga) inserted into the right iliac fossa should be performed by the radiologist or surgeon. Having a pediatric surgeon involved in the nonoperative reduction improves success. The surgeon can assist the radiologist in decision-making and can handle a perforation or other emergency should one occur.[2]

Delayed repeat enemas have become common and significantly decreased surgical intervention rates. Researchers have reported a 50% chance of successful reduction with each repeated attempt, if there is evidence of partial reduction at a previous attempt. It is thought that partial reduction allows for bowel and mesenteric edema to subside, which facilitates a subsequent reduction. Time intervals range from 30 minutes to several hours with no established standard of practice.[10] Authors of a retrospective study of almost 700 children with successful pneumatic (air) reductions suggest that pneumatic reduction attempts can be safely repeated up to four times (five total attempts) to avoid the need for surgical intervention.[14]

The use of sedation or general anesthesia for pediatric patients undergoing nonoperative reductions is controversial. Resistance from a child with no sedation or general anesthesia can decrease the chance of a successful reduction.[15,16] This raises the question of how best to manage the airway and to minimize aspiration risks in a child having sedation or general anesthesia for a nonsurgical procedure. A lack of research related to the anesthetic management of children having nonoperative intussusception reductions has resulted in no current standardization of care.[17]

ANESTHETIC MANAGEMENT

PREOPERATIVE EVALUATION

Frequently, anesthesia providers have no involvement with a child with an intussusception event until the decision is made to proceed with surgical intervention. At that point, the anesthesia provider should conduct a thorough preoperative evaluation. Because intussusception is a type of bowel obstruction, focal points are similar to those for other pediatric bowel obstruction emergencies.

Pertinent Labs

Hematology and electrolyte profiles should be evaluated in all intussusception patients. Liver and renal function, coagulation status, serum albumin level, and blood type/cross-matching should be added for those who have signs of dehydration, third-space fluid shifting or hypovolemia. The correction of abnormal metabolic processes should ideally happen before proceeding with anesthesia and surgery; however, because of the emergent nature of bowel perforation or impending necrosis, the child may not be optimized on arrival to the OR.[18]

ANESTHETIC TECHNIQUE

Intraoperative Management

As with most obstructive bowel disorders, aspiration prophylaxis with a rapid sequence induction (RSI) and a cuffed endotracheal tube (ETT) is recommended. Delaying a surgical procedure will often not reduce aspiration risks and can increase the risk of complications.[18] The use of preoperative US to assess gastric volume in children can be helpful, but more study in this area is needed.[17,19] With the availability of sugammadex, the use of rocuronium 1.2 mg/kg is a safe alternative to the potentially life-threatening hyperkalemia that can result in children from succinylcholine.[20]

The use of cricoid pressure during RSI has been questioned in adults and children. Authors of a Cochrane systematic review concluded that cricoid pressure may not be necessary to safely perform RSI and that potential risks of cricoid pressure include vocal cord closure or impaired visualization of the larynx, which can lead to repeated intubation attempts, failed intubation, or the need for a surgical airway.[21] In children specifically, authors from a national pediatric emergency airway registry reported that cricoid pressure during tracheal intubation was not associated with a lower regurgitation rate.[22] As with other intra-abdominal procedures, Trendelenburg positioning and insufflation during laparoscopy increases aspiration risks. Airway management with a laryngeal mask airway or uncuffed ETT should be avoided.[18] There is widespread agreement that children who have undergone general anesthesia with a full stomach and associated increased aspiration risk should be extubated awake.[23] An NG tube may be in place on arrival to the OR. If not, the surgeon may request one to help with surgical exposure. The decision of whether to leave the NG tube in place postoperatively will depend on the anticipated level of early postoperative GI function.

> **BOX 101.4 CLINICAL PEARLS**
>
> - Intussusception requires emergent treatment.
> - Symptoms can mimic other gastrointestinal disorders, delaying diagnosis.
> - Most are reduced nonsurgically, usually without sedation or GA.
> - Contraindications for nonsurgical reduction include full thickness bowel necrosis and prematurity.
> - When nonsurgical interventions fail, surgical reduction is required.
> - Preoperative preparation includes hematological and electrolyte profiles and fluid resuscitation.
> - The GA plan should include rapid sequence induction and awake extubation.
> - Surgical reduction can be accomplished with laparotomy or laparoscopy.
> - Consider intraoperative and postoperative opioid sparing adjuncts.
>
> GA, general anesthesia.

After securing the child's airway, the choice of intraoperative and postoperative anesthetic agents should be based on the patient's clinical presentation, the surgical approach being used and the anesthesia provider's preference. Opioids, acetaminophen, nonsteroidal anti-inflammatory medications and surgeon-administered local anesthetics are commonly used adjuncts for pediatric abdominal procedures.[18] In the absence of sepsis, regional techniques, such as epidural infusion and transabdominus plane (TAP) block, can provide analgesia and decrease the risk of opioid-induced ileus. Opioid-sparing strategies can be especially advantageous for those children who may not tolerate large doses of opioids, such as infants and children with obstructive sleep apnea or respiratory disease.[24]

Intraoperative anesthesia management can be difficult in children who have not been optimized preoperatively or have progressed to a necrotic bowel scenario. Ischemic bowel during the early portion of the procedure and reperfused bowel later can release mediators that lead to hemodynamic instability. In addition, sepsis and hypovolemia can lead to postinduction instability. Inotropic and vasopressor support may be required.[18]

Several surgical approaches may be used for the reduction of an intussusception. The intussusceptum is located in the ascending colon of more than 70% of patients.[25] Open laparotomy is usually done with a right transverse incision above or below the umbilicus.[2,10] In recent years, laparoscopic procedures have grown in popularity. With the classic laparoscopic approach, a port inserted at the umbilicus is used to create the pneumoperitoneum. Additional ports are placed under direct vision, commonly in the left iliac fossa and the epigastrium, which allows access to the right iliac fossa area of the abdomen.[2] Single-incision laparoscopic surgery (SILS) is a newer laparoscopic technique using an umbilical entry that allows a 360° view and access without multiple trocar sites. If reduction is not successful, a transabdominal bimanual reduction can be attempted. The SILS incision is extended superiorly and inferiorly to accommodate the surgeon's finger. When the intussusceptum is palpated, the surgeon uses the other hand to apply external pressure and to reduce the obstruction. Complete reduction can be confirmed by exteriorizing the affected bowel segment through the umbilical incision.[25]

Disadvantages exist, however, with the laparoscopic approach. When nonoperative enema attempts have been made to reduce the obstruction, the resultant dilated bowel loops can obscure the view and limit working space for the surgeon. In addition, because an indication for surgical reduction is the presence of necrotic bowel tissue, conversion to an open procedure for bowel resection may be required.[10] A right hemicolectomy with end-to-end anastomosis is most common. Stoma formation is usually not necessary unless a perforation has led to significant peritoneal contamination.[2] Laparoscopy offers a diagnostic advantageous when the etiology of the intussusception is unknown and/or confirmation of pathological lead points is needed.[10]

Complications/Emergencies

Recurrence of intussusception does occur unfortunately. The recurrence rate with enema reduction has been reported as high as 20%, while the recurrence rate after surgical reduction is 1% to 3%. The overall recurrence rate is approximately 13%, with almost 50% of those occurring during the first postreduction week. Risk factors for recurrence include an age greater than 2 years, symptoms for more than 48 hours, a lack of rectal bleeding, telescoping on the right side, the presence of a pathological lead point, and no history of infection.[26,27] C-reactive protein (CRP) levels rise with tissue damage and inflammatory processes such as those seen with intussusception events. A CRP level great than 0.5 mg/dL can be considered a predictive indicator for recurrence.[27] Dexamethasone used as an adjunct to enema reduction may lower recurrence rates when compared to enema reduction alone; however, high-level evidence is lacking, and more research is needed.[28] The treatment of a recurrent intussusception is generally the same as that of the primary event.[26]

KEY REFERENCES

Complete references for this chapter are online and available at https://connect.springerpub.com/content/book/978-0-8261-3875-0/part/part04/toc-part/ch101.

2. Bradshaw CJ, Johnson PR. Intussusception. *J Paediatr Child Health*. 2018;28(5):222–226. doi:10.1016/j.paed.2018.03.005
3. Laquerre JN. Intussusception: sonographic findings to fluoroscopic reduction in pediatrics. *Radiologic Technology*. 2020;91(4):380–384.
4. Lampl BS, Glaab J, Ayyala RS, et al. Is intussusception a middle-of-the-night emergency? *Pediatr Emerg Care*. July 2017 doi:10.1097/pec.0000000000001246
5. Boston Children's Hospital. Intussusception. Accessed September 20, 2020, from http://www.childrenshospital.org/conditions-and-treatments/ conditions/i/intussusception.
10. Beasley SW. The 'ins' and 'outs' of intussusception: where best practice reduces the need for surgery. *J Paediatr Child Health*. 2017;53:1118–1122. doi:10.1111/jpc.13738
11. Binkovitz LA, Kolbe AB, Orth RC, et al. Pediatric ileocolic intussusception: new observations and unexpected implications. *Pediatr Radiol*. 2018;49(1):76–81. doi:10.1007/s00247-018-4259-9
14. Ma G, Lillehei C, Callahan MJ. Air contrast enema reduction of single and recurrent ileocolic intussusceptions in children: patterns, management and outcomes. *Pediatr Radiol*. 2020;50:664–672. doi:doi.org/10.1007/s00247-020-04612-5
18. Hansen TG, Henneberg SW, Lerman J. General abdominal and urologic surgery. In: Coté CJ, Lerman J, Anderson BJ, eds. *A Practice of Anesthesia for Infants and Children*. Elsevier; 2019:669–672.
25. Chang PC, Duh Y, Fu Y, et al. Single-incision laparoscopic surgery for idiopathic intussusception in children: comparison with conventional laparoscopy. *J Pediatr Surg*. 2019;54(8): 1604–1608. doi:10.1016/j.jpedsurg.2018.07.010
28. Gluckman S, Karpelowsky J, Webster AC, McGee RG. Management for intussusception in children. *Cochrane Database Syst Rev*. 2017;6.

CHAPTER 102

Laparoscopic Surgery

Nathan S. Jones

INDICATIONS/CONTRAINDICATIONS

The laparoscopic approach has been used in pediatric surgery since the early 1990s, with the use of laparoscopy increasing in the last 15 to 20 years. Laparoscopic surgery affords the benefits of smaller incisions, better wound cosmesis, reduced postoperative pain, and shorter hospital length of stay.[1-4] Although the laparoscopic approach is less invasive than traditional laparotomy, the anesthetic management presents its own unique set of challenges due to the use of carbon dioxide for abdominal insufflation and the implementation of steep surgical positions (e.g., Trendelenburg and reverse Trendelenburg), which are sometimes necessary for optimal surgical visualization.[5] Despite these challenges, the laparoscopic technique has become the method of choice for many pediatric surgical procedures.[6]

A contraindication to laparoscopic surgery will pertain to the patient's ability to tolerate the adverse effects of pneumoperitoneum. Patients with congenital heart disease, pulmonary hypertension, and hemodynamic instability deserve special consideration, and the benefits of laparoscopy must be balanced with the potential negative sequelae.[7-9]

SPECIAL CONSIDERATIONS AND CONCERNS

Due to its nontoxic, inert, and inflammable properties, carbon dioxide is the preferred gas used to create pneumoperitoneum, but it is not without consequence.[10] The physiological changes that occur during carbon dioxide insufflation are well-documented in the literature and summarized in **Table 102.1**.

NEUROLOGICAL SYSTEM

During laparoscopy, intracranial pressure (ICP) is increased due to the increase in cerebral blood flow related to hypercarbia-induced vasodilation. ICP will further increase in the Trendelenburg position. Caution must be exercised in any patient with an intracranial mass or other cause of increased ICP. There appears to be no change or only mild decrease in cerebral oxygenation during pneumoperitoneum.[11,12] A decrease in cerebral oxygenation is potentially attributable to increased ICP or decreased cardiac output (CO).

TABLE 102.1	Physiological Changes During Carbon Dioxide Pneumoperitoneum		
System	Variable	Effect	Cause
Neurological	ICP	Increased	Increased CBF Trendelenburg position
	CBF	Increased	Hypercarbia
	Cerebral oxygenation	Decreased or no change	Increased ICP Decreased CO
Respiratory	Diaphragm position	Cephalad displacement	Increased IAP
	FRC	Decreased	Increased IAP
	Lung compliance	Decreased	Increased IAP
	Airway resistance	Increased	Increased IAP
	Minute ventilation	Decreased	Increased IAP
Cardiovascular	Venous return	Increased or decreased	Degree of IAP Head position
	MAP	Increased	Hypercapnia Neuroendocrine response
	CO	Increased or decreased	Degree of IAP Head position
	SVR	Increased	Increased IAP Catecholamine release
	Cardiac rhythm	Bradyarrhythmia	Vagal stimulation
	Blood pressure	Hypotension	Decreased IAP Decreased venous return Abdominal desufflation
Renal	Renal blood flow	Decreased	Increased IAP
	Urine output	Decreased	Increased IAP ADH secretion

ADH, antidiuretic hormone; CBF, cerebral blood flow; CO, cardiac output; FRC, functional residual capacity; IAP, intra-abdominal pressure; ICP, intracranial pressure; MAP, mean arterial pressure; SVR, systemic vascular resistance.

RESPIRATORY SYSTEM

At baseline, younger pediatric patients have decreased functional residual capacity (FRC), high pulmonary closing capacity, and a high rate of oxygen consumption that predisposes them to atelectasis and hypoxemia during laparoscopy.[13] With abdominal insufflation, the increase in intra-abdominal pressure (IAP) causes cephalad displacement of the diaphragm. This diaphragmatic elevation further decreases FRC, increases airway resistance, decreases compliance, and can cause atelectasis. Decreased FRC, when combined with atelectasis, can result in ventilation/perfusion (V/Q) mismatch and hypoxemia.[2,4,5] Recruitment maneuvers can be used to improve atelectasis and gas exchange. Likewise, ventilator changes are often necessary after abdominal insufflation to limit peak airway pressure and increase minute ventilation to normalize end-tidal carbon dioxide ($ETCO_2$).

CARDIOVASCULAR SYSTEM

Intra-abdominal pressure and patient position are key variables that affect cardiovascular function during laparoscopy. A slower rate of gas insufflation and a lower IAP can minimize the adverse effects of pneumoperitoneum. With low IAP (less than 10 mm Hg), venous return is increased due to displacement of blood from the splanchnic bed. Trendelenburg positioning also facilitates venous return. At IAP greater than 15 mm Hg, venous return is decreased due to compression of the inferior vena cava along with collateral vessels. The decrease in venous return can result in hypotension and decreased CO. These effects are exacerbated by reverse Trendelenburg positioning.[2,14] Mean arterial pressure (MAP) can increase with pneumoperitoneum due to catecholamine release and resultant sympathetic stimulation. Likewise, a pneumoperitoneum-induced increase in systemic vascular resistance (SVR) is multifactorial and includes compression of vasculature from IAP and circulating catecholamines. The peritoneal stretching and stimulation that accompanies insertion of the Veress needle or abdominal insufflation can result in vagal stimulation and profound bradycardia. Emergent desufflation may be required in this scenario.[4] With rapid desufflation, the sudden reduction in IAP also decreases SVR and venous return, and can result in hypotension.[15]

RENAL SYSTEM

Increased IAP has both direct and indirect renal effects. The pneumoperitoneum directly compresses the renal parenchyma, resulting in decreased blood flow through the renal vein, resulting in decreased urine output. Additionally, compression of the renal parenchyma stimulates increased secretion of antidiuretic hormone (ADH), which contributes to oliguria.[2]

ANESTHETIC MANAGEMENT

PREOPERATIVE EVALUATION

A thorough preoperative evaluation is necessary to understand patients' history and physiology, which might place them at higher risk of complications during a surgical procedure. As mentioned earlier, pneumoperitoneum and steep head-up (reverse Trendelenburg) or head-down (Trendelenburg) positions are the major concerns for hemodynamic or respiratory changes during laparoscopy. These concerns might mitigate the benefit of smaller incisions in patients with congenital heart disease.[8] The decrease in preload and potentially decreased CO related to pneumoperitoneum and/or reverse Trendelenburg position are elevated risks for patients with congenital heart disease. Consultation with a pediatric cardiologist and intraoperative anesthesia care by anesthesia providers who have experience with this patient population is warranted.[4] In healthy children, routine preoperative labs are not required for laparoscopic surgery.

PREOPERATIVE PHARMACOLOGY

Depending on the age and demeanor of the child, preoperative pharmacological anxiolysis may be indicated. The goal of premedication is to achieve anxiolysis without respiratory depression. Fortunately, distraction techniques or use of child life services can reduce the need for anxiolytic medication.[4]

ANESTHETIC TECHNIQUE

Intraoperative Management

There is no dedicated anesthetic technique for laparoscopic surgery in children. Inhalation and IV routes for induction are both appropriate, assuming patients have complied with fasting guidelines and are not at elevated risk for aspiration of gastric contents. There is, however, controversy related to the use of nitrous oxide for induction. Nitrous oxide can increase the risk of postoperative nausea and vomiting (PONV) and cause bowel distention, potentially obscuring the surgical view and increasing postoperative pain.[4,16]

The gold standard for airway management is the endotracheal tube, though the use of a laryngeal mask airway has also been reported.[17,18] Atropine should be available in the event of bradycardia due to vagal nerve stimulation by pneumoperitoneum.[2]

BOX 102.1 CLINICAL PEARLS

- Have atropine available for abdominal insufflation, although emergent desufflation may be required if profound bradyarrhythmias or asystole occurs.
- Pay close attention to the ventilator during abdominal insufflation and position changes and make adjustments as necessary.
- Place an orogastric tube to decompress the stomach and increase surgical visibility.
- Ensure the patient is properly secured to the table if steep position changes are anticipated. Prior to the start of surgery, it is prudent to test these positions and to assess for patient shifting or sliding.
- During steep head-down positioning, endobronchial intubation can occur. Be vigilant of increased airway pressure and decreased SpO_2.
- If robotic-assisted laparoscopy is anticipated, access to the patient can be quite limited. Ensure the airway is secure; IV lines are padded and flowing well; and extension tubing is used as necessary.

Anesthesia can be maintained with either volatile agents or IV medications. Neuromuscular blocking drugs are commonly administered for tracheal intubation and to optimize surgical conditions. Placement of an orogastric tube is appropriate to decompress the stomach, increase intra-abdominal visibility and minimize needle injury.[2] Pain management should be multimodal, appreciating the potential for visceral pain due to the irritation of the peritoneum because of abdominal insufflation.[19]

Pressure-control ventilation is often used during laparoscopy to optimize ventilation and minimize atelectasis. The peak inspiratory pressure will likely need to be increased after abdominal insufflation to achieve an adequate tidal volume. Respiratory rate can be adjusted to increase the minute ventilation and to maintain an acceptable $ETCO_2$. Upon desufflation, careful attention is required to decrease the inspiratory pressure in order to avoid a drastic increase in tidal volume and resultant overdistention of the lungs (Box 102.1).

Complications and emergencies are noted in Table 102.2.

POSTOPERATIVE CARE

Postoperative care after laparoscopy includes multimodal pain management including acetaminophen, nonsteroidal anti-inflammatory drugs, and opiates. Laparoscopic surgery has been identified as a risk factor for PONV, so using antiemetic drugs is warranted for this surgery.[4]

TABLE 102.2 Potential Complications of Laparoscopic Surgery

Complication	Causes	Signs and Symptoms	Action/Treatment
Bradycardia	• Vagal nerve stimulation due to pneumoperitoneum	• Slower heart rate	• Communication with surgeon • Desufflation • Atropine
Hypotension	• Elevated IAP • Trendelenburg position • Hypovolemia • Bleeding	• Decreased blood pressure	• Confirm IAP is acceptable • Reduction in anesthetic depth • Fluid management • Position change

(continued)

TABLE 102.2	Potential Complications of Laparoscopic Surgery (continued)		
Vascular injury	• Veress needle or trocar insertion	• Acute hypotension • Tachycardia	• Call for help • Preparation for conversion to open procedure • Bolus fluids • Vasoactive medications • Consider transfusion
Venous CO_2 gas embolism	• CO_2 gas enters venous circulation • Misplacement of needle during insufflation • Transection of vessels during surgical dissection	• Sudden rise in $ETCO_2$ • Tachycardia • Hypotension • Hypoxemia • Cyanosis • Mill-wheel murmur • Embolism confirmed by transesophageal echocardiogram	• Notify surgeon • Call for help • Desufflation • FiO_2 1.0 and hyperventilation • Left lateral, head-down position • Consider placement of central venous catheter to aspirate CO_2 from right heart
Capnothorax	• CO_2 gas enters mediastinum from peritoneum	• Palpable SC emphysema • Hypercarbia • Reduced breath sounds • Increased airway pressure • Hypoxia • Hypotension	• Notify surgeon • Call for help • Desufflation • FiO_2 1.0 and hyperventilation • Needle decompression (for tension capnothorax)

CO_2, carbon dioxide, $ETCO_2$, end-tidal carbon dioxide, FiO_2, fraction of inspired oxygen; IAP, intra-abdominal pressure.

CASE STUDY: Laparoscopic Appendectomy

CLINICAL SCENARIO

A 13-year-old male presents to the emergency department with 2 days of right lower quadrant abdominal pain, anorexia, vomiting, and diarrhea. An ultrasound of the appendix shows perforated appendicitis, and he is scheduled to undergo laparoscopic appendectomy.

SPECIAL CONSIDERATIONS

Given the patient's history of vomiting, rapid-sequence induction is indicated. If the patient is volume depleted and a higher IAP is used for insufflation, decreased venous return could manifest as profound hypotension. Be prepared to administer crystalloids for volume resuscitation. Efficient and clear communication with the surgeon is essential, and it might be necessary to decrease the IAP.[14]

APPROACHES TO CARE

Evidence-Based Approaches to Care

In the course of an appendectomy, the surgeon may request a head-down, left-tilt positioning for the optimization of the surgical view. Head-down positioning combined with pneumoperitoneum will lead to cephalad displacement of the diaphragm. Additionally, increased airway pressures, decreased lung compliance, and decreased tidal volume can occur, as can endobronchial intubation. Ventilator changes are often necessary (e.g., change to pressure-control mode and increase in respiratory rate) to minimize peak airway pressure and hypercarbia.[2,20]

COMPLICATIONS

Bradycardia, hypotension, vascular injury, venous gas embolism, and capnothorax are potential complications of laparoscopy.[21-24] The causes and treatments of these complications are outlined in **Table 102.2**.

KEY REFERENCES

Complete references for this chapter are online and available at https://connect.springerpub.com/content/book/978-0-8261-3875-0/part/part04/toc-part/ch0102.

2. Muñoz CJ, Nguyen HT, Houck CS. Robotic surgery and anesthesia for pediatric urologic procedures. *Curr Opin Anaesthesiol.* 2016;29(3):337–344. doi:10.1097/ACO.0000000000000333

4. Spinelli G, Vargas M, Aprea G, et al. Pediatric anesthesia for minimally invasive surgery in pediatric urology. *Transl Pediatr.* 2016;5(4):214–221. doi:10.21037/tp.2016.09.02

5. Neira VM, Kovesi T, Guerra L, et al. The impact of pneumoperitoneum and trendelenburg positioning on respiratory system mechanics during laparoscopic pelvic surgery in children: a prospective observational study. *Can J Anaesth.* 2015;62(7):798–806. doi:10.1007/s12630-015-0369-0

8. Chu DI, Tan JM, Mattei P, et al. Outcomes of laparoscopic and open surgery in children with and without congenital heart disease. *J Pediatr Surg.* 2018;53(10):1980–1988. doi:10.1016/j.jpedsurg.2017.10.052

14. Mishra P, Gupta B, Nath A. Anesthetic considerations and goals in robotic surgery: a narrative review. *J Anesth.* 2020;34(2):286–293. doi:10.1007/s00540-020-02738-2

CHAPTER 103

Posterior Sagittal Anorectoplasty

Kimberly Stumpf and Joseph Tobias

INDICATIONS/CONTRAINDICATIONS

Anorectal malformations, such as Hirschsprung's disease, mega colon, imperforate anus or atresia, and malalignment of the colon to the anus, or no anus at all, result from various disruptions in the normal embryological development of the fetus in utero. Some of these malformations require interventions immediately after birth, while others will be medically managed until the child is a few months old when surgery can be performed to correct the underlying condition. Several malformations require a two-step surgical procedure, with creation of a colostomy initially to allow the surgical correction of the underlying condition time to heal. Once the repair is healed, the colostomy is reversed, typically occurring a few weeks or months later. A commonly used surgical technique used to correct these malformations is posterior sagittal anorectoplasty or posterior sagittal anorectoplasty (PSARP). *Pullthrough* is another common term used.

A PSARP may bypass the need for a colostomy.[1] This procedure is performed by an experienced pediatric colorectal surgeon with the patient in prone, jack-knife position. Ideally, the procedure is performed in prone position only; however, there is always a chance that scar tissue from prior procedures may limit the surgeon's access to obtain enough healthy bowel from the rectal/prone approach, thereby requiring that the patient is turned supine followed by an abdominal incision to provide access to additional healthy bowel tissue.

SPECIAL CONSIDERATIONS

Some special considerations for these cases include intraoperative fluid management, postoperative pain management, temperature regulation, vascular access, and positioning. Each of these is discussed in this chapter.

ANESTHETIC MANAGEMENT

PREOPERATIVE EVALUATION

Patients presenting for PSARP often have complex medical histories and require a thorough preoperative evaluation. Patients with colorectal abnormalities may have associated congenital anomalies including *VACTERL* association,[2] which includes *v*ertebral defects, *a*nal atresia, *c*ardiac defects, *t*racheal-*e*sophageal fistula (TEF), *r*enal anomalies, and *l*imb abnormalities (Box 103.1). Many patients presenting for PSARP have sacral and vertebral anomalies which may include misshapen or fused vertebrae. It is imperative this is vetted preoperatively as it may limit the ability to place a single-injection caudal epidural injection or an epidural catheter for postoperative pain management. If an epidural catheter cannot be placed, other modes of types of regional anesthesia (transversus abdominis blocks, quadratus lumborum (QL) blocks) or pain management (patient-controlled analgesia [PCA] and nurse-controlled analgesia [NCA]) may be utilized.

Cardiac involvement may vary from life-threatening problems (ductal-dependent obstructive right- or left-side lesions)

BOX 103.1 VACTERL ASSOCIATION

V: vertebral defects

A: anal atresia

C: cardiac defects

TE: tracheal-esophageal fistula

R: renal anomalies

L: limb abnormalities

that may require correction at birth to minor defects such as atrial septal or ventricular septal defects that require follow-up or surgical intervention at a later time. Given the potential for associated congenital heart disease (CHD), patients should have a preoperative echocardiograph to identify CHD and help guide the anesthesia team's perioperative goals, including hemodynamic and fluid management. Whether there is associated CHD or not, especially in younger patients, perioperative fluid management may be complicated by the need for a preoperative bowel prep and its associated volume losses. In such cases, preoperative IV access and hydration may be indicated.

The kidneys and the collecting systems can be misshapen or solitary, which may lead to renal insufficiency or failure. Ultrasound evaluations may be obtained and routine monitoring of renal function (electrolytes, blood urea nitrogen, serum creatinine) indicated based on the patient's status. In patients with underlying renal dysfunction or anatomical malformations, medications known to have potential deleterious effects on renal function, such as ketorolac, may be avoided. At our institution, we do not routinely administer ketorolac if the patient has a solitary kidney.

Limb anomalies include poorly developed extremities and/or missing digits. This may lead to difficulty with IV catheter placement. As a full-body prep is generally performed, placing IV lines in the upper extremities may become challenging if there are poorly developed limbs.

Pertinent Labs

Baseline laboratory evaluations may include chemistry panels and a complete blood count (CBC). In general, these cases do not involve large blood losses; however, if the patient has had multiple previous procedures, scar formation and adhesions may require surgical dissection and blood loss. Based on these concerns, a preoperative type and screen may be required. This is often drawn after induction of anesthesia to avoid the need for an additional preoperative venipuncture and pain.

PREOPERATIVE PHARMACOLOGY

Anxiety is frequent in toddlers and older children in this patient population as it is not uncommon for colorectal patients to require repeat visits to the operating room (OR) for various procedures. Preoperative anxiolysis can be provided by oral midazolam (.5 mg/kg) if there is no IV access. Perioperative involvement of a child life specialist is also suggested and beneficial. The child life specialist can meet the patient during the initial workup prior to the day of surgery, allowing them to build rapport. On the day of surgery, the child life specialist can accompany the patient to the OR and allow the patient to play with a tablet, listen to music, or play with age-appropriate toys as a means of distraction. These techniques can be very beneficial in making the child's experience of coming to the OR a positive one, as these patients may require multiple trips to the OR for procedures such as exam under anesthesia (EUA) to check for strictures and possibly injection of botulinum toxin injection.

Intraoperative Management

These patients are often admitted the night before their procedure to have a nasogastric feeding tube placed and their bowel prep administered. The bowel prep may lead to nausea, vomiting, or issues of intolerance of the prep. Therefore, a rapid-sequence induction (RSI) may be indicated. Communication with the surgeon is suggested to discuss the use of neuromuscular blocking agents (NMBA) for induction and during the procedure. If the anal sphincter needs to be identified with a nerve stimulation, it may not be appropriate to use a long-acting NMBA. Alternatively, residual neuromuscular blockade can be reversed with sugammadex if available.

Patients with an associated TEF often require surgical intervention during the neonatal period. As a result, associated or residual airway anatomical changes due to scarring or stenosis may dictate the need to downsize the endotracheal tube (ETT). For term neonates, a 3.0-mm cuffed ETT may be used, but uncuffed tubes should be available as needed. Outside the neonatal period, standard formulas are used to judge ETT size (age divided by 4 plus 3.5 when using a cuff). Regardless of the size of the ETT, a leak should be present with the cuff down and the cuff inflated to 20 cmH_2O to seal the airway.

Given the duration of these procedures and the need for intraoperative fluid resuscitation, many of these procedures are optimally performed with two IV catheters. These are preferably placed in the upper extremities as a full-body prep including the legs and feet may be performed. If necessary, the saphenous vein or a foot can be used, and the IV and tubing prepped in with the operative site. Anesthesia providers should be aware that this IV catheter cannot be used until prepping into the sterile field is accomplished. When the patient is prone, they are placed on a hip roll and ankle rolls, which may lead to obstruction of the IV catheter if it is in the foot. The sterile field can also make troubleshooting a challenge.

In younger patients, IV access should be in place to allow preoperative fluid replacement (the 4–2–1 rule for maintenance fluid) while completing the prep. However, additional fluid resuscitation is frequently required intraoperatively to replace ongoing blood loss, third-space losses, and residual deficit. Options for fluid replacement include isotonic crystalloid fluids (Normosol®, lactated Ringer's, normal saline) or colloids such as 5% albumin. These fluids can be administered in boluses of 10 mL/kg and repeated based on heart rate and blood pressure responses, as well as ongoing assessment of intraoperative losses. Although there are limited data available to demonstrate differences in postoperative outcomes, our practice includes administration of colloids in preference to crystalloids to limit tissue edema.

Temperature management should start prior to the patient's arrival at the OR. The OR should be warmed, and an underbody Bair Hugger should be placed on the OR table, with plastic drapes set aside or a blanket on top of the bed. The Bair Hugger should be turned on high temperature, which will help to pre warm the table before the patient's arrival. Once the patient is on the OR table, the Bair Hugger should be decreased to medium so as not to cause burns, especially to smaller patients, and the patient should be kept covered for as long as possible to maintain their core body temperature. Once the OR staff starts the full-body prep, the patient's temperature will drop. Once the patient is fully prepped and the surgical drapes are up, it is helpful to attach the clear plastic Bair Hugger drapes to the surgical drapes above the head (**Figure 103.1**). This will form a tent to keep the patient warm, yet not stick to the patient if they are turned from supine to prone and back throughout the case. Other techniques to help with the patient's temperature include using a heat and moisture exchangers (HME) in the anesthesia circuit, along with low-flow fresh gas flows. As the patient's temperature is stable after the start of the case, the room temperature can be adjusted.

An opioid-sparing technique is often utilized for longer procedures ranging from 4 to 8 hours or longer. This allows the anesthesia provider to limit opioid administration throughout the procedure. While evidence-based medicine is somewhat limited in the pediatric population, adult

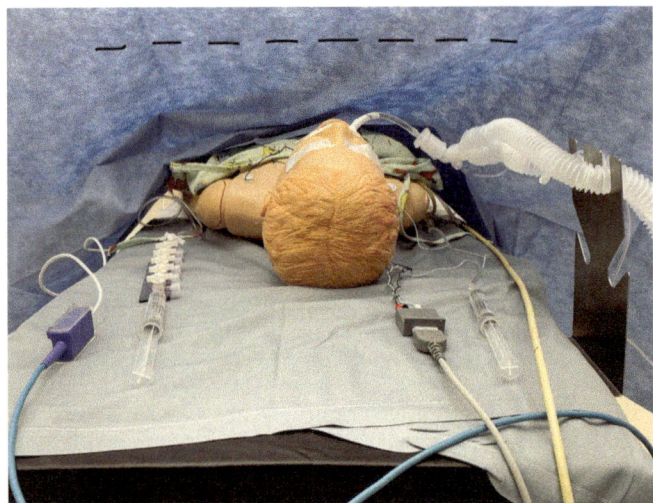

Figure 103.1: Head of the bed setup. Supine patient positioning, keeping the lines/tubes/drains in an organized manner. The black dotted line indicates placement for Bair Hugger drapes, allowing for positioning the patient supine/prone throughout the case without the drapes sticking to the patient.

Source: Courtesy of Kimberly Stumpf, MSN, CRNA.

studies have demonstrated a decrease in opioid-related adverse effects, including nausea, vomiting, and ileus.[3] An opioid-sparing technique may help in a more rapid return of bowel function. These techniques have also become more popular recently given the significant increase in substance and opioid abuse.

The modified enhanced recovery after surgery (ERAS) protocol that is used for our patients includes the following:

- **ketamine:** Bolus of 0.5 mg/kg (maximum 50 mg) with an infusion of 0.25 to 0.5 mg/kg/hr, discontinuing 1 hour before the end of the case
- **dexmedetomidine:** bolus of 0.5 mcg/kg with an infusion of 0.5 mcg/kg/hr, decreasing to 0.3 mcg/kg/hr toward the end of the case, discontinuing close to the end of the procedure
- **lidocaine for patients more than 2 years of age who are not receiving regional anesthesia:** bolus of 1 mg/kg with an infusion of 1 to 1.5 mg/kg/hr (maximum 120 mg/hr), discontinuing 1 hour before the end of the case
- **fentanyl:** 1 to 4 mcg/kg as needed. Often administered at the beginning of the case while additional IV access is obtained, and boluses of the infusion medications can be established
- **hydromorphone:** may be given if needed at the end of the case until the NCA/PCA can be set up and started. These procedures can be painful depending on the amount of work done by the surgeon, especially if an abdominal incision is needed
- **volatile agent (sevoflurane or isoflurane):** usually at 0.5 to 1 minimum alveolar concentration (MAC) based on the patient's age. If the abdomen is opened, an epidural catheter can be placed after the procedure (possibly beforehand if opening is anticipated) with the infusion started during the case or postoperatively and
- **IV fluids (isotonic):** administration includes hourly maintenance as well as replacement for third-space losses and blood loss

If an epidural is planned at the end of the case, a lidocaine infusion is not used intraoperatively. If the epidural is placed at the end of the case, IV opioids may be required to provide analgesia until the epidural sets up. If the epidural is placed before the procedure starts, use extra caution when flipping the patient under the drapes and start the infusion as soon as possible to allow for the best setup and patient comfort level during and after the procedure.

Special Techniques and/or Equipment

At Nationwide Children's Hospital (Columbus, Ohio), an ERAS protocol has been developed and instituted for bariatric patients by Amanda Craver, CRNA, Brian Hall, CRNA, Sarah Rutletdge, CRNA, Vidya Raman, MD, and Marc Michalsky, MD. This protocol has been modified and adapted for extensive colorectal procedures. Oral acetaminophen is administered preoperatively (10 mg/kg to a maximum of 1 g) to initiate pain management prior to any painful surgical stimulus. If oral administration is not feasible, IV acetaminophen is administered. Perioperative gabapentin is also part of the perioperative opioid-sparing technique, with oral administration prior to anesthetic induction. Although somewhat conflicting, adult and pediatric studies have suggested its role in postoperative pain management aids in decreasing the amount of postoperative narcotic required for pain management.[4] Gabapentin has been noted to have analgesic properties and may be effective in treating acute, chronic, and neuropathic pain. The dose used at our facility is 10 mg/kg (maximum dose of 600 mg) by mouth, using the liquid formulation given via the nasogastric tube that was used for the bowel prep. Potential concerns with use of gabapentin include perioperative sedation and hemodynamic effects, including intraoperative hypotension.

Clinical Pearls

The colorectal service is often assisted by urology and OB/GYN (for female patients). Urology may place the patient in a lithotomy position to perform cystoscopy and place ureteral stents, which affords the colorectal surgeon a landmark when working in the abdomen. While the hope is to avoid damaging the ureters, should trauma occur intraoperatively, it can be recognized and addressed during the procedure. The stents are typically removed at the end of the procedure.

OB/GYN may be involved if a patient is known to have a cloacal malformation or any other reproductive concerns. The patient is then taken out of lithotomy and a full-body prep is performed, including placing 1,000 drapes around the upper chest and wrapping the legs per colorectal protocol. The patient is then flipped prone. A Foley catheter will be placed in the sterile field. The scrub nurse will often empty the syringe that is attached to the Foley and notify the anesthesia provider of the patient's urine output. This may be difficult to measure initially as urology performs a cystoscopy to place the ureter stents. This is done using fluid to inflate the bladder. The anesthesia provider should take this into consideration with the first measurements.

Complications/Emergencies

Repositioning from supine to prone under the drapes can be very challenging for all parties involved. The most crucial part of the repositioning process is the communication between the head of the bed (anesthesia and nurses) and the surgical team (surgeons and scrub). During this time, the anesthesia provider cannot see the lower half of the patient. A count-out is called and the patient is flipped. Organization is key at this time as flipping carries the risk of inadvertent tracheal extubation (Box 103.2, Figure 103.2). Clear, closed-loop communication is essential.

BOX 103.2 COMPLICATIONS AND EMERGENCIES IN POSTERIOR SAGITTAL ANORECTOPLASTY

Some pointers for flipping the patient to prone position include the following:

- Clearly label each IV line, including the size, location, and if it is the infusion or the push line. Tape the ETT to the right side of the patient's face. When positioning prone, keep the head turned to the patient's right side as this will keep the ETT to the top when the patient is prone and easily accessible. Disconnect ECG lines, temperature probe, and blood pressure cuff cable, and if it makes you more comfortable pause your infusions and disconnect and properly cap off your IV lines as well. Beware if you have an epidural in place. It is ideal to have it secured over the patient's right shoulder. The last thing to disconnect is the ETT but leave the pulse oximeter connected for monitoring. Keep the patient on 100% oxygen before the flip. Have assistance, room nurses or other anesthesia personnel on each side of the upper part of the bed.

- We have found it useful to always turn the patient's right side up and over. When turning back supine, again flip with the patient's right side up and over. This keeps the ETT from going under the patient and hitting the bed, risking dislodgment.

- Vocalize what you are doing at the head of the bed. Remember, the surgeon cannot see you. Confirm your upper body assistants and lower body personnel are ready. Count out loud and clearly, "flipping the patient's right side up and over. I'm disconnecting my ETT. Flip on 3. 1, 2, 3—flip."

- The assistants will help in positioning the arms up right into a superman position and placing the chest roll simultaneously to the flip (**Figure 103.2**). A Z-Flo fluidized positioner is placed under the head with the head, turned to the patient's right. Vocalize after the flip, "Connecting the ETT and verifying placement." It is important to remember to check for bilateral breath sounds with patient positioning. Once confirmed, let the surgeon know that all is stable up top and they can continue with the procedure. It is this closed-loop communication that will ultimately keep the patient safe. If any issues arise, such as accidental extubation, it will be addressed immediately. your ETT placement is verified, reconnect all your IV infusions, tubes, and monitors.

- Once everything is stable at the head of the bed, perform a walk around to make sure that the patient's extremities are padded appropriately on the surgical side of the drapes. This includes a hip roll and an ankle roll. Confirm pressure is not being placed from the Foley catheter or the syringe. For male patients, confirm that their genitals are free from the hip roll. If a foot IV is in place, confirm that it continues to work or have the surgical team reposition the extremity.

ETT, endotracheal tube.

POSTOPERATIVE CARE

Following emergence and tracheal extubation, the patient is transported to the postanesthesia care unit (PACU), where care is transferred after a situation, background, assessment, recommendation hand off. The anesthesia pain team will set up the initial orders the use of a PCA/NCA or the epidural infusion to be started in PACU. This team continues to round on the patient and manage the PCA/NCA or the epidural infusion until pain control is transitioned to oral medications.

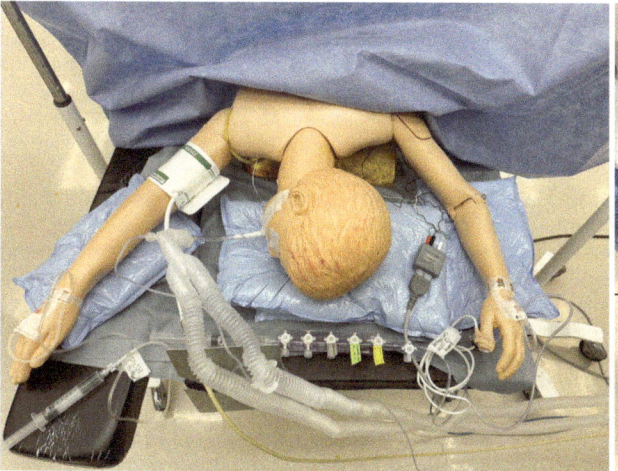
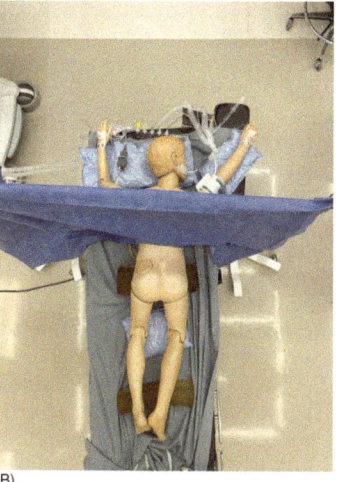

(A)   (B)

Figure 103.2: Prone positioning. Prone positioning of the patient, keeping the lines organized. The endotracheal tube (ETT) and epidural are taped to patient's right side. The patient's right side always flips up and over, limiting the risk of dislodgment of ETT. Arms are in a superman position and padded, and the neck neutral with the head turned right, watching for downward pressure on the ears and eyes.

Source: Courtesy of Kimberly Stumpf, MSN, CRNA.

CASE STUDY: A 5-Year-Old Presenting for Revision Posterior Sagittal Anorectoplasty

CLINICAL SCENARIO

A 5-year-old male presents to the Center for Colorectal and Pelvic Reconstruction (CCPR) at Nationwide Children's Hospital with a history of Hirschsprung's disease complicated by persistent colo cutaneous fistulas. The patient reported to the hospital the day before his redo-PSARP for placement of a soft nasogastric (NG) tube and bowel prep. The patient's history included a colostomy creation and pull-through in June to August 2018. In November and December 2018, the patient had an exploratory laparotomy with lysis of adhesions and drainage of an intra-abdominal abscess. He now presents for a second opinion after having multiple complications after prior procedures. The patient weighed 21.6 kg, with no known drug allergies. Aside from the colorectal complications, the patient was otherwise healthy without any other comorbidities or VACTERL history. He is toilet-trained for urine but would have stool accidents four to five times per week, especially if the bowel movements were loose; however, he could go up to 3 days without bowel movements at all. His cystogram before his redo-PSARP showed a large bladder for his age. His chemistry panel was normal, while his complete blood count showed a hemoglobin of 11.0 g/dL (normal reference range: 11.5–13.5 g/dL).

SPECIAL CONSIDERATIONS

The patient had an MRI before the procedure, which showed a lot of inflammation and multiple areas containing persistent colo cutaneous fistulas. Because of this, the general surgery team was included in the planning of the procedure. On the day of surgery, the patient was held nil per os for 8 hours. IV hydration was provided during the bowel prep. Preoperatively, gabapentin (100 mg) was administered via the NG tube as part of the opioid-sparing technique.

APPROACHES TO CARE

The preoperative plan after consultation with the surgical team was an epidural catheter for postoperative pain control. The patient was brought to the operating room (OR) with a member of the child life team present. An anesthesia time-out was performed to verify the patient's identity, weight, allergies, surgical procedure, and anesthesia plan. He was positioned supine on the OR table and was pre oxygenated. Anesthesia was induced with propofol (100 mg), fentanyl (1 mcg/kg), and lidocaine (1 mg/kg). Rocuronium (1 mg/kg) was administered to facilitate tracheal intubation after discussion with the surgeon regarding use of a neuromuscular blocking agent. The patient was atraumatically intubated with a Miller 2 blade, grade 1 view, using a 5.0-mm ETT with a leak sealed to 20 cmH$_2$0. Once the airway was secured, a second IV was placed and blood sent for a type and cross. After anesthetic induction, an epidural catheter was placed at the beginning of the case and the infusion started. The patient was turned to a left lateral position for epidural placement. The epidural catheter was placed at the T8–T9 vertebral level. After a negative test dose of 1.5% lidocaine with 1:200,000 epinephrine, the infusion was started. The epidural infusion was properly labeled and secured over the patient's right shoulder to help keep the lines organized when turning the patient prone/supine throughout the case. The patient was then returned to supine position and placed in lithotomy position. A cystoscopy and the placement of ureteral stents were performed by the urology service as landmarks for the general and colorectal surgeons.

A bolus dose of ketamine (.5 mg/kg) was followed by an infusion at .5 mg/kg/hr. A bolus dose of dexmedetomidine (.5 mcg/kg) was followed by an infusion at .5 mcg/kg/hr. A lidocaine infusion was not used as the epidural catheter contained .2% ropivacaine with clonidine, which was started at 4 mL/hr. During the case, the ketamine infusion was decreased to .25 mg/kg/hr. With approximately 1 hour left in the procedure, the ketamine was discontinued, and the dexmedetomidine was decreased to .3 mcg/kg/hr.

The patient was taken out of lithotomy where the full-body prep was performed by the surgical scrub and OR nursing staff. Once the patient was fully prepped, the legs wrapped per the protocol, and the OR drapes secured to the anesthesia poles, the surgeon came in to assist in flipping the patient to the prone position. Anesthesia prepared the patient by administering 100% oxygen, disconnecting the ECG monitors and blood pressure cable, and taking the NG off suction. With closed-loop communication, anesthesia confirmed with all staff members that the patient would be turned right side up. It was called out, "disconnecting ETT, turn on 3; 1, 2, 3—turn. Reconnecting the ETT, ventilating the patient (bilateral breath sounds verified by auscultation). You may proceed with the procedure".

The patient was placed back on the ventilator, the monitors were reattached, and the lines padded and secured. During the flip, while the patient was elevated, the OR nursing staff who were assisting at the head of the bed placed a chest roll. It was confirmed that neck alignment was neutral, with the head turned to the patient's right. The ears and eyes were examined for any pressure points and were appropriately padded. The anesthesia provider then did a walk around the bed to confirm positioning in the field was appropriate. This was the process each time the patient was turned during the procedure.

(continued)

CASE STUDY: A 5-Year-Old Presenting for Revision Posterior Sagittal Anorectoplasty (*continued*)

Dexamethasone and ondansetron were administered for prophylaxis against postoperative nausea and vomiting. Rocuronium was redosed based on the train-of-four during the procedure. Albumin 5% was administered at two separate times for volume resuscitation to replace blood loss and third-space losses (250 mL each time), 3 hours apart. Normosol-R was placed on a pump with the infusions as a carrier fluid. A total of 237 mL administered during the procedure. Lactated Ringer's was used as a bolus/push line, with a total of 550 mL administered.

Due to the extensive nature of the procedure, an SPY technique was used which allows the surgeon to see the blood flow of the bowel using indocyanine green. Anesthesia diluted the indocyanine green per pharmacy protocol and administered 1.1 mg with a rapid flush, which allowed the surgeon to confirm the healthy bowel that was being used for the procedure. This caused a brief false drop in the patient's pulse oximeter, which was expected. Per the surgeon's request, a 14-French NG was placed for postoperative bowel decompression.

At the end of the case, the patient was turned supine. He was breathing spontaneously with airway reflexes intact after reversing residual neuromuscular blockade with sugammadex (2 mg/kg with 4/4 twitches) and documentation of return of normal neuromuscular function with the train-of-four. The patient's trachea was extubated when he was following commands of eye-opening and moving arms toward his head. He was responsive and talking appropriately, denying pain. The patient was transported to the postanesthesia care unit and then admitted to the inpatient ward with his epidural infusion intact. The epidural infusion was discontinued on postoperative day 3 after he was tolerating oral medications. He was discharged home on postoperative day 5.

Evidence-Based Approaches to Care

An opioid-sparing anesthesia technique, as discussed earlier, was used during this procedure in addition to a thoracic epidural infusion. Due to the nature of excessive fistulas, an ileostomy was created by the surgical team to allow the bowel to heal after being repaired. This was then reversed 5 weeks later in a brief operative procedure with the use of a quadratus lumborum block to provide postoperative analgesia.

COMPLICATIONS

While there are risks involved with this procedure, including blood loss, ETT dislodgment, IV infiltrations, and surgical complications, among others, there were no complications that arose during this procedure. Blood products were not administered, IVs were monitored closely, vitals remained stable, the epidural catheter was infused without issues, and further intervention was not needed as the block set up well. At the end of the procedure, the patient awoke without issues and remained comfortable with the postoperative epidural infusion.

REFERENCES

1. Davis P, Cladis F, Motoyama E. *Smith's Anesthesia for Infants and Children*. Elsevier. 2011.
2. VACTERL Association: MedlinePlus Genetics. *MedlinePlus, U.S. National Library of Medicine*. 2020. medlineplus.gov/genetics/condition/vacterl-association
3. Zhu A, Benzon H, Anderson T. Evidence for the efficacy of systemic opioid-sparing analgesics in pediatric surgical populations. *Anesth Analg*. 2017;125(5):1569–1587. doi:10.1213/ANE.0000000000002434
4. Buck M. Gabapentin Use in Postoperative and Neuropathic Pain in Children. *Pediatric Pharmacotherapy University of Virginia Children's Hospital*. 2016. https://med.virginia.edu/pediatrics/wp-content/uploads/sites/237/2015/12/Feb16_Gabapentin_Ped-Pharmaco.pdf

CHAPTER 104

Pilonidal Cyst

Nathan S. Jones

INDICATIONS/CONTRAINDICATIONS

Pilonidal sinus disease is a chronic inflammatory skin condition typically occurring in the natal cleft of the buttocks. The exact etiology of the disease is not completely understood, although the presence of hair in the natal cleft is thought to play a key role. Accordingly, the term *pilonidal* is derived from the words *pilus* and *nidus*, meaning "hair" and "nest," respectively. Pilonidal sinus disease mostly affects adolescents and young adults, with risk factors, including obesity, hirsutism, deep natal cleft, sedentary occupation, poor hygiene, and familial predisposition.[1-4] Patients with an acute abscess will present to the surgical setting for incision and drainage under anesthesia.[5] Unfortunately, pilonidal sinus disease can be recurrent, with patients requiring multiple anesthetics. There are no absolute anesthetic contraindications to pilonidal surgery; however, patient comorbidities should be considered and optimized when possible.

SPECIAL CONSIDERATIONS AND CONCERNS

Patients with an acute pilonidal abscess can present to the surgical setting with severe pain that may be exacerbated in the sitting position. Every effort should be made to allow the patient to assume a position of comfort to minimize exacerbations of pain. Given the potentially embarrassing location of the wounds, privacy and professionalism are paramount in the perioperative setting. Patients with recurrent pilonidal sinus disease who have previously required surgery may be understandably anxious. An investigation of the patient's fears and expectations is warranted.

ANESTHETIC MANAGEMENT

PREOPERATIVE EVALUATION

As obesity is a known risk factor for pilonidal sinus disease, anesthesia providers should be sure to vet the presence of known comorbidities, such as obstructive sleep apnea (OSA), restrictive lung disease, diabetes mellitus, and hypertension. Exploring the presence of these disease processes when performing a preanesthetic history and physical examination is key to ensuring delivery of safe and effective anesthetic care.[6] In a patient with OSA, inquiry into patient use of a continuous positive airway pressure (CPAP) or bilevel positive airway pressure (BiPAP) device, as well as device settings, can inform expectations for postoperative ventilation requirements.

PREOPERATIVE PHARMACOLOGY

A patient presenting for urgent irrigation and drainage of a pilonidal abscess may have rapid onset of severe pain.[2] Preoperative analgesia might be prudent to facilitate the patient's comfort, cooperation, and transition from a stretcher to the operating table. Pharmacological anxiolysis may also be indicated with an anxious patient.

ANESTHETIC TECHNIQUE

Intraoperative Management

There is no single anesthetic technique for pilonidal sinus or abscess surgery. General anesthesia is commonly used, but monitored anesthesia care, local anesthesia with sedation, epidural anesthesia, and spinal anesthesia have also been reported in the management of pilonidal sinus disease.[7-12] There are risks associated with each technique. If general anesthesia is desired, recall that overweight patients placed supine for induction will have a decrease in functional residual capacity (FRC), increased work of breathing, a restrictive lung pattern, and a predisposition to hypoxemia.[6] Additionally, transferring overweight patients from supine to prone position can be a challenge and may require the assistance of additional staff members. Studies have reported success with allowing the patient to position themselves in the prone position prior to induction of anesthesia. Once anesthetized, a laryngeal mask airway (LMA) can be inserted with the patient in the prone position with the head turned to the side. This technique reduces the personnel required for patient positioning and shortens the time from incision to induction.[13-16] If this technique is utilized, a stretcher should always be immediately available should the patient need to be emergently placed in the supine position.

Should local infiltration be the primary plan, anesthesia providers should be cognizant that the level of anesthesia provided might not be sufficient to provide a painless operation, and repeated doses of local anesthesia may increase the risk of toxicity. When considering local anesthesia with sedation or neuraxial anesthesia with sedation, ensure the patient is able to cooperate with positioning, both preoperatively and intraoperatively (Box 104.1).

Complications

Anesthesia complications during pilonidal sinus surgery may result from the prone position. To reduce the risk of complications related to the prone position, it is recommended to ensure adequate supportive padding, avoid stretching the brachial plexus nerves by keeping the humerus anterior to the thoracic cage, and avoid direct pressure on the orbits. Additionally, anesthesia providers should ensure rescue airway devices are readily available.[17] In the event of a dislodged endotracheal tube in the prone position, using an LMA has been described as a rescue device as it can be inserted while the patient remains prone.[15,16]

BOX 104.1 CLINICAL PEARLS: PILONIDAL CYST

- Perform a thorough preoperative history and examination to identify comorbidities such as obstructive sleep apnea.
- In the preoperative area, provide anxiolytic and analgesic medications, as necessary.
- If a prolonged need for positive pressure ventilation is anticipated, supine induction with endotracheal intubation is prudent.

POSTOPERATIVE CARE

Recovery in the supine position might be uncomfortable due to the location of the surgical site. Therefore, it is imperative that anesthesia providers ensure the patient has received adequate analgesia. Multimodal analgesia is advantageous.[18] The patient can be repositioned to their side or a "bump" can be added using blankets or a pillow under one hip in order to relieve pressure off the sacrococcygeal area.

CASE STUDY: An Overweight Adolescent Male With Pilonidal Abscess

CLINICAL SCENARIO

A 16-year-old male, weighing 115 kg, 70 inches tall (body mass index 35), presents to the preoperative area for incision and drainage of an acute pilonidal abscess. The patient is in the lateral position on the stretcher and states that he is unable to lie supine due to severe pain. When asked about his medical history, he reports having obstructive sleep apnea and has been prescribed continuous positive airway pressure, which he does not wear because he does not like the way it feels. He denies other medical history. He tells you that he had this same pilonidal cyst surgery about 1 year ago and woke up with severe pain in the recovery room.

SPECIAL CONSIDERATIONS

Given the patient's severe pain and large body habitus, a supine induction with transfer to prone position might be burdensome. While maintaining his privacy and keeping him covered below the waist with a loose sheet, it is reasonable to ask him to position himself prone on the operating room table. It is important to test his surgical position prior to induction and correct any discomfort he feels related to paresthesia, numbness, restricted movement, or pressure on bony prominences.[19]

APPROACHES TO CARE

Evidence-Based Approaches to Care

After application of standard monitors, the patient is asked to turn his head to the side facing the anesthesia machine for pre oxygenation. Following IV induction, an appropriately sized laryngeal mask airway (LMA) is placed easily on the first attempt.[14] Due to the patient's history of pain in the recovery room following his previous surgery, multimodal analgesia is indicated as it utilizes multiple, simultaneous mechanisms of pain control while minimizing the side effect profile on any one drug. Acetaminophen, a nonsteroidal anti-inflammatory drug, a local anesthetic, and opiates are all components of the patient's multimodal analgesic plan.[18]

COMPLICATIONS

Laryngospasm, bronchospasm, airway dislodgment, and vomiting have all been described with the use of LMA in the prone position. These complications, however, do not always require management in the supine position. Medications can be administered via the IV (propofol, succinylcholine) or inhalation (albuterol) routes while the patient remains supine. If an LMA or endotracheal tube becomes dislodged while the patient is in the prone position, the LMA has been described as a rescue device and may be inserted while the patient remains prone.[15,16] If the patient regurgitates, turning the patient supine and proceeding with endotracheal intubation might be necessary.[14]

KEY REFERENCES

Complete references for this chapter are online and available at https://connect.springerpub.com/content/book/978-0-8261-3875-0/part/part04/toc-part/ch0104.

1. Young T. Understanding pilonidal disease. *Wounds UK.* 2019;15(3):48–53.
2. Kallis MP, Maloney C, Lipskar AM. Management of pilonidal disease. *Curr Opin Pediatr.* 2018;30(3):411–416. doi:10.1097/MOP.0000000000000628
6. Samuels PJ, Sjoblom MD. Anesthetic considerations for pediatric obesity and adolescent bariatric surgery. *Curr Opin Anaesthesiol.* 2016;29(3):327–336. doi:10.1097/ACO.0000000000000330
14. Gable A, Whitaker EE, Tobias JD. Use of the laryngeal mask airway in the prone position. *Ped Anesth Crit Care J.* 2015;3(2):118–123. doi:10.14587/paccj.2015.24
17. Kwee MM, Ho Y-H, Rozen WM. The prone position during surgery and its complications: a systematic review and evidence-based guidelines. *Int Surg.* 2015;100(2):292–303. doi:10.9738/INTSURG-D-13-00256.1
18. Beverly A, Kaye AD, Ljungqvist O, Urman RD. Essential elements of multimodal analgesia in enhanced recovery after surgery (ERAS) guidelines. *Anesthesiol Clin.* 2017;35(2):115–143. doi:10.1016/j.anclin.2017.01.018

CHAPTER 105

Cholecystectomy

Mary J. Scott-Herring and Aileen Mendez

INDICATIONS/CONTRAINDICATIONS

Cholecystectomy is the surgical removal of the gallbladder and is considered the standard of care for cholecystitis. Cholecystectomy is generally the preferred approach over medical treatment.[1] Cholecystitis, simply defined, is an inflammation of the gallbladder. Cholecystitis is not as common in children as it is in adults, with just 1.3 pediatric cases occurring in every 1,000 adult cases.[1] The rise of pediatric obesity, however, has led to an increased incidence of cholelithiasis (gallstones) among children and adolescents. In fact, current literature suggests that the risk of cholelithiasis is four times higher in obese children and is the cause of approximately 8% to 33% of cases of pediatric cholelithiasis.[2] Given this alarming trend, more cholecystectomies are now being performed in the pediatric patient population, accounting for approximately 4% of all cholecystectomies being performed.[1,3]

The incidence of cholecystitis in younger children is essentially equal among males and females, although the incidence among females increases with the onset of puberty. No preponderance of cholecystitis has been found in one racial demographic compared with another, although North American Pima Indians and Scandinavians may be at higher risk.[4]

In addition to obesity, there are several risk factors for pediatric gallbladder disease, including use of certain medications (cephalosporins or diuretics), coexisting conditions (sickle cell disease or various hemolytic conditions, Crohn's disease, renal failure, gallbladder cancer), abdominal surgery (ileal resection), trauma, sepsis, pregnancy, long periods of fasting, weight loss, low-calorie diets, congenital and biliary anomalies, and biliary pseudolithiasis.[4-7] Furthermore, newborns who are premature are at an increased risk of cholelithiasis if they receive prolonged total parenteral nutrition in the neonatal period or if they have coexisting congenital heart disease or gastrointestinal syndromes.[8] See Box 105.1 for the risk factors associated with pediatric gallbladder disease.

The presenting signs and symptoms of cholecystitis are not different between adults and children, although they may be more difficult to discern in children. Patients present with a constellation of symptoms such as right upper quadrant pain, pain radiating to their back, abdominal bloating, a loss of appetite, fever, nausea, vomiting, positive Murphy's sign, Boas's sign, biliary colic, and/or chronic abdominal pain.[4]

While not the only approach, a laparoscopic technique is considered the gold standard when performing a cholecystectomy.[8,9] Larger medical facilities in particular are 1.4 (1.3, 1.7) times more likely to employ a laparoscopic technique when compared with smaller facilities. In fact, a recent study reviewed 78,578 pediatric cholecystectomy cases and found that 88.1% were performed laparoscopically, with 11.9% performed via an open technique.[9]

There are only a few relative contraindications to performing a cholecystectomy, such as severe intestinal adhesions or severe cardiopulmonary compromise.[3] It should be noted that surgical removal of asymptomatic gallstones is not the current standard practice. The sole exception is for children with sickle cell anemia as laparoscopic cholecystectomy is currently recommended for this population even when the gallstones are not causing issues to prevent future complications.[4]

> **BOX 105.1 PEDIATRIC GALLBLADDER DISEASE RISK FACTORS**
>
> - Cephalosporins
> - Diuretics
> - Sickle cell disease
> - Hemolytic conditions
> - Abdominal surgery
> - Trauma
> - Ileal resection
> - Crohn's disease
> - Sepsis
> - Pregnancy
> - Renal failure
> - Fasting
> - Weight loss
> - Dieting
> - Congenital or biliary abnormalities
> - Biliary pseudolithiasis
> - Prematurity
> - Total parenteral nutrition
> - Coronary heart disease
> - Gastrointestinal syndromes

SPECIAL CONSIDERATIONS AND CONCERNS

Pediatric patients may present without the traditional findings, making a thorough history and physical essential. Of note, patients with sickle cell anemia are twice as likely as the general population to develop cholelithiasis, with approximately 20% to 40% of all cases of pediatric gallstones being attributed to hemolytic disease.[4] It is imperative this patient population remains properly hydrated and normothermic and receives adequate pain management to avoid crisis. Ideally, these patients should receive IV hydration at a rate 1.5 times the normal maintenance dose.[1]

ANESTHETIC MANAGEMENT

PREOPERATIVE EVALUATION

Patients should be appropriately NPO per the American Society of Anesthesiologists guidelines. Preoperatively, IV fluids should be administered to achieve euvolemia as determined by standard pediatric calculations. Children with

> **BOX 105.2 KEY ASSESSMENT POINTS: CHOLECYSTECTOMY**
>
> - Assess for loose dentition
> - Address anxiety concerns
> - Discuss pain management plan
> - Review preoperative labs
> - Administer antiemetics
> - Consider comorbidities

underlying disease processes should be carefully evaluated to determine the extent of their comorbid health status and any impact it may have on their anesthetic plan. This includes, but is not limited to, children with various hemolytic conditions such as sickle cell disease. In addition, patients with obstructive sleep apnea, congenital heart defects, preexisting pulmonary pathologies, and/or elevated intracranial pressures require a thorough evaluation before proceeding as the positioning during surgery may exacerbate physiological disturbances (Box 105.2).[10]

Pertinent Labs

Depending on the status and acuity of the patient, labs are not always indicated. If available, complete blood count, liver function test, and urinalysis should be reviewed for abnormal results.[4]

PREOPERATIVE PHARMACOLOGY

Pediatric patients presenting for cholecystectomy often report preoperative anxiety in addition to pain due to cholelithiasis. It may be appropriate to administer an anxiolytic in addition to an opioid such as fentanyl. As a high percentage of acute cholecystitis cases are complicated by bacterial colonization, anesthesia providers should maintain a low threshold for administering antibiotic therapy prior to incision.[1]

ANESTHETIC TECHNIQUE

Intraoperative Management

As with all patients, standard monitoring should include oxygen saturation, ventilation, circulation, and temperature monitoring. Patients with cholecystitis or cholelithiasis often present with complaints of nausea and vomiting and should be considered to have a full stomach. IV access should be obtained preoperatively to facilitate rapid sequence induction. Rapid sequence intubation induction agents such as propofol and either succinylcholine or rocuronium should be considered with active vomiting. Cuffed endotracheal tubes (ETT) are preferred due to the decreased compliance and increased peak inspiratory pressures needed to achieve adequate alveolar ventilation during insufflation.

A second large-bore peripheral IV should be placed following induction should there be a need for volume resuscitation during the procedure. After the patient is asleep, anesthesia providers may opt to decompress the stomach by placing an orogastric or nasogastric tube. If the patient did not void prior to surgery, a urinary catheter may be placed to empty the bladder, although this is being done less frequently on a routine basis to reduce the risk of genitourinary trauma and urinary tract infections.[11]

Routine antiemetics such as dexamethasone and ondansetron should be administered, and for pain management the anesthesia provider may consider IV acetaminophen 15 mg/kg, ketorolac, dexmedetomidine, and/or appropriately dosed weight-based opioids. Historically, morphine was avoided as it was thought to cause spasmodic effects on the sphincter of Oddi,[1] but this is not seen in practice. To limit opioid-induced sequelae, a multiple modal approach is suggested, incorporating dexmedetomidine, local anesthetics, acetaminophen, and nonsteroidal anti-inflammatory agents such as ketorolac.

If a laparoscopic approach is employed, carbon dioxide (CO_2) will be used to insufflate the abdomen. While surgeons attempt to keep the pneumoperitoneum pressure low to mitigate undesired sequelae, anesthesia providers should be aware that excessive insufflation pressures can result in cardiovascular and respiratory compromise, pneumomediastinum, or pneumothorax.[12] Suggested insufflation pressures range from 6 to 8 mm Hg in infants and from 10 to 12 mm Hg in children and should not exceed 15 mm Hg.[12] CO_2 is rapidly absorbed and the peak end-tidal carbon dioxide ($ETCO_2$) is greater in infants than in children. There is an inverse relationship between age and the rate of CO_2 absorption which is attributed to a thinner peritoneum and fat deposits in babies compared with older children; the longer the surgery, the higher the $ETCO_2$, requiring an increase in minute volume from 50% to 100% to maintain physiological pH (Table 105.1).[12]

Table 105.1 Anesthetic Management of a Laparoscopic Cholecystectomy		
Preoperative	**Intraoperative**	**Postoperative**
IV access	General anesthesia	Pain management
Premedicate	Cuffed endotracheal tube	Opioids
Anxiety: midazolam, dexmedetomidine	Second PIV	Acetaminophen
Pain: opioids	Antiemetics	Ibuprofen
ERAS considerations	Dexamethasone	Ketorolac
Scopolamine for age >12	Ondansetron	Early ambulation
	Pain management	Early diet advancement
	Opioids	
	Acetaminophen	
	Ketorolac	
	Euvolemia	
	Normothermia	
	Forced-air warmer	
	Fluid warmer	
	Local anesthetic to port sites	

ERAS, enhanced recovery after surgery; PIV, peripheral IV line.

Special Techniques and/or Equipment

There is scant literature evaluating pediatric enhanced recovery after surgery (ERAS) protocols, although some benefit has been suggested.[13] It has been offered that ERAS protocols result in a significantly increased rate of same-day discharge for pediatric patients following elective laparoscopic cholecystectomies without an associated increase in ED visits or readmissions.[14]

Although some regional anesthesia options are described in the literature for adult patients, pediatric cholecystectomies most commonly undergo general anesthesia with an ETT. For postoperative pain management, regional anesthesia may be considered; however, the results are mixed.[10] While injection of local anesthetic at the port sites has been reported to be as effective as paravertebral blocks, abdominal wall nerve blocks have demonstrated shorter hospital stay when compared with patients infiltrated with local anesthetic.[15] In matched-group studies comparing the impact of infiltration with paravertebral blocks, patients who received a paravertebral block required less intraoperative narcotics, although no significant difference in pain scores was observed during the first 8 hours postoperatively.[15,16] Ultimately, there is no consensus regarding the efficacy of regional anesthesia for analgesia following cholecystectomy in the pediatric population.

Clinical Pearls

When issues arise during surgery, consider the influence of patient positioning, as well as insufflation, that may impact the patient's physiological and hemodynamic status intraoperatively.[10] Positions such as a steep Trendelenburg can decrease pulmonary compliance and functional residual capacity and increase the likelihood of the ETT entering the right mainstem bronchus and triggering a bronchospasm. Increased intra-abdominal pressure in the Trendelenburg position, along with increased systemic vascular resistance (SVR) and increased partial pressure of carbon dioxide ($PaCO_2$), may also increase intracranial pressure to unsafe levels, predisposing patients with ventriculoperitoneal shunts to harm. Patients with ventriculoperitoneal shunts should have their device evaluated before surgery. Increased abdominal pressure may also decrease renal blood flow, impacting renal function and creatinine clearance. Hence, care should be taken to not fluid-overload the patient.[12] Reverse Trendelenburg positioning may also be used intraoperatively, which may also result in hypotension. See Chapter 102, "Laparoscopic Surgery," for further information regarding potential complications secondary to insufflation.

Complications/Emergencies

There is a risk of massive bleeding from Veress-type needle insertion or vessel injury, potentially requiring the surgeon to emergently open the patient's abdomen to obtain hemostasis. Also, excessive pneumoperitoneal pressures may cause cardiac and respiratory depression, hypothermia, pneumothorax, SC emphysema, and/or endobronchial intubation.[12]

Although not a common occurrence, the anesthesia provider should be aware of the possibility of gas embolism. Cardiovascular collapse due to intravascular CO_2 may occur when the insufflation pressure is greater than the venous pressure. This phenomenon can force those gas bubbles into the venous circulation. Physiologically, children with patent foramen ovale (PFO) are more susceptible to experiencing gas emboli. In practice, more adverse events occur as the intra-abdominal pressures increase. There are resultant decreases in pulmonary and thoracic compliance, vital capacity, functional residual capacity, and closing volumes, resulting in a ventilation-perfusion (V/Q) mismatch and hypoxemia.

POSTOPERATIVE CARE

Most patients undergoing cholecystectomy are safely extubated in the operating room and recover in the postanesthesia care unit afterward. Postoperative pain generally arises from the incision sites, retained gas in the abdomen, shoulder pain (referred from the diaphragm), or from positioning-related pain from the stretch placed on the patient's back and shoulder. Studies have supported the use of local anesthetics along incision sites and incorporating a multimodal technique including acetaminophen, nonsteroidal anti-inflammatory medications, and opioids.[12]

KEY REFERENCES

Complete references for this chapter are online and available at https://connect.springerpub.com/content/book/978-0-8261-3875-0/part/part04/toc-part/ch105.

7. Rothstein DH, Harmon CM. Gall bladder disease in children. *Semin Pediatr Surg.* 2016;25:225–231. doi:10.1053/j.sempedsurg.2016.05.005

9. Babb J, Davis J, Tashiro J, et al. Laparoscopic versus open cholecystectomy in pediatric patients: a propensity score-matched analysis. *J Laparoendosc Adv Surg Tech.* 2020;30(3). doi:10.1089/lap.2019.0655

12. Cote CJ, Lerman J, Anderson BJ, et al. *A Practice of Anesthesia for Infants and Children.* 6th ed. Elsevier; 2019

14. Yeh A, Butler G, Strotmeyer S, et al. ERAS protocol for pediatric laparoscopic cholecystectomy promotes safe and early discharge. *J Pediatr Surg.* 2020;55(1):96–100. doi:10.1016/j.jpedsurg.2019.09.053

18. Khurmi N, Gorlin A, Misra L. Perioperative considerations for patients with sickle cell disease: a narrative review. *Can J Anaesth.* 2017;64:860–869. doi:10.1007/s12630-017-0883-3

SECTION I: Gastrointestinal Procedures

CHAPTER 106

Endoscopy and Colonoscopy

Ashley J. Austin and Judith M. Lewis

INDICATIONS/CONTRAINDICATIONS

Endoscopic procedures in pediatric patients are key to the diagnosis and management of numerous gastrointestinal (GI), biliary, and liver conditions.[1] Upper endoscopies and colonoscopies are the most common endoscopic procedures performed in infants and children. Endoscopic procedures for pediatric patients are primarily diagnostic or therapeutic in nature, whereas adult colonoscopies are typically done for screening of colorectal malignancies.[1] The European Society of Gastrointestinal Endoscopy (ESGE) and European Society for Paediatric Gastroenterology Hepatology and Nutrition (ESPGHAN) Guideline Summary (2017) has outlined the indications and contraindications to pediatric esophagogastroduodenoscopy (EGD) and colonoscopy. Indications for EGD in infants and children can be classified by the functional purpose, being either diagnostic or therapeutic in nature. Common indications for a diagnostic EGD include weight loss, failure to thrive, dysphagia, odynophagia, abdominal pain with concern for organic disease, chronic gastroesophageal reflux disease (GERD), surveillance of Barrett's esophagus, ingestion of a caustic substance, recurrent vomiting of unknown origin, hematemesis, chronic diarrhea of unknown origin, hematochezia, and suspected graft-versus-host disease.[2] Therapeutic EGDs are frequently indicated for placement or replacement of a percutaneous endoscopic gastrostomy (PEG) tube, duodenal tube, or percutaneous jejunostomy tube, dilation of esophageal strictures, removal of foreign body, food impaction, hemostasis, perforation, achalasia, polypectomy, and esophageal varices.[2]

Contraindications to EGD include diagnosis of perforation and peritonitis in a toxic patient,[2,3] with relative contraindications being coagulopathy, partial or complete bowel obstruction, abdominal or iliac aortic aneurysm, recent digestive surgery, prematurity, recent food intake, and severe thrombocytopenia.[2] Anesthesia providers should be aware that connective tissue disorders, such as Ehlers–Danlos syndrome type IV and Marfan's syndrome, are also associated with an increased risk of perforation.[4]

In general, children have EGDs three times more often than colonoscopies. Indications and contraindications to colonoscopy in infants and children can also be classified as diagnostic or therapeutic. Indications for diagnostic colonoscopy include unexplained anemia, unexplained chronic diarrhea, rectal bleeding, unexplained failure to thrive, suspected graft-versus-host disease, complications following intestinal transplantation, investigation of radiological stricture, and polyposis syndromes.[2] Therapeutic colonoscopy is frequently performed for dilation of strictures, removal of foreign body, treatment of hemorrhagic lesions, polypectomy, and reduction of sigmoid volvulus.[2] Finally, the varied epidemiology of pediatric GI disease may necessitate the need for urgent or emergent endoscopy or colonoscopy.[5]

Contraindications to colonoscopy in infants and children include recent colonic perforation, recent intestinal resection, toxic megacolon, and cardiopulmonary instability.[2] Neutropenia and coagulopathy are considered relative contraindications. Ultimately, the benefits of information gained or therapeutic intervention of pediatric EGD or colonoscopy must outweigh the risks of proceeding.[4]

Pediatric endoscopies have historically been performed by pediatric gastroenterologists in specialized centers, as well as nonpediatric endoscopists in collaboration with pediatricians.[2] Lack of cooperation in the pediatric population necessitates these procedures to be done under parenteral sedation or general anesthesia.[4,6] A fundamental variation between adult and pediatric endoscopy practice is the routine tissue sampling done in children, even in the absence of gross abnormalities.[7] In the pediatric population, the risks of exposure to repeated anesthetics and endoscopies outweigh the risks of biopsy obtainment.[7] Furthermore, several studies have demonstrated difficulty of ruling out advanced disease based on endoscopic visualization of the upper GI tract of children, deeming biopsies during upper endoscopy necessary.[7]

SPECIAL CONSIDERATIONS AND CONCERNS

Special considerations and concerns for endoscopy and colonoscopy are noted in **Box 106.1**.

ANESTHETIC MANAGEMENT

PREOPERATIVE EVALUATION

A complete preanesthetic evaluation, including a review of a current history and physical (H&P), should be conducted.[8,9] The airway evaluation should also include assessment for the presence of loose teeth, piercings, and/or large tonsils. Loose teeth or piercings can inadvertently become dislodged by the endoscope and enter the airway. Enlarged tonsils may cause obstructive apnea and should be examined by the physician prior to induction of anesthesia.[9]

Adherence to proper fasting guidelines should be verified. Any risk factors that increase the likelihood of reflux or esophageal dysfunction should be considered. Stomach and bowel insufflation during the procedure can potentially increase the probability of reflux.[8] Risk factors that may increase the incidence of adverse outcomes during an EGD or colonoscopy include sepsis, dehydration, shock, electrolyte disturbances, and organ dysfunctions, such as respiratory conditions (acute and chronic), cardiac disease, neurological conditions, liver dysfunction, and/or renal dysfunction.[7]

Pertinent Labs

Routine laboratory tests are not indicated in healthy children scheduled for outpatient EGD and/or colonoscopy, but, may be indicated based on the patient's medical history and presence of comorbidities.[8] If an inhalation mask induction is planned, lab work can typically be drawn following induction of anesthesia, during IV catheter placement.[10]

> **BOX 106.1 SPECIAL CONSIDERATIONS AND CONCERNS FOR ENDOSCOPY AND COLONOSCOPY**
>
> - The airway is shared with the endoscopist during the EGD, increasing the risk of airway compromise.
> - Observe for any airway compromise throughout the procedure, but especially during insertion and removal of the endoscope (airway obstruction, partial or complete laryngospasms due to light plane of anesthesia or secretions, loss of airway control, hypoventilation, apnea, and dislodged teeth).
> - Airway equipment and emergency medications should be readily available.
> - Positioning: Both EGD and colonoscopy may be performed with the patient in the left lateral decubitus position with knees bent. The lateral position can facilitate drainage of secretions. Additionally, both procedures can be done in the supine frog-leg position, which optimizes airway management for the anesthetist.
> - Patients may be mildly hypovolemic due to fluid shifts following the bowel preparation.
> - The stomach should be deflated by the endoscopist prior to the end of the EGD in order to reduce bloating and discomfort during the postoperative period.
>
> EGD, esophagogastroduodenoscopy.

PREOPERATIVE PHARMACOLOGY

Patients scheduled for a colonoscopy will have received a bowel preparation prior to the day of the procedure. The method of bowel preparation is dependent on age. In infants who are solely bottle- or breastfed, small volume enemas and a clear liquid diet for 12 to 24 hours are typically adequate preparations. In older children and adolescents, a solution of polyethylene glycol and electrolytes (PEG-ELS) produces an osmotic diarrhea. A minimal risk of dehydration exists due to the limited transmural flux of water and sodium.[4]

ANESTHETIC TECHNIQUE

Intraoperative Management

Airway management during pediatric EGD can be achieved via placement of an endotracheal tube, placement of a laryngeal mask airway (LMA), or avoidance of airway instrumentation and placement of supplemental oxygen. The endoscope may cause upper airway obstruction by causing compression of the trachealis muscle. Therefore, tracheal intubation is recommended to maintain airway patency in specific circumstances, such as procedures with increased risk of bleeding (i.e., injection of varices), abnormal airway anatomy, severely obese children, and infants weighing less than 10 kg. If intubated, the anesthesia provider should also stabilize the endotracheal tube to prevent inadvertent endotracheal tube movement during scope insertion, advancement, and removal, and the child should be extubated fully awake.

An LMA can also be utilized for airway management during an EGD, with a variety of techniques commonly employed. One approach is to place the LMA, deflate the cuff, then have the endoscopist place the scope, being sure to reinflate the cuff of the LMA once in place. An alternative approach to LMA placement is to topicalize the larynx, place the endoscope, and then place the LMA (one size smaller than appropriate weight-based size) following insertion of the endoscope. Alternatively, in cases deemed appropriate, the airway can be managed without instrumentation using supplemental oxygen via a nasal cannula with end-tidal carbon dioxide ($ETCO_2$) monitoring or procedural oxygen mask (POM).

Inhalation induction and placement of IV are followed by maintenance with either sevoflurane, intermittent boluses of propofol (1–1.5 mg/kg IV boluses), or propofol infusions.[10] Propofol is an ideal primary anesthetic during EGDs and/or colonoscopies in children and adolescents.[11] Benefits include rapid and clear-headed recovery and reduced incidence of postoperative nausea and vomiting. Inherent risks associated with use of propofol include compromised airway control. Furthermore, propofol can have pharmacodynamic and pharmacokinetic variability, exaggerated when used in conjunction with additional medications such as short-acting opioids. Some patients can remain awake with seemingly appropriate weight-based dosing, while patients who are dosed with smaller dosing can become apneic, requiring ventilatory support. Additionally, reflexive coughing and subsequent laryngospasm can result from the airway instrumentation of an inadequately sedated patient. Titration to adequate sedation level is imperative.[11]

EGDs are brief procedures typically not requiring an infusion. Adjuncts of fentanyl (1 mcg/kg IV) or remifentanil have also been reported. While the addition of an opioid is not necessary if the patient is deeply anesthetized with sevoflurane or propofol, it may aid in blunting airway reflexes. When both an endoscopy and a colonoscopy are scheduled, alternative opioids such as alfentanil or remifentanil can serve as an adjunct to reduce the overall amount of propofol required for the duration of the case. All infusions should be titrated to maintain a balance of comfort and adequate respiration.[10]

Special Techniques and/or Equipment

The use of a nasal cannula with $ETCO_2$ monitoring or a POM can both be utilized with a spontaneously breathing patient during an endoscopy. The POM maximizes oxygen reserve, monitors $ETCO_2$ levels, limits the risk of hypoxia during sedation, and provides an insertion point for the scope. Ideally, procedural interruptions due to hypoxia are minimized when a POM is utilized. The POM is available in sizes appropriate for adolescent children but is not currently available in smaller sizes.

Pediatric gastroenterologists and anesthesia providers face unique pandemic-related challenges as endoscopic procedures are considered high risk for COVID-19 transmission. An unintended benefit of utilizing a POM is the simultaneous reduction of aerosolization and potentially infectious particles such as COVID-19.[12] In addition to aerosolization and fecal shedding of SARS-CoV-2, the virus causing COVID-19, children are more likely to be asymptomatic or have only mild disease, making it challenging to identify patients who may be infected with the virus without definitive testing. The use of a POM may help limit spread during endoscopy. While it may not prevent all airborne particle transmission, use of a POM provides a mechanical barrier to transmission of airborne pathogens from coughing during and after upper endoscopy and should be utilized by anesthesia providers when appropriate.

Clinical Pearls

The most stimulating portion of the EGD is the insertion of the endoscope into the esophagus. Anesthesia providers may be asked to provide a jaw thrust or flex the head forward to facilitate insertion of the endoscope. Additionally, the patient may be positioned in the left lateral position or supine to promote scope advancement. Each is associated with unique airway concerns. The lateral position can facilitate drainage of excess secretions out of the mouth as opposed to collection into the oropharynx, whereas the supine position ensures convenient access to the airway.

COMPLICATIONS/EMERGENCIES

Endoscopic procedures are deemed safe in children, with complication rates associated with both diagnostic EGD and colonoscopy in pediatric patients very low. Data published from the Pediatric Clinical Outcomes Research Initiative note the overall complication rate during EGDs to be 2.3%, which includes a specific risk of bleeding (.3%) and respiratory issues (1.5%). Interventional procedures are associated with greater risk than diagnostic procedures, with complications during colonoscopy reported to be 1.1%.[13]

A large retrospective review from a single children's hospital monitored perforation rates of 21,345 cases over an 11-year period. The esophageal perforation rate was .014% and the intestinal perforation rate was .028%.[4] Ehlers–Danlos syndrome type IV and Marfan's syndrome are associated with increased risk of perforation. Prompt diagnosis of a perforation is imperative as delayed diagnosis beyond 24 hours is associated with an increased mortality rate of 25% to 50%.[14]

A clinical report from the North American Society for Pediatric Gastroenterology, Hepatology & Nutrition (NASPGHAN) endoscopy committee identified factors that increase a patient's risk for adverse events include cardiopulmonary disease, compromised intestinal luminal wall integrity, coagulopathies, compromised immune systems, and craniofacial or anatomical airway abnormalities. Najafi et al.[6] identified young age to be a critical risk factor due to the increased vulnerability of the population as well as the significant comorbidities warranting endoscopic procedures.

POSTOPERATIVE CARE

If intubated, the patient should be extubated awake in the procedure room prior to transfer to the postanesthesia care unit. Following extubation or in patients with a POM or nasal cannula, the patient can be positioned in the supine position or placed in the lateral position with the head of the bed raised about 30 degrees during recovery until the patient fully awakens. Pain management depends on the procedure performed and the patient's comorbidities. While often not a painful procedure, a variety of analgesics may be employed, including acetaminophen 10 to 15 mg/kg PO, 15 mg/kg IV, or 35 to 40 mg/kg PR, morphine .05 to .1 mg/kg IV, fentanyl .5 to 1 mcg/kg, or potentially hydromorphone .01 to .015 mg/kg IV.

KEY REFERENCES

Complete references for this chapter are online and available at https://connect.springerpub.com/content/book/978-0-8261-3875-0/part/part04/toc-part/ch106.

1. Barakat MT, Triadafilopoulos G, Berquist WE. Pediatric endoscopy practice patterns in the United States, Canada, and Mexico. *J Pediatr Gastroenterol Nutr.* 2019;69(1):24–31. doi:10.1097/mpg.0000000000002310
2. Tringali A, Thomson M, Dumonceau J-M, et al. Pediatric gastrointestinal endoscopy: European Society of Gastrointestinal Endoscopy (ESGE) and European Society for Paediatric Gastroenterology Hepatology and Nutrition (ESPGHAN) Guideline Executive summary. *Endoscopy.* 2017;49(01):83–91. doi:10.1055/s-0042-111002
3. Kay M, Barry J, Wyllie R. Colonoscopy, polypectomy and related techniques. In: *Pediatric Gastrointestinal and Liver Disease.* 6th ed. Elsevier Health Science; 2020:639–659.
4. Kay M, Bhesania N, Wyllie R. Esophagogastroduodenoscopy and related techniques. In: *Pediatric Gastrointestinal and Liver Disease.* 6th ed. Elsevier Health Science; 2020:613–638.
7. Lightdale JR, Acosta R, Shergill AK, et al. Modifications in endoscopic practice for pediatric patients. *Gastrointest Endosc.* 2014;79(5):699–710. doi:10.1016/j.gie.2013.08.014
8. Jaffe RA, Schmiesing CA, Golianu B, et al. 13.2 Out of operating room procedures—pediatric; upper and lower GI endoscopy. In: *Anesthesiologist's Manual of Surgical Procedures.* Wolters Kluwer; 2020:1725–1727.
10. Lerman J, Coté CJ, Steward DJ. Anesthesia outside the operating room. In: *Manual of Pediatric Anesthesia: With An Index of Pediatric Syndromes.* Springer; 2016:519–521.
13. Lightdale JR, Fishman DS, Thomson M, et al. Pediatric endoscopy and high-risk patients: a clinical report from the NASPGHAN endoscopy committee. *J Pediatr Gastroenterol Nutr.* 2019;68(4):595–606. doi:10.1097/MPG.0000000000002277

CHAPTER 107

Manometry Placement, Esophageal Dilatation, and Botulinum Toxin Injection

Jennifer B. Mills and Jeanie Skibiski

INDICATIONS/CONTRAINDICATIONS

ESOPHAGEAL MANOMETRY

The rate of esophageal motility disorders among pediatric patients continues to rise, especially in premature and low-birth-weight infants.[1] Esophageal motility disorders involve dysfunction of the esophagus and result in complaints of dysphagia, heartburn, and/or chest pain.[2] Esophageal motility disorders can be primary in nature (e.g., achalasia, diffuse esophageal spasm, and eosinophilic esophagitis) or secondary to a systemic disorder that is causing esophageal dysmotility (e.g., systemic sclerosis and Chagas disease). If a motility disorder is suspected, high-resolution esophageal manometry (HREM) should be performed to measure intraluminal pressure activity in the gastrointestinal tract.

Achalasia is a rare neurogenic esophageal motility disorder characterized by esophageal peristalsis and a lack of lower esophageal sphincter (LES) relaxation during swallowing.[3] The symptoms of achalasia include slowly progressive dysphagia (difficulty swallowing) and regurgitation of undigested food. Diffuse esophageal spasm is characterized by nonpropulsive and hyperdynamic contractions. Symptoms often include chest pain and dysphagia, although esophageal spasm can also cause severe pain without dysphagia. Eosinophilic esophagitis is a chronic immune-mediated disease of the esophagus that can cause reflux-like symptoms, dysphagia, and food impaction.

HREM can be performed to evaluate patients presenting with complaints of dysphagia, heartburn, regurgitation, choking with feedings, or chest pain. It may also be indicated in patients who have undergone a Nissen fundoplication to evaluate for obstruction. HREM is an adaptation of conventional manometric hardware that basically employs an increased number of pressure sensors spaced closely together. The standard manometry utilizes four to eight pressure sensors spaced at 3- to 5-cm intervals, whereas HREM employs 24 or 36 sensors spaced in 1-cm increments.[2] The data generated by HREM can then be used to better interpret manometric data (Figure 107.1).

Together with esophageal pressure topography (EPT), which creates averages between each sensor, HREM has standardized the assessment of esophageal motility. The Chicago classification system uses a hierarchical classification scheme and provides a standardized approach for analysis and categorization of abnormalities. This can be utilized to interpret manometric findings and facilitate diagnosis of esophageal motility disorders. Table 107.1 reviews the Chicago classification.

A newer approach employs an endoluminal functional imaging probe (EndoFLIP) and utilizes impedance planimetry to assess the distensibility and mechanical properties of the esophagus.[6] As the esophagogastric junction's distensibility is often decreased in achalasia, use of an EndoFLIP probe can aid in the assessment of contractility and distensibility of the esophagus, including repetitive antegrade or retrograde contractions. This approach has proved beneficial as it can detect achalasia patients with relatively low integrated relaxation pressures, which has historically been difficult to diagnose using HREM.[7] Despite using the same technology, an EsoFLIP probe differs slightly from an EndoFLIP probe as an EsoFLIP provides therapeutic dilation, which can be useful in the management of patients with esophageal stenosis.[6] An EndoFLIP is solely a diagnostic device.

Generally, there are no contraindications to esophageal manometry, although pressure measurements are most accurate in a cooperative patient who can swallow.

ESOPHAGEAL DILATION

Esophageal stenosis is a clinical condition defined by a fixed narrowing of the esophagus and can be either congenital or acquired in nature. Congenital esophageal stenosis (CES) is a rare condition that occurs in 1 out of every 25,000 to 50,000 live births. It is characterized by an intrinsic narrowing of the esophagus secondary to congenital malformation of the esophageal wall architecture. CES can be divided into three pathohistological types: tracheobronchial remnants (TBR), fibromuscular thickening or fibromuscular stenosis (FMS), and membranous webbing or esophageal membrane (EM). Both dilation and surgery are routinely employed in the treatment of CES, with the choice of treatment dependent on the

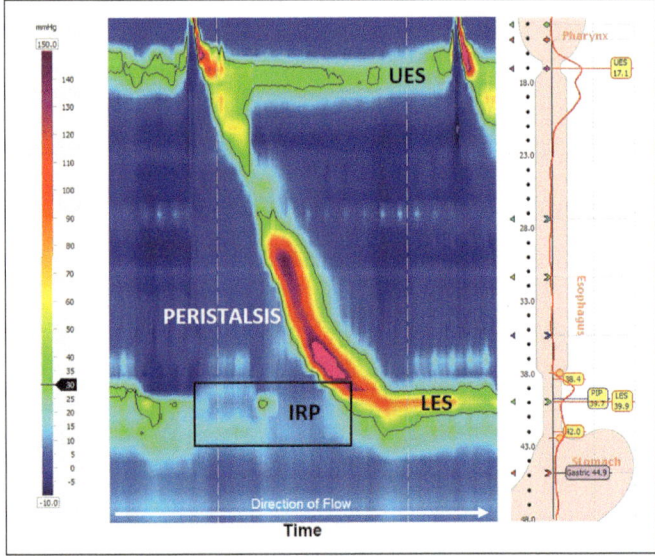

Figure 107.1: Example of a high-resolution manometry with esophageal pressure topography.

LES, lower esophageal sphincter; PIP, peak inspiratory pressure.

Source: From Mari A, Patel K, Mahamid M, et al. Achalasia: Insights into diagnostic and therapeutic advances for an ancient disease. *Rambam Maimonides Med J.* 2019;10(1):e0008. doi:10.5041/RMMJ.10361.

Table 107.1	Chicago Classification for Esophageal Pathology	
Chicago Classification	**Esophageal Pathology**	**Treatment Recommendations**
I (classic achalasia)	100% failed peristalsis	All treatments are effective
II (achalasia with esophageal compression)	100% failed peristalsis Esophageal pressurization occurs, high relaxation pressure	Pneumatic dilation
III (spastic achalasia)	No normal peristalsis, premature contractions	Peroral endoscopic myotomy or laparoscopic Heller myotomy

Sources: From Kahrilas PJ, Pandolfino JE. Treatments for achalasia in 2017: How to choose among them. *Curr Opin Gastroenterol.* 2017;33(4):270–276. doi:10.1097/MOG.0000000000000365; Torresan F, Ioannou A, Azzaroli F, Bazzoli F. Treatment of achalasia in the era of high-resolution manometry. *Ann Gastroenterol.* 2015;28(3):301–308.

Table 107.2	Common Classification of Esophageal Injury Score
Endoscopic Grade	**Esophageal Injury**
0	Normal, no injury
I	Mucosal edema, erythema
IIa	Noncircumferential and superficial ulceration with white plaques, friability, erosions, hemorrhage, blisters, exudates
IIb	Grade IIa lesions plus deep or circumferential lesions
IIIa	Small or scattered areas of necrosis
IIIb	Extensive or circumferential necrosis
IV	Perforation before or during endoscopy

Sources: From Kurowski JA, Kay M. Caustic ingestions and foreign bodies ingestions in pediatric patients. *Pediatr Clin North Am.* 2017;64(3):507–524. doi:10.1016/j.pcl.2017.01.004; Uygun I. Caustic oesophagitis in children: prevalence, the corrosive agents involved, and management from primary care through to surgery. *Curr Opin Otolaryngol Head Neck Surg.* 2015;23(6):423–432. doi:10.1097/MOO.0000000000000198.

pathological features of the stenosis. Dilation can be achieved using either fixed diameter dilators or expanding balloon dilators.[8,9]

Acquired esophageal strictures in children are often due to either caustic ingestion or are functional in nature, such as with epidermolysis bullosa or eosinophilic esophagitis.[8] Strictures are the most common complication after caustic ingestion and typically occur within 1 to 2 months after exposure.[10,11] The most common presenting symptoms in children following caustic ingestion are vomiting, drooling, refusal or difficulty swallowing, abdominal pain, and oropharyngeal burns or ulcerations.[11] The extent of injury secondary to caustic ingestion depends on the concentration and pH of the substance, as well as the total area injured and the length of time of the exposure.[11] It is reasonable to monitor asymptomatic children; however, those demonstrating symptoms must be scoped to determine the extent of injuries.[10–12] Ideally, endoscopy should be performed 12 to 24 hours postingestion under general anesthesia with a protected airway to facilitate grading of the severity of injury.[11] Table 107.2 reviews the scoring commonly used to classify esophageal injury. Esophageal strictures may also be at the site of surgical anastomosis following reconstructive surgery.[9]

Most esophageal dilations in the pediatric population are performed under general anesthesia for patient comfort and, when necessary, to protect the airway.[8,9]

BOTULINUM TOXIN INJECTION

Botulinum toxin injection is considered an effective and low-risk procedure for short-term symptom relief in patients with achalasia and spastic esophageal motility disorders. Eight different types of botulinum toxins have been described, with type A being the first approved by the Food and Drug Administration for direct muscle injection to alleviate muscle spasms due to excess central neural activity or muscle spasm.[13] Botulinum toxin is a potent inhibitor of the release of acetylcholine from the nerve endings. Injecting botulinum toxin has the potential to counteract otherwise unopposed LES contraction, thereby lowering LES pressure by disrupting or weakening the LES.

Botulinum toxin injection may be used in multiple sites to treat gastrointestinal motility symptoms in children. Motility disorders that benefit from botulinum toxin injection include cricopharyngeal achalasia and esophageal achalasia, as well as gastroparesis. Defecation disorders, such as Hirschsprung's disease and internal anal sphincter achalasia, have also been reported to benefit from botulinum injection.[13]

Compared with both pneumatic dilation and myotomy, botulinum toxin injection has clearly shown to have been at a disadvantage with respect to therapeutic efficacy. Nonetheless, botulinum toxin injection has several advantages, such as ease of technique, safety, ease of return to work, and higher success rate in vigorous achalasia, when compared with pneumatic dilation and surgical myotomy. Unfortunately, the response to esophageal-directed botulinum toxin injection is variable depending on the severity of the underlying motility disorder and is not beneficial to all. Therefore, it has been suggested that this technique should be preferentially reserved for patients with significant comorbidity or for patients who are on a waiting list for surgery or who are refusing other forms of treatment.

SPECIAL CONSIDERATIONS AND CONCERNS

All children with motility disorder present the potential risk of aspiration. This is especially true for children with a history of gastroparesis or obstruction. The Eckardt Symptom Score (ESS) is the gold standard self-report assessment used to evaluate the symptoms, stages, and efficacy of treatment in patients with achalasia. It attributes points (0–3 points) to the frequency of dysphagia, regurgitation, retrosternal pain, and weight loss. Scores greater than 4 indicate treatment failure and potentially greater risk of aspiration during induction of general anesthesia.[14]

ANESTHETIC MANAGEMENT

PREOPERATIVE EVALUATION

A full examination prior to induction of anesthesia is essential as many patients presenting with motility disorders are dehydrated and/or exhibit signs and symptoms of malnourishment. It is not uncommon for children who have not yet undergone a diagnostic workup to exhibit symptoms of malnutrition or be underweight. Common signs of malnourishment include an overly thin appearance, cachectic, sunken eyes, prominent clavicles, edema, and abdominal swelling. Signs of dehydration include dry skin and mucous membranes, dry tongue, decreased skin turgor, and orange-tinged palms and soles as evidence of carotenemia in anorexia nervosa, lanugo hair, amenorrhea in pubescent females, heart murmur, and hypotension.

In addition to assessing the extent of malnutrition and the severity of gastroesophageal reflux, anesthesia providers should vet the impact of malnutrition on other systems. Malnutrition is a complex metabolic disorder that involves inflammatory and neurohumoral mediators and affects virtually every organ system. The inability or altered ability to regulate salt and fluid can lead to overhydration or dehydration.

Anesthesia providers should also be aware that frequently patients presenting for botulinum injection are poor surgical candidates. It is imperative that the preanesthetic assessment vet any history of prematurity and/or cardiac disease that may necessitate the need for prolonged or more acute monitoring postoperatively.

Pertinent Labs
Routine labs are generally not indicated for any of the procedures discussed in this chapter; however, assessing electrolyte and albumin levels preoperatively may be warranted in patients presenting with severe weight loss and failure to thrive or those who are severely malnourished.

PREOPERATIVE PHARMACOLOGY
Patients presenting for HREM, esophageal dilation, and/or botulinum injection may be taking a variety of medications that anesthesia providers should be aware of. For example, they may be prescribed calcium antagonists to block esophageal contraction or nifedipine sublingually before meals.[5] Children with esophageal strictures are often on proton pump inhibitors for treatment of esophagitis and may be applying mitomycin C topically as its antifibroblastic activity may be helpful in the treatment of strictures.[9] Systemic and intralesional corticosteroids have also been used to treat symptoms in children.[9]

Prior to HREM, prokinetics, narcotics, and anticholinergics are typically held 48 hours prior to test. Patients may also present with vagal nerve stimulators (VNS), which impact esophageal motility. The risks and benefits associated with disabling the VNS prior to anesthesia should be considered on an individual basis.[2] Patients with cardiac anomalies or hematological/oncological abnormalities may require prophylactic antibiotics as determined by the underlying disease process.

ANESTHETIC TECHNIQUE

Intraoperative Management
While manometry is best done with an awake cooperative patient, sedation or general anesthesia may be used to facilitate HREM catheter placement. Should sedation or general anesthesia be utilized, the risk of aspiration should be considered when determining the sedation or anesthesia plan. This especially holds true for children with gastroparesis or obstructive symptoms. If anesthesia is necessary, intubation with an endotracheal tube may facilitate catheter placement, as well as protect against inadvertent aspiration. It should be noted that HREM catheters are usually placed nasally in children older than 4 months, but may be placed orally in premature infants. Children with craniofacial abnormalities or small infants may have the catheter passed orally as well. In most instances, endoscopy or fluoroscopy will be used to guide HREM catheter placement if the patient is receiving sedation or general anesthesia.

Historically, there was concern regarding the potential detrimental impact anesthetic medications may have on esophageal motility and subsequently HREM. As such, opioids have been avoided in the past due to the presumed effect on motility. A recent study by Tariq et al.,[15] however, reported that fentanyl used for sedation during HREM catheter placement had no impact on measurements following catheter placement. Likewise, oral midazolam has been reported to have minimal to no effect on the LES pressure. This has greatly changed clinical practice by again allowing the use of commonly used medications. Should sedation or anesthesia be used for HREM catheter placement, it is recommended that testing does not commence sooner than 2 to 4 hours post sedation or anesthesia to ensure residual impact from the medications used.

General anesthesia is not always indicated or necessary in HREM catheter placement, however. In many institutions, the HREM catheter is passed nasally into the esophagus in an awake patient. To ease HREM catheter placement, local anesthetics may be used to anesthetize the nasopharynx and oropharynx.

Most esophageal dilations in the pediatric population are performed under general anesthesia for patient comfort and to ensure the airway is protected during the procedure.[8,9] It is not uncommon to encounter an increase in peak inspiratory pressure (PIP) due to insufflation of the stomach, which decreases lung compliance during the procedure, especially in younger children.[16] Increases in PIP may also be attributed to stress on the trachea following balloon inflation.[16] Likewise, balloon inflation may be associated with transient tachycardia, and occasionally reflexive bradycardia due to vagal stimulation if the patient is not adequately anesthetized.[16]

Anesthesia providers should be aware that pharyngeal and/or laryngeal edema or swelling may be present following a caustic ingestion due to fumes or splashing of caustic agents into the upper airways. This can create challenges with endotracheal intubation if the airway is compromised.[12] It is recommended that equipment to manage a difficult airway be readily available prior to induction of anesthesia.

Botulinum toxin injection requires no special anesthetic techniques. Subsequently, the approach to anesthesia for botulinum toxin injection will be determined by the patient's overall health and presenting comorbidities. In patients with motility disorders, botulinum toxin is typically injected at the LES under direct vision during a routine endoscopy with a sclerotherapy needle in four different quadrants.

In most instances, a total of 80 to 100 units are injected in equal, divided doses.[17]

Anesthesia providers should remain cognizant that the metabolic and physiological changes accompanying malnutrition can significantly alter response to anesthetics. Any decrease in the total circulating albumin has wide implications for drug administration and volume of distribution. Likewise, protein deficiency may reduce drug metabolism as a result of decreased microsomal enzyme activity and altered cytochrome P450/nicotinamide adenine dinucleotide phosphate–dependent transport mechanisms. In severe cases, decreased transformation of compounds that are hepatically detoxified may lead to pathological responses requiring dosage alteration.

Standard monitors, as described by the American Society of Anesthesiologists, should be employed in all the procedures described and patients should have at least one well-running peripheral IV catheter. While these are all typically brief procedures, patients with malnutrition may have impaired temperature regulation mechanisms, and active warming techniques should be considered. Care should be given to patient positioning to avoid pressure sores. Perhaps most importantly, it is imperative that higher risk procedures only be performed in facilities with adequate support rather than nonoperating room locations or ambulatory surgery centers.[18]

Complications/Emergencies

The most common complication following esophageal dilation is bleeding, while perforation is the most serious complication.[8] Anesthesia providers should be aware that the incidence of esophageal perforation is higher in children during dilation of congenital esophageal strictures as opposed to other types of esophageal strictures.[9]

Botulinum injection is primarily associated with minor pain; however, rash and allergic reaction, bowel perforation, and incidental paralysis of the vocal cords have all been reported.[13]

POSTOPERATIVE CARE

As there is little to no pain associated with any of the procedures discussed in this chapter, postoperative care is largely supportive. The primary complaints following the previously described procedures are sore throat and hoarseness, both of which are relatively time-limited in nature. As transient chest pain may occur in approximately 4.4% of patients presenting for botulinum injection, nurses in the postanesthesia care unit should ensure pain is adequately controlled and not negatively impacting respiratory function.[7] While bleeding and perforation are very rare, it is important to closely monitor the patient in the immediate postoperative period following esophageal dilatation and botulinum injection. Postoperatively, signs and symptoms of sepsis may indicate perforation, which would require emergent intervention.[11]

CASE STUDY: A 4-Year-Old With Status Post Ingestion

CLINICAL SCENARIO

A 4-year-old boy ingested an unknown alkaline cleaning substance in his family's dairy farm after mistaking it for milk. Initial treatment was sought at a local facility, although the child ultimately presented to a pediatric referral center for subsequent treatments.

SPECIAL CONSIDERATIONS

The patient was scheduled for serial esophageal balloon dilations (EBD) once every 2 weeks under general anesthesia. Due to the frequency of procedures, parental presence at induction was allowed to reduce anxiety and encourage cooperation.

APPROACHES TO CARE

Sevoflurane and nitrous oxide were introduced via face mask. After he was anesthetized, a peripheral IV catheter was placed and propofol was administered. The airway was then secured with an endotracheal tube. This allowed the gastroenterologist the ability to assess the extent of esophageal scarring and healing, and introduce balloon dilation. Dilation proceeded without incident intraoperatively and no complications were noted postoperatively.

Evidence-Based Approaches to Care

Alkaline substances commonly cause esophageal strictures, leading to dysphagia, while acidic substances commonly cause pyloric strictures, leading to gastric outlet obstruction.[11] Alkaline substances are often colorless and odorless[11] while strong acids are bitter in taste and often spit out by the child but if swallowed are more likely to damage the stomach rather than the esophagus.[11,12] Acidic ingestions lead to coagulation necrosis and eschar formation, limiting mucosa penetration.[12] Alkaline ingestions are associated with worse esophageal injuries as compared with acidic ingestions.[10]

Strong alkalines in crystal form tend to lodge in the proximal esophagus, while liquid alkalines can cause injuries to the upper, middle, and lower sections of the esophagus.[12] Alkaline ingestions will penetrate the mucosal tissue and induce liquefactive necrosis, which destroys the epithelium, submucosa, and occasionally muscular layers.[8,11,12] It is possible for damage to continue underneath formed eschars.[8,12] Mucosal injury begins within minutes of caustic ingestion, with necrosis and hemorrhagic congestion secondary to the formation of thrombosis in the small vessels witnessed in the first 24 hours. These events typically continue the next several days. Approximately 4 to 7 days later mucosal sloughing, bacterial invasion, granulation tissue, and collagen deposition occur, followed by neovascularization and scar formation that result in strictures.[12]

Long-term outcomes in children with caustic esophageal stricture include repeat EBD. In some children, an esophageal stent is an option for refractory esophageal stricture. Surgery is indicated if the stricture is so severe that dilation is unsuitable or if esophageal perforation occurs during

(continued)

CASE STUDY: A 4-Year-Old With Status Post Ingestion (*continued*)

dilatation. In a series reported by Geng et al., 42 children with a mean age of 44 months underwent 168 esophageal balloon dilatation procedures with a 60.5% success rate. Successful dilatation was correlated with shorter segment stricture length. In patients who failed EBD, esophageal stents or gastrostomy tubes were placed.[19]

Of note, most ingestions by children are accidental, while ingestions by adolescents and adults are more likely to be intentional.[11,12] Interestingly, patients who have a history of caustic ingestion are at an increased risk of developing esophageal cancer, often three to four decades after the initial insult.[11]

KEY REFERENCES

Complete references for this chapter are online and available at https://connect.springerpub.com/content/book/978-0-8261-3875-0/part/part04/toc-part/ch107.

3. Sharp NE, St Peter SD. Treatment of idiopathic achalasia in the pediatric population: a systematic review. *Eur J Pediatr Surg.* 2016;26(2):143–149. doi:10.1055/s-0035-1544174

7. Ghiselli A, Bizzarri B, Ferrari D, et al. Endoscopic dilation in pediatric esophageal strictures: a literature review. *Acta Biomed.* 2018;89(8-S):27–32. doi:10.23750/abm.v89i8-S.7862

11. Uygun I. Caustic oesophagitis in children: prevalence, the corrosive agents involved, and management from primary care through to surgery. *Curr Opin Otolaryngol Head Neck Surg.* 2015;23(6):423–432. doi:10.1097/MOO.0000000000000198

13. van Lennep M, van Wijk MP, Omari T, et al. Clinical management of pediatric achalasia. *Expert Rev Gastroenterol Hepatol.* 2018;12(4):391–404. doi:10.1080/17474124.2018.1441023

17. Lightdale JR, Liu QY, Sahn B, et al. Pediatric endoscopy and high-risk patients: a clinical report from the NASPGHAN endoscopy committee. *J Pediatr Gastroenterol Nutr.* 2019;68(4):595–606. doi:10.1097/MPG.0000000000002277

SECTION J: Hematological Procedures

CHAPTER 108

Splenectomy

Paula J. Belson

INDICATIONS/CONTRAINDICATIONS

The spleen performs many physiological functions, including filtration of blood cells and protection against infection. Filtration and removal of nuclear remnants and excess cell membrane of immature erythrocytes by the splenic sinusoids maintain normal erythrocyte morphology.[1] Abnormal and aged red blood cells are filtered and removed by macrophages and other cells of the reticuloendothelial system. Phagocytosis and antibody production are facilitated in the white pulp of the spleen. The spleen also has a role as a reservoir for platelets. Despite its many physiological functions and contributions to maintain homeostasis, the spleen is not essential for life.

Removal of the spleen may be indicated due to trauma or a host of pathophysiological conditions (Table 108.1). Splenectomy significantly increases red cell survival and reduces the severity of anemia and jaundice.[2] Patients with immune thrombocytopenia (ITP, formerly referred to as idiopathic thrombocytopenic purpura), hereditary spherocytosis (HS), thalassemia, sickle cell anemia, and hemolytic anemias complicated by symptomatic splenomegaly, hypersplenism, and frequent transfusions may require a splenectomy.[3] However, splenectomy is usually reserved for the most severe cases. For example, splenectomy is recommended for patients with sickle cell disease that have had two acute splenic sequestration crises and/or massive splenomegaly or symptomatic hypersplenism.[4] In patients with HS, splenectomy is indicated in those transfusion-dependent or with severe anemia.[4] Additional indications include splenic cysts, abscesses, or masses, and symptomatic splenomegaly and hypersplenism associated with leukemia.

The spleen is the most frequently injured abdominal organ in children.[1] Approximately 90% of patients with a splenic injury can be treated nonoperatively, and rates of splenectomy

Table 108.1	Conditions Requiring Splenectomy		
Condition	**Pathophysiology**	**Indications**	**Effectiveness**
Hereditary spherocytosis	Rare genetic disorder producing spherical erythrocytes (spherocytes) susceptible to premature destruction in the spleen. Splenomegaly, severe anemia, hyperbilirubinemia, reticulocytosis, fatigue, and abdominal pain result	Moderate-to-severe disease, transfusion-dependent, severe anemia, splenomegaly	Very effective, strongly recommended. Can do partial splenectomy
Sickle cell disease	Sickled erythrocytes cannot readily pass through spleen and must be ingested by macrophages. Repeated splenic sequestration resulting in splenomegaly, critical anemia, significant abdominal pain, and splenic infarctions	Excessive transfusion requirement. History of two acute splenic sequestration crises, massive splenomegaly, symptomatic hypersplenism	No evidence that splenectomy increases hemoglobin level, decreases hemolysis, or improves patients' survival. Can do partial splenectomy
Immune thrombocytopenia	Autoimmune-mediated acquired bleeding disorder resulting in increased destruction and decreased production of platelets	Reserved for chronic, severe ITP	Very effective, response rate 80%
Thalassemia	Hereditary disorder causing abnormalities in red blood cell structure and hemoglobin synthesis resulting from a defect in erythropoiesis. Accelerated destruction of defective red blood cells. Need for repeated blood transfusions	Extreme transfusion requirement, symptomatic splenomegaly	Palliative does not influence underlying defect
Traumatic spleen rupture	Secondary to motor vehicle accident or other trauma	Nonoperative management and splenic preservation is standard of care; however, some will still require splenectomy	Mortality varies depending on severity of injury
Splenic abscess, cyst, or tumor	Benign or malignant, vascular, lymphoid and nonlymphoid tumors (hemangioma, lymphangioma, lipoma, Hodgkin's disease, non-Hodgkin's disease)	Depends on size, pathology, and patient symptoms. Many may have splenomegaly, abdominal pain, anemia, thrombocytopenia	Variable. May be partial or total splenectomy

have been found to be higher at nontrauma or adult trauma centers than pediatric trauma centers.[5] Nonoperative treatment has become the standard of care and is associated with better outcome, shorter hospital length of stay, and decreased need for blood transfusion.[5] However, hemodynamic instability and severe splenic damage causing hemoperitoneum may ultimately require splenectomy despite nonoperative treatment.

SPECIAL CONSIDERATIONS AND CONCERNS

Overwhelming postsplenectomy infection (OPSI) is a risk due to the role of the spleen in immune competence and blood filtration.[4] While the risk is rare (4.4% in children under the age of 16 years), mortality is as high as 38% to 70%.[1] The risk of postsplenectomy infections varies due to indication for surgery (intermediate risk in HS and higher risk in other inherited anemias), patient's age, and time since splenectomy was performed, with highest risk during the first year following surgery.[4] The risk of sepsis remains increased for up to 10 years postsplenectomy and probably remains elevated for life.[6] Children younger than age 5 are at highest risk of OPSI; thus, splenectomy should not be performed before this age if possible. Those with underlying immunodeficiency, such as leukemia, are also at increased risk and have a high mortality rate.[6] Children should receive *Haemophilus influenzae* type b (Hib), pneumococcal, and meningococcal vaccines at least 2 weeks prior to splenectomy. In addition, the American Academy of Pediatrics recommends antimicrobial prophylaxis with penicillin V for at least 1 year following splenectomy.

Emergency splenectomy is rarely performed, as conservative nonoperative treatment is preferred even in traumatic spleen injury. With the advent of thrombopoietin receptor agonists in the treatment of ITP, the incidence of severe refractory thrombocytopenia and persistent hemorrhage requiring emergent splenectomy is now rare.[7] Rates of splenectomies among patients with ITP have consistently declined over time especially in those younger than 5 years of age.[8] While an effective treatment in children with ITP (80% response rate), splenectomy is irreversible, with short- and long-term complications and lifelong risks of asplenia.[8,9]

A partial splenectomy may be indicated to allow for maintenance of normal immune function, especially in patients less than 6 years of age. Patients with sickle cell disease requiring multiple transfusions and those with HS and splenomegaly may benefit from a partial splenectomy, decreasing the need for transfusions and episodes of splenic sequestration, respectively. Partial splenectomy can be considered when moderate improvements in hemoglobin and reticulocytes are required, while total splenectomy is more likely to be required in severe disease.[10] Splenic regrowth will occur, and a salvage splenectomy may be required later, but the benefit is the delay in loss of immune function as a young child.[1]

ANESTHETIC MANAGEMENT

PREOPERATIVE EVALUATION

As patients presenting for splenectomy may be chronically ill, it is imperative that anesthesia providers perform a thorough

---

BOX 108.1 KEY ASSESSMENT POINTS

History of red blood cell and/or platelet transfusions

History of infections

History of corticosteroid use (ITP)

Presplenectomy antibiotic prophylaxis and immunizations

Hematologist recommendations regarding medical therapy and platelet transfusion requirement for platelets <30,000/mm³

Discontinuation of any platelet-inhibiting medication

ITP, immune thrombocytopenia.

Source: From Adams TL, Latham GJ, Eisses MJ, et al. Essentials of hematology. In: Cote C, Lerman J, Anderson B, eds. *A Practice of Anesthesia for Infants and Children.* 6th ed. Elsevier; 2019.

---

preoperative evaluation (Box 108.1). Patients being treated with chemotherapeutic agents may present with neurological, cardiac, and/or pulmonary comprise. Deficits, both centrally and peripherally, may ensure secondary to the administration of chemotherapeutic agents. Cardiac function may be impaired secondary to ongoing medical treatment with cardiotoxic agents, such as doxorubicin. Should there be a history of cardiac compromise, an ECG should be reviewed preoperatively to further evaluate the cardiac status and a cardiology consult may be warranted. Pulmonary function may be impaired due to left lower lobe atelectasis, depending on the size of the child's spleen. Chemotherapeutic agents may also result in hepatoxicity, impacting the liver's ability to metabolize medications commonly administered during the course of a general anesthetic.

Pertinent Labs

Laboratory tests that should be performed preoperatively include complete blood count, prothrombin time, partial thromboplastin time, bleeding time, platelet count, electrolytes, blood urea nitrogen, and creatinine.[1] An electrolyte panel, albumin, and liver enzymes are also recommended. Type and cross-match should be done due to potential for large blood loss intraoperatively. Thrombocytopenic patients may require platelet transfusion preoperatively. Patients with sickle cell anemia will require preoperative transfusion or exchange transfusion to reduce the percentage of hemoglobin S.

PREOPERATIVE PHARMACOLOGY

If the patient has been receiving long-term corticosteroids preoperatively, such as in ITP, they should be continued perioperatively to avoid adrenal insufficiency. A stress dose of hydrocortisone should be given prior to induction. Preoperative vaccinations should be administered at least 2 weeks prior to surgery as per OPSI guidelines. Premedication with oral or IV midazolam is recommended.

ANESTHETIC TECHNIQUE

Intraoperative Management

The majority of splenectomies are performed laparoscopically with or without robotic assistance. Transumbilical single-incision laparoscopic surgery (SILS) is often utilized and is beneficial as it leaves no scar but can be challenging with enlarged spleens.[11] Perioperative spleen embolization can be performed to improve the safety of laparoscopic splenectomy for splenomegaly.[11] An open splenectomy may be required; however, laparoscopic has become the standard approach and is associated with shorter hospital stay, fewer perioperative transfusions, and similar overall rate of complications and surgical time.[12] Contraindications to laparoscopic approach include inability to tolerate general anesthesia, portal hypertension with cirrhosis of the liver, and severe uncorrected coagulopathy.[1] The laparoscopic approach may be technically difficult to perform in those with massive splenomegaly and may lead to conversion to an open approach. Intraoperative bleeding is the primary indication for conversion from laparoscopic to an open approach.[1]

General endotracheal anesthesia (GETA) is standard for laparoscopic splenectomy. Nitrous oxide should be avoided to prevent bowel distention although evidence is conflicted.[13] If the patient is at risk of aspiration, a rapid sequence induction can be performed. Muscle relaxation is recommended to provide optimal surgical operating conditions. A cuffed endotracheal tube is preferred to ensure adequate ventilation during abdominal insufflation. A urinary catheter should be placed to empty the bladder and a nasogastric tube to decompress the stomach. A modified right lateral decubitus position with a small bump under the right flank is used for the lateral approach, which improves exposure and reduces risk of injury to the splenic capsule.[1] An anterior approach or supine position may be beneficial when a concomitant laparoscopic cholecystectomy will be performed, as in patients with sickle cell anemia or HS.[1]

Attention to the respiratory and cardiovascular effects of pneumoperitoneum during laparoscopic removal of the spleen is necessary (Box 108.2). Increased abdominal pressure causes decreased diaphragmatic excursion. Over time, this leads to atelectasis and ventilation/perfusion mismatch. Increased carbon dioxide levels may be difficult to control with mechanical ventilation. Trendelenburg position further decreases functional residual capacity and lung compliance especially in smaller children. Cephalad movement of the carina may cause endobronchial intubation and venous return may be impaired causing decreased cardiac output; however, these effects are most pronounced in infants who rarely will require splenectomy. Decreased compliance in the lower lung (right lateral decubitus position) occurs under anesthesia with positive pressure ventilation and paralysis due to displacement of the relaxed diaphragm and the downward gravity force of the mediastinum.[14] Attention to intra-abdominal pressure (normally 15 cmH$_2$O), airway pressures, bilateral breath sounds, and changes in positioning is essential to detect intraoperative issues.

While significant blood loss during splenectomy is unusual, two large-bore peripheral IV lines should be established (Box 108.3). Intraoperative bleeding is higher in the laparoscopic approach versus open and is the primary indication for conversion to open splenectomy.[1] An arterial and/or central line are not routine unless indicated due to the patient's underlying condition. A forced-air warming blanket should be used to prevent hypothermia.

Due to the increased incidence of postoperative nausea and vomiting with laparoscopic surgery, ondansetron and dexamethasone should be given intraoperatively. Pain management can be provided by IV acetaminophen and ketorolac with or without intraoperative narcotics. Epidural anesthesia is not necessary with the laparoscopic approach, and infiltration of the port sites with local anesthetic is effective. If open splenectomy is performed, an epidural catheter can be placed for postoperative pain management in those without bleeding issues. Awake extubation in the operating room at the end of the procedure is routine.

BOX 108.2 CLINICAL PEARLS: SPLENECTOMY

- Platelets, if needed, should ideally be transfused after the clamping of the splenic artery.[2]
- Children with HS will often undergo concurrent cholecystectomy, especially those with symptomatic gallstones, as there is potentially an increased risk of intrahepatic choledocholithiasis following splenectomy.[4]
- Partial splenectomies are sometimes performed because they allow for the retention of some immune function against bacterial infections, especially in younger children.[2]
- As for all surgeries in patients with sickle cell disease, careful perioperative attention to hydration, pain management, and temperature regulation are necessary to avoid triggering a sickle cell crisis.

HS, hereditary spherocytosis.

BOX 108.3 COMPLICATIONS/EMERGENCIES

- Bleeding
- Portal vein thrombosis
- Thrombocytosis
- Splenosis
- Overwhelming postsplenectomy sepsis
- Pleural effusion, pneumonia, pneumothorax (secondary to diaphragmatic injury)
- Subphrenic abscess
- Wound infection
- Pancreatic, gastric, or colon injury
- Missed accessory spleen with recurrence of hematological disorder
- Deep vein thrombosis

Sources: From Landmann A, Calisto JL, Scholz S. Laparoscopic splenectomy. In: Walsh DS, ed. *The SAGES Manual of Pediatric Minimally Invasive Surgery*. 2017;593–607. doi:10.1007/978-3-319-43642-5_44; Stork A, Garcia L. Open splenectomy for disease. In: Hoballah, JJ, ed. *Operative Dictations in General and Vascular Surgery*. 2017:403–404. doi:10.1007/978-3-319-44797-1_117.

POSTOPERATIVE CARE

The nasogastric tube should remain in place following surgery to allow for gastric decompression. Postoperative nausea and vomiting are common following laparoscopic procedures and multimodal therapy is standard of care.[13] Postoperatively, the child's diet can be advanced as tolerated. The laparoscopic approach to splenectomy allows for decreased pain and minimal postoperative ileus leading to a shorter hospital stay.[1] Pain after laparoscopic surgery consists of incisional, visceral/deep abdominal, and referred shoulder pain.[13] Multimodal pain therapy consisting of opioids, nonsteroidal anti-inflammatory drugs (NSAIDs), and local anesthetics is recommended. NSAIDs, however, should be avoided in those with bleeding risks (e.g., ITP). Corticosteroid coverage should continue postoperatively for those patients on previous therapy. Patients are usually ready for discharge on postoperative day 1 or 2.

Complete blood counts (hemoglobin and platelets) should be monitored postoperatively. There is potential for thrombocytosis and patients should be followed by hematology. The risk of infection remains postoperatively.

KEY REFERENCES

Complete references for this chapter are online and available at https://connect.springerpub.com/content/book/978-0-8261-3875-0/part/part04/toc-part/ch108.

1. Landmann A, Calisto JL, Scholz S. Laparoscopic splenectomy. In: Walsh DS, ed. *The SAGES Manual of Pediatric Minimally Invasive Surgery.* 2017;593 -607 doi:10.1007/978-3-319-43642-5_44

2. Adams TL, Latham GJ, Eisses MJ, et al. Essentials of hematology. In: Cote C, Lerman J, Anderson B, eds. *A Practice of Anesthesia for Infants and Children.* 6th ed. Elsevier; 2019:217-238.

4. Iolascon A, Andolfo I, Barcellini W, et al. Recommendations regarding splenectomy in hereditary hemolytic anemias. *Haematologica.* 2017;102(8):1304–1313. doi:10.3324/haematol.2016.161166

6. Luoto TT, Pakarinen MP, Koivusalo A. Long-term outcomes after pediatric splenectomy. *Surgery.* 2018;159(6):1583 -1590. doi:10.1016/j. surg.2015.12.014

10. Guizzetti L. Total versus partial splenectomy in pediatric hereditary spherocytosis: a systematic review and meta-analysis. *Pediatr Blood Cancer.* 2016;63(10):1713-1722. doi:10.1002/pbc.26106

SECTION K: Oncological Procedures

CHAPTER 109

Mediastinoscopy and Mediastinal Mass Resection

Barry Swerdlow

INDICATIONS/CONTRAINDICATIONS

Mediastinoscopy is usually employed to biopsy tissue for diagnostic purposes, although limited thymectomies, resection of mediastinal cysts, and a few other therapeutic procedures have been performed using this approach.[1] Furthermore, while mediastinal tissue sampling in adults increasingly has relied on endobronchial ultrasound-guided techniques, mediastinoscopy remains the primary method for such evaluation in pediatric patients.[2]

Mediastinoscopy involves the insertion of a rigid fiberoptic videoscope (mediastinoscope) into the prevascular mediastinum. Most commonly, it is performed either via a small incision above the manubrium through a potential plane between the pretracheal fascia and the trachea (known as a cervical mediastinoscopy [CM]), or less often, via a small parasternal incision (known as an anterior mediastinoscopy [AM]) that allows access to the aortopulmonary window through the interchondral space.

SPECIAL CONSIDERATIONS AND CONCERNS

Relative contraindications for CM include the presence of a tracheostomy, severe kyphosis, cervical spine disease with limited neck extension, severe tracheal deviation, or previous recurrent laryngeal nerve (RLN) injury; relative contraindications for both CM or AM include prior mediastinoscopy, radiotherapy, or mediastinitis in the surgical area, coagulopathy, superior vena cava (SVC) syndrome, ascending aortic aneurysm, or significant pulmonary hypertension.[3]

ANESTHETIC MANAGEMENT

PREOPERATIVE EVALUATION

Induction of general anesthesia (GA) can be associated with disastrous consequences in children with anterior or superior ("prevascular") mediastinal masses (AMMs), therefore preoperative evaluation of these patients based on history, physical examination, and imaging studies provides crucial information related to risk stratification. A history of significant position-related dyspnea (usually orthopnea), stridor, or cyanosis places the patient at higher risk of airway compromise during GA.[4] Mild, moderate, and severe orthopnea translate, respectively, as being able to lie supine despite some cough or pressure sensation, being able to lie supine for limited periods only, and not being able to lie supine due to mass-effect symptoms. Furthermore, preoperative identification of provocative positions and positions of maximum comfort allows providers to avoid the former and return to the latter if conditions under anesthesia worsen ("rescue positions").

Likewise, imaging studies serve a key role in identifying children at risk for GA, with a computed tomography scan cross-sectional area (CSA) of <70% of normal or bronchial compression being associated with GA-related airway adverse events, and CT findings of vascular compression or echocardiographic (ECHO) evidence of tamponade correlating with adverse hemodynamic events during GA (Table 109.1).[4,5] Surgery can proceed with GA for low-risk patients, but patients of intermediate or high risk first should be managed by a multidisciplinary team that considers the possibilities of extrathoracic tissue diagnosis not requiring GA, or preoperative use of steroids and/or radiation therapy to optimize mediastinal physiology even in the absence of a pathological diagnosis.[6] Unfortunately, this algorithm is often complicated, especially in infants and young children, by the inability to provide an adequate history and the need for sedation to obtain adequate imaging (with associated additional hazards).[5,7] Partly for these reasons, there is an increased risk of AMM complications in small infants.[5] Other factors that contribute to morbidity in the latter population include smaller intrathoracic volumes and hence more extensive compression due to growing masses, and inability to perform biopsies with IV sedation, which is an option for older children.[8]

When GA is planned for a child with an AMM, there are multiple important considerations (Box 109.1). If possible, AMM patients should be managed in the main operating room, potentially with extracorporeal bypass capability (if preinduction use of extracorporeal membrane oxygenation (ECMO) is planned; "cardiopulmonary bypass standby" is not an option as cannulation cannot be performed in an adequately timely manner once untoward mass effects occur.[8] Optimally, procedures should be timed to allow for a maximum number of support personnel to be present.[4] Premedication is best avoided to minimize the likelihood of an adverse event in an uncontrolled environment, and children are maintained in the position of maximum comfort (minimum symptoms) through the induction process. Preinduction placement of age-appropriate large-bore IV catheter (including lower extremity access in the presence of SVC syndrome) is important, as well as an arterial line if possible.

Volume loading should be considered prior to anesthetic induction in the setting of vascular or cardiac compromise, and vasoactive agents need to be readily available to prevent circulatory collapse. The thoracic surgeon (who should be an experienced bronchoscopist) and appropriate equipment for rigid bronchoscopy and sternotomy must be present and immediately available in the operating room at the time of induction.

ANESTHETIC TECHNIQUE

Intraoperative Management

Anesthesia for all mediastinoscopic procedures involves common considerations, although patients with AMMs have additional specific issues. With the exception of children from the latter population, these surgeries are usually performed as same-day discharge procedures under GA using a single-lumen endotracheal tube with strict neuromuscular

Table 109.1	Risk Stratification of Children With Anterior Mediastinal Masses	
	Symptoms	Imaging Findings
Low risk	None	No airway compression No vascular or cardiac compression
Intermediate risk	Mild to moderate postural symptoms (see text)	Tracheal compression <70% No bronchial compression
High risk	Orthopnea, stridor, or cyanosis	Tracheal compression >70% Bronchial compression Great vessel compression Tamponade

Notes: Imaging should consist of computed tomography esophagography (CTE) to assess airway and vessels; transthoracic echocardiogram (TTE) to assess heart. Any of the findings in the intermediate-risk or high-risk categories are sufficient to stratify a patient accordingly.

BOX 109.1 ANESTHETIC CONSIDERATIONS FOR MEDIASTINOSCOPY

Preoperative

- Exclude tracheobronchial, vascular, or cardiac mass effects, and paraneoplastic syndromes.
- Confirm no surgical contraindication to procedure (see text).
- Confirm no severe limitation of neck extension.
- Verify availability of cross-matched blood.

Intraoperative

- Establish large-bore IV access (in lower extremity with SVC syndrome).
- Place pulse oximeter probe on right hand for early detection of innominate artery compression.
- Place blood pressure cuff on left upper extremity.
- Consider the use of an arterial line. Preferential location for an arterial line is the left radial artery.
- Consider electroencephalographic monitoring in patients with poor collateral cerebral perfusion.
- Perform general anesthesia with a single-lumen endotracheal tube.
- In the absence of a prevascular mediastinal mass, ensure strict neuromuscular blockade.
- Design anesthesia for same-day discharge.

Postoperative

- Evaluate patient for signs of recurrent laryngeal nerve injury, tracheal injury, or neck hematoma.
- Evaluate chest x-ray to exclude mediastinal hemorrhage, phrenic nerve injury (elevated hemidiaphragm), pneumothorax, or pneumomediastinum.

SVC, superior vena cava.

BOX 109.2 MANAGEMENT OF CHILDREN WITH ANTERIOR MEDIASTINAL MASSES REQUIRING GENERAL ANESTHESIA FOR MEDIASTINOSCOPY

Preinduction

- Schedule elective procedures when maximum support personnel are present.
- Perform procedure in main operating room whenever possible.
- Consider advisability and feasibility of extracorporeal bypass with preinduction femoral cannulation.
- Avoid premedication.
- Maintain optimal patient position throughout preinduction and induction phases of anesthesia.
- Have adequate personnel immediately accessible to alter patient's position rapidly if needed.
- Thoracic surgeon with rigid bronchoscope set up for use in the operating room during induction.
- Establish age-appropriate large-bore IV access; a lower extremity site should be used with SVC syndrome.
- Place an arterial line if possible.

Induction and Maintenance

- In cases of vascular or cardiac compression, consider volume loading prior to induction.
- Maintain spontaneous ventilation throughout induction, maintenance, and emergence.
- Consider using CPAP during induction.
- Employ NMB only if mandated by surgery, and only after an endotracheal tube (ideally armored) is placed distal to area of maximal tracheobronchial compression and manually delivered positive pressure ventilation is demonstrated to be adequate.
- If NMB is performed, use small titratable doses of short-acting relaxants.

Postoperative

- Monitor for airway and hemodynamic compromise.

CPAP, continuous positive airway pressure; NMB, neuromuscular blockade; SVC, superior vena cava.

blockade to minimize the risk of inadvertent patient movement and associated injury. In the absence of the aforesaid mass-associated pathology or other contraindications, premedication is acceptable; and after application of standard monitors, anesthesia is induced in an age-appropriate fashion considering the specific patient circumstances.

A number of anesthesia induction agents (volatile anesthetics, propofol, ketamine, or dexmedetomidine) may be utilized with equivalent safety, with the paramount concerns being the maintenance of spontaneous ventilation, at least until after an endotracheal tube (ETT) is passed beyond the area of tracheobronchial compression and maintenance of hemodynamic stability.[4,9] In the rare case where muscle relaxation is absolutely required, ventilation via the ETT should first gradually be assumed manually and use of small doses of short-acting neuromuscular blocking agents should be employed only after such positive pressure ventilation has been demonstrated to be feasible.

For CM, after tucking arms, the operating room table is rotated 90°, a transverse roll is placed under the shoulders, and with the patient's head at the end of the table, the neck is maximally extended with care to avoid inadvertent patient extubation. Short- or ultra-short-acting anesthetics are employed, and usually patients are extubated in the operating room prior to transfer to the postanesthesia care unit.

Definitive resection of mediastinal masses, although a much less common procedure than mediastinoscopy, involves the same anatomy with potential injury of similar critical structures. Surgical techniques include thoracoscopy with or without robotic instrumentation, thoracotomy, median sternotomy, or combined methods, such as supraclavicular incision-sternotomy-anterior thoracotomy ("trap-door approach") or bilateral anterior thoracotomy ("clamshell approach").[10] Selection of the optimal approach varies according to the location, type, and anatomic involvement of the mediastinal mass. In high-risk cases where cardiopulmonary compromise is severe, such as with thymectomy and/or definitive mass resection, preemptive (including preinduction) femorofemoral cannulation for ECMO should be considered. The added safety value of ECMO in this setting must be weighed against the likelihood of increased bleeding complicating mass resection once extracorporeal bypass is initiated.[10]

THYMECTOMY

Thymectomy is an example of a mediastinal mass resection that deserves special mention because of its association with myasthenia gravis. Indications for thymectomy in children include (a) thymoma, (b) early-onset anti-acetylcholine receptor positive myasthenia, (c) progressive weakness with myasthenia, and (d) non-thymoma-related autoimmune myasthenia failing treatment.[11] There are three separate surgical options for thymectomy: transcervical, trans-sternal, and thoracoscopic (robotic and nonrobotic).[11,12]

Children with severe myasthenia undergoing thymectomy are routinely stabilized preoperatively with plasmapheresis, IV immunoglobulin therapy, and corticosteroids.[12] Thereafter, their maintenance dose of pyridostigmine is given on the day of surgery. Neuromuscular blocking agents are employed with caution in these patients, although the availability of sugammadex has improved the safety of pharmacological paralysis in this setting.

DEFINITIVE MASS RESECTION

Like thymectomy patients, children with masses in the anterior and superior (prevascular) mediastinum undergoing diagnostic mediastinoscopy or definitive resection require separate consideration, as they present unique challenges for anesthesia providers.[5,13] These challenges most commonly relate to compression of the tracheobronchial tree or of cardiovascular structures that may occur preoperatively and may be exacerbated by GA. The overall risk of anesthesia-related complications with an AMM in children has been reported to range between 9% and 20%, and even patients without symptoms on preoperative evaluation have developed catastrophic mass-effect problems, including death.[4,5]

COMPLICATIONS/EMERGENCIES

The ability to rapidly manage intraoperative complications is a key feature of successful anesthetic planning in AMM patients undergoing GA. If worsening tracheobronchial compression occurs, the child immediately should be placed in a "rescue position." When no such position has been identified preoperatively, consideration should be given to placing the patient prone to minimize gravitational mass effects on the cardiopulmonary system. If possible, the child is then allowed to awaken. Otherwise, the trachea should be intubated and the ETT advanced past the obstruction. Alternatively, a rigid bronchoscope can be inserted beyond the area of maximal compression, potentially into a main stem bronchus, and used for oxygenation. After adequate resuscitation, an airway exchange catheter may be delivered through the bronchoscope and an ETT introduced over the catheter once the bronchoscope is withdrawn. If these attempts are inadequate or if hemodynamic compromise is progressive, performing an immediate sternotomy with surgical elevation of the mass is indicated.[5]

There are three major reasons for exaggerated airway compression after induction of GA in these patients: (a) tracheobronchial diameters decrease when lung volumes decrease, (b) bronchial smooth muscle relaxes, and (c) absence of spontaneous ventilation eliminates the transpleural pressure gradient that normally distends the airways during inspiration.[5] This compression has a dramatic effect on airflow (Poiseuille's law) and passing an ETT past the point of airway collapse may not be possible, especially if the obstruction occurs in the distal trachea or in a main stem bronchus. Similarly, GA-associated venodilation, together with increased vascular compression associated with loss of muscle tone and assuming the supine position, may result in critical reduction in right heart return and hemodynamic collapse in patients with venous obstruction or ongoing tamponade who are dependent on higher-than-normal venous pressures to maintain their stroke volumes.

Excluding mass effect issues associated with GA, significant complications with mediastinoscopy result from hemorrhage, innominate artery compression (CM), bradycardia associated with tracheal or great vessel traction, recurrent laryngeal nerve (CM) or phrenic nerve injury (AM), tracheobronchial laceration, esophageal or thoracic duct trauma (CM), venous air embolism (CM), and/or pneumothorax. Hemorrhage may be relatively minor and controlled via the mediastinoscope with packing and electrocautery. In these situations, placing the patient in a head-up position or using relative hypotension may be of value. More significant hemorrhage potentially requiring massive transfusion may necessitate either emergent sternotomy or thoracotomy.[3] The likelihood of specific vessel injury depends on the approach (CM vs. AM), with the aorta and pulmonary arteries being more vulnerable during AM. Need for one-lung ventilation or cardiopulmonary bypass is possible depending on the source of hemorrhage. When the innominate vein or SVC needs repair, lower extremity IV access is critical to prevent loss of volume resuscitation and pharmacology into the surgical field.

Partial or complete innominate artery compression with potential cerebral ischemia may occur during CM in which the

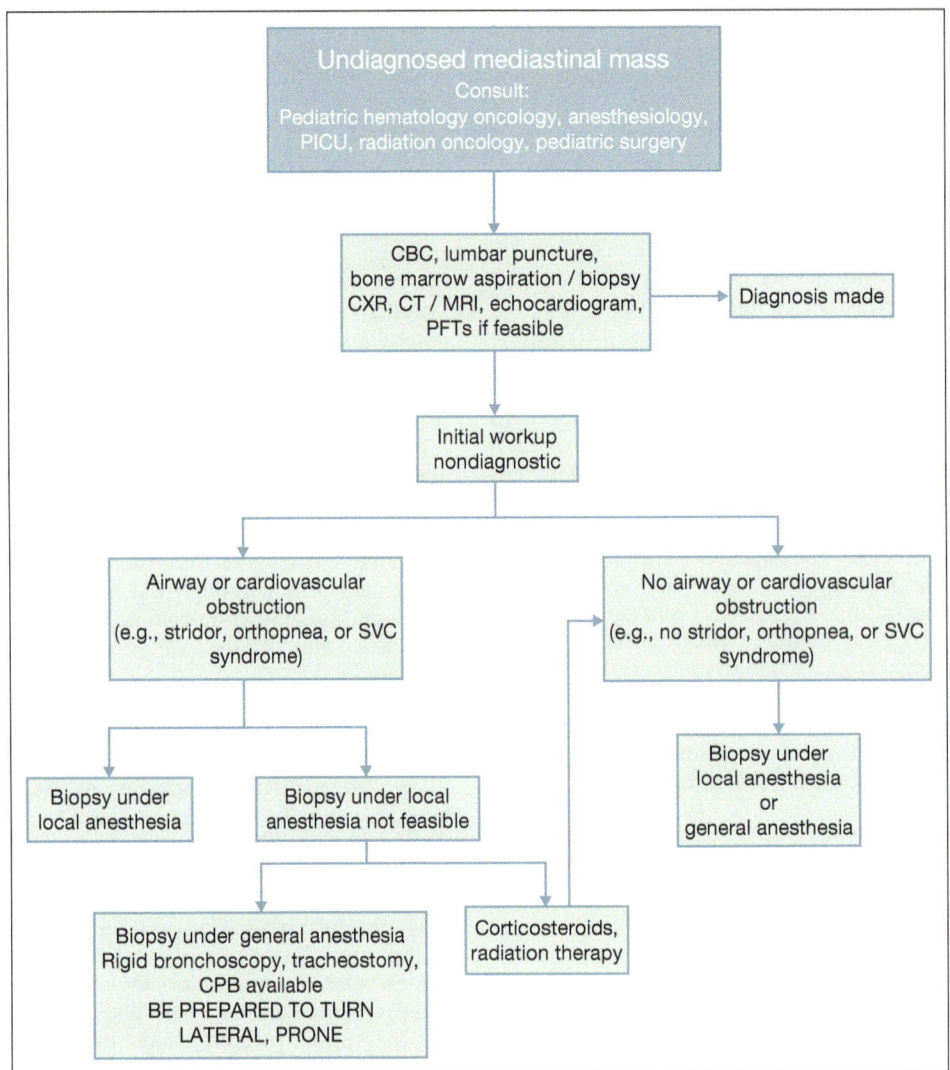

Figure 109.1: Algorithm for management of the child with a mediastinal mass.

CBC, complete blood count; CPB, cardiopulmonary bypass; CXR, chest x-ray; PFTs, pulmonary function tests; PICU, pediatric intensive care unit; SVC, superior vena cava.

Source: From McEwan A. Anesthesia for children undergoing heart surgery. In: Cote CJ, Lerman J, eds. *A Practice of Anesthesia for Infants and Children.* 4th ed. Elsevier; 2009: Fig. 15.13, p. 291.

scope passes dorsal to this vascular structure. Placement of the pulse oximeter probe on the patient's right hand allows for early detection of such a complication, and electroencephalographic monitoring may be considered in children with compromised collateral cerebral circulation.[3] Blood pressure determinations should employ the left upper extremity for this reason.

POSTOPERATIVE CARE

Postoperatively, the patient is awoken and transferred to the postanesthesia care unit (PACU). While in PACU, a chest x-ray (CXR) should be obtained to assess for development of a pneumothorax. In addition, it is imperative to monitor for hemodynamic compromise, including monitoring for hematoma development, which may result in compression of the airway.

APPROACHES TO CARE

Given an extrathoracic source of diagnostic tissue, and with clinical and CT evidence for airway compromise, the patient is scheduled for a cervical lymph node excision using local anesthesia and IV sedation. After the patient positions themselves comfortably in the left lateral decubitus position, standard American Society of Anesthesiologists monitors are employed, oxygen is administered via nasal cannula, and a dexmedetomidine–remifentanil infusion provides adequate sedation for the procedure. Anesthetic dose is titrated to a spontaneous respiratory rate of 8 to 12 breaths per minute. Tissue pathology reveals a diagnosis of T-cell lymphoblastic lymphoma. See **Figure 109.1** for an approach to the child with a mediastinal mass.

CASE STUDY: Patient With Anterior Mediastinal Mass

CLINICAL SCENARIO
A 13-year-old boy presents with a persistent, nonproductive cough of 3 weeks' duration, associated with low-grade fevers, night sweats, and generalized malaise. His pediatrician obtained a CXR that revealed a large anterior mediastinal mass. You are asked to consult as part of a multidisciplinary team to determine the optimal diagnostic approach.

SPECIAL CONSIDERATIONS
On detailed history, the patient notes that he sleeps on two pillows but is able to be flat for 5 to 10 minutes before getting short of breath, especially if he lies prone or on his left side. He has been increasingly fatigued with exercise but denies syncopal or presyncopal events. In the sitting position, his blood pressure is 112/66 with 5 mm Hg pulsus paradoxus, pulse 88 regular, respiratory rate 18 breaths per minute sitting, and oxygen saturation on room air 98%. There is no facial swelling or cyanosis, his breathing is unlabored without stridor, and his chest is clear to auscultation. Nontender right anterior cervical lymphadenopathy is present.

The patient's preoperative complete blood count and comprehensive metabolic panel are within normal limits. A chest CT (with and without IV contrast) obtained with the patient in the prone position reveals a large mass occupying the prevascular and visceral mediastinal spaces with no evidence for vascular compromise but with compression of the right mainstem bronchus. TTE is normal with a minimal anterior pericardial effusion, and no evidence for cardiac tamponade.

KEY REFERENCES

Complete references for this chapter are online and available at https://connect.springerpub.com/content/book/978-0-8261-3875-0/part/part04/toc-part/ch109.

3. Hartigan PM. Mediastinoscopy. In: Hartigan PM, ed. *Practical Handbook of Thoracic Anesthesia*. Springer; 2008:323–333. doi: 10.1007/978-0-387-88493-6
4. Pearson JK, Tan GM. Pediatric anterior mediastinal mass: a review article. *Sem Cardiothorac Vasc Anes*, 2015;19(3):248–254. doi: 10.1177/1089253215578931
5. Brenn BR, Hughes AK. The anesthetic management of anterior mediastinal masses in children: a review. *Int Anes Clin*. 2019;57(4):e24–e41. doi: 10.1097/aia.0000000000000247
8. Trifa M, Burrier C. Anesthetic management of anterior mediastinal masses in children. In: Lalwani K, Cohen IT, Choi EY, Raman VT, eds. *Pediatric Anesthesia: A Problem-Based Learning Approach*. Oxford University Press; 2018. doi: 10.1093/med/9780190685157.001.0001

CHAPTER 110

Lumbar Puncture
Barry Swerdlow

INDICATIONS/CONTRAINDICATIONS

Indications and contraindications for the performance of lumbar puncture (LP) in pediatric oncology are listed in Box 110.1.[1-3] In children with cancer, in contrast with the general pediatric population, intrathecal (IT) chemotherapy is often delivered by repeat LP in an ambulatory setting, and there is an increased prevalence of thrombocytopenia related both to disease processes and antineoplastic drugs. For example, patients with acute lymphoblastic leukemia (ALL) require an LP for initial diagnosis and then repeat LPs for IT methotrexate and/or cytarabine administration.[4] With the exception of some diagnostic purposes, LPs are performed for pediatric oncology patients largely as outpatient procedures.

> **BOX 110.1 INDICATIONS AND CONTRAINDICATIONS FOR LUMBAR PUNCTURE IN THE PEDIATRIC ONCOLOGY PATIENT**
>
> **Indications**
> - Diagnosis of CNS involvement of malignancy
> - Diagnosis of CNS infection
> - Diagnosis of subarachnoid hemorrhage when clinically suspected with negative imaging studies
> - Diagnosis of demyelinating processes
> - Delivery of IT chemotherapy
>
> **Contraindications**
> - Increased intracranial pressure (absolute contraindication)
> - Bleeding diathesis
> - Cardiopulmonary instability (related to position for procedure)
> - Soft tissue infection at puncture site
> - Epidural abscess
> - Status epilepticus
> - Anatomic spinal column abnormalities

> **BOX 110.2 COMPLICATIONS OF LUMBAR PUNCTURE**
> - Traumatic lumbar puncture
> - Cerebral herniation
> - Epidural or subdural hematoma
> - Postdural puncture headache
> - Spinal nerve injury
> - Infection
> - Backache
> - Persistent cerebrospinal fluid leak
> - Epidermoid spinal cord tumor

SPECIAL CONSIDERATIONS AND CONCERNS

Traumatic lumbar puncture (TLP) represents the most common complication of performing an LP in children, and it is most often due to overly deep insertion of the needle with laceration of the vertebral venous plexus.[1] When peripheral blood contaminates cerebrospinal fluid (CSF) derived from LPs, diagnosis of central nervous system (CNS) pathology may be obscured and/or adequate treatment impeded; for example, TLP in children with ALL is associated with underdiagnosis of CNS involvement, inadequate instillation of IT chemotherapy, and worsened event-free survival.[4] Modifiable risk factors for TLP in pediatric ALL patients include platelet count, interval between successive LPs (a shorter interval is associated with a higher incidence of TLP), and proceduralist experience.[4] Interestingly, type of anesthesia was not considered as a potential variable for TLP in this latter study, and all LPs were performed under deep sedation.

Also, while a coagulopathy represents a relative contraindication for this procedure, it should be noted that LPs have been performed in pediatric oncology patients with platelet counts less than 10,000/mm[3] without problem,[3,5] and prophylactic platelet transfusions are not routinely recommended in this setting.[6] Nevertheless, thrombocytopenia clearly is a risk factor for TLP in pediatric ALL patients (Box 110.2).[4]

Several other complications are associated with LPs, though they are less common. Spinal hematoma may occur in patients with bleeding diatheses and most frequently presents with back pain as well as symptoms and signs consistent with cauda equina syndrome. A low index of suspicion, with prompt imaging and timely surgical decompression, is critical to prevent permanent neurological injury. The incidence of postdural puncture headache (PDPH) after LPs in children has been estimated at between 5% and 15%, and often is neglected.[3,7] Standard measures limiting PDPH in adults may not apply to pediatric patients, including using smaller needle sizes or atraumatic needles, alignment of the needle bevel parallel to the long axis of the spine, reinserting the stylet before needle withdrawal, or bed rest, although epidural blood patch has proven to be an effective treatment of PDPH and other consequences of intracranial hypotension in children much as in adults.[2,8,9] Traumatic nerve root injury may occur during LPs, with resultant radicular symptoms, especially in the setting of general anesthesia (GA) in which nerve laceration is rendered relatively insensible. Epidermoid spinal cord tumor formation represents a rare, delayed complication of LPs likely due to inadvertent epidermoid tissue transplantation into the spinal canal during LP performance without a tight-fitting stylet.[3]

Because anesthesia providers at times also may perform LPs in the pediatric oncology population, in addition to indications, contraindications, and complications, they should understand a number of nuances related to technique beyond the usual admonitions associated with prudent performance of this procedure. In patients with difficult anatomy, especially when requiring repeat LPs, use of ultrasound guidance markedly improves success rates, and offers some advantages over fluoroscopy.[10] Both topical analgesia with a eutectic mixture of local anesthesia (EMLA) cream and/or needle-free injected lidocaine significantly improve pain management for children with cancer requiring LPs.[11-13] Of note, multiple studies have demonstrated that repeat LPs are accompanied by substantial anxiety and fear that is remembered by pediatric patients for years after their cancer treatment ends.[14] Appropriate anesthesia for LPs in this setting not only likely mitigates these unfortunate results, and but it also improves success rate and diminishes the incidence of TLP.[3]

ANESTHETIC MANAGEMENT

PREOPERATIVE EVALUATION

Because increased intracranial pressure is an absolute contraindication for LP due to the risk of cerebral herniation, neuroimaging should be performed prior to LP whenever there is a clinical suspicion of intracranial mass effect, such as with unexplained impaired consciousness or focal neurological findings, including cranial nerve palsies, papilledema, and abnormal posturing, or with bradycardia with hypertension.[3]

ANESTHETIC TECHNIQUE

Intraoperative Management

The objectives in providing adequate analgesia and sedation for LPs in these children are to minimize pain, prevent adverse psychological events, and facilitate a successful procedure. Many of these children have indwelling central venous access, including implanted ports, and meticulous attention should be given to aseptic technique when accessing these devices for drug delivery. In this context, different pharmacological regimens for IV sedation have been shown to be equally efficacious and safe, including procedural administration of propofol alone, propofol with fentanyl, midazolam with fentanyl, dexmedetomidine, and ketamine, provided adequate monitoring and intervention are employed.[15-17] Use of short-acting agents is prudent since these procedures most often are performed as outpatients. Nitrous oxide has been advocated as a safe and effective analgesic, but concern has been raised regarding the additive effect of methotrexate chemotherapy and nitrous oxide with respect to inhibition of methionine synthetase and related adverse neurological events.[18-20]

GA may also be employed with LPs in pediatric oncology patients (both inhalational and IV inductions are used depending on the specific patient circumstances), and outcomes with GA are similar to sedation, including the frequency and severity of adverse events.[17] If IT methotrexate or cytarabine is planned or there is a history of postoperative nausea or vomiting, prophylactic ondansetron should be administered provided there is no contraindication.[21,22] A potential consideration in choosing between conscious sedation and GA is the possible negative effect of repeat GA on intellectual development in children under the age of 3 years.[16] Some data suggest that offering children a choice of GA, conscious sedation, or no anesthesia may limit the emotional trauma associated with LPs in children with cancer, particularly because some of these children associate GA with death.[14] With a subset of patients, a minimum of anesthesia may be particularly efficacious if procedures are planned with good child and parental preparedness, and parents are allowed to accompany the child to the procedure area and to remain with the child during awakening.[23] Non-pharmacological adjuncts including distraction techniques, guided imagery, and hypnosis may be useful.[24]

Special Techniques and Equipment

Since LPs are most often performed outside the operating room complex (e.g., in clinics, on the wards, or in radiology), providing sedation or GA for these procedures involves considerations common to all remote anesthesia. Additional personnel and resources are often located at a distance, and as a result, extra vigilance is necessary to ensure safe delivery of anesthesia, including the availability of redundant systems and the provision for relatively infrequent problems (Box 110.3).[23,24]

Complications/Emergencies

Fortunately, serious anesthesia-related complications are rare.[17] Optimal design of either sedation or GA includes planning for the absence of child movement during the procedure, rapid onset and offset of anesthesia to allow for early discharge if applicable, minimal airway obstruction if sedation is planned, ability to rapidly titrate drug to effect, and minimal postoperative nausea/vomiting.[21]

BOX 110.3 PREANESTHESIA CHECKLIST FOR LUMBAR PUNCTURE OUTSIDE THE OPERATING ROOM

- Preanesthesia evaluation as for all operating room patients including verification of patient preparation and fasting, as well as a preoperative history and focused examination
- Absence of procedural contraindication (see Box 110.1)
- Informed consent for the procedure and for anesthesia
- A warm, well-lit procedure room with standard operating room electrical outlets and easy communication to the operating room or its equivalent
- Adequate support personnel
- Standard ASA monitors including an ECG, pulse oximetry, end-tidal carbon dioxide, blood pressure, and temperature monitors
- Primary and secondary oxygen sources
- Set up to provide positive pressure ventilation
- Functional suction apparatus with appropriate suction devices
- Airway supplies including oxygen masks, nasal cannula, face masks, oropharyngeal airways, laryngeal mask airways, endotracheal tubes, and laryngoscope blades
- Standard anesthesia cart containing medications (including resuscitation drugs) and supplies
- Equipment to maintain patient temperature (including blankets and forced-air warmer)
- Functional infusion pumps
- Resuscitation cart with defibrillator
- Equipment to transport child safely to an appropriate postanesthesia recovery area

ASA, American Society of Anesthesiologists.

POSTOPERATIVE CARE

Following the LP, the patient should be transported either to the postanesthesia care unit or returned to same day surgery for postanesthesia monitoring, based on institutional protocol. Quite often, pediatric oncology patients presenting for LP will receive therapeutic medications following the LP, based on their diagnosis and treatment protocol. Therefore, it is imperative that the patient's central line or mediport remained accessed to facilitate oncological therapy.

CASE STUDY: Fearful Child With Acute Lymphoblastic Leukemia for Diagnostic Lumbar Puncture

CLINICAL SCENARIO

An inpatient, 10-year-old boy with recently diagnosed ALL is scheduled for a diagnostic LP. The child was admitted for workup of symptoms related to failure to thrive, weight loss, and fatigue. The patient has no medical history of significance, and there is no family history of problems with surgery or anesthesia. The procedure will be performed by the pediatric oncology fellow in the ward procedure room on the next day.

SPECIAL CONSIDERATIONS

During the preoperative visit, both the patient and his parents are very anxious about the procedure. The boy's weight is 30 kg, and his vital signs are unremarkable. Physical examination is notable for diffuse nontender anterior lymphadenopathy, a clear chest, normal cardiac examination, and mild hepatomegaly. His complete blood count shows a hematocrit of 28.5%, white blood cell count of 51,000/mm^3, and platelet count of 75,000/mm^3. Other laboratory studies are normal. The child desires to be completely asleep for the LP, and the parents concur, as they recently had a suboptimal experience with a bone marrow procedure performed with conscious sedation. Informed anesthesia consent is obtained.

APPROACHES TO CARE

One hour prior to the procedure, EMLA cream 2.5 g is applied over the LP area and covered with an occlusive dressing, and the child receives a dose of oral midazolam 0.5 mg/kg. At the appropriate time, he is transported to the procedure room escorted by his parents. After application of standard American Society of Anethesiologists monitors, an antecubital 22-gauge IV catheter is started and procedural sedation is induced with IV fentanyl 1 mcg/kg and propofol 2.0 mg/kg. The patient is then placed in the left lateral decubitus position in an orientation suitable for his LP, oxygen is delivered by facemask, spontaneous ventilation is maintained, and additional intermittent boluses of 0.5 to 1 mg/kg of propofol are administered to avoid motion during the procedure. Following the procedure, the patient is transported to a monitored postanesthesia recovery area on the ward, where he awakens uneventfully in the presence of his parents.

KEY REFERENCES

Complete references for this chapter are online and available at https://connect.springerpub.com/content/book/978-0-8261-3875-0/part/part04/toc-part/ch110.

1. Bonadio W. Pediatric lumbar puncture and cerebrospinal fluid analysis. *J Emerg Med*. 2013;46(1):141–150. doi:10.1016/j.jemergmed.2013.08.056
14. Maslak K, Favara-Scacco C, Barchitta M, et al. General anesthesia, conscious sedation, or nothing: decision-making by children during painful procedures. *Pediatr Blood Cancer*. 2019;66(5):e27600. doi:10.1002/pbc.27600
17. Meneses CF, de Freitas JC, Castro CG, et al. Safety of general anesthesia for lumbar puncture and bone marrow aspirate/biopsy in pediatric oncology patients. *J Pediatr Hematol Oncol*. 2009;31(7):465–470. doi:10.1097/MPH.0b013e3181a974a1
23. Lerman J, Cote CJ, Steward DJ. Anesthesia outside the operating room. In: *Manual of Pediatric Anesthesia: With An Index of Pediatric Syndromes*. 7th ed. Springer; 2016:507–521. doi:10.1007/978-3-319-30684-1_18
24. Farrell T. Procedural sedation: anesthesia and sedation of children away from the OR. In: Sims C, Weber D, Johnson C, eds. *A Guide to Pediatric Anesthesia*. 2nd ed. Springer; 2020:453–463. doi:10.1007/978-3-030-19246-4_27

CHAPTER 111

Neuroblastoma Resection

Paula J. Belson

INDICATIONS/CONTRAINDICATIONS

Neuroblastoma is the most common extracranial solid tumor in children, accounting for 7% of all childhood cancers.[1] It is an embryonal malignancy of the sympathetic nervous system, derived from neural crest cells that normally form the sympathetic nervous system and adrenal medulla. The tumor is typically intra-abdominal but can be located anywhere where neural crest cells are found including intrathoracic or cervical. One third of abdominal tumors arise from the adrenal glands. The adrenal glands are located in the retroperitoneal space adjacent to the superior pole of the kidneys, thus renal involvement is common.

Most patients with neuroblastoma have metastatic disease at the time of diagnosis, and imaging is crucial in determining the presence or absence of risk factors and stage of disease.[2] Presentation is commonly a palpable abdominal mass, pain, and fullness. Fever, weight loss, and lymphadenopathy can be nonspecific signs. Symptoms may arise from pressure on surrounding organs or structures (e.g., kidney, liver, or spine) or metastasis. Cervical or thoracic tumors can cause respiratory symptoms and Horner syndrome (unilateral ptosis, anhidrosis, and miosis).[3] Spinal cord compression can result from tumors arising from the paraspinal ganglion.[4] Hypertension can occur due to excess catecholamine production.[5] Urinary catecholamines are present in over 90% of patients.[5] Neuroblastoma often spreads to the orbital bones causing periorbital ecchymoses, proptosis, and visual impairment.[3] Additional sites of metastases include bone marrow and cortical bone, lymph nodes, dura, and liver.[4] Prognosis is related to age, stage of tumor, and pathological type.

Surgery is often necessary initially to establish a diagnosis, as well as after neoadjuvant chemotherapy for resection of tumor. Tumors with favorable biology and no distant metastasis in those less than 18 months of age can often be treated with surgery alone. Those with less favorable tumor biology, metastasis, and larger size tumors often need chemotherapy, radiation, and/or hematopoietic stem cell transplantation (HSCT) prior to surgical resection. Surgical resection can be laparoscopic or via a laparotomy or thoracotomy. If spinal cord compression is present, a laminectomy may be required.

SPECIAL CONSIDERATIONS AND CONCERNS

Staging of neuroblastomas follows two protocols. The International Neuroblastoma Staging System (INSS) depends on tumor resectability, lymph node involvement, and metastasis (Table 111.1). The International Neuroblastoma Risk Group Staging System (INRGSS) bases staging on radiological findings (Table 111.2). Preoperative staging of neuroblastoma is determined by the presence or absence of image-defined risk factors (IDRFs). IDRFs are surgical risk factors that may increase morbidity of a surgical resection.[2] Risk classification is assigned based on extent of metastasis and presence of IDRFs and has been validated to be predictive of survival.[6]

ANESTHETIC MANAGEMENT

Anesthetic plans for children with cancer must take into consideration the possible direct effects of the tumor and surgical procedure, toxic effects of chemotherapy and radiation, drug–drug interactions with recent medications, current pain levels, and psychological status of the child and family.[7] Children undergoing treatment for cancer can be very ill and vulnerable to mild physiological changes. Potential complications in children undergoing cancer therapy include sepsis, multiorgan failure, coagulopathy, thromboembolism, tumor lysis syndrome, and respiratory and cardiac compromise.[8] Children with neuroblastoma may have anemia, renal involvement including obstruction of urinary flow or compression of renal vasculature, and rarely an anterior mediastinal mass.[9] Immunosuppression secondary to HSCT and/or T-cell therapy may also be present.

PREOPERATIVE EVALUATION

A thorough preoperative evaluation should include a review of the child's history, physical examination, concurrent illnesses, and prior anesthesia exposures and reactions (Box 111.1). Medication allergies, fasting times, and family history of anesthetic complications should be considered as always. Oncological treatment protocol information, including cumulative chemotherapy and radiation therapy doses and side effects, should be reviewed. Patients who have received chemotherapy (especially doxorubicin) should have an echocardiogram and possible cardiology consult. Particular attention should be paid to the organ systems involved with the tumor. Children with large abdominal masses may have tachypnea and decreased respiratory reserve. Intestinal compression from the tumor may increase the risk of gastric aspiration. Hypertension, flushing, diaphoresis, and palpitations may be present in those with a catecholamine-secreting tumor. Patients with a history of chronic diarrhea from vasoactive peptides secreted by the tumor may present with dehydration and electrolyte abnormalities including hypokalemia.[5]

Pertinent Labs

Laboratory studies should include a complete blood count (CBC) due to the potential for blood loss. Anemia is common, occurring in 51% to 74% of children with newly diagnosed neuroblastoma.[10] Neutropenia and thrombocytopenia are also a direct effect of myelosuppression due to cancer, bone marrow involvement, and chemotherapy/radiation.[10] Neutropenia less than 1,000 cells/mm^3 is associated with an increased risk of infection and can be accompanied by fever.[10] Besides chemotherapy and radiation therapy, thrombocytopenia can be caused by tumor invasion in the bone marrow, infection, intravascular coagulation, platelet sequestration or dysfunction, and dilutional thrombocytopenia.[10] Thrombocytopenia less than 40,000 to 50,000 mL^{-1} may require platelet transfusion prior to surgical resection.[10]

Table 111.1	Impact of Anesthetic Agents
International Neuroblastoma Staging System	
Stage	**Definition**
1	Localized tumor with complete gross resection, with or without microscopic residual disease; ipsilateral lymph nodes negative for tumor microscopically
2A	Localized tumor with incomplete gross resection; ipsilateral nonadherent lymph nodes negative for tumor microscopically
2B	Localized tumor with or without complete gross resection; ipsilateral nonadherent lymph nodes positive for tumor. Enlarged contralateral lymph nodes must be negative microscopically
3	Unresectable unilateral tumor infiltrating across the midline, with or without regional lymph node involvement; or localized unilateral tumor with contralateral regional lymph node involvement; or midline tumor with bilateral extension by infiltration (unresectable) or by lymph node involvement
4	Any primary tumor with dissemination to distant lymph nodes, bone, bone marrow, liver, skin and/or other organs (except as defined by stage 4S)
4S	Localized primary tumor (as defined for stage 1, 2A, or 2B), with dissemination limited to skin, liver, and/or bone marrow (limited to infants <1 yr of age and bone marrow with <10% tumor cell involvement)

Source: From Whittle SB, Smith V, Doherty E, et al. Overview and recent advances in the treatment of neuroblastoma. *Expert Rev Anticancer Ther.* 2017;17(4):369–386. doi:10.1080/14737140.2017.1285230.

Table 111.2	International Neuroblastoma Risk Group Staging System
Stage	**Definition**
L1	Localized tumor not involving vital structures as defined by the list of IDRFs[a] and confined to one body compartment
L2	Localized tumor with the presence of one or more IDRFs
M	Metastatic disease (except stage MS)
MS	Metastatic disease in children younger than 18 months of age at diagnosis with metastasis limited to the skin, liver, and/or bone marrow

[a]IDRF: Ipsilateral tumor extension within two body compartments: neck and chest; chest and abdomen; abdomen and pelvis. Infiltration of adjacent organs/structures: pericardium, diaphragm, kidney, liver, duodenopancreatic block, and mesentery. Encasement of major vessels by tumor: vertebral artery, internal jugular vein, subclavian vessels, carotid artery, aorta, vena cava, major thoracic vessels, branches of superior mesenteric artery at its root and the celiac axis, and iliac vessels. Compression of trachea or central bronchi. Encasement of brachial plexus. Infiltration of portohepatic or hepatoduodenal ligament. Infiltration of the costovertebral junction between T9 and T12. Tumor crossing the sciatic notch. Tumor invading renal pedicle. Extension of tumor to base of skull. Intraspinal tumor extension invading more than one third of the spinal cord, leptomeningeal space is obliterated, or spinal cord, magnetic resonance imaging (MRI) signal is abnormal.[2]

IDRFs, image-defined risk factors.

Source: Modified from Dasgupta R, Billmire D, Aldrink JH, Meyers RL. What is new in pediatric surgical oncology? *Curr Opin Pediatr.* 2017;29(1):3–11. doi:10.1097/MOP.0000000000000439.

BOX 111.1 KEY ASSESSMENT POINTS

Signs/Symptoms
- Abdominal mass
- Anorexia/weight loss
- Fever
- Vomiting, diarrhea
- Abdominal tenderness
- Hypertension
- Bone/joint pain
- Proptosis and periorbital ecchymosis

BOX 111.2 PREOPERATIVE LABS

- Hemoglobin
- Hematocrit
- Platelet count
- Absolute neutrophil count
- Electrolyte panel
- PT/PTT/INR
- Liver function: AST, ALT, albumin
- Renal function: BUN, serum creatinine

ALT, alanine aminotransferase; AST, aspartate aminotransferase; BUN, blood urea nitrogen; INR, international normalized ratio; PT, prothrombin time; PTT, partial thromboplastin time.

Platelet count should be rechecked post-transfusion. In children, 10 mL/kg platelets should increase the platelet count by 50,000 to 100,000 mL^{-1}. In those with a normal platelet count and no history of bleeding, preoperative coagulation studies may not be necessary. However, if significant blood loss is likely, they may be beneficial.

Patients with adrenal or renal tumor involvement should have a preoperative serum chemistry, creatinine, and blood urea nitrogen.[11] Neuroblastoma patients can have hypercalcemia. Tumor lysis syndrome can cause hyperkalemia, hyperphosphatemia, and hypocalcemia.[12] Hepatic and renal function tests are routinely monitored during cancer therapy, and recent results should be reviewed. Blood urea nitrogen and serum creatinine should be examined in patients with possible renal or ureteral compression to rule out acute renal dysfunction.[12]

The presence of increased urinary catecholamines indicates excess neurohumoral production and can result in intraoperative hypertension in 25% of patients.[5] Patients with catecholamine-secreting neuroblastomas should have preoperative alpha-adrenergic and beta-adrenergic blockade to avoid blood pressure lability during intraoperative tumor manipulation.[5] A recent ECG, as well as any pertinent pulmonary test results, should be readily available.

Preoperative imaging is vital to surgical preparation and determination of the approach technique. Imaging provides the position and size of the tumor as well as information regarding extension into surrounding vascular structures, lymph nodes, soft tissue, or organs.[13]

PREOPERATIVE PHARMACOLOGY

Corticosteroid therapy is commonly incorporated into many treatment protocols for cancer. They are utilized for their antiemetic, cytotoxic, and immunosuppressive properties.[8] Anesthesia providers should continue corticosteroid therapy perioperatively, with stress-dose steroids often recommended preoperatively to patients who have received high-dose steroids within the past 2 months.[9] Due to their tumor and immune suppression effects, however, perioperative administration of steroids should be discussed with the oncology team prior to administration.

Neuroblastomas, like pheochromocytomas, arise from neural crest cells and may be catecholamine secreting. Patients presenting with hypertension should be screened for increased levels of serum or urine catecholamines or their metabolites. Hypertension can also be caused by renal artery compression from the tumor itself. Patients with neuroblastoma, hypertension, and elevated catecholamine levels may require preoperative blood pressure control similar to the management of pheochromocytoma.[5] Combined alpha- and beta-adrenergic blockade to control blood pressure and heart rate and prevent intraoperative hypertensive crisis is typically achieved with phenoxybenzamine and labetolol.[14]

ANESTHETIC TECHNIQUE

Surgical approach for neuroblastoma will depend on tumor location and presence of IDRFs. Abdominal tumors may be excised via laparotomy, either from a suprapubic transverse approach or median umbilical, while others may require a retroperitoneal approach. Minimally invasive surgery (MIS) has been found to be feasible and safe in pediatric patients with malignant abdominal tumors.[15] MIS has many advantages over traditional open surgery, such as reduction in postoperative pain, decreased hospital stay, smaller incision, and reduced surgical complications.[15] Laparoscopic MIS is also feasible and effective for initial diagnostic exploration, allowing for tumor biopsy under direct visualization and adequate tissue procurement for diagnostic and prognostic analysis.[16] Laparotomy is preferred if complete resection of the tumor is uncertain or when vascular control may be difficult.[17]

Children with adrenal neuroblastoma may require an adrenalectomy. Depending on tumor size and vascular involvement, this may be performed either laparoscopically or open. Benefits of laparoscopic approach include smaller incision with clear visualization of anatomic structures, less trauma, and faster postoperative recovery with reduced hospitalization time.[13] However, if the tumor is found to surround or infiltrate important blood vessels or organs, ruptures intraoperatively, or severe hemorrhage or organ damage occurs, the procedure may need to be converted to open laparotomy.[13] Open laparotomy is often technically more difficult since the adrenal gland is located in the retroperitoneum. Tumor recurrence and 5-year survival rates were found to be similar in either approach.[13]

For thoracic neuroblastoma, a thoracotomy may be required. A minimally invasive approach to excise neuroblastomas located in the thorax may also be utilized. Lateral thoracotomy and median sternotomy are the most common approaches to mediastinal masses.[18] Patients with intraspinal lesions may require neurosurgical resection via laminoplasty. Intraspinal extension of the tumor occupying more than one third of the spinal canal is considered an IDRF.[19] Signs of neurological impairment including motor deficit, neurogenic bladder, and paraplegia may be present preoperatively. Surgical decompression of the spine with laminectomy prior to chemotherapy and surgical resection of the tumor may be needed.

Intraoperative Management

General anesthesia (GA) with endotracheal intubation and control of ventilation with standard anesthetic monitors is required for excision of neuroblastoma. The addition of arterial or central venous access is dependent on the extent of tumor size and location, anticipated blood loss, the presence of catecholamine-secreting tumor, and hemodynamic involvement. Large-bore peripheral IV access, fluid warmers, and preparation of blood products for transfusion should be obtained for potential massive blood loss. IV catheters should be placed in the upper extremities if possible, especially if there is tumor involvement of the inferior vena cava and the possible need for cross-clamping to avoid large blood loss. Rapid sequence induction may be warranted for young infants with a large abdominal mass and subsequent increased intra-abdominal pressure. Neuromuscular blockade is recommended to facilitate surgical exposure in abdominal cases but may need to be avoided if somatosensory and

---

BOX 111.3 CLINICAL PEARLS: NEUROBLASTOMA RESECTION

- The addition of a caudal, lumbar, or thoracic epidural for postoperative pain relief is recommended.
- While there is no evidence to support the use of regional anesthesia over GA, the addition of a neuraxial block may mitigate the neuroendocrine response to surgical stress associated with immune system suppression and a heightened risk of infection.[20]
- Combined GA and epidural analgesia for pediatric oncological surgery allows for decreased use of opioids and/or volatile anesthetics and may help lessen the immunological and inflammatory stress response. Nonetheless, this approach has not yet been found to reduce metastasis rates.[21]

GA, general anesthesia.

BOX 111.4 COMPLICATIONS/EMERGENCIES

- Intraoperative hemorrhage
- Tumor rupture
- Vascular injury
- Damage to surrounding organs, such as kidneys, ureters, or diaphragm
- Air embolism (laparoscopic approach)
- SC emphysema (laparoscopic approach)

Source: From Yao W, Dong K, Li K, et al. Comparison of long-term prognosis of laparoscopic and open adrenalectomy for local adrenal neuroblastoma in children. Pediatr Surg Int. 2018;34(8):851–856. doi:10.1007/s00383-018-4294-5.

motor evoked potential monitoring is planned. Insertion of an orogastric or nasogastric tube for stomach decompression prior to resection, especially with the laparoscopic approach, is recommended. Urinary catheter placement is typically performed.

Strict aseptic technique is vital in all cancer patients especially if currently neutropenic, as immunocompromised patients are at high risk of postoperative infection. This includes line placement, medication administration, strict adherence to medication expiration times (especially for propofol), avoidance of the administration of rectal medications, and assurance of appropriate perioperative protective isolation if necessary. Prophylactic antibiotics should be administered at least 30 minutes prior to skin incision.

The potential for significant intraoperative blood loss and need for replacement should be anticipated. Compression from the tumor may cause venous obstruction, and in advanced stages, hepatic enlargement, making the potential for massive rapid blood loss a significant risk.[9] Significant hypotension may occur after tumor removal necessitating fluid administration and an alpha-adrenergic agonist, such as phenylephrine. While uncommon, severe intraoperative hypertension from catecholamine-secreting neuroblastomas has been reported.[22-24] Labetolol is effective in treating intraoperative hypertension from tumor manipulation but may cause paroxysmal hypertension and heart failure in patients who did not receive preoperative alpha-adrenergic blockade.[5] To help maintain euvolemia and hemodynamic stability throughout the surgical procedure, third-space losses can be replaced with 5% albumin.

Special Techniques and/or Equipment
Excision of cervicothoracic or mediastinal tumors may require a double lumen endotracheal tube (ETT) or a single-lumen ETT with a bronchial blocker for intubation if surgical approach is via thoracotomy.[25] Neural monitoring may be required for tumors located near nerve roots and for laminoplasty.

POSTOPERATIVE CARE
Following neuroblastoma excision, patients should be extubated at the completion of surgery as long as there were no intraoperative complications or excessive blood loss and fluid replacement. Routine postoperative care and hospital admission for pain control are expected. Follow-up by the pain management team for epidural infusion or patient-controlled IV analgesia is recommended for nonlaparoscopic procedures. Postoperative hematocrit, venous or arterial blood gas, and chest x-ray are routine. Patients typically stay hospitalized for a few days or until they have sufficient pain control and have returned to full oral intake.

KEY REFERENCES
Complete references for this chapter are online and available at https://connect.springerpub.com/content/book/978-0-8261-3875-0/part/part04/toc-part/ch111.

2. Dasgupta R, Billmire D, Aldrink JH, Meyers RL. What is new in pediatric surgical oncology? *Curr Opin Pediatr.* 2017;29(1):3–11. doi:10.1097/MOP.0000000000000439
3. Whittle SB, Smith V, Doherty E, et al. Overview and recent advances in the treatment of neuroblastoma. *Expert Rev Anticancer Ther.* 2017;17(4):369–386. doi:10.1080/14737140.2017.1285230
5. Hansen TG, Henneberg SW, Lerman J. General abdominal and urologic surgery. In: Cote C, Lerman J, Anderson B, eds. *A Practice of Anesthesia for Infants and Children.* 6th ed. Elsevier; 2019:669–689.
7. Latham GJ. Anesthesia for the child with cancer. *Anesthesiol Clin.* 2014;32(1):185–213. doi:10.1016/j.anclin.2013.10.002
8. Latham GJ, Greenberg RS. Anesthetic considerations for the pediatric oncology patient-part 1: a review of antitumor therapy. *Paediatr Anaesth.* 2010;20(4):295–304. doi:10.1111/j.1460-9592.2010.03257.x
10. Latham GJ, Greenberg RS. Anesthetic considerations for the pediatric oncology patient-part 2: systems-based approach to anesthesia. *Paediatr Anaesth.* 2010;20(5):396–420. doi:10.1111/j.1460-9592.2010.03260.x
12. Latham GJ, Greenberg RS. Anesthetic considerations for the pediatric oncology patient-part 3: pain, cognitive dysfunction, and preoperative evaluation. *Paediatr Anaesth.* 2010;20(6):479–489. doi:10.1111/j.1460-9592.2010.03261.x

SECTION L: Genitourinary Procedures

CHAPTER 112

Circumcision

Dawn Elizabeth Bent and Sharifah Wilson

INDICATIONS/CONTRAINDICATIONS

While rates vary according to geographic area, socioeconomic status, religious affiliation, insurance coverage, hospital type, and racial and ethnic group, it is estimated that approximately 80% of males in the United States are circumcised (Box 112.1). The prevalence of circumcision makes it one of the most commonly performed genitourinary procedures among male pediatric patients. Multiple techniques can be utilized to perform a circumcision, which entails the surgical excision of the foreskin or prepuce from the tip of the penis.[1] A variety of special devices, such as the Gomco clamp, Plastibell, and Mogen clamp, are commonly used with infant patients, and the Shang clamp is frequently employed for adult males requiring circumcision.[2] Additionally, the procedure can be performed utilizing a freehand, dorsal slit, or sleeve surgical technique, with the dorsal slit technique being the preferred approach in patients with phimosis or paraphimosis.

The dorsal slit technique involves identification of the corona of the glans, followed by a surgical excision extending 75% of the distance from the meatal opening to the corona. The preputial skin is then be held perpendicular from the shaft of the penis and excised at its base. After first reapproximating the frenulum, the remaining cut edges of the foreskin are closed with multiple sutures. Cauterization may be required to control bleeding.[1]

The United States is the only country in the developed world where the majority of male infants are circumcised for nonreligious reasons. Symptomatic changes in the foreskin, such as pain, redness, and swelling commonly lead parents to seek medical attention.[4] Indications for circumcision include pathological phimosis, balanitis xerotica obliterans (BXO), and paraphimosis. With phimosis, the preputial opening is too narrow, thereby preventing exposure of the glans.[2] If untreated, scarring may ensure, which may further restrict the opening of the preputial ring.[2] BXO is a chronic disease that results in progressive sclerosing inflammatory dermatosis of the glans penis, foreskin, and at times the urethra. The sclerotic changes secondary to BXO result in meatal stenosis, urethral stricture, recurrent urinary tract infections, and urinary retention prompting medical intervention.[2] Paraphimosis is a rare occurrence where the foreskin remains stuck in the retracted position resulting in painful constriction of the glans.[5] Paraphimosis is considered a true urological emergency.[3,5]

Contraindications to circumcision can be either absolute or relative. Absolute contraindications include prematurity, anomalies of the penis, such as epispadias and hypospadias, congenital megaprepuce, chordee of the penile shaft, and penoscrotal webbing.[3] Relative contraindications include buried penis, jaundice, and patients with any bleeding diathesis.[3] While medical indications for circumcision require that a surgeon performs the procedure under some form of anesthesia, the procedure may be performed by a community leader from a mosque or synagogue if being done for cultural or religious reasons.[2] It is imperative, however, that patients with bleeding diathesis only have their circumcision performed by a surgeon.[3]

ANESTHETIC MANAGEMENT

PREOPERATIVE EVALUATION

The preoperative evaluation for circumcision is summarized in Box 112.2.

PREOPERATIVE PHARMACOLOGY

It is important to assess the child's mental health during the preoperative period. The pediatric patient requiring surgery may exhibit separation anxiety, general anxiety, and fear and it is not uncommon for a child older than 1 year to require an anxiolytic medication preoperatively.[6] The most common anxiolytic premedication used is oral midazolam, with doses ranging from 0.25 to 0.75 mg/kg.[6] Commonly employed premedications are listed in Appendix C, "Preoperative Pharmacology."

BOX 112.1 SPECIAL CONSIDERATIONS AND CONCERNS

- There is much debate about the risk and benefit of routine circumcision in infant males.
- The American College of Obstetricians and Gynecologists reports a reduced risk of urinary tract infections, HIV, sexually transmitted disease, and penile carcinomas in the circumcised male.

Source: From Prabhakaran S, Ljuhar D, Coleman R, et al. Circumcision in the paediatric patient: a review of indications, technique and complications. *J Paediatr Child Health.* 2018;54(12):1299–1307. doi:10.1111/jpc.14206.

BOX 112.2 KEY ASSESSMENT POINTS

- Birth history
- Health history (respiratory health high importance)
- Patient anesthesia history
- Family history of problems with anesthesia
- Surgical history
- Any history of bleeding disorders or clotting abnormalities
- History of familial bleeding disorders
- NPO status
- Allergies and any medications

Pertinent Labs

Laboratory work is not routinely ordered prior to a circumcision, however, checking a hemoglobin level may be indicated in the preterm neonate and infants under the age of 6 months.[7] Clotting studies should be collected when indicated by patient medical history.[7]

ANESTHETIC TECHNIQUE

Intraoperative Management

There is no gold standard regarding anesthesia for circumcision, as various anesthetic techniques can be employed, including local, regional, and/or general anesthesia (GA; Box 112.3).[4] A discussion regarding the patient's plan of care should occur between the anesthesia and surgical teams prior to the start of the procedure to help guide development of the anesthetic plan. When choosing an anesthetic plan, the patient's history, duration of surgical procedure, and the risk of anesthesia to the patient should be considered.[8] The most common anesthetic for circumcision is GA with a laryngeal mask airway (LMA) and a dorsal penile nerve block (DPNB).[7]

The DPNB is usually performed by the surgeon given the proximity of the block site to the surgical field. Surgeons may prefer to perform the DPNB following completion of the procedure to prevent distortion of the surgical field.[1] The surgeon may also perform a ring block in conjunction with the DPNB to optimize pain control as the DPNB may fail to anesthetize the ventral aspect of the penis.[8] Should the plan be to perform DPNB at the end of the procedure, it is important an adequate depth of anesthesia be achieved prior to surgical incision or stimulation to prevent a laryngospasm. Additional common analgesic interventions include morphine (0.05–0.1 mg/kg IV), ketorolac (0.5 mg/kg IV), acetaminophen preoperatively (10–15 mg/kg orally or 30–40 mg/kg rectally), and acetaminophen (10–15 mg/kg IV intraoperatively).[4] At the end of the procedure, a compression dressing may be placed on the penis to aid in hemostasis. If there are no contraindications, a deep emergence may help prevent postoperative complications, such as bleeding due to agitation and pain.[8]

Special techniques are summarized in Box 112.4.

Complications

About 0.5% of cases with postoperative bleeding return to the operating room.[2] While rare, undiagnosed coagulation disorders may result in intraoperative blood loss requiring resuscitation or the need to transfer blood products.[7]

BOX 112.3 COMMON ANESTHETIC TECHNIQUES

- GA with LMA
- GA with ETT
- GA with LMA and DPNB
- GA with ETT and DPNB
- GA with LMA and caudal epidural

DPNB, dorsal penile nerve block; ETT, endotracheal tube; GA, general anesthesia; LMA, laryngeal mask airway.

Source: From Cafer A, Kucukosman G, Ozkocak-Turan I. Anesthesia methods used by anesthetic specialists for circumcision cases. *Saudi Med J.* 2017;38(1):75–81. doi:10.15537/smj.2017.1.15632.

BOX 112.4 REGIONAL ANESTHESIA TECHNIQUES FOR CIRCUMCISION

DPNB: commonly performed at the surgical field by surgeon and provides good analgesia[8]

- **Position:** supine position (subpubic approach)[9]
- **Equipment:** syringe, short-bevel 23-gauge needle and 30 mm length, local (bupivacaine 0.25%–0.5% or ropivacaine 0.2%) without epinephrine due to terminal dorsal penial arteries.[9] Dose is typically 0.1 mL/kg with a max dose of 5 mL per side.[9]
- **Technique:** The lateral sides of the penis are marked just below both pubic ramus (0.5 cm for infants and 1 cm for children).[9] Penis is held downward, and the needle is directed slightly medial and caudal during insertion.[9] When the needle passes through the Scarpa's fascia, there is a notable "pop."[9]
- **Complications:** Bleeding and hematomas are the most common complications associated with penile nerve blocks.[9] When giving local, it is important to know the correct dosing as local toxicity is always a possible complication.[9]

Caudal epidural anesthesia: most frequently used regional anesthetic in pediatrics[10]

- **Position:** lateral decubitus or prone with small roll for placement under iliac crest[10]
- **Equipment:** IV needle, IV catheter[10]
- **Technique:** Locate the posterior superior iliac spine. Palpate the cornu of the sacral hiatus.[10] Advance needle about 45 degrees until a "pop" is detected as the needle is inserted into the sacrococcygeal ligament.[10] Once in the ligament, the needle angle at the skin is positioned parallel to the sacrum and needle or catheter is advanced within the caudal canal in a cephalad direction.[10] Local of choice is injected.
- **Complications:** Possible complications include cardiac arrest following intravascular or intraosseous injection, infection, neural injury, and hematoma.[10] Patients may experience delayed and lower extremity movement and urinary retention.[10]

DPNB, dorsal penile nerve block.

Postoperatively, the patient may need to return to the operating room to resolve a host of potential complications, such as a trapped penis, redundant foreskin, recurrent phimosis, preputial adhesions, meatal stenosis, urethrocutaneous fistula, or glandular necrosis.[2]

POSTOPERATIVE CARE

Postoperatively, the patient is transferred to the postanesthesia care unit (PACU) for further care. Care in the PACU focuses on ensuring respiratory and hemodynamic stability, as well as ensuring the patient has adequate analgesia. Prior to discharge, it is important that the patient's parents understand the postoperative instructions relating to care of the surgical site as offered by the surgeon.

CASE STUDY: Circumcision With a Laryngeal Mask Airway and Dorsal Penile Nerve Block

CLINICAL SCENARIO

An 11-month-old infant boy weighing 13 kg is scheduled for a circumcision with general anesthesia. Prior to surgery, anesthesia consent was obtained, however, caudal epidural was refused by the parents.

APPROACHES TO CARE

Anesthesia is induced with a combination of inhaled nitrous/oxygen/sevoflurane. Once asleep, a 22-gauge IV line is placed in patient's hand and 35 mg of propofol is administered. An LMA #2 is inserted without difficulty and the patient is maintained inhaled sevoflurane and 30% FiO_2. A multimodal approach to pain management is utilized, consisting of 130 mg of IV acetaminophen and 6.5 mg of ketorolac. Following completion of the procedure, the surgeon performs a DPNB with 6 mL of 0.25% bupivacaine. A compression dressing is applied, and the patient is placed on 100% FiO_2. A deep emergence is performed with the LMA removed without incident. The patient is transported to PACU with 6 L of oxygen delivered via a Mapleson. There were no complications and no pain noted in PACU.

REFERENCES

1. Wang X, Dong C, Beeko D, et al. Dorsal penile nerve block via perineal approach, an alternative to a caudal block for pediatric circumcision: a randomized controlled trial. *J BioMed Res.* 2019;2019:1–7. doi:10.1155/2019/6875756
2. Chan I, Wong K. Common urological problems in children: prepuce, phimosis, and buried penis. *Hong Kong Med J.* 2016;22(3):263–269. doi:10.12809/hkmj154645
3. Prabhakaran S, Ljuhar D, Coleman R, Nataraja R. Circumcision in the paediatric patient: a review of indications, technique and complications. *J Paediatr Child Health.* 2018;54(12):1299–1307. doi:10.1111/jpc.14206
4. Nguyen T, Kraft E, Nasrawi Z, et al. Avoidance of general anesthesia for circumcision in infants under 6 months of age using a modified Plastibell technique. *Pediat Surg Int.* 2019;35(5):619–623. doi:10.1007/s00383-019-04452-x
5. Bragg B, Leslie S. Paraphimosis. In: *StatPearls*. StatPearls Publishing; 2020.
6. Dave NM. Premedication and induction of anaesthesia in paediatric patients. *Indian J Anaesth.* 2019;63(9):713–720. doi:10.4103/ija.IJA_491_19
7. Eroglu E, Sozmen BO, Kayiran SM, et al. Evaluation of coagulation tests before newborn circumcision: is it necessary? *Blood Coagul Fibrinolysis.* 2016;27(2):160–162. doi:10.1097/MBC.0000000000000399
8. Cafer A, Kucukosman G, Ozkocak-Turan I. Anesthesia methods used by anesthetic specialists for circumcision cases. *Saudi Med J.* 2017;38(1):75–81. doi:10.15537/smj.2017.1.15632
9. Mcphee AS, McKay AC. Dorsal penile nerve block. In: *Statpearls*. Statpearls Publishing; 2019
10. Wiegele M, Marhofer P, Lonnqvist A. Caudal epidural blocks in paediatric patients: a review and practical considerations. *Br J Anaesth.* 2019;122(4):509–517. doi:10.1016/j.bja.2018.11.30

CHAPTER 113

Hypospadias Repair

Megan Gdowski, Renee Pederson, and Audrey Rosenblatt

INDICATIONS/CONTRAINDICATIONS

Hypospadias is a congenital anomaly in which the opening of the urethral meatus is malpositioned along the ventral side of the penis.[1] Hypospadias is the second-most common genitourinary congenital anomalies in males, affecting nearly 1 in every 200 to 300 male newborns.[2] The preoperative meatal position is used to classify the type and severity of hypospadias, of which there are three general categories: distal/anterior, middle/midshaft, and proximal/posterior.[3] Nearly all variants of hypospadias are associated with chordee or a downward curvature of the penis.

The more proximal the location of the urethral meatus, the more significant the degree of chordee.[4] Distal hypospadias (**Figure 113.1**) is the most common and most mild form of the defect accounting for 70% of all cases.[5] With a distal hypospadias, the meatus is found just below the rounded end, or glans, of the penis. A middle or midshaft hypospadias (**Figure 113.2**)

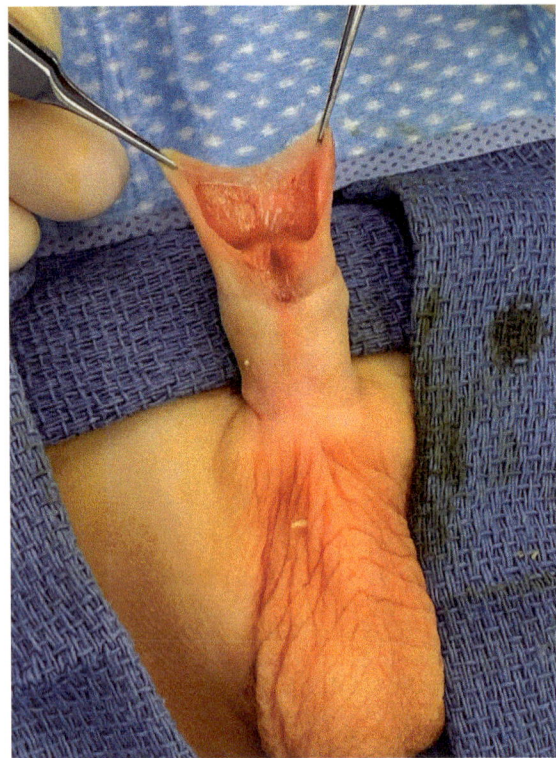

Figure 113.1: Distal hypospadias.

Source: Courtesy of Edward Gong, MD, Lurie Children's Hospital of Chicago.

occurs when the urethral meatus is found along the middle to lower portion of the shaft of the penis. Proximal hypospadias, the most severe manifestation, occurs when the meatus is located at the scrotum or perineum. Proximal hypospadias is often associated with inguinal hernia, cryptorchidism, and other renal anomalies.[6,7] The complexity of the proximal

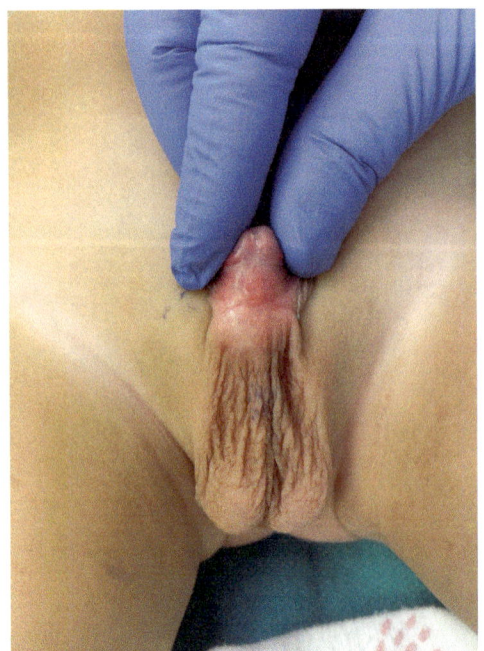

Figure 113.2: Middle or midshaft hypospadias.

Source: Courtesy of Edward Gong, MD, Lurie Children's Hospital of Chicago.

hypospadias may require an endocrine evaluation to rule out disorders of sex development as well as a genetics consultation to investigate chromosomal anomalies.[6] Hypospadias is generally diagnosed at birth and surgical correction, if indicated, should be completed within the first 2 years of life.[8]

The goals of surgical hypospadias repair are the achievement of desired cosmetic appearance, and functional urinary and reproductive health.[6] Concerns considered when repairing hypospadias include abnormal urinary stream, curvature causing difficulty with intercourse, fertility issues secondary to impaired sperm deposition, and dissatisfaction with penile appearance.[2] Resolving chordee and reconstructing the urethra to the tip of the penis facilitate a controlled stream of urinary and ejaculative flow.[4] In some cases of distal hypospadias with straight urinary stream and mild to no chordee present, repair may be performed by choice for cosmetic reasons rather than functional improvement.

The main components of a hypospadias repair include correction of chordee, urethroplasty, glanuloplasty, and skin coverage.[4] Chordee is addressed by performing a penoplasty, which excises chordee and straightens the penis. Urethroplasty reconstructs the urethra to promote forward flow of urine and semen.[6] Glanuloplasty is often coupled with meatoplasty to create a new urethral opening and make the glans more cone shaped. Finally, skin coverage with or without grafts may be necessary to close the surgical site. Many surgical techniques exist to facilitate repair; however, the three most commonly performed techniques include tubularized incised plate urethroplasty (TIP), transverse preputial island flap (TPIF), and inner preputial inlay or buccal mucosa graft.[4,6] The surgical approach varies by severity of underlying defect and degree of chordee and can be performed in one-stage or two-stage procedures. A decision to perform a single or staged procedure depends on the degree of curvature and the health of the urethral plate or tissues that would have normally created the urethra.[6] A two-staged approach is usually necessary if the defect requires an incision in the urethral plate for chordee correction, which is then followed by the urethroplasty at a later date.[4] A staged repair is most often seen with a proximal hypospadias. See Table 113.1 for details on surgical techniques.

Complication rates are related to the degree of hypospadias and complexity of repair.[9,10] Notable complications following repair include bleeding or hematoma formation, wound infection, skin and flap necrosis, urethral stricture formation, urethrocutaneous fistula formation, meatal or urethral stenosis, cosmetic dissatisfaction, and voiding dysfunction.[11] Glans dehiscence is the most common short-term complication seen after urethroplasty repair, attributed to tension at the closure site or pressure from a urethral stent or urinary catheter.[4] The more common long-term complications include urethral fistula and stricture formation.[6] These rarely resolve on their own and often require surgical intervention. Although surgical approach may vary, anesthetic management for this wide variety of surgical techniques is remarkably uniform.

ANESTHETIC MANAGEMENT

PREOPERATIVE EVALUATION

Children presenting for hypospadias repair are usually 6 to 18 months of age and often otherwise healthy. The preoperative assessment includes a routine review of systems, as well as any notable events during the perinatal period. Unless the patient has associated medical conditions, preoperative labs

Table 113.1	Surgical Techniques for Hypospadias Repair		
	TIP	**TPIF**	**Inner Preputial Inlay Graft or Buccal Mucosa Graft**
Indications	• Distal and midshaft hypospadias • Little to no ventral curvature • Healthy and adequately sized urethral plate • Most commonly performed procedure	• Midshaft hypospadias with less than 30-degree curvature but urethral plate too narrow • Proximal hypospadias and second-stage repairs • Ventral components of penis (foreskin, urethral plate) are deficient enough to necessitate additional tissue	• Same as TPIF • Redo procedures • Often used when there is poor blood supply to local tissues or deficiency of local skin flaps to use
Method	• Neourethra is translocated to the tip of the glans to create an orthoptic neomeatus	• Urethral plate is preserved as the posterior urethral wall • Flap from inner preputial skin along native blood supply is used to create the anterior wall of neourethra • Native blood supply remains intact	• Tissue removed from donor site inner prepuce or buccal mucosa and transferred to host bed where revascularization is required

TIP, tubularized incised plate urethroplasty; TPIF, transverse preputial island flap.

Sources: From Daboos M, Helal AA, Salama A. Five years' experience of double faced tubularized preputial flap for penoscrotal hypospadias repair in pediatrics. *J Pediatr Urol.* 2020;16(5):673.e1–673.e7. doi:10.1016/j.jpurol.2020.07.037; Loloi J, Harrington S, Boltz S, Decter RM. Ingrafts in hypospadias surgery: longer-term outcomes. *Journal of pediatric urology.* 2020;16(5):555.e1–555.e5. doi:10.1016/j.jpurol.2020.04.030.

are generally not needed. Box 113.1 includes a general summary of considerations for hypospadias repair.

Key Assessment Points

There are three key areas of focus when organizing the anesthetic plan for hypospadias repair.

Anatomy of Sacral Spine

If a caudal epidural block is planned, the sacral spine must be evaluated for the presence of sacral dimple or an abnormal gluteal crease. Sacral dimples are estimated to be present in 2% to 4% of all newborn infants.[12] This is of significance because on rare occasions, sacral dimples are associated with underlying occult incomplete spinal fusion, such as tethered cord, spinal cord lipoma, dermal sinus tract, lipomyelomeningocele, and diastematomyelia.[13] Although these assessments are often done by the pediatrician during routine childhood assessments and the surgeon during a presurgical consultation, the anesthesia provider should perform their own assessment during physician examination. A simple sacral dimple, defined as midline less than 5 mm in diameter and less than 25 mm from the anus, has a less than 0.34% probability of an underlying occult spinal dysraphism.[14] Lesions located entirely within the gluteal crease are much less likely to be contiguous with the dura and often found to be a normal variant. Concern is raised when accompanied by skin stigmata, such as a sacral hair patch, hemangioma, or atypical sacral dimple.[13]

Recent or Current Upper Respiratory Infection

The presence of an upper respiratory infection (URI) may place the child at an increased risk of perioperative respiratory adverse events.[15] While timely repair is required to achieve typical cosmetic appearance and functional urinary and

---

BOX 113.1   CONSIDERATIONS FOR HYPOSPADIAS REPAIR

- Intubation and controlled ventilation
  - Length of procedure
  - Spontaneous ventilation increases the movement of penis due to abdominal movement; surgeons may prefer or request positive pressure ventilation
- Preferred age for repair is 6–18 months
- Penile tourniquets are used to decrease surgical bleeding—low risk of hemorrhage
- Standard anesthesia concerns for young child apply
  - Postextubation croup
  - NPO times
  - Warming measures
- Buccal mucosa grafting requires oral cavity access
  - Obtained from either cheek or upper/lower lip
- Operative time dependent on hypospadias variant.
- Placement of postoperative urinary stent or catheter
  - Distal urethral repair—urinary stent or catheter omitted
  - Proximal and midshaft repair—urinary stent or catheter placed
    - Windowed double diaper to prevent fecal contamination of surgical site
- Urethral instrumentation or catheterization (if needed) should be performed by urology in the postsurgical period due to concerns for repair integrity

reproductive health, repair may be safely delayed until the risk of bronchial hyperreactivity has resolved.[16] Particularly, given a typical patient's young age, duration of procedure, and need for intubation, it may be prudent to postpone surgical intervention. Hallmarks of URI, such as cough, fever, malaise, and the presence of increased nasal mucous production in the week leading up to surgery, and acute signs of URI on physical examination, such as wheezing, rhonchi, productive cough, and lethargy, are indicators to delay the surgical procedure.[16] See Chapter 3, "Preoperative Evaluation and Testing" for additional information regarding URI assessment and when to reschedule surgery.

Bleeding or Clotting Disorders

Hypospadias is not associated with coagulopathies beyond the risk in the general population, but anytime neuraxial anesthesia is performed, a careful history of bleeding or clotting disorders should be performed. Patients with known coagulopathies will need presurgical clearance and management recommendations from their hematologist. For hypospadias repair, this should include consideration of the risks and benefits when planning caudal block and neuraxial anesthesia.

PREOPERATIVE PHARMACOLOGY

While infants and toddlers will not recall surgery, children older than age 1 are more prone to separation anxiety and may benefit from a sedative premedication with a primary goal of anxiolysis. It is important to note that some hypospadias repairs may be completed in a series of staged procedures, requiring the child to return for a second completion surgery. Anesthesia providers should consider the use of an anxiolytic to facilitate stress reduction and promote a positive patient experience. Frequently used anxiolytics include midazolam (oral or intranasal administration) or dexmedetomidine (intranasal administration). If clonidine is a planned additive to the neuraxial block, appreciate the compounding sedative effects of premedication.

ANESTHETIC TECHNIQUE

INTRAOPERATIVE MANAGEMENT

General anesthesia is required for hypospadias repair and is typically maintained with the volatile anesthetic agent sevoflurane. Following induction of anesthesia, the airway can be managed via tracheal intubation or placement of a laryngeal mask airway. Placement of an endotracheal tube should be considered if there is a potential need for access to the oral cavity for a buccal mucosa graft.

Caudal epidural blockade is the predominant regional anesthesia technique and the routine practice of many anesthesia providers.[11] In recent years, there has been concern that caudal anesthesia during hypospadias repair increases the risk of surgical complications, however, this has been steadily refuted in the literature by multiple retrospective reviews of males undergoing hypospadias repair reporting that common anesthetic techniques have minimal impact on perioperative complications.[11,17-19] Regional anesthetic adjuncts allow for opioid-free or opioid-sparing anesthesia techniques and enhanced and extended pain relief in the postoperative period.[21] Caudal epidural blockade may be performed as a single injection preprocedure, postprocedure, or both depending on the length of the surgical procedure.[21]

Table 113.2 Local Anesthetic for Caudal Blockade

Local Anesthetic	Caudal to Level T10	Caudal to Level T6
Bupivacaine 0.125%	0.5 mL/kg	1 mL/kg
Bupivacaine 0.25%		
Ropivacaine 0.1%		
Ropivacaine 0.2%		

Special considerations:
- Use of local anesthetic at lower concentrations decreases occurrence of motor blockade while providing adequate sensory blockade
- Addition of clonidine (1–2 mcg/mL) may extend duration of action upward of 3 hours

Caudal blockade is very safe with low incidence of complications.[22] Rare complications include neurological sequelae (incidence of 2.4:10,000) and local anesthetic systemic toxicity (incidence of 0.76:10,000) with three of seven overall occurrences being related to single-shot caudal blocks.[22] For long-duration procedures, placement of a caudal catheter allows for repeated epidural dosing. There are no differences in complication rates for either repeated single-injection caudal blocks or catheter placement.[22] See Table 113.2 for a guide to local anesthetic choices.

If neuraxial anesthesia is contraindicated, other regional anesthetics to consider include dorsal penile nerve block (DPNB) or pudendal nerve block. The use of alternative blocks may warrant opioid use for procedural analgesia as blockade of the dorsal penis nerves with the DPNB does not anesthetize the ventrum of the penis, scrotum, or perineum.[23] In addition, these authors observe surgeon preference at their institution to perform DPNB only at the end of the procedure necessitating IV opioid administration for surgical analgesia. Surgical correction commonly requires degloving the penis to complete repair, which can increase the vascular uptake of the local anesthetic from a penile block, particularly since epinephrine must be avoided.

POSTOPERATIVE CARE

At the conclusion of the surgical procedure, the penis will be wrapped with a mildly compressive dressing to control swelling and promote hemostasis.[4] A urinary stent or catheter is typically placed for procedures involving middle shaft and proximal hypospadias (Figures 113.3 and 113.4). This aids in urethral healing and prevents urinary retention and may remain in place for up to 2 weeks.

Depending on the severity of hypospadias and complexity of the surgical procedure, repair may be completed as a same-day outpatient surgery or may warrant short-stay admission for observation. In the postoperative period, anticipate the need for additional analgesia as the regional anesthetic block recedes. Surgeons may prescribe oral hydrocodone/acetaminophen for postoperative pain. However, alternating oral acetaminophen and ibuprofen is common practice. IV or oral ketorolac use is surgeon dependent. Bladder relaxants, such as oxybutynin, may be prescribed for children who are toilet trained. The use of postoperative antibiotics while a urinary stent or catheter is in place is no longer customary as recent studies are unclear about antibiotics providing proven benefit.[4,20]

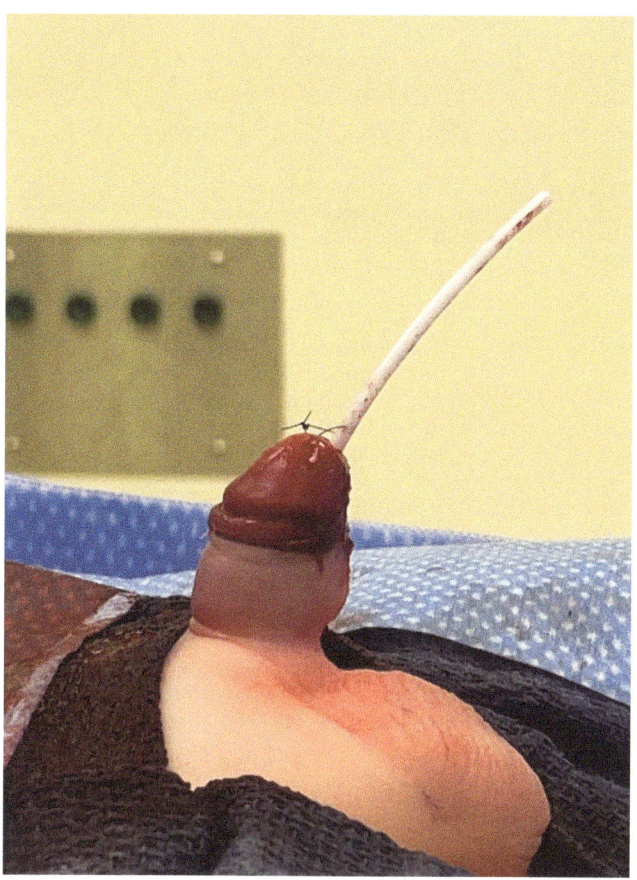

Figure 113.3: Urinary stent.
Source: Courtesy of Edward Gong, MD, Lurie Children's Hospital of Chicago.

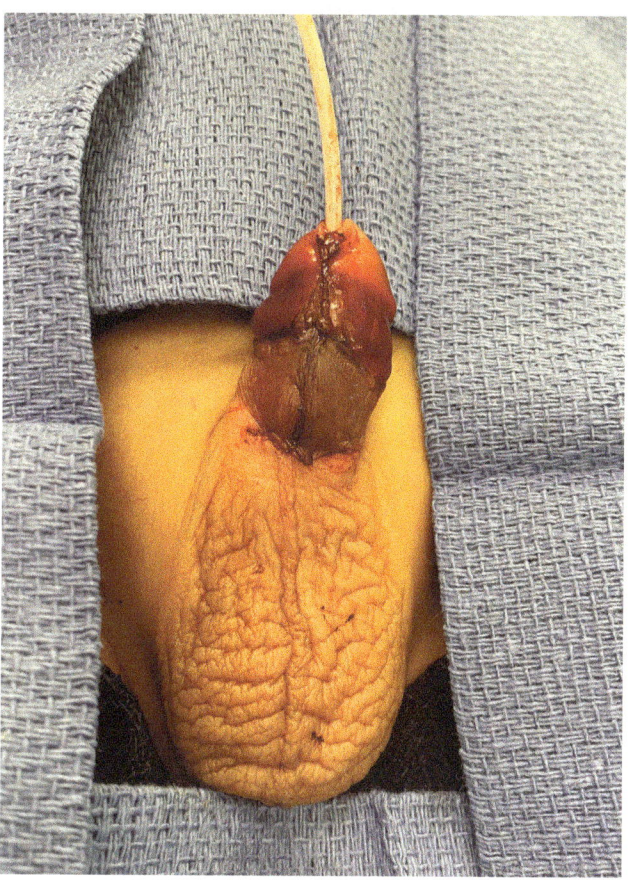

Figure 113.3: Urinary stent.
Source: Courtesy of Edward Gong, MD, Lurie Children's Hospital of Chicago.

CASE STUDY: 4-Year-Old Boy Presenting for Hypospadias Revision With Buccal Mucosal Graft

CLINICAL SCENARIO

A 15-kg 4-year-old boy presents for hypospadias revision with buccal mucosal graft. He was born full term after an uncomplicated pregnancy. His medical history includes reactive airway disease, innocent heart murmur, urethral fistula, emergence delirium, and proximal hypospadias. His surgical history includes three penile surgeries, two-stage hypospadias repair, and urethral calibration and fistula repair. Home medications include albuterol PRN during respiratory illnesses. He is appropriately NPO. He is watching videos on his tablet when you enter the room. He engages appropriately but declines trial separation, insisting his mom come with him to select a mask flavoring.

APPROACHES TO CARE

The parents are consented for general anesthesia and a single-injection caudal possibly twice depending on length of surgery. Based on his anxiety and history of emergence delirium, a child life specialist (CLS) is consulted to help normalize the surgical experience for him, and a premedication of midazolam 0.5 mg/kg oral syrup is ordered. He is given his premedication. After 10 minutes, he is appropriately sedated and easily separates from his parents with the support of the CLS.

The child chooses a seated induction. The CLS supports the patient through induction. The anesthesia provider positions the child in a cross-legged position (crisscross applesauce) with his back against her chest. ECG, pulse oximeter, and blood pressure monitors are placed prior to induction as the patient is tolerant. She holds the mask from the bottom with her left hand out of his line of vision. Her right arm is free to adjust the anesthesia machine and to wrap around the patient and hold him safely. General anesthesia is induced via an inhalation induction technique with 4 L nitrous oxide, 4 L oxygen, and 8% sevoflurane. After he loses consciousness, the anesthesia provider and nurses place him in the supine position. The nitrous is turned off. A 22-gauge IV is placed in his

(continued)

CASE STUDY: 4-Year-Old Boy Presenting for Hypospadias Revision With Buccal Mucosal Graft (*continued*)

hand. Rocuronium 0.6 mg/kg IV is administered to facilitate intubation. Given his history of reactive airway disease, ensuring adequate depth of anesthesia prior to airway instrumentation is important to prevent bronchospasm and 2 mg/kg propofol IV is given as well. The patient is intubated with a Mac 2 blade and a 4.5 cuffed endotracheal tube. The endotracheal tube is secured and bilateral breath sounds are confirmed with an air leak at 20 cmH$_2$O. The endotracheal tube is secured in the right corner of the mouth with surgical access to the bottom lip. The child is then positioned in the left lateral position, and a single-shot caudal is performed with 15 mL 0.2% ropivacaine with epinephrine 1:200,000.

Anesthesia is maintained with sevoflurane titrated to effect, air, and oxygen. The caudal epidural covers all surgical stimuli below T10. When the buccal graft is removed, fentanyl 1 mcg/kg IV and acetaminophen 10 mg/kg IV are administered. Patient is paralyzed with rocuronium titrated with train-of-four twitches for the duration of the procedure. To prevent pressure injury, his elbows and heels are padded with gel positioners, and every hour the patient's head is adjusted and his scalp briefly massaged.

The surgical duration is 5.5 hours. At around 5 hours, the patient is becoming more responsive to surgical stimulus as the epidural begins to recede. Prior to emergence, the single-shot caudal is repeated and 0.1% ropivacaine with epinephrine 1:200,000 is administered. Due to the history of emergence delirium and the oral surgical site, fentanyl 1 mcg/kg IV and dexmedetomidine 0.3 mcg/kg IV are titrated in to ensure a smooth emergence. Neuromuscular blockade is reversed with a combination of IV neostigmine and glycopyrrolate. The patient is emerged from anesthesia in the operating room, and the trachea is extubated. He is breathing appropriately and resting comfortably. The patient is administered oxygen by simple face mask and taken to the postanesthesia recovery room. Morphine 50 mcg/kg IV times 3 doses are ordered for postoperative pain, as well as telemetry monitoring, until the patient meets requirements for phase 2 recovery.

KEY REFERENCES

Complete references for this chapter are online and available at https://connect.springerpub.com/content/book/978-0-8261-3875-0/part/part04/toc-part/ch00113.

4. Morrison CD, Cheng EY. Hypospadias repair. In Gosain AK, Chung KC, eds. *Operative Techniques in Pediatric Plastic and Reconstructive Surgery.* Wolters Kluwer; 2020:447–457.
6. Long CJ, Zaontz MR, Canning DA. Hypospadias. In Partin AW, Dmochowski RR, Kavoussi LR, Peters CA, eds. *Campbell-Walsh-Wein Urology.* 12th ed. Elsevier; 2021:905–948.
10. Pohl HG, Rana S, Sprague BM, et al. Discrepant rates of hypospadias surgical complications: a comparison of U.S. News & World Report and Pediatric Health Information System® data and published literature. *J Urol.* 2020;203(3):616–623. doi:10.1097/JU.0000000000000554
21. Taenzer AH, Hoyt M, Krane EJ, et al. Variation between and within hospitals in single injection caudal local anesthetic dose: A report from the pediatric regional anesthesia network. *Anesth Analg.* 2020;130(6):1693 -1701. doi:10.1213/ANE.0000000000004447
25. Daboos M, Helal AA, Salama A. Five years' experience of double faced tubularized preputial flap for penoscrotal hypospadias repair in pediatrics. *J Pediatr Urol.* 2020;16(5):673.e1–673.e7. doi:10.1016/j.jpurol.2020.07.037
26. Loloi J, Harrington S, Boltz S, Decter RM. Ingrafts in hypospadias surgery: longer-term outcomes. *J Pediatr Urol.* 2020;16(5):555.e1–555.e5. doi:10.1016/j.jpurol.2020.04.030

CHAPTER 114

Orchidopexy

Heena Pranav and Megha Kanjia

INDICATIONS/CONTRAINDICATIONS

Cryptorchidism is defined as the absence of one or both testes in the normal scrotal position. The undescended testicles may be found in the normal line of descent, including the abdomen, inguinal canal, and the external ring just proximal to the scrotum; however, they also may be found in an ectopic position. On initial presentation and physical examination, the testes will be noted to not be in the scrotum. The location of the undescended testes may be palpable (cryptorchid) or nonpalpable (absent). The undescended testicle is usually associated with a hernia but can also rarely be associated with malignancy (**Figure 114.1**).[1,2]

Unrepaired cryptorchidism is associated with degeneration of the testes, impaired fertility, increased risk of germ cell tumors, and the psychological stigma associated with an empty scrotum. Thus, surgical correction is indicated to improve testicular function, reduce testicular malignancy, provide cosmetic benefits, and reduce risk of hernia or torsion.[1]

In infants, observation is indicated for the first 6 months to allow for potential spontaneous testicular descent. Surgery is recommended after 6 months but preferably by 12 months.[1] Spontaneous descent is less likely to occur after 6 months of age. An orchidopexy is an outpatient surgical procedure performed to repair undescended testicles or cryptorchidism and place them into the scrotal position. Additionally, it was found that testicular growth was restored after early orchidopexy at 9 months of age.[1]

Repair of palpable undescended testis entails either an orchidopexy performed via either a scrotal or inguinal

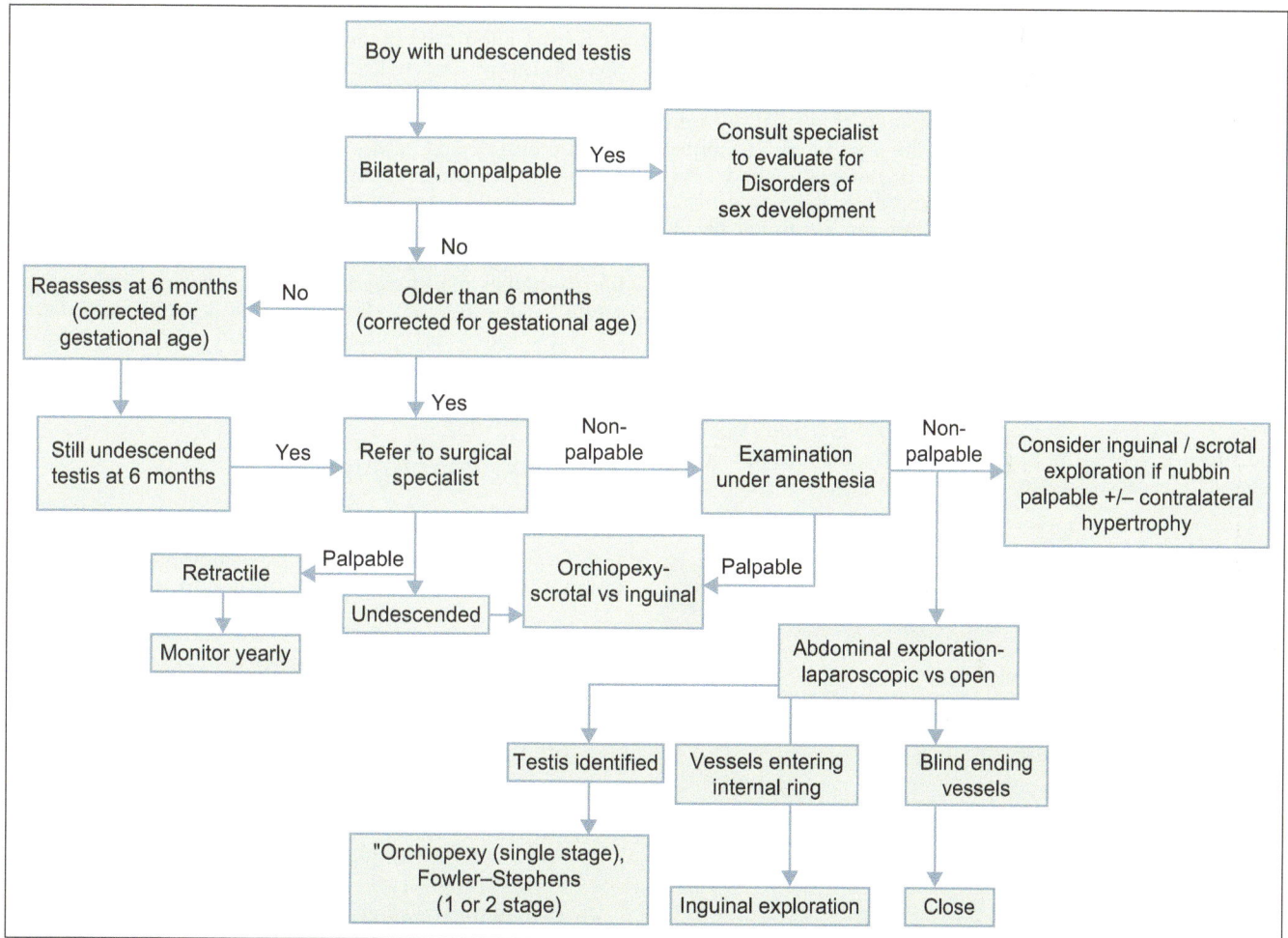

Figure 114.1: American Urological Association cryptorchidism guidelines for evaluation and treatment of cryptorchidism.

Source: From Kolon TF, Herndon CDA, Baker LA, et al. Evaluation and treatment of cryptorchidism: AUA guideline. *J Urol.* 2014;192(2):337–345. doi:10.1016/j.juro.2014.05.005.

approach. The surgical approach for the scrotal orchidopexy involves an incision on the superior scrotal border, which allows the testis to be identified and brought into the scrotal position. Should an inguinal surgical approach be utilized, a low transverse open incision will be made at the inguinal crease to facilitate identification of the testis. Once identified, the testis is mobilized and brought down to the scrotal position.

Should the testis be nonpalpable, an examination under anesthesia followed by abdominal exploration (diagnostic laparoscopy) is warranted. If the testis is found, it is either removed or surgically placed in the scrotum in a laparoscopic or open approach. Correction can be accomplished via a staged orchidopexy, autotransplantation of the testis, or the Fowler–Stephens procedure.[1] The Fowler–Stephens procedure takes advantage of the vasculature between the spermatic arteries in the cord to facilitate correction of the undescended testis. Because of this collateral blood flow, high ligation of the testicular vessels can preserve the testicular blood supply and improve mobility, thereby allowing the testicle to be transplanted to the scrotum.[2] During the first stage of the Fowler–Stephens procedure, the vessels are dissected, and the testicle is brought as close to the scrotum as possible. The second stage of surgery, which occurs 1 to 2 years later, moves the testicle to the remaining distance into the scrotum. The waiting period allows the blood supply to enlarge and form collateral circulation to supply the testicle.[3]

SPECIAL CONSIDERATIONS AND CONCERNS

Cryptorchidism may occur as an isolated abnormality in an otherwise healthy patient, or it may be associated with other congenital abnormalities, such as prune belly syndrome, posterior urethral valves, neural tube defects, gastroschisis, and microcephaly.[1] Box 114.1 includes an additional list of congenital anomalies associated with an increased risk of cryptorchidism.

ANESTHETIC MANAGEMENT

PREOPERATIVE EVALUATION

Patients who present for orchidopexy are generally healthy. The surgical procedure is determined by the location of the testes. Undescended testes are more common in premature infants than full-term infants. The incidence of one undescended testicle is 33% in preterm infant males compared to 3% in full-term males.[2] Thus, it is important to review the patient's neonatal history and any residual complications from prematurity during the preoperative evaluation. Additionally, a number of congenital syndromes are associated with undescended testicles and include Noonan syndrome, Prader–Willi syndrome, cloacal exstrophy, and Down syndrome as seen in Box 114.2.[2]

PREOPERATIVE PHARMACOLOGY

Orchidopexy is most commonly performed between the ages of 6 and 12 months of age. Around 9 to 12 months of age, children begin showing signs of stranger anxiety and parental separation may be challenging; therefore, ample consideration should be given to anxiolysis. As the majority of these surgeries occur in the outpatient setting, patients are unlikely to have an IV catheter prior to induction. Therefore, options for preoperative anxiolytic medications would include oral, IN, SC, IM, or rectal administration. Oral may be the most common route of administration; however, other options should be considered for various patient populations. Midazolam, ketamine, and dexmedetomidine are the most commonly utilized premedication. Additionally, child life specialists may be of assistance with older toddlers and grade school–aged children who may benefit from distraction techniques and games in the perioperative period. For additional information regarding the management of anxiety and anxiolysis, please refer to Chapter 131, "Pediatric Pain Management."

ANESTHETIC TECHNIQUE

Intraoperative Management

Induction of general anesthesia can occur either via an inhalational mask induction or IV induction, with inhalation

---

BOX 114.1 CONGENITAL ANOMALIES ASSOCIATED WITH INCREASED RISK OF CRYPTORCHIDISM

- Prune belly syndrome
- Posterior urethral valves
- Neural tube defects
- Cloacal exstrophy
- Gastroschisis
- Microcephaly
- Arthrogryposis
- Omphalocele
- Congenital diaphragmatic hernia

BOX 114.2 CONGENITAL SYNDROMES ASSOCIATED WITH UNDESCENDED TESTICLES

Noonan syndrome
Prader–Willi syndrome
Down syndrome
OEIS syndrome (cloacal exstrophy)

OEIS, omphalocele-exstrophy-imperforate anus-spinal defects.

BOX 114.3 CLINICAL PEARLS: ORCHIDOPEXY

- Patients in this age group may require anxiolytic premedication.
- Up to 33% of these patients may be ex-preterm infants.
- Associated congenital anomalies should be given consideration.
- Anesthetic management should consider some kind of regional anesthetic as a part of multimodal pain management.

induction being the most common technique given the typical age of patients presenting for an orchidopexy. Following induction, the airway can be managed with either placement of a laryngeal mask airway (LMA) or intubation with an endotracheal tube (ETT). If an inguinal surgical approach is planned, use of an LMA or ETT is appropriate. However, if the patient is having an abdominal exploration via a laparoscopic approach, intubation with an ETT is recommended. Standard monitors and a single IV catheter are sufficient for this procedure. Use of active warming devices, such as a forced-air warming blanket, should be considered given the age of patients typically presenting for an orchidopexy.

Anesthesia can be maintained with volatile anesthetic agents. Attention to adequate depth of anesthesia is necessary especially when the surgeon puts traction on the testis or spermatic cord, as this may trigger laryngospasm if the airway is unprotected. Anesthesia providers should consider administering an IV bolus of propofol or increase the inspired concentration of volatile anesthetic agent to deepen the plane of anesthesia during this phase of surgery. Additionally, use of caudal blockade may reduce the response to traction on the spermatic cord. Accordingly, pin should be managed in a multimodal fashion, incorporating the use of nonsteroidal anti-inflammatory drugs (NSAIDs), acetaminophen, and opioids coupled with regional anesthesia to provide adequate analgesia in the postoperative period.

Special Techniques and/or Equipment
A variety of regional techniques can be employed to provide postoperative analgesia (Table 114.1).

A caudal blockade is the most common technique used to provide postoperative analgesia in children undergoing infraumbilical surgery. It is typically performed following induction and intubation. The two most commonly used local anesthetics are 0.2% ropivacaine and 0.25% bupivacaine, with dosing of 1 mL/kg providing adequate coverage for infraumbilical surgery. One major limitation of this approach is the relatively short duration of analgesic action owing to a single injection. Thus, adjuvants, such as dexmedetomidine, ketamine, clonidine, or opioids, are frequently added to the local anesthetics in order to improve analgesic efficacy and duration of block.[4] Dexmedetomidine 1 mcg/kg added to 0.2% ropivacaine in a caudal prolongs postoperative analgesia 1.4-fold.[5] Dexmedetomidine 1 mcg/kg added to 0.25% bupivacaine extends postoperative analgesia duration by 2.5- to 3-fold compared with bupivacaine alone.[6] IV dexamethasone (0.5 mg/kg) has also been shown to prolong analgesic duration of caudal anesthesia.[7]

Other options are available if caudal blockade is contraindicated. An ilioinguinal nerve block is a peripheral nerve block that provides sensory blockade to the lower abdominal wall and can provide pain control for inguinal approach orchidopexy.[8] Spinal anesthesia has also been described in infants and is being increasingly utilized for short outpatient procedures. Concerns regarding neurotoxicity of anesthesia in the pediatric population have led to an increased use of spinal blockade in the pediatric population as an alternative to general anesthesia. A recent retrospective case series explored the use of spinal anesthesia in infants 1 to 14 months of age for outpatient urological procedures, such as orchidopexy, and found the overall anesthesia time, surgical time, and length of stay in the postanesthesia care unit were shortened in patients who received spinal anesthesia compared to those who received general anesthesia.[9]

Complications/Emergencies
Orchidopexy is generally a safe procedure; however, it is important to be aware that traction and manipulation of the spermatic cord and testicle somewhat increase the incidence of intraoperative bradycardia and laryngospasm.[10] As a result, a deeper level of anesthesia is required to preclude untoward events. The need for a deeper plane of anesthesia, however, can be lessened by the use of intraoperative nerve blocks or regional anesthesia as can the risk of bradycardia and laryngospasm.

POSTOPERATIVE CARE
Considerable postoperative pain and a high incidence of nausea and vomiting have been reported in patients undergoing orchidopexy.[11] While procedures involving the testes pose an independent risk of postoperative nausea and vomiting (PONV), the incidence is increased with opioid administration. It is important to administer PONV prophylaxis intraoperatively and use a multimodal pain management strategy to help with postoperative pain control. An observational multicenter cohort study done in the United Kingdom looked at the prevalence of pain at home and its consequences following orchidopexy and found that pain at home is a significant problem with a high rate of pain lasting longer than previously thought. Moreover, approximately 20% of patients required a prescription for opioids on discharge.[10]

Table 114.1	Advantages and Disadvantages of Various Regional Anesthesia Techniques		
Regional Technique	Pro	Con	Medication
Caudal	Complete infraumbilical sensory blockade	Often a blind procedure, can be inadequate with scrotal traction	Bupivacaine, ropivacaine + additives
Spinal	Complete sensory blockade	Can be technically challenging. Parents may not be amenable	Bupivacaine, ropivacaine
Ilioinguinal	Peripheral block	May not allow for complete sensory coverage	Bupivacaine, ropivacaine

CASE STUDY: 8-Month-Old Male Undergoing Orchidopexy

CLINICAL SCENARIO
An 8-month-old male presents for inguinal approach orchidopexy. He was born at 32 weeks via vaginal birth. He is otherwise healthy. On physical examination, he was found to have undescended palpable testis. His parents are concerned because this is his first anesthetic. They are particularly concerned about his pain following surgery.

SPECIAL CONSIDERATIONS
This patient was born 32 weeks, premature. On preoperative evaluation, it is important to evaluate if this child has any sequelae of prematurity, paying particular attention to the length of neonatal intensive care unit stay, the need for intubation, and any respiratory issues since birth.

APPROACHES TO CARE
Evidence-Based Approaches to Care
This patient would benefit from general anesthesia with an LMA with a regional block for postoperative pain control. Caudal blockade has been found to provide prolonged postoperative pain control. Adding additional adjuvants, such as clonidine for dexmedetomidine, has been found to prolong the duration of sensory blockade and is recommended.

KEY REFERENCES

Complete references for this chapter are online and available at https://connect.springerpub.com/content/book/978-0-8261-3875-0/part/part04/toc-part/ch114.

1. Barthold JS, Hagerty JA. Etiology, Diagnosis, and Management of the Undescended Testis. In *Campbell-Walsh Urology*. 12th ed. Elsevier; 2016.
2. Williams RK, Lauro HV, Davis PJ. Anesthesia for general abdominal and urologic surgery. *Smith's Anesthesia for Infants and Children*. 9th ed. Elsevier; 2016:789–816.
3. Zeigler LN, Modes KB, Deshpande JK. Anesthesia for pediatric urological procedures. *Gregory's Pediatr Anesth*. 2020;813–833. doi:10.1002/9781119371533.ch32
10. Williams G, Bell G, Buys J, et al. The prevalence of pain at home and its consequences in children following two types of short stay surgery: A multicenter observational cohort study. *Paediatr Anaesth*. 2015;25(12):1254–1263. doi:10.1111/pan.12749

CHAPTER 115

Cystoscopy

Dusty C. Pourciau

INDICATIONS/CONTRAINDICATIONS

Cystoscopy is a common procedure usually performed under general anesthesia in the pediatric population that utilizes a rigid or flexible fiberoptic scope to visualize the inside of the bladder and urethra. During a cystoscopy, a cystoscope is inserted into the urethra, allowing the urologist to evaluate a number of structures, including the urethra, bladder, and ureters. Most cystoscopes have multiple channels allowing for instillation of irrigation and the insertion of instruments to be utilized during the procedure. Common indications for cystoscopy include hematuria, urethral/ureteral strictures, bladder calculi, ureterocele, hydronephrosis, and bladder tumors. Contraindications to cystoscopy are few but may include the inability to pass the cystoscope beyond urethral stricture.

ANESTHETIC MANAGEMENT

PREOPERATIVE EVALUATION

Prior to undergoing cystoscopy, all patients should receive a thorough preanesthetic evaluation with a specific focus on symptoms related to dysfunction of the genitourinary system. As the presenting symptoms may be secondary to or part of genetic syndrome, it is imperative that anesthesia providers vet the overall health of the patient to ensure there are no additional abnormalities that may impact the ability to deliver a safe, effective anesthetic.

Pertinent Labs

For routine cystoscopy on otherwise healthy pediatric patients, preoperative labs are usually not required. In patients with hydronephrosis, strictures or urosepsis, consider obtaining preoperative complete blood count (CBC) and chemistry panel to ensure there are no existing electrolyte abnormalities or renal dysfunction.

PREOPERATIVE PHARMACOLOGY

Preoperative sedation may be appropriate for anxious patients. Anxiolytics commonly utilized include midazolam (PO, IV), dexmedetomidine (IV, IN), ketamine (IM, IV, IN), or fentanyl (IV, IN). Prior to administration of these medications, anesthesia providers should establish there are no factors that would preclude the case from moving forward, such as acute illness or *nil per os* violation.

ANESTHETIC TECHNIQUE

Intraoperative Management

In the pediatric population, cystoscopy is most frequently performed with the patient under general anesthesia. Anesthesia can be induced either with an inhalational or IV technique, depending on the patient's age, overall health, and comorbidities. Following induction, anesthesia is typically maintained with volatile anesthetic agents. Airway management can be accomplished via mask, nasal cannula, laryngeal mask airway (LMA), or endotracheal tube (ETT).[1] The method of airway management selection should mirror the criteria used in adult patients.

Standard monitors, as defined by the American Society of Anesthesiologists, should be employed to monitor the patient throughout the procedure. Temperature management may be difficult if large amounts of irrigation are used, especially with smaller pediatric patients. Forced air and fluid warmers, as well as warming the operating room, may be necessary to maintain the patient's temperature. Typically, only one IV catheter is required given intraoperative blood loss and third-space/evaporative fluid loss for cystoscopy is minimal.

Patients are commonly moved to the foot of the bed to allow the urologist better access to the patient. Anesthesia providers should be prepared to extend the breathing circuit and add necessary extensions to IV fluid lines. For smaller patients, the increase in dead space associated with extending the breathing circuit can increase inspired CO_2. In addition to being moved to the foot of the bed, patients are commonly placed in lithotomy or frog-leg position based on their size and age. Caution should be taken with positioning to decrease the risk of nerve injury or injury to the hips. During the procedure, lasers may be utilized to break apart calculi. If lasers are used, appropriate eye protection for both the patient and personnel in the room is imperative.

> **BOX 115.1 CLINICAL PEARLS: CYSTOSCOPY**
>
> - Injections of indigo carmine during the procedure result in darkening of the urine and can aid in the identification and evaluation of the ureteral orifices.
> - Indigo carmine administration can have both hemodynamic and respiratory effects (e.g., decrease in cardiac output, transient decrease in pulse oximetry reading) for which the anesthesia provider should be ready to address.

Pain following cystoscopy is typically minimal. Anesthesia providers should consider employing a multimodal approach to pain management, with the use of acetaminophen, nonsteroidal anti-inflammatory drugs, and lidocaine jelly routinely proving to provide sufficient analgesia. Depending on the patient's medical history and the procedure being performed, oxybutynin may be indicated to stave off bladder spasms. Caudal anesthesia can also be used for both intraoperative and postoperative pain management.[2] Opioids are rarely required for the procedure itself.

Anesthesia providers should ensure that an adequate depth of anesthesia has been achieved prior to insertion of the cystoscope as urethral manipulation can elicit a laryngospasm as a result of the Breuer–Lockhart reflex.[3] In addition, it is important to recognize that caring for patients presenting with strictures can be especially challenging as they may have developed urosepsis, placing them at higher risk of perioperative anesthesia complications.[4]

During the procedure, the surgeon may request IV injection of indigo carmine (Box 115.1).

Complications/Emergencies

Although rare, a number of complications are associated with cystoscopy. Bladder perforation can result from direct injury by the cystoscope or instruments or secondary to retained irrigation, leading to increased cystic pressure. Signs and symptoms of bladder perforation include hematuria, lower abdominal pain, nausea, vomiting, anuria, or fever. The treatment course includes immediate open repair of the bladder. Should an urgent open repair be required to address bladder perforation, anesthesia providers should be aware the patient may require supportive treatment due to hemodynamic instability.

Although rare in the pediatric population, fluid reabsorption during cystoscopy can be significant and could cause symptoms similar to transurethral resection of prostate (TURP) syndrome seen in adult patients. Signs and symptoms can include seizures, confusion, visual disturbances, cerebral edema, nausea, vomiting, or restlessness. Treatment is composed of supportive therapy, as well as the need for admission for further observation. Throughout the procedure, anesthesia providers should monitor the amount of irrigation administered versus the amount of irrigation removed to the best of their abilities. Theoretically, the two volumes should be approximately equal to minimize the likelihood of retained irrigation and complications, such as bladder perforation.

POSTOPERATIVE CARE

Postoperative care of cystoscopy patients is largely dependent on the patient's comorbidities. Healthy patients who require minor interventions are often discharged home the same day and require little to no postoperative pain control. Patients who require significant intervention or who are hemodynamically unstable will be admitted for inpatient observation, possibly in the intensive care unit when warranted.

REFERENCES

1. Sanket B, Ramavakoda C, Nishtala M, et al. Comparison of second-generation supraglottic airway devices (i-gel versus LMA ProSeal) during elective surgery in children. *AANA J.* 2015;83(4):275–280.
2. Weigele M, Marhofer P, Lonnqvist P. Caudal epidural blocks in paediatric patients: a review and practical considerations. *Br J Anaesth.* 2019;122(4):509–517. doi:10.1016/j.bja.2018.11.030
3. Hernandez-Cortez E. Update on the management of laryngospasm. *JACCOA.* 2018;8(6):1–6. doi:10.15406/jaccoa.2018.08.00327
4. Liang X, Huang J, Xing M, et al. Risk factors and outcomes of urosepsis in patients with calculous pyonephrosis receiving surgical intervention: a single-center retrospective study. *BMC Anesthesiol.* 2019;19(61):1–8.

CHAPTER 116

Urolithiasis

Angela Milosh and Sarah Milligan

INDICATIONS/CONTRAINDICATIONS

Urolithiasis is a disease that is relatively rare in children, although the incidence is rising particularly among females.[1] The etiology behind the increased incidence is unclear but is postulated to be a combination of factors, including body habitus, fluid status, dietary habits, the environment, and better diagnostic imaging. Children with renal calculus, or kidney stone disease, are at an increased risk of recurrence; nearly 50% of patients who develop kidney stone disease as a child will have a recurrence within 3 years.[2] As such, these patients are likely to require ongoing care for management of this chronic disease into adulthood.

In adults, renal calculi are predominantly composed of calcium oxalate (75%–80%), followed by struvite (10%–20%), calcium phosphate (5%), and uric acid (5%).[3] In children, most renal calculi are calcium-based (oxalate, phosphate, and mixed oxalate–phosphate). Struvite, cysteine, uric acid, xanthine, and dihydroxyadenine stones are less common.[4] Metabolic abnormalities in children that predispose to stone formation include hypercalciuria, hyperoxaluria, hypocitraturia, cystinuria, and hyperuricosuria. Renal calculi prevention in patients with these conditions most often consist of fluid and dietary management but may also include pharmacological therapy.

SPECIAL CONSIDERATIONS AND CONCERNS

The treatment of urolithiasis in children includes medical expulsion therapy or surgical management. Medical expulsion therapy usually consists of pharmacological treatment to dilate the ureter combined with adequate hydration. The use of alpha-blockers (tamulosin or doxazosin) and calcium channel blockers (nifedipine) has demonstrated usefulness in promoting spontaneous ureteral stone passage in patients with favorable stone size and location.[5]

When expulsion therapy is not indicated, or has failed to lead to stone passage, there are surgical treatment options. The majority of stones can be managed with extracorporeal shock wave lithotripsy (ESWL), ureteroscopy (URS), and percutaneous nephrolithotomy (PCNL). Open surgical treatment is usually reserved for cases in which there are structural abnormalities, a large burden of infective or staghorn stones, or large bladder stones.[6]

Due to the higher risk of recurrence in children with metabolic abnormalities, these patients will undergo multiple repeated imaging and interventions. Imaging often includes the use of fluoroscopy. Children are particularly vulnerable to the cumulative effects of ionizing radiation, due to longer life expectancy and greater sensitivity of developing tissues to the effects of radiation. Additionally, these procedures in pediatric patients usually require general anesthesia. Exposure to multiple anesthetics during childhood is also a potential concern for neurotoxicity.[7]

ANESTHETIC MANAGEMENT

PREOPERATIVE EVALUATION

Preoperative evaluation should focus on physiological alterations related to the disorder, treatment, and presenting pathology (Box 116.1). Depending on the type and location of the renal calculi, these patients may be at risk of acute renal injury if there is obstructive pathology. As part of the surgical workup, preoperative evaluation will typically include a urinalysis, basic metabolic panel, magnesium, phosphorus, and uric acid.[7] Other laboratory studies may be indicated based on medical status.

> **BOX 116.1 KEY ASSESSMENT POINTS**
>
> - Children with urinary stones may have an underlying metabolic disorder, increasing their risk of stone recurrence.
> - Patients may be taking alpha-blockers or calcium channel blockers to facilitate spontaneous stone expulsion.
> - Preoperative diuretics are commonly prescribed for patients with metabolic disorders to prevent stone formation.

> **BOX 116.2 COMPLICATIONS/EMERGENCIES**
>
> - Hemorrhage
> - Fever
> - Ureteral injury
> - Urinary tract infection
> - Hydrothorax
> - Colonic injury
> - Seizures (dilutional hyponatremia)

PREOPERATIVE PHARMACOLOGY

Depending on the cause of the renal calculi, as well as any attempted medical expulsive therapy, patients may be on one or more different medications for management of their condition. These medications may include alpha-blockers, calcium channel blockers, diuretics, alkali agents, thiol-containing agents, allopurinol, or pyridoxine. See **Table 116.1** for commonly prescribed maintenance medications.[4,7]

ANESTHETIC TECHNIQUE

Intraoperative Management

Pediatric patients undergoing surgical treatment for urinary stones most often require general anesthesia. For cystoscopy, URS, and ESWL, anesthesia induction and maintenance are routine. The airway can be maintained by either facemask or supraglottic airway. Tracheal intubation is not required, unless indicated by the patient's comorbidities. A deep plane of anesthesia is required to prevent laryngospasm due to urethral stimulation by cystoscope insertion. For patients undergoing ESWL therapy, deep sedation may be an option.[8] Open or laparoscopic surgical techniques will most often require general anesthesia with endotracheal intubation to facilitate adequate ventilation and minimize unnecessary movement.

Based on the 2019 guidelines from the American Urological Association, single-dose antibiotic prophylaxis is indicated for URS stone removal, PCNL, and open or laparoscopic stone surgery. Prophylactic antibiotics are not indicated for ESWL, as long as the preprocedural urinalysis is negative for infection.[9]

Potential complications from surgical intervention include hemorrhage, fever, ureteral injury, urinary tract infection, hydrothorax, and colonic injury.[7] Seizures from dilutional hyponatremia have been reported in the literature.[10]

Complications and emergencies are noted in **Box 116.2**.

POSTOPERATIVE CARE

For patients undergoing cystoscopy or URS, opioids are rarely required for postoperative pain management. However, the risk of postoperative nausea and vomiting is increased in patients undergoing URS or PCNL, indicating a need for antiemetic prophylaxis.[11]

KEY REFERENCES

Complete references for this chapter are online and available at https://connect.springerpub.com/content/book/978-0-8261-3875-0/part/part04/toc-part/ch116.

2. Tasian GE, Kabarriti AE, Kalmus A, Furth SL. Kidney stone recurrence among children and adolescents. *J Urol.* 2017;197(1):246–252. doi:10.1016/j.juro.2016.07.090
7. Tasian GE, Copelovitch LA. Management of pediatric stone disease. In: Partin AW, ed. *Campbell-Walsh-Wein Urology.* Elsevier; 2021:853–870.
8. Cevik B, Tuncer M, Erkal KH, et al. Procedural sedation and analgesia for pediatric shock wave lithotripsy: a 10 year experience of single institution. *Urolithiasis.* 2018;46(4):363–367. doi:10.1007/s00240-017-0992-z
9. Lightner DJ, Wymer K, Sanchez J, Kavoussi L. Best practice statement on urologic procedures and antimicrobial prophylaxis. *J Urol.* 2020;203(2):351–356. doi:10.1097/JU.0000000000000509
11. Williams RK, Lauro HV, Davis PJ. Anesthesia for general abdominal and urologic surgery. In: Davis PJ, Cladis FP, eds. *Smith's Anesthesia for Infants and Children.* Elsevier; 2017:789–816.

Table 116.1	Pharmacological Treatment of Metabolic Abnormalities
Abnormality	**Treatment**
Hypercalciuria	Potassium citrate Thiazides
Hypocitraturia	Potassium citrate Bicarbonate
Hyperoxaluria	Potassium citrate Pyridoxine Neutral phosphate Magnesium
Hyperuricosuria	Potassium citrate Bicarbonate Allopurinol
Cystinuria	Tiopronin Penicillamine Captopril

CHAPTER 117

Pyeloplasty

Sarah Milligan and Angela Milosh

INDICATIONS/CONTRAINDICATIONS

Ureteropelvic junction (UPJ) obstruction is the most common antenatal cause of hydronephrosis.[1] If left untreated, hydronephrosis can restrict urinary flow and ultimately result in irreversible damage to the kidney. UPJ obstruction is usually caused by either intrinsic stenosis of the proximal ureter or extrinsic compression by an accessory renal artery (Figure 117.1; Baskin[1]). The initial diagnosis tool is renal ultrasound.[2] Surgery is indicated when the patient presents with pain, renal calculi, infection, and/or increasing grade of hydronephrosis.[1] If radiological studies indicate the presence of hydronephrosis during pain, but the hydronephrosis resolves when symptoms subside, surgery is indicated. Children who are symptomatic usually require operative intervention.[1] If a patient has a solitary kidney with UPJ obstruction, surgery needs to be considered earlier to preserve the function of the kidney.[2] Pyeloplasty is the surgical correction of UPJ stenosis, which entails the excision of the portion of the ureter with the stricture and re-anastomosed to the renal pelvis[3] (Figure 117.2).

Contraindications to surgery include pyelonephritis and asymptomatic patients with stable renal function. Children who present with an infection need to be treated with antibiotics and clear of symptoms prior to pyeloplasty.[1] If the infection does not resolve, a percutaneous pyelostomy tube should be placed to relieve obstruction.[1] Additionally, asymptomatic patients who have stable renal function and improvement in hydronephrosis over the period of observation are contraindicated for surgical intervention.

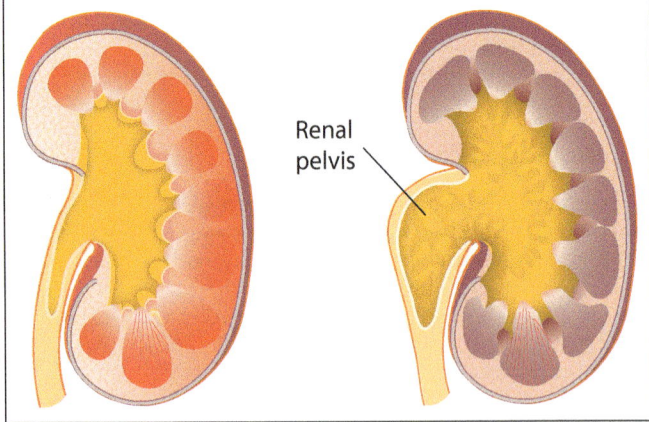

Figure 117.1: Example of enlarged renal pelvis/hydronephrosis due to ureteropelvic junction obstruction.

CHARGE syndrome has been associated with UPJ obstruction. Patients with CHARGE syndrome can present with C—coloboma ocular, H—heart defects, A—choanal atresia, R—retardation of growth, G—genitourinary anomalies, and E—ear abnormalities. For more information regarding CHARGE syndrome, please refer to Chapter 28, "CHARGE Syndrome."

In addition, a thorough assessment of renal function of all patients presenting for pyeloplasty should be completed as untreated hydronephrosis can result in kidney failure.[4] In patients with two kidneys, the unaffected kidney should provide filtration to compensate for the obstructed ureter.

Pertinent Labs

Blood urea nitrogen (BUN) levels, serum creatinine, creatinine clearance, and electrolytes are indicated.[5] Urinalysis is performed to assess for infection.

ANESTHETIC MANAGEMENT

PREOPERATIVE EVALUATION

A comprehensive review of all body systems should be performed prior to the anesthetic to determine any preexisting conditions or syndromes associated with UPJ obstruction.

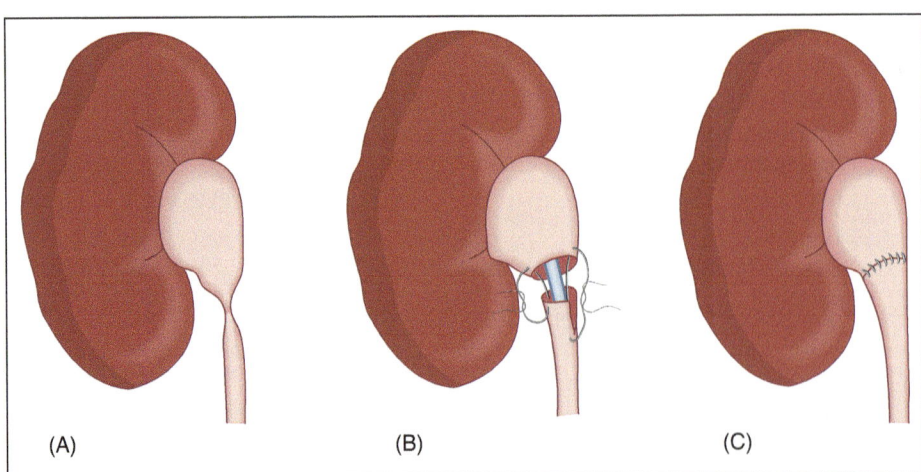

Figure 117.2: Dismembered pyeloplasty. Also referred to as Anderson–Hynes pyeloplasty.

PREOPERATIVE PHARMACOLOGY

Preoperative oral or IV midazolam should be administered to decrease anxiety if indicated.

ANESTHETIC TECHNIQUE

Intraoperative Management

General endotracheal anesthesia is required for pyeloplasty. Mask or IV induction of anesthesia is appropriate. One to two IV lines are placed for fluid management. Blood loss should be minimal, as well as hemodynamic changes, therefore an arterial line is not indicated.[3]

The patient will typically be placed in the lateral/flank position.[6] An anterior subcostal approach may also be used with the patient supine.[2] In the lateral position, an axillary roll is placed to prevent brachial plexus injury.[6] Lateral positioning can create a ventilation perfusion mismatch and cause dependent lung atelectasis. This will cause an increase in dead space throughout the surgical procedure.[7] The endotracheal tube may migrate in the lateral flexed position, therefore tube position must be verified following patient positioning.[7]

A flank, dorsal, or subcostal incision is made during an open technique. Additionally, a robotic or laparoscopic technique may be used.[2] A urinary catheter may be left in place for 24 to 48 hours, and a Penrose drain may be placed and removed within 7 to 10 days.[2]

POSTOPERATIVE CARE

Pain management after pyeloplasty is important for pediatric patients. Intraoperatively, fentanyl, morphine, and hydromorphone can be used for pain management. Adjuncts, such as dexmedetomidine, ketamine, and acetaminophen, are also indicated. Various regional anesthesia techniques can be performed while the patient remains anesthetized to optimize postoperative pain control and reduce overall opioid requirements. Possible regional techniques include caudal epidural, as well as ultrasound-guided peripheral nerve blocks, such as transversus abdominal plane (TAP) blocks and quadratus lumborum blocks. TAP blocks reliably cover T10 to L1 and may cover the subcostal region of T9.[8] Quadratus lumborum blocks can be performed to more reliably cover T4 to L1.[9] Quadratus lumborum blocks also provide somatic and visceral pain relief, whereas TAP blocks provide somatic relief only. For more information regarding peripheral nerve blocks, please refer to Chapter 131 in this text. In addition to pain management, the patient should be observed for signs and symptoms of infection, bleeding, urinary obstruction, and urinary leak.

KEY REFERENCES

Complete references for this chapter are online and available at https://connect.springerpub.com/content/book/978-0-8261-3875-0/part/part04/toc-part/ch117.

1. Baskin LS. Congenital ureteropelvic junction obstruction. *UpToDate*. https://www-uptodate-com.ccmain.ohionet.org/contents/congenital-ureteropelvic-junction-obstruction?search=congenital%20ureteropelvic%20junction&source=search_result&selectedTitle=1~30&usage_type=default&display_rank=1. Accessed 1 July 2020.
2. Carr MC, Snyder HM, III Urinary tract obstruction. In: Ziegler MM, Azizkhan RG, Allmen D, Weber TR. eds. *Operative Pediatric Surgery, 2e*. McGraw Hill; 2014. https://accesspediatrics-mhmedical-com.ccmain.ohionet.org/content.aspx?bookid=959&sectionid=53539634
6. Littlejohn J, Reed AJ, Cereda M. Anesthetic considerations for genitourinary and renal surgery. In: Longnecker DE, Mackey SC, Newman MF, et al. eds. *Anesthesiology, 3e*. McGraw Hill; 2017. https://accessanesthesiology-mhmedical-com.ccmain.ohionet.org/content.aspx?bookid=2152&sectionid=164237349
7. Butterworth IV JF, Mackey DC, Wasnick JD. eds. *Morgan & Mikhail's Clinical Anesthesiology, 6e*. McGraw Hill; 2018. https://accessanesthesiology-mhmedical-com.ccmain.ohionet.org/content.aspx?bookid=2444&sectionid=193561783

BOX 117.1 COMPLICATIONS/EMERGENCIES

Intraoperative
- Bleeding
- Pneumothorax
- Injury to surrounding organs/tissue

Postoperative
- Urinary leakage
- Stricture formation
- Infection

CHAPTER 118

Lower Urinary Tract Reconstruction

Heather J. Rankin, David B. Joseph, and Ching Man Carmen Tong

INDICATIONS/CONTRAINDICATIONS

Lower urinary tract reconstructive surgery is performed for a wide spectrum of congenital urological diseases in the pediatric population, often in children who have chronic renal insufficiency and had previously undergone intra-abdominal surgeries. The overarching goals of lower urinary tract reconstruction are to preserve renal function, minimize urinary tract infections (UTIs), and establish urinary continence. Patients requiring these surgeries are often complex, with multiple comorbidities and anatomical abnormalities, and are thus at high risk of perioperative complications. Anesthetic management of these complex patients can be challenging and generally requires judicious planning and use of multimodal pain control and goal-directed hemodynamic therapy. Close communication within a multidisciplinary team involving urologists, anesthesia providers, nursing staff, and physical therapists is necessary for postoperative success and accelerated recovery.

SURGICAL PROCEDURES

Ureteral Reimplantation

Vesicoureteral reflux (VUR), or abnormal retrograde flow of urine from the bladder to the upper urinary tract, is a relatively common condition encountered by pediatric urologists. When clinically correlated with febrile UTI, VUR can lead to renal scarring and chronic renal insufficiency, defined as reflux nephropathy. VUR should not be considered a pathological entity on its own; rather, it is a marker of a heterogenous condition involving the entire urinary tract.

VUR has traditionally been categorized into primary or secondary reflux. Primary VUR refers to the anatomical and functional abnormality of the vesicoureteral junction, resulting in the weakness of the flap–valve antireflux mechanism. In these children, the intravesical segment of the ureter is shortened, and the ureteral orifice is displaced laterally in comparison with the normal length and position at the base of the bladder. Secondary VUR describes an acquired condition associated with increased intravesical pressures due to abnormal bladder function or bladder outlet obstruction. Typically, correcting the bladder dysfunction resolves the associated VUR.

The most common clinical presentation of children with VUR is febrile UTI. The American Academy of Pediatrics Guidelines recommend that children with recurrent febrile UTIs or abnormal renal ultrasound after the first febrile UTI should undergo a voiding cystourethrogram (VCUG).[1] VCUG remains the gold-standard imaging study to diagnose VUR. The grading tool devised by the International Reflux Study Committee (**Figure 118.1**) is the most commonly used system to determine the severity and prognosis of VUR.[2]

The most common indication for surgical repair of VUR is recurrent breakthrough UTIs despite antibiotic prophylaxis or medical noncompliance. Other relative indications for corrective intervention include persistent high-grade reflux, VUR associated with other anatomical abnormalities such as ureteral duplication, or presence of new renal scar, renal growth delay, or reflux nephropathy. In these cases, surgery is a reasonable option for children older than 12 months of age.

Surgical Technique

VUR can be corrected with the traditional open repairs described in the following or as a minimally invasive procedure performed cystoscopically as an outpatient utilizing injection of a ureteral bulking agent. The choice of the procedure is based on multiple factors related to the clinical scenario, leading up to correction, patient characteristics, and the anatomical pathophysiology of the distal ureter and trigone.

Cystoscopy is often performed prior to open reimplantation to evaluate bladder appearance and condition. If acute cystitis is found during endoscopy, most surgeons opt to delay open surgery until completion of antibiotic treatment. Upon completion of cystoscopy, the patient is then positioned supine with a rolled towel or gel roll placed behind their upper sacrum to raise the lower pelvis and hips.

A Pfannenstiel skin incision is made approximately one fingerbreadth above the pubic symphysis. After incising the SC tissue and Scarpa's fascia, the anterior rectus sheath is opened and rectus flaps are created. The rectus muscle is then separated through the linea alba, and the space of Retzius

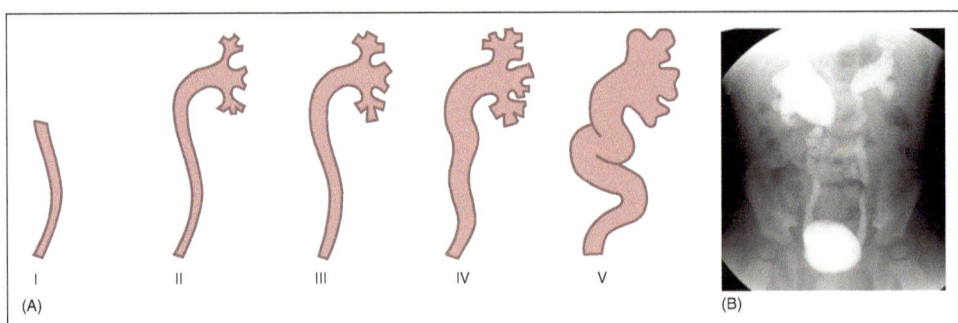

Figure 118.1: (A) Classification of vesicoureteral reflux as described by the International Reflux Study Committee.
(B) A voiding cystourethrogram demonstrating right grade V and left grade IV vesicoureteral reflux in a 3-year-old boy.

is entered bluntly. At this point, a self-retaining abdominal retractor, such as the Denis-Browne, is assembled to aid in retraction and exposure. If an intravesical approach is performed, the anterior bladder wall is incised longitudinally and moist sponges are packed into the bladder dome to flatten the posterior bladder wall and elevate the ureteral orifices into the operative field. The ureters are then intubated with a 5-French feeding tube, and the mucosal and muscular attachments of the ureter are dissected away, with care taken to avoid devascularization and injury. Adequate length has been reached once the ureter can reach the opposite bladder wall. From here, a variety of techniques have been described to reimplant the ureter. The Cohen cross-trigonal technique is perhaps the most popular technique used by most urologists for intravesical reimplantation. Popularized in 1974, this method creates a submucosal tunnel along the posterior bladder wall across the trigone toward the opposite ureteral orifice. An effective antireflux flap valve mechanism is developed by a tunnel length of at least three to four times the diameter of the ureter. The ureter is secured to the newly created ureteral orifice circumferentially, and the prior muscular and mucosal defects from the old orifice are closed. Prior to closure of the bladder, the feeding tube is passed up the new ureteral orifice to ensure patency of the ureter and to rule out inadvertent ureteral kinking.

If an extravesical approach is pursued, then instead of incising the anterior bladder, the bladder is retracted medially to expose and mobilize the ureter posterior to the bladder to the level of the ureterovesical junction. The serosal and muscular layers of the detrusor are incised along the course of the ureter and detrusor flaps are created. The bladder is often partially distended to aid in this dissection. The ureter is then laid down along the tunnel, and the detrusor flaps are closed over the ureter. An advantage of an extravesical approach is the reduced risk of postoperative hematuria and bladder spasms, but approximately 20% of children develop transient bladder dysfunction and urinary retention.[3]

Postoperatively, a urethral catheter is left in the bladder for overnight drainage. Most patients are discharged on postoperative day 1 after demonstrating tolerance of ambulation and oral intake. The success rate for either approach nears 100% in the hands of an expert urologist.[4] Postoperative evaluation typically involves a combination of urinalysis, a review of bladder and bowel habits, and renal sonograms, with routine blood pressure measurements and serum creatinine levels for those with renal scarring or insufficiency.

Augmentation Cystoplasty

Bladder reconstructive procedures are performed in children who are unable to store urine safely or empty the bladder in an efficient manner. The majority of children will require enlargement of the bladder through augmentation. Compromised bladder and sphincteric dysfunctions are often seen in children with central nervous system diseases such as spina bifida, multiple sclerosis, or spinal cord injury, as well as congenital conditions like bladder exstrophy. Children with spina bifida make up the majority of pediatric patients undergoing this surgical intervention. The primary goals of augmentation cystoplasty are to protect the upper urinary tract, preserve renal function, and promote urinary continence.

Meticulous preoperative evaluation and counseling for patients considering augmentation reconstruction are vital to postoperative success and longevity of the augmented segment. Patients and parents should be willing to commit to lifelong clean intermittent catheterizations (CICs), as well as frequent renal imaging and function studies. Because of this, augmentation surgery should not be pursued until the child has the physical and mental maturity to care for themselves.

Typically, preoperative assessment involves urodynamic bladder testing for assessment of noncompliant bladder associated with high intravesical pressures and VUR. These children also undergo renal assessment with serum creatinine levels, ultrasound imaging, and even radioisotope renal scans when there is concern for renal insufficiency or scarring. Baseline bowel function should also be ascertained as postoperative bowel dysfunction can occur in up to 50% of patients[5] when using an intestinal segment for augmentation. A comprehensive presurgical evaluation will allow the surgeon to tailor and choose the most appropriate donor segment for the patient.

Surgical Technique

Various donor tissues can be used to augment the bladder, including the ileum, colon, ureter, and stomach. The choice of donor segment depends primarily on the patient's disease process, comorbidities, prior surgeries, baseline renal function, and ability to tolerate metabolic derangements from urine absorption by the donor mucosa. The advantages and disadvantages of various donor sites are illustrated in **Table 118.1**.

Ileocystoplasty has become the most common intestinal segment used for augmentation. The mobility, abundant source of small intestine, predictable blood supply, and compliance of the rearranged tissue make the ileum an ideal donor segment to use. Once the intraperitoneal cavity is entered, care is taken lysing intra-abdominal adhesions that have formed from prior surgeries, such as ventriculoperitoneal shunt placement and revisions that often occur in the spina bifida population. A 20- to 40-cm segment of the ileum approximately 25 cm proximal to the ileocecal valve is selected. Avoiding the ileum adjacent to the ileocecal valve prevents malabsorption of vitamin B12 and bile salts. The segment chosen should have adequate mesentery length to reach the native bladder in the pelvis without tension. The bowel segment is then divided and an ileoileostomy is performed. The isolated ileal segment is copiously irrigated, detubularized on the antimesenteric border, and reconfigured into a U, S, or W shape. The reconfiguration effectively maximizes volume, capacity, and compliance, as well as reduces bowel peristaltic activity.

The native bladder is opened and clamshelled from the bladder neck anteriorly to the trigone posteriorly. The generous incision allows for an easier bowel-to-bladder anastomosis and prevents the native bladder from reforming and turning the bowel segment into a narrow-necked "hour-glass" deformity. If the bladder is particularly small and heavily trabeculated, an additional incision along the coronal plane is made to reconfigure the native bladder into a "star" appearance. The bowel segment is anastomosed to the bladder using absorbable suture.

Children undergoing bladder augmentation need to perform a CIC, with preference given to catheterizing through the native urethra. This becomes difficult for some boys because of a posterior urethral false passage and for girls who are nonambulatory. In these situations, a catheterizable channel can be fashioned from the bowel, appendix, or ureter. The bladder will be drained with a combination of urethral, channel, and suprapubic catheters. Additional peritoneal drains may be used.

Postoperatively, urinary drainage catheters remain in place for several weeks. The patient is instructed to begin daily bladder irrigations soon after surgery to prevent mucus

Table 118.1 Advantages and Disadvantages of Donor Segments for Augmentation Cystoplasty

Donor Segment	Advantages	Disadvantages
Stomach	Minimal mucus or stone formation Suitable for those with impaired renal function Not affected by short bowel syndrome or pelvic irradiation	Hematuria-dysuria syndrome Hypochloremic hypokalemic metabolic alkalosis
Ileum	Large quantity available Predictable blood supply Very compliant	Mucus/stone formation Higher risk of infections Vitamin B12 deficiency and risk of diarrhea if most distal ileum is used
Colon	Large diameter (i.e., capacious and compliant reservoir) Well-defined blood supply Ileocecal valve can be used as a continence mechanism	Worsened diarrhea if using ileocecal valve Potential risk of malignant transformation (adenocarcinoma) Mucus/stone formation Higher risk of infections
Ureter	Preservation of native urothelium Avoids use of bowel Full-thickness ureter does not shrink over time Can be performed extraperitoneally	Requires a very dilated ureter to a non functioning kidney
Auto augmentation	Preservation of native urothelium Avoids use of bowel Extraperitoneal procedure Does not preclude future augmentation enterocystoplasties	Success rate variable Theoretical increased risk of bladder rupture Segment can shrink over time

buildup and stone formation. Prior to removal of the final suprapubic tube, the patient must demonstrate proficiency with intermittent self-catheterization. Oftentimes, cystogram is performed to illustrate complete healing of the bowel/bladder anastomosis and absence of extravasation along the suture line. In children with mild to moderate VUR prior to surgery, postoperative VCUG typically demonstrates spontaneous resolution, eliminating the need for ureteral reimplantation at the time of bladder augmentation.[6,7]

Aside from the morbidity listed in Table 118.1, a major, potentially life-threatening complication following enterocystoplasty is spontaneous bladder perforation. A frequently linked cause is noncompliance to timely intermittent catheterizations, although vascular compromise to the bowel wall has also been demonstrated to be a contributing factor.[8,9] Diagnosing spontaneous perforation is challenging due to nonspecific symptoms, such as nausea or vomiting, oliguria, and diffuse abdominal pain. Patients should be properly counseled and have a high index of suspicion when these symptoms arise. A CT cystogram is typically required to help diagnose a spontaneous perforation. Immediate exploratory laparotomy is required if the bladder leak is substantial, supplemented with broad-spectrum antibiotics and maximal urinary leakage with suprapubic tube and urethral catheter drainage.

ANESTHETIC MANAGEMENT

PREOPERATIVE EVALUATION

A standard preoperative assessment with physical and airway assessment, documentation, and anesthesia consent should be completed, with special considerations taken into account for bladder reconstructive patients. Anesthesia providers should thoroughly vet the presence of comorbidities, in particular any cardiac or pulmonary concerns that may warrant an evaluation from a specialist. Likewise, it is imperative that electrolyte or renal deficiencies are explored prior to induction of anesthesia as they may have a profound impact on anesthetic management and mandate alterations to the plan. As there may be a potential for blood loss necessitating blood transfusion, preoperative lab work should be completed and reviewed with blood products available as indicated.

PREOPERATIVE PHARMACOLOGY

This patient population may have recurrent operative room visits and subsequently have a heightened level of preoperative anxiety. Administering anxiolytic medications may be warranted, with the most commonly used being midazolam (.3–.5 mg/kg with a typical maximum of 15 mg orally or .1 mg/kg intravenously with a typical maximum of 2 mg) or intranasal dexmedetomidine (1–2 mcg/kg).

ANESTHETIC TECHNIQUE

Intraoperative Management

Induction may be performed via either an inhalation induction or an IV induction. If the patient is entering the operating room as an outpatient without a previous IV catheter placed, an inhalation induction may be preferred. This often reduces patient anxiety about an IV catheter being placed awake and offers the anesthesia provider a calm patient with the benefit of vasodilation due to sevoflurane. If the patient prefers an IV induction or is an inpatient with an IV catheter in place, an IV induction may be performed.

Typically, only one peripheral IV line is needed in patients presenting for these procedures; however, depending on the anesthesia provider's choice of maintenance, an additional IV catheter may be desired if infusions are being utilized. An arterial line may be considered for several reasons, including extensive comorbidity history, particularly cardiac, a procedure potentially involving blood loss requiring transfusion, or a procedure that will last greater than 8 hours in a patient where repetitive noninvasive blood pressures would be less preferable than an arterial line.

Volatile agents and a total IV anesthetic can both be utilized and are based largely on provider preference. A muscle relaxant is typically used to aid the surgeon and works well when regional anesthetic techniques are part of the anesthesia plan. Maintaining normothermia in patients is imperative as patients who become hypothermic may have alterations in medication metabolism, clotting, postoperative shivering, cardiac alterations, and increased surgical site wound infections.[10,11] Normothermia may be maintained by a variety and combinations of devices such as forced-air warmers, fluid warmers, heat and moisture exchangers (HMEs), and increased room temperatures. As urinary catheters are often placed during bladder reconstruction surgery, anesthesia providers should be in frequent communication with the surgeon in order to assess output. Accurate urine output becomes difficult to monitor when the bladder is open and the urine is in the surgical field. Fluid administration may need to be altered based on output.

At times, the anatomy of complex urological patients is difficult for the surgeon to visualize. The anesthesia provider may be asked to administer methylene blue or Omnipaque to assist the surgeon's visualization via cystoscopy or fluoroscopy. Additionally, furosemide may also be requested with increased IV fluids.

Anesthesia providers should be aware that most patients presenting for bladder reconstruction surgeries have a health history including spina bifida with a repaired myelomeningocele. These patients have latex sensitivity, and although most equipment used in pediatric anesthesia is latex-free, equipment should be verified prior to use.

Special Techniques and/or Equipment
Regional Anesthesia

Regional anesthesia techniques continue to increase in popularity in pediatric patients. For bladder reconstruction procedures, a number of regional techniques can be performed with the most common administration of local anesthetics administered in the lumbar epidural or caudal region with a onetime administration bolus or with a continuous infusion after successful catheter placement. The caudal approach may be utilized more often as there is a reduced chance of risk of injury to the spinal cord or spinal tap and is a simple technique to learn. Local anesthetics such as lidocaine, ropivacaine, bupivacaine, or levobupivacaine can be infused with additives such as narcotics or clonidine. In some instances, a surgeon may desire the local anesthesia infusion to continue for several days. In this case, the lumbar area is superior to the caudal area as the caudal site can have higher rates of infection.[12] Epidural infusions have been reported after genitourinary reconstruction surgery of neonates following bladder exstrophy repair.[12] Regional anesthesia may be contraindicated in bladder reconstruction patients who have a history of myelomeningocele, sacral dimple, tethered cord, or other lumbar spine or regional abnormalities.

If an extended catheter is requested, a tunneled catheter can be placed.[13] Monitoring of local anesthetic blood levels postoperatively should be considered if the local anesthesia infusion is in place for more than several days. Added clonidine may provide an additional benefit of sedation postoperatively and can be beneficial to patients in traction after bladder exstrophy repair with pelvic osteotomies.

The transversus abdominis plane (TAP) block is another regional technique that has been successfully used for genitourinary procedures. Under ultrasound guidance, anesthesia providers can inject local anesthetic in the plane between the transversus abdominis and the internal oblique and can also place an indwelling catheter to deposit local anesthetic for several days postoperatively. Continuous infusions of .2% ropivacaine over a 48-hour period following renal transplant have demonstrated a significantly lower incidence administration of postoperative narcotics.[14]

A variant of the TAP block, as described by Blanco,[15] is the quadratus lumborum (QL) block, which can be used for lower abdominal surgeries such as bladder reconstructive surgeries. Utilizing ultrasound, the QL muscle is identified and a number of different areas can be blocked depending on the placement of the local anesthetic.[16] A recent study comparing caudal anesthesia and QL block in conjunction with general anesthesia for pediatric patients undergoing ureteral implantation found lower doses of narcotics utilized postoperatively in the group with the QL block during the first 24 hours.[17] Due to higher complications with neuraxial anesthesia, TAP and QL blocks may be utilized more in the future. For more information regarding regional anesthetic techniques, please refer to Chapter 30, "Pediatric Pain Management," the section on regional anesthesia.

If regional anesthesia is avoided or contraindicated, a multimodal pain management approach, including acetaminophen, nonsteroidal anti-inflammatory drugs (NSAIDs), dexmedetomidine, ketamine, and opioids, may be utilized to reduce overall opioid use.

Opioid Usage and Enhanced Recovery After Surgery

The opioid crisis is changing the way many anesthesia providers and surgeons handle intraoperative and postoperative pain. Specific to pediatric patients, nearly double the rates of opioid prescription poisonings have occurred,[18] with focus being put on more multimodal ways of controlling pain and emphasis on less opioids being prescribed.

Enhanced recovery after surgery (ERAS) is a newer multidisciplinary concept that takes coordination from the team throughout the perioperative period. ERAS planning starts weeks prior to the surgical date. Research suggests that the use of ERAS in patients undergoing lower urinary tract reconstruction procedures reduced postoperative complications such as readmission, length of stay, and narcotic use. While there has been research on ERAS dating back to the late 1990s,[19,20] there is little research on pediatric patients. A multicenter group has developed a prospective study titled Pediatric Urology Recovery After Surgery Endeavor (PURSUE) to explore ERAS in pediatric urology patients using pathways created in the adult general surgery urology literature.[21] The pathway utilizes a multidisciplinary team involving pediatric anesthesiology, nursing, physical therapy, and pediatric urology to standardize postoperative care and minimize physiological stress brought on by surgery. See **Box 118.1** for a summary of ERAS goals. For more information regarding ERAS in pediatrics, please refer to Chapter 31, "Enhanced Recovery After Surgery."

However, varied outcomes have been found with regard to postoperative opioid prescription patterns for pediatric patients who experience bladder reconstruction. Hecht et al.[22] actually found an increased number of opioid prescriptions

> **BOX 118.1** ERAS GOALS IN LOWER URINARY TRACT RECONSTRUCTION
>
> **Preoperative Goals**
> - Surgical planning and counseling with parents/patients regarding ERAS protocol and postoperative expectations and recovery
> - Clear liquids with carbohydrate load 2 hours prior to surgery
> - Avoidance of aggressive bowel prep the day before surgery
>
> **Intraoperative Goals**
> - DVT prophylaxis
> - Use of both general and regional anesthesia, such as epidurals and TAP blocks
> - Guideline-recommended, culture-sensitive prophylactic antibiotics
> - Maintenance of normothermia and normovolemia
> - Multimodal pain control in an effort to minimize intraoperative opioid use
> - Avoidance of excessive drains
>
> **Postoperative Goals**
> - Avoidance of postoperative nasogastric tube
> - Early introduction of oral feeds with ice chips or clear liquids the night of surgery
> - Early mobilization with assistance by physical therapy
> - Continuation of multimodal pain control
> - Tight control of nausea and emesis with antiemetic medications
>
> DVT, deep vein thrombosis; ERAS, enhanced recovery after surgery.

given to patients who were on an ERAS protocol in their facility despite a significantly shorter length of stay and no significant differences in the opioid prescription days and total morphine equivalents. Significantly more urology residents prescribed higher morphine dosed by weight than pediatric urology fellows, suggesting improvement can be made to the protocol as the opioid prescription was not standardized. Suggested reasons for increased prescribing include possible fear of postoperative pain after discharge and a shorter length of stay in the hospital or fear of inability to obtain opioids after discharge.

POSTOPERATIVE CARE

After the surgery is complete and the anesthetic choice discontinued, the vast majority of patients will be extubated and taken to the postanesthesia care unit (PACU). Depending on the surgical procedure and patient health history, the patient may be discharged from the PACU to a regular floor or may

CASE STUDY: Bladder Augmentation in a Child With Spina Bifida

CLINICAL SCENARIO

A 10-year-old 40-kg boy with spina bifida, a myelomeningocele closed postnatally, and a ventriculoperitoneal (VP) shunt had been followed by the comprehensive spina bifida clinic since infancy. He is compliant on intermittent catheterizations every 4 hours and has not responded to oral antimuscarinic medications or intravesical botulinum toxin injections. Urodynamic testing revealed he had a small bladder capacity, poor detrusor compliance, and incompetent bladder neck. The decision was made to proceed with bladder augmentation surgery and a bladder neck sling placement with an enhanced recovery after surgery (ERAS) protocol utilized. The family was educated on the ERAS protocol preoperatively, which included an aggressive oral bowel regimen up to the night prior to surgery.

APPROACHES TO CARE

Evidence-Based Approaches to Care

The day of surgery, the patient presented to preoperative surgery unit and a preoperative assessment was performed. His allergies included latex and vancomycin sensitivity. The family reported no anesthesia complications with his previous surgeries, including the myelomeningocele closure, VP shunt placement and revision, and tonsillectomy and adenoidectomy. There is no reported family history of problems with anesthesia, muscle diseases, or bleeding disorders. The family reported a history of allergic rhinitis and denied other health problems with the child. Medication regimen included nitrofurantoin, oxybutynin, and cetirizine. On examination, the child had S1S2 and clear breath sounds on auscultation, with a Mallampati class 2 airway examination.

Midazolam 10 mg was administered orally 30 minutes prior to transfer to the operating room. Standard monitors were applied and anesthesia was induced with nitrous oxide and sevoflurane. A 20-gauge peripheral IV line was easily placed in the dorsum of the left hand, and lidocaine 60 mg, propofol 100 mg, fentanyl 25 mcg, and rocuronium 30 mg were administered. He was easily intubated with

(continued)

CASE STUDY: Bladder Augmentation in a Child With Spina Bifida (*continued*)

a 5.5 cuffed endotracheal tube (ETT) and then subsequently underwent augmentation ileocystoplasty and bladder neck sling. Euvolemia was maintained with 5 to 10 mL/kg/hr of crystalloids. Anesthesia was maintained with volatile agent at .8 MAC, a dexmedetomidine infusion, ketamine, rocuronium, ondansetron, and IV acetaminophen administered on closing. A suprapubic tube and a urethral Foley catheter were placed at the end of the procedure to maximally drain the bladder. Total anesthesia time was about 7 hours. After the surgical procedure was completed, a ultrasound-guided bilateral transversus abdominis plane block was performed with 16 mL .2% ropivacaine (.4 mL/kg maximum of 20 mL/side) injected uneventfully. For emergence, sugammadex was administered to reverse muscular blockade, and the patient was extubated and taken to the PACU.

Postoperatively, pain was well controlled with scheduled acetaminophen and ketorolac, with opioids for breakthrough pain, including morphine for the first 24 hours, then transitioning to oral oxycodone. The patient was allowed ice chips the night of the surgery. On postoperative day 1, the patient was placed on a clear liquid diet which was advanced as tolerated. Physical therapists were consulted to assist in early postoperative mobilization. An antiemetic medication ondansetron was prescribed and given on an as-needed basis. He was instructed to irrigate his bladder twice daily to prevent mucus buildup. He stayed in the hospital for 5 days and was discharged home without complications.

COMPLICATIONS

Approximately 1 year after surgery, he presented to the ED with an acute onset of abdominal pain and nausea. He reportedly had been diligent with intermittent catheterizations at home. His physical examination was notable for diffuse abdominal pain and his laboratory studies revealed an elevated serum creatinine level and leukocytosis with a left shift. CT cystogram revealed contrast extravasation from the posterior aspect of the bladder. He was emergently taken to the operating room for exploratory laparotomy, washout, repair of bladder perforation, and suprapubic tube placement. His anesthesia evaluation was not changed from his previous surgery. Anesthesia management consisted of a rapid sequence induction as the patient had eaten a full meal reportedly 2 hours before acute onset of pain, including lidocaine, propofol, fentanyl, and succinylcholine. After successful intubation, anesthesia was maintained with volatile agent, fentanyl, and rocuronium. IV acetaminophen was given on closing and the muscle relaxant reversed with sugammadex. He was extubated and taken to the PACU, where he was admitted postoperatively for broad-spectrum IV antibiotics and pain control. Postoperative pain was controlled again with scheduled acetaminophen and nonsteroidal anti-inflammatory drugs, with opioids for breakthrough pain. He was discharged several days later with his bladder maximally drained through the suprapubic tube. Three weeks after the surgery, a cystogram demonstrated recovery of the perforation with no contrast extravasation.

---

need a higher acuity monitored care in the ICU or a step-down unit. Unique patient condition may require postoperative intubation, particularly after a long surgery, if large fluid volume shifts occurred, or if underlying pulmonary comorbidities such as prematurity and bronchopulmonary dysplasia are present.

KEY REFERENCES

Complete references for this chapter are online and available at https://connect.springerpub.com/content/book/978-0-8261-3875-0/part/part04/toc-part/ch118.

7. Simforoosh N, Tabibi A, Basiri A, et al. Is ureteral reimplantation necessary during augmentation cystoplasty in patients with neurogenic bladder and vesicoureteral reflux? *J Urol*. 2002;168(4 Pt 1):1439–1441. doi:10.1097/01.ju.0000029978.56171.bd

14. Farag E, Guirguis MN, Helou M, et al. Continuous transversus abdominis plane block catheter analgesia for postoperative pain control in renal transplant. *J Anesth*. 2015;29(1):4–8. doi:10.1007/s00540-014-1855-1

16. Akerman M, Pejčič N, Veličkovič I. A review of the quadratus lumborum block and ERAS. *Front Med*. 2018;5:44. doi:10.3389/fmed.2018.00044

21. Rove KO, Strine AC, Wilcox DT, et al. Design and development of the pediatric urology recovery after surgery endeavor (PURSUE) multicentre pilot and exploratory surgery. *Br Med J*. 2020;10(11):e039035. doi:10.1136/bmjopen-2020-039035

Section M: Orthopedic Procedures

CHAPTER 119

Spinal Fusion

Jason Perry, Abigail Monnig, and Ramsey S. Sabbagh

INDICATIONS/CONTRAINDICATIONS

Children may experience a spectrum of spinal deformities, including congenital anomalies, neuromuscular disorders, skeletal dysplasia, and idiopathic disorders. These may be the result of disorders of the neuromuscular system or the result of trauma. In addition, deformities may be progressive in nature, with the patient experiencing further physiological compromise over time. Among the most encountered spinal deformities in children are scoliosis and kyphosis.

SCOLIOSIS

Scoliosis is defined as a complex three-dimensional rotational deformity of the spine characterized by a lateral curvature of the spine greater than 10 degrees. Most often there is no identified cause of scoliosis in children, with the diagnosis then becoming idiopathic scoliosis. Idiopathic scoliosis can subsequently be categorized by the age at which it is detected: infantile (younger than 3 years), juvenile (younger than 9 years), and adolescent (older than 10 years).

Adolescent idiopathic scoliosis (AIS) is the most common type of pediatric spinal deformity. Although the etiology of AIS is unclear, several theories exist, including genetic factors, hormonal factors, growth abnormalities, and more. Two major classification systems exist for AIS, the King–Moe classification system and Lenke's classification. The King–Moe classification system divides the curves into five types based on their number, flexibility, and deviation from the midline (Figure 119.1). Lenke's classification considers three key attributes: the curve type, the deviation of the lumbar curve from the mid-sacral line, and the sagittal profile of the curve (Figure 119.2). Lenke's classification results in 42 types. Options for treatment of AIS include observation for curves less than 25 degrees, bracing for curves 25 to 40 degrees, and surgery for patients with curves greater than 40 degrees (if immature), or 50 degrees (if mature). The most common surgical intervention is posterior spinal correction and fusion.

Scoliosis can also be congenital in nature, with an abnormal curvature of the spine developing before birth. Congenital spinal deformities typically develop during the embryological period of intrauterine development in the first 6 weeks of life. Congenital scoliosis anomalies are divided into failures of formation, failures of segmentation, or mixed anomalies. Most curves are progressive and will require surgical treatment. However, nonprogressive curves account for 25% of congenital scoliosis cases and may be managed nonsurgically.

Neuromuscular scoliosis results from a disruption in central nervous system (CNS) pathways that coordinate muscle activity. There are two subtypes: neuropathic (i.e., cerebral palsy, spina bifida, or spinal muscular atrophy) or myopathic (muscular dystrophies such as Duchenne's muscular dystrophy). Significant comorbidities often exist in this group, including mental retardation, nutritional deficits, contractures, and more.

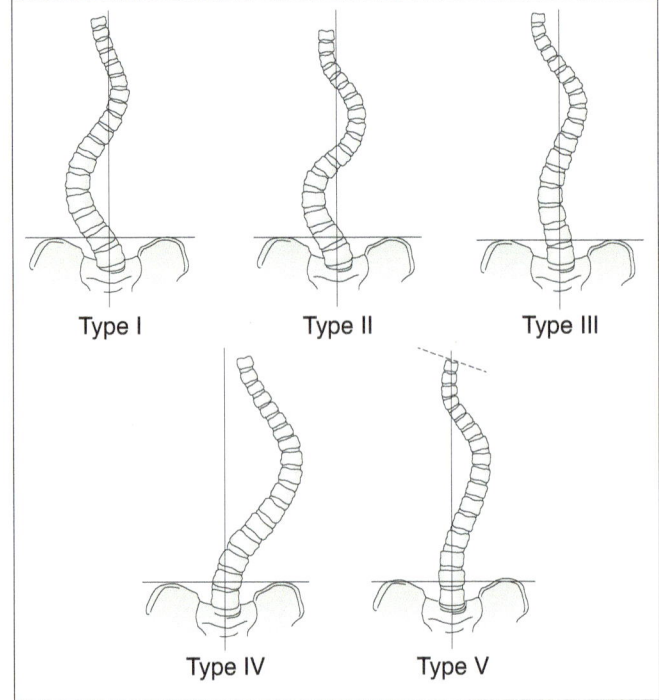

Figure 119.1: King–Moe classification.

L, lumbar; L-MT, lumbar-main thoracic; MT, main thoracic; PT, proximal thoracic; TL, thoracolumbar.

KYPHOSIS

Kyphosis is defined as an exaggerated roundback deformity of the thoracic or thoracolumbar spine that measures greater than 40°. While this can occur at any age, it is common in adolescence and is often seen in conjunction with poor posture and carrying heavy schoolbags, which can lead to stretching of the ligaments and muscles that support the vertebrae.

Scheuermann's kyphosis is a structural deformity associated with thoracic wedged vertebral bodies, and presents in late childhood. Most often, Scheuermann's kyphosis has a benign course. Surgical treatment is reserved for curves greater than 75 degrees in mature patients, those who have progressed despite brace treatment, and in patients whose pain is unresponsive to nonoperative measures. Anterior release and fusion, followed by a posterior spinal fusion, has been proposed to avoid loss of correction.[1,2] Congenital kyphosis is less common than scoliosis but can lead to far worse consequences if left untreated. Anesthesia providers should be aware, however, that the risk of neurological insult may be higher in patients with congenital spinal deformities.

MANAGEMENT OF SPINAL DEFORMITIES

Nonoperative treatment of neuromuscular scoliosis consists mostly of bracing to slow progression and postpone the need

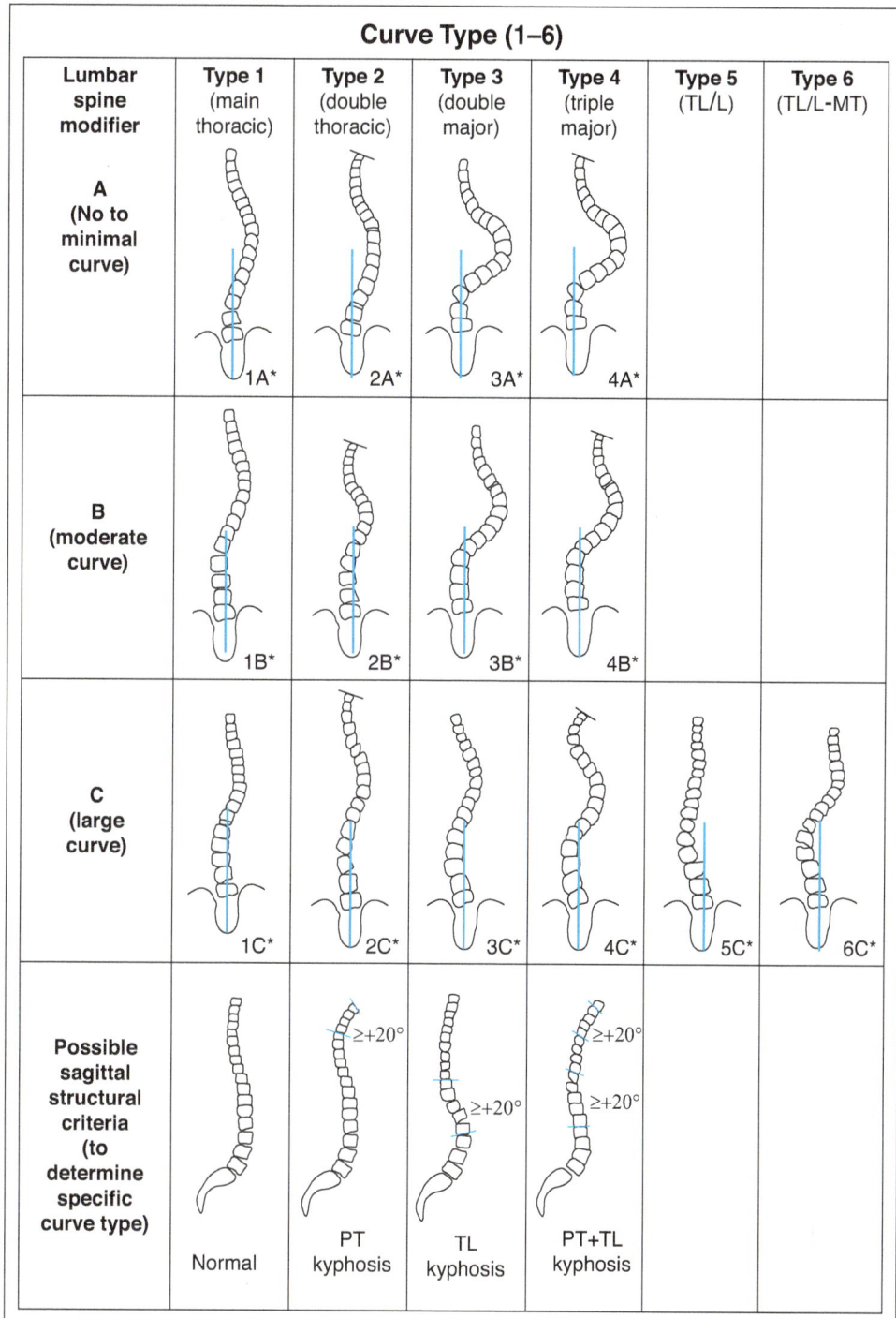

Figure 119.2: Lenke's classification of adolescent idiopathic scoliosis.
L, lumbar; L-MT, lumbar-main thoracic; MT, main thoracic; PT, proximal thoracic; TL, thoracolumbar.

for surgery. However, neuromuscular scoliosis is almost always progressive, and by the adolescent growth spurt surgical stabilization is usually necessary.

Depending on the patient's age and severity of scoliosis, surgical insertion of growing rods and/or vertical expandable prosthetic titanium ribs (VEPTR) may be indicated. In younger patients, growing rod placement may be used initially to correct the scoliosis by placing two rods, one on each side of the spine. Strong spinal anchor points are made at both ends of the scoliotic curve and connected to these rods.[3] The growing rods are then periodically lengthened to allow for growth of the spinal column. When the child has finished growing, a definitive spinal fusion will be performed.

VEPTR are placed in younger patients with rib anomalies that result in thoracic insufficiency. If the child's thorax is unable to support appropriate lung growth, thoracic expansion and stabilization surgery, followed by repetitive distraction with a rib-based growth-promoting system, may be warranted to prevent progression of restrictive lung disease.[4]

Spinal fusion is a definitive treatment to halt further progression of scoliosis. After sufficient growth of the thorax and lungs has occurred, the spine is stabilized by removing the joints between the vertebrae where scoliosis is present. Instrumentation, including rods, can be attached to the spine via hooks, wires, and pedicle screws to fix the spine internally in the corrected position. The vertebrae are then decorticated and bone graft is placed, ultimately fusing over time.

In some instances, such as a large curve (>75 degrees) or severe kyphosis, an anterior release may be performed in conjunction with or prior to a posterior spinal fusion. In recent years, novel anterior instrument devices have been developed to treat scoliotic curves solely via anterior instrumentation and fusion techniques. This is usually achieved via a thoracoscopic approach, although thoracotomy or abdominal approaches have been used for anterior release.

SPECIAL CONSIDERATIONS AND CONCERNS

Complex medical histories and comorbidities can be challenging to manage in patients with neuromuscular and congenital scoliosis. Among children with congenital scoliosis, up to 35% have concomitant neurological malformations, 25% have some form of congenital heart malformation, and 20% have urological anomalies, along with other musculoskeletal abnormalities.[5] Additionally, among children with neuromuscular scoliosis, restrictive lung disease is common. Anesthesia providers should also be aware that multiple diseases associated with neuromuscular scoliosis have an increased incidence of airway-related anomalies, mandating they be prepared to manage a difficult airway during and immediately after induction of anesthesia.

ANESTHETIC MANAGEMENT
PREOPERATIVE EVALUATION

A well-communicated, multidisciplinary approach is paramount to successful preparation of pediatric patients presenting for spinal fusion. Most institutions mandate preoperative screening on an outpatient basis well before the scheduled surgical date to ensure the patient is optimized prior to surgery.

During the preoperative evaluation, it is imperative anesthesia providers gather a thorough medical history and perform comprehensive physical assessment as the severity of curvature can be indicative of perioperative complications. For example, a curvature greater than 75 degrees secondary to scoliosis or greater than 90 degrees due to kyphosis correlates with increased surgical complications.[3] Likewise, bleeding disorders, such as Von Willebrand's disease, should be identified.

Spinal cord and nerve root injuries occur in 0.26% to 1.75% of all surgeries for idiopathic scoliosis. Since some of the most devastating complications of spine surgery involve paralysis or sensory loss, a baseline motor and sensory examination is paramount. While complications are uncommon for surgically managed AIS, a high body mass index (BMI) can cause an increased likelihood of suffering wound complications, readmission, reoperation, and longer hospital stays in patients undergoing surgery for idiopathic scoliosis.

The presence of significant comorbidities should be vetted as congenital and neuromuscular scoliosis are risk factors for serious complications, including major blood loss and nerve injury. The reported overall perioperative complication rate in patients with neuromuscular scoliosis undergoing surgical intervention is as high as 33%.[6] In patients with neuromuscular scoliosis, preoperative evaluation should include radiographic evaluation of the spine, as well as cardiac, pulmonary, psychological, and laboratory assessment. In patients with neuromuscular scoliosis secondary to Duchenne's muscular dystrophy, congenital myopathy, and myotonic dystrophy type 1, cardiac evaluation is of utmost importance.[3] Preoperative cardiac evaluation includes a thorough clinical examination, ECG, echocardiogram, and in cases of rhythm disorders, Holter monitoring.[3] Due to the severity of the spinal deformity in many neuromuscular scoliosis patients, preoperative echocardiography can prove technically difficult and further cardiac evaluation may be indicated via multigated cardiac radionuclide ventriculography or cardiac MRI.[7]

Regardless of the etiology of the spinal deformity, the patient's pulmonary status should be evaluated and optimized. It is imperative anesthesia providers review pulmonary function test (PFT) results as a history of pulmonary issues is associated with higher risk of postoperative respiratory complications.[7,8] In addition, it is recommended to check preoperative range of motion and positions of comfort as a decreased range of motion can cause challenges with positioning intraoperatively. Patients should also be assessed for any preexisting weakness, pain, or neuropathies.

In some patients with insufficient body weight for undergoing surgery or a nutritional deficiency, a period of nasogastric feeding may be necessary prior to surgery as poor perioperative nutritional status is associated with an increase in surgical complications, including infection.[3,6] As such, supplemental iron, folate, and/or erythropoietin may be warranted.[9] Additionally, routine evaluation of gastroesophageal reflux should be performed to mitigate potential perioperative respiratory complications.

The preoperative evaluation is also an opportunity for anesthesia providers to discuss with the patient and their family the risks and potential complications associated with the planned surgery. This includes the potential for blood loss, nerve injury, postoperative facial edema, and injury to the patient's teeth, lips, and tongue from motor-evoked potentials (MEPs). Equally as important, it is an opportunity to convey the measures that will be taken to prevent such complications from occurring. This time also provides the opportunity to set realistic expectations.

The information gathered collectively during the preoperative screening appointment can be complied in a prebrief summary. The authors' institution employs a prebrief process which allows concerns and expectations to be communicated among all members of the multidisciplinary team. The surgical and anesthesia teams, in addition to the operating room staff, receive the prebrief a week prior to scheduled spinal fusions, detailing key information for the surgical case. This includes information such as prior surgical or anesthetic complications (previous loss of intraoperative neuromonitoring (IONM) potentials, difficult vascular access, or difficult airway), the requested antibiotics, and the need for cell saver, an arterial line, and/or central venous catheter. The prebrief process is again reviewed with the surgeon, anesthesia team, and operating room staff the morning of surgery (**Box 119.1**).

Pertinent Labs

The most important complication that necessitates preoperative laboratory evaluation is the high likelihood of massive blood loss during posterior spinal fusion for

> **BOX 119.1 KEY ASSESSMENT POINTS FOR SPINAL FUSION**
>
> - Body mass index: Is the patient obese?
> - Motor and sensory examination: Establish a baseline prior to spine surgery.
> - Pulmonary function testing: In patients with a scoliotic deformity or neuromuscular disease.
> - Cardiac evaluation: In certain syndromic patients (ECG, echocardiogram).
> - Radiographic evaluation: In patients with fractures or spinal deformities.

pediatric scoliosis. Preoperative laboratory testing should include hemoglobin, hematocrit, and platelet count, as well as prothrombin time and international normalized ratio (INR). A renal panel should be considered if there are comorbidities impacting electrolyte levels. In addition, due to the difficulty of performing preoperative echocardiography in patients with severe spinal deformities, additional laboratory testing for cardiac-related pathology may be necessary, including brain natriuretic peptide and creatine kinase.[7]

PREOPERATIVE PHARMACOLOGY

Pediatric patients may be premedicated with a short-acting benzodiazepine, midazolam, in order to reduce preoperative anxiety and stress. To reduce blood loss and transfusion of allogenic blood products in surgeries in which massive blood loss is a concern, patients may be administered preoperative iron, erythropoietin, and autologous blood, or even undergo blood salvage, during which blood lost during surgery is reinfused to the patient. Acute normovolemic hemodilution may be used to mitigate the effects of blood loss by storing the patient's blood prior to surgery, replacing it with crystalloid solution, and then readministering the stored blood during surgery as needed.

ANESTHETIC TECHNIQUE

Intraoperative Management

Intraoperative management will depend on the type of surgery, as well as any comorbidities present (Table 119.1). In pediatric patients undergoing spine surgery, arterial oxygen saturation, end-tidal carbon dioxide, electrocardiographic patterns, core temperature, and urine output must all be recorded intraoperatively. Invasive blood pressure monitoring is used for spinal fusions and initial growing rod insertions. Conversely, an arterial line is typically not required for growing rod revisions.

Most, if not all, procedures will also need two peripheral IV catheters. If significant blood loss is not expected, as in growing rod revisions, a single well-functioning IV catheter may be acceptable, keeping in mind that the entire anesthetic may be reliant on that single IV. Point-of-care testing, such as an iStat, is often useful throughout spinal surgeries to assess changes in electrolytes and volume status.

Patients undergoing scoliosis surgery should be positioned and padded in a manner that avoids extreme pressure points, and all extremities should be maintained in a neutral position to avoid peripheral nerve injury. Likewise, it is imperative to avoid compression of the chest and abdomen, which can result in hypotension, hemodynamic instability, and high airway pressures/difficulty with ventilation. Most commonly, these patients are placed in a Relton–Hall frame, or a related variant, wherein four padded supports are arranged in V-shaped pairs, with the upper pair supporting the thorax and the lower pair supporting the pelvis. In children with severe deformities, distributing the weight of the arms in a fashion that avoids ulnar nerve injury can prove difficult.

In the prone position, postoperative vision loss is a serious, uncommon complication, occurring in about 3 in 10,000 prone cases.[10] Therefore, it is important the eyes are free of pressure when prone. The use of a prone pillow or headrest with a mirror allows for frequent monitoring of the eyes while in prone position. The etiology varies and includes ischemic optic neuropathy, retinal artery occlusion due to direct pressure on the globe, and cortical blindness due to injury to the visual cortex secondary to hypoperfusion.[11] Blood loss greater than 1,000 mL and a length of surgery greater than 6 hours are also associated with postoperative vision loss.[12] Anesthesia providers should ensure adequate oxygenation and perfusion pressure to the optic nerve by maintaining adequate blood volume (hematocrit [HCT] >30) and avoiding hypotension and hypovolemia to reduce the likelihood of postoperative vision loss.

While in prone position, it is equally important to ensure the endotracheal tube (ETT) does not kink or become occluded, dislodged, or inadvertently advanced. Anesthesia providers should have the ability to assess the face and ETT throughout the case of the ETT. However, it is important to be aware of the location of the needles used for IONM during surgery to prevent inadvertent needle sticks.

Thoracic insufficiency is common in neuromuscular scoliosis. With this and other comorbidities, such as chronic lung disease, ventilation can be difficult in prone position. This can especially be true when surgeons are exerting force when placing instrumentation. Pulmonary complications are more common in patients with neuromuscular scoliosis. It is imperative anesthesia providers ensure optimal positioning and securement of ETT to prevent any kinking or dislodgment of ETT. Ventilation settings should be optimized to adequately ventilate patients throughout the intraoperative course. Preoperative PFTs should be reviewed, as severe restrictive lung disease with decreased vital capacity is a risk factor for increased pulmonary complications.[7] A history of pneumonia, the presence of gastrostomy tube, and low transferrin levels

Table 119.1 Basic Anesthetic Considerations for Pediatric Spinal Surgery

Type of Surgery	Access	Invasive Monitoring	Antifibrinolytics	Intraoperative Neuromonitoring	Anesthetic Technique
Spinal fusions	2 PIVs	Arterial line	TXA and cell saver	Yes	TIVA
Growing rod insertions	2 PIVs	Arterial line	None	Yes	TIVA
Growing rod adjustment or lengthening	2 PIVs	None	None	Yes	TIVA

PIV, peripheral intravenous catheter; TIVA, total IV anesthetic: TXA, tranexamic acid..

were associated with respiratory complications postoperatively following spinal fusion.[8] Additionally, patients with a tracheostomy had a strong trend for postoperative respiratory complications.[8] Additionally, achieving lung isolation by double-lumen endobronchial intubation or a bronchial blocker is crucial in an anterior release or anterior spinal fusion, yet can introduce additional ventilation challenges.[13]

Typically, all pediatric spinal surgeries will require IONM, and subsequently, a total IV anesthetic (TIVA) or a combined technique, limiting the use of volatile anesthetic agents to a level no greater than ½ MAC. The technique of choice is typically institution-specific and thus it is important to discuss the anesthetic technique with the neuromonitoring team prior to induction of anesthesia. TIVA is often achieved via infusions of propofol and remifentanil, especially in the pediatric population. All volatile anesthetics produce dose-related reductions in amplitude and increases in latency of the somatosensory-evoked potentials (SSEP).[14] It is also known that MEPs are more readily assessed than SSEPs in children less than 6 years, assuming the use of a permissive anesthetic.[15]

Propofol can usually be started at 200 to 250 mcg/kg/min, and remifentanil can be started at 0.1 to 0.3 mcg/kg/min. The propofol infusion rate can be decreased in 30- to 60-minute intervals as guided by EEG monitoring feedback. Avoiding bolus dosing of propofol is important to maintain a steady anesthetic depth is important in maintaining a steady anesthetic depth without negative affecting IONM. Remifentanil can be increased periodically at particularly stimulating portions, such as incision. Other potentially safe agents include dexmedetomidine, but again institutional protocols and streamlining the anesthetic choice will be important.[16,17]

While remifentanil offers excellent intraoperative pain management, it lacks any postoperative benefit. It is recommended that a multimodal pain management should be employed, including use of IV acetaminophen 10 to 15 mg/kg, IV ketorolac 0.5 mg/kg up to 15 mg (if no contraindications), and opioids (morphine or hydromorphone and possibly methadone) titrated near the end of the procedure. Administration of diazepam 0.05 mg/kg (in appropriate patients) once the patient is awake, extubated, and responding to simple commands can help stave off pain related to muscle spasms secondary to surgical dissection.

Some degree of hypotension is common during pediatric spinal fusion. Most commonly, sustained hypotension is related to hypovolemia. Anesthesia providers should consider evaporative losses due to large surgical exposure. Administration of crystalloid, albumin 10 mL/kg administration, and autologous cell saver are all viable options to replete volume loss. For hemoglobin levels less than 8 g/dL, packed red blood cell (PRBC) administration should be considered, as well as calcium gluconate for low ionized calcium levels. Phenylephrine infusion is commonly used to maintain mean arterial pressure (MAP). During the instrumentation phase of spinal surgeries, the MAP is often increased artificially using vasopressors. Ephedrine and phenylephrine boluses can be employed, although a phenylephrine infusion may be required. It is often best to have the infusion set up prior to the start of surgery if there is an expectation of use.

Predictors of massive transfusion during scoliosis surgery include number of fused vertebrae, BMI, and Cobb angle. Patients with low BMI and severe scoliosis requiring a large number of fused vertebrae are more likely to suffer excessive blood loss. Since transfusion during spine surgery is associated with poorer clinical outcomes, a thorough evaluation of the patient's preoperative nutritional status and severity of disease should be performed.

Patients with neuromuscular scoliosis have seven times greater risk of greater than 50% blood loss of total blood volume compared with those without neuromuscular disease.[7] However, blood loss can be significant in any major spine surgery. Severe scoliosis, including larger curves (Cobb angle >70 degrees), increasing levels fused, and the need for osteotomies are associated with increased operative time and blood loss.[18,19] Methods to reduce blood loss include permissive hypotension and use of antifibrinolytics.

Intraoperative hemostasis may be monitored through point-of-care testing for hemoglobin/hematocrit level, as well as thromboelastography (TEG), for coagulation status.[20] While spectrophotometry may be useful for continuous monitoring of hemodynamic status in high-risk patients, it is less accurate than point-of-care testing.[20] Pharmacologically induced controlled hypotension has been demonstrated to decrease perioperative blood loss, although it simultaneously decreases end-organ perfusion. Therefore, this is not a technique used in the pediatric population. In fact, for spine surgery the patient is kept normotensive during the dissection phase and the blood pressure is then elevated to a goal MAP of 70 to 80 when hardware is placed. Antifibrinolytics (aminocaproic acid, tranexamic acid) have been shown to significantly reduce intraoperative blood loss and need for blood transfusion in spine surgery, without increasing intraoperative or postoperative complications.[21] While the most effective dose has been debated, high-dose tranexamic acid has been shown to be effective and other studies have shown benefit from antifibrinolytics regardless of dose.[21]

Special Techniques and/or Equipment

There are several assessment techniques that have been described through the years to assess for neurological injury during spinal fusion. The Stagnara wake-up test was the first form of neuromonitoring available for scoliosis surgery and continues to be the gold standard.[22] The wake-up test involves partially awakening the patient intraoperatively to test their motor function and maintains utility today as a method of confirming signal changes identified through modern neuromonitoring.

IONM is an important tool for anesthesia providers managing a scoliosis spine surgery as it allows for early detection of a neural injury. Moreover, while some studies find that consistent and reliable IONM in patients with neuromuscular disease is difficult and arguably unreliable, multimodal IONM has been demonstrated to be both sensitive and specific in detecting intraoperative neurological injuries during spinal surgery.[23,24] Hence, IONM is the most widely employed comprehensive method for detecting intraoperative neurological injuries through the combined techniques of SSEP, transcranial motor-evoked potentials (tcMEPs), neurogenic motor-evoked potentials (nMEPs), spontaneous electromyography (sEMG), and triggered electromyography (tEMG).[29] Table 119.2 demonstrates the inherent strengths and weaknesses of the components of various intraoperative monitoring techniques.

SSEP allows for continuous monitoring throughout the surgery, but cannot detect motor changes and requires temporal summation for detection of a signal change, which results in delayed detection. While MEPs do not allow for continuous monitoring, they are sensitive to detection of motor deficits and spinal cord ischemia. Electromyography (EMG) has a high rate of false-positive alarms but provides real-time

Table 119.2 Intraoperative Multimodal Neuromonitoring

Modality	Anatomy	Not Addressed	Anesthetic Concerns	Temporality	Risks
Wake-up test	Gross motor function	Nerve roots and sensation	Use only short-acting reversible agents	Single point, difficult to repeat	Self-extubation, delayed warning, missed deficit
SSEP	Ascending pathways: dorsal column proprioception and vibration	Focal motor and nerve roots	Muscle relaxants helpful. Volatile anesthetics inhibit SSEP monitoring. No dose-related barbiturate inhibition	Continuous, 3–5 min summation	Missed focal motor and nerve root injury, up to 16 min delay to warning
tcMEP	Anterior spinal grey of descending pathways	Sensation and complex motor movement	Precludes use of neuromuscular blockade. Highly sensitive to inhalation inhalation	Single point, easily repeated	Concern for patient movement
nMEP	Whole cord with significant antidromic column component	Nerve roots	Inhalation anesthetic is acceptable, precludes use of neuromuscular blockade if compound muscle action potentials are being recorded	Single point, easily repeated	Possible lack of true motor data
sEMG	Nerve root (assessment in selected myotomes)	Sensation and anterior descending motor pathways	Precludes use of neuromuscular blockade, sensitive to temperature changes. Inhalation anesthetic is okay	Continuous	High false-positive rate
tEMG	Nerve root (stimulator/pedicle screw to end muscle)	Sensation and anterior descending motor pathways	Precludes use of neuromuscular blockade, inhalation anesthetic is okay, less sensitive for thoracic pedicle screws than for lumbar pedicle screws	Single point, easily repeated	High false-positive rate

The characteristics of the various components of intraoperative multimodal neuromonitoring. SSEP indicates somatosensory-evoked potentials; tcMEP, transcranial motor-evoked potentials; nMEP, neurogenic motor-evoked potentials; sEMG, spontaneous electromyography; tEMG, triggered electromyography.

nMEP, neurogenic motor-evoked potential; sEMG, spontaneous electromyography; SSEP, somatosensory-evoked potential; tcMEP, transcranial motor-evoked potential; tEMG, triggered electromyography.

Source: Modified from Charalampidis A, Jiang F, Wilson JR, et al. The use of intraoperative neurophysiological monitoring in spine surgery. *Global Spine J*. 2020; 10(1 Suppl.):104S–114S.

information about the nerve root and may be combined with SSEP to improve specificity.[29]

The combination of IONM with the wake-up test for confirmation of neurological insults constitutes a modern and effective method for ongoing evaluation of neurological injury during scoliosis surgery.

Clinical Pearls

The authors' institution treats spinal fusion and instrumentation as an "SSI case," or a surgical site infection case. Institutional guidelines are maintained for infection control and prevention. Appropriately prescribed and dosed antibiotics are given prior to incision. Fraction of inspired oxygen (FiO_2) greater than 60% prior to incision is maintained throughout the surgery. The patient's core body temperature should be greater than 35.5°C prior to incision and throughout the surgery. Sterile technique is used with arterial line placement and with central line placement, if indicated. All peripheral IV catheters and arterial lines are appropriately scrubbed with chlorhexidine prior to access. In addition to appropriate operating room attire, a hood and shoe coverings are also worn by all staff. Traffic through the operating room is also kept to a minimum. An evidence-based, multidisciplinary approach to infection prevention is vital and has been shown to decrease the rate of surgical site infections following spinal fusion with instrumentation.[25]

Complications/Emergencies

Major Blood Loss

Anesthesia providers must be prepared to administer blood products for anemia and coagulopathies. For all spinal fusion surgeries, a type and screen must be performed preoperatively and two units of PRBCs should be readily available. Additionally, the use of antifibrinolytics and autologous blood can be considered to minimize the need for blood transfusion. Institutions where pediatric spinal fusions are performed should have the ability and training in place treat major blood loss and to perform massive transfusion.[26] Additionally, best-practice guidelines for perioperative treatment of blood loss during spinal fusion should be maintained institutionally.[27]

Loss of Evoked Potentials

The loss of evoked potentials intraoperatively is considered a sentinel event. While institutional protocols may vary, it is imperative a clearly delineated algorithm be readily available to guide care should this occur.

POSTOPERATIVE CARE

Postoperative care focuses on pain management, respiratory function, nutrition, and increasing mobility. Postoperative pain is dictated by the multifactorial relationship of genetic, physiological, and psychological determinants with the somatosensory alterations related to nerve injury and inflammation. Therefore, a multimodal approach to postoperative pain is most appropriate. Options for postoperative pain control include acetaminophen, nonsteroidal anti-inflammatory drugs, gabapentin, opioids, and patient-controlled analgesia. As previously mentioned, obese patients with surgically managed musculoskeletal conditions require special consideration in the preoperative, perioperative, and postoperative setting. The combined effect of obstructive sleep apnea and obesity has been demonstrated to increase sensitivity to opioids; therefore, care must be taken when dosing.

All types of scoliosis surgery result in a postoperative decrease in lung volumes and pulmonary function like those encountered in thoracic and abdominal surgery. These values take 1 to 2 months to return to baseline, with a nadir of 3 days for forced vital capacity (FVC) and forced expiratory volume in 1 second (FEV_1). Due to the high likelihood of respiratory compromise in scoliosis patients, preoperative pulmonary assessment is essential. Depending on the severity of curvature, these patients may experience restrictive pulmonary function at baseline. In one study, a vital capacity of less than 60% was determined to be predictive of prolonged postoperative mechanical ventilation, likely due to an impaired ability to cough, thereby predisposing the patient to respiratory complications. Another study found that pediatric patients with a preoperative vital capacity of less than 40% who were undergoing spine surgery were safely able to be discharged home despite short-term respiratory complications. Daily respiratory therapy, including physiotherapy, intermittent positive-pressure breathing, mechanical cough assistance, and in some patients, the introduction of a tracheostomy prior to surgery, may constitute several means of minimizing respiratory complications in patients with neuromuscular scoliosis.[3] After undergoing surgical intervention, the scoliosis patient may also have worsening of reflux postoperatively secondary to a straightened torso.[3]

Patients with neuromuscular scoliosis tend to have increased risk of postoperative complications, including postoperative anemia and respiratory complications. The risk of prolonged postoperative ventilation in neuromuscular scoliosis is higher than in other types of scoliosis due to the additive effect of both the structurally mediated decrease in tidal volume associated with severe scoliosis and the neuromuscular dysfunction of the laryngeal, pharyngeal, and respiratory muscles, leading to an increased risk of aspiration, inadequate cough, and diminished respiratory effort. These patients often require monitoring postoperatively in the ICU.

CASE STUDY: A Teen With Idiopathic Scoliosis for Posterior Spinal Fusion

CLINICAL SCENARIO

A 14-year-old otherwise healthy male with adolescent idiopathic scoliosis presents for posterior spinal fusion at T2–L4 with spinal monitoring. The patient had no previous surgeries or anesthesia. Preoperative imaging revealed a curvature of 59 to 64 degrees in the thoracolumbar region. Preoperative workup including pulmonary function tests, resting ECG, and neurological examination were all normal.

APPROACHES TO CARE

The patient was premedicated with midazolam 2 mg and underwent IV induction with lidocaine 50 mg, fentanyl 100 mcg, and propofol 230 mg. Infusions of remifentanil 0.3 mcg/kg/min and propofol 250 mcg/kg/min were started immediately following induction of anesthesia. Oral endotracheal intubation, arterial line placement, and a second large-bore IV access were obtained prior to positioning. The patient was then prepared for positioning. The eyes were lubricated and protected with Tegaderm, a tooth guard and bilateral blocks were utilized, and a prone pillow was used to avoid pressure on the eyes, mouth, nose, and ears. Surgical team was present prior to final positioning.

The patient remained hemodynamically stable throughout the dissection phase of the surgery, with an estimated blood loss of 1 L. Phenylephrine infusion was begun to increase mean arterial pressures to a goal of 70s during the instrumentation phase of the surgery. One autologous blood transfusion of 300 mL was administered near the end of instrumentation. Total estimated blood loss (EBL) was estimated to be 1,200 mL. Arterial blood gases throughout the surgery were notable for a downtrend in HCT to a nadir of 30 and a final HCT of 32. The patient made 1 L of urine. The procedure was otherwise uneventful.

Toward the end of the surgery, hydromorphone 2 mg was titrated to respiratory rate. He was given IV acetaminophen approximately 3 hours before the end of surgery. He awoke and was given diazepam 1 mg IV before transfer to the postanesthesia care unit (PACU). In the PACU, IV ketorolac 15 mg was administered. He remained comfortable in the PACU but had escalating pain on postoperative day (POD) POD 0 to POD 1. Some newer evidence now suggests other pain regimens that could have potentially improved this patient's pain. These modalities include intraoperative methadone and the potential for epidural rather than patient-controlled analgesia (PCA).

Evidence-Based Approaches to Care

Uncontrolled pain is a common complication of major orthopedic surgery, including spinal fusion. Multimodal pain management regimens can lead to improved patient satisfaction, earlier mobilization, shorter hospital stays, and lower postoperative pain scores.[28–30] The authors' institution has recently employed an updated pain pathway based on more recent literature, as outlined in Table 119.3. Note that our institution is not currently using gabapentinoids as there is mixed evidence regarding effectiveness. Additionally, there are increasing reports of abuse potential. Epidural analgesia or intrathecal morphine has been shown to be safe and equally effective alternative to PCA, although not commonly employed at our institution.[31–34] We are currently not routinely using lidocaine or ketamine infusions. However, it may be reasonable to consider these adjuncts in patients who are opioid-tolerant.

(continued)

CASE STUDY: A Teen With Idiopathic Scoliosis for Posterior Spinal Fusion (*continued*)

Table 119.3 Pain Management Plan for Spinal Fusion in Idiopathic Scoliosis

Modality	Components	Comments
Preoperative	• Education, anxiety risks, behavioral modifications, and so forth	Weak evidence to support this, but potential benefit outweighs any risk
Intraoperative	• Propofol and remifentanil infusions • Methadone 0.1–0.2 mg/kg (max 10 mg) • Ketorolac 0.5 mg/kg/dose (max 15 mg) • IV acetaminophen 15 mg/kg/dose (max 1,000 mg) • Epidural 0.1%–0.25% bupivacaine 5–10 mL + morphine 30–50 mcg/kg or intrathecal morphine 9–15 mcg/kg	• Potential concerns of opioid hyperalgesia, most commonly used modality • Pediatric dosing studies needed, decreases postoperative opioid consumption • Low-dose ketorolac safe and effective • Cost-effectiveness of IV versus PO not established • Safe and effective alternative to PCA
POD 0	• PCA hydromorphone 5 mcg/kg demand doses with 10 mcg/kg PRN breakthrough dose q4h or epidural 0.0625%–0.125% bupivacaine 4–10 mL/hr with hydromorphone/morphine • Acetaminophen 15 mg/kg IV or PO q6h • Ketorolac 0.5 mg/kg IV q6h for 8 doses alternating with APAP • Diazepam 0.05 mg/kg (max 5 mg) IV q4h PRN muscle spasms • Methocarbamol 15 mg/kg (max 1,000 mg) q8h IV • Zofran for nausea/vomiting, nalbuphine for pruritus • Other: ice packs, breathing techniques/massage	
POD 1	• If PCA: start oxycodone 0.1 mg/kg PO q4h scheduled and discontinue PCA if tolerating PO meds • If epidural: continue epidural • Continue ketorolac until 8 doses have been reached • Switch other meds to PO on the same schedule as above • Start bowel regimen • Other: regular diet, walk 3×/d, PT, spirometer 10×/hr while awake	
POD 2	• Continue PO pain medications • Discontinue epidural catheter if present • Continue nonpharmacological adjuncts • Discharge to home if adequate pain control with PO meds • Transition oxycodone to PRN at discharge	

APAP, acetaminophen; PCA, patient-controlled analgesia; POD, postoperative day; PT, physical therapy.

KEY REFERENCES

Complete references for this chapter are online and available at https://connect.springerpub.com/content/book/978-0-8261-3875-0/part/part04/toc-part/ch119.

3. Mary P, Servais L, Vialle R. Neuromuscular diseases: diagnosis and management. *Orthop Traumatol Surg Res*. 2018;104(1S):S89–S95. doi:10.1016/j.otsr.2017.04.019

4. Hasler CC. Early-onset scoliosis: contemporary decision-making and treatment options. *J Pediatr Orthop*. 2018;38(Suppl. 1):S13–S20. doi:10.1097/BPO.0000000000001184

8. Luhmann SJ, Furdock R. Preoperative variables associated with respiratory complications after pediatric neuromuscular spine deformity surgery. *Spine Deform*. 2019;7(1):107–111. doi:10.1016/j.jspd.2018.05.005

26. Sono T, Fujibayashi S, Izeki M, et al. Decreased rate of surgical site infection after spinal surgery with instrumentation using bundled approach including surveillance and intrawound vancomycin application. *Medicine (Baltimore)*. 2018;97(34):e12010. doi:10.1097/MD.0000000000012010

30. Seki H, Ideno S, Ishihara T, et al. Postoperative pain management in patients undergoing posterior spinal fusion for adolescent idiopathic scoliosis: a narrative review. *Scoliosis*. 2018;13:17. doi:10.1186/s13013-018-0165-z

31. Shah AS, Guidry R, Kumar A, et al. Current trends in pediatric spine deformity surgery: multimodal pain management and rapid recovery. *Global Spine J*. 2020;10(3):346–352. doi:10.1177/2192568219858308

CHAPTER 120

Knee Ligament Reconstruction

Eric Wall and James S. Furstein

INDICATIONS/CONTRAINDICATIONS

Over the past two decades there has been a revolution in the surgical treatment of anterior cruciate ligament (ACL) injuries in skeletally immature patients, which was rarely performed over fears of growth plate damage. For patella instability, medial patellofemoral ligament (MPFL) reconstruction has largely supplanted less effective medial capsular plication, medial muscle advancement, and lateral release procedures. While these surgeries are mostly performed through minimal incisions, they often create maximal pain secondary to drilling of bone tunnels and the harvest of hamstring, patellar, or quadriceps autografts.

ACL RECONSTRUCTION

Young athletes with complete ACL tears who wish to return to their sports are indicated for ACL reconstruction. The bulk of recent studies shows that active children who do not undergo ACL reconstruction soon after injury are more prone to meniscal tears and chondral injury than those who have early surgical stabilization.[1] This is especially true for children who have repeat give-way instability episodes after an ACL tear. Young athletes place much more demand on their knee than adult athletes, mainly due to the extensive time they spend practicing and competing in their sports, often over 200 hours per high school season. Soccer and basketball produce the highest risk of ACL tears in female high school sports per athletic exposure and football for males.[2] The peak age of ACL tears occurs during adolescence for both males and females.[3] Children who tear their ACL and are nonathletic may undergo a trial of physical therapy and bracing. Any episode of give-way would indicate surgery in this group.

An open growth plate is not a contraindication to an ACL reconstruction, but the sports surgeon must adapt the adult technique to minimize risk to the femoral and tibial growth plates of the knee. Meniscal tears are frequently associated with ACL tears. In children, these tears usually warrant repair due to their high healing rate and prevention of future arthritis. Flipped bucket-handle tears and other complex tears may require an open incision located over the medial or lateral knee, which may need to be considered in the regional anesthetic plan. Patients who are noncompliant or not able to participate in postoperative physical therapy may be a relative contraindication to ACL surgery.

MPFL RECONSTRUCTION

Patella dislocation incidence also peaks during the adolescent years. A first-time traumatic dislocation that reduces back to normal position and is not associated with an osteochondral fracture is indicated for a trial of physical therapy rehabilitation, even though there is up to 71% risk of recurrent dislocation.[4] Trochlea dysplasia, opposite knee instability, female sex, younger age, and high patella increase the risk of recurrence.[5] About one third of traumatic patellar dislocations are associated with an osteochondral fracture in children and about half of these may need an open repair.[6] A repairable osteochondral fracture (seen on MRI) serves as an indication for surgery after a first-time traumatic patellar dislocation. After a second patellar dislocation, the patient is at a much higher risk of future dislocations, and most recurrent patellar dislocations are considered an indication for surgical stabilization.

Like ACL reconstruction surgery, an open growth plate should be avoided when placing the femoral tunnel. Knee growth disturbance has rarely been reported after MPFL reconstruction surgery and can be minimized by placing the femoral tunnel just distal to the femur growth plate with fluoroscopy guidance.

SPECIAL CONSIDERATIONS AND CONCERNS

Anesthesia providers should tailor their regional anesthetics to the type of graft the surgeon chooses. The three most common grafts for ACL reconstruction are the hamstring, patella, and quadriceps tendon autografts. Allografts (cadaver grafts) are popular in adult ACL reconstruction, but due to their high retear rate in children they are usually avoided in patients younger than 20 years. For MPFL reconstruction, the hamstring and quadriceps tendon are the most commonly harvested autografts. Allografts are also popular due to their comparable success with autografts. It is important to confirm the type of graft the surgeon will be using, along with their surgical procedure, before performing regional anesthesia to ensure the harvest site is adequately anesthetized.

Before placing regional anesthesia for ACL or MPFL reconstruction, it is prudent to have the surgeon perform their exam under anesthesia (EUA) just after induction. The surgeon's preoperative history, physical examination, and image review are key to making a diagnosis of ACL or MPFL injury, but each is associated with a rate of error. The EUA is key to confirming the correct diagnosis. If the EUA is normal for an ACL or for patella stability, the surgeon may abort the reconstructive procedure or elect to perform only a diagnostic arthroscopy and not the preoperatively planned reconstructive procedure. Placing the block after an EUA surgical plan change avoids a potentially unnecessary or unwarranted insensate extremity.

MPFL reconstruction is the primary surgery for traumatic patella dislocation in otherwise normal patients. Other procedures such as tibial tubercle osteotomy, femur or tibia osteotomy, proximal quadricepsplasty, medial muscle advancement, lateral retinacular release or lengthening, trochlear groove deepening, and medial soft tissue reefing may be indicated in congenital, syndromic, or neuromuscular patients. These adjunctive procedures may require different regional anesthesia techniques. Osteotomies with their risk of compartment syndrome may make surgeons nervous about regional anesthesia masking a compartment syndrome. Hence, it is always a good practice to communicate with the surgeon prior to the surgical procedure and/or performing regional anesthesia.

> **BOX 120.1 KEY ASSESSMENT POINTS FOR KNEE LIGAMENT RECONSTRUCTION**
>
> - Coexisting injuries
> - Current level of pain
> - Current pain management regimen
> - Mechanism of injury
> - Presence of existing neuropathies
> - Presence of strength and motor deficits

ANESTHETIC MANAGEMENT

PREOPERATIVE EVALUATION

Prior to anesthesia, all patients should receive a thorough history and physical to vet the presence of any comorbid conditions that may impact the anesthetic plan. In addition, special attention should be given to the injured lower extremity scheduled for surgical repair. As regional anesthesia will likely be incorporated in the pain management plan, it is imperative anesthesia providers determine the patient's current level of pain, inciting factors, current pain management regimen, presence of numbness, and if there are any motor or strength deficits as compared with the noninjured extremity. Understanding the preoperative state is key to developing a safe regional anesthesia plan (Box 120.1).

Pertinent Labs

No labs are needed preoperatively unless mandated by comorbid conditions.

PREOPERATIVE PHARMACOLOGY

Administration of an anxiolytic, such as midazolam, may be indicated preoperatively.

In recent years, there has been a growing interest in expanding multimodal analgesia practices in pediatric anesthesia. Preoperative administration of cyclooxygenase-2 inhibitors, gamma-aminobutyric acid (GABA) analogs, and acetaminophen has been shown to reduce the use of opioids postoperatively. Cyclooxygenase-2 inhibitors may reduce postoperative pain, opioid use, postoperative nausea and vomiting, and recovery room length of stay.[7] While preoperative administration has become standard prior to ACL reconstruction, anesthesia providers should avoid the use of cyclooxygenase-2 inhibitors if the patient has a history of renal insufficiency. Likewise, pregabalin, a gamma-aminobutyric acid analog, has been offered to be a valuable adjuvant to multimodal analgesic regimens that can significantly reduce early postoperative pain in patients undergoing ACL reconstruction.[8] Pregabalin inhibits voltage-gated calcium influx at the nerve terminals, which in turn reduces the release of excitatory neurotransmitters and gradually attenuates central sensitization of the dorsal horn neurons, thereby preventing hyperalgesia. The use of pregabalin should be avoided if there is a history of suicidal ideation. Acetaminophen should be avoided in the presence of hepatic impairment.

ANESTHETIC TECHNIQUE

Intraoperative Management

ACL and MPFL reconstruction is typically performed under general anesthesia. The induction of anesthesia usually occurs via an IV induction, although an inhalation mask induction is acceptable in younger children who do not have a peripheral catheter in place. Should NPO status be insufficient, a rapid sequence induction may be indicated. A single large-bore peripheral IV catheter capable of volume resuscitation is sufficient for both ACL and MPFL reconstruction as blood loss is anticipated to be minimal. Standard monitors, as recommended by the American Society of Anesthesiologists (ASA), are often adequate as invasive monitoring is seldom indicated.

While the airway can be managed with either a laryngeal mask airway (LMA) or an endotracheal tube (ETT), anesthesia providers should consider the length of the scheduled procedure and comorbid conditions that may impact airway management when determining the most appropriate means of airway management.

Nondepolarizing neuromuscular blocking agents may be used to facilitate intubation and patient positioning. In most instances, it is not necessary to redose neuromuscular blocking agents throughout the procedure. Prophylactic antibiotics, such as cefazolin or clindamycin, should be administered prior to surgical incision. Anesthesia providers may administer short- and long-acting narcotics, such as fentanyl and morphine or hydromorphone, in conjugation with nonnarcotic medications, such as acetaminophen, for pain management. Regional anesthesia is commonly employed to temper postoperative pain. It should be noted that regional anesthesia techniques will not stave off spasms at the hamstring autograft donor site. As such, administering methocarbamol or diazepam should be considered.

Tourniquets are commonly used during ACL and MPFL reconstruction to afford the surgeon an unencumbered view of the surgical field. Common complications associated with use of a tourniquet include muscle, nerve, vascular, or skin damage, as well as increased core body temperature and a theoretical increase in the risk of deep vein thrombosis right after cuff release.[9] Pediatric patients are more sensitive to pressure and time threshold for tourniquet use, and this should be taken into consideration to avoid tissue damage.[10] Therefore, it is recommended that the tourniquet not be set to a pressure greater than 100 mm Hg higher than the patient's systolic blood pressure at the time of inflation. Tourniquet inflation time should also not exceed 120 minutes. Limiting tourniquet inflation pressure and time minimizes the likelihood of tourniquet-related complications. Anesthesia providers should also be aware that sudden reperfusion after deflation of the tourniquet may cause a slight decrease in blood pressure and a rapid increase in carbon dioxide levels.

Special Techniques and/or Equipment

The management of postoperative pain following ACL and MPFL reconstruction is achieved using a variety of analgesic regimens, which are often based on both surgeon- and anesthesia provider-specific preferences. Even though there remains no gold standard, regional anesthesia remains the primary treatment for postoperative pain after ACL and MPFL reconstruction.

Femoral nerve blockade has long been regarded as the gold standard for providing analgesia to the anterior aspect of the thigh and knee. Concerns related to the lack of motor strength in the lower extremity associated with use of a femoral nerve block have driven providers to look for alternative approaches. In recent years, continuous adductor canal blocks have emerged as an appealing alternative to a continuous femoral nerve block as they produce a predominantly sensory nerve block of the saphenous nerve with limited motor involvement. While a femoral nerve block affects all four quadriceps muscles, the only motor nerve traversing the adductor canal is the nerve to the vastus medialis muscle, thereby allowing an adductor canal block to preserve quadriceps muscle strength.[11] Concerns regarding analgesic efficacy, however, lead many pediatric anesthesia providers to employ femoral nerve blockade as opposed to an adductor canal block. Regardless of the regional anesthesia technique used, ACL and MPFL reconstruction is a painful surgical procedure associated with severe pain for several days postoperatively. Anesthesia providers should consider the use of an indwelling continuous perineural infusion catheter to extend analgesia postoperatively.

Key factors to consider when formulating a pain management plan also include the autograft technique utilized, being either bone–patellar–tendon–bone, hamstring autograft, or allograft, and the severity of pain associated with each of these techniques. Remaining cognizant of these factors affords the discerning anesthesia provider the ability to target pain sites specifically and to do so for an adequate duration such that rebound pain can be averted. To date, sciatic nerve blockade has been reported to reduce hamstring donor site pain most reliably; however, there remains no consensus as to the duration of action required to effectively control donor site pain throughout the postoperative period.[12,13]

Several clinical trials suggest the addition of sciatic block following total knee arthroplasty (TKA) improves postoperative analgesia; however, the extent of the role sciatic block plays in pain control remains undetermined.[14] While a different surgical procedure, much of the pain experienced by patients during the postoperative period is similar to that of patients undergoing knee ligament reconstruction due to the anatomical areas disrupted during surgery. Ben-David et al.[14] reported that following TKA, pain scores were greatly reduced in patients receiving an indwelling continuous perineural infusion catheter when compared with those who received only a single-injection sciatic nerve block. Wegener et al.[15] investigated whether the addition of sciatic nerve block to continuous femoral nerve blockade would shorten the time-to-discharge readiness following TKA. Although no impact on time-to-discharge readiness was appreciated, a distinction in postoperative pain control was noted, as a single-injection sciatic nerve block reduced severe pain on the day of the surgery, whereas continuous sciatic nerve block reduced moderate pain during mobilization on the initial 2 postoperative days.

While both single-injection sciatic nerve block and continuous sciatic nerve blockade alleviate pain the day of surgery, only continuous sciatic nerve blockade can reduce pain on subsequent postoperative days. Proponents of continuous sciatic nerve block assert that the extended duration of analgesia afforded using an indwelling continuous perineural infusion catheter improves overall pain control postoperatively and reduces the need for supplemental pain medications.[16] Ganesh and Cucchiaro's[16] contention that the duration of action of single-injection sciatic nerve block may fail to outlast the pain arising from the hamstring donor site has prompted some clinicians to employ indwelling continuous perineural infusion catheters.

The use of indwelling continuous perineural infusion catheters is not without its detractors, however. Advocates of single-injection sciatic nerve block, which can last up to 24 hours or longer, note that in adult studies sciatic nerve block offered significant advantages in pain control only during the initial 24 hours following knee surgery.[15] Furthermore, concerns regarding increased risk of falls, decreased active knee movement, and masking of a compartment syndrome

> **BOX 120.2 CLINICAL PEARLS: KNEE LIGAMENT RECONSTRUCTION**
>
> - Know the surgeon's graft choice for reconstruction and discuss block plan before doing block (patellar, hamstring, quadriceps, or allograft tendon).
> - The surgeon's EUA may affect the procedure, especially for patellar stabilization. For blocks performed under anesthesia, have the surgeon do EUA after induction but prior to block.
> - Osteotomies may be performed in conjunction with patella stabilization and may preclude a block out of fear of masking a compartment syndrome.
>
> EUA, exam under anesthesia.

preclude routine use of indwelling continuous perineural infusion catheters by many clinicians.[17] Not only are these potential risks undesirable, but they can also be costly should they occur and may require further medical or surgical intervention to correct.

Infiltration of the interspace between the popliteal artery and the capsule of the posterior knee (IPACK) block has been introduced as an alternative to the sciatic nerve block. The IPACK block has been reported to provide posterior knee analgesia through blockade of terminal branches innervating the posterior knee capsule while sparing the tibial and peroneal nerves. The risk of neural and vascular injury remains with the use of an IPACK block due to the presence of the popliteal vessels and the tibial and peroneal nerves near the posterior capsule (Box 120.2). While further studies are required to establish their benefit and safety profile, IPACK blocks may represent a significant advance in providing analgesia to the posterior aspect of the knee.[18]

Complications/Emergencies

Excessive blood loss is rarely a concern with pediatric ACL and MPFL reconstruction as tourniquets are frequently used. Arterial or vein injury is also extremely rare, but there is a higher risk of vessel injury with posterior cruciate and multiligament reconstructions.

POSTOPERATIVE CARE

Perioperative pain management of children and adolescents undergoing ACL and MPFL reconstruction typically uses a multimodal approach, combining acetaminophen, nonsteroidal anti-inflammatory drugs (NSAIDs), opioids, antispasmodics, and regional anesthesia.[19] Acetaminophen acts through several different mechanisms, including the cyclooxygenase (COX), endocannabinoid, serotonergic, and nitric oxide synthesis pathways, to achieve analgesia.[20] NSAIDs act to reduce prostaglandin synthesis by inhibiting the COX pathway, thereby decreasing tissue inflammation and producing analgesic effects.[21] In surgeries in which moderate to severe postoperative pain is expected, opioids are an appropriate therapy.[19]

Pediatric patients are routinely discharged home with indwelling continuous perineural infusion catheters without significant complication.[22] Although discharging patients with an insensate extremity remains controversial and puts greater emphasis on patient/guardian selection, data suggest that the risk of injury to these patients is relatively minimal.[23,24] Furthermore, patients with indwelling continuous perineural infusion catheters do not fall more frequently than either patients without indwelling continuous perineural infusion catheters or other surgical patients.[25] Appropriate patient selection and thorough patient education prior to discharge have also been key to success.[26] Although the potential for complication exists with any procedure, studies in large cohorts of pediatric patients discharged with indwelling continuous perineural infusion catheters have failed to highlight the severe complications reported in adult studies as only minor side effects have been commonly noted in the pediatric population.[27]

Regardless of the regional anesthesia technique employed (single-injection or indwelling continuous perineural infusion catheter), the patient should be advised not to put weight on the insensate extremity and to always use crutches when walking to preclude fall or injury. It is also imperative the patient guards against catheter dislodgment every time they transfer or ambulate. The caregiver should be properly educated on care of the indwelling continuous perineural infusion catheters, the signs and symptoms of local anesthetic toxicity, and catheter removal. In addition, they should be informed how to contact an anesthesia provider should questions or concerns arise.

A clearly delineated postoperative pain management plan should be discussed with the patient and their caregiver. A key part of the plan entails the transition to oral medications and ultimately a weaning plan to prevent long-term use and reliance on opioid analgesics.

CHAPTER 121

Mehta Cast Application

Aaron Sundberg

INDICATIONS/CONTRAINDICATIONS

Early-onset scoliosis (EOS) is one of the most challenging conditions that pediatric orthopedic surgeons face in our world today. Over the years, there have been multiple techniques employed to help children overcome this condition, each with various advantages and disadvantages. While several spinal implants that accommodate growth exist, such as growing rods, vertical expandable prosthetic titanium rib (VEPTR), and MAGnetic Expansion Control (MAGEC), these techniques have high complication rates, require multiple expansion procedures, and have been shown to result in unintended autofusion in nearly 90% of patients. Serial casting, however, has proved to be a valuable option in treating children with EOS, as many children realize complete correction and for others surgery is successfully delayed to a more opportune time or later age.

The serial casting technique for EOS relies on the principle of guided growth, with the goal being improvement of the deformity due to the continued growth afforded by the cast. It should be noted that although serial casting has been associated with complete resolution of deformity in patients with infantile idiopathic scoliosis (IIS), the goal of casting is not necessarily complete cure. Rather, casting can be an effective tactic to delay surgical treatment with growing instrumentation in patients with severe scoliosis or other orthopedic deformity.

Joseph Risser was one of the first to develop an elongation–derotation technique to address scoliosis. In 1964, French orthopedic surgeons Cotrel and Morel pioneered the elongation–derotation–flexion (EDF) casting technique, which improved on Risser's technique by addressing a third component.[1] The EDF cast corrects the spine three-dimensionally by applying forces in longitudinal, transverse, and rotatory directions and is custom-made for each patient. The idea behind serial EDF casting is that while the casts are made to allow for spinal growth, the casts can prevent the progression of the spinal deformity.

While many cases of IIS resolve spontaneously, in part due to the rapid development of trunk and motor control in the neonate, curves with documented progression require intervention to stave off further detriment. Most notably, marked pulmonary constriction and even early death can occur in the most severe cases.

In 1975, Min Mehta developed the idea of serial casting, changing casts every 8 to 12 weeks to accommodate growth of the child. This was a new application of the EDF technique, as it had not previously been employed to address IIS. Soon after adapting this technique, however, Mehta reported that 69% of patients realized complete resolution by an average age of 3.5 years, thanks to the early intervention. Given the success of Dr. Mehta's casting technique, it has become the preferred noninvasive treatment for IIS and EOS in patients between the ages of 12 months and 4 years.

SPECIAL CONSIDERATIONS AND CONCERNS

While children presenting for Mehta cast application typically receive a general anesthetic, the need for general anesthesia has been challenged. A recent study examined the outcomes of 129 patients who underwent serial casting for IIS. Of the cases reviewed, 92 (76%) received general anesthesia during casting procedures, while 29 (24%) remained awake. Patients in the awake cohort experienced significantly greater first-in-cast correction of the major curve, as well as significant improvement in thoracic spine height.[2] While the rate of curve progression between the groups was reported to be similar, the rate of casting success was ultimately found to be higher in the awake cohort (72%) as compared with the asleep cohort (48%).[2]

The outcomes of this study have led some to question the need for general anesthesia. This is especially germane given the concern in recent years about the impact repeated exposure to volatile anesthetics may have on the developing brain. Relative to this patient population, disease severity, a non idiopathic diagnosis, and longer length of follow-up have all been found to be associated with an increase in anesthesia needs. In fact, patients with EOS who are treated by Mehta casting will be exposed to volatile anesthetics in excess of 3 hours prior to 3 years of age.[3]

Anesthesia providers, however, must also consider the patient's degree of anxiety, developmental level, and existing comorbidities when developing an anesthetic plan. Not all patients will tolerate the application of a Mehta cast without general anesthesia. Accordingly, when developing a plan to address IIS and EOS, a conversation should occur between the surgeon, the anesthesia provider, and the patient's guardian to determine the most appropriate course of action.

ANESTHETIC MANAGEMENT
PREOPERATIVE EVALUATION

The preoperative assessment of patients presenting for Mehta cast application is similar to patients presenting for spinal fusion (see Chapter 119, "Spinal Fusion"). Given the likelihood of respiratory compromise in patients with scoliosis, a thorough pulmonary assessment preoperatively is essential. Depending on the severity of curvature, patients may experience restrictive pulmonary function at baseline. It is also imperative anesthesia providers review all imaging and orthopedic clinic notes to ascertain the severity of scoliosis. Profound curvature of the spine may predispose the patient to both cardiac and pulmonary impairment. A vital capacity of less than 60% is predictive of prolonged postoperative mechanical ventilation, likely due to an impaired ability to cough, thereby predisposing the patient to respiratory complications.[4] It is worth noting that patients presenting for Mehta cast application will likely not have undergone pulmonary testing given their age. Nonetheless, data from older patients with scoliosis can be used as a guide. Anesthesia providers should be assured, however, that pediatric patients with a preoperative vital capacity of less than 40% who undergo spine surgery are generally able to be discharged home despite short-term respiratory complications.[5] Special consideration, however, should be given to moving forward in patients presenting with an active or recent upper respiratory tract infection as respiratory efforts may be further hindered following cast application.

As patients generally undergo Mehta cast application several times, anesthesia providers should review prior anesthetic records and note any challenges with intubation, ventilation, or hemodynamics that may have occurred.

PREOPERATIVE PHARMACOLOGY

While premedication is not mandated by the procedure, pediatric patients may benefit from administration of a short-acting benzodiazepine, such as midazolam, to reduce preoperative anxiety and stress.[6] Anesthesia providers should consider any comorbidities, as well as the potential impact on respiratory function, prior to administration.

ANESTHETIC TECHNIQUE
Intraoperative Management

General anesthesia is routinely employed to facilitate Mehta cast application and is typically maintained with volatile anesthetic agents. In most instances, patients will not have an indwelling peripheral IV catheter prior to surgery. Hence, an inhalation mask induction is the most used technique to induce anesthesia. While the airway can be managed via tracheal intubation with an endotracheal tube (ETT) or placement of a laryngeal mask airway (LMA), placement of an ETT is recommended. Airway pressures often transiently increase during cast application, requiring increased pressures to maintain adequate ventilation and prevent atelectasis formation. This may prove more challenging should an LMA be used as opposed to an ETT. Following intubation, a soft bite block should be placed to protect the patient's tongue, as well as the ETT, once the patient has been placed in traction. While the use of a neuromuscular blocking agent may not be necessary to facilitate intubation, their use should be discussed with the orthopedic team prior to induction of anesthesia as it may facilitate correction.[7]

Standard monitors, as described by the American Society of Anesthesiologists, should be employed. A single well-running peripheral IV catheter is sufficient, although anesthesia providers should consider the laterality and location of placement to limit interference from the IV fluid tubing during cast placement. The patient's head should be wrapped with a blue towel to protect their face while in traction during cast application (Figure 121.1).

Once vascular access is established and the patient is intubated, a body stockinette is placed over the trunk and the patient is transitioned to the frame for cast application. The patient is supported by two horizontal metal bars, one under the shoulders and the other sustaining the pelvis. Halter traction is applied from both the head and foot ends of the casting frame. The patient's head is put into a halter strap and attached to the pulley at the head of the frame (Figure 121.2). Two pelvic straps are then wrapped around the waist overlying the body stockinette and connected to the pulley at the foot end of the casting frame.

Towels or a roll can be placed on the child's abdomen temporarily to ensure adequate room for stomach expansion and respiratory excursion once the cast is complete. Several layers of plaster of Paris are then applied for correction. Axial correction (elongation) of the spine is obtained with traction. Simultaneous posterolateral compression and rotation (derotation) are

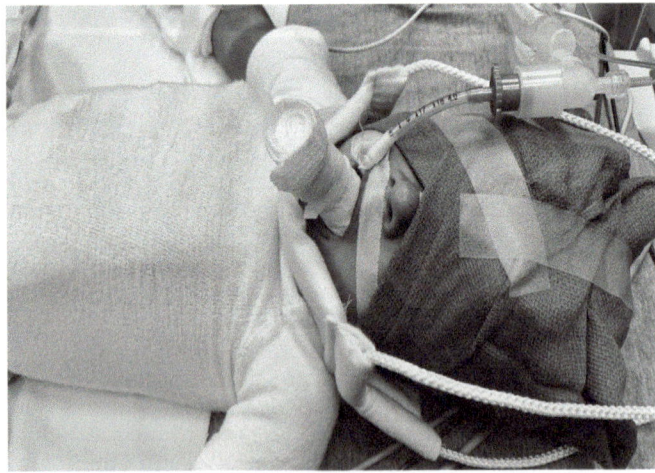

Figure 121.1: Oral protection and head wrap.

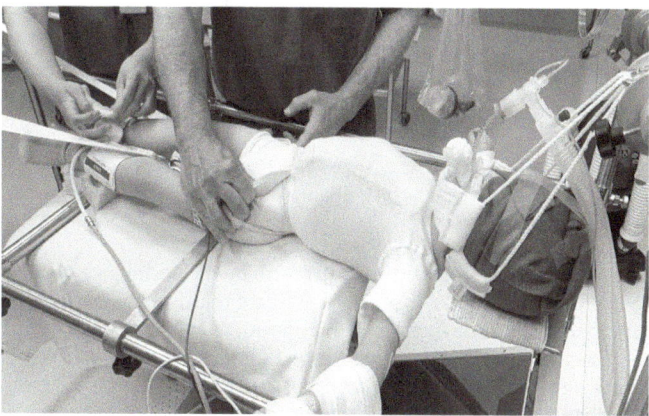

Figure 121.2: Positioning on the frame.

BOX 121.2 COMPLICATIONS/EMERGENCIES: MEHTA CAST APPLICATION

- Low rate of complication
- Most common: minor skin lesions
- Increased peak inspiratory pressures may increase up to 106% above baseline and persist somewhat higher than baseline into recovery
- Rare: ventilatory problems following cast application (typically resolved after cast removal) and subclavian vein thrombosis (caused by lack of care in trimming the cast in the axillary regions)
- Desaturation during casting due to inadequate ventilation

obtained with a band surrounding the apex of the spinal curvature (convex side). Should the patient have a double curve, a second band can be applied in the opposite direction and side, at the level of the convexity of the second curve. Manual lateral compression (flexion) is applied while the plaster is still malleable. Once the plaster of Paris is hardened, it can be reinforced with synthetic fiberglass. Once the fiberglass has hardened, a thoraco abdominal window is cut to obtain a decompression of the anterior abdomen (stomach and bowels) and a better expansion of the thoracic cage, and the towels or the roll placed on the child's abdomen can be removed (Box 121.1).

Anesthesia providers should consider manual ventilation and 100% fraction of inspired oxygen (FiO_2) until the chest towels are removed during trimming to ensure optimal ventilation and to prevent atelectasis.[8] While not a painful procedure, analgesics such as fentanyl or acetaminophen should be considered to relieve discomfort secondary to spinal manipulation. The entire procedure typically takes 45 to 60 minutes to complete.

Special Techniques and/or Equipment

A Risser trolley or a Cotrel's frame is often used to facilitate Mehta cast placement. The frame has one or two horizontal bars to support the patient, as well as pulleys with ratcheting mechanisms attached to the ends to allow the application of traction. The frame allows support of the patient's head, shoulders, sacrum, and legs via traction and/or support of the bars. Most frames also have a mirror positioned below the patient to facilitate cast application.

Complications/Emergencies

Complications and emergencies are summarized in Box 121.2.

BOX 121.1 CLINICAL PEARLS: MEHTA CAST APPLICATION

- Place a soft bite block following intubation to protect the patient's tongue and the endotracheal tube while traction is applied.
- Be sure to support the patient's head until all straps are secured and full traction is applied.
- Hand-ventilate the patient until the towels between the patient and the Mehta cast are removed to ensure adequate ventilation and prevent atelectasis.
- Cover the patient's face with towel during trimming to protect their face.

POSTOPERATIVE CARE

Following extubation, the patient should be transferred awake to the postanesthesia care unit (PACU). Typically, the cast will be petaled, which entails application of moleskin, padding, and tape over all rough edges to prevent abrasions secondary to the cast. This process typically takes 10 to 15 minutes, and the patient may benefit from administration of additional sedation, typically IV dexmedetomidine, midazolam, or fentanyl.

As this is a painless procedure, the focus of assessments in the PACU should be on respiratory function and support. Additionally, altered neurovascular assessments and/or derangements in hemodynamics may indicate a cast that is too tight or impeding circulation.

REFERENCES

1. Cotrel Y, Morel G. La technique de IE. DF dans la correction des scolioses. *Rev Chir Orthop Reparatrice Appar Mot.* 1964;50:59–75.
2. LaValva SM, MacAlpine EM, Kawakami N, et al. Awake serial body casting for the management of infantile idiopathic scoliosis: is general anesthesia necessary? *Spine Deform.* 2020;8(5):1109–1115. doi:10.1007/s43390-020-00123-3
3. Baky FJ, Milbrandt TA, Flick R, Larson AN. Cumulative anesthesia exposure in patients treated for early-onset scoliosis. *Spine Deform.* 2018;6(6):781–786. doi:10.1016/j.jspd.2018.05.001
4. Yuan N, Skaggs DL, Dorey F, Keens TG. Preoperative predictors of prolonged postoperative mechanical ventilation in children following scoliosis repair. *Pediatr Pulmonol.* 2005;40(5):414–419. doi:10.1002/ppul.20291
5. Payo J, Perez-Grueso FS, Fernandez-Baillo N, Garcia A. Severe restrictive lung disease and vertebral surgery in a pediatric population. *Eur Spine J.* 2009;18(12):1905–1910. doi:10.1007/s00586-009-1084-8
6. Frizzell KH, Cavanaugh PK, Herman MJ. Pediatric perioperative pain management. *Orthop Clin North Am.* 2017;48(4):467–480. doi:10.1016/j.ocl.2017.06.007
7. Canavese F, Botnari A, Dimeglio A, et al. Serial elongation, derotation and flexion (EDF) casting under general anesthesia and neuromuscular blocking drugs improve outcome in patients with juvenile scoliosis: preliminary results. *Eur Spine J.* 2016;25(2):487–494. doi:10.1007/s00586-015-4100-1
8. Dhawale AA, Shah S, Reichard S, et al. Casting for infantile scoliosis: the pitfall of increased peak inspiratory pressure. *J Pediatr Orthop.* 2013;33(1):63–67. doi:10.1097/BPO.0b013e318264936f

CHAPTER 122

Shoulder Surgery

Ramsey S. Sabbagh, James S. Furstein, and Shital N. Parikh

INDICATIONS/CONTRAINDICATIONS

Glenohumeral joint instability is the most common indication for shoulder surgery in the adolescent population. Glenohumeral instability can be multidirectional in nature (bilateral, atraumatic origin) or unidirectional (unilateral, traumatic origin). Additional less frequent indications include infection, fracture, acromioclavicular joint separation, rotator cuff tear, hemarthrosis secondary to hemophilia, and brachial plexus palsy. Currently it is recommended that patients under the age of 13 years with shoulder instability trial longitudinal conservative therapy prior to undergoing surgery; however, primary operative intervention may be necessary in adolescent athletes with traumatic unidirectional instability for whom an expeditious return to sport is a priority.[1] The risk of recurrence of a first-time subluxation or dislocation in an adolescent patient after conservative treatment is commonly regarded to be greater than 60%, and many will eventually require labral or capsular surgical intervention for unidirectional instability despite adequate physical therapy and rehabilitation.[2]

For adolescent patients with atraumatic multidirectional shoulder instability, the preferred initial management is a minimum of 6 months of physical therapy, particularly in patients with laxity caused by underlying collagen disorders.[3–5] Only after a longitudinal course of conservative therapy should surgical intervention be considered in patients with atraumatic multidirectional shoulder instability.

In adolescent and adult patients alike, unidirectional shoulder instability most commonly occurs in the anterior direction.[6,7] The most common lesion responsible for anterior instability is an anterior capsulo labral tear, also known as Bankart lesion. While surgical intervention is an appropriate course of action for adolescent patients with anterior shoulder instability, studies demonstrate higher rates of recurrence after surgical intervention in the adolescent population than in the adult population.[5] Nevertheless, in surgically managed adolescent patients with anterior shoulder instability, the overall rate of recurrence is still lower than for nonoperative management, especially in patients with more mature bone.[8] Surgical intervention is also highly effective for adolescent patients with posterior shoulder instability. Posterior instability is usually due to a posterior labral tear from a direct loading injury, such as from bench press, pushups, or wrestling injuries.[9,10]

Early surgery is indicated for adolescent patients presenting with a history of anterior shoulder dislocation in the presence of an impaction fracture of the posteromedial humeral head (largely engaging a Hill–Sachs lesion), the presence of a large anterior glenoid fragment, or for an irreducible dislocation.[11] Thankfully, most fractures around the shoulder in pediatric and adolescent patients can be treated conservatively. Open fractures, fractures with skin tenting, associated neurovascular injury, and fractures with intra-articular displacement, however, are absolute indications for operative intervention.[6,12] Polytrauma, severe fracture displacement or angulation, head trauma, or fractures in pediatric patients with neuromuscular disease constitute relative indications for operative fracture fixation.[12]

Since children under the age of 13 years rarely sustain complete acromioclavicular joint disruptions, conservative treatment typically produces excellent results.[13] Nevertheless, in adolescents with more skeletally mature bone, management corresponds to the severity of the separation. Disruption of the acromioclavicular and coracoclavicular ligaments with displacement of the clavicle (Rockwood types IV–VI) warrants surgical intervention.[14]

Although rare, septic arthritis of the shoulder is an absolute indication for operative intervention.[5,15] Septic arthritis is typically seen following neonatal septicemia or from a hematogenous infection in older children. Arthroscopic glenohumeral irrigation and debridement is the preferred index procedure for septic arthritis, with mainstay open debridement reserved for instances of recurrent joint infection.[5,16] Arthroscopic subtotal synovectomy is indicated for recurrent hemarthrosis secondary to hemophilia after trialing conservative therapy, although the need for such surgery has decreased due to optimization of medical management.[17,18] Open synovectomy should be performed with caution as it is associated with loss of motion, especially in the pediatric population.[17] Serial nerve surgeries or tendon transfers are indicated for children who sustain obstetric brachial plexus injuries that are recalcitrant to physical therapy and splinting.[19]

Patients should not undergo elective shoulder surgery when there is an active infection of the skin overlying the surgical site. General contraindications to arthroscopic shoulder surgery include a severely ankylosed shoulder, heterotopic ossification, and substantial overlying soft tissue injury.[5] Underlying bone dysplasia may impede the field of view during arthroscopy and consequently increase the risk of chondral damage.

Patient noncompliance to initial conservative management for shoulder instability is considered a relative contraindication to surgical intervention.[5] Patients with uncontrolled or partially controlled seizures have significantly higher failure rates after shoulder stabilization surgery. Hence, medical management should be optimized to control seizures before surgical treatment is considered. Shoulder stabilization surgery is also contraindicated in voluntary anterior dislocators.[20]

SPECIAL CONSIDERATIONS AND CONCERNS

A potential barrier to shoulder arthroscopy in the pediatric population is the size of the joint space. Limitations in arthroscopic visualization and instrumentation may affect the surgeon's ability to perform a procedure, especially in small children.[5] Additionally, pediatric anatomy may vary enough to warrant individualized portal placement.

Other factors that make shoulder arthroscopy in the pediatric population challenging include conditions such as cerebral palsy or arthrogryposis that often result in limited range of motion, which may restrict manipulation during surgery.

A child's ability to comply with postoperative instructions should guide intervention. Very young or developmentally delayed patients may not be able to follow directions to the same extent as an adult. Therefore, limb casting may be useful in restricting injurious or risky behavior involving the operative shoulder in patients too young to comply but comes at the cost of early mobilization.

Physeal damage can have dramatic consequences and result in growth arrest of the affected extremity. As such, traction should be used sparingly during shoulder surgery in order to prevent stress across the growth plate. Instrumentation and implant placement involving the physis should also be minimized.[5] Local anesthetic and/or glucocorticoid joint injections are best avoided in pediatric patients due to chondrotoxicity and the risk of physeal damage.[21,22] Similarly, thermal devices and fluids harbor a risk of intraoperative physeal damage that can lead to early growth plate closure and should be used sparingly in children and adolescents.[23]

ANESTHETIC MANAGEMENT

PREOPERATIVE EVALUATION

As with all patients, a detailed preoperative evaluation should be performed prior to initiation of general anesthesia. Patients presenting following trauma may have limited neck and jaw range of motion and require a thorough assessment to discern the likelihood of difficulty with securing the airway intraoperatively. In pediatric patients undergoing operative management for a brachial plexus injury, a thorough preoperative evaluation of their respiratory history is warranted. Specifically, the integrity of the phrenic nerve should be determined via ultrasonography of diaphragmatic movement.[19]

PREOPERATIVE PHARMACOLOGY

Many pediatric and adolescent patients presenting for shoulder surgery are anxious about the forthcoming surgical procedure. In most cases, an anxiolytic can be administered (either orally or intravenously if an IV access has been established) preoperatively to anxiety levels. Anxiolytics and narcotics should be administered with caution to those with a history of sleep-disordered breathing, obesity, or other concerning comorbidity that may impact the ability to maintain spontaneous ventilation and/or respiration.

ANESTHETIC TECHNIQUE

Intraoperative Management

Induction of anesthesia is typically achieved via an IV induction, followed by intubation with an endotracheal tube (ETT). Standard monitors, as recommended by the American Society of Anesthesiologists (ASA), are often adequate for shoulder arthroscopy and shoulder repair as invasive monitoring is seldom indicated. To better monitor perfusion to the brain, the blood pressure cuff should be placed on the arm as opposed to the lower extremity. A single large-bore peripheral IV catheter capable of volume resuscitation is sufficient as blood loss is anticipated to be minimal.

Pediatric patients undergoing shoulder surgery may be positioned in either the lateral decubitus position (LDP) or the beach chair position (BCP). The BCP is a popular choice for shoulder arthroscopic procedures due to ease of setup, minimal strain on the brachial plexus and other neurovascular structures, good intra-articular visualization, and ease of conversion to an open approach if necessary.[24,25] For smaller children, a bump may be required to raise the child's sitting height to gain adequate shoulder access. It is imperative that the head and neck remain neutral throughout the position and surgery to prevent devastating sequelae. Despite efforts to ensure neutral alignment, anesthesia providers should be aware that the BCP is associated with rare but devastating side effects. Gravitational effects of head elevation on cerebral perfusion may lead to hypotension, bradycardia, and ischemic damage to neurological structures.[5,26] Anesthesia providers should also be aware that there is an increased risk of venous air embolism when in the semisitting position or BCP.

The LDP may also be used as it allows for easier circumferential glenohumeral joint access than the BCP, avoids BCP-related obstructed visualization of the inferior aspect of the joint, and most importantly is not associated with cerebral hypoperfusion.[5,24] Regardless of the position and surgical approach employed, care should be taken in order to avoid iatrogenic phrenic nerve palsy secondary to repeated manipulation or transection.[27] Likewise, all pressure points should be padded and there should not be extraneous pressure on the patient's eyes.

Acute postoperative pain after shoulder surgery is believed to originate predominantly from the surrounding muscles, either as a direct result of surgical trauma or from reflex muscle spasm.[28] All the motor, and most of the sensory, innervation of the shoulder is supplied by the brachial plexus.[29] In particular, the axillary and suprascapular nerves provide key innervation to the supraspinatus, infraspinatus, deltoid, and teres minor muscles, as well as the skin of the shoulder.[29] The axillary nerve derives from C5 and C6, whereas the suprascapular nerve derives from spinal segments C4, C5, and C6. The origin of these two nerves innervating the shoulder explains why a brachial plexus block at the interscalene level successfully abates pain following surgical shoulder reconstruction.

Interscalene brachial plexus blockade is commonly performed to provide relief of postoperative pain following surgical shoulder repair. This technique has proved to be a reliable means of reducing the required doses of intraoperative and postoperative opiates and effectively delaying postoperative pain, as well as hastening patient discharge and increasing patient satisfaction.

While regional anesthesia has traditionally been performed prior to surgery with the hope that preemptive analgesia will most effectively abate postoperative pain, it has been argued that sensitization to pain can be attributed to many factors, not solely the nociceptive battery associated with incision and subsequent intraoperative events.[30] In fact, it has been offered that the duration of action and effectiveness of the treatment modality may play a more important role than the actual timing of the treatment delivered.[31] Accordingly, interscalene catheters are commonly placed to manage postoperative pain following shoulder surgery and left in situ for 48 hours postoperatively. Pediatric anesthesia providers may also opt to perform an interscalene block at the conclusion of the surgical procedure but prior to emergence from anesthesia as opposed to prior to induction of anesthesia. Not only will this theoretically extend the duration of analgesia postoperatively, but it may also promote maintenance of cerebral perfusion pressure intraoperatively.

Special Techniques and/or Equipment

Ultrasound-guided interscalene block is commonly employed to abate postoperative pain. Although performing interscalene brachial plexus blockade while the patient is under general anesthesia has historically been reported as being an unsafe practice in adults, despite its safety and efficacy, of this approach. Moreover, it has been argued that performing interscalene blockade while the patient is under general anesthesia is perhaps more effective than when performed in an awake patient.[3]

Under ultrasound guidance, the cervical roots of the brachial plexus are readily identified in the lateral portion of the neck as they lie in the interscalene groove, positioned between the anterior and middle scalene muscles. The nerves appear hypoechoic and can be traced distally to the clavicle, where the trunks and/or divisions of the brachial plexus can be found tightly bundled and positioned slightly superiorly and lateral to the subclavian artery.

Local anesthesia can be injected under real-time visualization following a negative aspiration. If a single-injection block is performed, local anesthesia is deposited adjacent to C5 C6 within the fascial plane, but not within the epineurium. Should a continuous peripheral nerve catheter be placed, the catheter will be placed under ultrasound guidance, with the tip of the catheter being placed immediately adjacent to the nerve bundle after the local anesthesia has been deposited. The technique for block placement does not differ between the preemptive and postoperative regional anesthesia, only the timing in relation to the surgical procedure. For additional information regarding regional anesthesia in children and adolescent patients, please refer to Chapter 131 in this text.

Postoperative Care

Postoperatively the patient should be extubated and transferred to the postanesthesia care unit (PACU). While the patient is in the PACU, the primary points of concern are the patient's respiratory function and reported levels of pain. If an interscalene block was performed, the phrenic nerve may have been inadvertently anesthetized, resulting in temporary loss of diaphragmatic function on the ipsilateral side. Likewise, forceful injection of local anesthetic or injection of an excessive volume while performing an interscalene block may result in Horner's syndrome. Horner's syndrome presents as a combination of symptoms, namely, miosis, ptosis, and anhidrosis. The recurrent laryngeal nerve may be impacted, as well as lead to hoarseness. Prior to discharge from the PACU, it is imperative to ensure there are no derangements in respiratory function.

It is also important to review the pain management plan with the patient and their caregiver prior to discharge. The operative arm should be in a sling to prevent deleterious movement that may not be detected due to having an insensate extremity. Likewise it is important to convey that prolonged periods of heat or cooling devices may lead to thermal injury in an insensate extremity. As a single-injection interscalene block will typically not last beyond 24 hours with the use of adjunctive medications, it is important to have a plan in place to manage transitional pain as the analgesia afforded by an interscalene block subsides.

KEY REFERENCES

Complete references for this chapter are online and available at https://connect.springerpub.com/content/book/978-0-8261-3875-0/part/part04/toc-part/ch122.

8. Shanmugaraj A, Chai D, Sarraj M, et al. Surgical stabilization of pediatric anterior shoulder instability yields high recurrence rates: a systematic review. *Knee Surg Sports Traumatol Arthrosc.* 2021; 29(1):192–201. doi:10.1007/s00167-020-05913-w
16. Brown DW, Sheffer BW. Pediatric septic arthritis: an update. *Orthop Clin North Am.* 2019;50(4):461–470. doi:10.1016/j.ocl.2019.05.003
18. van Vulpen LFD, Holstein K, Martinoli C. Joint disease in haemophilia: pathophysiology, pain and imaging. *Haemophilia.* 2018;24(February):44–49. doi:10.1111/hae.13449
19. Grossman JAI, Price A, Chim H. Complications in surgery for brachial plexus birth injury: avoidance and treatment. *J Hand Surg.* 2018;43(2), 164–172. doi:10.1016/j.jhsa.2017.11.008
20. Domos P, Lunini E, Walch G. Contraindications and complications of the Latarjet procedure. *Shoulder Elbow.* 2018; 10(1):15–24. doi:10.1177/1758573217728716
21. Kreuz PC, Steinwachs M, Angele P. Single-dose local anesthetics exhibit a type-, dose-, and time-dependent chondrotoxic effect on chondrocytes and cartilage: a systematic review of the current literature. *Knee Surg, Sports Traumatol, Arthrosc.* 2018;26(3):819–830. doi:10.1007/s00167-017-4470-5
25. Xinning L, Eichinger JK, Hartshorn T, Zhou H, Matzkin EG, Warner JP. A comparison of the lateral positions for shoulder surgery: advantages and complications. *J Am Acad Orthop Surg.* 2018;23(1):18–28. doi:10.5435/JAAOS-23-01-18

CHAPTER 123

Fasciotomy

Carrilee Powell and Ramsey S. Sabbagh

INDICATIONS/CONTRAINDICATIONS

Compartment syndrome is a serious condition that occurs when the tissue pressure within a confined space builds to dangerous levels. Bleeding, swelling after an injury, anabolic steroid use, constricting bandages, or the reestablishment of blood flow after blocked circulation can lead to increased intracompartmental pressure that impedes venous flow when the fascia is no longer able to accommodate further expansion. The resulting venous congestion further increases intracompartmental pressure and has the potential to limit arterial blood flow if the intracompartmental pressure reaches dangerous levels. The disruption of blood ultimately deprives the tissues of oxygen and nutrients and can lead to irreversible muscle ischemia, rhabdomyolysis, and tissue necrosis.[1] Compartment syndrome can be either acute or chronic in nature.

ACUTE COMPARTMENT SYNDROME

Children are at an increased risk of developing acute compartment syndrome (ACS) due to the high muscle bulk to compartment size ratio, which limits the ability of the enclosed fascial space to accommodate for inflammation and damage. Pediatric ACS typically occurs in children between the ages of 10 and 14 years of age, with the incidence among males is four times that of females.[2]

Pediatric ACS most commonly occurs following an injury to the leg or forearm, although it can involve the hand, foot, or buttock.[1] Causes of pediatric ACS include fractures, trauma, surgery, vascular compromise, constrictive dressings or casts, burns, and infections. If a patient has a displaced fracture, it should be reduced immediately to minimize swelling as fractures account for 85% of pediatric ACS cases. Supracondylar humeral fractures and surgical repair of forearm fractures with intramedullary nails are the most common causes of forearm compartment syndrome.[2] Tibial fractures account for 40% of pediatric ACS and are the most common cause of lower extremity ACS, typically affecting the anterior and deep posterior compartments[3] (Figure 123.1).

In the absence of a fracture, ACS can develop from blunt trauma or crush injuries. Patients undergoing surgery are also at risk of postoperative ACS related to surgical swelling or positioning. Vascular etiologies of ACS include an IV infiltration injury, arterial cannulation injury, reperfusion event after an arterial injury, thrombosis, and spontaneous bleeding event(s) related to anticoagulation or bleeding disorders. Poor positioning is equally as culpable. For example, prolonged lithotomy positioning during urological, gynecological, or general surgery procedures places the patient at risk of lower extremity compartment syndrome. It has been offered that the postoperative diagnosis of ACS may be delayed if a thoracic epidural was placed for pain control and therefore should be avoided in patients at high risk of developing postoperative ACS.[1]

A host of other causes of ACs are known to exist that anesthesia providers should be aware of. Placement of a constrictive cast or dressing can also induce an external pressure that reduces the compliance of the underlying compartments. When recognized, the cast of dressing should be immediately removed to relieve pressure as removal of constrictive casts or dressings can reduce compartmental pressure by 65% to 85%.[2] Full-thickness burns result in fluid shifts, edema, and eschars causing tissue construction and increased intracompartmental pressures. Infections, as well as insect and animal bites, cause localized swelling and fluid buildup either within or around a compartment that can result in increased compartmental pressure.[1,4]

Regardless of the etiology, ACS requires immediate recognition and emergent treatment. This most commonly includes a fasciotomy to minimize the risk of serious complications to the affected area or limb.[2]

Diagnosis of ACS

Patients with ACS typically present with symptoms within 24 hours of the initial injury but can present as late as multiple days following the injury. Diagnosis of compartment syndrome is made based on a detailed history and physical examination in conjunction with intracompartmental pressures if indicated. Diagnosing ACS in children can prove to be challenging, as they may not be able to articulate their symptoms. Adults with ACS typically describe the six Ps: pain, paresthesia, paresia, pallor, poikilothermia, and pulselessness. A study by Livingston et al. found that the majority of patient presents with two to three symptoms. Of those found to have ACS, 85% present with pain that is often described as severe, deep, and burning out of proportion to the injury and worsens with passive stretch of muscles.[2,4]

The six Ps are less reliable in the diagnosis of ACS in children due to inability to communicate; therefore, many practitioners utilize the three As: anxiety, agitation, and increased analgesia requirement (Box 123.1; Gottlieb et al.[2]). Increased analgesic requirement often occurs before anxiety and agitation, which can be very telling of the development of compartment syndrome.[1] Following a history, the anesthesia provider should perform a physical examination of the affected area to assess for motor and sensory deficits.

Palpation of compartments will be performed to assess for tenderness as well as passive stretching to assess for correlation between stretching and pain. Palpation of extremity pulses should be performed to assess vascular status. The absence of a palpable pulse may indicate a vascular injury or late diagnosis of ACS and places the patient at higher risk of detrimental outcomes.[1]

Although ACS is typically diagnosis by the described methods earlier, it may be confirmed with direct intracompartmental pressure measurements. Providers can utilize either a handheld intracompartmental pressure monitor or arterial line transducer set up to measure intracompartmental pressure. Normal intracompartmental pressure in children is 13 to 16 mm Hg. Diagnosing ACS is made if the intracompartmental pressure is 30 to 40 mm Hg or if the difference between compartment pressure and diastolic blood pressure is less than 30 mm Hg.[2] Many children will not tolerate compartment measurements, as it is painful. Therefore, many

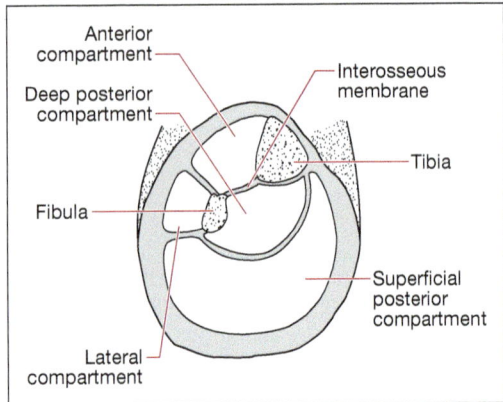

Figure 123.1: Four major compartments of the lower extremity.

Source: From Brown DP, Freeman ED, Cuccarullo SJ, et al. Musculoskeletal Medicine. In: Cuccarullo SJ, ed. *Physical Medicine and Rehabilitation Board Review.* 4th ed. Springer; 2019:Fig. 4.114.

children are diagnosed with ACS based on history and physical assessment.[1]

CHRONIC EXERTIONAL COMPARTMENT SYNDROME

Chronic exertional compartment syndrome (CECS) is most commonly reported in athletes, specifically those in running sports, and is believed to be a transient ischemia that occurs during exercise. Strenuous exercise increases IM pressure impeding neuromuscular blood flow within a specific compartment. Patients who have CECS may initially be misdiagnosed as the symptoms in CECS are very vague. Patients will commonly report a bilateral pain that is achy, dull, full, cramping, or pressure within a specific location of the lower leg that occurs during exercise without a history of trauma or injury. Patients may report the pain begins consistently after a certain amount of time of running or distance into a run.

Generally, patients with CECS are not able to run through the pain though they experience resolution of the pain within an hour of stopping exercise. Occasionally, patients may report additional symptoms, such as paresthesias and transient foot drop. Initially, a patient with CECS may undergo conservative treatment consisting of rest when pain occurs, but ultimately, the gold standard is a decompressive fasciotomy.[5]

MANAGEMENT OF COMPARTMENT SYNDROME

An emergent fasciotomy is indicated immediately following the diagnosis of ACS to release pressure in the affected compartment and restore perfusion. A fasciotomy consists of surgical incisions of the affected compartments to release pressure. If not managed immediately, muscle ischemia can result in permanent necrosis within 4 to 8 hours of onset of elevated intracompartmental pressures.[1,3] Delayed surgical intervention can result in irreversible damage, including loss of limb function, contracture,

amputation, and death.[1,2] Multiple compartments may require decompression. Excision of nonviable tissue should be performed. If an ACS patient presents with a fracture, the fracture should be reduced and stabilized with internal fixation.

Following fasciotomy, the incisions are typically left open for about a week with placement of a wet to dry dressing or vacuum-assisted device for temporary closure. Evaluation of the site occurs every 24 to 72 hours following surgery to perform dressing changes and determine if additional debridement is indicated. Eventually, the patient will return to the operating room for incision closure once no more debridement is warranted. Split-thickness skin grafts may be utilized during closure.[1]

ANESTHETIC MANAGEMENT

PREOPERATIVE EVALUATION

In children presenting with musculoskeletal trauma, anesthetic management should begin with a review of all existing injuries sustained by the patient. Bleeding, volume status, and the urgency of the orthopedic surgery should be evaluated, and the risk of aspiration during a non-fasted anesthetic induction should be weighed against the danger of delayed surgical intervention.[6] Pediatric fractures of the pelvis often encompass complex decision-making with respect to the timing and staging of surgery and anesthesia. While the incidence of pelvic fractures in children younger than age 13 is merely 0.01%, the mortality is a staggering 10.20% due to the high rates of concomitant polytrauma and subsequent life-threatening complications.[7]

ACS may be difficult to diagnose in children and a detailed history and physical examination should be performed to determine the presence and extent of injury to the limb. The physical examination should include evaluation of the affected extremity with notation of any existing numbness, tingling, pain, discoloration, edema, and range of motion.

Pertinent Labs

ACS patients are at risk of rhabdomyolysis, hyperkalemia, and renal failure therefore a review of pertinent labs should include electrolytes, renal function tests, and acid–base status. Rhabdomyolysis can occur in up to 40% to 50% of patients with compartment syndrome. An elevated creatinine kinase greater than 1000 U/mL or presence of myoglobinuria can be indicative of rhabdomyolysis. Patients with myolysis are at risk of acute renal failure and should be monitored for alterations in kidney function. Dialysis may be warranted depending on severity.[2]

PREOPERATIVE PHARMACOLOGY

Administration of an anxiolytic, such as midazolam, may be indicated preoperatively.

ANESTHETIC TECHNIQUE

Intraoperative Management

The procedure will most commonly be performed under general anesthesia with an endotracheal tube. Depending on NPO status, a rapid sequence induction may be indicated. Prophylactic antibiotics, cefazolin or clindamycin, should be administered prior to surgical incision. The majority of patients with compartment syndrome can undergo an anesthetic maintained on sevoflurane and the administration of neuromuscular blocking agents if indicated. Alterations to anesthetic plans may be indicated for additional traumatic injuries and specific patient comorbidities.

Anesthesia providers may administer short- and long-acting narcotics, such as fentanyl and morphine or hydromorphone in conjugation with nonnarcotic medications, such as

---

BOX 123.1 THREE A'S IN DIAGNOSING ACUTE COMPARTMENT SYNDROME IN PEDIATRIC PATIENTS

- Anxiety
- Agitation
- Increased analgesia requirement

acetaminophen, for pain management. Caution should be utilized with the administration of ketorolac due to the risk of renal impairment potentially associated with ACS. Regional anesthesia should be avoided as it may mask postoperative evaluation of the extremity. A consult for the acute pain service should be considered to manage postoperative pain with a patient-controlled analgesia pump (PCA pump).

Upon conclusion of surgical intervention, the patient should be extubated awake and transferred to the post anesthesia care unit (PACU) for recovery with subsequent hospital admission for continued surgical team observation of the affected area.

Special Techniques and/or Equipment

Tourniquets are commonly used in the surgical management of musculoskeletal injuries affecting the extremities due to the advantages and ease of "bloodless surgery." Sudden reperfusion after deflation of the tourniquet may cause a slight decrease in blood pressure and a rapid increase in CO_2 associated with a transient increase in cerebral blood volume, which may have serious consequences in patients with an already raised intracranial pressure. Common complications associated with the use of a tourniquet include muscle, nerve, vascular, or skin damage, as well as increased core body temperature and a theoretical increase in the risk of deep vein thrombosis right after cuff release.[8] Pediatric patients are more sensitive to pressure and time threshold for tourniquet use, and this should be taken into consideration to avoid tissue damage.[9]

Clinical Pearls

Regional anesthesia is traditionally discouraged in clinical settings where the development of ACS is a concern as sensory and motor nerve blockade may mask postoperative evaluation of the extremity and symptoms of ACS. ACS can be difficult to detect in an adult patient after a peripheral nerve block due to a compromised sensory and motor examination. The "five Ps" of compartment syndrome (pain, paresthesia, paralysis, pallor, and pulselessness) are unreliable in children, and instead, the three As (agitation, anxiety, and analgesia requirements) are demonstrated to be more useful clinical signs of ACS[10] (Box 123.1).

POSTOPERATIVE CARE

The primary foci of postoperative care are frequent assent of the impacted extremity, pain management, and monitoring for signs and symptoms of rhabdomyolysis.

Postoperatively, it is imperative to monitor for signs of continued and/or progression ACS. This will largely be guided by employing the five Ps and three As to direct frequent assessment. Should there be acute changes, the orthopedic team should be notified immediately. Chronic changes may be indicative of reoccurrence of the need to modify the postoperative pain and rehabilitation protocols.

Postoperative pain management typically entails a multimodal approach, combining acetaminophen, nonsteroidal anti-inflammatory drugs (NSAIDs) if there is no concern for renal impairment, opioids, and antispasmodics.[6] Acetaminophen acts through several different mechanisms including the cyclooxygenase (COX), endocannabinoid, serotonergic, and nitric oxide synthesis pathways to achieve analgesia.[11] NSAIDs act to reduce prostaglandin synthesis by inhibiting the COX pathway, thereby decreasing tissue inflammation and producing analgesic effects.[12] In surgeries in which moderate-to-severe postoperative pain is expected, opioids are an appropriate therapy.[6] Due to concerns over the safety of tramadol and codeine in children aged 12 to 18 with obesity, sleep apnea, or severe lung disease, in 2017 the Food and Drug Administration restricted the use of codeine and tramadol in this demographic.[13] When able to tolerate a diet, oxycodone is the opioid of choice for pediatric patients postoperatively. They are transitioned from IV to oral opioids when tolerating a diet.

One of the most common considerations for a patient with traumatic ACS is rhabdomyolysis, which can occur in up to 40% to 50% of patients with compartment syndrome. An elevated creatinine kinase greater than 1000 U/mL or presence of myoglobinuria can be indicative of rhabdomyolysis. Patients with rhabdomyolysis are at risk of acute renal failure and should be monitored for alterations in kidney function. Dialysis may be warranted depending on severity.[2]

REFERENCES

1. Gresh M. Compartment syndrome in the pediatric patient. *Pediatr Rev.* 2017;38(12):560–564. doi:10.1542/pir.2016-0114
2. Gottlieb M, Adams S, Landas T. Current approaches to the evaluation and management of acute compartment syndrome in pediatric patients. *Pediatr Emerg Care.* 2019;36(6):432–437. doi:10.1097/01.pec.0000562132.21902.89
3. Mortenson SJ, Orman S, Testa EJ, et al. Risk factors for developing acute compartment syndrome in the pediatric population: a systemic review and meta-analysis. *Eur J Orthop Surg Traumatol.* 2020;30:839–844. doi:10.1007/s00590-020-02643-0
4. Livingston K, Glotzbecker M, Miller PE, et al. Pediatric non-fracture acute compartment syndrome. *J Pediatr Orthop.* 2016;36(7):685–690. doi:10.1097/bpo.0000000000000526
5. Vajapey S, Miller TL. Evaluation, diagnosis, and treatment of chronic exertional compartment syndrome: a review of current literature. *Phys Sportsmed.* 2017;45(4):391–398. doi:10.1080/00913847.2017.1384289
6. Wu JP. Pediatric anesthesia concerns and management for orthopedic procedures. *Pediatr Clin North Am.* 2020;67(1):71–84. https://doi:10.1016/j.pcl.2019.09.006
7. Galos D, Doering TA. High-energy fractures of the pelvis and acetabulum in pediatric patients. *J Am Acad Orthop Surg.* 2020;28(9):353–362. doi:10.5435/JAAOS-D-19-00082
8. Wilton NC, Anderson BJ. Orthopedic and spine surgery. In *A Practice of Anesthesia for Infants and Children* (6th ed.). Elsevier Inc., 2019. doi:10.1016/B978-0-323-42974-0.00032-X
9. Tredwell SJ, Wilmink M, Inkpen K, McEwen JA. Pediatric tourniquets: analysis of cuff and limb interface, current practice, and guidelines for use. *J Pediatr Orthop.* 2001;21(5):671–676. doi:10.1097/00004694-200109000-00023
10. Bae DS, Kadiyala RK, Waters PM. Acute compartment syndrome in children: contemporary diagnosis, treatment, and outcome. *J Pediatr Orthop.* 2001;21(5):680–688. doi:10.1097/01241398-200109000-00025
11. Przybyła GW, Szychowski KA, Gmiński J. Paracetamol – An old drug with new mechanisms of action. *Clin Exp Pharmacol Physiol.* 2021;48(1):3–19. doi:10.1111/1440-1681.13392
12. Gupta A, Bah M. NSAIDs in the treatment of postoperative pain. *Curr Pain Headache Rep.* 2016;20(11). doi:10.1007/s11916-016-0591-7
13. US Food and Drug Administration. FDA restricts use of prescription codeine pain and cough medicines and tramadol pain medicines in children; recommends against use in breastfeeding women. FDA Drug Safety Communication; 2019. https://www.fda.gov/Drugs/DrugSafety/ucm549679.htm

CHAPTER 124

Slipped Capital Femoral Epiphysis Surgery

Carrilee Powell

INDICATIONS/CONTRAINDICATIONS

Slipped capital femoral epiphysis (SCFE) is the most common hip disorder in children 8 to 15 years of age. SCFE is characterized by a displacement of the capital femoral epiphysis from the femoral neck through the physeal plate. More specifically, the epiphysis, or head of the femur, slips posterior and inferior to the femoral neck at the growth plate, which is the weaker area of bone as it has not yet developed. While the etiology of SCFE is often believed to be multifactorial, it most often occurs during a period of rapid growth. SCFE may also be associated with trauma, although the condition most commonly develops gradually over a period of weeks to months without associated injury.

The overall incidence of SCFE is reported to be 10.8 cases per 100,000 children. Although the average age at the time of diagnosis varies by gender, males are typically diagnosed between the age of 12 and 14 years of age and females diagnosed between the age of 11 and 12 years. SCFE is far more prevalent in males than females, with a ratio of approximately 1.5 to 1.[1] Approximately one-half of children presenting with SCFE are obese, with weights frequently at or above the 95th percentile. Additional risk factors for SCFE include a family history of SCFE and an endocrine or metabolic disorder, such as hypothyroidism or hyperthyroidism.

While SCFE is most often unilateral in nature, approximately 10% to 20% of patients will present with bilateral SCFE. Furthermore, of those presenting with unilateral SCFE, 10% to 20% will develop SCFE in the contralateral hip during adolescence.

The diagnosis of SCFE in children is often a delayed or missed diagnosis, as the symptoms can be vague. A thorough physical history and examination, as well as radiographs, guide the diagnosis of SCFE. The two hallmark features of SCFE are pain in the hip and an altered gait. In addition to these key symptoms, children will complain of generalized pain in the groin, thigh, or knee regions and difficulty with ambulating. Symptoms are generally worse with physical activity and relieved by rest, and may be acute, chronic, or intermittent in nature. The classic presentation is that of an obese adolescent without other risk factors and a complaint of nonradiating, dull, aching pain in the hip, groin, thigh, or knee without a history of trauma. As there are multiple hip disorders that can impact children, the diagnosis of SCFE is likely to be missed at the initial visit if hip pain is absent. Table 124.1 summarizes important differential diagnoses to consider for children presenting with hip pain.

SCFE can be classified based on intensity and the duration of symptoms. The four prevailing patterns of presentation include pre-slip, acute, acute on chronic, and chronic. Pre-slip SCFE refers to patients presenting with pain but without discernible displacement of the epiphysis. When compared to the asymptomatic hip, however, x-ray will demonstrate a widening of the proximal femoral physis. Children presenting with acute SCFE often report a traumatic event followed by symptoms lasting less than 3 weeks. Symptoms often include an external rotational deformity and limited motion of the hip, as well as the inability to bear weight on the affected extremity. Active motion of the hip is severely limited by muscle spasm, and the patient complains of intense pain with any attempt at passive motion. A joint effusion is usually present, although metaphyseal remodeling is absent. These patients should bear weight on the affected extremity until they receive definitive treatment to avoid further negative sequelae. Acute or chronic SCFE occurs when a patient with an extended history of symptoms and signs of chronic SCFE presents with an acute increase in pain and a loss of motion of the affected hip. The most frequent presentation is chronic SCFE, which is characterized by vague, intermittent symptoms over a protracted period lasting longer than 3 weeks.

Once SCFE has been diagnosed, it is important to determine if the condition is stable or unstable as this will further guide management. Patients with stable SCFE may present with limping, while unstable SCFE patients will be unable to

Table 124.1 Differential Diagnosis of Hip Pain in Children

Condition	Typical Age	Duration	Clinical Features	Diagnosis
Transient synovitis	3–10	Acute	Refusal to bear weight, recent viral illness, hip held in abduction and external rotation, possible fever	Normal inflammatory markers, radiographs, ultrasound
Slipped capital femoral epiphysis	11–15	Acute or chronic	Pain in hip, groin, thigh, or knee in obese adolescent	Bilateral hip radiographs
Legg–Calvé–Perthes disease	3–12	Chronic	Gradual onset, decreased internal rotation of hip, pain referred to thigh or knee	Hip radiographs or MRI
Septic arthritis	All	Acute	Fever, refusal to bear weight, pain with range of motion, warmth surrounding joint	Elevated inflammatory markers, joint aspiration, radiographs
Malignancy	All	Acute or chronic	Pain worsens at night or not related to activity, systemic symptoms, possible fever	Radiographs, laboratory abnormalities

Source: From Slipped Capital Femoral Epiphysis. https://aneskey.com/slipped-capital-femoral-epiphysis.

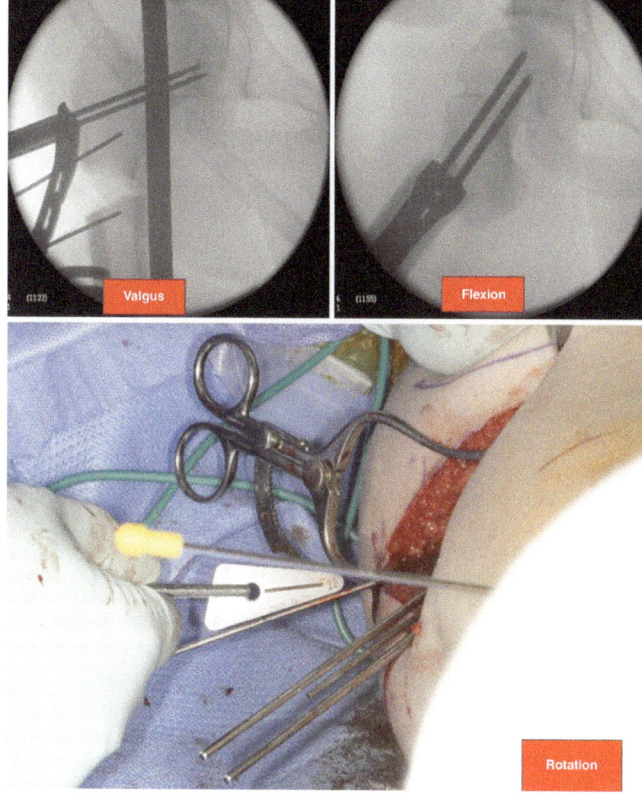

Figure 124.1: Surgical repair of slipped capital femoral epiphysis (SCFE).
Source: From Balasubramanian B, Alshryda S, Madan S. Slipped capital femoral epiphysis. In: Alshryda S, Howard J, Huntley J, Schoenecker J, eds. *The Pediatric and Adolescent Hip*. Springer; 2019. doi:10.1007/978-3-030-12003-0_8.

ambulate.[1] While a history of trauma is rare with stable SCFE, trauma may be present with unstable SCFE.[2] Confirmation of an SCFE diagnosis will be made with bilateral hip x-rays, including an anteroposterior and frog-leg views. If the SCFE is unstable, additional films of cross-table lateral view will be performed to determine the extent of the slip. The degree of slip noted on x-ray can range from mild to moderate and severe.[1]

Following diagnosis, the child will require surgical intervention to prevent further slippage and additional damage or complications. The surgical approach to this condition is relatively noninvasive and entails the placement of screws or pins percutaneously (**Figure 124.1**). If not surgically repaired, SCFE can lead to avascular necrosis, loss of cartilage, femoroacetabular impingement (FAI), and early osteoarthritis. The sequelae worsen with delays in diagnosis and/or surgical repair, so making an early diagnosis and intervention are key. Surgical repair most commonly involves in situ fixation with a screw or pins. Occasionally, the patient may have to undergo a hip dislocation with realignment and fixation or proximal femoral osteotomy.[3]

SPECIAL CONSIDERATIONS AND CONCERNS

Childhood obesity is highly prevalent in the United States, affecting 17% of all children.[4] Since most patients with SCFE are clinically obese, weight-related comorbidities must be considered during the surgical and anesthetic management of patients undergoing percutaneous pinning of the hip.[2] Therefore, a comprehensive preoperative evaluation of the obese pediatric patient is a necessity and includes an evaluation for sleep-disordered breathing (SDB) due to concern for higher rates of respiratory adverse effects, including oxygen desaturation, airway obstruction, laryngospasm, oversedation, and the need for escalation in care.[5,6]

SCFE can also be related to endocrine abnormalities including hypothyroidism, growth hormone supplementation, hypogonadism, and panhypopituitarism. It is recommended that children diagnosed with SCFE outside the age rages of 8 to 15 years or those who are underweight should undergo an endocrine evaluation prior to surgery.[1]

ANESTHETIC MANAGEMENT

PREOPERATIVE EVALUATION

A detailed preoperative history and physical examination should be performed prior to surgery, with a concerted effort placed on identifying comorbidities related to obesity and endocrine disorders. In addition, anesthesia providers should be sure to document any report of numbness, tingling, pain, and/or weakness in the affected extremity. Discussion of analgesic medications previously taken should occur, with special attention to the timing of the last dose of nonsteroidal anti-inflammatory drugs (NSAIDs). Patients with unstable SCFE may present for urgent surgical repair, and NPO time should be assessed.

Patients diagnosed outside the anticipated age ranges based on gender, as well as those diagnosed within age range norms who are underweight, should be evaluated for endocrine and/or renal disorders prior to surgery. The possible associated conditions of concern include hypothyroidism, panhypopituitarism, hypogonadism, growth hormone disorders, and renal osteodystrophy. Pediatric patients with hypothyroidism can be challenging to manage under general anesthesia as they may have an exaggerated response to surgical stimulation, may be hemodynamically unstable during anesthesia, may have pronounced depression from sedative drugs, or may experience a delayed emergence from anesthesia. Patients with growth hormone disorders may be short in stature and have decreased or deficient bone growth. Collectively, this can result in increased difficulties with airway management and endotracheal intubation. In addition, they may have abnormalities associated with glucose metabolism.

Renal osteodystrophy is a form of metabolic bone disease that is characterized by bone mineralization deficiency due to electrolyte and endocrine abnormalities. Patients present with abnormalities of serum calcium, phosphate, and parathyroid hormone (PTH) levels.

Pertinent Labs

Routine laboratory work is not necessary, however, may be warranted based on the presence and severity of coexisting diseases. Should endocrine disorders be present, preoperative laboratory evaluation should be based on the current recommendations relating to the coexisting condition.

PREOPERATIVE PHARMACOLOGY

Prior to transport to the operating room, administration of an anxiolytic, such as midazolam, may be useful in reducing anxiety and aiding in separation from family.

ANESTHETIC TECHNIQUE

Intraoperative Management

Surgical repair of SCFE requires a general anesthetic with an endotracheal tube. Induction of anesthesia can be achieved via an inhalation mask induction or IV induction depending on the child's NPO status, aspiration risk, and additional comorbidities. A rapid sequence induction may be required for those patients with an unstable SCFE presenting for urgent repair or when the NPO time is inadequate.

The use of standard monitors, as recommended by the American Society of Anesthesiologists, is appropriate for this surgery. Invasive monitoring is not necessary as blood loss is anticipated to be minimal for patients undergoing an in situ fixation. As such, a single well-running peripheral IV catheter will suffice in most instances. Anesthesia providers should be aware, however, that if more invasive repair is indicated, blood loss may be larger.[7]

Depending on the patient's body habitus, mask ventilation and intubation can be challenging. Compared with normal-weight children, obese children have an increased incidence of difficult mask ventilation (7.4% vs. 2.2%, respectively), difficult laryngoscopy (1.3% vs. 0.4%), and postoperative airway obstruction.[5] It recommended that adequate time be allowed for preoxygenation prior to induction of anesthesia and attempts at intubation. Use of a "ramped" position may improve the view of the larynx during laryngoscopy compared with a standard "sniff" position.

Anesthesia will typically be maintained on sevoflurane throughout the procedure, as general anesthesia and the use of muscle relaxation in obese children are known to result in atelectasis, severe respiratory mechanics alterations, and increased hypoxemia risk. Accordingly, use of a protective ventilation strategy is reasonable to maintain oxygenation, normocapnia, and to avoid lung damage when controlled ventilation is required. This includes the use of tidal volumes (6–8 mL/kg IBW) and levels of oxygen (FiO_2 0.5–0.8) to prevent reabsorption atelectasis and oxygen toxicity, positive end-expiratory pressure (PEEP), and the use of intermittent recruitment maneuvers.[5]

Underlying obstructive sleep apnea associated with obesity may make postoperative opioid use problematic. In addition, many patients with SCFE present with baseline pain due to the nature of the injury. Therefore, implementing multimodal pain management strategies should be utilized to combat intraoperative and postoperative pain. Anesthesia providers may elect to administer short- and long-acting opioids, such as fentanyl and morphine or hydromorphone perioperatively. Caution with opioids should be taken in those patients with obesity and/or a history of SDB. Nonopioid medications, including acetaminophen and/or NSAIDs, should be incorporated in the analgesic plan. NSAIDs should be avoided in patients with bleeding disorders and used with caution in those with significant blood loss. A discussion should occur with the surgeon prior to administration of NSAIDs due to the potential impact on bone formation. Central or peripheral regional techniques have been used successfully for postoperative pain management as well.

Patients are often positioned on either a fracture or radiolucent table to facilitate the use of x-ray or fluoroscopy during the procedure to guide and confirm screw and pin placement. As many patients presenting for SCFE repair are obese, positioning can be challenging. It is imperative that anesthesia providers ensure all pressure points are appropriately padded.

Prior to emergence, the administration of antiemetics will aid in reducing the risk of postoperative nausea and vomiting.

Complications/Emergencies

Complications following SCFE include avascular necrosis (degeneration of the femoral head), chondrolysis (rapid onset of painful arthritis), and impingement. Avascular necrosis occurs secondary to the interruption of the blood supply to the femoral head and is more likely to occur in patients with unstable SCFE. Should this occur, a gradual and very painful collapse of the bone and the articular cartilage covering the bone ensues. Without this smooth cartilage, bone rubs against bone, leading to painful arthritis in the joint. Depending on the extent of damage secondary to avascular necrosis, additional hip surgery may be needed.

Chondrolysis is a rare but serious complication of SCFE in which the articular cartilage on the surface of the hip joint degenerates very rapidly, leading to pain, deformity, and permanent loss of motion in the affected hip. While the etiology is not fully understood, it is believed chondrolysis results from inflammation in the hip joint. As with avascular necrosis, patients may require additional surgery should the patient not have full range of motion in the hip.

Impingement within the hip joint may occur secondary to placement of the screw used to stabilize the SCFE. FAI may occur secondary to remodeling of the femur and/or socket. Surgeries, including screw removal, arthroscopy, or open reconstruction, may be needed should the patient complain of persistent pain or limited range of motion in their hip.

POSTOPERATIVE CARE

Upon conclusion of surgical intervention, the patient will be extubated awake and transferred to the postanesthesia care unit for recovery. While postoperative pain is generally mild, patients may require additional doses of IV and/or oral opioids and nonopioid analgesics for pain control. Opioids should be administered with caution in obese patients to limit opioid-related respiratory depression. NSAIDs, such as ketorolac, are effective analgesics in this patient population if not contraindicated by coexisting disease. If significant pain persists postoperatively, the acute pain service should be consulted to guide pain management. As atelectasis formation correlates with body weight and may be sustained into the postoperative period, supplemental oxygen may be necessary and recruitment maneuvers should be encouraged.

Patients are typically admitted overnight to the hospital for continued observation following surgical repair. Following discharge, patients will be monitored for an extended period as avascular necrosis may not present for 12 to 18 months postoperatively.

REFERENCES

1. Peck DM, Voss LM, Voss TT. Slipped capital femoral epiphysis: diagnosis and management. *Am Fam Physician.* 2017;95(12):797–784.

2. Aprato A, Conti A, Bertolo F, Masse A. Slipped capital femoral epiphysis: current management strategies. *Orthop Res Rev.* 2019;47–54. doi:10.2147/ORR.S166735

3. Kyriakos P, Dimitrios S, Starvos S, et al. Non-traumatic infantile slipped capital femoral epiphysis following an epileptic seizure – a case report. *J Orthop Case Rep.* 2019;9(5):35–38. doi:10.13107/jocr.2250-0685.1522

4. Sanyaolu A, Okorie C, Qi X, et al. Childhood and adolescent obesity in the United States: a public health concern. *Glob Pediatr Health.* 2019;6:doi:10.1177/2333794X19891305.

5. Chidambaran V, Tewari A, Mahmoud M. Anesthetic and pharmacologic considerations in perioperative care of obese children. *J Clin Anesth.* 2018;45:39–50.

6. Scalzitti NJ, Sarber KM. Diagnosis and perioperative management in pediatric sleep-disordered breathing. *Pediatr Anesth.* 2018;28(11):940–946.

7. Wu JP. Pediatric anesthesia concerns and management for orthopedic procedures. *Pediatr Clin North Am.* 2020;67(1):71–84. http://doi.org/10.1016/j.pcl.2019.09.006

CHAPTER 125

Pediatric Amputation

Motaz Awad, Soroush Merchant, Alexandra Szabova, and Kenneth R. Goldschneider

INDICATIONS/CONTRAINDICATIONS

The anesthesia provider will occasionally care for patients undergoing amputation or posttraumatic amputation-related procedures. Overall epidemiological data are poorly documented in the literature, but the reasons for amputation often include trauma, congenital deformity, oncological diagnoses, and infection. When caring for patients presenting for amputation, anesthesia providers should be prepared to manage multiple comorbidities, such as multitrauma and intoxication in the trauma victim, sepsis in the infection group, coagulopathy and chemotherapy effects in the oncology patient, and related airway, pulmonary, or cardiac defects in the patient with congenital limb deficiencies. The balance of this chapter focuses on the unique aspects of amputation management, with a specific focus on phantom pain and its prevention.

SPECIAL CONSIDERATIONS AND CONCERNS

It is imperative that anesthesia providers recognize that postamputation neurological phenomena following amputation are varied in nature and can include residual limb pain, phantom limb pain, and phantom limb sensations and apply to any amputated body part. Residual limb pain is pain localized to the remaining limb and is also referred to as stump pain.[1] Phantom limb pain is any painful sensation localized to the lost limb, whereas phantom sensations include nonpainful sensations (e.g., movement, sense of limb presence). Phantom limb pain and associated sensations are neuropathic findings resulting from supraspinal, spinal, and peripheral mechanisms, including reorganization of the somatosensory cortex, dorsal horn sensitization due to deafferentation, and peripheral nerve regeneration with abnormal activity.[2] Interestingly, some of these neurophysiological processes are similar to those seen in complex regional pain syndrome (CRPS).[3] In contrast, residual limb pain can be postsurgical nociceptive, neurogenic, prosthogenic, arthrogenic, ischemic, referred, infectious sympathetically mediated, or from abnormal residual limb tissue, and each should be evaluated and treated as indicated.[4]

The presence of any preoperative pain, regardless of the site, increases the risk of phantom limb pain in children and chronic postsurgical pain in general.[5,6] Therefore, perioperative pain management should focus on treating preoperative pain. This is best accomplished when a multimodal analgesic approach is utilized, one that includes regional anesthesia and pharmacological therapies that specifically target multiple receptors throughout the nociceptive system. For elective surgery, the pain service should be involved well in advance of surgery to optimize analgesic conditions and provide pain education to both the patient and their family. As inadequate intraoperative analgesia has been associated with chronic postsurgical pain, it is important anesthesia providers ensure pain is adequately managed throughout all perioperative phases.[7] Timelines for phantom limb pain interventions are shown in Figure 125.1 and Figure 125.2.

ANESTHETIC MANAGEMENT

PREOPERATIVE EVALUATION

The pain service should be involved prior to elective, semi-elective, or urgent surgery so that any preoperative pain can be adequately treated. The earlier multimodal preemptive analgesic therapies are implemented, the more effective they may be. Furthermore, educating the patient and their family about phantom phenomena, preemptive analgesia, and perioperative pain management is essential in setting realistic postoperative expectations and allaying fears. In addition, it is important the anesthesia provider convey to the family that complaints of phantom sensations and pain are not psychosomatic or factitious in nature. While there is no literature to provide a protocol for amputation education, it is widely believed to be an important aspect of care in planned amputations.[8]

There are certain scenarios in which amputation is not certain but remains a possibility, as in cases of aggressive infections or thromboembolic disease. In these cases, it is equally important that all approaches to managing phantom pain are discussed with the patient and their family preoperatively and appropriate consent is obtained, thereby allowing implementation during the intraoperative phase if indicated (Table 125.1). When amputation is emergent or traumatic, preemptive analgesia may not be possible. However, the same analgesic modalities, including regional, pharmacological, and nonpharmacological therapies, should be utilized aggressively intra- and postoperatively whenever patient clinical status allows.

PREOPERATIVE PHARMACOLOGY

Preemptive or preventive analgesia theoretically serves to prevent the establishment of central sensitization that may be caused by incisional and inflammatory injuries, including pain in the postoperative setting.[9] Therefore, it is important that preemptive analgesia be employed to temper preoperative pain, irrespective of the location of origin of the pain. Therapies commonly employed to provide preemptive analgesia include regional anesthesia and pharmacological treatments. Peripheral and neuraxial nerve blockade reliably provide postoperative pain relief, and by effectively treating acute postoperative pain, regional anesthesia may indirectly reduce chronic pain.[7] Some studies support the use of epidural analgesia to reduce phantom limb pain, particularly when preemptive analgesia is started earlier in the perioperative phase (i.e., 48 hours instead of 24 hours before surgery).

A host of pharmacological therapies, such as patient-controlled analgesia and gabapentin, should be considered when developing a preemptive analgesic plan.[10,11] The administration of vitamin C has been shown to reduce the incidence of

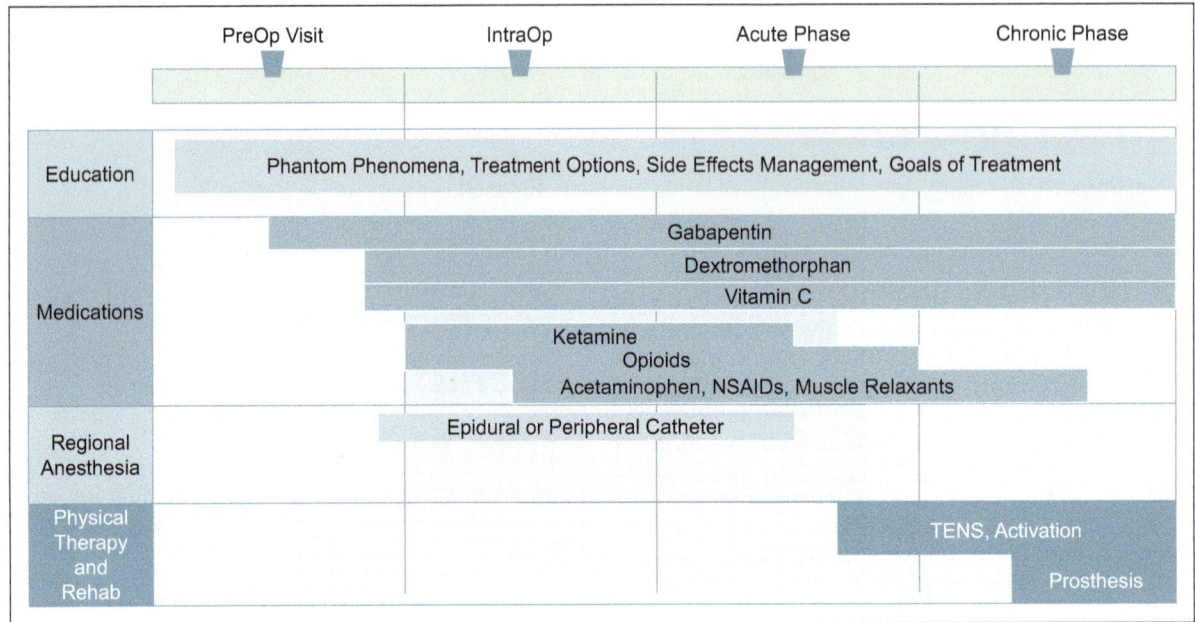

Figure 125.1: Phantom pain treatment timeline for planned amputation.
NSAIDs, nonsteroidal anti-inflammatory drugs; TENS, transcutaneous electrical nerve stimulation.

CRPS after radius fracture[12] and should be considered when anticipating phantom limb pain (Table 125.1). This is based on theoretical similarities between the conditions and the innocuous nature of ascorbic acid. At our institution, vitamin C is started in the preoperative period and continued after.

Anxiety in particular plays a role in amplifying acute and chronic pain and should be addressed in the preoperative setting. Please see Chapter 131, "Pediatric Pain Management," which addresses the role of anxiety in perioperative pain and its management.

ANESTHETIC TECHNIQUE

Intraoperative Management

Anesthesia for amputation typically involves general anesthesia with placement of an endotracheal tube (ETT). Large-bore IV access should be secured in the event volume resuscitation, blood transfusion, or the administration of vasopressor medications are needed. Should significant blood loss or hemodynamic instability be anticipated, placement of an arterial line may be warranted.

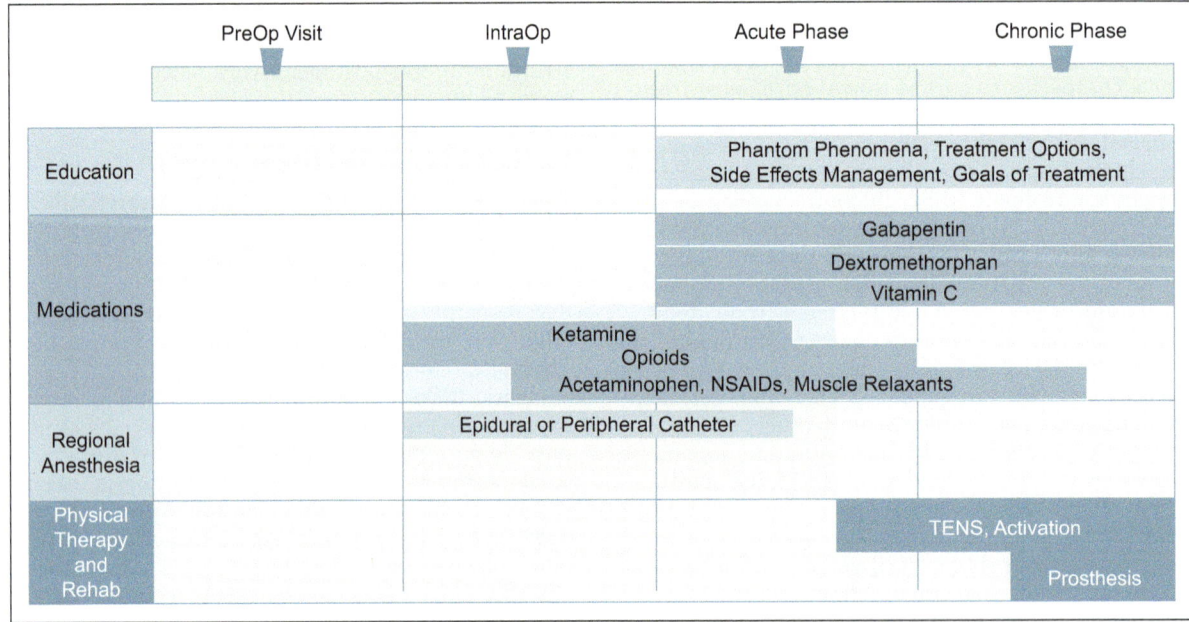

Figure 125.2: Phantom pain treatment timeline for unplanned amputation.
NSAIDs, nonsteroidal anti-inflammatory drugs; TENS, transcutaneous electrical nerve stimulation.

Table 125.1	Preoperative Medications to Prevent Phantom Limb Pain	
Drug	Dose	Comments
Gabapentin	Start at 10 mg/kg/day, divided into three doses	Dose is typically increased by 10 mg/kg/day every 3–5 days to a final dose of 30 mg/kg/day. As gabapentin takes weeks to provide full effect, this medication is typically started days in advance of elective surgery.
Dextromethorphan*	30 mg BID to start and titrate to 60 mg BID as needed	Risk of serotonin syndrome when used with SSRIs or drugs that increase serotonin levels. Use with caution in these patients.
Vitamin C[a]	500–1000 mg daily	No studies directly evaluating benefit in reducing phantom limb pain but proved to be beneficial for CRPS, a condition sharing neurophysiological phenomena with phantom pain.

[a]Dosing for patient <12 years unknown; dosing based on weight-based extrapolation. Monitor for side effects.
CRPS, complex regional pain syndrome; SSRIs, selective serotonin reuptake inhibitors.

If not yet initiated, a peripheral nerve block or epidural catheter should be placed with a bolus of local anesthetic administered and continuous infusion started prior to surgical incision. A bolus of ketamine should be administered prior to incision, followed by a continuous ketamine infusion.[11,13] Not only does this aid with intraoperative analgesia, but postoperatively, the analgesia these medications offer also reduces the incidence of phantom limb pain. To ensure adequate intraoperative and postoperative analgesia, further multimodal analgesia medications should be utilized, such as acetaminophen, nonsteroidal anti-inflammatory drugs (depending on coagulation status), opioids, and diazepam.[14]

POSTOPERATIVE CARE

Continuation of a multimodal analgesic strategy is key in the postoperative period. If amputation was emergent or traumatic with no time for placement of a peripheral nerve block or epidural catheter prior to surgery, this should be done as soon as possible. Postoperatively, ketamine infusions should continue, as should systemic opioid therapy with patient-controlled analgesia being a viable means of delivery. Gabapentin should be administered throughout the postoperative period and anesthesia providers may consider the addition of additional anti-neuropathic pain medications (e.g., amitriptyline). Dextromethorphan has demonstrated analgesic efficacy when given postoperatively[11] and is a staple of the authors' phantom pain regimen, based on long-term, empiric experience. Depending on the nature of the residual limb pain, medications used for phantom limb pain may also target residual limb pain.

Nonpharmacological therapies for phantom limb pain are numerous and include graded motor imagery, biofeedback, and meditation.[14] Graded motor imagery (aka mirror complex regional pain syndrome therapy) is a fascinating approach that involves visual and motor training protocol to reintegrate expected and perceived sensation to reduce phantom pain and can be effective.[15] Chronic postsurgical pain can be influenced by psychological factors including anxiety, depression, and poor coping skills.[7] Therefore, psychological therapies play a crucial role in perioperative pain management. Therapies, such as cognitive behavioral therapy and hypnotherapy, have proved to play a key role in postoperative pain management.[16] Additionally, pain psychology and counseling services should be offered to all patients, since anxiety, depression, and coping skills may have a role in the development of phantom limb pain postoperatively.

KEY REFERENCES

Complete references for this chapter are online and available at https://connect.springerpub.com/content/book/978-0-8261-3875-0/part/part04/toc-part/ch125.

2. DeMoss P, Ramsey LH, Karlson CW. Phantom limb pain in pediatric oncology. *Front Neurol.* 2018;9:219. doi:10.3389/fneur.2018.00219
6. Wilkins KL, McGrath PJ, Finley GA, Katz J. Phantom limb sensations and phantom limb pain in child and adolescent amputees. *Pain.* 1998;78(1):7–12. doi:10.1016/s0304-3959(98)00109-2
11. Alviar MJ, Hale T, Dungca M. Pharmacologic interventions for treating phantom limb pain. *Cochrane Database Syst Rev.* 2016;10(10):CD006380. doi:10.1002/14651858.CD006380.pub3
12. Aïm F, Klouche S, Frison A, et al. Efficacy of vitamin C in preventing complex regional pain syndrome after wrist fracture: a systematic review and meta-analysis. *Orthop Traumatol Surg Res.* 2017;103(3):465–470. doi:10.1016/j.otsr.2016.12.021
13. Wang X, Yi Y, Tang D, et al. Gabapentin as an adjuvant therapy for prevention of acute phantom-limb pain in pediatric patients undergoing amputation for malignant bone tumors: a prospective double-blind randomized controlled trial. *J Pain Symptom Manage.* 2018;55(3):721–727. doi:10.1016/j.jpainsymman.2017.11.029

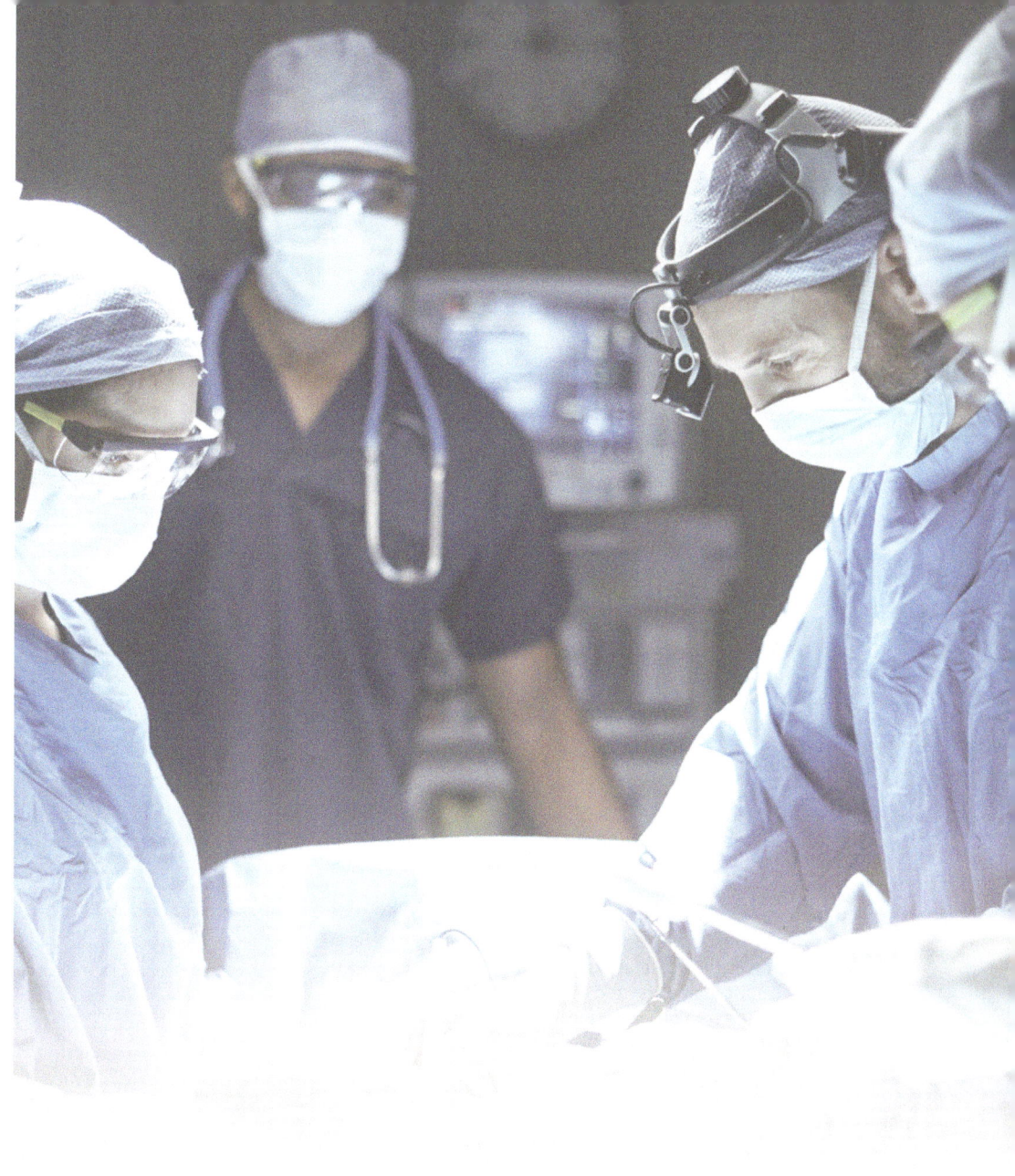

PART V

SPECIAL TOPICS IN PEDIATRIC ANESTHETIC CARE

CHAPTER 126

Malignant Hyperthermia

Dorothea L. Connolly and Jennifer Raynor

LEARNING OBJECTIVES

- Define *malignant hyperthermia* (MH) genetics and *pathophysiology*.
- Review how to identify MH-susceptible children.
- Describe the clinical features and diagnosis of MH.
- Describe anesthesia for the MH susceptible.
- Discuss current MH testing methods and resources available to practitioners and affected families.

INTRODUCTION

Malignant hyperthermia (MH) is a rare pharmacogenetic disorder of skeletal muscle. When a susceptible individual is exposed to volatile anesthetic agents or the depolarizing muscle relaxant succinylcholine, a life-threatening hypermetabolic process can occur.[1] In rare cases, an MH crisis may be associated with environmental heat, vigorous exercise, or stress.[1] Current MH presentations can be insidious due to the use of modern halogenated agents and IV anesthetic medications, neuraxial techniques, routine monitoring of end-tidal carbon dioxide ($ETCO_2$), and early discontinuation of triggering agents.[2] For these reasons, early recognition of an MH crisis may be difficult.[3] However, increased understanding of the pathophysiology, clinical manifestations, and treatment of MH has decreased mortality from 80% 30 years ago to <5% in 2006.[1]

EPIDEMIOLOGY

Although the exact prevalence is unknown, MH is thought to affect 1 in 2,000 to 3,000 individuals varying geographically.[1] The incidence is estimated between 1 in 10,000 and 250,000 general anesthetics, with patients requiring three anesthetics on average before triggering an event.[1] MH occurs more frequently in males than in females (2:1) and affects all ethnic groups.[1,4] The mean age of all MH reactions is 18 years of age, though more than half of all reactions occur in patients less than 15 years of age.[1] MH exhibits variable penetrance with susceptible individuals exposed to, on average, three uncomplicated anesthetics before experiencing a crisis event.[1]

PATHOPHYSIOLOGY

MH was first described by Denborough in 1962 as an autosomal dominantly inherited disorder,[5] however, it has since been found to occur de novo.[6] During an MH, there is uncontrolled release of myoplasmic Ca^{2+}, which is the hallmark of malignant hyperthermia. The most prominent cytosolic Ca^{2+} elevation results from the freeing of stored sarcoplasmic Ca^{2+} mediated by ryanodine receptor type 1 (RyR1). While volatile anesthetics stimulate Ca^{2+} release via RyR1, succinylcholine acts indirectly by activating the nicotinergic acetylcholine receptor (nAChR), a nonspecific cation channel, resulting in continuous local depolarization. The depolarization can trigger propagated action potentials and will further activate the dihydropyridine receptors (DHPRs, $Ca_v1.1$) leading to the gating of both Ca^{2+} release from the sarcoplasmic reticulum via ryanodine receptor type 1 (RYR1) and L-type Ca^{2+} current from the extracellular space (Figure 126.1).

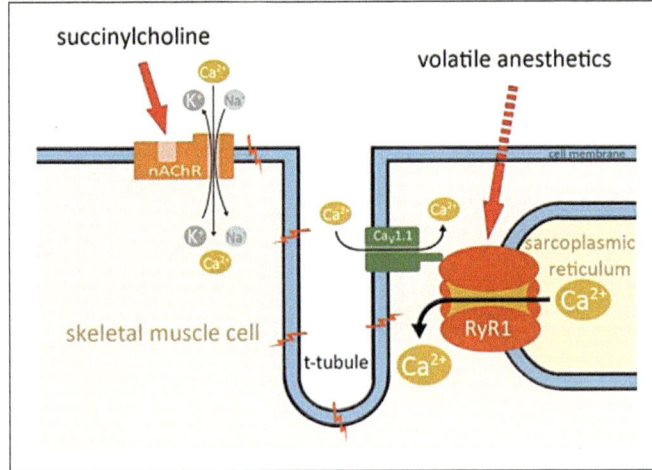

Figure 126.1: Effects of MH triggers on Ca^{2+} release.

MH, malignant hyperthermia; nAChR, nicotinergic acetylcholine receptor.

Source: From Klingler W, Heiderich S, Girard T, et al. Functional and genetic characterization of clinical malignant hyperthermia crises: a multi-centre study. *Orphanet J Rare Dis.* 2014;9(1):8. doi:10.1186/1750-1172-9-8.

IDENTIFICATION OF MALIGNANT HYPERTHERMIA-SUSCEPTIBLE CHILDREN

Identification of high-risk children or young adults typically occurs during the preanesthetic assessment and evaluation. Early identification remains the mainstay of prevention and enables anesthesia providers to plan a trigger-free anesthetic. Anesthesia providers should explore both patient and family anesthetic histories and review past anesthetic records when available. It is imperative that anesthesia providers maintain a high level of suspicion when anesthetic-related fevers or illness in patients or family members is reported. As MH testing is complex and may require high out-of-pocket expenses, definitive testing may not be available to confirm a suspected diagnosis.[8] Nonetheless, anesthesia providers must decide on relative risk and the need to administer a nontriggering anesthetic.[6]

A clinical grading scale was developed by Larach et al. (1994)[9] to help determine the likelihood of an actual prior MH event. The tool may aid the anesthesia provider in the anesthetic planning process without confirmed diagnostic testing (Table 126.1). Scores greater than 20 are likely for a past MH event, with scores over 50 strongly support diagnosis of MH.[10]

There are only a few confirmed myopathies that predispose patients to MH. These include King–Denborough

Table 126.1	Clinical Grading Scale for MH	
Process	**Indicator**	**Score**
I. Rigidity	• Generalized muscular rigidity (in absence of shivering due to hypothermia, or during or immediately following emergence from inhalational anesthesia)	15
	• Masseter spasm shortly following succinylcholine administration	15
II. Muscle breakdown	• Elevated creatine kinase >20,000 IU after anesthetic that included succinylcholine	15
	• Elevated creatine kinase >10,000 IU after anesthetic without succinylcholine	15
	• Cola-colored urine in perioperative period	10
	• Myoglobin in urine >60 mcg/L	5
	• Myoglobin in serum >170 mcg/L	5
	• Blood/plasma/serum K⁺ >6 mEq/L (in absence of renal failure)	3
III. Respiratory acidosis	• $PETCO_2$ >55 mm Hg with appropriately controlled ventilation	15
	• Arterial $PaCO_2$ >60 mm Hg with appropriately controlled ventilation	15
	• $PETCO_2$ >60 mm Hg with spontaneous ventilation	15
	• Arterial $PaCO_2$ >65 mm Hg with spontaneous ventilation	15
	• Inappropriate hypercarbia (in anesthesia provider's judgment)	15
	• Inappropriate tachypnea	10
IV. Temperature increase	• Inappropriately rapid increase in temperature	15
	• Inappropriately increased temperature >38.8°C (101.8°F) in the perioperative period	10
V. Cardiac involvement	• Inappropriate sinus tachycardia	3
	• Ventricular tachycardia or ventricular fibrillation	3
VI: Family history (used for MH susceptible)	• Positive MH family history in relative of first degree[a]	15
	• Positive MH family history in relative not of first degree[a]	5
VII. Other indicators that are not part of a single process	• Arterial base excess more negative than −8 mEq/L	10
	• Arterial pH <7.25	10
	• Rapid reversal of MH signs of metabolic and/or respiratory acidosis with IV dantrolene	5
	• Positive MH family history together with another indicator from the patient's own anesthetic experience other than elevated resting serum creatine kinase[a]	10
	• Resting elevated serum creatine kinase in patient with a family history of MH[a]	10

[a]These indicators should be used only for determining MH susceptibility.

MH, malignant hyperthermia; $PaCO_2$, partial pressure of carbon dioxide; $PETCO_2$, end-tidal partial pressure of CO_2.

Source: From Yang L, Tautz T, Zhang S, et al. The current status of malignant hyperthermia. *J Biomed Res.* 2020;34(2):75–85. doi:10.7555/JBR.33.20180089.

syndrome, central core disease, and multiminicore disease, Native American myopathy, and myopathies associated with *RYR1*, *CACNA1S*, and *STAC3*.[8] The most common diseases associated with MH susceptibility are those associated with known *RYR1*-associated phenotypes, known as the "ryanodinopathies" (Table 126.2). Less common loci of causality of MH susceptibility (approximately 2% of cases) are variants in the alpha-1 subunit of the dihydropyridine-sensitive L-type voltage-dependent calcium-channel receptor (*CACNA1S*), which are also part of the excitation–contraction complex located in skeletal muscle. MH susceptibility is associated with pathological variants in the *STAC3* gene, which is most commonly manifested as Native American myopathy. Anesthesia providers should be aware that nearly 50% of MH-susceptible individuals do not carry known variants in the aforementioned genes, underscoring the need for confirmation via muscle biopsy.[11]

Anesthesia providers should be aware that some myopathic conditions, such as Duchenne and Becker muscular dystrophy, have been associated with the development of fatal or life-threatening rhabdomyolysis with hyperkalemia following exposure to volatile anesthetic agents or succinylcholine (Table 126.3). This is not secondary to MH, however, as hypermetabolic symptoms, such as respiratory acidosis, metabolic acidosis, and excessive heat production are lacking.[12] Duchenne and Becker muscular dystrophy were historically associated with MH due to the increased likelihood of rhabdomyolysis and hyperkalemia after exposure to triggering anesthetic agents. Because of the potential for volatile anesthetic agents and succinylcholine to cause non-MH-related rhabdomyolysis and hyperkalemia in patients with Duchenne and Becker muscular dystrophy, it is often recommended these medications should be avoided in these populations despite multiple case reports citing safe administration.[12]

Table 126.2 Phenotypes Associated With MH Susceptibility

Phenotype	Clinical Characteristics	Genotype	Association With MH
Normal	No apparent muscle symptoms	Dominant *RYR1* or (dominant and recessive) *CACNA1S* variants	Based on clinical MH episodes in patient or family and findings of pathogenic *RYR1* variants
CCD	Congenital myopathy characterized by nonspecific motor developmental delays and weakness and varying degrees of clinical involvement and progression	Dominant (and heterozygous *de novo*) *RYR1* variants	Based on presence of *RYR1* variants and pedigree analyses of families with CCD and MH episodes
Multiminicore myopathy	Congenital myopathy characterized by generalized muscle weakness and amyotrophy, which may progress slowly or remain stable; may have ophthalmoparesis	Recessive *RYR1* and recessive *CACNA1S* variants	Reports of MH episodes in these patients
Congenital myopathy with cores and rods	Varying degrees of severity of hypotonia during infancy	Most typically dominant *de novo RYR1* variants, as well as variants in *NEB*, *ACTA1*, and *TPM2*	Compound heterozygosity (triplet of *RYR1* variants in one allele and fourth *RYR1* variant on the other allele) resulted in a complex phenotype of malignant hyperthermia and core myopathy
Centronuclear myopathy	Muscle weakness that may begin at birth and affect different muscle groups; may have ophthalmoparesis	Variants in *DNM2*, *MTM1*, *BIN1*, *CCD78*, *DNM2*, *TTN*, *SPEG*, and *RYR1*	MH episodes likely only in patients with *RYR1* variants (and possibly *CACNA1S*, though these patients also typically have cores) and not in other subtypes. There are no reports of MH in patients with centronuclear myopathy, but precautions are advisable because of possible *RYR1* variant before genetic testing is performed
Congenital fiber type disproportion	Nonprogressive or slowly progressive myopathy with weakness and hypotonia during infancy. Clinical features include failure to thrive, developmental delays of gross motor skills, limb weakness, joint contractures, and scoliosis	Variants in *ACTA1*, *SEPN1*, *LMNA*, *RYR1*, *MYH7*, *CACNA1S*, or *TPM3*	One study reported between 10% and 20% of congenital fiber-type disproportion is caused by variants in *RYR1*. There are no reports of MH in patients with congenital fiber-type disproportion, but precautions are advisable because of possible *RYR1* variant before genetic testing is performed
KDS	Congenital myopathy characterized by skeletal abnormalities and dysmorphic features	Reported cases of KDS with and without variants in *RYR1*	Multiple reports of MH in patients with KDS. Subsequent findings of *RYR1* variants in KDS patients
Periodic paralysis	Periods of extreme muscle weakness or paralysis based on fluctuating serum potassium levels	Variants in *RYR1*, *CACNA1S*, or *SCN4A*	Consider MH susceptible if *RYR1*, *CACNA1S*, or unknown genotype
Nemaline rod myopathy	Primarily proximal muscle weakness, delayed motor development beginning in early childhood, variable in severity and progression	Mainly associated with variants in *ACTA1*, *NEB*, *TPM3*, *TPM2*, *TNNT1*, and *CFL2*. Rarely associated with *RYR1*	Consider MH susceptible if *RYR1* or unknown genotype
Native American myopathy	Myopathy characterized by congenital weakness, arthrogryposis, cleft palate, ptosis, myopathic facies, short stature, kyphoscoliosis, and talipes deformities	Variants in the *STAC3* gene	Case reports and pedigrees reporting association with MH
Idiopathic hyperCKemia	Persistent elevations in serum creatine kinase levels without evidence of other neuromuscular diseases	Associated with many different entities, such as undiagnosed Duchenne, variants in *CAV3*, *RYR1*, and others	Reports of patients with hyperCKemia and *RYR1* variants have developed clinical MH

CCD, central core disease; KDS, King-Denborough syndrome; MH, malignant hyperthermia.

Source: From Litman RS, Griggs BS, Dowling JJ, Riazi S. Malignant hyperthermia susceptibility and related diseases. *Anesthesiology.* 2018;128(1):159–167. doi:10.1097/ALN.0000000000001877.

Table 126.3	Disease Associated With Non-MH-Induced Rhabdomyolysis		
Disease	**Clinical Characteristics**	**Genetics**	**Association With MH**
DMD	Progressive proximal muscular weakness with cardiac involvement	Dystrophin (DMD) variants (X-linked)	No association with MH, but fatal and life-threatening hyperkalemia reported with administration of succinylcholine and volatile agents
Becker muscular dystrophy	Less severe form of muscular dystrophy than Duchenne; characterized by muscle wasting and weakness at variable ages	Dystrophin (DMD) variants (X-linked)	No association with MH, but fatal and life-threatening hyperkalemia reported with administration of succinylcholine and volatile agents
CPT2 deficiency	Recurrent episodes of rhabdomyolysis triggered by prolonged exercise, fasting, or febrile illness	Variants in *S113L, P50H, Q413fs-F448L*	One report of a child with CPT2 deficiency who developed rhabdomyolysis after exposure to a volatile anesthetic agent. In a population of MH-susceptible individuals, none had CPT2 deficiency
Merosin-deficient congenital muscular dystrophy	Congenital muscular dystrophy characterized by muscle weakness apparent at birth	Recessive variants in *LAMA2*	One report of an MH-like episode after a non-triggering anesthetic. There is no evidence of a link to MH susceptibility

CPT2, carnitine palmitoyltransferase type 2; DMD, Duchenne muscular dystrophy; MH, malignant hyperthermia; Non-MH, nonmalignant hyperthermia.
Source: From Litman RS, Griggs BS, Dowling JJ, Riazi S. Malignant hyperthermia susceptibility and related diseases. *Anesthesiology*. 2018;128(1):159–167. doi:10.1097/ALN.0000000000001877.

Mitochondrial disorders, Noonan syndrome, arthrogryposis, osteogenesis imperfecta (prone to intraoperative hyperthermia), and neuroleptic malignant syndrome are not associated with MH and do not require the use of nontriggering anesthetic techniques.[12]

CLINICAL PRESENTATION, TREATMENT, AND DIAGNOSIS

CLINICAL PRESENTATION OF MALIGNANT HYPERTHERMIA

MH can occur during anesthesia at any time, including in the early postoperative period.[1] The most common presenting symptoms of MH include unexplained increasing $ETCO_2$ despite adjustment in minute ventilation, sinus tachycardia, muscle rigidity, and rapidly increasing body temperature >38.8°C.[8] Anesthesia providers must keep in mind the increase in $ETCO_2$ may be gradual due to the decreased use of succinylcholine, as well as the minute ventilation adjustments made by the anesthesia provider.[1] Masseter muscle rigidity (MMR) can be an early sign of MH. While MMR develops in approximately 1% of children receiving succinylcholine in the absence of generalized muscle rigidity, it should subside after the succinylcholine is metabolized.[6] If it does not, MH should be considered and further investigated.[6] Hyperthermia can manifest as an early or late sign, with increases in temperature of 1°C to 2°C every 5 minutes typical.[1]

Unexpected hyperkalemia can develop rapidly during an MH crisis leading to life-threatening arrhythmias. Additional complications include renal failure and disseminated intravascular coagulation (DIC), with the latter the most frequent cause of MH-related deaths.[6]

TREATMENT OF MALIGNANT HYPERTHERMIA

The hypermetabolic state of MH can lead to a combined metabolic and respiratory acidosis, cardiac arrhythmias, renal failure, and death if untreated.[10] Morbidity and mortality of an MH event are directly related to early identification and timely treatment initiation. If MH is suspected, the anesthesia provider should transition to a nontriggering anesthetic and immediately add a charcoal filter and increase the fresh gas flow to 10 LPM to remove the presence of remaining volatile anesthetic agents.

Dantrolene sodium, a specific agonist for MH, should be administered within 15 minutes of the decision to treat a crisis according to the Malignant Hyperthermia Association of the United States (MHAUS).[3] Dantrolene is a hydantoin derivative that directly interferes with muscle contraction by inhibiting calcium ion release from the sarcoplasmic reticulum, possibly by binding to RYR-1. The initial dose is 2.5 mg/kg, repeated every 5 minutes until reversal of the reaction occurs or a total dose of 10 mg/kg is reached. Over 20 years of data gathered by the North American Malignant Hyperthermia Registry suggest that every 15-minute delay in the time to dantrolene sodium administration is associated with an increased risk of complications or death of 7.8%.[3]

Additional supportive measures include the administration of sodium bicarbonate for the treatment of metabolic acidosis. Calcium gluconate, or calcium chloride if central venous access is available, as well as insulin (0.1 units/kg to a maximum of 10 units) and dextrose (0.5–1 g/kg), can be administered for correction of hyperkalemia. In addition, the patient can be actively cooled in an effort to decrease the rising temperatures secondary to the hypermetabolic state. Anesthesia providers should obtain laboratory work, including blood gas, creatinine kinase, and electrolytes to further guide care (**Figure 126.2**).

DIAGNOSIS OF MALIGNANT HYPERTHERMIA

The diagnosis of MH should be based on a combination of clinical diagnosis and supporting laboratory tests. The caffeine halothane contracture test (CHCT) is the gold standard for establishing the diagnosis of MH. The CHCT requires a skeletal muscle biopsy from the patient's thigh to assess muscle contractile properties upon exposure to ryanodine receptor agonists (e.g., caffeine and halothane). The tissue needs to be tested soon after it is obtained at 1 of 30 MH muscle biopsy testing centers worldwide; 4 of which are in the United States, with another in Canada. Abnormally high

> **Malignant Hyperthermia**   ↑ Temp ↑ HR ↑ CO_2 acidosis
>
> - Get MH Cart, dantrolene, and help
> - Notify team and stop procedure, if possible
> - Stop volatile anesthetic, succinylcholine.
> - Attach charcoal filter. Turn O_2 flow to 10 L / min
> - Hyperventilate patient to reduce $ETCO_2$
>
> **MH hotline 1-800-644-9737**
>
> - Give dantrolene 2.5 mg / kg IV, rapidly, through large bore IV if possible, every 5 min until symptoms resolve. May need up to 10 mg / kg (if no response at this dose, consider alternative diagnoses)
>   - Dantrium/Revonto: Assign dedicated person to mix these formulations of dantrolene (20 mg / vial) with 60 mL non-bacteriostatic sterile water
>   - Ryanodex: 250 mg is mixed with 5 mL non-bacteriostatic sterile water
>
> - Transition to non-triggering anesthetic
> - Give sodium bicarbonate 1-2 mEq / kg IV for suspected metabolic acidosis
> - Cool patient:
>   - Apply ice externally to axilla, groin and around head
>   - Infuse cold saline IV
>   - NG and open body cavity lavage with cold water
>   - Stop cooling when temperature < 38 °C
>
> - Hyperkalemia treatment:
>   - Calcium gluconate 30 mg / kg IV or calcium chloride 10 mg / kg IV;
>   - Sodium bicarbonate 1-2 mEq / kg IV;
>   - Regular insulin 0.1 units / kg IV (MAX 10 units) and dextrose 0.5-1 g / kg IV
>
> - VT or afib treatment: Do NOT use calcium channel blocker; give amiodarone 5 mg / kg
> - Send labs: ABG or VBG, electrolytes, serum CK, serum/urine myoglobin, coagulation
> - Place urinary catheter, maintain UO > 2 mL / kg / hr
> - If cardiac arrest occurs, begin CPR & consider ECMO, see 'Cardiac Arrest' card
> - If no response after 10 mg / kg dantrolene, consider other dx: sepsis, NMS, serotonin synd., myopathy, pheochromocytoma
> - Call ICU to arrange disposition. For post-acute management, see: http://www.mhaus.org
>
> Revision Mar 2018

Figure 126.2: Malignant hyperthermia critical event checklist.

ABG, arterial blood gas; afib, atrial fibrillation; CK, creatinine kinase; dx, diagnosis; ECMO, extracorporeal membrane oxygenation; ETCO2, end-tidal carbon dioxide; HR, heart rate; ICU, intensive care unit; MH, malignant hyperthermia; NG, nasogastric; NMS, neuroleptic malignant syndrome; UO, urine output; VBG, venous blood gas, VT, ventricular tachycardia.

Source: From PediCrisis Critical Events Checklists. Society for Pediatric Anesthesia. 2018. https://www.pedsanesthesia.org/critical-events-checklist.

levels of contractile force indicate MH susceptibility, with the test having a sensitivity close to 100% (false negatives are rare) and specificity of approximately 80% (approximately 20% false positives).

Genetic testing may also be performed, exploring the presence of variants in the *RYR1* gene. The presence of pathogenic variant in *RYR1* gene is diagnostic for MH susceptibility. At this time, however, not all proven MH-susceptible individuals have been found to carry a pathogenic variant. The sensitivity of the genetic test depends on several factors, including the population selected and the methodology of the testing utilized. Sensitivity for ideal test candidates (family history of MH plus either positive in vitro contracture test or an MH event) is approximately 60%.[14,15] Once a pathogenic variant is found, family members can have targeted genetic testing for the familial pathogenic variant; if found, the individual is considered MH susceptible and a muscle biopsy for contracture testing can be avoided.

Unfortunately, both the CHCT and the genetic test are expensive and not always covered by insurance. Neither test is recommended as a screening tool for MH susceptibility. Therefore, careful examination of patient and family medical and anesthetic history often determines the need for further testing.

ANESTHESIA FOR THE MALIGNANT HYPERTHERMIA-SUSCEPTIBLE PATIENT

Known MH-susceptible patients can safely receive anesthesia by utilizing nontriggering agents, such as opioids, propofol, or nitrous oxide. Prior to the start of anesthesia, it is imperative that the anesthesia machine is properly prepared. Charcoal filters are placed on the anesthesia circuit's inspiratory and expiratory limbs to avoid residual volatile agent from reaching the patient. While the use of charcoal filters precludes the need to flush the machine with high-flow oxygen, institutional protocols will vary.[6] In addition, many anesthesia providers take further precautions including taping over the volatile agent vaporizers to prevent unintentional use or simply removing the vaporizers from the machine entirely.

When utilizing a nontriggering technique to provide anesthesia to a child, oral premedication, such as midazolam and/or topical anesthetics, to potential peripheral IV sites facilitates the transition to the operating room. In the operating room, inhaled nitrous oxide can be used to enhance IV placement. The use of total IV anesthesia (TIVA) can be achieved with a bolus of propofol for the induction of anesthesia followed by a continuous infusion of propofol (150–250 mcg/kg/min). The TIVA anesthetic can be augmented with various MH-safe drugs, opioids, dexmedetomidine, ketamine, and local anesthetics.[8]

All MH-susceptible patients should have close monitoring of core temperature and minute ventilation throughout the procedure. Assuming there are no signs or symptoms of MH, typical postanesthesia care unit and day-surgery discharge criteria apply. A thorough review of signs and symptoms of MH should be incorporated in discharge teaching, and the parents should be informed of the need to bring their child to the hospital if fever or urine discoloration develops.[6]

RESOURCES

Malignant Hyperthermia Association of the United States

The MHAUS was formed in 1981 to educate medical practitioners and act as a resource for families affected by MH. MHAUS serves two essential functions, as a 24-hour consultation hotline (1-800-644-9737) and an informational website (www.MHAUS.org), for providing information and resources to the medical community as well as the public.[6]

Muscle Biopsy Testing Centers

Toronto General Hospital
Malignant Hyperthermia Investigation Unit
Eaton 3-323
200 Elizabeth St.
Toronto, Ontario M5G 2C4
PH: (416) 340-3128
EMAIL: sheila.riazi@uhn.ca

Uniformed Services University of the Health Sciences
Bethesda, MD (Military & Civilian)
LCDR Michael Lee MC, USN
CAPT Dale F. Szpisjak MC, USN (back up)
Department of Anesthesiology
PH: (301) 295-3140
EMAIL: MHLab@usuhs.edu

UC Davis MH Biopsy Testing Center
Sacramento, CA
Timothy Tautz, MD
PH: (916) 734-2431
EMAIL: tjtautz@ucdavis.edu

University of Minnesota
Minneapolis, MN
Paul A. Iaizzo, PhD
PH: (612) 624-7912 or -3959
EMAIL: iaizz001@umn.edu

Wake Forest Baptist Medical Center
Winston-Salem, NC
Sherry Meacham
PH: (336) 716-7194
EMAIL: smeacham@wakehealth.edu

KEY REFERENCES

Complete references for this chapter are online and available at https://connect.springerpub.com/content/book/978-0-8261-3875-0/part/part01/toc-part/ch126.

3. Malignant Hyperthermia Association of the United States and the North American. (2019, Winter). A genetic test or muscle biopsy: which is right for you? *The Communicator, 37 Number 1.* Sherbourne, New York, USA.
8. Ellinas H, Albrecht M. Malignant hyperthermia update. *Anesthesiol Clin.* 2020;38(1):165–181. doi:10.1016/j.anclin.2019.10.010
10. Yang L, Tautz T, Zhang S, et al. The current status of malignant hyperthermia. *J Biomed Res.* 2020;34(2):75–85. doi:10.7555/JBR.33.20180089
11. Larach MG. A primer for diagnosing and managing malignant hyperthermia susceptibility. *Anesthesiology.* 2018;128(1):8–10. doi:10.1097/ALN.0000000000001879
12. Litman RS, Griggs BS, Dowling JJ, Riazi S. Malignant hyperthermia susceptibility and related diseases. *Anesthesiology.* 2018;128(1):159–167. doi:10.1097/ALN.0000000000001877
13. PediCrisis Critical Events Checklists. *Society for Pediatric Anesthesia.* 2018. https://www.pedsanesthesia.org/critical-events-checklist

CHAPTER 127

Neonatal Emergencies

Carrilee Powell and Vera Winograd-Gomez

> **LEARNING OBJECTIVES**
>
> - Identify potential surgical emergencies anesthesia providers may encounter when caring for the neonatal patient.
> - Understand the pathophysiology of the identified neonatal surgical emergencies.
> - Formulate an appropriate anesthetic plan for each neonatal surgical emergency reviewed.

CONGENITAL DIAPHRAGMATIC HERNIA

PATHOPHYSIOLOGY AND CLINICAL MANIFESTATIONS

Congenital diaphragmatic hernia (CDH) is a condition that results when intra-abdominal organs extrude into the thoracic cavity through a defect in the diaphragm interfering with normal lung development. The incidence of CDH ranges from 0.8 to 5 per 10,000 live births, with a slight male dominance and a lower incidence of isolated CDH among African American patients.[1,2] Despite significant advances in the diagnosis and management of CDH, morbidity and mortality remain high.[3,4]

The cause of CDH largely remains unclear and is currently thought to be multifactorial, with a majority of cases having an isolated diaphragmatic defect presenting with pulmonary hypoplasia and persistent pulmonary hypertension of the newborn.[5,6] Although most cases seem to be sporadic, genetic associations are becoming more and more common. CDH is present in a variety of syndromes such as CHARGE (coloboma, heart, atresia choanae, retardation, genital, and ear), Cornelia de Lange, Beckwith–Wiedemann, Fryns, Apert, Pentalogy of Cantrell, Goldenhar sequence, and VACTERL (vertebral, anal, cardiac, tracheoesophageal, renal, and limb).[7] Trisomies 13, 18, 21, Tetrasomy p12, and monosomy X are the most common aneuploidies associated with CDH.[8,9] However, despite the possible genetic basis for a great number of CDHs, genetic evaluation, including whole-exome sequencing, is usually normal. If there is no family history, risk of recurrence is minimal.[10]

Other theories involve environmental factors as the main cause of CDH. Rodent models have consistently shown vitamin-A pathways to be significantly involved in the origin of CDH.[11] Low retinol and retinol-binding protein levels have been found in cord blood of neonates presenting with CDH, it remains unclear if this is a cause–effect or an associated, confounding finding.[12]

The embryological basis of CDH remains controversial. The diaphragm begins to form simultaneously with the lungs and gastrointestinal tract around 4 weeks' gestation and is fully formed by 12 weeks.[13] Diaphragmatic closure begins with the ventral (membranous) component enveloping the esophagus, vena cava and aorta to fuse with the foregut mesentery to form the posterior and medial portions of the diaphragm. Pleuro-peritoneal canals close when all the membranous portions of the diaphragm fuse together and complete diaphragmatic closure is usually complete by 9 weeks' gestation.[14]

There is significant controversy surrounding the exact chain of events that leads to herniation of abdominal viscera into the thoracic cavity. One theory hypothesizes that delayed closure of the pleuroperitoneal canals (beyond 8–10 weeks) or early rotation and settling of the midgut (before 10 weeks) would cause midgut to herniate into the pleural cavity. Some rat models showed that this theory was caused not because of a delay in closure of the pleuroperitoneal canal but was due to a defect in the formation of the pleuroperitoneal fold, a much earlier event, typically occurring around 4 weeks of gestation.[15] An alternate theory is that lung hypoplasia might be the primary cause.[16] If there is a disturbance in the formation of the lung bud, posthepatic mesenchymal plate formation will be altered resulting in a defective diaphragm. Rat models have shown that impaired formation of the posthepatic mesenchymal plate leads to a diaphragmatic defect.[17] Regardless of the basis, a defect in the diaphragm causes the abdominal viscera to herniate and results in impaired lung development. The defect also causes abnormal fetal breathing movements causing an alteration in the stretch-induced lung maturation process.[15]

More than half of all CDH cases are diagnosed via ultrasound at a mean gestational age of 24 weeks.[18] Other diagnostic tools, such as three-dimensional ultrasound, fetal echocardiography, and MRI are used mainly to evaluate for severity and outcome predictors of CDH. It is usually easier to diagnose left-sided CDH due to the presence of a heterogeneous mass composed of stomach and/or intestines. Right-sided CDH, in contrast, may be extremely difficult to diagnose if the only organ that herniates is the liver. Indirect signs may be of use when diagnosing CDH, especially right-sided hernias. These include shift in the cardiac axis, identification of the gall bladder, and Doppler evaluation of hepatic vasculature. MRI is useful in detecting the position of the liver but especially in the estimation of lung volume.[19] Using adjunct diagnostic tools is of use in detecting associated malformations as cardiac and neural tube defects affect the long-term outcome of children with CDH.[8] Once diagnosed, patients should be referred to tertiary care centers with expertise in handling CDH patients and extracorporeal membrane oxygenation (ECMO).

The most common defect associated with CDH is Botchdalek's (posterolateral) hernia, accounting for more than 95% of cases, 80% of which are left sided.[15,20] In approximately 2% of cases, CDH is bilateral. Morgagni (anterior) and paraesophageal hernias are rarer versions of this disease. Interestingly, trisomy 21 is the most frequent genetic abnormality associated with Morgagni hernia.[15]

Herniation of abdominal organs into the pleural cavity leads to a combination of lung immaturity and hypoplasia that ultimately causes persistent pulmonary hypertension. This is frequently associated with, and aggravated by, right ventricular hypertrophy and left ventricular underdevelopment resulting in ventricular dysfunction.[21,22] Lung hypoplasia occurs ipsilateral to the herniation with variable degrees of affection to the contralateral lung. Hypoplasia was initially thought to be caused by direct compression caused by abdominal organs. However, recent rat models have shown a possible two-hit event in which bilateral hypoplasia results from an initial insult during organogenesis followed by ipsilateral lung compression caused by the herniated organs. This theory explains the significant variability found on the contralateral lung.[23]

In CDH, there is a reduction of pulmonary vasculature with a reduction in the vessel-to-lung ratio. Additionally, medial hyperplasia and peripheral extension of the musculature into arterioles is a key finding of the pulmonary vascular remodeling phenomenon found in CDH. Reducing the pulmonary vasculature and vascular remodeling contributes to the irreversible component of primary pulmonary hypertension.[24,25] The reversible component of persistent pulmonary hypertension of the newborn (PPHN) is due to altered vasoreactivity. This alteration is caused by an altered autonomic innervation (increased sympathetic, decreased parasympathetic), an imbalance between vasodilator and vasoconstrictor factors, and/or impairment of the endothelium-induced relaxation of pulmonary arteries.[26–28]

Ventricular dysfunction is frequently associated with CDH. Altered pulmonary vasculature, in addition to the normal physiological changes of postnatal circulation, results in pulmonary hypertension and may ultimately lead to right ventricular dysfunction. Left ventricular anomalies are also found in infants with CDH.[29] Reduced left ventricular output has been documented in infants with both right- and left-sided CDH. However, left-sided CDH has been associated with significantly lower left ventricular mass when compared to other causes of PPHN.[30] Reduced left ventricular mass leads to functional left ventricular hypoplasia resulting in increased left atrial pressure and pulmonary venous hypertension.[31]

There are three main outcome predictors in CDH: presence of associated anomalies, especially heart disease; the extent of lung hypoplasia; and the position of the liver.[18] The prognosis of CDH is better in the absence of associated anomalies. This has been confirmed by population-wide studies, which report higher survival for isolated CDH compared to CDH associated with additional anomalies.[1,32] The timing of diagnosis seems to be related to severity at presentation with CDH diagnosed before 25 weeks, presenting with worse lung hypoplasia and more severe PPHN. However, it is unclear if this is independently related to the gestational age at diagnosis or if smaller defects are harder to detect in earlier ultrasounds.[33]

Metkus et al.[34] described the lung-to-head ratio (LHR) that results when comparing the contralateral lung with the head circumference. Variability on gestational age and low inter-center reliability lead to the description of the observed to expected LHR (O/E LHR, found by dividing the observed LHR by the expected ratio for gestational age), which was shown to be independent of gestational age.[35,36] LHR is often used with liver herniation to predict outcome. LHR over 1.35 has a 100% survival whereas LHR under 0.6 has no survival. Alternatively, O/E LHR under 25% is considered severe CDH with 100% mortality in cases with O/E LHR under 15% and liver herniation. Liver herniation (liver-up) is also associated with worse prognosis. Liver herniation is predictive not only of overall survival but also of ECMO, with figures ranging between 74% and 100% survival with liver-down compared to 45% to 56% survival with liver-up. Likewise, need for ECMO was independently predicted by liver herniation (25% liver-down vs. 80% liver-up).[34,37,38]

SPECIAL CONSIDERATIONS AND CONCERNS

Although the perinatal management of CDH is beyond the scope of this chapter, there are some aspects anesthesia providers should consider. The prenatal administration of either corticosteroids or phosphodiesterase inhibitors has shown promising results in rat models, however, there is no evidence to date of benefit in humans.[39,40] Prenatal surgical management using tracheal occlusion seems promising. In a lamb model of CDH, occlusion of the fetal trachea led to an acceleration of lung growth. A randomized trial of hysterotomy-guided fetal endoscopic tracheal occlusion performed in humans, however, yielded no changes in survival when compared to standard postnatal care.[41] More recently, meta-analyses have reported increased survival rates at 30 days and 6 months in patients with severe CDH undergoing fetal tracheal occlusion despite an increased risk of premature membrane rupture and decreased gestational age.[42] A new, minimally invasive procedure via fetoscopy, termed percutaneous fetal endoluminal tracheal obstruction (FETO), is being subjected to multiple randomized clinical trials with results expected in late 2020/early 2021 (see www.totaltrial.eu or clinicaltrials.gov NCT00763737).

Infants who are born with bilateral lung hypoplasia or severe unilateral compromise are symptomatic immediately at birth. Patients should be referred to a tertiary care center immediately upon prenatal diagnosis. The classic triad of CDH consists of dyspnea, cyanosis, and apparent dextrocardia. Physical examination shows a bulging chest with diminished breath sounds, scaphoid abdomen, right-displaced heart sounds, and bowel sounds in the chest. A plain chest radiograph shows mediastinal shift, bowel gas in the chest, and alterations at the right costophrenic angle. Infants born before 33 weeks' gestation, under 1000 g, or have an alveolar-to-arterial oxygen gradient above 500 rarely survive.[43] However, over the last few decades, antenatal diagnosis, increasing expertise in neonatal stabilization, appropriate timing of surgery, ECMO, and, especially, avoiding ventilator-induced lung damage have greatly improved outcomes for children with severe CDH.[44]

The optimal mode of mechanical ventilation for children with CDH is not known. Many centers initiate conventional mechanical ventilation for respiratory support, adjusting peak inspiratory pressure (PIP), positive end-expiration pressure (PEEP), and respiratory rate to optimize ventilation. A randomized trial comparing conventional mechanical ventilation (CMV) and high-frequency oscillatory ventilation (HFOV) showed no statistically significant difference in mortality or bronchopulmonary dysplasia. However, patients randomized to CMV were ventilated for fewer days, had shorter duration of vasoactive drugs, and less often required ECMO support, sildenafil, or nitric oxide as compared to children ventilated by HFOV. Of note, CMV parameters in the study included low PEEP of 3 to 5 cmH_2O and low PIP (20–25 cmH_2O).[45]

Invasive blood pressure monitoring is paramount to hemodynamic monitoring and management. Both preductal and postductal saturations and heart rate should be continuously monitored as end-organ perfusion is the goal of hemodynamic monitoring in infants with CDH. Due to right-to-left shunting associated with PPHN, preductal and postductal saturation variance may exist. Anesthesia providers should be aware that the absence of a preductal and postductal saturation difference does not rule out pulmonary hypertension. In some patients with CDH, an initial improvement in oxygenation may be observed (referred to as "honeymoon" period), with a subsequent deterioration in oxygenation parameters.[46] An echocardiogram is the best noninvasive method of evaluating ventricular function and pulmonary pressures and should be performed within the first 24 hours of life. If preductal saturations fall below 85%, hemodynamic management and ventilation adjustments should be pursued prior to initiating any therapy. The CDH consortium recommends maintaining normal blood pressure levels if the preductal saturation levels are between 80% and 95%.[47] When ventilation adjustments and hemodynamic management are not sufficient, there are several therapeutical options to optimize end-organ perfusion.

Inhaled nitric oxide (iNO) is the first agent of choice for treatment of pulmonary hypertension in neonates above 34 weeks' gestation as it relaxes pulmonary vascular smooth muscle cells with a selective pulmonary vasodilator effect. The criteria for initiation of iNO depend on the severity of PPHN as assessed by the oxygenation index (OI = mean airway pressure × FiO_2 × $100/PaO_2$). It is worth noting that patients with CDH may be more resistant to iNO, with iNO potentially only being effective following ECMO.[48] However, even in the setting of respiratory failure without CDH, the long-term benefits of iNO compared to other interventions are controversial. In a Cochrane review, iNO improved outcome by reducing the need for ECMO but the response was not related to presence or absence of pulmonary hypertension. In fact, not only were outcomes not improved in infants with CDH, but they also seem to be slightly worse.[49] Nevertheless, iNO remains an important therapeutic tool in patients with CDH, even if only as a bridge to ECMO. Some suggest a short trial of iNO should always precede ECMO, while no clinical marker predicts response to iNO, sometimes an infant responds dramatically. Prostaglandin I2 or sildenafil may also serve as rescue therapy in the setting of severe pulmonary hypertension associated with CDH.[50,51]

The evolution in the role of ECMO support for infants with CDH has gone from apparently improving survival[52] to showing short-term benefits without clear improvement in long-term outcomes.[53] Many suggest that improved outcomes have been the result of improved cardiorespiratory interventions with minimal ventilation-induced lung trauma and delayed surgery and not because of ECMO.[54,55] Thus, in many centers, the frequency of ECMO in CDH has decreased over the last few years. The criteria for ECMO vary and no selection criteria seem to accurately predict survival. However, the CDH EURO consortium consensus statement established the following criteria for initiating ECMO[56]:

- Acidosis with pH <7.15 and lactate >5 mmol/L despite optimal ventilation
- Inability to maintain preductal SaO_2 >85% or postductal SaO_2 >70%
- PIP >28 cmH_2O or mean airway pressure >17 cmH_2O is needed to achieve SaO_2 >85%.
- Systemic hypotension resistant to fluid or inotropic resuscitation and leading to urine output <0.5 mL/kg/hr for 12 to 24 hours
- OI >40 for 4 to 6 hours or "consistently present"

Similar criteria are used across the United States although some centers replace OI with inability to wean from FiO_2 1.0 in the first 48 hours of life. Furthermore, patients must have completed 34 weeks' gestation, weigh more than 2 kg, have no significant intracranial hemorrhage (greater than grade 1), and have no other congenital or chromosomal abnormalities.[57]

ANESTHETIC MANAGEMENT

Although many centers now approach CDH repair via a minimally invasive approach, open repair still remains a common technique. There is significant controversy surrounding the benefits of minimally invasive techniques over open repair. Although the benefits of each are beyond the scope of this chapter, the anesthesia provider must be familiar with the differences in perioperative management for each type of repair. First and foremost, a variety of inclusion/exclusion criteria for thoracoscopic repair have been described. However, the limiting factor for thoracoscopic repair of CDH is persistent pulmonary hypertension. Therefore, the following have been widely accepted as adequate exclusion criteria[58]:

- pCO_2 at birth >60 mm Hg
- iNO during the first 24 hours of life
- Bidirectional left-to-right shunt
- Intrathoracic stomach on plain radiograph
- OI >30
- FiO_2 >0.5
- Congenital heart disease (some centers do not consider this an exclusion criterion)

Another significant factor to consider is the need to insufflate carbon dioxide in order to collapse the ipsilateral lung during thoracoscopic surgery. This represents a significant CO_2 load and may not be hemodynamically tolerated. Thoracoscopic repair is associated with higher incidence of significant acidosis and hypercarbia as well as an apparent increase in complications and reintervention rates.[59] Regardless of the approach, surgery should be delayed until the patient's cardiorespiratory status has been optimized. This includes a normal arterial pressure (for gestational age) and stable readings for at least 12 hours, preductal SaO_2 >85% (preferably >90%), no acidosis, and normal urine output. The goals of ventilation in the operating room (OR) resemble those in the preoperative period with special emphasis on avoiding ventilation-associated lung injury (small tidal volume, minimal PEEP ranging 2–4 cm H_2O, permissive hypercapnia maintaining pH >7.25). If sudden decompensation occurs, differential diagnosis includes pulmonary hypertension crisis and contralateral pneumothorax. Close attention should also be placed on temperature regulation. Hypothermia increases oxygen consumption that, in the setting of marginal cardiorespiratory function, may lead to inadequate oxygen delivery and acidosis; this in turn increases pulmonary vasoconstriction and worsens oxygen saturation. Hypothermia also increases pulmonary vascular resistance and may worsen right-to-left shunting. The selection of anesthetic agents and intraoperative management depends on the cardiorespiratory status of the patient, the setting of the intervention (NICU or OR), and the plans for perioperative ventilatory support.

ANESTHETIC TECHNIQUE: CDH ANESTHETIC MANAGEMENT

Preoperative Management

- Naso- or orogastric tube for stomach decompression
- Avoid bag-mask ventilation
- Intubation and ventilation with permissive hypercapnia
- Pre-incision broad-spectrum antibiotics

Intraoperative Management

- Right upper extremity pulse oximeter (preductal SpO_2 >90%)
- Left upper extremity or lower extremity (postductal) pulse oximeter
- Central venous access

- Arterial cannulation
- If available, low-concentration sevoflurane may aid in pulmonary vasodilation
- High-dose opioids (50 mcg/kg rentanyl) or low-concentration sevoflurane with moderate dose of opioids (10–20 mcg/kg fentanyl)
- Protective ventilation (PEEP 2–4 cmH$_2$O, peak pressures <25 cmH$_2$O)
- Nondepolarizing muscle relaxant
- Close temperature monitoring and active warming
- Consider iNO or ECMO for refractory pulmonary hypertensive crisis

Postoperative Management

- Consider opioid-sparing analgesic techniques (regional anesthesia) for postoperative pain
- Continue postoperative protective ventilation

SACROCOCCYGEAL TERATOMA

PATHOPHYSIOLOGY AND CLINICAL MANIFESTATIONS

Sacrococcygeal teratomas (SCTs) are one of the most common congenital tumors, ranging in incidence from 0.25 to 1 per 10,000 live births, with a female:male prevalence of 4:1.[60] SCTs are tumors derived from pluripotential cell lines consisting of all three germ layers. Perinatal mortality is high (up to 40%) when the tumor is diagnosed prenatally. Usually, prenatal death arises from anemia from hemorrhage into the tumor or tumor rupture, high output cardiac failure, dystocia, or preterm labor due to polyhydramnios.[61] While the majority of SCTs are benign at birth, up to 70% of tumors become malignant before 1 year of age and may recur as malignant SCTs after resection.[62] SCTs develop from the tip of the coccyx with variable amount of internal or external extension. Histologically, they are classified into mature, immature, or malignant teratoma, with this classification being useful to predict recurrence rates but not to predict long-term outcomes.[63,64]

SCTs are usually diagnosed by prenatal ultrasound and present at birth as a skin-covered tail mass. Multiple associated malformations may occur in up to 45% of patients with SCT. Most of these associated anomalies are anorectal and genital malformations. Other anomalies have been described including spinal dysraphism, meningocele, vertebral anomalies, and sacral agenesis.[65,66] Tumor markers may be elevated in up to 70% of patients with malignant SCTs. Usually, alpha-fetoprotein (derived from yolk-sac components) or beta human chorionic gonadotrophin (beta hCG) is elevated. Thus, serum levels of both should be evaluated during the diagnostic period to rule out malignant components. As in other tumors producing these hormones, serial follow-up of serum levels is helpful to monitor for tumor relapse.

The most widely accepted classification of SCT was described by the American Academy of Pediatrics Surgery section and divides tumors into four subtypes.[67] Type I SCTs are predominantly external with minimal internal component; type II are present externally but are predominantly intrapelvic; type III have a small external component with significant pelvic mass extending into the abdominal cavity while type IV SCTs are presacral with no external component.

SPECIAL CONSIDERATIONS AND CONCERNS

Surgical treatment entails removal of both the tumor and coccyx. Incomplete resection is the main cause for recurrence. Therefore, complete removal of both tumor and coccyx is paramount.[64] Only malignant SCTs benefit of post-resection chemotherapy. Platinum-based chemotherapy has been used in patients with large tumors before surgical resection to reduce tumor volume.[68] Large teratomas are usually supplied by the middle sacral artery and branches of the internal iliac. These tumors may present with significant shunting and may pose risk of massive intraoperative hemorrhage. In some cases, preoperative embolization is useful to reduce blood loss and allow faster and safer resections.[69] In utero treatment options include open fetal surgery, endoscopic laser, or radiofrequency ablation. Depending on tumor size and systemic compromise, ex utero intrapartum treatment procedure may be selected to allow resection under placental support.

ANESTHETIC MANAGEMENT

Anesthetic management for tumor resection in the neonatal period requires the anesthesia provider to understand neonatal physiology and be prepared for cardiovascular instability, hypothermia, massive transfusion, and coagulation dysfunction. Death during resection is not unusual and results from massive hemorrhage, coagulopathy, hypothermia, and cardiopulmonary instability. For large tumors, central venous access, invasive blood pressure monitoring, and adequate IV access are essential.

ANESTHETIC TECHNIQUE: SACROCOCCYGEAL TERATOMA ANESTHETIC MANAGEMENT

Preoperative Management

- Assessment for coagulopathy, platelet dysfunction, and congestive heart failure
- Guarantee blood product availability. Significant blood loss should be expected

Intraoperative Management

- Central venous access (for large-sized tumors)
- Arterial cannulation
- Two large-bore IV catheters
- Prone precautions
- Inhalational or IV induction
- Maintenance inhalational anesthesia with opioid supplement
- Close temperature monitoring and active warming
- Blood loss should be expected, be prepared for massive transfusion

Postoperative Management

- Extubation depends on associated underlying anomalies and hemodynamic instability

OMPHALOCELE AND GASTROSCHISIS

PATHOPHYSIOLOGY AND CLINICAL MANIFESTATIONS

The most common abdominal wall defects in neonates are gastroschisis and omphalocele. Omphalocele is a centrally located abdominal wall defect characterized by herniation of abdominal viscera including the small and large intestines, liver, spleen, and sometimes the gonads through the umbilical ring.[70,71] The herniated viscera in omphalocele is covered and protected by a membrane made up of Wharton's jelly, peritoneum, and amnion.[71]

The incidence of omphalocele is estimated to be 4 cases per every 10,000 live births.[72] During the sixth week of fetal development, the fetal midgut is rapidly developing due to abdominal cavity inability to accommodate growth of the midgut herniates through the umbilical ring. Approximately 4 weeks later, at 10 weeks of gestation, the abdominal cavity has expanded, and the midgut returns to the abdominal cavity. In a patient with an omphalocele, the midgut fails to return to the abdominal cavity.[73]

Omphalocele has an associated anomaly rate of up to 88% cases. Omphalocele is most commonly associated with trisomies 13, 18, and 21. Trisomy 18, Edwards syndrome, accounts for up to 80% to 90% of the trisomy diagnosis associated with omphalocele.[74] About 20% to 30% of infants with omphalocele have an associated congenital heart defect, most frequently an atrial septal defect, ventricular septal defect, or tetralogy of Fallot.[9,71] Other associated anomalies include Beckwith–Wiedemann syndrome, neural tube defects, defects of the genitourinary tract, and pulmonary hypertension.[75] Maternal risk factors for the development of omphalocele include extremes of maternal age and maternal obesity.[74]

In comparison to omphalocele, gastroschisis is typically a smaller abdominal wall defect with abdominal viscera herniation occurring to the right of the umbilical cord with no protective sac. Contents of herniation in gastroschisis are typically limited to intestine but occasionally may include the liver and gonads.[70] The lack of the protective sac exposes the intestines to the amniotic fluid causing inflammation of fetal intestines, thickening of the mesentery, and matting of the bowel.[72]

The incidence of gastroschisis is reported as about 4 cases per every 10,000 live births.[72] Gastroschisis is more commonly reported in male neonates.[70] Similar to omphalocele, gastroschisis occurs 6 to 10 weeks after contraception but etiology of the development of gastroschisis is unknown with multiple different proposed theories. Skarsgard et al. suggested multiple theories including failure of ventral fusion of the lateral body folds, amniotic membrane rupture at the base of the umbilical cord, weakness of paraumbilical tissue with right umbilical vein regression, or the vitelline artery undergoing a vascular incident leading to infarction and necrosis at the umbilicus base.[76] Maternal risk factors for the development of gastroschisis include young maternal age, smoking, recreation drug use, alcohol consumption, the use of decongestants and aspirin, exposure to toxins, and low body mass index.[70,72] Delivery of an infant with gastroschisis is seven times more likely to occur in women under the age of 20 years.[72]

In contrast to omphalocele, gastroschisis is typically an isolated lesion with associated anomalies rarely reported (Table 127.1). Anomalies reported with gastroschisis are usually

Table 127.1	Comparison of Gastroschisis to Omphalocele	
	Gastroschisis	**Omphalocele**
Defect	Abdominal wall defect to the right of umbilical cord Involves intestine, with rare involvement of liver and gonads Bowel does not have a protective sac therefore bowel is exposed to amniotic fluid causing inflamed, thickened, and matted bowel	Centrally located abdominal wall defect Involves small and large intestines, liver, spleen, and gonads Viscera covered by protective sac
Incidence	4:10,000 live births More common in males	4:10,000 live births

Pathogenesis	Multiple proposed theories:
	    Failure of ventral fusion of the lateral body folds
	    Amniotic membrane rupture at the base of the umbilical cord
	    Weakness of paraumbilical tissue with right umbilical vein regression
	    Vitelline artery vascular incident leading to infarction and necrosis
		Midgut herniates at 6 weeks' gestation and fails to return to abdominal cavity at 10 weeks' gestation

Risk Factors	Young maternal age (<20 yrs) Smoking Recreational drug use Alcohol consumption Decongestants Aspirin Exposure to toxins Low BMI	Extremes of maternal age Maternal obesity
Associated Anomalies	Rare	Commonly associated anomalies Trisomies 13, 18, and 21 Congenital heart defects Beckwith–Wiedemann syndrome Neural tube defects Defects of genitourinary tract Pulmonary hypertension

BMI, body mass index.

related to the gastrointestinal tract, most commonly intestinal atresia in 10% to 15% of the cases.[70] Chromosomal abnormalities are only reported in about 1.2% of gastroschisis cases.[76]

Omphalocele and gastroschisis are almost always diagnosed on a prenatal ultrasound allowing for delivery planning and preparation. Additionally, the presence of elevated maternal serum alpha-fetoprotein levels warrants further evaluation for gastroschisis.[72] After diagnosis of omphalocele on ultrasound, further workup, including an amniocentesis and fetal echocardiography, is warranted to identify additional anomalies. The decision for a vaginal delivery or cesarean section remains controversial. Factors to determine mode of delivery include size of defect, presence of protective sac, presence of herniated liver, and known associated anomalies.[70,76] Physicians may decide to deliver a gastroschisis infant earlier around 37 weeks of gestation to limit bowel exposure and damage to the amniotic fluid environment.[70]

Patients with gastroschisis and omphalocele will require surgical repair to return the abdominal viscera to the abdominal cavity and closure of the abdomen. Gastroschisis repair is typically performed within the first day of life but may be taken to the OR emergently if perfusion to the bowel is threatened. Repairing an omphalocele is not as urgent as gastroschisis unless the sac has ruptured, which will prompt surgical repair within the first few hours of life.[70]

SPECIAL CONSIDERATIONS AND CONCERNS

Preoperative management of an infant with gastroschisis and omphalocele focuses on protection of the herniated viscera, fluid resuscitation, temperature regulation, respiratory support as indicated, and bowel decompression.[70] It is imperative to protect and cover the exposed viscera to prevent further damage to intestine, insensible fluid loss, and heat loss. The exposed defect should be covered with saline-soaked gauze, and the lower half of the infant's body can be placed in a clear plastic bag. Vigilant care should be taken to support the viscera and prevent further injury, twisting, or compression to the intestines and liver.[75,76]

Infants with abdominal wall defects and exposed viscera are highly susceptible to significant fluid loss and hypothermia, especially with gastroschisis or ruptured omphalocele.[70] Infants can experience significant insensible and evaporative fluid losses from exposed bowel that can be 2.5 times greater than a healthy newborn.[72] Hypovolemia can result in significant hypotension with potential detrimental cardiovascular effects. Therefore, it is imperative to cover the exposed viscera and obtain IV access to allow for fluid resuscitation of the infant. IV fluids containing dextrose should be started to achieve euvolemia.[71] Poddar et al.[70] report that maintenance fluids containing sodium chloride and 10% dextrose at a rate of 80 mL/kg/day in addition to fluid boluses of crystalloid or albumin may be required to achieve and maintain euvolemia.[70] Adequate fluid resuscitation should be determined by stability of hemodynamics, urine output, and capillary refill.[76] Caution with inotrope administration should be taken if the patient has not adequately been fluid resuscitated as myocardium damage may occur.[73]

A large surface area-to-body weight, lack of insulating SC fat, and underdeveloped ability to shiver in response to cold make all infants susceptible to hypothermia. Infants with omphalocele and gastroschisis are more prone to hypothermia with their exposed bowel. The infant is at high risk of heat loss during transport to the OR and should be transported in a warmed incubator. To prevent intraoperative hypothermia, the operating ambient temperature should be warmed, the infant should be placed on a warming mattress or underbody forced-air warmed, all fluids both IV and surgical irrigation should be warmed, and the anesthetist should utilize heated and humidified inhaled gases.[73]

After birth, an infant with omphalocele or gastroschisis may require intubation and mechanical ventilation. Abdominal wall defects, especially large defects, may cause reduced chest capacities and pulmonary hypoplasia. Infants may also present with pulmonary hypertension and require mechanical ventilation and pulmonary vasodilators.[77] Lung protection ventilation strategies are typically employed.[73]

A nasogastric or orogastric tube should be placed after delivery and prior to repair to allow for intestine decompression.[70] Additional preoperative preparation should include a full set of labs and abdominal and chest x-rays. Infants with omphalocele may require more preoperative evaluation compared to gastroschisis because of the higher rate of associated anomalies with omphalocele. An echocardiogram should be performed to evaluate for presence of pulmonary hypertension or congenital heart defects. Up to 57% of infants with omphalocele may develop pulmonary hypertension after birth.[71] Pulmonary vasodilators may be indicated in patients found to have pulmonary hypertension.[77] A genetics consult may be warranted for chromosomal analysis especially if the infant displays dysmorphic features. A renal ultrasound may also be performed to look for kidney abnormalities.[71]

ANESTHETIC MANAGEMENT

Infants are at high risk of cardiovascular and respiratory decompensation on induction and should be fully monitored. If the infant is not yet intubated prior to arriving in the OR, a rapid sequence intubation will need to be performed to minimize the risk of aspiration. Prior to induction, the infant's nasogastric or orogastric tube should be placed on suction to allow continued bowel decompression. Infants are prone to rapid desaturation on induction due to reduced functional residual capacity (FRC) and high metabolic rate, therefore the infant should be preoxygenated for at least 60 seconds.[73] After induction, additional vascular access may need to be obtained, including intravascular and arterial access.

The infant's hemodynamic status will guide appropriate anesthetic management, but the infant can typically be maintained on a low concentration of sevoflurane, air, oxygen, and muscle relaxation. To prevent bowel distention, nitrous oxide should be avoided. If postoperative mechanical ventilation is planned, IV fentanyl or morphine can be administered. In the presence of hemodynamic stability, analgesia can also be maintained with a single-shot caudal block. Maintenance fluids containing dextrose and sodium chloride will be continued intraoperatively. Surgical exposure of the bowel increases third-space and evaporative losses intraoperatively and administration of 10 to 20 mL/kg of crystalloid and colloid may be warranted. Blood loss should be monitored closely with administration of blood products as indicated.[70]

The repair and closure of the abdominal wall defects depend on size of defect and abdominal cavity and the infant's ability to tolerate return of the herniated viscera to the abdominal cavity. Options for repair and closure include a primary (single stage) repair, a staged repair, or a silo placement with delayed closure. A primary repair can usually be performed in defects that are smaller than 5 cm and do not contain liver. During a primary repair, the intestine will be completely reduced and returned to the abdominal cavity with fascial closure. Infants with defects greater than 5 cm, a herniated liver, an abdominal cavity that is too small to accommodate the viscera, or those with severe pulmonary hypoplasia or pulmonary hypertension will typically undergo a staged repair or silo placement with delayed closure. With a staged repair, the infant will return to the OR multiple times to slowly reduce the herniated viscera return to the abdomen allowing the infant's abdominal cavity time to enlarge and accommodate for the reduced viscera. During a staged repair, the defect may be covered with a synthetic or biological mesh bridge for protection, or a silo may also be utilized.[71]

A silo made of silastic or Teflon coating can be placed in the NICU or the OR as either a primary technique for reduction of viscera to the abdominal cavity or in conjunction with a staged surgical closure. A silo utilizes gravity to aid in the gradual reduction of the herniated viscera to the abdominal cavity. The silo is placed over the entire herniated defect, sutured to the infant's skin of fascia, elevated above the abdomen, and undergoes tightening and reduction every 12 to 24 hours for up to 10 days.[70] Upon reduction of all herniated viscera, the infant will undergo surgical closure of the fascia and skin in the OR. Silo reduction in the NICU can be performed on both awake and sedated neonates.[71,76]

The major concern during any reduction of herniated viscera to the abdominal cavity is increased intra-abdominal pressure that can potentially lead to abdominal compartment syndrome, difficulty, or inability to ventilate the patient, impaired organ perfusion, and altered hemodynamics. Intragastric pressure should be measured and monitored during repair and closure. An intragastric pressure greater than 20 mm Hg is typically a contraindication to abdominal closure.[78] During the abdominal repair, bladder pressure can be transduced through a foley catheter to assess for potential abdominal compartment syndrome. Abdominal compartment syndrome is a potentially life-threatening situation effecting ability to ventilate, perfusion to vital organs and lower extremities, and possible mesenteric ischemia. Abdominal compartment syndrome requires immediate surgical intervention to open the abdomen.[70]

Intraoperatively, it is imperative that anesthesia providers monitor for respiratory compromise caused by increased intra-abdominal pressure and elevation of the diaphragm. Impending respiratory compromise can be signified by a significant increase in peak airway pressure, reduced tidal volume, or desaturation. Indicators of respiratory compromise will delay abdominal reduction and closure until the abdominal cavity is able to accommodate the viscera. After reduction and repair, the majority of infants will require mechanical ventilation therefore returning to the NICU intubated, sedated, and paralyzed. Additionally, the infant requires postoperative monitoring for increased intra-abdominal pressure and subsequent effects.[70]

Increased intra-abdominal pressure can reduce cardiac output, cause hypotension with impaired organ perfusion, and potential cardiovascular collapse. Yaster et al.[78] discussed a study that reported a 20% cardiac output reduction and a 20% to 40% reduction in gastrointestinal and renal blood flow when intra-abdominal pressures exceeded 15 to 20 mm Hg. Poor capillary refill, cool extremities, and administration of inotropic medications may signify impending cardiovascular collapse. Patients with an intragastric pressure greater than 20 mm Hg may demonstrate a significant increase in central venous pressure (CVP), oliguria, or anuria.[78]

Survival rates of omphalocele and gastroschisis are approximately 90%. Survival depends on severity and complexity of the abdominal wall defect and associated anomalies.[72]

ANESTHETIC TECHNIQUE: GASTROSCHISIS AND OMPHALOCELE ANESTHETIC MANAGEMENT

Preoperative Management

- Protection of the herniated viscera
- Assessment of fluid and electrolyte status with resuscitation as indicated
- Temperature regulation and active warming
- Respiratory support as indicated
- Naso- or orogastric tube for bowel decompression
- Evaluation of labs, chest x-ray, and echocardiogram (if indicated)
- Assessment for additional anomalies

Intraoperative Management

- Rapid sequence intubation for airway securement
- Establishment of adequate vascular access including peripheral IV and an arterial line
- Fluid resuscitation for large third-space and evaporative losses
- Vigilant monitoring of increased intra-abdominal pressure and potential subsequent effects of abdominal compartment syndrome, difficult ventilation/ high peak pressures, impaired organ perfusion, and altered hemodynamics

Postoperative Management

- Depending on the size of the defect, surgical repair, and hemodynamics, the infant may stay and require continued mechanical ventilation with paralysis and sedation
- Continued monitoring for increased intra-abdominal pressure

NECROTIZING ENTEROCOLITIS

PATHOPHYSIOLOGY AND CLINICAL MANIFESTATIONS

Necrotizing enterocolitis (NEC) is a life-threatening intestinal condition that primarily affects premature and low birth weight infants leading to infant morbidity and mortality. The pathogenesis of NEC is believed to be multifactorial but not clearly defined. Severe NEC causes ischemia of the intestine and increased mucosal permeability leading to eventual development of a systemic inflammatory response and sepsis.[79]

The primary risk factors for NEC are prematurity and low birth weight. There is an inverse relationship between onset of NEC and gestational age. NEC will typically present around the fourth week of life in premature infants after the initiation of enteral feedings. In comparison, full-term or near full-term infants will develop symptoms of NEC during the first week of life in the absence of enteral feedings. Infants who are full-term with a normal birth rate only represent about 10% of the total reported NEC cases and typically have lower mortality rates. An inverse relationship also exists between birth weight and risk of developing NEC. Infants with birth weights of less than 1,000 to 1,500 grams have higher risk of developing NEC.[80] Another risk factor of developing NEC is congenital heart disease. Full-term infants diagnosed with a congenital heart disease have a higher risk for the development NEC related to impaired intestinal blood flow after feeding and administration of vasoactive medications.[81]

The pathogenesis of NEC is unclear and believed to be multifactorial, with contributing factors of immature intestinal barrier, alteration of bacterial colonization, and formula feedings. Although infant formula contains a similar caloric and nutrient supply similar to human milk, the infant formula lacks the ability to promote immune function, mucosal integrity, and intestinal tract function and may impair bacterial growth due to a higher intestinal pH. Formula feeding is also associated with increased intestinal stasis and increased intestinal permeability.[79,81]

Clinical presentation of NEC ranges on a spectrum of severity. Gastrointestinal presentation of NEC includes abdominal distension, abdominal tenderness, feeding intolerance, emesis, high gastric residuals, and blood stools. Other symptoms include lethargy, temperature instability, apnea, hypotension, and bradycardia. NEC may initially be misdiagnosed as sepsis.[80] Progression of the disease may present abdominal wall edema, erythema, or discoloration, crepitus, and/or a palpable abdominal mass.[80,81]

Abdominal radiographs are the standard for NEC diagnosis and utilized to evaluate the need for surgical intervention. Pneumatosis intestinalis or pneumoperitoneum is the hallmark finding of NEC. Portal venous gas, bowel wall thickening, and fixed bowel loops may also be present on radiographs. Serial abdominal x-rays are obtained every 6 to 12 hours to follow the progression of the disease. Patients with NEC may also experience altered laboratory values including thrombocytopenia, neutropenia, increased leukocyte, hyponatremia, metabolic acidosis, and increased lactate. Labs are obtained every 12 to 24 hours.[81]

Traditionally, NEC was diagnosed and staged based on Bell's Criteria for the Diagnosis of Necrotizing Enterocolitis. Bell's criteria, developed in 1970s, took into consideration systemic, radiographic, and abdominal signs for the diagnosis and staging of NEC. Knell et al.[81] report that the utilization of Bell's criteria leads to overdiagnosis of NEC and has fallen out of favor.

SPECIAL CONSIDERATIONS AND CONCERNS

After diagnosis of NEC, the majority of infants undergo medical management prior to surgical intervention. It is reported that mortality rates are lower for medically managed NEC, 21%, compared to 35% mortality rates in surgically managed NEC.[79] NEC medical management includes bowel rest, holding enteral feedings, placement of a nasogastric or orogastric tube for gastric decompression, placement of central IV access, typically a peripherally inserted central catheter (PICC), the administration of broad-spectrum antibiotics, and parenteral nutrition. Administration of large amount of IV fluids may be indicated for fluid resuscitation because infants with NEC experience high third-space losses due to systemic inflammatory responses. Vasopressors and blood products will be administered as indicated. Insertion of an endotracheal tube with mechanical ventilation may be necessary due to the combination of premature lungs and abdominal distension leading to limited pulmonary reserve and function.[80] NEC can lead to rapid decompensation therefore providers will frequently monitor the clinical status of the infant, including physical examination, lab values, abdominal radiographs, and other indicated tests to monitor for signs of decompensation.[81] The duration of medical management is dependent on clinical status of the patient or indication for surgical intervention.

It is estimated that one third to one half of infants who develop NEC will require surgical intervention.[80] The two main surgical indications include pneumoperitoneum indicating an intestinal perforation or clinical deterioration after maximal therapy. Surgical options include a peritoneal drain and an exploratory laparotomy. Peritoneal drains may be placed at the bedside and utilized as a temporary treatment measure for infants who are unstable to undergo an exploratory laparotomy as a primary treatment. The goal of the drain is to reduce contamination and create a controlled fistula to drain gas, pus, and fecal contents from the abdomen. A small incision is made in the right upper quadrant of the abdomen. Typically, the abdomen is irrigated with saline until it is cleared, and then a Penrose drain is inserted through the incision.[79,81]

An exploratory laparotomy via a supraumbilical incision allows for assessment of the bowel for necrosis or perforation, management of abdominal contamination, and resection of necrotic or injured bowel as necessary. Some patients may require creation of a stoma A silo may be placed if the patient required a return trip to the OR for a second look. During surgical intervention, some infants may be found to have the most severe form of NEC, NEC totalis, which has high morbidity and mortality rates as almost the entire intestine is necrotic with no viable intervention option available.[80]

There are a variety of anesthetic considerations for infants undergoing an exploratory laparotomy for NEC. First, it is important to identify the infant's overall physiological development, especially if they are premature, as they may have immature development. Premature infants may exhibit immature lungs with limited pulmonary reserve. Lung function may be further inhibited by abdominal distention decreasing functional residual capacity and impeding adequate ventilation. Decompression of the stomach should be utilized before and during the intraoperative period. Infants with NEC may exhibit altered laboratory values, such as acidosis and coagulopathies, temperature instability, and hemodynamic instability requiring vasopressors. Dopamine is the vasopressor of choice as it can improve intestinal perfusion. Fluid management during the intraoperative period may be challenging due to third-space losses and bleeding.[81]

The mortality rates of infants with NEC can be as high as 40%. Those infants who survive will go on to face lifelong challenges due to the multisystem organ effect of NEC 50% to 70% of infants who require surgical intervention experience postoperative complications, including wound dehiscence, strictures, infections, compartment syndrome, stoma complications, and short gut syndrome.[80,81] NEC is the leading cause of short gut syndrome in children. Short gut syndrome occurs when the bowel remaining after surgical resection is too short or too damaged, causing malabsorption and inability to meet the patient's caloric demand. Patients with short gut syndrome experience high stool loss, acidosis, and dehydration.[79,80] The nutritional deficiencies these infants experience may lead to growth delays. Additionally, patients may experience motor and cognitive delays.[80]

ANESTHETIC MANAGEMENT

ANESTHETIC TECHNIQUE: NECROTIZING ENTEROCOLITIS ANESTHETIC MANAGEMENT

Preoperative Management

- Evaluation of serial abdominal x-rays every 6 to 12 hours to monitor progression of disease
- Assessment of electrolytes and fluid status with resuscitation as indicated
- Naso- or orogastric tube for bowel decompression

- Placement of endotracheal tube with mechanical ventilation as indicated
- Placement of central IV access as indicated
- Administration of vasopressors and antibiotics as indicated

Intraoperative Management

- Placement of endotracheal tube with a rapid-sequence induction (RSI) if not placed prior to arrival
- Establishment of adequate vascular access—peripheral and central venous access and arterial line
- Naso- or orogastric tube for bowel decompression
- Monitoring and management of altered laboratory values, such as acidosis and coagulopathies
- Close temperature monitoring and active warming
- Administration of vasopressors as indicated (dopamine vasopressor of choice) to maintain hemodynamic stability

Postoperative Management

- Depending on stability and hemodynamics of the infant, they may return to the NICU requiring mechanical ventilation, paralysis, and sedation

HYPERTROPHIC PYLORIC STENOSIS

PATHOPHYSIOLOGY AND CLINICAL MANIFESTATIONS

Hypertrophic pyloric stenosis (HPS) is a medical condition that often necessitates infants undergoing surgery within the first few months of life.[82] Pyloric stenosis develops as the pyloric muscle progressively hypertrophies until gastric outlet obstruction occurs. Infants with HPS typically present between 2 and 12 weeks of life with a history of progressive non-bilious projectile vomiting.[83] Recurrent vomiting and dehydration will cause a hypochloremic, hypokalemic metabolic alkalosis necessitating adequate fluid and electrolyte resuscitation. Pyloric stenosis is a medical emergency that requires fluid and electrolyte correction and stabilization prior to surgical intervention.[84]

Pyloric stenosis is reported to occur in 2 to 5 per 1,000 live births, affecting males four times as often as females.[84] HPS is reported to have strong familial tendencies even with distant relatives, although the incidence among African and Asian infants is considerably lower. There is no definitive etiology of pyloric stenosis, but it is believed that it may be multifactorial with both genetic and environmental factors. It has been suggested that the nitric oxide pathway may play a role in the development of HPS. A deficiency of nitric oxide synthase, which is responsible for pyloric sphincter relaxation, may cause pylorospasm and eventually pyloric muscle hypertrophy.[83] Both maternal and infant risk factors have been suggested in the development of HPS. Maternal risk factors include young maternal age, smoking, hyperthyroidism, use of quinolone antibiotics and intranasal decongestants, and high prepregnancy body mass index. Infant risk factors include bottle-feeding, erythromycin and azithromycin use in the first 2 weeks of life, and pesticide exposure, with infants who bottle-feed being 4.6 times more likely to develop pyloric stenosis compared to breastfed infants.[83]

Diagnosis of HPS is made with presentation of recurrent projectile vomiting and hypochloremic, hypokalemic metabolic alkalosis. Additional clinical presentation may include dehydration, lethargy, poor feeding, and weight loss.[84] Although the infant is experiencing projectile vomiting after feeding, they may appear hungry or want to feed again shortly after vomiting.[85] On physical examination, the child may appear dehydrated, and the hypertrophied pyloric muscle is often readily palpated, frequently being described as an "olive" mass in the abdomen. Palpation of the "olive" is considered diagnostic with a 99% positive predictive value. Ultrasound allows for earlier diagnosis and treatment of HPS and can be performed by both surgeons and emergency medicine physicians. The diagnosis of HPS on ultrasound will be made when the pyloric muscle thickness, length, and diameter are greater than normal values.[85]

SPECIAL CONSIDERATIONS AND CONCERNS

Prior to surgical intervention, it is imperative that the infant undergo adequate fluid and electrolyte resuscitation. Recurrent vomiting results in dehydration with depletion of chloride, potassium, sodium, and hydrogen ions, hence the presentation of hypochloremic, hypokalemic metabolic alkalosis.[83] Late identification or inappropriate resuscitation of fluid and electrolytes status in infants with HPS can have a detrimental effect on perfusion and lead to an acidosis.[85] Fluid and electrolyte resuscitation will be based on the patient's individualized presentation and laboratory values. Craig et al.[86] reported that the optimal laboratory values for surgical intervention are pH 7.3 to 7.45; Cl- 95 to 112 mmol/L; base excess −4 to 2.5 mmol/L; and K+ 3.5 to 5.5 mmol/L. It has been suggested that patients should be maintained on a continuous infusion of 5% dextrose in 0.45% saline with or without potassium at 1.5 times calculated maintenance rate.[82] Additionally, the administration of a 20 mL/kg sodium chloride bolus with a subsequent recheck in laboratory values is warranted. Anesthesia providers should be aware that additional 20 mL/kg sodium chloride boluses may be indicated based on patient status and chloride and bicarbonate levels. It is recommended that a 60-minute break should occur between the administration of every bolus.[86]

An alternate fluid resuscitation plan entails the administration of 150 mL/kg/day of 0.45% or 0.9% sodium chloride with 5% dextrose and 10 to 20 mmol/L of potassium chloride.[83] Once HCO_3^- values <25 mmol/L, the maintenance rate can be decreased to 100 mL/kg/day. Additional 10 to 20 mL/kg boluses of 0.9% sodium chloride can be administered as indicated. In the majority of infants with HPS, the fluid and electrolyte correction can be completed within 24 hours and the infant will be prepared for surgery.[83] Electrolyte abnormalities on initial presentation are predictive of longer hospital length of stay in infants, more fluid resuscitation, and increased frequency of labs with HPS.[82]

Once the patient has been adequately fluid resuscitated with electrolyte replace, the patient will be taken to the OR for a pyloromyotomy, which can be performed, open or laparoscopic. A pyloromyotomy can be performed via an open or laparoscopic approach to divide the avascular portion of the hypertrophic pyloric muscle.[84] Traditionally, an open approach was utilized via an incision in the right upper quadrant, but eventually to minimize scarring, the incision was transitioned to a circumumbilical skin crease incision.[87] In the early 1990s, a laparoscopic technique was introduced that included insertion of a laparoscope in the umbilicus with a stab incision of the hypoepigastrium. Electrocautery or an arthrotomy knife was utilized to perform the pyloromyotomy. Depending on surgeon preference, both the open and laparoscopic techniques are employed in today's practice.[83] Administration of antibiotics is a debated topic and may depend on center or surgeon preference.[87] After pyloric muscle division, but prior to closure, the surgeon may request the anesthesia provider to fill the abdomen with air. This is done for two reasons, first to ensure there is no leak at the myotomy site and second to demonstrate air movement into the duodenum. Surgical postoperative complications from a pyloromyotomy are reported to occur in 4.6% to 12% of patients and include an incomplete pyloromyotomy, mucosal perforation, wound infection, and persistent nonbilious vomiting.[83]

ANESTHETIC MANAGEMENT

Although infants presenting of a pyloromyotomy are NPO appropriate, they remain at high risk of pulmonary aspiration during anesthesia induction due to their gastric outlet obstruction and potential large gastric residual. Infants may or may not arrive to the OR with a nasogastric tube in place. Placement of a nasogastric tube prior to arrival in the OR remains controversial and may vary depending on institution.[83] Regardless of nasogastric tube placement prior to arrival in the OR, the infant should undergo gastric suctioning, via a multiorifice nasogastric or orogastric tube, prior to induction of anesthesia, to aspirate as much gastric contents as possible and reduce the risk of aspiration. Even after gastric suctioning prior to induction of anesthesia the infant remains a high risk for aspiration as gastric fluid residual volumes can remain up to 4.8 mL/kg.[87] Ultrasound assessment of gastric contents in infants with pyloric stenosis can be useful in estimating gastric content volume.[88] Gastric suctioning is performed on an awake infant with typically a 14 French multiorifice suction catheter in various positions, including supine, left lateral, and right lateral, to maximize removal of gastric contents.[86] Awake gastric suctioning can prove to be very stressful to the infant and an anticholinergic may be administered prior to the start of suctioning.

Following gastric suctioning, an RSI is routinely performed to secure the airway and minimize risk of aspiration. RSIs can prove to be challenging in infants as they are known to have a limited oxygen reserve, leading to rapid desaturation, bradycardia, and potential cardiac arrest.[89] Adequate preoxygenation prior to the RSI is imperative as it is reported that in infants 1 month of age, desaturation can occur within 6.6 seconds of apnea with inadequate preoxygenation.[84] To decrease the risk of desaturation, providers may opt to perform a modified RSI providing ventilation utilizing pressure no greater than 10 to 12 cmH$_2$O. The majority of infants presenting for a pyloromyotomy will be induced with propofol and either succinylcholine or rocuronium. Although succinylcholine is associated with a quicker onset and shorter duration of action, it is associated with possible bradycardia and acute rhabdomyolysis, which could cause hyperkalemia, ventricular dysrhythmias, and cardiac arrest in children with myopathies yet to be diagnosed. Rocuronium has longer duration of action, which may outlast the pyloromyotomy, which has 29-minute mean duration of surgery time, but the availability of sugammadex allows for prompt reversal of nondepolarizing neuromuscular blocking agents.[84] The anesthetic is primarily maintained with sevoflurane.[83] Infants should be extubated fully awake after demonstration of adequate ventilation.[86]

A major anesthetic concern of a pyloromyotomy is postoperative apnea caused by the metabolic alkalosis. The primary function of the central chemoreceptors is to regulate respiratory activity and is influenced by concentrations and changes in hydrogen ions in cerebrospinal fluid (CSF). Although systemic metabolic alkalosis is corrected preoperatively, alkalosis may persist in CSF postoperatively as equilibration of pH between plasma and CSF takes multiple hours.[86] The administration of opioids for analgesic control increases the risk of postoperative apnea in an infant following a pyloromyotomy. Administration of nonopioids, such as acetaminophen alone, has proved to be successful in postoperative pain control following a pyloromyotomy without the risk of increased respiratory depression.[90] Acetaminophen has a proven safe profile in infants and can be administered orally postoperatively, IV, or rectally. The systemic absorption of rectal acetaminophen has proven to be unpredictable; therefore, the initial dose of rectal acetaminophen requires a higher dose at 40 mg/kg to achieve the desired plasma levels. In addition to the administration of acetaminophen, surgeon infiltration of local anesthesia at the surgical site or use of regional anesthesia, such as a caudal block, can reduce or eliminate the need for opioid administration.[91] Following a pyloromyotomy, an infant should be placed on apnea and pulse oximetry monitoring for at least 12 hours.[86]

ANESTHETIC TECHNIQUE: HYPERTROPHIC PYLORIC STENOSIS ANESTHETIC MANAGEMENT

Preoperative Management

- Correction of acid–base and electrolyte disturbances
- Fluid resuscitation as indicated

Intraoperative Management

- Gastric suctioning in supine, left lateral, and right lateral positions in the awake infant prior to induction
- Adequate preoxygenation with an RSI
- Avoidance of narcotic administration for analgesia to prevent postoperative apnea. Administration of nonopioids, such as acetaminophen, for pain control
- Awake extubation at the end of the procedure

Postoperative Management

- Avoidance of narcotic administration
- Apnea and pulse oximetry monitoring for at least 12 hours following surgery

BILIARY ATRESIA

PATHOPHYSIOLOGY AND CLINICAL MANIFESTATIONS

Biliary atresia (BA) is a rare but severe disease of the intrahepatic and extrahepatic biliary tree causing inflammation and fibrosis with consequential cholestasis and eventual hepatic damage.[92] If BA is left untreated, it will progress to cirrhosis and end-stage liver failure resulting in death within the first 2 years of life. BA has proved to be the most common cause of liver transplantation in children, representing 45% of liver transplants in children.[93]

There is a wide range of BA incidence from 1:5,000 to 1:19,000 live births. The incidence of BA has proven to be geographical with higher BA incidences reported in Asian and African populations, with lower incidences reported in Europe and North America.[94] The incidence of BA in the United States is reported to be 4.5 cases per 100,000 children.[93] BA is more likely to occur in female infants compared to male infants.[92]

The pathogenesis and etiology of BA are unknown but are believed to be multifactorial. It has been suggested that contributing factors to BA may be infectious viruses, toxins, immune, or genetic.[93] Cholangiopathies can be caused by viruses of the liver and hepatobiliary tree, including reovirus, rotavirus and cytomegalovirus (CMV). It has been reported that at the time of diagnosis that 60% of BA patients had CMV DNA.[94] Although BA may have a genetic component, it is rare to see a report of familial BA cases even with identical twins.[92]

A diagnosis of BA may not occur immediately after birth, as physiological jaundice is a common finding in many neonates. If jaundice persists after 14 days in full-term infants or 21 days in premature infants, the child should undergo further testing to determine if BA is present. In addition to jaundice, clinical presentation includes pale stool that can range from white to beige, dark urine from the excretion of water-soluble bilirubin conjugates, coagulopathy, and failure to thrive. Late clinical finding of BA includes ascites and hepatosplenomegaly.[95] Early identification and diagnosis of BA is imperative to improve outcomes with immediate intervention. Diagnosis of BA may not be made until 6 to 12 weeks of life after other causes of cholestasis have been ruled out. Diagnosis is typically made with a percutaneous liver biopsy.[92]

SPECIAL CONSIDERATIONS AND CONCERNS

Shortly after diagnosis of BA the infant should undergo the Kasai hepatic portoenterostomy (HPE) to restore bile flow and drainage. HPE is a palliative surgical treatment that has the potential to preserve the native liver and delay or prevent the need for liver transplantation. This is achieved with the removals of the extrahepatic biliary system and replacing it with a Roux-en-Y jejunal anastomosis that is directly connected to the portal section of the liver. HPE is typically performed in an open laparotomy fashion, but some sites are now utilizing a laparoscopic approach. The age at which the infant undergoes an HPE determines the success of the procedure. Earlier BA intervention with an HPE is believed to lead to more successful and optimal outcomes, with HPE intervention occurring prior to 45 to 60 days of life for best results. A successful HPE is determined by clearance of jaundice with native liver survival. Sundaram et al.[96] discussed that if jaundice is cleared within 3 months of HPE, there is a 75% to 90% 10-year transplant free survival rate. Comparatively, there is only a 20% 3-year survival transplant-free rate in children who are not cleared of jaundice following an HPE. Evaluation for liver transplants should occur in infants with persistent bile flow obstruction and jaundice 3 months after HPE with the goal of transplant by 6 to 9 months of age.[96] Bezerra et al.[92] report that at least 50% of patients who have undergone HPE will require a liver transplant by the age of 2 years and older and 75% who have had successful palliation following HPE will require a liver transplant before 20 years of age. Once placed on the transplant wait list, infants with BA typically have a wait time of 90 days in the United States. To reduce wait time and potential mortality, living donor transplants are also an option.[96]

ANESTHETIC MANAGEMENT

Children undergoing an HPE will require a general anesthetic with an endotracheal tube. Vascular access typically includes two peripheral IV catheters, although the infant may already have a PICC placed. Arterial lines may be warranted if indicated by hemodynamic instability or need for frequent laboratory monitoring. Medications undergoing biliary excretion should be avoided. Pain control can be provided through administration of IV opioid or insertion of an epidural catheter. Phelps et al.[97] compared epidural analgesic to no epidural with opioid analgesics in infants undergoing HPE and found that those infants with epidural analgesic had lower requirement for opioids in the first 96 hours following the HPE. Additionally, those infants with epidurals for an HPE were more likely to be extubated in the OR than those who received only opioids.[97] Extubation of the infant is the goal at the end of the Kasai procedure.

Following an HPE and preservation of the native liver, many children will experience issues with poor growth, developmental delay, biliary cirrhosis, portal hypertension, and cardiomyopathy. Poor growth occurs in children with chronic liver disease due to deficiencies of fat-soluble vitamins, fat malabsorption, and increased metabolic rate. BA patients have a 29% greater energy expenditure compared to healthy children. The majority of patients with BA have some degree of portal hypertension. Patients with portal hypertension may exhibit ascites, esophageal and gastrointestinal varices, and splenomegaly, increasing morbidity and mortality. Approximately 90% of children with varices will require an endoscopic intervention and about 30% will experience an episode of variceal bleeding. Children with varices may require band ligation, sclerotherapy, and/or blood transfusions. Infants with BA may develop cardiomyopathy with findings of left ventricle and septum hypertrophy, impaired left ventricle relaxation during diastole, hyperdynamic left ventricle contraction, prolonged QTc, and reduction in cardiac response to stressors. A study discussed by Kilgore and Mack[94] reported that 70% of BA patients younger than the age of 2 years had abnormal echocardiogram findings including increased left ventricle wall thickness and increased left ventricular mass, and 30% of patients had abnormalities in structure in function.

DUODENAL ATRESIA

PATHOPHYSIOLOGY AND CLINICAL MANIFESTATIONS

Duodenal atresia is a congenital condition characterized by duodenal obstruction presenting with bilious or nonbilious vomiting within the first 24 to 48 hours of life, characteristically, after the first feeding. It is one of the most common cases of fetal bowel obstruction and is associated with polyhydramnios. The incidence of duodenal obstruction ranges from 0.5 to 2 per 10,000 live births and is often associated with other congenital anomalies, such as cystic fibrosis, Down syndrome, and midline defects, such as esophageal atresia and imperforate anus.[98] Duodenal atresia is an obstruction of the duodenum, generally distal to the ampulla of Vater in the second portion of the duodenum. Errors in duodenal recanalization during the 8th to 10th week of embryological life are the main cause of duodenal atresia. However, the exact cause of this altered recanalization is unknown.[99]

Patients characteristically present with projectile-like vomiting after the first oral feeding and may simulate HPS. Bilious vomiting usually differentiates duodenal atresia from pyloric stenosis, although in some cases, the duodenal stenosis may be proximal to the ampulla of Vater and nonbilious vomiting may be present.

Diagnosis may occur via prenatal ultrasound with the characteristic "double bubble" sign in which the sonographer will see the normal fluid-distended stomach followed by a smaller but enlarged "second bubble" that is the obstructed part of the duodenum. Neonatal diagnosis may be either via ultrasound or plain abdominal radiograph. In cases in which doubt remains, barium contrast may be administered via naso- or orogastric tube. A small amount of barium is placed to confirm obstruction and then suctioned to prevent aspiration. This study is useful to differentiate duodenal atresia from midgut volvulus since the latter requires emergent surgery.[100]

SPECIAL CONSIDERATIONS AND CONCERNS

Treatment of duodenal atresia involves gastric decompression via nasogastric suction and surgery to correct the obstruction. Duodenoduodenostomy is the procedure of choice and may be performed either by open or laparoscopic approach, although laparoscopic duodenoduodenostomy may be technically challenging. Possible complications of this bypass include impaired duodenal motility, megaduodenum, and gastric reflux.[101]

ANESTHETIC MANAGEMENT

Anesthetic considerations are similar to that of patients presenting with bowel obstructions of other etiologies. These include airway management of a full stomach, assessment of fluid status, cardiorespiratory evaluation, and treatment of possible sepsis. Gastric contents are often incompletely emptied by NG or orogastric tube suction, and the risk of aspiration is significant, particularly during induction. Marked abdominal distension may interfere with ventilation through impaired diaphragmatic excursion. Endotracheal intubation of infants with normal airway may be accomplished with an RSI.

Intraoperative considerations are similar to those of NEC and intestinal obstruction with special emphasis placed on adequate fluid management. Monitoring heart rate, blood pressure, and urine output is a basic requirement to evaluate fluid status and needs. Invasive monitoring, including central access and arterial cannulation, is reserved for patients with significant cardiorespiratory instability.[102]

Postoperatively, patients usually require continued NG drainage and may require total parenteral nutrition. Oral feeds are usually started in low amounts once output through the NG tube has stopped or decreased significantly.

ANESTHETIC TECHNIQUE: DUODENAL ATRESIA ANESTHETIC MANAGEMENT

Preoperative Management

- Evaluation of the degree of bowel obstruction
- Assessment of the fluid and electrolyte status

Intraoperative Management

- Airway RSI
- Balanced anesthesia with low-dose inhalational agent supplemented with opioid
- Neuromuscular blocking agent
- Close temperature monitoring and active warming
- Central venous access and arterial cannulation reserved for patients with cardiorespiratory instability

Postoperative Management

- Extubation depends on associated underlying anomalies and hemodynamic instability
- Patients may require total parenteral alimentation, broad-spectrum antibiotics for sepsis, and/or cardiovascular support
- Consider opioid-sparing analgesic techniques (regional anesthesia) for postoperative pain

KEY REFERENCES

Complete references for this chapter are online and available at https://connect.springerpub.com/content/book/978-0-8261-3875-0/part/part01/toc-part/ch127.

74. Khan FA, Hashmi A, Islam S. Insights into embryology and development of omphalocele. *Semin Pediatr Surg.* 2019;28(2):80–83. doi:10.1053/j.sempedsurg.2019.04.003

75. Gonzalez KW, Chandler NM. Ruptured omphalocele: diagnosis and management. *Semin Pediatr Surg.* 2019;28(2):101–105. doi:10/1053/j.sempedsurg.2019.04.009

77. Duggan E, Puligandla PS. Respiratory disorders in patients with omphalocele. *Semin Pediatr Surg.* 2019;28(2):115–117. doi:10.1053/j.sempedsurg.2019.04.008

81. Knell J, Han SM, Jaksic T, Modi BP. Current status of necrotizing enterocolitis. *Curr Probl Surg.* 2019;56(1):11–38. doi:10.1067/j.cpsurg.2018.11.005

84. Swenker D, van der Kniff-van Dortmont A, Candel AG, et al. Neuromuscular blocking agents and rapid sequence induction for laparoscopic pyloromyotomy: impact on time to extubation and perioperative complications. *Euro J Pediatr Surg.* 2019;30(5):440–446. doi:10.1055/s-0039-1692656

90. Mclaughlin C, Squillaro AI, Ourshaliman S, et al. The association between opioids use and outcomes in infants undergoing pyloromyotomy. *Clin Ther.* 2019;41(9):1690–1700. doi:10.1016/j.clinthera.2019.07.002

97. Phelps HM, Robinson JR, Chen H, et al. Enhancing recovery after Kasai portoenterostomy with epidural anaglesia. *J Surg Res.* 2019;243:354–362. doi:10.1016/j.jss.2019.05.059

CHAPTER 128

Trauma

Timothy P. Grannell and Kelly Moon

> **LEARNING OBJECTIVES**
> - Understand the ways in which pediatric trauma patients present differently in comparison to adult trauma patients.
> - Recall details related to the anesthetic management of abdominal, thoracic, neurological, and burn trauma in pediatric patients.

INTRODUCTION

Trauma is defined as an injury to living tissue cause by an extrinsic agent. As trauma is often preventable and frequently predictable, it is subject to the same epidemiology as any disease that affects all age groups. Unfortunately, in the pediatric population, traumatic injuries remain a major cause of death. It has been reported that in recent years, more than 11,000 children and adolescents 0 to 18 years of age die of unintentional and intentional injuries (Centers for Disease Control and Prevention).

When caring for trauma victims, anesthesia providers must consider that children have unique age-related cardiovascular and pulmonary considerations when compared to adults. An understanding of these differences is essential to delivering safe, effective anesthetic care. Globally, there are physiological differences between adults and children, such as higher metabolic rates, decreased functional residual capacity (FRC), and a larger body surface area (BSA), that impact the pharmacokinetics and pharmacodynamics of many medications delivered during an anesthetic. These physiological variations have the potential to predispose children to such untoward events as hypoxemia, hypotension, and hypothermia. In addition, children's cardiac output is dependent on heart rate. For additional information regarding age-related physiological differences, please refer to Chapter 1, "Anatomy and Physiology of the Pediatric Patient."

TRAUMA MANAGEMENT

ASSESSMENT OF SHOCK

Following traumatic injury, shock often ensues. Shock is defined as a physiological state characterized by inadequate tissue perfusion, which results in decreased tissue oxygenation and decreased ability to meet metabolic demands. According to the Pediatric Advance Life Support (PALS) course, shock can be broken down into three stages. Shock can be classified as compensated, hypotensive (decompensated), or irreversible. Determining the state of shock is essential as it guides further management.

In compensated shock, the body's hemostatic mechanisms can compensate for diminished perfusion, and systolic blood pressure (SBP) is maintained within normal range for age. Commonly, the clinical presentation in this state is comprised of tachycardia, delayed capillary refill, and decreased urine output. In hypotensive or decompensated shock, the body's compensatory mechanisms are overwhelmed. Hypotension is late finding in most types of shock and may signal impending cardiac arrest. Although children typically maintain normal SBP even in the face of losing as much as 30% to 35% of their circulating blood volume, once hypotension develops, the child's condition can deteriorate rapidly. Irreversible shock occurs when progressive end-organ dysfunction leads to irreversible organ damage and death. In this state, tachycardia may change to bradycardia and the SBP decreases significantly.

Hypovolemia due to blood loss is the most common cause of shock in pediatric trauma. Unfortunately, the progression of shock is unpredictable. Therefore, it is imperative that the signs and symptoms of the various stages of shock are recognized early and followed by rapid intervention. It may take hours for compensated shock to progress to hypotensive shock but only minutes for hypotensive shock to progress to cardiac arrest.

FLUID MANAGEMENT

IV fluid resuscitation with isotonic fluid, such as lactated Ringer's or normal saline, should begin immediately. Prompt placement of reliable peripheral vascular access is key. The preferred venous access site during pediatric resuscitation is the largest and most accessible vein that does not require the interruption of resuscitation. Depending on the child's size, two large-bore peripheral IV catheters should be obtained. This can be difficult sometimes, especially in a critically ill infant or child. If peripheral IV access is not obtained promptly, IO access should be considered. IO cannulation is relatively simple and an effective way to administer emergency fluids to an unstable patient. IO access provides a noncollapsible venous access point through which any medication that can be given IV can be given. The main sites for IO placement are the proximal tibia, distal tibia, distal femur, and the anterior–superior iliac spine. Anesthesia providers should not place an IO cannula near fracture sites and/or previous IO attempts. In addition, be aware of patients with a history of fragile bones (e.g., osteogenesis imperfecta). In patients with compensated shock, a 20 mL/kg fluid bolus of warm isotonic crystalloid solutions should be administered. For adult-sized pediatric patients, 1 to 2 liters are commonly administered. The child's response during the initial fluid resuscitation should be used to make further therapeutic and diagnostic decision.

BLOOD TRANSFUSION

In children, a massive transfusion protocol (MTP) may be appropriate for patients who have profound hemorrhage or ongoing bleeding. However, the optimal volume trigger for initiating an MTP is unknown. Taking into consideration estimated circulating volumes, a weight-based approach that accounts for approximately half of a child's blood volume can be used to determine the transfusion volumes required once an MTP has been initiated (Tables 128.1 and 128.2).

Table 128.3 depicts Nationwide Children's Hospital (NCH) ongoing fluid resuscitation outline. NCH uses 40 mL/kg as the activation for point MTP.

Massive blood transfusions can result in hypocalcemia due to the chelation of calcium by the citrate preservative in packed red blood cells. As such, administration of calcium chloride 10 to 15 mg/kg centrally or calcium gluconate 30

Table 128.1	Estimated Circulating Blood Volumes
Neonate	85–90 mL/kg
Infant	75–80 mL/kg
Children	70–75 mL/kg
Adolescent/adult	65–70 mL/kg

mg/kg peripherally should be considered to correct potentially life-threatening hypocalcemia.

COGNITIVE AIDS

The initial management of a trauma patient, either adult or pediatric, should follow the standardized Advanced Trauma Life Support (ATLS) protocol (primary survey, resuscitation, and secondary survey) to ensure optimal patient outcomes. Early implementation of such cognitive aids has proven to optimize outcomes following trauma, especially when implemented during the "golden hour." The term *golden hour* refers to an early and critical period in the care of a trauma victim, during which evidence-based management has the potential to significantly increase patients' survival rate. A number of well-vetted pediatric-specific cognitive aids are readily available, many of which now have corresponding mobile apps to facilitate accessibility.

Table 128.2	Estimated Blood Transfusion Needs
<5 kg (neonate)	55 mL/kg
5–25 kg (infant)	50 mL/kg
25–50 kg (child)	45 mL/kg
>50 kg (adolescent)	40 mL/kg or 6 units of PRBCs

PRBCs, packed red blood cells.

ANESTHETIC MANAGEMENT
PREOPERATIVE EVALUATION

When possible, a thorough history and medical examination should be conducted prior to induction of anesthesia. At baseline, the pediatric population can present additional challenges as children may not be able to talk, they are overcome by fear, and/or they may have been separated from their families. Nonetheless, even in urgent situations, a brief history should be obtained when possible. The mnemonic AMPLE can be used to guide collection of key patient-related information (Box 128.1).

ANESTHETIC TECHNIQUE

Intraoperative Management
Induction of Anesthesia
A variety of medications can be used to safely induce anesthesia in trauma victims, with practices varying from facility to facility (Table 128.4). Ketamine has long been a staple when providing anesthesia to trauma victims as it will not decrease the systemic vascular resistance (SVR) to the same extent as other hypnotic agents. While propofol is routinely used to induce anesthesia, it has the potential to decrease the patient's SVR significantly. Therefore, it is prudent to use reduced doses of propofol (0.5–1 mg/kg) when caring for trauma victims or choose a different induction agent in hypotensive patients. Etomidate 0.1 to 0.2 mg/kg is considered a preferable induction agent in hypovolemic patients with a head injury as it provides hemodynamic stability while decreasing cerebral oxygen consumption. Neuromuscular relaxation sufficient to facilitate endotracheal intubation can be achieved in approximately 45 seconds with succinylcholine (1 mg/kg). Succinylcholine has long been considered the prototypical neuromuscular blocking agent to achieve swift intubating conditions. Its use, however, is contradicted in patients

Table 128.3	Nationwide Children's Hospital Fluid Resuscitation Outline
Patient is a "responder" (estimated <20% blood loss)	• Patient responds rapidly to the initial fluid bolus and remains hemodynamically stable upon completion of the initial bolus • No further bolus or immediate blood administration is indicated • There is currently no supported role for permissive hypotension in children after traumatic injuries

Patient is a transient responder (estimated 20%–40% blood loss)	• Patient responds to the initial fluid bolus but shows hemodynamic instability or signs of inadequate perfusion after the initial bolus is completed
	• Initiation of blood transfusion is indicated
	   ○ A maximum of 40 mL/kg warmed *isotonic* crystalloid may be given, including prehospital fluid
	   ○ If additional fluid resuscitation is required, warmed PRBCs should be administered (0–15 mL/kg/dose)
	   ○ Obtaining early thromboelastography is strongly recommended to guide further therapy

Minimal or no response (severe, >40% blood loss)	• Failure to respond to crystalloid and blood administration in the ED dictates the need for immediate operative intervention to control exsanguinating hemorrhage
	   ○ Refer to hospital policy number XI-45:16–MTP
	   ○ MTP should be activated after 40 mL/kg of PRBCs have been administered and there is presence of refractory hypotension and/or coagulopathy represented by INR >1.5 and platelets <50,000
	   ○ Early balanced blood product resuscitation with ratios 1:1:1 (PRBC, FFP and platelets) is strongly recommended

FFP, fresh frozen plasma; INR, international normalized ratio; MTP, massive transfusion protocol; PRBCs, packed red blood cells.

BOX 128.1	PREOPERATIVE EVALUATION MNEMONIC (AMPLE)
A	Allergies
M	Medications
P	Past medical history
L	Last oral intake
E	Event related to the injury

presenting with burns, spinal cord injury, or certain known neuromuscular diseases. Likewise, the use of succinylcholine is associated with malignant hyperthermia in pediatric patients. A viable alternate to succinylcholine is rocuronium, which is a nondepolarizing neuromuscular blocking agent that is not contraindicated in patients presenting with burns, spinal cord injury, or neuromuscular diseases.

Airway Management

Trauma victims may arrive to the ED with an endotracheal tube (ETT) in place. In this scenario, it is the anesthesia provider's duty to assess the airway to ensure appropriate ETT size and placement. If the child does need to be intubated, they should be given 100% oxygen prior to induction/intubation to denitrogenate the lungs. This will increase the patient's oxygen reserve and will ideally allow for a longer period of apnea without desaturation during intubation. Pediatric trauma patients should always be considered a full stomach and at high risk of aspiration during induction/intubation. In such scenarios, a rapid-sequence induction (RSI) is considered the gold standard of care.

There are several physiological variances that should be considered when intubating pediatric patients. Children have smaller oral cavities, coupled with a relatively large tongue and tonsils, thereby predisposing them to airway obstruction. The larynx in children is more cephalic and anterior making visualization during endotracheal intubation more difficult. In addition, children have short tracheas (5 cm long in infants and 7 cm long in an 18-month-old child). This puts them at a higher risk of unintentional placement of the ETT in the right mainstream bronchus or accidental extubation with any motion of the head. Infants and young children also have large occiputs, which naturally flex the neck in the supine position. This position may lead to airway obstruction and has the potential to exacerbate any unstable cervical spine injuries.

Ventilation

One of the most common causes of cardiorespiratory arrest is hypoventilation. Anatomically, children's ribs are positioned more horizontally. Therefore, with inspiration the ribs only move up, and not up and out, like the adult rib cage. In a spontaneous breathing child, this limits the capacity to increase their tidal volumes. Young children also tend to be diaphragmatic breathers as their respiratory muscles have fewer type 1 fibers, which can lead to exhaustion more quickly when compared to adults.

Respiratory rate varies with age. In addition, children have a higher oxygen demand resulting in higher respiratory rates. Young children do not tolerate long periods of apnea well as they have a high oxygen consumption rate, low FRC, and a rapid bradycardia response to hypoxia. Furthermore, infants and young children have smaller tidal volumes (6–8 mL/kg). It is imperative that anesthesia providers are aware that infants and young children are at an increased risk of iatrogenic barotrauma with overly aggressive artificial ventilation.

Circulation

Vital sign norms change as children reach various developmental milestones (Table 128.5). In general, a child's heart and respiratory rate are higher than that of an adult, with blood pressure being lower comparatively. The 5th percentile SBP for age can be approximated by the following formula for children 1 to 10 years of age: systolic pressure = 70 mm Hg + 2 × (age in years).

A child's physiological response to major trauma differs from that of an adult as they are able to maintain a near-normal blood pressure in the face of 25% to 30% blood volume loss. Anesthesia providers should be aware that hypovolemia due to blood loss is not a benign phenomenon, however, it is the most common cause of shock in the pediatric patient. Due to this physiological reserve in children, blood pressure may be maintained despite a significant loss of the circulating blood volume. Tachycardia is usually the first sign of frank hypovolemia in the child. Compensated shock occurs when there has been significant blood loss, but the blood pressure has been maintained by tachycardia and vasoconstriction. Clinically, subtle changes in the heart rate and extremity perfusion may signal impending cardiorespiratory failure. Therefore, the trauma patient who is cool and tachycardic should be considered to be in shock until proven otherwise. In infants, uncompensated shock with hypotension in the early stages is accompanied by tachycardia, which may change to bradycardia if blood loss continues unchecked.

Thermoregulation

Children have larger BSA to body mass ratio which predisposes them to larger heat and insensible fluid losses than adults. To help counter this, the metabolic rates of children are increased, mandating higher fluid and caloric requirements. Considerable efforts should be made to avoid hypothermia in trauma patients as it can complicate an already critical situation by worsening metabolic acidosis and exerting a negative inotropic effect on the heart. Increasing the ambient room temperature, using a radiant warmer, warming IV fluids and blood, and using warm and humidified inspired oxygen are all viable means of heat conservation.

NEUROTRAUMA

Pediatric head injuries are one of the most common traumatic lesions among pediatric patients. When a child presents with significant trauma to the brain, it is called a traumatic brain injury (TBI). TBI is the leading cause of death and disability in children. In general, children have thinner and more pliable skulls which afford less protection to the brain. Anatomically,

Table 128.4	Rapid Sequence Induction Medications for Trauma Patients at Nationwide Children's Hospital		
	Premedication	Sedation	Paralytic
Patients less than 1 yr of age	Atropine 0.02 mg/kg	Ketamine 1 mg/kg	Rocuronium 1 mg/kg
Patients greater than 1 yr of age		Ketamine 1 mg/kg	Rocuronium 1 mg/kg

Table 128.5 Normal Pediatric Vital Signs

Age	Heart Rate (beats/minute)	Blood Pressure (mm Hg)	Respiratory Rate (beats/minute)
Premature	110–170	SBP 55–75 DBP 35–45	40–70
0–3 mos	110–160	SBP 65–85 DBP 45–55	35–55
3–6 mos	110–160	SBP 70–90 DBP 50–65	30–45
6–12 mos	90–160	SBP 80–100 DBP 55–65	22–38
1–3 yrs	80–150	SBP 90–105 DBP 55–70	22–30
3–6 yrs	70–120	SBP 95–110 DBP 60–75	20–24
6–12 yrs	60–110	SBP 100–120 DBP 60–75	16–22
>12 yrs	60–100	SBP 110–135 DBP 65–85	12–20

DBP, diastolic blood pressure; SBP, systolic blood pressure.

Source: From Zeno R, Kosla J, Melnyk BM. Evidence-based assessment of children and adolescents. In: Gawlik KS, Melnyk BM, Teall AM, eds. *Evidence-Based Physical Examination: Best Practices for Health and Well-Being Assessment.* Springer; 2020:Table 4.1, p. 57.

infants and young children less than 8 years of age have a disproportionately larger head and weaker neck muscles. This results in a high center of gravity, as well a higher incidence of head and neck trauma. Infants also have skulls with open sutures and larger subarachnoid space. This does offer some benefit in the presence of a head trauma, however, it allows the skull to expand in the presence of an intracranial hematoma.

TRAUMATIC BRAIN INJURY ASSESSMENT

TBI can be classified as either primary or secondary. A primary TBI is one that is the direct result of trauma, such as brain contusion, diffuse axonal injuries, or intracranial hemorrhage (epidural, subdural, and/or subarachnoid). Secondary TBIs are those that appear hours to days after the initial traumatic event. These appear as a result of metabolic effects and may present as cerebral ischemia and edema. TBI can cause an elevated intracranial pressure (ICP), which can lead to devastating complications. Early recognition of elevated ICP and prompt treatment are key as these can prevent neurological sequelae and death. The normal range of cerebrospinal fluid (CSF) pressure in children is 12 to 28 cmH$_2$O (9–21 mm Hg) by lumbar puncture. A measured ICP greater than 20 mm Hg for 5 minutes or greater accompanied by signs and symptoms of an elevated ICP is often regarded as the threshold for treatment (Tables 128.6 and 128.7).

Signs and Symptoms of Elevated Intracranial Pressure

The signs and symptoms of elevated ICP are summarized in Box 128.2.

Glasgow Coma Scale

The Glasgow Coma Scale (GCS) is a commonly used tool to objectively assess the extent of impaired consciousness (Table 128.8). It is a simple, quick, and reliable way to determine the severity of a TBI. There are three key components to

Table 128.6 Neurotrauma Characteristics Based on Age

Newborns	• Delivery head injury • Intracranial hemorrhages • Cephalic hematoma • Subgaleal hematoma	• Caused by head compression and traction through the birth canal (vaginal delivery) with obstetric instruments. • A low birth weight and hypoxemia are risk factors for intracranial hemorrhage.
Infants	• Accidental head injury • Abusive head injury	• Caused by inappropriate childcare practices. • If mechanism of injury is not clear, careful consideration for diagnosis of child abuse is required. Abusive head injury is the most common cause of TBI-related hospitalization and death.
Toddlers and Schoolchildren	• Accidental head injury	• Caused by accidents increases as children develop motor ability. • With increase in use of child safety seats, the severity of injury and the mortality have dropped. • Pedestrian injury also increases in this age group.
Adolescents	• Bicycle and motorcycle-related accidents • Sports-related head injuries	• Awareness of prevention must be raised. • Trainers and players involved in contact sports (i.e., judo, rugby, or American football) will require education about concussion.

TBI, traumatic brain injury.

Source: From Araki T, Yokota H, Morita A. Pediatric traumatic brain injury: characteristic features, diagnosis, and management. *Neurol. Med. Chir.* 2017;57(2):82–93. doi:10.2176/nmc.ra.2016-0191.

Table 128.7 Structural Consideration in Pediatric Neurotrauma

Skin	• Scalp • Epidermis/dermis • Subcutaneous fat layer • Galea aponeurotica • Periosteum	• The younger a child is, the thinner and the poorer their ability to cushion against external forces. • Fragile and prone to blistering and tearing. • Easily retains water and microvascular breakdown causes SC hematoma. • Blood and exudate can accumulate beneath galea. • Cephalic hematoma can be calcified rarely.
Cranium	• Cranium	• The craniofacial ratio is at its greatest. Cranial sutures are loose and highly mobile. • Calvarium is soft and rich in bone marrow, connected with a periosteum, strongly attached to the bone cortex. Continuity of the skull tends to be well maintained. Bone fragments are less likely to occur.
Brain and nerve fibers	• Nerve fibers • Brain/cortical veins	• Undeveloped myelin sheaths, the water content per unit volume of brain tissue is high. Fibers are pliable and less prone to rupture. • Cerebral contusion by direct external force is high because of its softness. Easily extended with accelerated–decelerated motion and can cause subdural hematoma with disruption.
Neck and cervical spine	• Neck • Vertebrae	• Undeveloped neck muscle and poor head support. The fulcrum of the vertebral body is located in the upper cervical spine. • Ligaments and soft tissues are flexible and facets are flat. Vertebral body is prone to dislocation.

Source: From Araki T, Yokota H, Morita A. Pediatric traumatic brain injury: characteristic features, diagnosis, and management. *Neurol. Med. Chir.* 2017;57(2):82–93. doi:10.2176/nmc.ra.2016-0191.

the GCS: eye opening, verbal response, and motor response. A number can be assigned, based on a standardized rubric, for each of these components, with the GCS score being the sum of the three assessments. A low GCS has been shown to correlate with poor patient outcomes.

TRAUMATIC BRAIN INJURY TREATMENT

The goal of care for a pediatric patient with a TBI is to maintain cerebral perfusion. Due to an underdeveloped auto-regulatory mechanism for cerebral blood flow (CBF), children are particularly vulnerable to cerebral hyperemia, which can result in serious intracranial hypertension. Infants have a low mean arterial pressure with little reserve capacity to counter low blood pressure and hypoxia. This makes them susceptible to a fatal decrease in CBF. Cerebral perfusion can be adequately maintained by maintaining cerebral perfusion pressure (CPP). CPP is regulated by two opposing forces: mean arterial pressure and ICP. Normal CPP in adults ranges from 50 to 70 mm Hg. As children have a lower SBP, patients younger than 5 years old have a lower CPP at baseline. The treatment of TBI and/or elevated ICP needs to be managed appropriately to reduce the likelihood of secondary brain injury from hypoxia, ischemia, and cerebral edema while maintaining CPP.

Interventions to Manage Elevated Intracranial Pressure

Box 128.3 outlines interventions in the management of elevated ICP.

THORACIC TRAUMA

Thoracic trauma occurs in approximately 5% to 12% of children presenting with a traumatic injury. Despite this relatively low incidence, injury secondary to thoracic trauma is associated with a disproportionately high morbidity and mortality rate, much more than other types of injuries. Children have a compliant chest wall, and the thickness of the SC and muscular layers is reduced. This compliance allows significant injury to occur with few external signs of trauma. In addition, the mediastinum is much more mobile in children than adults, which accounts for the increased incidence of pneumothorax, hemothorax, and diaphragmatic rupture. Of note, rib fractures are less common and pulmonary injury is often present without bony disruption. Injuries associated with thoracic trauma include chest wall injury and intrapleural injuries, such as lung, heart, tracheobronchial, esophageal, or diaphragmatic injury.

PULMONARY CONTUSION

The most common injury with blunt thoracic trauma is pulmonary contusion, with a reported incidence over 50%. The presentation of pulmonary contusion can vary from uncomplicated findings seen on a chest x-ray to serious respiratory insufficiency. A pulmonary contusion can result in damage at the level of the alveoli with hemorrhage and edema, resulting in ventilation/perfusion mismatch, hypoventilation,

---

BOX 128.2 SIGNS AND SYMPTOMS OF ELEVATED INTRACRANIAL PRESSURE

Bulging anterior fontanel
Headache
Irritability
Nausea and vomiting
Seizures
Altered mental status
Lethargy
Poor oral intake
Papilledema
Cushing triad: hypertension, bradycardia, and respiratory depression

Table 128.8 Adapted Glasgow Coma Scale for Infants and Children

Eye Opening

Score	Infants and Children Younger Than 1 Yr	Infants Older Than 1 Yr
4	Open spontaneously	Open spontaneously
3	To loud noise	To verbal command
2	To pain only	To pain only
1	No response	No response

Motor Response

Score	Infants and Children Younger Than 1 Yr	Infants Older Than 1 Yr
6	Movements purposeful and spontaneous	Obeys commands
5	Localizes pain	Localizes pain
4	Flexion withdrawal to pain	Flexion withdrawal to pain
3	Flexion involuntary and abnormal (decorticate rigidity)	Flexion involuntary and abnormal (decorticate rigidity)
2	Involuntary extension (decerebrate rigidity)	Involuntary extension (decerebrate rigidity)
1	No response	No response

Verbal Response

Score	Birth–23 Mos	Children Aged 2–5 Yrs		Children Older Than 5 Yrs
5	Smiles, coos, cries, vocalizes	Appropriate words and phrases	Oriented and converses	
4	Cries	Inappropriate words; confused	Disoriented and converses	
3	Inappropriate crying and/or screaming	Cries and/or screams	Inappropriate words	
2	Grunts	Grunts	Incomprehensible, nonspecific sounds	
1	No response	No response	No response	

Note: Score is obtained by determining the score for each of the three criteria (eye opening, best motor response, and best verbal response) and adding them. 13–15 = mild head injury; 9–12 = moderate head injury; and <8 = severe head injury.
Source: From Christensen B. *Glasgow coma scale—pediatric.* 2014. https://emedicine.medscape.com/article/2058902-overview.

and hypoxia. Patients with pulmonary contusion may also develop pulmonary edema following excessive fluid resuscitation. Nonetheless, fluids should be provided during initial management as needed to support blood pressure and improve end-organ perfusion.

PNEUMOTHORAX

The second-most common injury following thoracic trauma is pneumothorax, which is observed as isolated injury in up to 37% of the cases. A small minor pneumothorax may present with no clinical symptoms. Conversely, a large pneumothorax can cause clinical symptoms that may overlap with those produced by lung parenchymal damage, such as tachypnea, respiratory distress, and decreased oxygen saturation levels. Patients with tension pneumothorax may present with respiratory distress, absent breath sounds, and jugular venous dissension and may have hemodynamic compromise from a lack of venous return. In young children, it may be difficult to assess for jugular venous distension and tracheal deviation. Needle decompression at the second intercostal space along the mid-clavicular line is typically performed to relieve the tension pneumothorax in patients who are unstable. Placement of a pigtail catheter, rather than thoracotomy tube, may be appropriate for smaller pneumothoraces. Thoracostomy tubes are indicated, however, when a hemothorax is present.

TRACHEOBRONCHIAL TREE INJURY

Tracheobronchial tree injuries occur in less than 3% of children presenting with thoracic trauma, however, death occurs in about one third of these cases. The mechanism of injury is anterior–posterior compression of the compliant pediatric chest wall, resulting in the sternum compressing the spine causing lateral displacement of the lungs and injuring the bronchi and/or trachea at the carina. Patients with a tracheobronchial tree injury may be asymptomatic initially, which can delay diagnosis. More obvious signs and symptoms include a pneumothorax, hemothorax, pneumomediastinum, hemoptysis, SC emphysema, and respiratory distress. In many instances, nonoperative management is indicated if the patient's respiratory status remains stable. Defining parameters include the ability to place an endotracheal tube beyond the site of injury, successful evacuation of the pneumothorax/hemothorax, and the injury involving less than a third of the tracheal diameter.

CARDIAC INJURIES

Commotio cordis is a disorder described in the pediatric population, mostly adolescents, that results from sudden impact

> **BOX 128.3 ELEVATED INTRACRANIAL PRESSURE MANAGEMENT**
>
> - Supplemental oxygen to keep SpO_2 >95%
> - Elevate head of bed to 30 degrees
> - Early reconnection of adequate ventilation
>   - Inadequate breathing or a GCS less than or equal to 8 requires early intubation
> - Patients who present with hypotension require fluid resuscitation or blood transfusion to maintain cerebral perfusion. Even a small loss of blood volume can lead to hemorrhagic shock in a newborn, infant, or toddler
> - IV mannitol 0.5–1 g/kg and/or 3% hypertonic saline 2–6 mL/kg (1–3 mEq/kg)
>   - Hypertonic saline has an advantage over mannitol in that it does not exacerbate hypovolemia due to osmotic diuresis. However, mannitol is often used because it works rapidly and has a sustained effect.
> - Normothermia should be maintained (<38°C)
> - Hyperventilation
>   - Maintaining PCO_2 25–30 mm Hg until clinical signs improve
>   - Hyperventilation with a $PaCO_2$ less than 35 mm Hg may cause cerebral ischemia as the result of decreased cerebral blood flow. Use caution applying hyperventilation in a hypotensive patient.
> - Hyponatremia must be avoided as this may worsen cerebral edema (serum sodium 135–145)
> - Prophylactic administration of anticonvulsant
>   - Children, particularly infants, have lower seizure thresholds and are at high risk of early seizures.
>
> GCS, Glasgow Coma Scale; $PaCO_2$, partial pressure of carbon dioxide; PCO_2, partial pressure of carbon dioxide; SpO_2, blood oxygen saturation level.

to the left anterior chest wall that causes cessation of normal cardiac function. The impact occurs during ventricular repolarization with a force sufficient to cause ventricular depolarization. The sudden focal distortion of the myocardium results in ventricular fibrillation. Baseball is the most common sport in which commotio cordis occurs. The child may have immediate dysrhythmias or ventricular fibrillation that is refractory to resuscitation efforts.

Cardiac tamponade presents when fluid, mostly blood, accumulates in the pericardial sac. This causes a restriction on the myocardium, leading to a decreased cardiac output and reduced venous return. It may manifest as Beck's triad (distended neck veins, muffled heart sounds, and reduced pulse pressure), which may be absent with hypovolemia. Cardiac tamponade also may cause pulseless electrical activity (PEA) in the absence of hypovolemia and tension pneumothorax.

Injuries to the great vessels and heart are rare in the pediatric population and occur less commonly than in adults. Children with thoracic aortic injury present with first rib and sternal fractures, paraplegia, upper extremity hypertension, or blood pressure differentials in extremities. Prompt operative management with either open or endovascular approaches and mandatory and aggressive blood pressure control should be implemented preoperatively.

ABDOMINAL AND SOLID ORGAN TRAUMA

Blunt injury accounts for approximately 90% of all pediatric trauma. Although injuries may range from mild to moderate in severity, when blunt force is applied to a child's small body, multisystem trauma often ensues as children have less fat, more elastic connective tissue, and a pliable skeleton, making abdominal and thoracic structures vulnerable. In addition, children have relatively compact torsos with smaller anterior–posterior diameters, thereby decreasing the overall area which the force of injury can be dissipated. As such, the force of impact is transmitted widely through a child's body resulting in multisystem injuries in as many as 50% of children after a significant trauma. Hence, the abdomen represents a site of "silent" hypovolemia, with abdominal trauma being the most common cause of unrecognized fatal injury in children.

Motor vehicle crashes, automobile versus pedestrian injury, and falls are the major causes of blunt abdominal injury in children. Bicycle injuries, all-terrain vehicle injuries, and child abuse also contribute to the incidence of abdominal trauma. The most common structures injured in pediatric abdominal trauma are solid organs, with the liver and spleen being the most frequently injured, followed by kidneys. This is due, in part, to the fact that children have larger viscera, especially the liver and spleen, which extend below costal margins. The liver and spleen in infants and toddlers are even less protected by the rib cage and are more prone to direct injury.

Mortality due to blunt abdominal trauma is rare, occurring in less than 1% of patients. Rather, mortality is directly related to the number and type of structures injured being less than 20% in isolated liver, spleen, kidney, or pancreatic trauma. Mortality rates increase to 20% if the gastrointestinal tract is involved and 50% if major vessels are injured.

Following injury, hypotension places the child at high-risk of further intra-abdominal injury. Children who do not respond to fluid resuscitation require direct operative intervention. A focused abdominal sonography for trauma (FAST) examination may be helpful in characterizing the injury in this situation. A FAST examination evaluates the abdomen for free intraperitoneal fluid, which often coincides with intra-abdominal injury. Those who become hemodynamically stable after fluid resuscitation should have an abdominal CT performed. CT remains the gold standard for diagnosing abdominal injuries. Although CT detects most abdominal injuries, only 5% of patients with abnormal findings go to surgery. Nonoperative management is successful in approximately 95% of patients. This often includes serial abdominal examinations, hematocrit measurement, bed rest, and potentially additional imagining studies.

BURN INJURY

Because of their unique pathophysiology, burn injuries are associated with an increase in morbidity and mortality in any patient. According to the American Burn Association, each year up to 600 children die from fire and burn injuries. Fires and burns are the leading cause of unintentional death in the home for children, with children under the age of 5 years of age being at the greatest risk.

The goals of initial patient management include preservation of overall homeostasis, resuscitation, and airway management. Anesthesia providers must be aware of the physiological stress a burn injury places on the body. Major burn injuries not only result in local damage from the injury but often result in multisystem injury. Inflammatory and vasoactive mediators, such as histamine, prostaglandins, and cytokines, are released causing systemic capillary leak, intravascular fluid loss, and large fluid shifts (Box 128.4).

> **BOX 128.4 PATHOPHYSIOLOGICAL MANIFESTATIONS OF BURN INJURY**
>
> - **Cardiovascular:** capillary leak; hypermetabolic state; interstitial edema; SIRS; myocardial depression; hypotension
> - **Respiratory:** airway edema; inhalation injury; CO poisoning; ARDS
> - **Gastrointestinal:** decreased gastric emptying; gastric ulceration and bleeding; possible bacterial translocation and sepsis
> - **Renal:** altered drug clearance; acute kidney injury
> - **Hepatic:** altered drug metabolism; coagulopathy
> - **Neuromuscular:** upregulation of acetylcholine receptors
> - **Immune:** decreased barrier function (skin and gut); immunosuppression
>
> ARDS, acute respiratory distress syndrome; CO, carbon monoxide; SIRS, systemic inflammatory response syndrome.

CLASSIFICATION OF BURN INJURY

Initial classification of burn injury involves both depth of the burn and the total BSA (TBSA) encompassed by the burn injury. Infants and young children have a smaller BSA than adults but will sustain a proportionally larger TBSA burn than an adult (See Chapter 87, "Burns," Figure 87.1 for Lund–Browder diagram to estimate TBSA in children with burns).

MANAGEMENT OF A BURN INJURY

Initial care and management of a severely burned child is like that following a major trauma, with primary and secondary surveys guiding care. Airway evaluation is a priority to ensure there is no airway compromise or issues with oxygenation and ventilation. Mouth opening may also be limited due to edema, pain, or the development of contractures.

Inhalation Injury

Predictors of significant inhalation injury and impending respiratory failure include stridor, wheezing, drooling, and hoarseness as they are all indicators of airway swelling and compromise. Inhalation injuries include upper airway edema from direct thermal injury aggravated by systemic capillary leak, bronchospasm from aerosolized irritant, small airway occlusion with sloughing end-bronchial debris, and a loss of ciliary function. Inhaled by-products of burning wood, plastic and other materials can also lead to carbon monoxide (CO) and cyanide (CN) poisoning. CO has a 250-fold affinity for hemoglobin as compared to oxygen, and shifts the oxyhemoglobin dissociation curve to the left, resulting in the impairment of oxygen delivery to the tissues. It is imperative that anesthesia providers recognize that standard pulse oximeters cannot distinguish between oxyhemoglobin and carboxyhemoglobin. Additionally, the partial pressure of oxygen (PaO_2) can be normal or high in patients receiving oxygen therapy, even with high levels of carboxyhemoglobin. Treatment of CO relies on administering 100% oxygen, which will decrease the half-life of carboxyhemoglobin from 4.5 hours to 50 minutes.

Thermoregulation

Measures to conserve body heat are essential for the infant and young child. Thermoregulatory responses are impaired. Burned skin is unable to retain heat and water, with the potential consequence of massive evaporative fluid losses and metabolic responses. Given the large surface area of an infant's or young child's head, the head should be covered to conserve body temperature during assessment and treatment.

Fluid Resuscitation

Fluid resuscitation is of the utmost importance during care of a burned child. Due to the high capillary leak into the interstitial space in the hours after a burn, a delay in fluid resuscitation may result in both acute renal failure and increased mortality. Peripheral IV access, away from burn sites, should be obtained promptly. Central venous access may be necessary due to the extent and areas burned. The type of fluid administered is generally an isotonic crystalloid, with the recommendation for the addition of dextrose to children under 20 kg to prevent the development of hypoglycemia. The Parkland formula is the most used fluid resuscitation guide. It recommends the use of isotonic crystalloid initially, with lactated Ringer's being preferred, and use of colloids 24 hours after injury (Box 128.5).

There are two other formulas that can be used, the Galvestron and Brooke formulas. No matter what formula is used, fluid resuscitation should be titrated to physiological endpoints (Table 128.9).

Pharmacological Considerations

Physiological changes, such as altered protein binding and decreased clearance, may occur after burn injuries altering the pharmacodynamic and pharmacokinetic properties of many drugs. Serum albumin, which mostly binds to acidic and neutral drugs, is decreased almost immediately after a major burn. Renal clearance is impaired initially due to hypotension and organ injury, while after 48 hours, hyperdynamic and hyper-metabolic states lead to increased clearance. Propofol clearance and volume of distribution are increased in patients with major burns during the hyperdynamic phase of the injury and can lead to decreased hypnotic effects.

A systemic upregulation of acetylcholine receptors and proliferation to extrajunctional locations have been noted.

> **BOX 128.5 PARKLAND FORMULA**
>
> - First 24 hours:
>   - Adults and children >20 kg
>   - Lactated Ringer's: 2–4 mL /kg/%BSA /24 hrs
>   - (Half in first 8 hours and the other half in following 16 hours)
>   - Colloid: none
> - If the patients develop hypotension, give 20 mL/kg crystalloid until normotension is achieved.
> - Second 24 hours, based on urine output:
>   - <1 mL /kg /hr: 20 mL/kgg crystalloid solution 1–3 mL /kg/hr: continue with Parkland formula
>   - > 3 mL/kg/hr: reduce to 2/3 of initial formula
> - Goal urine output varies depending on the age of the patient:
>   - Adults: 0.5 mL/kg/hr; children: 1 mL/kg/hr; infants: 1–2 mL/kg/hr
>
> BSA, body surface area.

Table 128.9	Indicators of Adequate Circulating Volume
Urine output	0.5–1.0 mL/kg/hr
Blood pressure	Within normal range for age. Can be normal even with hypovolemia
Heart rate	Variable. Can be high despite normovolemia
Central venous pressure	3–8 mm Hg Can be artificially altered by airway pressures, pleural or pericardial fluid or abdominal pressure
Fractional excretion of Na+	<1% (indicated hypovolemia)
BUN/Cr ratio	≥20 (indicates hypovolemia)
Echocardiogram/ultrasound	Normal stroke volume and ejection fraction
Base deficit	<5 (suggests hypoperfusion in the absence of carbon monoxide)

BUN, blood urea nitrogen; Cr, creatinine.

Hence, administration of succinylcholine is not recommended in patients 48 hours after burn injury. There is concomitantly a decrease sensitivity to the neuromuscular effects of non-depolarizing muscle relaxants (NDMRs). This is mainly from upregulation of acetylcholine receptors and increased binding to alpha1-acid glycoprotein (AAG) and enhanced renal and hepatic elimination of the NDMRs. An increased rocuronium dose of 1.2 to 1.5 mg/kg for RSI is recommended in patients with major burn injury.

Pain Management

Severe pain is a major consequence of burn injury. Anxiety and depression are confounding components in a major burn and can further decrease the patient's pain threshold. Opioid requirements are increased in burn-injured patients. Opioid tolerance makes pain management challenging throughout all phases of care. High-dose opioids are commonly used and require dosing that could far exceed standard recommendations. If a patient comes to the operating room with infusions of sedatives and narcotics, these infusions should be continued and not stopped; the infusions have been maintained to reach a steady state of effect. The use of ketamine has many potential advantages for induction and maintenance of anesthesia. Ketamine is associated with hemodynamic stability, preserving airway patency and reflexes as well as hypoxic and hypercapnic responses. Clonidine, dexmedetomidine, and methadone have been found be effective in the multimodal pain management approach for burn patients who have developed an opioid tolerance. For additional information regarding the anesthetic management of burn victims, please refer to Chapter 87, "Burns."

THE OTHER PATIENT

Pediatric anesthesia providers must understand that there is a second victim to consider when trauma occurs: the parents or guardians of the child. It is important to address both the acute injuries and the posttraumatic stress reactions of both the child and the parent. Hospitals that admit children who have experienced a trauma must be prepared to manage both the child and their family. Having a host of services immediately present and available helps minimize the psychological impact of the trauma to both parties. Key multidisciplinary team members should include social workers, child life specialists, psychiatrists, and chaplains. It should be noted that most children and their parents report at least one severe traumatic stress reaction during the first month after an injury. This is something anesthesia providers need to be aware of as these children often must return to the operating room multiple times to manage the injuries sustained during the trauma.

KEY TAKEAWAYS

- Due to the physiological differences (e.g., higher metabolic rate, decreased FRC, and larger BSA), pediatric trauma patients are more predisposed to hypoxemia, hypotension, and hypothermia.
- Shock in pediatric trauma has multiple stages with progression being unpredictable and hypovolemic shock being the most common. It is imperative that the anesthesia provider continually assess the patient and closely monitors the child's vital signs.
- Due to children having less fat, more elastic connective tissue and a pliable skeletal structure, the force of impact is transmitted throughout the whole body, resulting in multisystem injuries (e.g., abdominal, thoracic, head trauma).
- Abdominal trauma is the most common cause of unrecognized fatal injury in pediatrics. The abdomen represents a site of "silent" hypovolemia.

RESOURCES

ATLS algorithms (https://www.facs.org/quality-programs/trauma/atls)

Pedi Crisis 2.0 app (https://pedsanesthesia.org/pedi-crisis-app)

KEY REFERENCES

Complete references for this chapter are online and available at https://connect.springerpub.com/content/book/978-0-8261-3875-0/part/part05/toc-part/ch128.

3. American Academy of Pediatrics. *Management of pediatric trauma. Pediatrics.* 2016;138(2):1–9. doi:10.1542/peds.2016-1569
5. American Heart Association. Pediatric advanced life support provider manual, 2016.
15. Lee LK, Fleischer GR. Trauma management: unique pediatric considerations. In: Wiley JF, ed. *UpToDate.* 2020. https://www.uptodate.com/contents/trauma-management-unique-pediatric-considerations/print
18. McFadyen JG, Ramaiah R, Bhananker SM. Initial assessment and management of pediatric trauma patients. *Int J Crit Illn Inj Sci.* 2012;2(3):121–127. doi:10.4103/2229-5151.100888
24. Saladino RA, Conti K. Pediatric blunt abdominal trauma: Initial evaluation and stabilization. In: Wiley JF, ed. *UpToDate.* 2020. https://www.uptodate.com/contents/pediatric-blunt-abdominal-trauma-initial-evaluation-and-stabilization
27. Tobin JM, Barras WP, Bree S, et al. Anesthesia for trauma patients. *Mil. Med.* 2018;183(9/10):32–35. doi:10.1093/milmed/usy062

CHAPTER 129

Transplant Surgery

129.1: CARDIAC TRANSPLANTATION

Jamie W. Sinton and Zhe Amy Fang

The incidence of congenital heart disease (CHD) has been estimated at 6 in 1,000.[1] Although the incidence of heart failure is low, the cost and morbidity are high.[2] Heart failure is defined as a syndrome of impairment of ventricular filling or ejection of blood and consequent end-organ perfusion.[3] Common reasons for heart failure and indications for heart transplantation in children include CHD, cardiomyopathies (often acquired in myocarditis or chemotherapy), rhythm disorders, and Kawasaki disease.

INDICATIONS

Indications for cardiac transplantation in children differ from ischemia and hypertension in adults. The two most common indications for children presenting for heart transplant are CHD and cardiomyopathy. Examples of CHDs that qualify for hemodynamically significant diagnoses are Ebstein's anomaly, hypoplastic left heart syndrome, and atrial isomerism/heterotaxy (accessed from https://optn.transplant.hrsa.gov/news/pediatric-heart-allocation-policy-and-system-changes on 11/6/2020).

Cardiomyopathy diagnosis may be hypertrophic, dilated, or restrictive in nature. It may also be anthracycline induced, endocardial fibroelastosis, noncompaction, catecholamine induced, arrhythmogenic right ventricular cardiomyopathy, or metabolic. The spectrum of pathophysiology and severity dictates the anesthetic considerations.

HEART FAILURE

Heart failure is described variously; however, preservation or reduction in left ventricular systolic function is a common method. Heart failure with reduced ejection function (HFrEF) and heart failure with preserved ejection fraction (HFpEF) are final common pathways of heart failure. Heart failure may include one or both types.

HFrEF is systolic or pump failure. This may commonly be due to myocarditis, anthracyclines, or CHD. If HFrEF is decompensated with volume overload, there may be dependent edema, pulmonary edema, distention of neck veins, and an S3 due to resistance of the ventricular muscle during the early rapid-filling phase to accommodate a larger volume. An S4 sound is heard when a disproportionate amount of ventricular filling occurs late in diastole during the atrial kick and is due to pressure overload as in systemic hypertension or aortic stenosis; this may also be heard in heart failure.

HFpEF is also called diastolic heart failure and may exist alone as in hypertrophic cardiomyopathy or in addition to other cardiac conditions or single-ventricle disease. Again, an acute volume overload in a patient with acute worsening of HFpEF will also typically be associated with an S3.

Treatment of Heart Failure

Medical management of heart failure for the pediatric population is similar to adults, including diuretics, beta-blockers, angiotensin-converting-enzyme (ACE)/angiotensin receptor blockers (ARBs), afterload reduction, and/or inotropes. Mechanical circulatory support is offered in cases of pump failure in the form of short-term devices, such as Rotaflow or extracorporeal membrane oxygenation (ECMO). Intra-aortic balloon pump and Impella devices may be considered in teenagers. Durable, or long-term, mechanical support comprises ventricular-assist devices (VADs), such as Berlin EXCOR and HVAD, may also be present. Resynchronization therapy may be considered to optimize conduction.

Like adults, children with decompensated heart failure may present for cardiac transplantation with a VAD. These patients have increased risk of bleeding due to repeat sternotomy and anticoagulation. Adequate IV access and blood products should be made available.

ORGAN ALLOCATION

The United Organ Sharing Network assigns priority for transplant listing. This priority is geographic, as ischemic time should be limited to under 4 hours.

SPECIAL CONSIDERATIONS AND CONCERNS

Timing of cardiac transplantation attempts to minimize graft ischemic time. A panel of reactive antibodies (PRAs) can be used to predict graft acceptance by the host. In the pediatric population, ABO-incompatible heart transplants may be considered for neonates and infants younger than 1 year of age who have not developed ABO antibodies. The exact age cutoff for consideration for an ABO-incompatible heart transplant varies with institution and is dependent on antibody titers. For the anesthesia provider caring for children undergoing an ABO-incompatible heart transplant, particular attention must be paid to transfusion of blood products, as they must be compatible with both the donor and the recipient.

ANESTHETIC MANAGEMENT

Children presenting for heart transplantation range from arrival from home, well compensated with mechanical circulatory support, to acutely decompensated and critically ill. Medical optimization occurs during the heart transplant workup for listing and there is often little to be done following an offer for an organ. The anesthetic goals are focused on maintaining perfusion and oxygenation based on the patient's physiology.

Surgical dissection will be prolonged and bloody in children who are anticoagulated and who have had multiple previous sternotomies. With this population, prebypass transfusion is common.

MONITORING

Refer to Chapter 89, "Cardiac Surgery: On-Pump," for further information regarding cardiac, neurological, temperature, and coagulation monitoring. For children undergoing heart transplantation, the same considerations apply as for those undergoing cardiac surgery on-pump. Of note, serial lactate and venous oxygen saturation measurement may be especially relevant to this cohort.

CARDIOPULMONARY BYPASS

Activated clotting time (ACT) of at least 400 seconds (varies by institution) prevents clot formation in the bypass circuit. If the patient is already anticoagulated, heparin resistance or reduced need for additional anticoagulation may be present. Once on cardiopulmonary bypass (CPB), the cross-clamp is applied, and the native heart is often allowed to fibrillate until asystole is achieved while awaiting preparation of the donor heart. The heart and any mechanical-assist device that is present are explanted, and the graft is sewn in place. Aortic, pulmonary artery, vena cavae and left atrial cuffs are anastomosed. If there is a patent foramen ovale or any defect in the donor heart, it is repaired.

Weaning From Cardiopulmonary Bypass

Depending on the duration of cold ischemic time, the donor heart may or may not have functional impairment. Most heart transplants require inotropic support separating from CPB. Even if the donor heart has preserved function, the recipient often has elevated pulmonary artery pressures (PAPs) due to prolonged heart failure. Thus, the donor right ventricle will still have to pump against the recipient's pulmonary vascular resistance (PVR). This may complicate weaning from CPB and inhaled nitric oxide is often used. The patient's heart rate may be maintained by temporary epicardial pacing wires if needed.

It is important to understand that the new donor heart is denervated and will generally have a higher resting heart rate, blunted heart rate response to pain, light anesthesia, and hypovolemia. While the new heart will respond to circulating catecholamines, the response may be delayed. Furthermore, denervation implies that direct-acting inotropic agents will have the most response and vagal maneuvers will not have an effect on heart rate.

If ischemic time is prolonged, poor preservation has occurred, or there is primary graft nonfunction, temporary mechanical support may be initiated prior to leaving the operating room.

129.2: Liver Transplantation

Lori A. Aronson, Niekoo Abbasian, and Ximena Soler

INDICATIONS/CONTRAINDICATIONS

There are a multitude of causes for pediatric liver disease; categories include acute, chronic, cholestatic, metabolic, malignancy-related, toxicity, cirrhosis, and miscellaneous (Table 129.1). Extrahepatic biliary atresia (BA) at 30% to 40% is the most common etiology resulting in pediatric liver transplantation (PLT).[4,5] BA patients typically present with neonatal jaundice and require a Kasai portoenterostomy to improve biliary drainage. While curative for a small subset, most will go on to liver transplantation as young children. The need for retransplantation constitutes an additional 21% and fulminant hepatic failure (FHF) 14%. FHF has a particularly high mortality rate; risk factors contributing to poor outcome include grade 3 or 4 encephalopathy, younger age, more severe coagulopathy, ascites, and elevated total bilirubin.[6-8] Hepatoblastoma is the most common malignancy resulting in PLT, as this is the only treatment option for unresectable hepatoblastoma.[9]

Many etiologies of pediatric liver disease are associated with other organ dysfunctions unrelated to liver failure. Alagille syndrome is a form of intrahepatic biliary paucity secondary to inflammation with associated cardiac, renal, and skeletal abnormalities. Cardiac anomalies include varying degrees of pulmonary artery hypoplasia to complex CHD, such as tetralogy of Fallot. Of the metabolic pediatric liver diseases, alpha-1-antitrypsin deficiency and cystic fibrosis may have pulmonary comorbidities, whereas primary hyperoxaluria results in renal disease. Urea cycle defects, glycogen storage disease, and other inborn errors of metabolism may require special intraoperative fluids to maintain glucose, electrolyte, or acid–base homeostasis. If transplant is indicated secondary to malignancy, adverse effects of chemotherapy should be identified. Table 129.2 describes a small subset of pediatric liver diseases and associated multisystem involvement.

Table 129.1 Most Common Causes for Pediatric Liver Transplantation by Etiology of Liver Disease

Acute liver failure	Nontypeable hepatitis
Chronic liver disease	Biliary atresia
Malignancy	Hepatoblastoma
Metabolic liver disease	Alpha-1-antitrypsin deficiency
Miscellaneous	Retransplantation

SPECIAL CONSIDERATIONS AND CONCERNS

Liver failure affects a multitude of organ systems that contributes to perioperative complications: cardiac, pulmonary, renal, hematological, gastrointestinal, oncological, endocrine, neurological, and genetic.

The effects on the cardiovascular system typically include high cardiac output with an elevated resting heart rate but low systemic vascular resistance (SVR) and blood pressure. Cirrhotic cardiomyopathy (CC) may manifest as prolonged QTc on ECG and prolonged relaxation time, hyperdynamic state, ventricular hypertrophy to decreased contractility, left atrial enlargement, and diastolic and/or systolic dysfunction by transthoracic echocardiogram (TTE). More than two thirds of patients with BA have abnormal TTE,[10] and left ventricular mass index is more predictive than Pediatric End-Stage Liver Disease (PELD) of adverse events and peri-liver transplant death.[11] These patients usually have a blunted response to vasoactive medications and the only definitive treatment for CC is liver transplantation.

Pulmonary concerns include pulmonary edema, pleural effusion, restrictive lung disease secondary to ascites, hepatopulmonary syndrome (HPS) and portopulmonary hypertension (POPH). End-stage liver disease (ESLD) can lead to opposing pulmonary conditions: HPS is the triad of *hypoxemia* secondary to *intrapulmonary vascular shunting* from vasodilation with *liver disease* while POPH is a vasoconstrictive process resulting in increased PVR and possible right heart failure. Both have an incidence of 5% to 10% in pediatric liver patients. HPS severity is determined by pulse oximetry and partial pressure of oxygen

Table 129.2 Some Causes of Pediatric Liver Disease and Associated Organ Involvement						
Etiology of Pediatric Liver Disease	Cardiac	Pulmonary	Gastrointestinal	Renal	Musculoskeletal	Other
Alagille Syndrome	+			+	+	+
Alpha-1-Antitrypsin Deficiency	+	+	+			
Wilson Disease	+		+	+		+
Primary Hyperoxaluria	+			+	+	+
Cystic Fibrosis	+	+	+			
Glycogen Storage Disease (Type Ia)		+		+	+	+
Hepatoblastoma	+	+				+

(PaO_2) in room air. Diagnosis of shunting is made by saline contrast TTE ("bubble echo"), lung perfusion scan, or pulmonary angiography. A positive bubble study confirms agitated saline in the left heart with three to six cycles. Signs and symptoms include platypnea–orthodeoxia, cyanosis, clubbing, and spider hemangiomas.[12] POPH is defined as increased PAP and PVR with normal pulmonary capillary wedge pressure (PCWP). In adults, mean PAP (MPAP) >35 mm Hg markedly increases the risk of perioperative morbidity and mortality during liver transplantation.[13] The exact mean pulmonary artery pressure (MPAP) number in children is less clear. However, if present, optimizing with pulmonary vasodilators is indicated prior to PLT, and having inhaled nitric oxide intraoperatively is warranted.

Renal insult secondary to ESLD can be a mild increase in creatinine to those with hepatorenal syndrome (HRS) requiring renal replacement therapy and is associated with decreased survival if untreated and not transplanted.[14,15] Chronic exposure to cytokines, bacterial fragments, and endogenous vasopressin deficiency result in splanchnic vasodilation, low vascular resistance and poor kidney perfusion.[16] Optimizing renal function and electrolytes prior to LT and avoiding and/or aggressively treating precipitating factors are critical. HRS is also associated with CC thus necessitating a cardiac workup in patients with HRS. Renal replacement therapy can be continued intraoperatively, but concern for hypothermia exists in children.[17]

Hematological abnormalities secondary to ESLD include anemia, thrombocytopenia, prolonged prothrombin, activated prothrombin times and international normalized ratio (INR), and low fibrinogen, vitamin K-dependent factors (II, VII, IX, X) and proteins S, C and Z and Factor V.[18] While disseminated intravascular coagulation is rare, the baseline coagulopathy contributes to bleeding from ulcers and varices. Of note, some pediatric patients develop a prothrombotic state due to reduced antithrombin, protein C and S, or elevation in von Willebrand factor.[19] Esophageal varices from portal hypertension may complicate nasogastric (NG) tube placement or use of transesophageal echocardiogram. Hypersplenism contributes to thrombocytopenia from platelet sequestration. Gastrointestinal comorbidities include ascites, anorexia/malnutrition, hypoalbuminemia, delayed gastric emptying, and cholangitis. Treatment and optimization strategies should be employed through time of PLT.

ANESTHETIC MANAGEMENT

PREOPERATIVE EVALUATION

The preoperative anesthetic assessment needs to be mindful of the aforementioned topics: etiology of ESLD, associated comorbidities, additional medical and surgical history, and laboratory results. Furthermore, if possible, once your institution lists a patient for PLT, an anesthesia consult should be performed. This allows ample time to review the medical record and data gathered and order more tests as deemed necessary. Multidisciplinary communication during this time is critical to ensure accurate assessment and optimal management.

If this is a chronic patient, an annual anesthetic assessment to update data is reasonable. Regardless of the timing to PLT, additional attention should be paid to assessing any interval change in clinical status: worsening PELD, neurological deterioration, recent gastrointestinal bleeding or peritonitis, renal function, cardiac status, energy level, fatigue, nutritional state, and others. If medical intervention was indicated, reassessment is vital (e.g., MPAP after instituting pulmonary vasodilator therapy or oxygen requirement, and saturation with HPS).

If significant anesthetic concern exists for a patient, this needs to be discussed with the multidisciplinary team preoperatively. A complete and accurate preoperative anesthetic evaluation is vital to safe and effective intraoperative care. It is prudent, however, to anticipate coagulopathy, the risk of major fluid shifts, massive blood transfusion and its stress on the cardiac, pulmonary, and renal systems, and the metabolic derangements throughout the perioperative stages.

In addition to the cause of liver failure, a comprehensive medical and surgical history is indicated to identify common diseases of childhood. A surgical history, especially abdominal, can increase bleeding secondary to adhesions (e.g., failed Kasai, necrotizing enterocolitis) in coagulopathic patients and needs to be anticipated.

Many children with liver failure have growth delay or failure to thrive further contributing to the frailty of this patient population. Acidosis and electrolyte abnormalities are common and attempted to be optimized prior to anesthetic induction. Early mortality after PLT has been associated with pre-reperfusion metabolic acidosis, post-reperfusion hyperlactatemia, and hyperglycemia, which were exacerbated by malnutrition, hemorrhage, and massive transfusion.[20]

Pertinent Labs

Based on the many organ systems affected by ESLD, a variety of laboratory and evaluation studies need to be performed and reviewed prior to LT. Tests include blood group, antibody screening, virology studies, complete blood count (CBC), electrolyte and renal panel, liver enzymes, albumin, coagulation studies (prothrombin time (PT), activated partial thromboplastin time (aPTT), international normalized ratio (INR), and fibrinogen), thromboelastography (TEG), or rotational thromboelastography (ROTEM). TEG and ROTEM evaluate viscoelastic properties of clot in whole blood and can provide real-time assessment of clot strength and fibrinolysis. Additional evaluation includes chest radiograph, ECG (e.g., QTc, rhythm), TTE (within past 2 months or sooner if evidence of CC or HRS), and cardiac catheterization data (if present).

Given the emergence of SARS-CoV-2 and concerns for COVID-19, recommendations vary by transplant center. Candidates with active COVID-19 should be deferred from transplantation. After complete symptom resolution, one or two SARS-CoV-2 PCR tests should also be negative within 48 hours since shedding of the virus has been documented to occur after resolution of symptoms.[21]

ANESTHETIC TECHNIQUE

Intraoperative Management

Beginning with the induction of anesthesia, most patients receiving a PLT are considered "full-stomach" due to increased intra-abdominal pressure from ascites or organomegaly in addition to delayed gastric emptying. Therefore, a rapid sequence IV induction with cricoid pressure and intubation with a cuffed endotracheal tube is usually performed. The choice of induction agent should be based on the patient's hemodynamic status. After induction and intubation, adequate IV and intra-arterial access are obtained. IV access must be appropriate to accommodate rapid fluid and blood administration with possible utilization of a rapid infusion device. Upper extremity IV access is critical to the successful management of these patients, as the inferior vena cava (IVC) is clamped during part of the procedure and occasionally the aorta during hepatic artery anastomosis.[22] In children, a double or triple central venous catheter is placed for central venous pressure (CVP) monitoring while the other ports are utilized for vasoactive infusions.

Maintenance of anesthesia can be accomplished in numerous ways, with no single technique having proved to be better than others. More crucial than the specific technique utilized is ability to maintain hemodynamic stability, fluid resuscitation goals, temperature maintenance, and correction of metabolic and coagulation abnormalities during the procedure. Consequently, careful monitoring and availability of measures to maintain hemostasis, normothermia, and normovolemia are essential. Adequate point of care and stat laboratory assistance are necessary, with rapid analysis of basic electrolytes, glucose, arterial blood gases (ABGs), ionized calcium and magnesium levels, and coagulation profiles. Perioperative use of TEG or ROTEM allows for an accurate assessment of the quality of the clotting system in real time.[23] Common vasoactive infusions immediately available for most PLT include epinephrine, vasopressin or norepinephrine, and calcium chloride.

Stages of Surgery

The surgical procedure can be divided into three distinct stages, referred to as preanhepatic, anhepatic, and neohepatic stages. Each stage presents varying anesthetic concerns and requires cooperative communication.

Preanhepatic Stage

The preanhepatic phase includes dissection and isolation of the native liver. This stage is characterized by the potential for large blood loss secondary to the presence of coagulopathy and surgical bleeding during dissection of the diseased liver, especially in those patients with prior abdominal procedures and portal hypertension. Maintenance of low CVP may reduce venous bleeding during hepatectomy.[24] The major anesthetic issues during this stage are the maintenance of hemodynamic stability by adequate fluid/blood administration and correction of coagulation abnormalities. The use of citrate-rich blood products may result in the development of hypocalcemia and hypomagnesemia. These electrolytes should be monitored closely and replaced as necessary. This phase ends with the clamping of the IVC, portal vein, and hepatic artery and removal of the diseased liver.

Anhepatic Stage

Immediately on ligation of the hepatic artery and removal of the liver, the anhepatic phase begins. During this phase, while the IVC is clamped, there is a reduction in venous return. Most pediatric patients tolerate this due to adequate collateral blood flow that developed secondary to portal hypertension. Veno-veno bypass may be indicated for instability in children ≥20 kg.[22] The goals during this phase are fluid management and correction of coagulopathic and metabolic abnormalities that developed secondary to the anhepatic state and maintenance of normothermia. Judicious volume resuscitation is important for hemodynamic stability, as well as avoiding hepatic congestion that may result after reperfusion. The volume resuscitation should be directed by CVP, arterial blood pressure and waveform, and urine output. Vasopressors may need to be added to augment the mean arterial pressure (MAP). Prior to reperfusion, potassium should be in low-normal range and calcium and bicarbonate should be in high-normal range; hemoglobin should be maintained between 9 and 10 g/dL.[25] Sufficient blood volume expansion to raise CVP to 12 to 15 cmH$_2$O and hematocrit to 40% minimizes the development of hypotension on unclamping and prevents dilutional anemia.[26] The anhepatic stage extends until the time of reperfusion of the donor liver, where the hepatic artery and portal veins are unclamped.

Neohepatic Stage

Despite adequate preparation for reperfusion, there may still be hypotension, bradycardia, and dysrhythmias associated with unclamping the IVC, thus entering reperfusion and the neohepatic stage. The cause of this reperfusion syndrome appears to be multifactorial and includes inadequate volume resuscitation, inadequate flushing of cold storage solution, and release of vasoactive substances into central circulation, which can result in hyperkalemia, hypocalcemia, and acidosis.[22] Reperfusion is associated with an increase in cardiac output and decreased in SVR with a decline in blood pressure; vasopressor support may be required. Additionally, the sudden circulatory influx of this cold solution may lead to increased PAP and right ventricular dysfunction. Although rare, air or microthrombotic embolism may also occur with reperfusion. Surgically, the remainder of this neohepatic stage involves the hepatic artery anastomosis and creation of the biliary drainage. During this phase, fluid resuscitation continues but must be performed carefully to avoid fluid overload and graft congestion. As the new liver begins to function, many metabolic abnormalities begin to self-correct. Signs of a well-functioning graft include good hepatic arterial flow, early bile formation, increasing body temperature, improvement in coagulation status, and correction of acidosis.

Complications

Several common complications in children after PLT that require surgical revision or intervention, include hepatic artery thrombosis (HAT), portal vein thrombosis (PVT), primary graft nonfunction, and biliary complications.[27] HAT is the most common vascular complication after PLT at 8% with younger age, anastomotic anatomy, rejection, hypotension, and hypercoagulability as risk factors. PVT has an incidence of 4% to 10% in children, especially since the primary indication for transplant is BA with associated hypoplastic portal veins. Biliary complications, including leaks and strictures, are another 10%. Other complications are acute and chronic rejection, infection, and malignancy.

PLT has experienced many advances over the past few decades especially regarding patient and graft survival. This is largely due to advances in surgical techniques, immunosuppressive regimens and pre- and postoperative medical therapies. While pediatric patients, especially infants, continue to have a higher mortality than adults, survival after PLT is >85% at 1 and 5 years post-PLT.[5,27]

POSTOPERATIVE CARE

The majority of LT patients will be transferred to the intensive care unit (ICU) intubated and sedated. The postoperative course will be determined by the patient's preoperative medical condition, intraoperative course, and, most important, graft function. Fluid resuscitation and correction of metabolic abnormalities continue through ICU course. Of note, fast-tracking extubation is on the rise after PLT with a trend toward immediate intraoperative extubation with criteria varying by institution.[28,29]

129.3: KIDNEY TRANSPLANTATION

Amanda Ford and Jaclyn Ashline

INDICATIONS/CONTRAINDICATIONS

Unfortunately, there are a variety of renal conditions and related functional abnormalities that can result in end-stage renal disease. Depending on the severity and progression of the disease process, the patient may require dialysis or renal transplant. Specifically, conditions, such as Alport syndrome, polycystic kidney disease (PKD), hemolytic uremic syndrome, prune belly, vesicoureteral reflux (VUR), and congenital nephritic syndrome, can cause long-lasting kidney disease and result in the need for a kidney transplant. Pediatric kidney transplant recipients are more likely to need a transplant due to obstructive nephropathy or hypoplastic kidneys than their adult counterparts.

According to the United Network for Organ Sharing, in 2019 there were 760 kidney transplants performed across the United States on patients under 18 years of age.[30] Fortunately, survival rates for kidney transplant recipients are quite high, with improvements in donor screening and procurement, living donor utilization, and immunosuppressive medications all synergistically contributing to the improvement in survival rates. Kidneys considered for transplant may be from cadaveric donors or from living donors (related or nonrelated), although outcomes are improved with living donors as compared to cadaveric donors.[31]

While there are a few relative contraindications to a kidney transplant, these can vary slightly between transplant centers and surgeons. There are, however, some widely accepted absolute contraindications for kidney transplant in pediatric patients. These include recent malignancy, no family or social support, central vascular disease (e.g., aortoiliac), and/or significant cardiac disease.

SPECIAL CONSIDERATIONS AND CONCERNS

There are some unique size-related considerations related to performing kidney transplants in the pediatric population. In small children and infants, the allograft kidney is placed in the retroperitoneal space; however, in larger children, the allograft kidney is placed in the iliac fossa outside of the peritoneal cavity (similar to adult kidney transplants). Like adult kidney recipients, the diseased kidney is typically left in place across all age ranges.[31] Blood supply to the allograft kidney is typically achieved via the external iliac artery. In addition, the renal vein is anastomosed to the external iliac vein, and the ureter is anastomosed to the bladder after the allograft kidney is reperfused. In infants and smaller children, however, the renal vessels are often anastomosed to the aorta and IVC to ensure adequate blood supply.

ANESTHETIC MANAGEMENT

PREOPERATIVE EVALUATION

It is imperative that the anesthesia provider perform a thorough preoperative evaluation for the patients presenting for a kidney transplant. Anesthesia providers must consider specific systems that may be affected by the patient's deteriorated renal function. Many children in need of a kidney transplant due to renal disease present with a history of hypertension, fluid overload, anemia, failure to thrive, metabolic disturbances, altered acid–base and electrolyte status, and altered metabolism of medications. In an effort to limit the impact of fluid and electrolyte imbalances, it is preferred that the patient have dialysis within the past 24 hours prior to surgery.

Pertinent Labs

Prior to transplant, the patient will typically have full sets of laboratory studies, including coagulation studies, a metabolic panel, CBC, viral testing, and antibody testing. Further studies may be ordered by the nephrology or transplant team, such as an abdominal ultrasound, chest x-ray, urodynamic studies, ECG, and cardiac echocardiogram.

PREOPERATIVE PHARMACOLOGY

Premedication with anxiolytics, such as midazolam, can be given as clinically indicated. Medications that are renally excreted should be avoided during the perioperative phase. Commonly used medications for management of anesthesia during a kidney transplant are listed in **Table 129.3**.

There are four general categories of immunosuppressive agents (corticosteroids, antimetabolites, macrolides, antibodies), and most transplant patients will require some amalgamation of these during the perioperative phase.[32] Therefore, the anesthesia provider should ensure the following medications are readily available prior to inducing anesthesia as they will be needed throughout the surgery: methylprednisolone, alemtuzumab, diphenhydramine, famotidine, and IV acetaminophen. Corticosteroids (methylprednisolone, prednisone) are given to inhibit the production and release of interleukin-1. Alemtuzumab is a monoclonal antibody, which acts to specifically inhibit lymphocyte function. It should be noted that this combination is specific to the authors' facility and other surgeons/facilities may prefer other combinations of medications to modulate the patient's immune response.

Table 129.3	Common IV Bolus and Infusion Medications Needed During Preparation for a Pediatric Kidney Transplantation
Medication	Concentration
Propofol	10 mg/mL, 10 mL × 2
Fentanyl	50 mcg/mL, 1–5 mL
Rocuronium	10 mg/mL, 1–10 mL
Cisatracurium	2 mg/mL, 1–10 mL
Succinylcholine (for emergency use)	20 mg/mL, 10 mL
Atropine	0.4 mg/mL, 5 mL
Glycopyrrolate	0.2 mg/mL, 2 mL
Calcium Gluconate	100 mg/mL, 10 mL × 2
Epinephrine	10 mcg/mL OR 1 mcg/mL, 10 mL; infusion available
NaHCO$_3$	1 mEq/mL, 10–50 mL
Mannitol (25%)	50 mL bottle × 4
D5W	50 mL as carrier infusion
Dopamine	Infusion to be used after reperfusion
Norepinephrine	Infusion available
Methylprednisolone	Up to 1000 mg
Alemtuzumab (Campath)	100 mL infusion bag
Diphenhydramine	50 mg/mL, 1 mL
Famotidine	10 mg/mL, 1–5 mL
Acetaminophen (IV)	100 mg/mL
Cefazolin	Ciprofloxacin and/or vancomycin if penicillin allergy
Heparin	Infusion, 5 units/kg/hr

Note: Some of the medications and doses are facility specific; this should serve as a guideline only.

Table 129.4	Typical Anesthesia Setup and Considerations for Intraoperative Management of Pediatric Kidney Transplantation
Monitoring	Standard general anesthetic monitoring, CVP, arterial line (no femoral related to aorta/iliac clamping)
Lines	Central venous catheter (RIJ preferred) placed with ultrasound; two additional large-bore PIVs (upper extremities preferred related to clamping of IVC during procedure), arterial line
Fluid	D5W carrier for infusions; use normal saline (no lactated Ringer's solution), consider 5% albumin, cell saver and PRBCs in room
Antibiotics	Cefazolin, cipro, and vancomycin if penicillin allergy
Positioning	Supine, arms abducted on arm boards (<90 degrees)
Thermoregulation	Temperature probe placed for central measurement (e.g., esophageal, bladder); consider increasing room temperature, use underbody warming blanket and/or forced-air warming device on upper body (above nipple line) and lower extremities, IV fluid warmer, fluid-warming blanket on OR bed, wrap infant head in plastic if necessary

CVP, central venous pressure; IVC, inferior vena cava; OR, operating room; PIV, peripheral IV; PRBCs, packed red blood cells; RIJ, right internal jugular.

ANESTHETIC TECHNIQUE

Intraoperative Management

These patients should already have IV access for medication administration. If the patient does need a mask induction, nitrous oxide can be used for induction of anesthesia only. Induction should include a sedative/hypnotic (propofol and/or ketamine) and muscle relaxation (rocuronium or cisatracurium). Standard intubation should be performed, and additional lines (central, large-bore peripheral IV[s], arterial line) placed at this point. Be mindful not to place the noninvasive blood pressure (NIBP) and/or arterial line on the same extremity as an arteriovenous fistula. An NG tube will also be placed, along with esophageal temperature probe and bladder temperature monitor. The patient will be positioned with arms out at 90 degrees or straight (depending on the patient's size). Anesthesia should be maintained with inhaled anesthetic (isoflurane is first choice at our institution), additional dosing of muscle relaxant, and pain medication (fentanyl). Keep in mind that renally excreted medications may need to be redosed less frequently related to impaired renal function. After placement of lines, obtain baseline point-of-care laboratory studies: ABG, electrolytes, lactate, hemoglobin/hematocrit, glucose, +/– TEG. Repeat labs at the following intervals (add additional laboratory studies as patient condition warrants): every hour, prior to reperfusion, 5 minutes after reperfusion, and 30 minutes after reperfusion. Administer antibiotics after confirmation with the surgeon. Alemtuzumab (Campath) will be given either the evening before surgery (living donor) or at the time of surgery (cadaver donor). Premedicate prior to avoid reaction (rash, bronchospasm, fever, hypotension) with methylprednisolone 10 to 15 mg/kg, IV acetaminophen 15 mg/kg, diphenhydramine 1 mg/kg (max 50 mg), and famotidine 0.5 mg/kg (max 20 mg). If hypotension occurs with alemtuzumab administration, the anesthesia provider should slow the infusion but maintain administration of the medication. Use sodium bicarbonate or similar (THAM) to treat base deficit >5 mEq/dL.

Special Techniques and/or Equipment
Special techniques and equipment are summarized in Table 129.4.

Clinical Pearls
During the dissection phase of surgery, anesthesia providers should ensure the patient potassium level is less than 5 mEq/L prior to reperfusion to prevent cardiac arrhythmias. Anesthesia providers may consider administering insulin with dextrose, calcium gluconate, and/or albuterol to treat hyperkalemia. If hyperkalemia is resistant to standard

treatment modalities, consider pretreatment with epinephrine (0.5–1.0 mcg/kg) prior to reperfusion, which will help prevent a cardioplegic-like effect secondary to the perfusate released from the kidney. Prior to reperfusion, the anesthesia provider should consider administering methylprednisolone (10–15 mg/kg), mannitol (1 g/kg), and furosemide (following mannitol, 1 mg/kg).

There are several key physiological parameters that must be maintained during release of clamp and reperfusion. Anesthesia providers should increase the FiO_2 being delivered to maintain oxygen saturation > 95%. The patient's CVP should be maintained between 10 and 12 mm Hg during reperfusion. Hypotension (systolic blood pressure <90) can be treated with boluses of ephedrine (0.1 mg/kg) and epinephrine (0.5–1 mcg/kg), a dopamine infusion, or calcium chloride administered as a slow bolus as indicated (10 mg/kg).[31] Anesthesia providers should have all vasoactive infusions and bolus syringes are prepared and ready to administer. Most surgeons prefer the patient's MAP to remain 10 to 20 mm Hg above baseline following reperfusion.

Anesthesia providers should use caution with blood product administration and should discuss with the surgeon prior to administration, especially during the early phases of surgery. Typically, the goal for hematocrit is 24% to 26%. Blood will need to be drawn at 5 and 30 minutes after reperfusion to assess laboratory values. In extreme cases, therapeutic phlebotomy may be considered at the end of the procedure for those patients with increased hemoglobin and hematocrit levels (generally described as a hemoglobin level greater than 16 to 18 g/dL or a hematocrit greater than 50%, respectively). Acute polycythemia increases the risk of thrombosis, particularly renal vessel thrombosis. A heparin infusion may be initiated after reperfusion to further prevent clotting. Additionally, it is imperative that the anesthesia provider ensure that potassium levels are adequate for reperfusion.

Complications and Emergencies

In the immediate postoperative phase, kidney recipients are at risk of fluid overload, hemorrhage, renal artery and/or vein thrombosis, urinary tract infections, electrolyte abnormalities, acute rejection, and wound infection.[33] In addition, newly prescribed immunosuppressive medications can cause cytokine release, so the patient will be monitored for fever, headache, and hypotension. Patients should be monitored for delayed graft function, which can be defined in part by the need for dialysis within the first week after transplantation.

Rejection is primary reason for graft loss in older children, while vascular thrombosis is the most common reason in recipients younger than 2 years of age.[31] Long-term thrombosis related to polycythemia (posttransplant erythrocytosis) usually develops 8 to 24 months after graft placement, and spontaneously resolves in 25% of these patients within 2 years.[34] Lymphoceles (accumulation of lymphatic fluid) originate either from lymphatics of the allograft or from dissection of blood vessels in the recipient and occur in 1% to 10% of pediatric kidney transplant recipients. The lymphatic fluid can accumulate over the allograft and can cause urinary obstruction and/or venous obstruction (Figure 129.1). A lymphocele can be diagnosed with ultrasound and is treated by creation of a peritoneal window to allow the fluid to drain into the peritoneum and subsequently be absorbed.[32]

POSTOPERATIVE CARE

Most patients will tolerate extubation at the end of the procedure. Anesthesia providers should consider using regional anesthesia, such as transversalis abdominis plane (TAP) blocks. Epidural placement is typically avoided related to recent administration of heparin. Most often, pediatric kidney recipients are initially monitored in the ICU where fluid management and electrolyte management can be under tight scrutiny of the primary team. Typically, there is a fluid replacement protocol in place postoperatively that will be guided by the patient's urine output.

Kidney transplant recipients will be monitored on a short- and long-term basis for general vital sign measurements, CBC, serum electrolytes, liver enzyme levels, immunosuppressive agent trough levels (e.g., tacrolimus cyclosporine), renal ultrasonography, and nuclear renography. The long-term prognosis for pediatric kidney transplant recipients is positive. Unfortunately, long-term immunosuppression can increase the risk of malignancy, particularly lymphoma, perineal carcinoma, liver, and sarcomas. In addition, kidney recipients continue to be at risk of acute or chronic rejection. Should acute rejection occur, management typically entails short-term treatment with corticosteroids and/or antilymphocyte antibodies.[32]

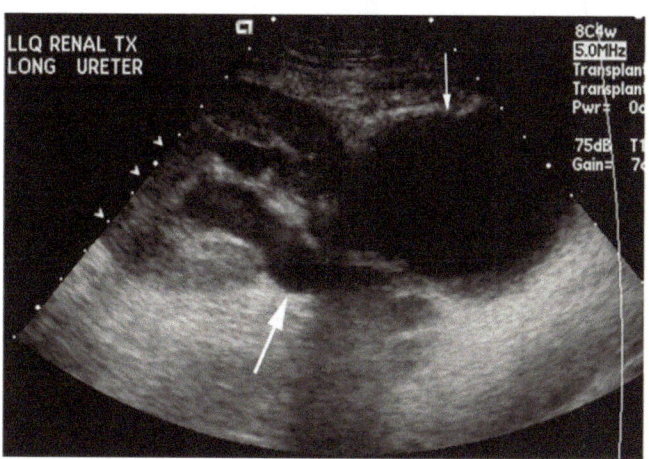

Figure 129.1: This ultrasound view of a transplanted kidney (left on image) with a lymphocele (thinner arrow). This lymphocele is compressing the ureter of the transplanted kidney, resulting in dilatation of the ureter (thicker arrow).

Source: From https://abdominalkey.com/imaging-of-the-renal-transplant-recipient.

129.4: TOTAL PANCREATECTOMY AND ISLET AUTOTRANSPLANTATION

Sean Barclay and Carrilee Powell

A total pancreatectomy and islet autotransplantation (TPIAT) is performed on patients with recurrent acute pancreatitis or severe chronic pancreatitis to provide pain relief when all other conservative medical and surgical options have failed. TPIAT is a surgical procedure in which the pancreas is completely resected, the islet cells are isolated, and then autotransplanted most commonly via the portal vein. The islet cells will engraft in the liver thus preserving beta cell mass and insulin secretory capacity to minimize or prevent diabetes.[35] This procedure is successful in alleviating pain, restoring quality of life, and providing insulin independence in greater than 40% of pediatric patients.[36]

PANCREATITIS

Pancreatitis is typically a progressively debilitating disease that impairs quality of life. Many patients with pancreatitis experience recurrent intractable pain that requires escalating doses of nonnarcotic and narcotic medications. Children will experience frequent hospitalization, recurrent school absences, low-self esteem, depression, and anxiety.[35]

Medical therapy and endoscopic interventions aimed at managing pancreatitis are attempted prior to surgical intervention. Medical therapies include pain management with nonnarcotic and narcotic medications, dietary changes, and pancreatic suppression via pancreatic enzyme therapy. Patients with ductal stones or strictures may also undergo endoscopic retrograde cholangiopancreatography (ERCP) procedures prior to surgical interventions. Patients who fail medical and endoscopic interventions may be candidates for surgical interventions, including drainage procedures and partial or full pancreatic resection. Those that undergo partial pancreatic resections may experience transient pain relief, but pain will recur in up to 50% of patients due to the full organ involvement of pancreatitis. Additionally, over time, these patients will develop exocrine and endocrine insufficiency.[36]

Chronic pancreatitis is a progressive inflammatory process of the pancreas with destruction of parenchyma, irreversible structural changes, and fibrosis. Patients with pancreatitis eventually develop both exocrine and endocrine insufficiency.[35] The pediatric population who develops pancreatitis is usually the result of a genetic predisposition. There are several mutations that occur with the most prevalent being the trypsinogen gene (*PRSS1*). *PRSS1* causes an inappropriate activation of trypsin inside of the pancreas therefore causing recurrent pancreatitis. Other mutations include *SPINK1*, the loss of trypsin inhibitor function, and *CFTR*, also known as the cystic fibrosis transmembrane receptor. *CFTR* reduces bicarbonate secretions, which in turn can contribute to intraductal obstruction and pancreatitis. There are also nongenetic causes of pancreatitis, including pancreas divisum, idiopathic disease, and trauma.[36] The incidence of chronic pancreatitis is 0.5% with a proven increase over the last 20 years.[37]

TOTAL PANCREATECTOMY AND ISLET AUTOTRANSPLANTATION

PREOPERATIVE EVALUATION

A TPIAT will be considered after failure to respond to medical and endoscopic interventions to provide long-term sustained pain relief and improvement in quality of life. Initial evaluation for a TPIAT involves a multidisciplinary approach including a transplant surgeon, gastroenterologist, endocrinologist, pain management, child psychologist, and a dietician. The team meticulously scrutinizes each case utilizing national guidelines and criteria to ensure each patient is a proper candidate for TPIAT. Eligibility criteria include (a) history of chronic or acute recurrent pancreatitis or imaging that is indicative of chronic pancreatitis, such as magnetic resonance cholangiopancreatography (MRCP) or endoscopic ultrasound, (b) failure to respond to medical or endoscopic treatment, (c) absence of medical or psychosocial contraindications, and (d) adequate beta cell function via C-peptide stimulation testing.[36,38]

SURGICAL APPROACH

TPIAT most commonly utilizes an open laparotomy to perform a total pancreatectomy, splenectomy, cholecystectomy, appendectomy, Roux-en-Y duodenojejunostomy and choledochojejunostomy, and the placement of a gastrojejunostomy (GJ) tube. A laparoscopic-assisted approach may be utilized by some surgeons.[39] To promote islet cell survival, it is imperative that the surgeons preserve blood flow to the pancreas for as long as possible to minimize warm ischemia time. Additionally, prevention of injury or spasm to pancreatic small vessels, preservation of the pylorus, and the use of a Roux-en-Y are important to prevent postoperative gastrointestinal complications, such as bile reflux gastritis. Patients undergoing TPIAT are at high risk of postoperative gastroparesis; therefore, a GJ tube will be placed to provide gastric decompression as needed and to facilitate enteral feeding. Bellin et al.[36] reported the duration of the entire surgical procedure, including islet isolation is 9.8 +/− 1.1 hours.

Following removal of the pancreas, the process of islet cell isolation begins. First, the pancreas is placed in a preservation solution where extraneous tissue is dissected off the organ. Next, the pancreas is transported to an off-site lab where a collagenase solution is infused through the pancreatic duct to aid in enzymatic digestion. In addition to chemical digestion, the pancreas will undergo mechanical digestion. A density gradient centrifuge is utilized for the separation process of islet. Following isolation, the islet cells must be examined for viability and quantified. Islet cell quantification is reported as total islet equivalents (IEQ) or IEQ per kilogram of body weight of the recipient (IEQ/kg). IEQ is the direct standardization of islet mass size as compared to medium-sized islet, 150 microns. Following islet isolation, the cells are placed in albumin that may include the addition of heparin to prevent islet cell aggregation. The islets will then be transported back to the operating room for transplantation. The entire islet isolation process is reported to take approximately 4 to 6 hours, during which time the surgeons continue to operate on the patient. There is a potential for downtime while waiting on the islet cells; however, the patient will remain under general anesthesia during this time.[36]

Upon return to the operating room, the islet cells will be infused via gravity into the portal vein while diligently monitoring patient hemodynamics and portal pressures. Occasionally, based on certain portal pressure or tissue volume constraints, the remainder of the islet cells is infused into either the peritoneal cavity, stomach subserosa, or an IM site.[36] The liver allows for islet cell neovascularization and engraftment in the hepatic sinusoids.[40] Additionally, the liver serves as an easy point of access and can accommodate large infusion volume. Some surgeons may elect to close the abdomen prior to islet transplantation and will transport the patient to interventional radiology when the islet cells are ready for a percutaneous portal vein infusion of islet cells.[38] It is estimated that 30% to 60% of islets infused are destroyed within 24 hours of transplantation, making it vital to prevent potential stressors to the islet cells.[41] Strategies to promote islet cell survival and engraftment are discussed later in this chapter.

ANESTHETIC MANAGEMENT

CASE PREPARATION

The setup for a TPIAT can be extensive as patients will undergo a general anesthetic that will last 10 hours or longer. Required vascular access will include multiple large-bore peripheral IV catheters, a central venous line, and an arterial line. A triple transducer is typically utilized to monitor arterial blood pressures, CVPs, and portal venous pressures. Patients will require frequent monitoring of laboratory values

Table 129.5	Total Pancreatectomy and Islet Autotransplantation Case Preparation
Access	• Two to three large-bore peripheral IVs with fluid warmers • Central venous line • Arterial line
Monitoring	• Arterial blood pressure • Central venous pressure • Portal venous pressure • Glucometer • ABG, electrolytes, hemoglobin, and hematocrit
Tubes / Drains	• Foley catheter • Nasogastric tube
Other	• 12–16 infusion pumps • Warming blanket or mattress • Fluid warmers • 2 units of packed red blood cell type and cross

ABG, arterial blood gas.

necessitating a glucometer and a device to monitor ABGs, electrolytes, and hemoglobin and hematocrit be readily available. Other necessary supplies and equipment include Foley catheter, NG tube, infusion pumps, and warming devices. Supplies and equipment for case preparation are outlined in Table 129.5. Administering greater than 10 continuous or intermittent infusions is common intraoperatively during a TPIAT as outlined in Table 129.6 with indications described throughout this section.

KEY ANESTHETIC CONCERNS

There are five primary anesthetic concerns for a TPIAT including intraoperative glucose control, fluid management, management of hemostasis, pain management, and management during islet cell infusion.

Table 129.6	Intraoperative Infusions for Total Pancreatectomy and Islet Autotransplantation
IV fluids	• Lactated Ringer's • D10 lactated Ringer's • PlasmaLyte A
Glucose management	• Insulin
Hemostasis	• Dextran 0.5 mL/kg (max 10 mL/hr) • Heparin 10 units /kg/hr
Vasoactives	• Dopamine
Pain medications	• +/− Lidocaine 20 mcg/kg/min • +/− Ketamine 0.2 mg/kg/hr • +/− Dexmedetomidine 0.2–0.7 mg/kg/hr
Antibiotics / antifungals (may vary by institution)	• Vancomycin • Meropenem • Fluconazole

Intraoperative Glucose Control

It is imperative to maintain strict glycemic control to maximize survival and engraftment of the islet cells. Hyperglycemia can cause islet cell damage and dysfunction through two mechanisms, which are direct injury to islet cells and inhibition of vascularization of islet cells.[35] Causes of intraoperative hyperglycemia include stress response from the procedure, lactate metabolism from IV fluids, and IV fluids containing dextrose that elevate the glucose infusion rate (GIR).[42] Intraoperative management entails monitoring blood glucose every 30 to 60 minutes prior to islet infusion with a goal blood glucose of 80 to 120 mg/dL. An insulin infusion will be started once the blood glucose is greater than 120 mg/dL and will be titrated to maintain the goal range of 80 to 120 mg/dL.[37] The patient will remain on the insulin postoperatively, eventually being transitioned to SC insulin.

Fluid Management

Maintenance of fluid rate will be calculated utilizing the standard "4–2–1" rule. Lactated Ringer's (LR) and dextrose 10 LR (D10LR) will be administered to maintain a GIR of 2 to 3 mg/kg/min. The calculation for GIR is Glucose Infusion Rate = (IV rate (mL/hr) * dextrose concentration (g/dL) * 1,000 (mg/g))/ (weight (kg) * 60 (min/hr) * 100 (mL/dL)). The LR and D10LR may be titrated based on the patient's blood glucose while administering the same overall calculated maintenance rate. The patient's baseline fluid deficit may not need to be replaced if they were admitted the day prior to preoperative fluids. There are large insensible losses due to the large open laparotomy. Consider a balanced IV crystalloid solution (normal saline, LR, Plasmalyte-A) and/or judicious albumin replacement. The goal CVP is 6 to 12 mm Hg.

Hemostasis

Large blood loss is possible with case reports of 350 to 1,200 mL of estimated blood loss during TPIAT surgery.[35] Causes of blood loss include extensive scarring of pancreas and abdomen, systemic heparinization prior to islet infusion, and splanchnic venous circulation congestion due to higher portal pressures. Coagulopathies, including platelet function inhibition and impaired coagulation cascade activation, may occur due to intraoperative hypothermia.[42] Therefore, it is imperative that anesthesia providers maintain adequate thermoregulation with the use of warming devices, such as forced-air warming devices, underbody water-warming mattress, warming device for IV fluids, and warmed irrigation fluids. Prior to administering blood products, it is important to discuss the risks and benefits of a transfusion with the surgical team. Allogeneic blood transfusions are associated with inflammation, which may affect the islet cells negatively.[43]

Pain Management

Management of pain in patients with chronic pancreatitis can prove to be challenging as many patients become opioid dependent and tolerant, with escalating dose requirements of nonnarcotics and narcotics as the disease progresses. Involving the hospital's acute pain service may be beneficial to establish an intraoperative and postoperative pain management plan.[40] A multimodal approach to pain control is often employed and options are outlined in Table 129.7. IV regimens often include fentanyl, morphine or hydromorphone, 1 mg/kg ketamine prior to incision, and methadone 0.1 mg/kg (max 5 mg) prior to incision. Continuous infusions utilized for pain management include lidocaine 20 mcg/kg/min for the first 8 hours of the procedure, ketamine 0.2 mg/kg/hr, which will continue

Table 129.7	Multimodal Analgesia Adjuncts for TPIAT Surgery
Bolus medications	Fentanyl
	Morphine or hydromorphone
	Ketamine
	Methadone
Infusions	Ketamine 0.2 mg/kg/hr
	Lidocaine 20 mcg/kg/min
	Dexmedetomidine 0.2–0.7 mg/kg/hr
Regional anesthesia	Bilateral paravertebral catheters (T8–9)
	Thoracic epidural
	Bilateral TAP catheters

TAP, transversus abdominis plane; TPIAT, total pancreatectomy and islet autotransplantation.

through the postoperative period, and dexmedetomidine 0.2 to 0.7 mg/kg/hr during the postoperative period.

A patient-controlled analgesia (PCA) infusion of hydromorphone may be ordered for the postoperative period, with eventual transition to oral analgesics.[44] The administration of IV acetaminophen may be avoided due to its formulation containing dextrose, which may alter blood glucose levels. Hutchins et al. discussed the use of regional anesthesia, specifically the placement of bilateral paravertebral catheters to manage surgical pain. The midline incision for a TPIAT typically involves dermatome levels T6 to T10–11 therefore authors placed bilateral paravertebral catheters at the T8-9 level for the first 7 days postoperatively. Hutchins et al.[44] demonstrated that utilization of bilateral paravertebral catheters with a continuous infusion for management of TPIAT-related pain decreased patients' total opioid consumption in the first 7 postoperative days. Placing a thoracic epidural is another option of regional anesthesia that can be utilized to manage pain with coverage of T6 to T10–11 dermatomes. Thoracic epidurals place patients undergoing TPIAT at higher risk of hypotension compared to the bilateral paravertebral catheters, which can be detrimental to the survival and function of the autotransplanted islet cells. A third option of regional anesthesia is bilateral subcostal TAP catheters to provide coverage of T6 to T10–11. Bilateral TAP catheters will only provide incision pain coverage while bilateral paravertebral catheters or a thoracic epidural will provide both incisional and visceral pain coverage. Caution should be taken with removing any catheter as TPIAT patients are on a heparin infusion postoperatively.[44]

Anesthesia Management During Islet Cell Infusion

Due to the autologous nature of the islet cell transplant, no immunosuppression is indicated.[35,41] The most common route of islet cell autotransplantation is a direct gravity infusion into portal circulation over 15 to 30 minutes.

Infusion of islet cells can initiate the coagulation cascade as well as inflammatory pathways.[40] Patients are at risk of instant blood-mediated inflammatory reactions (IBMIRs) within the first 6 hours following islet cell infusion. IBMIR occurs when the islet grafts come in direct contact with the portal blood leading to consumption of platelets and activation of the coagulation and complement cascades.[41] IBMIR can cause thrombosis as well as threaten islet function and integrity, resulting in islet cell destruction. Administering heparin and dextran sulfate prior to the initiation of islet cell infusion may minimize or prevent IBMIR.[38] Patients will be administered a total of 70 units/kg of heparin either IV or a combination of IV and mixed with the islet cells. The addition of heparin to the islet cell infusion will prevent islet cell clumping. The dose of IV heparin will be bolused immediately prior to the start of the islet infusion followed by a heparin infusion at 10 units/kg/hr until postoperative day 7. About 30 to 60 minutes prior to islet cell transplantation, the dextran sulfate infusion will be initiated at the rate of 0.5 mL/kg with a maximum rate of 10 mL/hr to minimize platelet aggregation.[44]

During islet infusion, it is imperative to monitor blood glucose, MAP, CVP, and portal venous pressure.[37] During this period, blood glucose levels are assessed about every 5 minutes with a goal of 80 to 120 mg/dL. Blood glucose results will direct titration of the insulin infusion and administration of bolused IV insulin may be necessary. Following the islet cell infusion, blood glucose levels should be checked every 5 to 15 minutes.

Patients are at risk of hypotension during the islet cell infusion, which can potentially threaten islet cell function and engraftment for two main reasons. First, infusion of the islet cells has the potential to cause an obstruction of portal flow leading to a decreasing venous return. Second, systemic hypotension may occur due to the substances released during islet infusion reducing SVR. The overall MAP goal is to prevent hypotension based on baseline and age-appropriate blood pressures for the patient. The patient may require a dopamine infusion and boluses of phenylephrine, epinephrine, and/or ephedrine to maintain an adequate MAP. Dopamine is typically the inotropic infusion of choice because of its mesenteric and renal vasodilator properties, but it may also improve islet cell perfusion.[42] CVP should be assessed every 5 minutes during the infusion with a goal of 6 to 12 mm Hg. Crystalloid and albumin should be administered as needed to maintain the CVP goal.

Portal pressure may transiently increase with islet infusion; therefore, it is necessary to obtain baseline and intermittent, every 5 minutes, portal venous pressures during islet cell infusion. Patients are at risk of portal hypertension throughout islet infusion, and if pressures greater than 25 mm Hg, the infusion will temporarily be paused and reassessed. The infusion will be resumed if portal pressures decrease. If portal pressures continue to remain elevated, the islet infusion into portal circulation will be halted and the remaining islets may be infused into an alternative site, such as the peritoneum or omentum.[38] Portal venous pressures greater than 26 mm Hg place the patient at risk of a PVT.[40] Pediatric patients have a 3% to 4% risk of partial or complete portal thrombosis.[35] PVT is typically caused by the islet cells causing a mechanical obstruction.[42] Systemic heparin will aid in the prevention of PVT. Postoperatively, the portal vein will be assessed by Doppler to assess for thrombosis.[37]

OUTCOMES

Engraftment and neovascularization of the autotransplanted islet cells can occur in 2 to 4 weeks but may take up to 3 months.[35,36] Beta-cell Dysfunction is common during this time especially if the patient experiences periods of hyperglycemia therefore insulin is necessary to maintain normal blood glucose levels and promote islet cell engraftment and survival.[36]

Patients will be transitioned from IV insulin to SC insulin with the eventual goal of insulin independence. Kotagal et al. demonstrated that at 90 days following TPIAT, pediatric patients demonstrated a simulated C-peptide level indicative of active beta-cell function with decreased insulin requirements.[37] Azahair et al. published that 50% of children will achieve insulin independence compared to 30% of adults.[35] Younger children are more likely to be successfully weaned off insulin compared to older children or adolescents.[36] The etiology for islet cell compensation during growth is unclear and it is unknown at this time if insulin independence will sustain into adulthood.[35,39] It is believed that even those on insulin therapy have partial islet graft function.[36]

The initial weaning of pain medications in patients with chronic pancreatitis can prove to be challenging, however, 50% to 80% of pediatric patients undergoing TPIAT are narcotic free at 1-year follow-up.[35] Azahair et al. reported that 89% of younger children achieved narcotic independence compared to 33% of adolescent patients. At follow-up, children reported a significant increase in quality of life, with approximately 75% of patients reporting quality of life as "good to excellent."[35] Children demonstrated an overall significant improvement in physical and mental health. Patients demonstrated improved school attendance, with a decrease in ED visits and hospitalization. It is believed that children have significantly better outcomes compared to adults in part because children typically experience shorter duration of disease, fewer endoscopic and surgical procedures, and typically produce a higher islet yield.[36]

KEY REFERENCES

Complete references for this chapter are online and available at https://connect.springerpub.com/content/book/978-0-8261-3875-0/part/part05/toc-part/ch129.

1. Hoffman JI, Kaplan S. The incidence of congenital heart disease. *J Am Coll Cardiol*. 2002;39(12):1809–1900. doi:10.1016/s0735-1097(02)01886-7
2. Nandi D, Rossano JW. Epidemiology and cost of heart failure in children. *Cardiol Young*. 2015;25(8):1460–1468. doi:10.1017/S1047951115002280
3. Yancy CW, Jessup M, Bozkurt B et al. 2013 ACCF/AHA guideline for the management of heart failure: a report of the American. *J Am Coll Cardiol*. 2013;62(16):e147–239. doi:10.1016/j.jacc.2013.05.019
5. Venick RS, Farmer DG, Soto JR, et al. One thousand pediatric liver transplants during thirty years: lessons learned. *J Am Coll Surg*. 2018:226:355–366. doi:10.1016/j.jamcollsurg.2017.12.042
11. Gorgis NM, Kennedy C, Lam F, et al. Clinical consequences of cardiomyopathy in children with biliary atresia requiring liver transplantation. *Hepatology*. 2019;69:1206–1218. doi:10.1002/hep.30302
12. Aldenkortt F, Aldenkortt M, Caviezel L, et al. Portopulmonary hypertension and hepatopulmonary syndrome. *World J Gastroenterol*. 2014;20:8072–8081. doi:10.3748/wjg.v20.i25.8072
18. Nacoti M, Corbella D, Fazzi F, et al. Coagulopathy and transfusion therapy in pediatric liver transplantation. *World J Gastroenterol*. 2016;22:2005–2023. doi:10.3748/wjg.v22.i6.2005
27. Cuenca AG, Kim HB, Vakili K. Pediatric liver transplantation. *Semin Pediatr Surg*. 2017;26:217–223. doi:10.1053/j.sempedsurg.2017.07.014
30. Organ Procurement and Transplantation Network. 2020. https://optn.transplant.hrsa.gov/data/view-data-reports/build-advanced
31. Davis PJ, Cladis FP. *Smith's Anesthesia for Infants and Children*. Elsevier. 2017;xv.
32. Hatch D. *Pediatric Kidney Transplantation*. 2019. https://emedicine.medscape.com/article/1012654-overview?src=iphone
33. Jaffe RA, Samuels SI, Schmiesing CA, Golianu B. *Anesthesiologist's Manual of Surgical Procedures*. Wolters Kluwer Health/Lippincott Williams; 2009.
34. Vlahakos D, Marathias K, Agroyannis B, Madias N. Posttransplant erythrocytosis, *Kidney Int*. 2003;63(4):1187–1194. doi:10.1046/j.1523-1755.2003.00850.x
35. Azhari H, Rahhal R, Uc A. Is total pancreatectomy with islet autotransplantation a reasonable choice for pediatric pancreatitis? *JOP*. 2015;16(4):335–341.
36. Bellin MD, Schwarzenberg SJ, Cook M, et al. Pediatric autologous islet transplantation. *Curr Diab Rep*. 2015;15(10):67. doi:10.1007/s11892-015-0639-9
37. Kotagal M, Slusher J, Ahmad S, et al. In-hospital and 90-day outcomes after total pancreatectomy with islet autotransplantation for pediatric chronic and acute recurrent pancreatitis. *Am J Transplant*. 2019;19(4):1187–1194. doi:10.1111/ajt.15150
38. Schrope B. Total pancreatectomy with autologous islet cell transplantation. *Gastrointestinal Endoscopy Clinics of North America*. 2018;28:605–618. doi:10.1016/j.giec.2018.05.003
39. Bellin MD, Forlenza GP, Majumder K, et al. Total pancreatectomy with islet autotransplantation resolves pain in young children with severe chronic pancreatitis. *J Pediatr Gastroenterol Nutr*. 2017;64(3):440–445. doi:10.1097/mpg.0000000000001314
40. Bondoc AJ, Abu-El-Haija M, Nathan JD. Pediatric pancreas transplantation, including total pancreatectomy with islet autotransplantation. *Semin Pediatr Surg*. 2017;26(4):250–256. doi:10.1053/j.sempedsurg.2017.07.004
41. Bellin MD, Gelrud A, Arreaza-Rubin G, et al. Total pancreatectomy with islet autotransplantation: summary of an NIDDK workshop. *Ann Surg*. 2015;261(1):21–29. doi:10.1097/SLA.0000000000001059
42. Manciu N, Beebe DS, Tran P, et al. Total pancreatectomy with islet cell autotransplantation: anesthetic implications. *J Clin Anesth*. 1999;11(7):576–582. doi:10.1016/s0952-8180(99)00100-2
43. Yoshimatsu G, Shahbazov R, Saracino G, et al. The impact of allogeneic blood transfusion on the outcomes of total pancreatectomy with islet autotransplantation. *Am J Surg*. 2017;214:849–855. doi:10.1016/j.amjsurg.2017.03.007
44. Hutchins J, Castro C, Wang Q, Chinnakotla S. Postoperative pain control with paravertebral catheters after pediatric total pancreatectomy and islet autotransplantation: a retrospective cohort study. *Pediatr Anesth*. 2016;26(3):315–320. doi:10.1111/pan.12840
45. *Indications/Contraindications*. https://www.med.unc.edu/surgery/transplant/patientinfo/KandP/indications-contraindications

CHAPTER 130

Fetal Surgery

LEARNING OBJECTIVES

- Understand the indications for minimally invasive fetal surgery.
- Discuss the anesthetic management for minimally invasive fetal surgery.
- Understand both maternal and fetal considerations with relation to EXIT (ex utero intrapartum treatment) procedures.
- Discuss the anesthetic management for EXIT procedures.

130.1: MINIMALLY INVASIVE FETAL SURGERY

Jagroop Parikh and Mario Patino

INTRODUCTION

Historically, congenital malformations have been treated with planned delivery at a tertiary care center followed by postnatal repair of the lesion.[1] With advances in both imaging and surgical technique, in addition to enhanced knowledge of fetal pathophysiology, some congenital malformations are now able to be repaired prenatally, which has been associated with improved fetal outcomes. Ultrasound technology has improved in quality and ability to now provide multidimensional images that enhance the sensitivity of diagnosing congenital malformations. The use of ultrasound is not reserved to prenatal assessment, as it is used intraoperatively to locate port site entry and placental location, monitor fetal heart rate, map placental vessels, and monitor umbilical artery blood flow, and to assess the amount of fluid in the uterus.

Fetoscopic surgery has decreased maternal morbidity when compared to open fetal surgery. A large retrospective study of 187 women undergoing intrauterine fetal intervention demonstrated significantly less maternal morbidity in relation to length of stay, intensive care unit admission, and need for transfusion, as compared to open fetal surgery. There was, however, no change between the groups in preterm rupture of membranes or preterm labor.[1]

Innovation in fetal therapy and the search for minimally invasive techniques is essential to continue to expand the benefits and reduce risk to pregnant women; however, formal clinical research can be challenging due to lack of numbers, limited animal models, and hesitancy of patients to consent to research involving their baby.

INDICATIONS/CONTRAINDICATIONS

Minimally invasive fetal surgery offers the ability to repair congenital malformations while minimizing the incidence of issues common after open fetal surgery: preterm labor and premature rupture of membrane (PROM). The ability to avoid these complications that make postpartum care problematic has led many surgeons to choose minimally invasive surgical techniques when appropriate.[2] Minimally invasive fetal surgery can be divided into two categories: fetoscopic techniques and needle-based. Fetoscopic procedures are performed using a single or multiple ports and trocars to gain entry into the amniotic cavity. Small endoscopes allow excellent visualization of fetal and placental structures while normal saline irrigation fluid is used to maintain uterine distension.[3] With this technique, the endoscope is inserted directly into the amniotic cavity using a trocar. Needle-based fetal techniques allow for aspiration of ascitic fluid, pleural effusion, cystic structures, or the bladder while leaving a shunt into the amniotic space.[4] This access is also used in fetal cardiac valvuloplasty and ablation procedures, such as radiofrequency ablation (RFA).

Examples of conditions especially amenable to minimally invasive fetal surgery include twin–twin transfusion syndrome (TTTS) for laser ablation of vessels and myelomeningocele repair. Additional congenital malformations, such as aortic or pulmonary stenosis (valvuloplasty), cyanotic heart disease (atrial septostomy), congenital diaphragmatic hernia (tracheal balloon occlusion), and twin-reversed arterial perfusion (TRAP) (RFA), are all now routinely repair via minimally invasive fetal surgery.[5] Other abnormalities prenatally diagnosed and treated with minimally invasive surgery include lower urinary tract obstruction, congenital diaphragmatic hernia repair, amniotic band syndrome, sacrococcygeal teratoma (SCT), congenital cystic adenomatoid malformations, and pleural effusions. Lower urinary tract obstruction is most often caused by posterior urethral valves (PUVs), urethral atresia, or prune belly syndrome.[4] With fetal intervention and relief of urinary obstruction, the resultant increased in amniotic fluid promotes lung development and maturity.

TWIN–TWIN TRANSFUSION SYNDROME

Prenatal repair of TTTS especially has seen significant improvements in success rates, largely due to the use of ultrasound in prenatal diagnosis and assessment. TTTS complicates 10% to 20% of monochorionic twin pregnancies and leads to a circulatory imbalance between the twins.[2] Clinical effects of TTTS are not seen until the second trimester. With TTTS, the recipient is often larger and at risk of cardiac overload with the donor typically smaller and hypoperfused. Both twins, however, are at risk of severe morbidity: the donor twin from hypoxic-ischemic injuries and growth restriction, and the recipient twin from cardiac decompensation and hydrops.[4] Disease severity is staged using Quintero staging and both clinical and ultrasonographic criteria (Table 130.1).

Following diagnosis, laser ablation is the technique of choice to correct this imbalance. A randomized control trial in Europe, named the Eurofetus trial, found that outcomes following fetoscopic laser photocoagulation for TTTS were improved when compared with the previous standard therapy of amnioreduction. This trial also demonstrated increased 6-month infant survival without major neurological morbidity.[1]

MYELOMENINGOCELE REPAIR

Myelomeningocele (MMC) is characterized by an incomplete closure of the neural tube leading to exposure of spinal

Table 130.1	Quintero Staging of Twin–Twin Transfusion Syndrome	
Stage	Ultrasound Parameter	Categorical criteria
I	MVP of amniotic fluid	MVP <2 cm in donor sac; MVP >8 cm in recipient sac
II	Fetal bladder	Unable to visualize bladder in donor twin after 60 mins
III	Umbilical artery, ductus venosus, umbilical vein Doppler waveforms	Absent or reversed umbilical artery diastolic flow, reversed ductus venosus a-wave flow, pulsatile umbilical vein flow
IV	Fetal hydrops	Hydrops in one or both twins
V	Absent fetal cardiac activity	Fetal demise in one or both twins

MVP, maximal vertical pocket.

Source: From Simpson L and Society for Maternal-Fetal Medicine (SMFM). Twin–twin transfusion syndrome. American Journal of obstetrics and gynecology. January 2013.

tissue. MMC is quite often associated with Arnold–Chiari II malformation, resulting in hydrocephalus and need for surgery to establish ventriculoperitoneal shunting of cerebrospinal fluid. Animal models of fetal MMC supported a two-hit hypothesis in which the first hit is the neural tube defect and the second hit is trauma to the exposed neural tissue while in utero.[2]

To assess the effectiveness of fetal surgery to correct MMC, the National Institutes of Health sponsored a multicenter randomized trial, the MOMS (management of myelomeningocele study) in which the outcomes following fetal MMC repair at 19 to 26 weeks' gestation were compared to those following postnatal repair (Table 130.2). The study concluded prior to its expected date as the results demonstrated that the outcomes following fetal MMC repair were significantly superior to those following postnatal repair. Fetal MMC repair not only reduced the need for ventriculoperitoneal shunting for hydrocephalus at 1 year of age, patients demonstrated improved motor function with the ability to walk at 30 months of age.[4] Disease morbidity, however, did remain high, and there were associated maternal complications with prenatal repair including spontaneous membrane rupture (46%), chorioamniotic membrane separation (26%), and placental abruption (6%).

ANESTHETIC MANAGEMENT

As the incision sites associated with minimally invasive fetal surgery are small, these procedures can often be performed under local anesthesia and maternal sedation. For maternal anxiolysis, IV midazolam followed by IV sedation is often administered. Most fetoscopic procedures involve manipulation of the placenta and umbilical cord and do not require fetal incision. Therefore, fetal anesthesia is rarely indicated for these procedures.[3] A mobile fetus could, however, displace the endoscope causing bleeding, fetal trauma, or compromised umbilical circulation.[2] Alternatively, if additional uterine manipulation is needed then regional anesthesia may be used. The choice of anesthetic is decided on after a conversation between the surgeon and anesthesia provider. Multidisciplinary fetal teams consisting of a fetal surgeon, maternal–fetal medicine (MFM), ultrasound tech, and anesthesia team trained in providing fetal anesthesia are critical to the delivery of quality care.

Table 130.2	Comparison of Outcomes of Minimally Invasive Myelomeningocele Repair and Open Fetal Surgery	
Outcome	MOMS Trial, Prenatal Surgery Cohort (n=78), n (%)	Case Series Review (n=51), n (%)
Aborted procedure	0	1 (2)
Chorioamniotic membrane separation	20 (26)	1 (2)
Maternal chorioamnionitis	2 (3)	4 (8)
Spontaneous membrane rupture / amniotic fluid leakage	26 (46)	43 (84)
Placental abruption	5 (6)	0
Mean GA at delivery (week +/− SD)	34.1 +/− 3.1	33 +/− 2.8
GA at birth <30 wks	10 (13)	9 (13)
GA at birth >35 wks	42 (54)	17 (23)
Perinatal deaths	2 (3)	4 (8)
Death within 1st yr of life	2 (3)	5 (7)
Postnatal recovery needed	N/A	20 (28)
Shunt within 1st yr of life	Criteria met: 51 (65) Shunt placed: 31 (40)	32 (45)
Chiari decompression surgery needed	1	3 (4)

GA, gestational age; MOMS, management of myelomeningocele study; N/A, not applicable.

Source: From Graves C, Harrison M, Padilla B. Minimally invasive fetal surgery. *Clin Perionatol.* 2017 Dec;44(4):729–751.

PREOPERATIVE EVALUATION

Optimal anesthetic technique for fetal surgical procedures depends on the planned surgical approach, the extent of fetal surgical stimulation, and the maternal and fetal medical history.[6] Important things to consider with minimally invasive fetal surgery include the number, position, and size of port sites; anticipated placenta location; maternal risk factors; and the surgeon and patient preference. The preanesthetic evaluation focuses on the maternal medical history with focus placed on obstetric history, additional medical problems, medication allergies, anesthetic history, and current medications. A physical examination is performed with focus on the cardiovascular, pulmonary, airway examination, and back anatomy. For minimally invasive fetal procedures, a preoperative ultrasound is performed to garner information related to the gestational age of the fetus and placental location, which affects the anesthetic choice. After a discussion with the surgical team, a decision is made regarding the anesthetic technique. For the majority of these procedures, either a regional anesthesia technique or local anesthesia with sedation is chosen.

ANESTHETIC TECHNIQUE

Intraoperative Management

Most patients receive IV midazolam for anxiolysis prior to the operating room (OR), in addition to Bicitra® and metoclopramide for stomach acid neutralization and enhanced gastric emptying, respectively. For patients with an anterior placenta, a regional technique involving placement of a lumbar epidural or a combined spinal epidural (CSE) at the level of L3–4 is chosen. In this scenario, regional anesthesia helps temper discomfort related to manipulation of the uterus and maternal positioning in order to create a surgical window. The epidural is typically dosed with 2% lidocaine, in divided doses to avoid a precipitous drop in blood pressure, and titrated to obtain a T6 sensory level of anesthesia. The epidural catheter may be redosed for lengthy procedures or if the patient exhibits increased sensation and pain. A Foley catheter is placed prior to incision in the case of epidural or CSE placement. The epidural catheter is removed at the conclusion of the procedure.

The mother is also administered sedative medication throughout the procedure for anxiolysis. Infusions of both dexmedetomidine (0.2–0.6 mcg/kg/hr) and remifentanil (0.05 mcg/kg/min) are reasonable options for providing maternal sedation, with remifentanil having the additional advantage of crossing the placenta and causing fetal immobility. The dosages for each infusion listed are starting points and can be titrated as needed.

When a preoperative ultrasound shows a posterior placenta, the anesthetic technique of choice includes administration of local anesthetic at the port sites by the surgeon, as well as maternal sedation. As with patients with an anterior placenta, maternal sedation typically includes either a low-dose dexmedetomidine or remifentanil infusion. Pain management can be supplemented with 25 to 50 mcg of IV fentanyl if the mother is uncomfortable, although patients routinely do not need to be administered medications for control of postoperative pain.

During all procedures, the mother is monitored with standard American Society of Anesthesiologists monitors and placed in a supine position with left uterine displacement. An ultrasound is performed by the MFM physician and a surgical window is defined. This may entail repositioning the patient in lateral position to optimize access to the surgical window. The MFM performs ultrasound intermittently throughout the case to monitor fetal cardiac activity and umbilical blood flow. Use of ultrasound also allows for an assessment of amniotic fluid volume. At the end of the procedure, IV ondansetron should be administered and the patient is taken to the fetal care unit for recovery.

Tocolysis is essential after fetal surgery due to the elevated risk of preterm labor. The medication choice is determined by the MFM physician, taking into consideration potential maternal side effects. There are rare instances when the uterus begins to contract at the end of the procedure; therefore, it may be prudent to leave the epidural catheter in place postoperatively should delivery be imminent and unavoidable. Additionally, given the risk of postoperative pulmonary edema associated with the administration of tocolytics, IV fluids are limited to 1 liter for the entire case to prevent further complications.

Complications

Complications of minimally invasive fetal surgery include bleeding, amniotic fluid leak, chorioamniotic separation, chorioamnionitis, PROM, preterm birth, and fetal demise.[4] Per Graves et al.,[4] a systematic review of 1,376 minimally invasive procedures for TTTS, lower urinary tract obstruction, and TRAP sequence identified maximum instrument diameter and maximum number of ports as predictors of iatrogenic preterm PROM (PPROM).

130.2: Ex Utero Intrapartum Therapy Procedures

Jagroop Parikh and Mario Patino

INTRODUCTION

The EXIT procedure involves the performance of a maternal hysterotomy with the exposure of the fetus to perform a fetal intervention. This surgical approach maintains uteroplacental perfusion and uterine relaxation with a posterior clamping of the umbilical cord with the delivery of the newborn. In many instances, this surgical approach is employed to allow establishment of a secure airway prior to separation from the placenta. While a variety of indications exist, EXIT procedures ultimately enable surgeons the ability to avert potentially fatal neonatal emergencies in a controlled environment that optimize fetal outcomes.

INDICATIONS/CONTRAINDICATIONS

The indications for EXIT procedures can be classified as EXIT to airway, EXIT to resection, EXIT to extracorporeal membrane oxygenation (ECMO), and EXIT to separation.[8] The most common surgical approach, EXIT to airway, allows for surgical airway management while maintaining fetal support via uteroplacental flow. Fetal anomalies with potential significant airway involvement requiring EXIT to airway include extrinsic neck masses, such as lymphatic malformations, cystic hygroma, vascular malformations, cervical teratoma, neuroblastoma, thymic cysts, and goiter. Intrinsic airway obstruction, which leads to congenital high airway syndrome (CHAOS), such as laryngeal cyst, laryngeal atresia, tracheal stenosis and tracheal atresia, also often require EXIT to airway procedures. EXIT to resection is considered in the treatment of conditions exhibiting rapid-growth masses exerting significant effect on the fetus, such as congenital cystic adenomatoid malformation (CCAM) of the lung and

SCTs. A CCAM can cause significant pulmonary hypoplasia and mediastinal deviation, while the SCT can progress into high output heart failure. If untreated, most of these conditions can progress into a life-threatening hydrops. Indications for EXIT to ECMO include severe congenital diaphragmatic hernia and severe congenital heart disease. EXIT to separation has been occasionally reported in cases of conjoined twins.[9]

MULTIDISCIPLINARY TEAM INVOLVEMENT IN EXIT PROCEDURES

A multidisciplinary approach is essential in the perioperative management of an EXIT procedure. EXIT procedures require highly coordinated teamwork, with a strong emphasis on rigorous planning and excellent communication among all team members. A variety of providers from diverse clinical backgrounds are often involved, such as fetal maternal medicine, pediatric general surgery with specific training in fetal surgery, pediatric otolaryngology, pediatric anesthesia providers with experience in fetal anesthesia, pediatric radiology, pediatric cardiology, pediatric cardiac interventionism, pediatric neurosurgery, neonatology, nursing team from both the OR and from neonatology, genetic counseling, and a social worker.

A preoperative meeting with all members of the team is essential to review the fetal diagnostic studies, the severity of the disease process, any other fetal concerns or anomalies, and maternal concerns and comorbidities. The surgical plan must be established with input from all members of the team, with alternative plans clearly delineated. All concerns and questions raised by any member of the team must be immediately addressed and resolved. During the planning phase, assignment of tasks must be done in a manner that ensures simultaneous or sequential tasks are performed in an efficient, effective, and coordinated manner. In many instances, team members are invited to participate in a preoperative simulation that allows different approaches to be vetted, which offers the potential to reduce conflict, confusion, poor communication, and ineffective teamwork especially during the most critical parts of the EXIT procedure. Perhaps most important, the preoperative meeting must include a thorough discussion emphasizing the risks and benefits of the plan with the patient, allowing ample time to answer questions and obtain consent. When obtaining surgical and anesthesia consent, it is imperative that blood transfusion consent be obtained as well given the high probability of blood transfusion during an EXIT procedure.

SPECIAL CONSIDERATIONS AND CONCERNS

MATERNAL ANESTHETIC CONSIDERATIONS

It is important to maintain the principle of providing fetal therapy during an EXIT procedure that is of reasonable benefit to the fetus while minimizing maternal risk. Therefore, patient selection is critical before proceeding with an EXIT procedure as excessive maternal risk must be considered a contraindication. During the maternal evaluation, it is important to explore the presence of any comorbidities and the degree of severity of any comorbidities if present and to establish an optimization plan if necessary. Previous anesthesia records should be reviewed with a focus on airway management, difficulties with regional anesthesia, or any other noted complications. A complete physical examination, with emphasis on airway evaluation and examination of the patient's back in preparation of neuraxial anesthesia, should be performed. A review of preoperative studies, specifically the fetal ultrasound and fetal magnetic resonance imaging (MRI), is key as they may uncover incidental findings of maternal anomalies.

Maternal anesthetic considerations associated with an EXIT procedure are largely guided by the physiological changes that occur during pregnancy. This includes the risk of aspiration, which is highest during induction of anesthesia due to the increased levels of estrogen and progesterone, both of which decrease the lower esophageal tone. In addition, increased secretion of gastrin from the placenta increases overall gastric hydrogen secretion and the gravid uterus positioned over the gastrointestinal tract produces mechanical effects that increase the risk of aspiration. Hence, aspiration prophylaxis entails administration of a nonparticulate antacid, metoclopramide, and an H2 receptor antagonist, such as ranitidine.

There are multiple physiological changes during pregnancy that impact the airway including airway capillary engorgement, volume increases of the soft tissues surrounding the airway, and generalized airway edema. Therefore, anesthetic planning should include management of the airway with anticipation of the need for alternative intubation techniques and the need to implement the difficult airway algorithm.[10] The use of a small endotracheal tube (ETT) size, such as a 6.0 mm to 6.5 mm, is recommended. Increases in multiple coagulation factors and decreased production of antithrombin III and tissue plasminogen activator (tPA) increase the risk of thromboembolic events during the prothrombotic stage of pregnancy. Therefore, the use of compression pneumatic devices in the lower extremities during the perioperative care of these patients is strongly recommended. Aortocaval compression by the gravid uterus can compromise the venous return, cardiac output, and uteroplacental flow leading to fetal distress and acidosis. It is important to place a wedge underneath the mother to provide left uterine displacement, which aids in minimizing the deleterious effects of the aortocaval compression. As uteroplacental flow lacks the ability to autoregulate and is entirely dependent of uterine perfusion pressure, maneuvers such as this are necessary to ensure fetal blood supply throughout the procedure. In addition, the use of vasopressors is commonly required to maintain the uterine perfusion pressure.[11] A consideration when performing neuraxial anesthesia is the engorgement of the epidural veins secondary to increases in intra-abdominal pressure. Engorgement of the epidural veins may increase the incidence of intravascular epidural catheter placement.

FETAL ANESTHETIC CONSIDERATIONS

It is important to understand the presenting fetal anomaly, the natural history of the process, and the severity of the congenital malformation. In addition, it is important to have a sound understanding of the management options and the planned surgical approach, as well as the risks and benefits of the EXIT procedure to the fetus as opposed to postnatal intervention. The rapid improvement of the prenatal diagnostic tools, such as high-resolution ultrasound, different ultrasound modalities, and MRI, has made evaluation of fetal congenital malformations precise and plays a key role in preoperative planning prior to an EXIT procedure. It is important to review in detail the preoperative fetal studies, not just to identify the disease process and severity but to also evaluate the progression of the anomaly by comparing studies performed at different gestational ages. Other critical information to gather preoperatively includes the position of

Table 130.3 Average Fetal–Maternal Ratios of Common Medications

Medications	Fetal:Maternal Ratio
Halothane	0.7–0.9
Isoflurane	0.7
Nitrous oxide	0.83
Thiopental	0.4–1.1
Propofol	0.5–0.85
Diazepam	1–2
Midazolam	0.76
Morphine	0.61
Fentanyl	0.16–1.2
Remifentanil	0.29–0.88
Ephedrine	0.7
Vecuronium	0.06–0.11
Glycopyrrolate	0.22
Nitroglycerin	0.18
Phenylephrine	0.17
Dexmedetomidine	0.12

Notes: Medications with high ratios (>0.6) are associated with considerable transfer to the placenta. It is important to realize that given the molecular weight and the molecular structure, sugammadex has very low placental transfer.

BOX 130.1 LYMPHATIC MALFORMATION STAGING SYSTEM

Stage I: no evidence of polyhydramnios with free egress of amniotic fluid and clear visualization of the aryepiglottic folds and larynx

Stage II: lesions of the tongue or epiglottis present but with normal aryepiglottic folds without polyhydramnios

Stage III: lesions of the tongue or larynx; no visualization of the aryepiglottic folds without free egress of amniotic fluid along with polyhydramnios

Stage III: lesions are associated with lesions at risk of airway compromise at birth

Source: From American Pediatric Surgical Association. Prenatal Counseling Series - Fetal Neck Masses. 2018. https://eapsa.org/apsa/media/Documents/APSA-Fetal-Neck-Masses-Broch_FNL.pdf.

---

the placenta to guide patient positioning that facilitates access to the fetus. Preoperative fetal evaluation should also include karyotyping to rule out additional genetic abnormalities that require further counseling.

Determination of the fetal weight is key to allow for weight-based calculation of medications, including resuscitation drugs and transfusion needs. It is important to understand the potential effects any medication administered to the mother may have on the fetus. The transfer of medications through the placenta depends on the fetal:maternal gradient, as well as the degree of innate maternal protein binding, and the liposolubility, molecular weight, and degree of ionization of the medication administered (Table 130.3).

EXIT procedures are a viable means of repairing a variety of congenital malformations or facilitating the safe transition from uteroplacental flow to independent neonatal circulation. With EXIT to airway procedures, fetal neck lesions are the most common indication with most of these lesions diagnosed during a routine ultrasound. Important characteristics to evaluate are the anatomical location, growth pattern, presence of polyhydramnios, characteristics of the lesion, such as a solid or cystic mass, and the potential progression to hydrops. In the case of lymphatic malformations, it is important to evaluate the involvement of the tongue, larynx, and the aryepiglottic folds. A lymphatic malformation staging system has been developed to determine the degree of airway involvement with three grades of stages ranging from no polyhydramnios or involvement of tongue, larynx, or aryepiglottic folds to the most severe form with severe polyhydramnios with significant airway involvement and no visualization of the aryepiglottic folds (Box 130.1).[12]

Another important tool to determine the severity of a neck mass with the potential to a difficult airway is the evaluation of the tracheoesophageal displacement index (TEDI), which calculates the degree of esophageal and tracheal deviation from the spine (Figure 130.1). Specifically, the TEDI is calculated by adding the lateral and ventral displacement of the trachea and esophagus from the ventral aspect of the cervical spine of fetal MRI. A TEDI more than 12 mm indicates a complicated airway.[13] Other characteristics associated with more difficult airway management are severe polyhydramnios and the presence of a cervical teratoma. Therefore, fetus without polyhydramnios, with the etiology of the neck mass being different to a cervical teratoma and with a TEDI less than 12 mm, can be delivered without the need for an EXIT procedure.

Fetal airway management during an EXIT procedure may include direct laryngoscopy, rigid bronchoscopy, retrograde airway intubation, or tracheostomy. Total or partial excision of a tumor or mass, whether it be in the neck, such as a cervical teratoma; in the intrathoracic cavity, such as a CCAM of the lung; or the presence of an SCT, is another common indication for EXIT procedures. The severity of a CCAM is determined

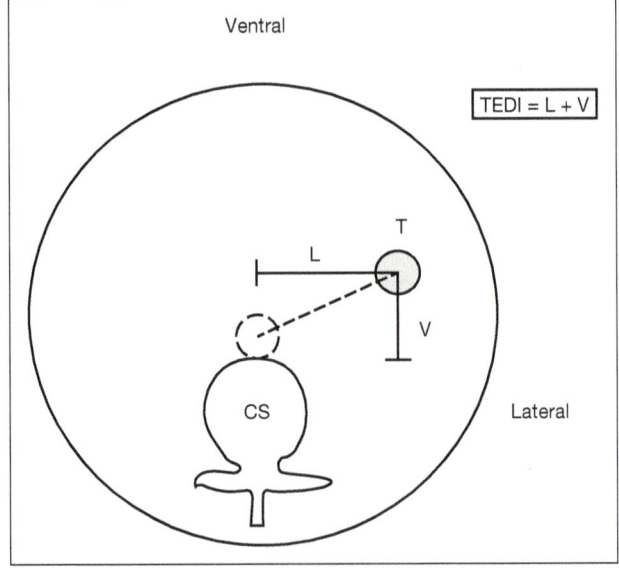

Figure 130.1: Tracheoesophageal displacement index (TEDI) evaluated with a fetal MRI.

> **BOX 130.2 STAGING OF SACROCOCCYGEAL TERATOMAS**
>
> - Type I: completely external, no presacral component
> - Type II: external component and internal pelvic component
> - Type III: external component and internal component extending into abdomen
> - Type IV: completely internal and no external component
>
> Source: From Bianchi DW, Crombleholme TM, D'Alton ME. *Fetology: Diagnosis and Management of the Fetal Patient.* McGraw-Hill; 2000.

using the CCAM volume ratio (CVR), which is calculated via ultrasound by dividing the volume by the head circumference. A CVR greater than 2 correlates with a high risk of developing hydrops, as well as the need for a fetal intervention.[14] SCTs are another congenital malformation that may require an EXIT to resection procedure. SCTs can lead to polyhydramnios, high-output heart failure, hemorrhage, and maternal mirror fetal syndrome. SCTs are usually diagnosed during a routine ultrasound. Once identified, additional testing is required to determine size, the solid and cystic component, vascular supply, and presence of calcifications. Staging of SCTs is largely based on the degree of extension of the lesion, taking into consideration if the lesion is external, invades the pelvis, invades the abdomen, or is solely internal (**Box 130.2**). The tumor volume to fetal weight ratio (TFR) is a key prognostic factor when evaluating SCTs. TFR is determined with ultrasound or MRI by dividing the total tumor volume by the estimated fetal weight before the 24th week of gestation. A TFR >0.12 is associated with 60% mortality and 80% incidence of hydrops. Other factors of poor prognosis in fetus with SCTs include a solid component, spinal canal involvement, high vascularity, rapid growth, heart failure, and hydrops. EXIT to resection for SCTs is especially indicated when there is a high risk of exsanguination secondary to the rupture of highly vascularized SCTs.[15-17] EXIT to ECMO can be performed for the fetus with severe congenital diaphragmatic hernia, although this is not common due to the unclear benefits.[18] Likewise, EXIT to ECMO for the fetus with severe cardiac disease is rarely performed in a life-threatening situation.

ANESTHETIC MANAGEMENT

PREOPERATIVE EVALUATION

A comprehensive preoperative evaluation prior to fetal surgery involves examination of both the mother and fetus. A focused evaluation of the mother preoperatively includes obtaining a medical history, a list of medications and allergies, an investigation of any previous anesthesia-related events, and a thorough physical examination. Due to the nature of maternal physiological changes associated with pregnancy, it is imperative that a focused physical examination includes assessment of the airway, heart, lungs, and back. The airway examination should clearly document Mallampati score, thyromental distance, and mouth opening. The back examination is important as an epidural will likely be placed to mitigate postoperative pain. Information collected about the fetus should include a review of fetal imaging that outlines the fetal defect and a fetal echocardiogram. The fetal echocardiogram will provide a baseline assessment of cardiac performance prior to intervention. The fetal echocardiogram will be repeated throughout the intraoperative period by the MFM or a fetal cardiologist to ongoing assessment of changes in fetal heart rate and/or contractility. Finally, the estimated fetal weight should be obtained. This will guide dosage of medication administration to the fetus should they be needed to maintain adequate fetal heart rate, provide pain relief, or produce fetal immobility.

The anesthetic management options should be discussed in detail with the mother, with ample time available to offer the opportunity to answer any questions the mother may have. In addition to general anesthesia, an epidural may be placed to provide postoperative analgesia. Epidural placement, including the associated risks and the use of multimodal therapies, should be discussed with the patient.

ANESTHETIC TECHNIQUE

Intraoperative Management

Prior to the start of the procedure, the mother should receive aspiration prophylaxis consisting of metoclopramide 10 mg IV and bicitra PO, as well as an IV anxiolytic (midazolam). There are two anesthesia techniques commonly employed for EXIT procedures: general anesthesia and regional anesthesia. A determining factor is the complexity of fetal defect and the time anticipated for fetal intervention. Should the plan entail general anesthesia, an epidural is placed at the level of T11–12 and dosed at the end of the procedure with 0.2% ropivicaine (10–15 mL) to provide postoperative pain control. After successful epidural placement, the patient is positioned supine with left uterine displacement. If general anesthesia is planned, a rapid sequence induction should be performed after adequate preoxygenation. Due to physiological changes associated with pregnancy, a smaller sized ETT should be used for intubation, commonly a 6.0 or 6.5 ETT. Difficult airway equipment including a laryngeal mask airway, C-MAC, or fiberoptic scope should be readily available. There are some EXIT cases, which are performed under regional anesthesia. In this scenario, a combined spinal epidural is placed at the beginning of the case and dosed with 12 to 14 mg of 0.75% bupivacaine. For EXIT procedures that involve a more complex repair or extended time on uteroplacental supply, general anesthesia for the mother is optimal to further control operating conditions, tackle hemodynamic changes, and avoid increased maternal anxiety.

Regardless of the anesthesia technique utilized, the patient should have two peripheral IV catheters and an arterial line placed prior to the start of the procedure. An arterial line that allows for continuous blood pressure monitoring, which is key during an EXIT procedure due to the elevated dose of volatile anesthetics, typically desflurane, is required to provide uterine relaxation when general anesthesia is the anesthesia technique employed. Commonly, the concentration of desflurane is increased to 10% to 12% to provide uterine relaxation. This elevated concentration, however, predisposes the patient to hypotension. Uterine relaxation is achieved with nitroglycerin boluses of 30 to 50 mcg or a nitroglycerin infusion if regional anesthesia is the technique employed. To mitigate issues related to hypotension, vasopressors are often used, either in incremental doses or as a continuous infusion, to combat the ensuing hypotension. The vasopressor of choice is phenylephrine; however, both phenylephrine and ephedrine have been used with success in correction of blood pressure. The surgeons

> **BOX 130.3 COMMONLY USED UTEROTONIC MEDICATIONS**
>
> - Oxytocin 20 units diluted in 1,000 mL LR or NS. Infusion of 5–10 IU/hr for 4 hours. A slow 3 IU bolus of oxytocin can be given after the delivery of the placenta. Avoid the administration of a rapid IV bolus that causes hypotension and may result in cardiovascular collapse.
> - Methergine 0.2 mg IM
> - Hemabate 250 mcg IM
>
> LR, lactated Ringer's; NS, normal saline.

> **BOX 130.4 POTENTIAL RISKS ASSOCIATED WITH EXIT PROCEDURES**
>
> Difficult airway
> Reflux and aspiration
> Amniotic fluid embolism
> Blood loss
> Failed regional technique
> Impaired uterine tone
>
> EXIT, ex utero intrapartum treatment.

continuously monitor the degree of uterine relaxation through manual touch to ensure optimal operating conditions are maintained throughout the procedure.

Due to the profound, and sometimes prolonged, uterine relaxation needed to perform the surgical intervention, the potential for profound blood loss exists. Communication with the surgical team is key to assess estimated blood loss and the potential need for blood transfusion. Fortunately, there is no limitation placed on the volume of IV fluids during EXIT procedures as the pregnancy is not going to continue and the fetus is going to be delivered. This is especially important as there is the potential for major fluid shifts and blood loss, albeit the likelihood is rare. In general, the anticipated blood loss is expected to be very similar, if not slightly higher, than that witnessed during a cesarean section.

Uteroplacental circulation is dependent on maternal perfusion, which is maintained throughout the intervention until surgical completion, at which point the cord is clamped and uterine tone becomes imperative. Uterotonic agents, which increase uterine contraction, are utilized to increase uterine tone at this time (Box 130.3).

Fetus Management

Estimated fetal weight is used to direct dosing of IM fetal medications, which is administered to the fetus upon exposure. This typical regimen includes atropine (20 mcg/kg), fentanyl (20 mcg/kg), and vecuronium (0.2 mg/kg) and ensures maintenance of fetal heart rate, pain control, and immobility. Some airway interventions performed while the fetus continues to receive placental support, thus they do not require the aforementioned combination of medications as they are relatively quick procedures. Intermittent ultrasound of the fetal heart is performed by the MFM to monitor fetal heart rate and direct any further intervention deemed necessary by the anesthesia provider. In some EXIT procedures involving more significant or complex intervention with the potential for fetal blood loss, a fetal cardiologist may be present to perform continuous fetal echocardiography to monitor cardiac filling, heart rate, and contractility. In cases where intervention is needed, the anesthesia provider will have access to a fetal peripheral intravenous catheter (PIV) placed by the surgeon in order to administer additional fluids or blood products (Box 130.4).

POSTOPERATIVE CARE

Epidural catheters are placed at the low thoracic level (T11–12) at the start of EXIT procedures to allow for dosing and control of postoperative pain. In some EXIT procedures, a CSE is placed at the L4–5 level, allowing for the epidural catheter to be dosed at the end of the procedure with an additional 0.2% ropivacaine and 3 to 4 mg of duramorph. Should the mother receive general anesthesia, the epidural catheter is dosed with 0.2% ropivacaine and 3 to 4 mg of duramorph at the end of the case when the mother is hemodynamically stable. Postoperative pain control should also include IV toradol 15 mg every 6 hours, alternating with IV acetaminophen 1,000 mg every 6 hours.

KEY TAKEAWAYS

- Fetal surgery is a growing subspecialty requiring unique anesthetic management administered by a specialty team.
- Minimally invasive fetal surgery is performed most commonly to treat TTTS using selective laser photocoagulation. The anesthetic plan for this subset of procedures is either regional anesthesia or maternal sedation with surgical administration of local skin infiltration.
- EXIT procedures require multiple teams to provide care for both the mother and fetus. Anesthetic management is focused on both maternal and fetal considerations.
- The success of fetal surgery is a direct reflection of communication among all specialty teams involved.

KEY REFERENCES

Complete references for this chapter are online and available at https://connect.springerpub.com/content/book/978-0-8261-3875-0/part/part05/toc-part/ch130.

1. Maselli K, Badillo A. Advances in fetal surgery. *Ann Transl Med*. 2016 Oct;4(20):394. doi:10.21037/atm.2016.10.34
5. Sviggum H, Kodali B. Maternal anesthesia for fetal surgery. *Clin Perinatol*. 2013 Sep;40(3):413–427. doi:10.1016/j.clp.2013.05.012
6. Hoagland M, Chatterjee D. Anesthesia for fetal surgery. *Paediatr Anaesth*. 2017 Apr;27(4):346–357. doi:10.1111/pan.13109
9. Bouchard S, Johnson MP, Flake AW, et al. The EXIT procedure: experience and outcome in 31 cases. *J Pediatr Surg*. 2002;37(3):418–426. doi:10.1053/jpsu.2002.30839
14. Cass DL, Olutoye OO, Cassady CI, et al. Prenatal diagnosis and outcome of fetal lung masses. *J Pediatr Surg*. 2011;46(2):292–298. doi:10.1016/j.jpedsurg.2010.11.004
18. Stoffan AP, Wilson JM, Jennings RW, Wilkins-Haug LE, Buchmiller TL. Does the ex utero intrapartum treatment to extracorporeal membrane oxygenation procedure change outcomes for high-risk patients with congenital diaphragmatic hernia? *J Pediatr Surg*. 2012;47(6):1053–1057. doi:10.1016/j.jpedsurg.2012.03.004

CHAPTER 131

Pediatric Pain Management

131.1: Regional Anesthesia

James Furstein, Nancy B. Samol, David L. Moore, and Marc Mecoli

LEARNING OBJECTIVES

- Describe the indications for regional anesthesia in the pediatric patient, as well as appropriate patient selection criteria.
- Enumerate the benefits of regional anesthesia for pain management, specifically as they apply to the pediatric population.
- Describe potential risks and complications of regional anesthesia in children along with current management strategies.

INTRODUCTION

The use of regional anesthesia for pediatric patients has evolved over the past several decades from a seldom performed technique to an integral aspect of clinical practice in pediatric facilities worldwide.[1] The rationale for this widespread evolution in practice is multifactorial, as there are a variety of inherent qualities that make regional anesthesia techniques both ideal and cost-effective.[1,2]

The use of regional anesthesia affords clinicians the ability to reduce, if not eliminate, the incidence of opioid-induced negative sequelae that routinely delay discharge following ambulatory surgery.[3] The ability to provide site-specific analgesia, coupled with the ability to reduce opioid requirements, ultimately has the potential to yield patients who are comfortable and symptom free in the immediate postoperative period. The improved patient outcomes experienced in the postanesthesia care unit (PACU) lend themselves to increased nursing efficiency, as fewer interventions are necessary, thereby reducing system delays and freeing up PACU resources.

Similarly, the time until discharge criteria is met indicates the length of time elapsed from the end of surgery until a patient is deemed ready for discharge home following surgery. As the length of this period varies among patients, it is often used as a measure when comparing analgesic efficacy.[4] The excellent analgesia afforded by regional anesthesia techniques, coupled with the reduction in opioid requirements, facilitates a swift, painless transition through the postoperative period.[2]

Regional anesthesia may also play a role in accelerating the healing process as well.[5] Compared with opioid analgesia, regional anesthesia has proved to improve postoperative analgesia, reducing overall opioid requirements and the associated nausea, vomiting, pruritus, and sedation.[6]

INDICATIONS/CONTRAINDICATIONS

While opioids have long been the mainstay of acute pain management, a multimodal approach to preventing and relieving pain has become widely accepted. Opioids elicit unwanted side effects such as nausea, vomiting, pruritus, somnolence, urinary retention, and hypoventilation.[7] The combination of nonopioid analgesics, local and regional analgesia, along with low-dose narcotics as needed, frequently minimizes these unwanted side effects. Therefore, there has been a concerted effort to incorporate regional anesthesia if there are no precluding factors.

Absolute contraindications to neuraxial anesthesia include patient or parent refusal, local infection at injection site, increased intracranial pressure, severe hypovolemia, severe coagulopathy, and an allergy to local anesthetics (LA,). The same contraindications apply to peripheral nerve blockade (PNB), with the exception of increased intracranial pressure. Relative contraindications include sepsis, neurological dysfunction, severe anatomic abnormalities, and tattoos at the site of injection. In addition, certain conditions may generate cause for consideration including skin lesions at the proposed site of injection, a severe systemic infection, severe thrombocytopenia, allergy to the LA, preexisting neurological injury or neuropathy in the nerve to be blocked, and patient and/or parental refusal. A bandage, brace, or cast on the operative limb and, while not a strict contraindication, requires increased monitoring for signs of compression or decreased perfusion postoperatively.

SPECIAL CONSIDERATIONS AND CONCERNS

ANATOMIC CONSIDERATIONS

Without question, significant anatomic and physiological variations exist between adults and children that impact the provision of regional anesthesia. Children are smaller than adults, requiring greater precision through slow movements and fine adjustments of the needle when advancing to the targeted injection site. Needle length and the depth of the targeted nerve also change with age. The volume of distribution, rate of bone growth and ossification, and termination of the spinal cord and dural sac, with reference to the bony spine, all change from infancy to adolescence and impact drug dose, needle location, and landmark identification using ultrasound.

Conversely, there are benefits that can be attributed to anatomic variations in children. For instance, neural structures are more readily anesthetized in pediatric patients due to having a thinner myelin sheath, short intermodal distance, and small fiber diameter. The loose connective tissue around neuraxial structures and nerve sheaths also allows for a more pronounced spread of LA following injection, as well as easing advancement of indwelling nerve catheters for continuous PNB.[8]

COMBINED GENERAL AND REGIONAL ANESTHESIA

While performing regional anesthesia on deeply sedated or anesthetized adults has long been debated, there is substantially less debate among pediatric anesthesia providers regarding the same practice in children. Challenges with patient cooperation and communication constitute the major difference in approach to performing regional anesthesia in adults versus children. In adults, the use of regional anesthesia while awake or mildly sedated allows for feedback regarding pain or paresthesia, which may signify a nerve injury.[9] The concern when performing regional anesthesia in children who are lightly sedated or under general anesthesia is the potential for unrecognized catastrophic neurological sequelae, possibly due to needle-phobia, poor patient cooperation, or the inability of the patient to reliably report paresthesia.[9,10] Nonetheless, performing regional anesthesia on patients under general anesthesia remains the standard practice for most pediatric anesthesia providers.

In fact, pediatric anesthesia providers will assert that performing regional anesthesia on patients under general anesthesia provides the ideal environment. As regional anesthesia depends on the accuracy of needle guidance and the injection of local anesthesia in relation to the targeted nerve, having an immobile patient is arguably paramount.[11] General anesthesia also eliminates anxiety, pain, and fear of needle insertion in an awake child, thereby allowing for placement in an unimpeded, proficient manner. Recent practice advisory guidelines issued by the American Society of Regional Anesthesia offer that the benefit of ensuring a cooperative and immobile infant or child may outweigh the risk of performing neuraxial regional anesthesia in pediatric patients undergoing general anesthesia or heavy sedation. Moreover, a recent multicenter study found that in 100,000 pediatric nerve blocks, there was no additional risk observed when placing blocks under general anesthesia. As with any case, however, it is recommended that anesthesia providers develop an individualized anesthetic plan that ensures the delivery of safe, effective care.

ANESTHETIC MANAGEMENT
PREOPERATIVE EVALUATION

As with any anesthetic, a thorough history and physical should be attained prior to performing regional anesthesia. In addition to garnering information about the mechanism of injury, current level of pain, and inciting and abating factors, the presence of transient or persistent neuropathy should be vetted. In addition, anesthesia providers should inquire about the current analgesic regimen being employed (**Box 131.1**).

When discussing analgesic options, all available pain control modalities should be discussed with both the child and parent(s), and they should be involved with development of the pain management plan. While children suffer postoperative pain (POP) in the same fashion as adults, fear, anxiety, coping mechanisms, and social support should be considered when developing an analgesic plan.[12] Additionally, aligning patient and family expectations with achievable and realistic goals fosters optimal pain-related outcomes and patient satisfaction. Often, patients are under the impression that regional anesthesia will prevent any pain upon awakening from surgery, which may not be a realistic expectation based on the surgery being performed. Aligning goals and expectations will better prepare the patient for the postoperative course and optimize patient outcomes.

When considering the use of regional anesthesia, anesthesia providers should be aware that an insensate extremity may increase anxiety or distress postoperatively. A child 6 years of age, for example, may become distressed to the point of being inconsolable by the lack of sensation over large areas of their body.[13] Therefore, it is imperative anesthesia providers consider psychological aspects and thoroughly prepare patients when planning pain management interventions.

LOCAL ANESTHETICS

Regional anesthesia, whether neuraxial or PNB, requires the use of LA alone or conjunction with an adjunct to prolong or increase efficacy of a block. LAs are highly effective but can be dangerous should maximum recommended doses be exceeded. LAs block sodium channels, thereby interrupting the propagation of nerve impulses. Unfortunately, this action is not limited to the sodium channels of nerve tissue involved in pain transmission. Systemic absorption of LA may block sodium channels in the central nervous or cardiovascular system, leading to seizures, tachyarrhythmias, and death from apnea or cardiovascular collapse.[10]

Before administering LA to young children, some important pharmacodynamic principles must be kept in mind: (a) when continuous infusions are employed, there is a potential for toxicity stemming from the prolonged elimination half-lives of LA; (2) LAs decrease the seizure threshold in those with seizure disorders; (3) decreased albumin and alpha-1-acid glycoprotein serum levels in infants decrease binding of LA and therefore increase blood concentrations of the free drug, again increasing the potential for toxicity.[14] While administering a low LA dose has been recommended to test proper needle or catheter location before full LA administration, it is not practical or sensitive to the proper location in children as most peripheral nerve blocks are performed under anesthesia or deep sedation. Additional arguments opposing the use of a low-test dose in children include (a) detection of accidental intravascular or intraosseous injection is not reliable during anesthesia or deep sedation,[15] (b) LA toxicity is extremely rare in pediatrics when the drug dose guidelines are followed and the procedure is performed properly, and (c) the intrinsic properties of ropivacaine eliminate the need for the addition of epinephrine as an adjunct.

Bupivacaine and ropivacaine remain the most used LA for regional analgesia in pediatric patients. Bupivacaine possesses the least desirable toxicity profile among the amide LA, with the ratio of cardiotoxic to convulsant dose being lower than that for most other LA. Moreover, cardiotoxicity secondary to bupivacaine is quite refractory to treatment. Despite these adverse properties, it remains the most used drug for regional anesthesia in infants and children. The toxic plasma concentration of bupivacaine is 4 µg/mL. The maximum single bolus of bupivacaine is 2.5 to 3.0 mg/kg, and the maximum infusion rate is 0.4 to 0.5 mg/kg/hr in older infants and children and 0.2 to 0.25 mg/kg/hr in neonates. Most reports of serious adverse effects secondary to bupivacaine have been associated with doses more than the recommended maximum dose.

BOX 131.1 REGIONAL ANESTHESIA: KEY ASSESSMENT POINTS

- Comorbid medical conditions
- Current analgesic regimen
- Current level of pain
- Current medications
- Inciting and abating factors
- Mechanism of injury
- Presence of transient or persistent neuropathy

Ropivacaine, an enantiomerically pure LA with the same potency as bupivacaine, is rapidly becoming the LA of choice for regional anesthesia as it possesses the same pharmacokinetic profile as racemic bupivacaine, with less risk for cardiotoxicity and less motor blockade. Additionally, 0.2% ropivacaine is equianalgesic to 0.25% bupivacaine giving it a safer therapeutic index.[16] Loading doses of 0.2% ropivacaine for epidural anesthesia in infants and children range from 0.5 to 0.85 mL/kg. Concentrations in epidural injections range from 0.2% to 0.25% in a volume of 1 mL/kg. In caudal, lumbar, or thoracic epidural anesthesia, comparable concentrations, and volumes of ropivacaine or bupivacaine produce equivalent analgesia.[17]

As no method of administering a test dose has proved infallible, slow incremental dosing with constant monitoring and observation remains the standard of safe administration.

REGIONAL ANESTHESIA TECHNIQUES

Neuraxial Analgesia

Since August Bier performed the first spinal block in 1898, the central nervous system (CNS) has been utilized as a target for anesthesia and pain control. For many years, the most common regional anesthesia technique in pediatric patients was the injection of local anesthesia in the neuraxial area. Of the types of neuraxial anesthesia, epidural block by caudal route is by far the most popular technique in pediatric patients, followed by lumbar route, thoracic route, and rarely spinal block.[18,7] While epidural analgesia is effective, its utility is limited in regard to outpatient surgery, as it must be discontinued prior to patient discharge, thereby limiting its ability to provide lasting analgesia in the postoperative period.

Benefits of neuraxial anesthesia include improved POP control, decreased intraoperative anesthetic requirements, a blunted adverse physiological response to surgery, earlier ambulation postoperatively, decreased opioid requirement and side effects, and decreased hypercoagulable events.[19] Neuraxial anesthesia is not without risk, however, as neurological injury from trauma, infection, ischemia, hypotension, seizures, and cardiac arrest are all a concern.[17] Ultimately, with the rise in popularity of ultrasound-guided PNB techniques, the use of neuraxial anesthesia has decreased.[20]

Caudal Epidural

Caudal epidurals are indicated for surgical procedures of the pelvis, bladder, perineum, genitalia, and lower extremities. Examples include orchidopexy, major hypospadias repair, unilateral ureteral reimplantation, and club foot repair.[21,22]

Caudal epidurals are not routinely performed in older children and are reserved for use in younger children for a number of reasons. The size of the roots that comprise the sciatic nerve impedes penetration of LA; thus, more distal structures may not be adequately anesthetized. In addition, older children are difficult to carry if motor block persists and prevents ambulation. It should be noted that although it is more difficult to find the caudal space in older patients due to thickening of the sacrococcygeal ligament, caudal epidurals have been performed in adults.

While caudal analgesia failure rate varies among institutions, it has been reported to be as high as 20%.[23] Caudal anesthesia is achieved by injecting LA into the distal or caudal end of the epidural space, approached at the lower end of the bony spine. Typically, the point of access, the sacral hiatus, is found approximately 5 cm cephalad from the coccyx. The distance from skin to the epidural space can be estimated to be 10 mm + (2 × age in mm). The needle should pass midline in the space between the sacral cornua, at nearly a 45-degree angle. Resistance is encountered as the needle passes through the sacrococcygeal ligament. Once loss of resistance is achieved, LA is injected incrementally. Depending on institutional practice, a test dose may be given. If the test dose is negative, then fractionated dosing of the LA is completed.

Most caudal epidurals utilize a single-injection technique; however, if the length of surgery is greater than 3 hours, a second injection consisting of half the original dose may be performed postoperatively to prolong analgesia. LA can also be continuously infused through caudal catheters. Caudal catheters are often inserted in neonates for major abdominal, thoracic, or cardiovascular surgery. The use imaging during catheter advancement facilitates accurate catheter placement and patient safety.[24] The options for imaging include fluoroscopy, nerve stimulation, x-ray with contrast, or ultrasound. The advantage of ultrasound is immediate feedback, equipment availability, ease of use, and no radiation exposure. The disadvantage is poor imaging because of smaller bony windows in children and adults.

Adjunct medicines can also be added to prolong the duration or density of blockade. Neostigmine, ketamine, and midazolam have all been injected with variable success. The most utilized adjuncts to prolong pain control are clonidine, dexmedetomidine, fentanyl, and morphine. The recommended dose of clonidine is 1 to 3 mcg/kg, as higher doses do not improve pain control but increase somnolence.[25] The dose for caudal morphine dose is 50 mcg/kg.[26] Anesthesia providers should be aware that care must be taken when epidural and IV opioids are administered together as respiratory depression can occur as long as 18 hours after epidural administration.

Lumbar/Thoracic Epidurals

Lumbar and thoracic epidurals are commonly utilized for major orthopedic, abdominal, thoracic, pectus bar placement, and fetal surgeries. In contrast to caudal epidurals, these routes use a catheter and infusion and rarely as a single injection. Table 131.1 lists the catheter tip location to provide analgesia for somatic innervation. The insertion point for

Table 131.1 Epidural Levels for Various Surgeries

Surgery Location (Visceral Spinal Segmental Levels)	Epidural Catheter Level
Heart (T1–5)	T5–6
Lungs (T2–4)	T4–5
Esophagus (T5–6)	T6–7
Stomach (T6–10)	T10–11
Liver and gallbladder (T6–10)	T10–11
Pancreas and spleen (T6–10)	T10–11
Small intestine (T9–10)	T10–11
Large intestine (T11–12)	T12–L1
Kidney and uterus (T10–L2)	T12–L1
Adrenals (T8–L1)	T10–11
Testis or ovaries (T10–L2)	T11–12
Urinary bladder (T11–L2)	T12–L1
Uterus (T10–L1)	T12–L1

abdominal/pelvic surgery is L4–5, located between the posterior superior iliac spine, along the pelvic rim. For thoracic surgery, the ideal insertion point is at the level of T6, located approximately at the distal aspect of the scapula. Increasingly, epidurals are being inserted at varying levels to best provide analgesia based on incisional location.

Before injection of a LA solution, the needle or catheter is aspirated for signs of blood or cerebrospinal fluid (CSF). Because a negative aspirate may not guarantee correct needle or catheter position, a test dose is administered using LA and epinephrine in a concentration of 1:200,000 to mark an intravascular injection.[15] The patient is then observed for any one of the following symptoms during 60 seconds after injection: increase in heart rate by 10 beats per minute or more, increase in systolic blood pressure by 10% or more, or increase in T-wave amplitude by 25% or more.

Rather than using a single medication for epidural infusion, multiple drugs are frequently infused simultaneously to better control pain via different mechanisms of action. When drugs are combined, care must be taken to observe the toxicity limits of both drugs. As LA toxicity is a more immediate concern when bolus dosing the epidural, strict adherence to the dosing guidelines is important. Opioid toxicity, specifically respiratory depression, is more common than LA toxicity but appears less immediate. Narcotic additives can vary with the clinical scenario.[27] For instance, more epidural spread is often desirable for abdominal procedures, while less spread is useful for thoracic procedures. Therefore, the more lipophilic fentanyl is useful for thoracic epidurals, and the more hydrophilic hydromorphone to lower thoracic and abdominal procedures. Clonidine, an alpha-2 agonist that results in a central sympathetic blockade and analgesia, represents an excellent choice for patients at risk for neuraxial opioid toxicity; clonidine can be used for single-injection caudal epidurals or mixed with infusions for catheters (Table 131.2).[27]

The use of intrathecal opioids is uncommon in children but is occasionally used for postoperative analgesia following urological, orthopedic, or general surgery. The intrathecal space is accessed by a 22-G or 25-G spinal needle inserted through the lower lumbar (L2–4) intervertebral spaces. Patients receiving intrathecal opioids should be followed by the pain service and monitored for respiratory depression and level of consciousness. Postoperatively, the use of adjunct analgesics must be tightly controlled to minimize inadvertent IV–intrathecal narcotic synergy. In addition to hypotension, potential complications of intrathecal opioids include urinary retention, pruritis, nausea, and emesis.[28]

Peripheral Nerve Blockade

PNB has become increasingly popular as a technique to manage acute POP management. PNB provides a viable alternative to IV opioids or neuraxial analgesia. Peripheral techniques offer better analgesia with fewer side effects than IV techniques. Peripheral techniques offer better target sensory and motor block than neuraxial analgesia, which typically results in minimal sympathetic block and hemodynamic disturbances, and less risk of catastrophic complications such as spinal hematomas and abscesses.[29] Additionally, compared with neuraxial analgesia, PNB is well suited for outpatient surgery.

The advent of novel ultrasound-guided PNB techniques have led to widespread use of PNB in pediatric anesthesia given the increases in safety and efficacy ultrasound guidance affords. In addition to the upper and lower extremity PNBs commonly employed when caring for adult patients, thoracic and truncal PNB have become commonplace. PNB techniques such as thoracic paravertebral, erector spinae plane, quadratus lumborum, transversus abdominus plane, and rectus sheath blocks are routinely employed. The recent rise of interest in thoracic and truncal peripheral nerve blocks has served to provide regional anesthesia to many who might not previously have been candidates.[20] As epidural anesthesia is typically avoided in patients with a history of tethered spinal cord, myelomeningocele, and previous spine surgery or paraplegia, thoracic and truncal blocks can often prove to be a viable means of providing excellent analgesia. Table 131.3 describes indications for common regional blocks in children along with LA dosing and potential complications.

Special Techniques and/or Equipment
Recommended Equipment

Real-time bedside visualization of anatomy by ultrasound visualization now permits anesthesia providers to perform PNB on anesthetized patients, promoting regional anesthesia in pediatric pain management. Ensuring facile placement of PNB requires several key pieces of equipment be present prior to the start of each procedure. At the minimum, a high-frequency linear array and low frequency curved array should be available to optimize identification of anatomy under ultrasound guidance. Nerve block needles, preferably hyperechoic needles, should be available in a variety of lengths to accommodate variance in individual body habitus and specific nerve location. When placing a peripheral nerve block catheter, dressing supplies will be needed. Several manufacturers produce kits that contain all the supplies requisite for peripheral nerve catheter placement.

To ensure patient safety, standard monitors as recommended by the American Society of Anesthesiologists should be utilized. In addition, oxygen, suctioning capability, and pillows or padding for positioning should be on hand. Additional supplies that should be readily available include sterile drapes, gloves and gowns, ultrasound lubricant and probe sleeves, and LA. It is also advisable to confirm the availability of a LipidRescue™ kit, in addition to the LipidRescue™ protocol, as part of the preprocedure checklist in the event of an intravascular injection.

Table 131.2	Epidural Dosing
Epidural Infusion Rate Based on Local Dosage/Epidural Narcotic Dosage	
Thoracic and sub-umbilical epidurals	0.2 mg/kg/hr
Supra-umbilical and low thoracic epidurals	0.3 mg/kg/hr
Maximum rate (institution dependent)	0.4–0.5 mg/kg/hr
*Remember, if 0.1% bupivacaine is used, the above guidelines convert to mL/kg/hr.	
Epidural Narcotic Dosing	
Fentanyl	1–2 mcg/mL (0.5 mcg/kg/hr)
Dilaudid	5–10 mcg/mL (1–3 mcg/kg/hr)
Stadol	4–5 mcg/mL (1–2 mcg/kg/hr)

Table 131.3 Common Peripheral Nerve Block in Pediatric Anesthesia

Nerve Block	Location of Surgery	Potential Complication
Adductor canal	Knee	Intravascular injection
Ankle block (saphenous, sural, tibial, superficial peroneal, and deep peroneal nerves)	Foot	Intravascular injection, transient paresthesias
Axillary	Elbow, forearm, hand	Intravascular injection
Erector spinae plane	Thorax, breast, abdomen	Rare, pneumothorax
Fascia iliaca	Hip surgery, femur	Intravascular injection
Femoral nerve	Thigh, femur, knee	Intravascular injection; persistent strength deficits
Infraclavicular	Elbow, forearm, hand	Intravascular injection, pneumothorax
iPACK	Knee	Intravascular injection
Interscalene	Shoulder, upper arm	Spinal cord injury, intrathecal injection, pneumothorax, vertebral artery puncture, phrenic nerve blockade, Horner syndrome
Lumbar plexus	Hip, fractures femoral head/shaft, knee	Hematoma in muscle sheath, retroperitoneal space, or kidney; epidural spread
PECS	Breast	Intravascular injection, pneumothorax
Popliteal	Ankle, foot	Intravascular injection
Rectus sheath	Umbilicus	Rare, hematoma
Saphenous nerve	Sensory medial lower leg, knee	Motor weakness with large volume; intravascular injection
Sciatic nerve	Knee, leg, ankle, foot	Intravascular injection
Supraclavicular	Arm below shoulder, elbow, forearm, wrist, hand	Pneumothorax, phrenic nerve blockade, intravascular injection
Thoracic paravertebral	Thorax, breast, abdomen	Intravascular injection, pneumothorax, hypotension
Transversus abdominis plane	Abdomen, inguinal region	Rare

Note: Locations and complications for common peripheral nerve blocks used in orthopedic procedures. Modified from Wu et al (J. P. Wu, 2020), data from Greensmith JE, Murray WB. Complications of regional anesthesia. *Curr Opin Anaesthesiol.* (2006)19(5):531–537. et al. (Greensmith & Murray, 2006); Flack S (Flack & Lang, 2017); and Gray AT. *Atlas of ultrasound-guided regional anesthesia* e-book. Elsevier Health Sciences; 2018. (Gray, 2018).

Single Injection versus Continuous Infusion
Over the past decade, pediatric ambulatory surgery centers have followed in the footsteps of their adult counterparts and found success in discharging patients with indwelling continuous nerve block catheters. A variety of infusion pumps are available to facilitate the continuous or intermittent infusion of LA. By incorporating continual follow-up, PNB can safely continue for 2 to 3 days postoperatively, which is considered to be the most painful period of convalescence. This approach to pain management has proved to provide statistically better analgesia at rest and during activity for 48 to 72 hours postoperatively with less nausea, sedation, and pruritus but, not surprisingly increased motor block when compared with opioid-based analgesic regimens.[29,6]

Complications/Emergencies

While performing PNB under general anesthesia continues to generate concern for an increased risk of complications, regional anesthesia in children carries an extremely low rate of complications or adverse effects.[30] The widespread use of single-injection and continuous PNB is associated with few complications, with the overall complication rate of approximately 1:1000 blocks. Most complications are attributed to technique employed rather than performing PNB with the child under general anesthesia. Moreover, long-term adverse sequelae or medicolegal actions from these complications is exceedingly rare.[31]

Infectious complications secondary to PNB are exceedingly rare.[32] To date, there have been no reports in the literature of infection following single-injection PNB. Although rare, transient symptoms of bacteremia have been reported in the literature following the use of PNB catheters. In the literature, there is consensus that a major risk factor to PNB catheter infection is duration of catheter use. Most cases of reported, bacteremia symptoms resolve on removal of the catheter and no long-term sequelae were reported.

The potential for serious complication per 10,000 peripheral nerve blocks performed is estimated to be 0 to 2.6 deaths, 0.3 to 4.1 cardiac arrests, 0.5 to 4.8 neurological injuries, and 3.9 to 11.2 seizures. While neurological injury is often one of the most feared complications following PNB, it should be noted that it is often difficult to determine how much of a neurological deficit, if any, is attributable to the use of an indwelling PNB catheter, as all surgical procedures are associated with a variable incidence of nerve injury regardless of the use of continuous PNB. Potential complications include LA toxicity, hemorrhagic complications, neurological complications, and infectious complications. In addition, further potential complications include infusion pump malfunction, skin irritation or allergic reaction secondary to dressing

Table 131.4	Local Anesthetic Systemic Toxicity Presenting Symptoms		
Presenting Symptoms and Signs			
Prodrome	Major CNS		Major CV
• Hypertension • Metallic taste • Tachycardia • Tinnitus	• Agitation/ confusion • Coma • Obtundation • Seizure		• Asystole bradycardia/ heart block • Hypotension • Ventricular tachycardia or fibrillation

CNS, central nervous system; CV, cardiovascular.

Source: https://www.apsf.org/article/local-anesthetic-systemic-toxicity-last-revisited-a-paradigm-in-evolution/.

material, unintentional catheter dislodgement, or fluid leakage at the insertion site of a PNB catheter.

Neuraxial analgesia is associated with an increased incidence of complications compared with that of PNB, being six times more frequent.[31] Compared with epidural catheters, PNB catheters are associated with a lower incidence of complications, as most complications associated with PNB catheters result from mechanical problems with the catheter rather than harmful sequelae. While the utilization of ultrasound has the potential to decrease the likelihood of injuries such as intraneural injection, intravascular injection, or pneumothorax, this benefit is only appreciated after skill with ultrasound-guided techniques are established.

With any regional anesthetic technique, LA systemic toxicity (LAST) is a concern. While rare, it is estimated to occur at a rate of approximately 1 per 1000 peripheral nerve blocks. Hypoxia, acidosis, preexisting heart disease, extremes of age, frailty, and conditions that cause mitochondrial dysfunction, and liver or kidney disease can increase the risk of LAST by depressing LA metabolism or disposition. LAST provokes a variable array of CNS and cardiovascular signs and symptoms (Table 131.4).

The initial resuscitation of LAST differs from standard as the focus is on reversing the underlying toxicity rather than or in addition to sustaining coronary perfusion. An infusion of a lipid emulsion has proven effective in treating LAST by accelerating the redistribution of LA, specifically moving drug away from sensitive organs such as the brain and heart to reservoir organs. It is imperative anesthesia providers ensure the availability of both lipid emulsion and the LipidRescue™ protocol prior to performing regional anesthesia.

POSTOPERATIVE CARE

The dramatic increase in the use of regional anesthesia in children to abate POP has redefined POP management protocols, with regional anesthesia being a standard of care for many surgeries. It is important that both the patient and caregiver are properly educated about the care of an insensate extremity and the signs and symptoms of LAST prior to discharge. Although discharging patients with an insensate extremity remains controversial, it has proved to be a safe and effective strategy provided proper education occurs with the risk of injury being relatively minimal.[33] This approach does however place greater emphasis on patient/guardian selection preoperatively.[2]

> **KEY TAKEAWAYS**
>
> - Regional anesthesia affords clinicians the ability to reduce, if not eliminate, the incidence of opioid-induced negative sequelae.
> - Although declining in popularity, neuraxial analgesia can safely and effectively provide perioperative analgesia.
> - The advent of ultrasound-guided peripheral nerve block techniques has become commonplace in pediatric anesthesia.
> - Patient selection and proper education are key to the success of regional anesthesia.

131.2: Patient-Controlled Analgesia Use in Pediatrics

Daniela Herrera

> **LEARNING OBJECTIVES**
>
> - Identify the indications and contraindications for patient-controlled analgesia (PCA) use in pediatric patients.
> - Indicate the advantages and disadvantages of PCA use in pediatric patients.
> - Understand how a PCA pump can be programmed for opioid medication dosing.
> - Recognize other options for pediatric patients unable to utilize a PCA independently.

INTRODUCTION

The delivery method of opioids via patient-controlled analgesia (PCA) in the pediatric population has become an acceptable and safe standard of analgesia, particularly in the postoperative period.[34] With adequate patient monitoring, such as the use of cardiopulmonary monitors, and regularly updated policies, protocols, and guidelines, PCAs can safely be utilized with pediatric patients to achieve adequate and stable pain control. PCA use allows small incremental IV bolus doses of opioids to be self-administered by the patient utilizing a microprocessor pump. Opioid delivery occurs when the patient presses a button. Safeguards can be programmed to preclude delivery prior to a predetermined time interval. Microprocessor pumps also allow for delivery of continuous IV opioid medications, in addition to storing key information, such as the amount and timing of delivered medication, to facilitate titration of dosing.

INDICATIONS

Indications for PCA use are not reserved for only the postoperative period as management of moderate to severe pain can include PCA use, especially when there will be an ongoing unavailability of the PO route, such as in a case of acute pancreatitis.[35] Patients must be able to understand the cause-and-effect relationship between the presence of pain, activation of the PCA dosing button, and subsequent pain relief.[36] Anesthesia providers must assess patients prior to initiation of a PCA to ensure they are developmentally appropriate and have the capacity to understand the cause-and-effect relationship. It is generally accepted that otherwise healthy children aged 7 years or older should be able to appropriately utilize a PCA. Prior to initiation, all patients must be educated on how to properly activate the demand dose button when they are in pain, stressing the importance of not waiting for severe pain to occur prior to utilizing the PCA. Anesthesia providers should solicit and document confirmation that the patient understands the importance of utilizing the demand dose function prior to anticipated painful stimuli and that they are the only party responsible for pushing the demand dose button before initiating PCA use. Contraindications to a PCA may include developmentally delayed children depending on the cognitive level of the child, the inability to push a button due to either weakness or restraints, or the patient's desire not to assume responsibility for their own personal pain management.

ADVANTAGES AND DISADVANTAGES

Aside from the clear advantages of self-administration and self-control over pain management with PCA use, there are many benefits associated with this delivery method. One of the primary advantages is that PCA use allows for achieving a steady opioid blood level that is self-regulated within a therapeutic range. Using a PCA also allows the patient to titrate opioid administration to effect more rapidly when compared with reliance on nurse-administered medications, thus eliminating possible wait times or delays in receiving the medication compared with as needed (PRN) or even around-the-clock (ATC) scheduled dosing. With acute variations in pain, such as in hemorrhagic cystitis, the availability of an easily accessible demand dose of opioid can assist in reducing anxiety and increasing patient satisfaction with overall pain control. The PCA pump's ability to store memory on the amount, timing, and delivery of the opioid medication typically throughout a 24-hour period can also provide anesthesia providers valuable objective information that can be then utilized to make informed decisions regarding dosing and titration for improved efficiency and effect.

It should be noted that PCA utilization has not demonstrated an overall decrease in opioid use. Furthermore, the efficacy of PCA use can vary depending on the extent and degree of the invasiveness associated with a given surgery.[37] Continuous or basal rates can be added to PCA regimes, although there is evidence of an increase in overall opioid usage and an increase of side effects may occur without a significant impact on analgesic efficacy.[34,38] Fortunately, pediatric patients have an overall lower risk of serious adverse events associated with a continuous infusion in a PCA when compared with the adult population.[34] In addition, most acute pain and surgical procedures do not cause continuous pain, making a use of basal rate infusion often unnecessary. As with the administration of any opioid, particularly IV opioids, there can be untoward side effects. These side effects include nausea, vomiting, constipation, bowel dysfunction, urinary retention, pruritus, dysphoria, sedation, respiratory depression, bradypnea, and hypoxemia.

GUIDELINES FOR USE IN CLINICAL PRACTICE

Currently, there is insufficient and conflicting evidence to recommend the use of a specific opioid agent over another for the PCA.[34,39] It has been reported that opioid-related side effects in children and adolescents following the delivery of equianalgesic doses of morphine and hydromorphone via PCA are equivalent. Thus, opioid agent selection should be based on efficacy of past use and the ability to tolerate side effects. Typical opioids used for PCAs in pediatric patients include morphine, hydromorphone, or fentanyl. Dosing guidelines are weight based in the pediatric patient population. For obese patients, ideal body weight should be used to calculate appropriate dosing.

Typically, when programming a PCA pump use of a demand dose, which is the dose the patient self-administers by pressing a button, is employed as the staple means of delivery. To preclude administration to frequently or in unsafe intervals, a lockout interval can be programmed to prevent the patient from activating the pump until effect from the previous demand dose is achieved. This time typically corresponds to the time from IV injection to peak effect of the medication. Should a basal or continuous infusion be used, the dose utilized is generally equivalent to a single demand dose. This can be useful to provide more restful sleep for those with severe pain and/or those with chronic pain, such as in cancer or sickle cell disease. Basal rates are not indicated for those patients who are opioid naive, possess a history of respiratory problems, have a prior episode of sedation and/or hypoventilation with opioids, and/or currently use long-acting opioids, such as methadone or oxycontin.[38] The PCA pump should also have a maximum hourly dose programmed to reflect the demand, lockout interval, and addition of a basal rate if indicated.

SPECIAL CONSIDERATIONS

Because many pediatric patients are either physically or developmentally unable to utilize a PCA, a surrogate may be required to aid with PCA use. This commonly includes a caregiver, parent, or nurse. The American Society of Pain Management Nursing supports the use of authorized agent-controlled analgesia (AACA) to provide timely and effective pain management while promoting equitable care for vulnerable patient populations who are unable to utilize a PCA.[36] For AACA to be successful, anesthesia providers must designate a consistently available and competent individual or set of individuals to activate the demand dosing button in response to pain. These designated individuals must be appropriately educated not only on how to activate and utilize the pump but how to also assess the patient's pain. The authorized agents or individuals can either be nurses, parents, caregivers, family members, and/or a combination of a set of these. There has been no significant difference in outcomes when comparing complications associated with AACA to PCA in pediatric oncology patients as demonstrated by Anghelescu et al.,[40] who reviewed a cohort of patients spanning 2004 to 2010. As an extra measure of safety, AACA pumps typically have a longer lockout interval programmed so that the designated agent or individual does not have to feel the burden or need to push the demand dose as frequently.

RESOURCES
- www.aspmn.org
- www.pedsanesthesia.org

KEY TAKEAWAYS
- PCAs can be utilized in the pediatric population safely and effectively.
- For pediatric patients who are unable to utilize a PCA, an AACA should be considered a viable option to encourage equitable pain management.

131.3: Opioid-Free Anesthesia

Tyler A. C. Davis-Sandfoss and Andrew K. Davis-Sandfoss

LEARNING OBJECTIVES
- Identify the medications currently used for provision of opioid-free anesthesia.
- Describe the benefits associated with opioid-free anesthesia.
- Summarize suggested dosing regimens for nonopioid medications utilized in opioid-free anesthesia.

INTRODUCTION

Despite offering predictable and reliable analgesia, opioid administration is not without shortcomings as it is associated with a host of undesired side effects. Opioid-related sequelae such as postoperative nausea and vomiting (PONV), pruritus, sedation, and delayed return of bowel function can have a negative impact on patient outcomes and impede achievement of postoperative milestones. Therefore, it is prudent anesthesia providers consider alternative medications and novel approaches when managing pediatric pain in the perioperative period.[41]

In the past decade, there has been a growing interest in the use of nonopioid medications to provide analgesia for pediatric patients. When used in concert, nonopioid medications afford anesthesia providers the ability to deliver predictable, reliable, opioid-free anesthesia that confers significant benefit to pediatric patients, such as reductions in opioid-related side effects, improved perioperative and long-term subjective pain control, and objective decreases in perioperative agitation. Despite the efficacy and favorable side-effect profile of this technique, there remains a relative paucity of scientific studies exploring the use opioid-free anesthesia among the pediatric population. Ultimately, this chasm in the literature may be responsible for the overall decreased utilization of this technique with pediatric patients.[42] In this chapter, the use of several nonopioid medications key to the delivery of opioid-free anesthesia will be discussed.

NONOPIOID MEDICATIONS COMMONLY USED IN OPIOID-FREE ANESTHESIA

ACETAMINOPHEN

In the pediatric population, perioperative administration of acetaminophen has been shown to reduce opioid administration, acute postoperative agitation, and acute postoperative and long-term pain.[43] Furthermore, the use of acetaminophen can expedite oral intake after surgery and reduce the presence and incidence of postoperative fever.[44]

Mechanism of Action

While the exact mechanism is unknown, acetaminophen is thought to provide analgesia via numerous pathways involved in nociception. Activation of descending serotonergic pathways, antagonism of N-methyl-D-aspartate receptors, and blockade of substance-P and nitric oxide pathways impact the development of prostaglandins, and interactions with cannabinoid receptors are thought to contribute to acetaminophen analgesic efficacy.[45]

Dosing

Thoughtful administration and documentation of acetaminophen is necessary to prevent hepatic toxicity. Prior to administration, anesthesia providers should ensure that a total daily dosage of 75 mg/kg/day has not been exceeded (Table 131.5).

Contraindications

Acetaminophen should be administered with caution to patients with liver disease. Additionally, prolonged fasting or malnutrition, such as with anorexia, is considered as a risk factor for acetaminophen-induced hepatotoxicity.

CLONIDINE

Perioperative administration of oral clonidine has been shown to reduce POP, decrease the overall requirement of perioperative opioids, lessen PONV, and temper the incidence of emergence delirium in pediatric patients.[43] In addition to enteral and parenteral administration, clonidine may be added to the LA administered via regional anesthetic techniques to prolong the duration of the block.[45,46] While statistically or clinically significant hemodynamic derangements have not been observed in the pediatric population, the time spent in the PACU prior to meeting discharge readiness criteria may be extended if clonidine is administered intravenously.[46]

Mechanism of Action

Similar to dexmedetomidine, clonidine is an alpha-2-adrenergic receptor agonist that decreases transmission via sympathetic pathways in the peripheral and CNS. Although clonidine exhibits an approximate 200:1 affinity for alpha-2 receptors

Table 131.5	Overview of Acetaminophen Dosing Utilized in Opioid-Free Anesthesia	
IV	Rectal	PO
Children: 10–15 mg/kg per dose max dosing of 75 mg/kg/day	Loading dose: 40 mg/kg	10–12.5 mg/kg every 4 hours OR 15 mg/kg every 6 hours
Neonates (32–44 weeks postconceptual age): 60 mg/kg/day	Maintenance dose: 20 mg/kg every 6 hours	
Neonate (preterm, 28–32 weeks PCA): 45 mg/kg/day		

PCA, patient-controlled analgesia.
Sources: From Coté CJ, Lerman J, Todres ID. *A practice of anesthesia for infants and children* e-book. Elsevier Health Sciences; 2018; Birmingham PK, Tobin MJ, Fisher DM. et al. Initial and subsequent dosing of rectal acetaminophen in children: a 24-hour pharmacokinetic study of new dose recommendations. *Anesthesiology*. 2001;94(3):385–389. doi:10.1097/00000542-200103000-00005.

Table 131.6	Overview of Clonidine Dosing Utilized in Opioid-Free Anesthesia			
Single-Injection Caudal	IV	Intranasal	PO	
1–3 mcg/kg	3 mcg/kg * 20 min prior to end of surgery	4 mcg/kg * 30 min prior to induction of anesthesia	4 mcg/kg * Pre-operatively (more beneficial than 2 mcg/kg)	

Source: From Wright JA. An update of systemic analgesics in children. Anaesth Intensive Care Med. 2016;17(6):280–285. doi:10.1016/j.mpaic.2016.03.001; Afshari A. Clonidine in pediatric anesthesia: the new panacea or a drug still looking for an indication? Curr Opin Anaesthesiol. 2019;32(3):327–333. doi:10.1097/ACO.0000000000000724.

compared with alpha-1 receptors[47] paradoxical hypertension may be seen after administration.

Dosing

Weight-based clonidine dosing varies based on route of administration. Typical dosing parameters that have been described as part of a multimodal or opioid-free analgesic regimen are summarized in Table 131.6.

Contraindications

Given the metabolism and excretion of clonidine by the hepatic and renal systems, dosing of clonidine should be reduced in the neonatal population given immaturity of hepatic and renal function leading to possible supratherapeutic drug levels.[45] Clonidine should also be avoided in patients with a history of bradycardia or atrioventricular heart block.

DEXAMETHASONE

Commonly utilized for prophylaxis against PONV, dexamethasone has also been shown to reduce perioperative pain.[43] When administered as an adjunct in multimodal strategies, dexamethasone effectively to reduces POP and opioid consumption after surgery.

Mechanism of Action

The mechanism by which dexamethasone provides analgesia is thought to occur at the cellular level, ultimately reducing the inflammatory response to surgical stimuli. As a glucocorticoid, dexamethasone reduces prostaglandin synthesis by inhibiting both phospholipase enzyme and cyclooxygenase type II. In addition, dexamethasone modulates the inflammatory response by inhibiting tumor necrosis factor, interleukin-1β, interleukin-6, c-reactive protein, and leukocyte receptors.[48] Collectively, the reduction in prostaglandin synthesis and modulation of the inflammatory response produces both analgesic and anti-inflammatory properties.

Dosing

The dosing of dexamethasone required to provide analgesia is higher than the dose commonly given to prevent PONV, with the doses of dexamethasone reported to provide analgesic benefit ranging based on from 0.4 to 1.0 mg/kg intravenously.[43] It has also been reported that intermediate dosing of 0.11 to 0.2 mg/kg provides significantly lower pain scores and opioid requirements, with no statistical difference in pain-related outcomes between the intermediate-dose group and doses greater than 0.2 mg/kg.[49]

Contraindications

Dexamethasone, being a corticosteroid, has the potential to increase a patient's blood glucose levels following administration and should be used with caution in patients who have diabetes.

DEXMEDETOMIDINE

Perioperative administration of dexmedetomidine has been shown to reduce emergence delirium, POP, perioperative opioid requirements, and PONV without statistically or clinically significant hemodynamic changes.[43] Prolongation of the time to meet criteria for extubation and an increase in PACU sedation have been noted with dexmedetomidine administration, especially when dexmedetomidine is administered immediately prior to emergence from general anesthesia. However, these clinically significant impacts have not been demonstrated if administration occurs immediately following induction of general anesthesia.[50]

Mechanism of Action

Similar to clonidine, dexmedetomidine is a selective alpha-2-adrenergic receptor antagonist. As opposed to clonidine, dexmedetomidine demonstrates a significantly greater affinity for alpha-2-adrenergic receptors.[45]

Dosing

IV bolus administration of up to 2.0 mcg/kg and IV infusions up to 1.0 mcg/kg/hr have been well described in the literature. Bolus administration of less than 0.5 mcg/kg has not been shown to provide clinical benefit.[50]

Contraindications

Like clonidine, dexmedetomidine should also be avoided in patients with a history of bradycardia or atrioventricular heart block and patients who are dependent on an elevated sympathetic tone, such as those in hypovolemic or cardiogenic shock.

DEXTROMETHORPHAN

Although not widely utilized, dextromethorphan may have a role in nonopioid anesthesia given its ability to reduce postoperative opioid requirements when administered in combination with ketamine, midazolam, and acetaminophen.[51]

Mechanism of Action

Dextromethorphan is a codeine analog that is similar in structure to other opioids but has minimal interaction with opioid receptors. Although not completely understood, dextromethorphan is thought to provide analgesia via NMDA-receptor and sigma-1 receptor antagonism.

Dosing

Typical dosing for dextromethorphan when utilized as part of a nonopioid analgesic technique is 1 mg/kg.[51]

Contraindications

Simultaneous use of dextromethorphan with nonselective monoamine oxidase inhibitors (MAO inhibitors) to avoid serotonin syndrome. As dextromethorphan contains aspartame, it should be used with caution in patients with phenylketonuria.

ESMOLOL

While typically utilized for its rapid impact on hemodynamics, esmolol can also be employed as part of an opioid-free anesthetic technique. Despite the paucity of research involving the use of esmolol for analgesia in pediatric patients, studies with adult patients have shown significant reduction in POP scores, analgesic use, and opioid administration when esmolol was administered.[52] It has been reported, however, to reduce emergence delirium in pediatric patients when administered in combination with lidocaine.[53]

Mechanism of Action
The exact mechanism by which esmolol provides analgesia is unclear, although it is thought to be secondary to modulation of the sympathetic component of the pain, that is, heart rate and blood pressure. By decreasing cardiac output, esmolol ultimately decreases hepatic blood flow, which may slow metabolism of other drugs that are hepatically metabolized, such as fentanyl.

Dosing
Typical loading doses range from 1.0 mcg/kg to 2.0 mg/kg, while infusion doses range from 5 to 500 mcg/kg/min.

Contraindications
Esmolol is contraindicated in patients with sinus bradycardia, sick sinus syndrome, atrioventricular heart block, heart failure, cardiogenic shock, and a history of pulmonary hypertension.[54] Concomitant administration of esmolol and calcium channel blockers should be avoided, as this may exacerbate hypotension and bradycardia.

GABAPENTINOIDS
The most frequently utilized gabapentinoids in opioid-free anesthesia protocols are gabapentin and pregabalin. Gabapentinoids have been shown to reduce POP scores and opioid consumption[43] without increasing time spent in the PACU.[55] Nonetheless, the efficacy of a single dose of gabapentinoid remains debated, as the reported reduction in POP scores has been shown to be minimal, questioning the clinical significance of their use in the perioperative period.[45]

Mechanism of Action
Gabapentinoids reduce neuronal excitability at primary afferent sensory neurons after tissue injury via decrease in release of neurotransmitters such as substance-P, glutamate, and calcitonin gene-related peptide.

Dosing
Gabapentin dosing varies widely, though studies have reported perioperative benefit from the administration of up to 15 mg/kg enterally preoperatively and up to 5 mg/kg three times daily postoperatively.

Contraindications
Gabapentinoids should be used with caution in patients with a history of myasthenia gravis, myoclonus problems, suicidal ideation, depression, or kidney disease impacting kidney function.

KETAMINE
Perioperative ketamine administration as a bolus, an infusion, or a combination thereof has been shown to decrease emergence delirium, POP, perioperative opioid administration, and the development of chronic pain in pediatric patients.[43,45]

Mechanism of Action
Ketamine exerts its analgesic effect via antagonism of N-methyl-D-aspartate (NMDA) receptors on secondary afferent neurons in the dorsal horn of the spinal cord. Antagonizing these receptors inhibits the voltage-dependent flow of ions, which results in reduction of central sensitization, wind-up, and chronic pain, making ketamine an excellent choice for the treatment of acute, chronic, and neuropathic pain. Ketamine has also been utilized for hyperalgesia and allodynia.[45]

Dosing
Depending on the indication for and setting of administration, dosing is highly variable. However, in provision of opioid-free anesthesia, suggested bolus doses range from 0.25 to 1.0 mg/kg, with infusion doses up to 1.0 mg/kg/hr. For additional information on specific dosing, please refer to Chapter 2, "Pharmacological Considerations for the Pediatric Patient."

Contraindications
Ketamine is contraindicated in patients with a history of uncontrolled hypertension or vascular aneurysm. In addition, the use of ketamine in patients with elevated CSF volumes remains controversial and not unanimously supported.

LIDOCAINE
Lidocaine has been shown to reduce postoperative opioid administration and PONV while expediting the time to postoperative ambulation.[56] There may also be benefit to IV administration of lidocaine in reduction of postoperative cough in the setting of recent upper respiratory infection.[57]

Mechanism of Action
The exact mechanism by which IV lidocaine provides analgesia is still under investigation. However, it has been postulated that lidocaine reduces the excitability of neurons in the dorsal horn of the spinal cord, thus reducing nociception.[58]

Dosing
In pediatric patients, 3.0 mg/kg/hr infused intraoperatively followed by 1.0 mg/kg/hr infused for 6 hours postoperatively has been reported to yield clinical benefit.[56]

Contraindications
Anesthesia providers should be cognizant that in patients who are taking medications that can precipitate methemoglobinemia, or if the patient has a hemoglobinopathy or another cause of anemia, methemoglobinemia can occur due to lidocaine metabolism to O-toluidine. However, this is more likely when very high doses are given.

MAGNESIUM
Magnesium, while an endogenous element with multiple roles in human physiology, may be administered exogenously as part of a nonopioid anesthetic regimen. Exogenous magnesium administration has been associated with reduction in inhalational anesthetic requirement, emergence delirium, and perioperative analgesic administration.[43,59]

Mechanism of Action
While the mechanism of action remains under investigation, magnesium is thought to exhibit its analgesic effects via impact on neurotransmitter release.

Dosing
Preferred doses vary widely. However, a 50 mg/kg bolus followed by an infusion of 15 mg/kg/hr has demonstrated clinically significant reduction in POP and emergence delerium.[43,59]

Contraindications

Caution should be utilized when administering magnesium to patients with known or suspected atrioventricular block, renal dysfunction, or neuromuscular diseases.

NONSTEROIDAL ANTI-INFLAMMATORY DRUGS

The administration of NSAIDs in the perioperative period has been associated with decreased opioid administration, improvement in pain scores, and reduction in PONV.[43] NSAIDs primarily studied for perioperative utilization are ibuprofen, ketorolac, diclofenac, and the selective COX-1 inhibitor celecoxib.

Mechanism of Action

NSAIDs are primarily thought to reduce systemic inflammation in response to tissue injury via inhibition of cyclooxygenase (COX) enzymes. Based on relative specificity for COX-1 and COX-2 enzymatic inhibition, NSAIDs have been associated with various consequential side effects, such as renal injury, gastrointestinal bleeding, and decreased platelet aggregation.

Dosing

Depending on route of administration and specific medication, dosing varies. Please refer to Table 131.7 for an overview of various dosing regimens.

Contraindications

NSAIDs should not be administered to patients with known gastrointestinal ulceration, severe cardiac failure, hepatic or renal dysfunction. Caution must be utilized with administration of NSAIDs to patients with suspected renal dysfunction given the role of prostaglandins in renal homeostasis. Aspirin administration to patients with underlying viral illness has been associated with Reye's syndrome. Non-steroidal anti-inflammatory drugs (NSAIDs) administration to patients with asthma associated with rhinosinusitis, nasal polyps, eczema, or allergies has also been associated with bronchospasm. Finally, when administering NSAIDs to patients with bony injuries, the risk of nonunion must be assessed.[45]

EMERGING TRENDS IN OPIOID-FREE ANESTHESIA IN PEDIATRICS

Although the association of perioperative opioid use has not been demonstrated to be a major risk factor for future opioid misuse among pediatric patients, there has been a trend to decrease opioid usage in pediatric surgeries. Several pediatric surgical populations in particular have garnered significant attention in the literature, with multiple studies investigating the safety and efficacy of opioid-free and opioid-sparing anesthesia techniques, namely, renal surgery, cardiac surgery, and adenotonsillectomy.

Opioid-free anesthetics incorporating regional anesthesia and nonopioid medications have recently been reported to promote improved patient outcomes following pediatric reconstructive urological surgery. Not only is pain well controlled, but the percentage of opioid-free days postoperatively can also increase significantly along with drastic reductions in the number of patients receiving opioids on the day of discharge.[60] Likewise, novel techniques such as erector spinae blockade afford anesthesia providers the ability to successfully provide opioid-free anesthetics for pediatric patients undergoing sternotomy for cardiothoracic surgery.[61]

Adenotonsillectomy is one of the most common pediatric surgical procedures in the United States, with more than 500,000 adenotonsillectomies performed annually.[62] Considered a painful procedure, analgesia regimens have long incorporated opioids to temper POP. Determining the optimal pain management regimen for pediatric adenotonsillectomy remains challenging, however, largely due to the higher prevalence of preexisting sleep-disordered breathing and obstructive sleep apnea in this patient population.[62] While there have been limited reports of opioid-free anesthesia for this population to date, judicious use of these nonopioid medications has repeatedly been reported to contribute to enhanced recovery and the avoidance of undesirable opioid-induced adverse effects.

Similarly, the use of dexmedetomidine, NSAIDs, and regional anesthesia for pediatric ambulatory surgeries has proven to minimize perioperative opioid administration, decrease the incidence of PONV, improve POP scores, and shorten the time to meeting discharge readiness criteria.[63] Given the success witnessed among the breadth of pediatric surgical populations, it is likely that opioid-free and opioid-sparing approaches will continue to evolve and will be applied to multitude of pediatric surgical populations with equal success.

Table 131.7	Overview of NSAID Dosing Utilized in Opioid-Free Anesthesia		
Celecoxib	**Diclofenac**	**Ibuprofen**	**Ketorolac**
PO: 6 mg/kg preoperatively followed by 3 mg/kg BID for 5 days postoperatively	PO: 1–2 mg/kg	PO: 20 mg/kg	IV: 0.5 mg/kg every 6 hours (15 mg maximum dosage)
	IV: 0.3 mg/kg		
	Rectal: 0.5 mg/kg	IV: 10 mg/kg	

Sources: From Zhu A, Benzon HA, Anthony Anderson T. Evidence for the efficacy of systemic opioid-sparing analgesics in pediatric surgical populations: a systematic review. *Anesth Analg.* 2017;125(5):1569–1587. doi:10.1213/ANE.0000000000002434; Standing JF, Tibboel D, Korpela R, Olkkola KT. Diclofenac pharmacokinetic meta-analysis and dose recommendations for surgical pain in children aged 1-12 years. *Paediat Anaesth.* 2011;21(3):316–324. doi:10.1111/j.1460-9592.2010.03509.x; Forrest JB, Heitlinger EL, Revell S. Ketorolac for postoperative pain management in children. *Drug Saf.* 1997;16(5):309–329. doi:10.2165/00002018-199716050-00003.

KEY TAKEAWAYS

- Given the known undesirable side effects of opioids, it is prudent pediatric anesthesia providers be knowledgeable of nonopioid medications commonly utilized to provide opioid-free anesthesia.

- Benefits directly related to the use of nonopioid medications for pain management include reductions in emergence delirium, PONV, requirement of rescue analgesics, and development of chronic pain.

- Benefits indirectly related to the use of nonopioid medications and minimization of opioid medications include decreased time to patients' ambulation and expedited oral intake postoperatively.

- Consideration and dosing adjustments should be made in the presence of underlying pathology that may alter the metabolism and excretion of certain medications.

131.4: Anxiety and Anxiolysis

David L. Moore

> **LEARNING OBJECTIVES**
> - Describe how anxiety impacts perioperative pain.
> - Apply techniques that impact pain and emergence delirium.
> - Recognize anxiety and its impact on pain.

INTRODUCTION

Surgery evokes a myriad of responses to POP. Obviously, the severity of POP is based, at least in part, on the amount of tissue trauma associated with the given procedure. The challenge for anesthesia providers, however, is to figure out why responses can vary so greatly between patients following the same surgery. One answer of course lies with the patient, with the reason for differing patient responses to pain being the presence of anxiety.

Anxiety has agency. For many, anxiety conveys a protective effect. Accompanied by high cognition, anxiety can also improve job performance.[64] Anxiety is also genetic with seemingly distinct pathways to the development of anxiety disorders in adolescence. Dr. Jerome Kagan, the Daniel and Amy Starch Research Professor of Psychology, Emeritus at Harvard University, was a key pioneer of developmental psychology who explored various facets of anxiety for over 50 years. He began his foray into better understanding anxiety by first examining infants as young as 6 months of age. Dr. Kagan's early research found that 20% of patients could be classified as "high reactors," with 40% being classified as "low reactors" based on their reaction to various noxious stimuli.[65] Interestingly, as he followed these infants longitudinally, the high-reactors became anxious adolescents. The low reactors, however, did not develop anxiety as they entered adolescence. Likewise, there was no crossing between the trajectory of each of the groups (i.e., none of the high reactors became "easygoing").[66] This early work provided the foundation for understanding the identification and ramifications of anxiety in the perioperative period.

MANIFESTATION OF ANXIETY IN THE PERIOPERATIVE PERIOD

Surgery causes stress in many patients, with anxiety developing as the internal reaction to stress or uncertainty.[67] *Stress* is defined as "uncertainty about what needs to be done to safeguard physical, mental or social well-being."[68] When there is a large disparity between expectations for external or internal events compared with actual experiences, uncertainty or "stress" can ensue in some patients due to the perception of a lack of control. Anxiety manifests as the reaction to stress and a perceived lack of control.[69] Patients who have little need for perceived control generally do not report anxiety preoperatively. Conversely, those patients with a high need for control tend to report high levels of anxiety preoperatively. Thus, anxiety appears to be directly correlated with need for control.[70]

ANXIETY AND POSTOPERATIVE PAIN

There is evidence that people with anxiety are physically more sensitive to various forms of stimulus.[71] Therefore, those with anxiety may not tolerate pain as well as someone who has no anxiety following the same painful event. In fact, there are multiple studies demonstrating an association between anxiety and POP.[72–78] Unfortunately, the specific nature of this relationship remains elusive. What is known, however, is that there appears to be an association between POP and pain catastrophizing. Pain catastrophizing is a subset of anxiety. A catastrophizing patient negatively projects the amount of pain they will have in the future, which results in reported pain intensity scores being higher and increased analgesic requirements.[73,74,79] The remainder of this chapter will discuss what is known to date regarding the assessment and treatment of anxiety in the perioperative period.

ASSESSMENT OF ANXIETY

TIMING OF ASSESSMENT

Proper timing of anxiety assessment is essential to the accurate identification of anxiety. Although assessments can theoretically be performed at any time, there are two timepoints in the perioperative period that are associated with statistically significant increases in anxiety: preoperatively and prior to discharge.[67] This should come as no surprise as both of these timepoints are associated with lack of control and uncertainty. The stress induced by a lack of control or uncertainty translates into anxiety, thus making these timepoints key moments for assessment.

ASSESSING ANXIETY

Anxiety is a complex issue that cannot be identified or quantified by a simple binary "yes/no" question.[80] Fortunately, there are multiple inventories, scales, and questionnaires that attempt to identify the cause. The tools all vary in nature but collectively attempt to discern if the anxiety is due to state anxiety, trait anxiety, and pain catastrophizing.

State anxiety is the most common driver of anxiety and occurs when a patient encounters a stressful situation in which they have little to no control (i.e., preoperatively before surgery or before leaving the hospital to go home).[81] This can be among the easiest causes of anxiety to treat as well, as once the needs of the "state" are addressed (patient is doing well postoperatively or patient is doing well at home), the anxiety is alleviated. Measuring clinical anxiety in a quick but relevant manner is difficult in a perioperative setting. There are, however, two scales that can be easily employed for measuring state or situational anxiety. They are the Numeric Rating Scale (NRS) and the Visual Analog Scale (VAS). The NRS is an 11-point scale, from 0 to 10, with zero indicating no anxiety to 10 indicating maximal anxiety.[82] If the patient has an anxiety score of 3 or above on the NRS, they should be considered anxious. The VAS for anxiety requires a 10-cm line, and the patient is asked to indicate where on the line their anxiety is located.[77] Similar to the NRS, 30 mm represents the threshold for anxiety.

Trait anxiety can be assessed by asking the patient if they typically have anxiety "all of the time/at home." This is a "yes/no" answer. While this is not validated, it is of historical interest to the anesthesia provider. If the patient answers "yes," they should then be asked if treatment is composed of medication use, counseling, or both.

Combined assessments can prove useful, as the presence of state anxiety can predict the incidence POP and the presence of trait anxiety is known to be associated with increased analgesic requirements.[72–74,76–78,83] The original anxiety assessment tool was the State-Trait Anxiety Inventory (STAI), which was first published in 1969 by Spielberger.[83] While considered the gold standard for anxiety assessment, it is inefficient for a busy clinical anesthesia practice. The Modified Yale Pediatric Anxiety Scale (MY-PAS) was originally published by Kain et al. in 1996 and then modified in 1997.[84] While a thorough tool that has proven to be effective in research, this too is inefficient for a busy anesthesia practice. An additional assessment tool is the Pain Catastrophizing Scale (PCS), which looks at catastrophizing as more of a link to intense pain.[85] It should be noted that the STAI and the PCS negatively correlate with age.[73] Quantitative sensory testing (QST) can also be performed to assess pain thresholds and pain intensity, which may help identify anxiety and anxiety related behaviors.[86]

ASSESSMENT INTERPRETATION

Incorporating anxiety assessment in the preoperative evaluation may help identify patients who will benefit from anxiolysis or those who might have challenges with managing pain postoperatively.

Anxious patients tend to have certain postoperative behaviors in common, often reporting high pain scores despite high opioid administration. Should a patient be identified as having anxiety preoperatively, it is imperative the anesthesia provider incorporate anxiolysis into the anesthetic plan.

False-Positive and False-Negative Tests

When inquiring about anxiety, you will encounter pediatric patients with a fairly stress-free childhood who are presenting for their first surgery. Commonly, these patients report they have no anxiety. This unwittingly may be false, as anxiety is best perceived during stress. If they have never experienced stress, they might not know they are anxious. These patients can have elevated pain intensity or decreased pain tolerance that manifests in severe POP that is only relieved by a combination of opioids and anxiolytics. This is the false-negative patient.

False-positive patients present with known trait anxiety and have received prior treatment for anxiety. This may entail counseling alone or in combination with drug therapy. When anxiety has been well treated, then a patient behaves similarly to patients who have no anxiety and can be considered resilient.

TREATMENT OF ANXIETY

Patients with profound anxiety are frequently unprepared for the surgical experience. Treatment depends on amount and type of anxiety and the temporal association with the surgery. Ideally, severely anxious patients should be in counseling with possible drug therapy preoperatively for the period of time necessary to achieve a desirable effect. Drug therapy regimens commonly include Selective serotonin reuptake inhibitors (SSRIs)/Serotonin-norepinephrine reuptake inhibitor (SNRI) such as Effexor, Prozac, and Cymbalta, among other medications. These medications take weeks to months to achieve effect, so immediate initiation of these medicines on the day of surgery would not be helpful.

DAY OF SURGERY: PREOPERATIVE TREATMENT

Overall, those needing perioperative anxiolytics benefit considerably when there is better recognition of anxiety. In addition, there are both external and internal stressors preoperatively that may be amenable to pharmacological or non-pharmacological techniques. Generally, there are three basic types of patients.

Type one: Patients who proceed to induction without administration of an anxiolytic, whether due to the lack of anxiety or the patient not liking the effect of anxiolytics. The latter gives anesthesia providers insight about the efficacy of nonpharmacological techniques, although admittedly nonpharmacological techniques will not help all patients who are anxious or poorly coping. For those patients who proceed to induction without receiving an anxiolytic, anesthesia providers often use instruction, distraction, and other techniques to reduce stress. Unfortunately, many patients (or their parents) choose to avoid an anxiolytic preoperatively only to later realize they cannot cope with the stress associated with surgery or parental separation.

Type two: Many patients recognize anxiety and request mitigation strategies. In this scenario, nonpharmacological methods do help. For many in this group, oral and IV premedications predominate and often prove beneficial. Midazolam and other benzodiazepines have an unparalleled success. Dexmedetomidine, an alpha-2 receptor antagonist, has also been proven to be useful as an anxiolytic preoperatively.

Type three: A patient in whom severe anxiety dominates and sedation worsens anxiety. This is the so-called paradoxical reaction. In this scenario, the patient has severe anxiety and therefore they "need" control. Sedation following administration of an anxiolytic, however, is perceived as loss of control resulting in the adverse reaction. In this situation, rapid loss of consciousness is desired.

While undesirable, a paradoxical behavior provides useful information as the patient is likely to have postoperative behavioral changes and emergence delirium, as well as higher amounts of POP. Anxious children are 6.5 times more likely to have emergence delirium than nonanxious patients.[78]

DAY OF SURGERY: INTRAOPERATIVE TREATMENT

Proper intraoperative management of anxiety helps prevent two recovery room issues: emergence delirium and excessive pain. To avoid these two issues, anesthesia providers should avoid unneeded anesthetics. As oral midazolam administered preoperatively can prolong emergence delirium, it is advisable to remove oral versed by orogastric or nasogastric tube (OGT/NGT).[87] Anesthesia providers should also consider minimizing long-acting anesthetics, such as volatile anesthetics and propofol infusions, as the accumulation may provoke anxious patients to have emergence issues postoperatively. Although frequently debated, the incidence of emergence delirium has been reported to be similar between following the administration of volatile anesthetics and a propofol infusion.[88] Techniques such as regional anesthesia, a nitrous-narcotic technique, or use of a dexmedetomidine infusion may help avoid emergence delirium by minimizing the need for long-acting anesthetics.[89-90]

DAY OF SURGERY: POSTOPERATIVE TREATMENT

There are multiple techniques that mitigate emergence delirium. First, as noted earlier, attempt to minimize the long-acting anesthetics. This allows the patient to emerge with increased mental clarity (and control) and be less prone to agitation. Second, promote a slow emergence with either dexmedetomidine or a bolus of propofol. This allows additional time for long-acting anesthetics to be metabolized and eliminated. Finally, counteract noxious stimuli. Frequently this entails the use of regional anesthesia, opioids, and other pain medications that are all known to decrease emergence delirium.[89-90]

Patients with anxiety may also have excessive pain out of proportion to the procedure performed. The best indication for this is a patient who has received a loading dose (0.1 mg/kg IV morphine or the equivalent) of opioid in the recovery room and still claims a pain score of 10 out of 10. This is secondary to anxiety and can be mitigated by the administration of midazolam or lorazepam. Interestingly, diazepam does not help this condition despite being a benzodiazepine.

POSTOPERATIVE PAIN

The presence of anxiety may increase the pain sensitivity postoperatively.[71] Therefore, for those with unsatisfactory pain control, an anxiolytic might be necessary to decrease the pain. If a patient has high pain scores and high opioid usage postoperatively, attempt to ascertain their level of anxiety. If a patient has known or presumed anxiety, consider treating them with 1 to 2 mg IV midazolam in the PACU or with low dose (10 mcg/kg, max 0.5mg) IV lorazepam every 6 hours. This not only treats the previously untreated anxiety, but it also subsequently normalizes opioid usage. Once the patient has been treated for a day or two with scheduled anxiolytics, change the anxiolytic schedule to "as needed" and wean them off the medication.

MANAGING ANXIETY BEYOND THE PERIOPERATIVE ENVIRONMENT

"To resolve uncertainty [stress], three processes play a crucial role: learning, attention, and habituation."[68] Learning helps to temper stress and anxiety by giving patients the information needed to decrease uncertainty. Attention is necessary for learning. These processes, specifically attention, explain the higher incidence of anxiety among patients diagnosed with attention-deficit/hyperactivity disorder (ADHD). Habituation is a form of tolerance. It decreases the emotional and physiological response of anxiety with experience and allows some patients to change their expectations to accommodate new learning or new experiences. This reduces the difference between expectations and experiences, thus reducing stress.

Anxious people have more difficulty decreasing stress compared with those who can habituate.[68] Anxiety becomes problematic when high stress occurs. It is important anesthesia providers recognize that the inability to decrease stress may be unrecognized by a patient until they are stressed. Therefore, while many pediatric patients deny having anxiety, they simply have not yet experienced the requisite level of stress to unveil their anxiety.

MANAGING ANXIETY BEYOND THE POSTOPERATIVE PERIOD

Since patients vary in the ability to cope, part of the anesthesia provider's job is to provide them the tools to deal with the stressors encountered during the perioperative period.

Step 1: Educate

Fear of the unknown or fear of change creates stress in pediatric patients. Establishing proper expectations can greatly help temper unrealistic expectations the patient might have in regard to their care.[91] Also, the patient's prior surgical experience, a form of knowledge, can help by decreasing anxiety related to the surgery by habituation.[68,75] This should be reinforced in the preoperative period.

Step 2: Surrender Some Control

Since anxiety is correlated with control, surrendering control to the patient (or family) may help decrease some of the stress and anxiety the patient is experiencing.[92] The use of PCA or patient-controlled epidural analgesia (PCEA) are both techniques that offer the patient a sense of control in managing their POP.[93] Surrendering control can also include involving the patient and their family in shared decision-making, such as family-centered rounds. Behavioral health can also teach patients cognitive behavioral therapy or other coping strategies, such as mindfulness or meditation, that have proved useful in generating a sense of control in patients.

Step 3: Medicate

Analgesics, LA, and anxiolytics can greatly decrease POP. Without question, anesthesia providers should employ a multimodal approach to pain management that incorporates opioids, nonopioid adjuncts, regional anesthesia, and LA to collectively optimize pain management. Regional anesthesia in particular has proved to be effective in greatly decreasing stress and ultimately POP. As anxiety is a multiplier of pain, it is imperative anesthesia providers incorporate anxiolytics in their pain control armamentarium when anxiety is interfering with pain management strategies.

KEY REFERENCES

Complete references for this chapter are online and available at https://connect.springerpub.com/content/book/978-0-8261-3875-0/part/part05/toc-part/ch131.

10. Lonnqvist PA. Toxicity of local anesthetic drugs: a pediatric perspective. *Paediatr Anaesth*. 2012;22(1):9–43. doi:10.1111/j.1460-9592.2011.03631.x
11. Marhofer P, Willschke H, Kettner SC. Ultrasound-guided upper extremity blocks: tips and tricks to improve clinical practice. *Paediatr Anaesth*. 2012;22(1):65–71. doi:10.1111/j.1460-9592.2011.03744.x
27. Szabova A, Sadhasivam S, Wang Y, et al. Comparison of postoperative analgesia with epidural butorphanol/bupivacaine versus fentanyl/bupivacaine following pediatric urological procedures. *J Opioid Manag*. 2010;6(6):401–407. doi:10.5055/jom.2010.0037
34. Cravero JP, Agarwal R, Berde C, et al. The Society for Pediatrid Anesthesia recommendations for the use of opioids in children during the perioperative period. *Pediatr Anesth*. 2019;29(6):547–571. doi:10.1111/pan.13639
35. Ousley R, Burgoyne LL, Crowley NR, et al. An audit of patient-controlled analgesia after appendicectomy in children. *Paediatr Anaesth*. 2016;26(10):1002–1009. doi:10.0000/pan.12964
36. Cooney MF, Czarnecki M, Dunwoody C, et al. American society of pain management nursing position statement with clinical practice guidelines: authorized agent controlled analgesia. *Pain Manag Nurs*. 2013;14(3):176–181. doi:10.1016/j.pmn.2013.07.003
37. Faerber J, Zhong W, Dai D, et al. Comparative safety of morphine delivered via intravenous route vs patient-controlled analgesia device for pediatric inpatients. *J Pain Symptom Manage*. 2017;53(5):842–850. doi:10.1016/j.jpainsymman.2016.12.328
38. Chou R, Gordon DB, de Leon-Casasola OA, et al. Management of postoperative pain: a clinical practice guideline from the American pain society, the American Society of Regional Anesthesia and Pain Medicine, and the American Society of Anesthesiologists' Committee on Regional Anesthesia, Executive Committee, and Administrative Council. *J Pain*. 2016;17(2):131–157. doi:10.1016/j.jpain.2015.12.008

42. King MR, Wu RL, De Souza E, et al. Nonopioid analgesic usage among pediatric anesthesiologists: a survey of Society for Pediatric Anesthesia members. *Paediatr Anaesth*. 2020;30(6):713–715. doi:10.1111/pan.13891
46. Afshari A. Clonidine in pediatric anesthesia: the new panacea or a drug still looking for an indication? *Curr Opin Anaesthesiol*. 2019;32(3):327–333. doi:10.1097/ACO.0000000000000724
50. Manning AN, Bezzo LK, Hobson JK, et al. Dexmedetomidine dosing to prevent pediatric emergence delirium. *AANA J*. 2020:88(5):359–364.
51. Alghamdi F, Roth C, Jatana KR, et al. Opioid-sparing anesthetic technique for pediatric patients undergoing adenoidectomy: a pilot study. *J Pain Res*. 2020;13:2997–3004. doi:10.2147/JPR.S281275
53. Ji JY, Park JS, Kim JE, et al. Effect of esmolol and lidocaine on agitation in awake phase of anesthesia among children: a double-blind, randomized clinical study. *Chin Med J*. 2019;132(7):757–764. doi:10.1097/CM9.0000000000000141
56. Batko I, Kościelniak-Merak B, Tomasik PJ, et al. Lidocaine as an element of multimodal analgesic therapy in major spine surgical procedures in children: a prospective, randomized, double-blind study. *Pharmacol Rep*. 2020;72(3):744–755. doi:10.1007/s43440-020-00100-7
60. Han DS, Brockel MA, Boxley PJ, et al. Enhanced recovery after surgery and anesthetic outcomes in pediatric reconstructive urologic surgery. *Pediatr Surg Int*. 2021;37(1):151–159. doi:10.1007/s00383-020-04775-0
62. Mann GE, Flamer SZ, Nair S, et al. Opioid-free anesthesia for adenotonsillectomy in children. *Int J Pediatr Otorhinolaryngol*. 2021;140:110501. doi:10.1016/j.ijporl.2020.110501
63. Franz AM, Martin LD, Liston DE, et al. In pursuit of an opioid-free pediatric ambulatory surgery center. *Anesth Analg*. 2021;132(3):788–797 doi:10.1213/ANE.0000000000004774
66. Kagan J. Perspectives on two temperamental biases. *Philos Trans R Soc Lond B Biol Sci*. 2018;373(1744):20170158. doi:10.1098/rstb.2017.0158
70. Hancock L, Bryant RA. Perceived control and avoidance in post-traumatic stress. *Eur J Psychotraumatol*. 2018;9(1):1468708. doi:10.1080/20008198.2018.1468708
71. Heathcote LC, Lau JY, Mueller SC, et al. Child attention to pain and pain tolerance are dependent upon anxiety and attention control: an eye-tracking study. *Eur J Pain*. 2017;21(2):250–263. doi:10.1002/ejp.920
80. Page MG, Watt-Watson J, Choiniere M. Do depression and anxiety profiles over time predict persistent post-surgical pain? A study in cardiac surgery patients. *Eur J Pain*. 2017;21(6):965–976. doi:10.1002/ejp.998
86. Roebuck GS, Urquhart DM, Knox L, et al. Psychological factors associated with ultramarathon runners' supranormal pain tolerance: a pilot study. *J Pain*. 2018;19(12):1406–1415. doi:10.1016/j.jpain.2018.06.003
89. Sabanovic Adilovic A, Rizvanovic N, Adilovic H, et al. Caudal block with analgosedation - a superior anaesthesia technique for lower abdominal surgery in paediatric population. *Med Glas*. 2019;16(2). doi:10.17392/1017-19
92. Worley NB, Hill MN, Christianson JP. Prefrontal endocannabinoids, stress controllability and resilience: a hypothesis. *Prog Neuropsychopharmacol Biol Psychiatry*. 2018;85:180–188. doi:10.1016/j.pnpbp.2017.04.004

CHAPTER 132

Enhanced Recovery After Surgery

Marc Mecoli

> **LEARNING OBJECTIVES**
> - Understand the key components of enhanced recovery after surgery paradigms.
> - Review sample protocols for a variety of pediatric surgical domains.

INTRODUCTION

Enhanced recovery after surgery (ERAS) is an evolving multidisciplinary approach that focuses on reducing stress, promoting functional recovery, and reducing complications following major surgery. First described over 20 years ago in adult colorectal patients, ERAS protocols incorporate evidence-based ideas that promote accelerated recovery and well-being following a variety of surgical procedures and patient groups. Implementing perioperative protocols based on ERAS strategies have shown to reduce hospital length of stay in a wide array of adult and pediatric surgical procedures.[1,2] The key tenets of the ERAS approach to surgical care are preoperative patient education, avoidance of prolonged fasting times, minimally invasive surgical approaches, use of nonopioid analgesics with a focus on regional techniques, maintenance of euvolemia and normothermia, nonroutine use of surgical drains and tubes, and early mobilization following surgery (**Box 132.1**).

> **BOX 132.1   KEY COMPONENTS OF ERAS**
>
> **Preoperative**
> - Avoidance of prolonged fasting
> - Fluid and carbohydrate loading
> - Avoidance of routine preoperative bowel preparation
> - Antibiotic and antithrombotic prophylaxis
>
> **Intraoperative**
> - Multimodal, opioid-sparing analgesia
> - Regional analgesia
> - Maintenance of euvolemic state
> - Maintenance of normothermia
>
> **Postoperative**
> - Nonroutine use of nasogastric tubes
> - Nausea and vomiting prophylaxis
> - Opioid-sparing analgesia
>
> ERAS, enhanced recovery after surgery.

PEDIATRIC ERAS

The ERAS Society has published perioperative guidelines for several adult surgical domains, including colorectal, major orthopedic, urological, and cardiac surgery.[3-6] These guidelines are comprehensive and include preoperative, intraoperative, and postoperative ERAS components. Unfortunately, there is paucity of similarly robust published guidelines available to guide care for pediatric surgical populations.[1] A recent review of enhanced recovery protocol cohort studies in pediatric patients undergoing gastrointestinal, urology, and thoracic surgery demonstrated that studies included six or fewer interventions compared with 20 recommended interventions in most adult ERAS Society guidelines.[7] However, there exists a plethora of reports on the effect of ERAS elements in isolation or in combination on the quality of recovery following a variety of surgical procedures.

GASTROINTESTINAL SURGERY

Multiple studies have demonstrated efficacy of enhanced recovery pathways in adult colorectal surgery.[8,9] In children, 19 key components for an ERAS pathway for adolescent colorectal surgery have recently been identified through surveys and expert opinion and notably excluded the recommendation to avoid bowel preparation and the use of insulin to control severe hyperglycemia.[10] Implementation of a pediatric ERAS pathway was shown to decrease opioid utilization and shorten time to full feeding in a cohort of adolescent patients with inflammatory bowel disease undergoing laparoscopic and open bowel surgery.[11]

A recent retrospective cohort study on pediatric colorectal surgery patients (n=98, 2–18 years) reported decreased opioid utilization, faster time to oral intake, reduced length of stay, and no increase in complications.[12] It was offered that the incorporation of preoperative education, preoperative carbohydrate loading, administration of gabapentinoids and celecoxib preoperatively, regional nerve block or epidural catheter placement, use of intraoperative ketamine and dexmedetomidine infusions, standardized intraoperative fluid management, and early mobilization on postoperative day (POD) 0 collectively yielded favorable results.[12]

Neonatal physiology makes certain aspects of the perioperative care in intestinal surgery unique. The ERAS Society recently published guidelines for neonatal intestinal surgery and are shown in **Figure 132.1**.[13] To date, these are the only guidelines published by this society specific to pediatric patients.

PECTUS EXCAVATUM REPAIR

Pectus excavatum is the most common congenital anomaly of the chest wall and can have effects on functional capacity and quality of life.[14] The minimally invasive Nuss procedure has

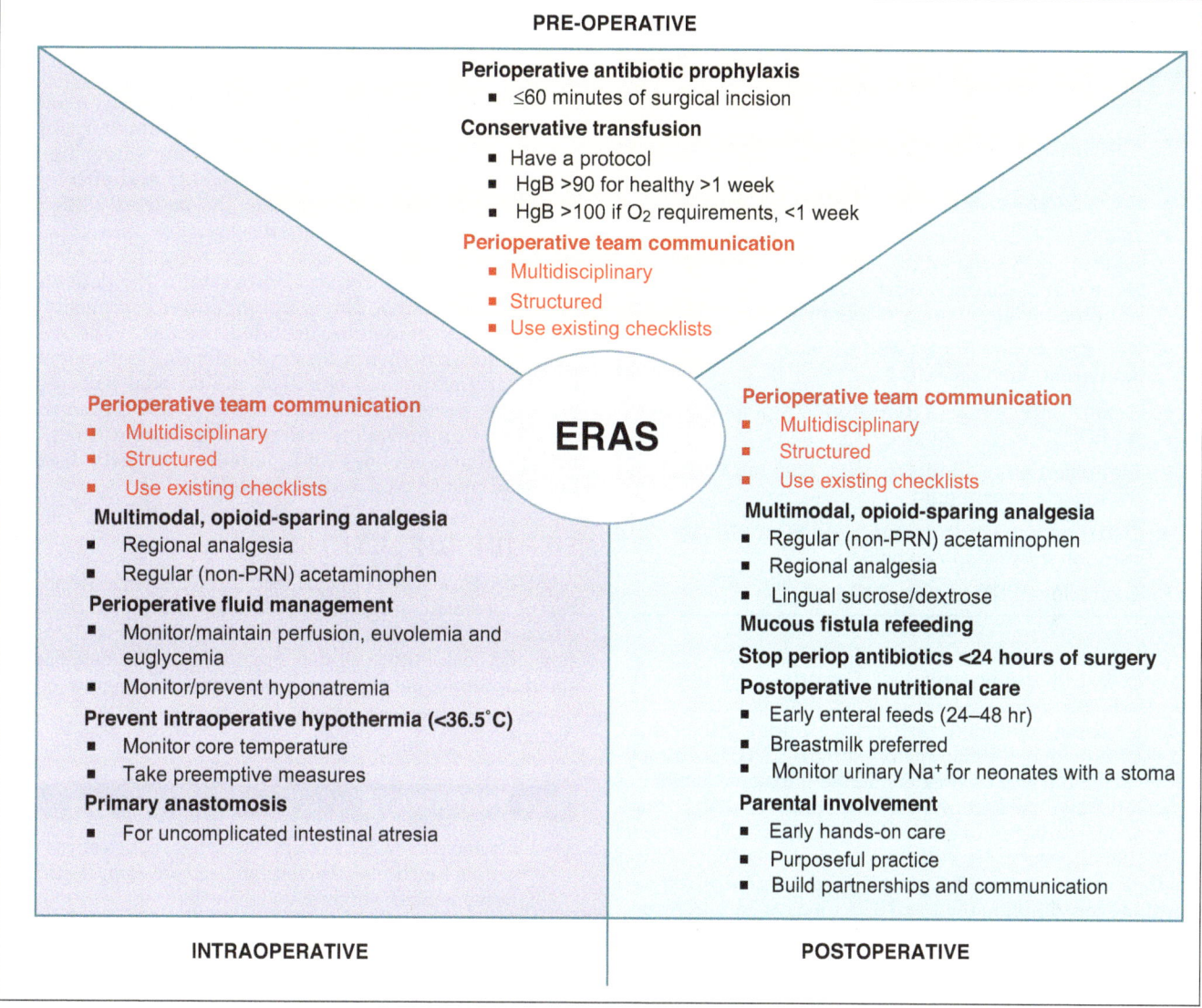

Figure 132.1: Components of ERAS Society approach for neonatal intestinal surgery ERAS, enhanced recovery after surgery.

ERAS, enhanced recovery after surgery; HgB, hemoglobin.

Source: From Brindle ME, McDiarmid C, Short K, et al. Consensus guidelines for perioperative care in neonatal intestinal surgery: enhanced recovery after surgery (ERAS®) society recommendations. *World J Surg.* 2020;44(8):2482–2492. doi:10.1007/s00268-020-05530-1.

become the standard surgical technique for repair of severe pectus excavatum.[14] For further information regarding the anesthetic management of pediatric patients undergoing surgical repair of a pectus excavatum, please refer to Chapter 97, "Pectus Excavatum Repair."

Adequate pain control and promotion of early mobilization are the mainstays of recovery following repair, and there is no consensus on how to best manage pain postoperatively. Enhanced recovery focused postoperative clinical pathway for pectus surgery targets early mobilization, frequent incentive spirometry, multimodal pain control including the use of regional techniques, and aggressive antiemetic and bowel regimens. Gurria and colleagues recently published a quality improvement study focused on the implementation of a standardized clinical pathway (n=350 patients) that resulted in postoperative length of stay reduction from 4.5 to 3.4 days.[15] Patient satisfaction and postoperative pain management were not compromised, and total patient charges decreased by 30%. Recently, at our institution, we have employed the use of erector spinae catheters for postoperative pain and opioid reduction. Current Cincinnati Children's Hospital Medical Center pain management regimen is shown in **Box 132.2**.

IDIOPATHIC POSTERIOR SPINAL FUSION

Surgical correction of idiopathic scoliosis is a major surgical procedure for adolescents. Postoperative pain, anxiety, and postoperative narcotic requirements and the resulting side effects inhibit functional recovery and early mobilization. A recent study examined outcomes following implementation of an enhanced recovery protocol for surgical correction

> **BOX 132.2** **PAIN MANAGEMENT REGIMEN FOLLOWING MINIMALLY INVASIVE PECTUS EXCAVATUM REPAIR**
>
> - Preoperative pregabalin 50–75 mg PO
> - Intraoperative methadone 0.1 mg/kg IV up to 5 mg
> - Intraoperative rib blocks performed by surgeon
> - Bilateral erector spinae catheters infusing ropivacaine 0.15% via infusion pumps. Catheters remain in place upon discharge and are removed at home by family on postoperative day (POD) 5
> - Acetaminophen IV q6h with transition to oral acetaminophen on POD 2
> - Ketorolac IV q6h with transition to oral ibuprofen on POD 2
> - Methocarbamol 15 mg/kg up to 1000 mg PO TID for muscle spasm pain
> - Diazepam 0.05 mg/kg up to 5 mg PO for breakthrough muscle spasm pain
> - Oxycodone PRN to start POD 1

of adolescent idiopathic scoliosis.[16] The primary tenets of the reported ERAS protocol included fasting time reduction, carbohydrate loading, multimodal analgesia, including paracetamol and nonsteroidal anti-inflammatory drugs (NSAIDS), intraoperative ketamine and dexmedetomidine infusions, avoidance of postoperative background narcotic infusions, early mobilization, and early removal of urinary catheters. For patients in the ERAS group, the authors found significantly shorter length of stay (4 days vs. 7 days in the control group), reduced morphine consumption (25% and 35% on days 2 and 3, respectively), and reduced pain intensity at rest and movement.

UROLOGICAL PROCEDURES

Urological surgery in pediatric patients includes a variety of complex intra-abdominal procedures that often involve primary bowel anastomosis such as bladder augmentation, creation of continent ileovesicostomy (Monti procedure), creation of continent appendicovesicostomy (Mitrofanoff procedure), and antegrade colonic enema (ACE) creation. These patients often have underlying neurogenic bowel and bladder and postoperative complications include ileus, stomal herniation, and wound infection.[17] Rove and colleagues recently published a report on implementation of an ERAS protocol in 13 patients undergoing reconstructive urological procedures including bowel anastomosis.[18] Protocol elements included no bowel preparation, preoperative oral carbohydrate loading, avoidance of opioids, regional anesthesia, no postoperative nasogastric tube, and early feeding. Protocol adherence improved after implementation, and complications were not increased. More recently, a multicenter prospective study has been initiated to examine protocol adherence and outcomes in pediatric patients undergoing complex urological procedures utilizing a structured ERAS pathway.[19]

CONGENITAL CARDIAC SURGERY

Enhanced recovery protocols have been studied in cardiac surgical patients, and the ERAS Society recently published evidence-based guidelines for perioperative care in adult cardiac surgical patients.[6] The mainstays of recommendations specific to cardiac surgery include the use of antifibrinolytics, perioperative glycemic control, goal-directed fluid therapy, perioperative opioid-sparing analgesia, avoidance of persistent hypothermia after cardiopulmonary bypass, early extubation, and the use of delirium screening tools. There are emerging reports on feasibility and effectiveness of enhanced recovery programs for patients undergoing surgery for congenital heart disease. Roy and colleagues recently published a report of reviewing the implementation of an enhanced recovery program in 155 patients (age >30 days to adulthood) undergoing lower complexity heart defects.[20] Key guidelines included the use of dexmedetomidine for emergence from anesthesia, implementation of an early extubation checklist, multimodal pain regimen guideline, postoperative nausea prophylaxis, preoperative nutritional optimization and reducing fasting times, early mobilization guidelines, and guidelines for early discontinuation of invasive lines and catheters.

FUTURE DIRECTIONS

ERAS programs are being utilized in a wide variety and number of pediatric surgical populations and show promising effects on various outcomes, including opioid use, length of stay, and cost. Future studies are warranted to better understand optimal quality metrics, adherence to program components, and impact on patient outcomes in pediatric surgery patients.

> **KEY TAKEAWAYS**
>
> - Early recovery after surgery pathways reduce stress, promote functional recovery, and reduce complications following major surgery.
> - Preoperative education, avoidance of prolonged fasting times, opioid reduction, utilization of reginal anesthesia, and maintenance of euvolemia and normothermia are key tenants of ERAS pathways.
> - ERAS programs are increasingly being utilized in a wide variety of pediatric surgical populations including colorectal, orthopedic, urological, chest wall, and cardiac.
> - Further data and research are needed to better elucidate optimal protocols in pediatric surgical patients.

RESOURCE

- Official ERAS Society website: https://erassociety.org/

KEY REFERENCES

Complete references for this chapter are online and available at https://connect.springerpub.com/content/book/978-0-8261-3875-0/part/part05/toc-part/ch132.

1. Rove KO, Edney JC, Brockel MA. Enhanced recovery after surgery in children: promising, evidence-based multidisciplinary care. *Paediatr Anaesth.* 2018;28(6):482–492. doi:10.1111/pan.13380
2. Ljungqvist O, Scott M, Fearon KC. Enhanced recovery after surgery: a review. *JAMA Surg.* 2017;152(3):292–298. doi:10.1001/jamasurg.2016.4952

7. Shinnick JK, Short HL, Heiss KF, et al. Enhancing recovery in pediatric surgery: a review of the literature. *J Surg Res.* 2016;202(1):165–176. doi:10.1016/j.jss.2015.12.051
10. Short HL, Heiss KF, Burch K, et al. Implementation of an enhanced recovery protocol in pediatric colorectal surgery. *J Pediatr Surg.* 2018;53(4):688–692. doi:10.1016/j.jpedsurg.2017.05.004
12. Purcell LN, Marulanda K, Egberg M, et al. An enhanced recovery after surgery pathway in pediatric colorectal surgery improves patient outcomes. *J Pediatr Surg.* 2021;56(1):115–120. doi:10.1016/j.jpedsurg.2020.09.028
13. Brindle ME, McDiarmid C, Short K, et al. Consensus guidelines for perioperative care in neonatal intestinal surgery: enhanced recovery after surgery (ERAS((R))) society recommendations. *World J Surg.* 2020;44(8):2482–2492. doi:10.1007/s00268-020-05530-1
15. Gurria JP, Simpson B, Tuncel-Kara S, et al. Standardization of clinical care pathway leads to sustained decreased length of stay following Nuss pectus repair: a multidisciplinary quality improvement initiative. *J Pediatr Surg.* 2020;55(12):2690–2698. doi:10.1016/j.jpedsurg.2020.08.009
16. Julien-Marsollier F, Michelet D, Assaker R, et al. Enhanced recovery after surgical correction of adolescent idiopathic scoliosis. *Paediatr Anaesth.* 2020;30(10):1068–1076. doi:10.1111/pan.13988
18. Rove KO, Brockel MA, Saltzman AF, et al. Prospective study of enhanced recovery after surgery protocol in children undergoing reconstructive operations. *J Pediatr Urol.* 2018;14(3):252.e1–252.e9. doi:10.1016/j.jpurol.2018.01.001
20. Roy N, Parra MF, Brown ML, et al. Initial experience introducing an enhanced recovery program in congenital cardiac surgery. *J Thorac Cardiovasc Surg.* 2020;160(5):1313–1321.e5. doi:10.1016/j.jtcvs.2019.10.049

CHAPTER 133

Operative and Anesthetic Care of the Patient With Chronic Pain

Soroush Merchant, Motaz Awad, Alexandra Szabova, and Kenneth R. Goldschneider

LEARNING OBJECTIVES

- The biopsychosocial model that governs chronic pain management can also be effectively applied to guide acute pain management.
- The patient on chronic opioids or opioid antagonist presents unique challenges to perioperative care.
- Patients with chronic pain have both cognitive-emotional and physical factors that need to be accounted for during preoperative planning as they can affect perioperative care.
- Anxiety is a common comorbidity present in patients with chronic pain and should be addressed.

INTRODUCTION

Knowing the basic concepts that underlie pain management is vital to best understanding and caring for the patient with chronic pain who presents to the operating room. While the *biopsychosocial model* of pain care is the conceptual umbrella term for how chronic pain is approached,[1] it can be directly applied to the management of acute pain as well. With this model, biologic pathology is seen as a facet of the pain experience but acknowledges that this is not the sole mechanism driving how the pain experience is perceived. The psychological and social interplay between the patient and their world combine to form the final pain experience. Thus, anything affecting one facet has the potential to improve or worsen the pain experience. For example, a patient presenting to the operating room with an ankle fracture may have sustained the injury while scoring the winning point in a tournament or as a result of being bullied. Despite the biological insult being the same, the psychosocial context differs greatly leading to variance in degree or severity of patient complaints of pain. This is similar to how anxiety can modify the pain experience (see Chapter 131, "Pediatric Pain Management," for information on anxiety and anxiolysis). In the chronic pain patient, the presence of pain, as well as the interplay amongst the psychosocial factors, typically have a considerably longer duration that results in the buildup of central sensitization. Thus, pain management following procedures in the operating room will require a holistic approach. This includes not only the typical acute pain modalities commonly employed but also extra time to build rapport, the use of anxiolytics, input from the chronic pain care team, the support of a child life specialist, and patience.

Another key concept of chronic pain management is that function is a key outcome that is perhaps even more important than actual pain relief. The rationale is twofold. Although not all pain will resolve, the patient needs to be able to live life to its fullest extent; in most cases, function needs to return to normal before chronic pain can resolve. Therefore, the general philosophy is to support and guide the patient to become as active as possible, which usually involves skilled psychologists and physical therapists as part of the pain management strategy. In the perioperative period, it is imperative anesthesia providers make every effort to prevent acute pain from derailing gains made in functional recovery as this can lead to setbacks in chronic pain management.

CARE OF THE PATIENT ON OPIOIDS FOR CHRONIC PAIN

Long-term opioid therapy, defined as daily or almost daily administration of an opioid for more than 90 days,[2] is used for only a small portion of pediatric chronic pain conditions (e.g., pain from sickle cell disease, epidermolysis bullosa, cancer and its sequellae). Despite its rarity, patients on long-term opioid therapy may present to the operating room. It is important that anesthesia providers understand the impact long-term opioid use can have on perioperative care and pain management.

TOLERANCE AND DEPENDENCE

Tolerance is a phenomenon that occurs following the administration of opioids on a regular interval, typically for at least a week. The result is a reduction in the maximum achievable effect or a right-shift in the dose-effect curve that mandates increased dosing to achieve the previously achieved effect. Acute desensitization of mu-opioid receptors is thought to be an initial step in the development of tolerance to opioids. Tolerance to various opioid-related effects, however, develops at different rates. This is termed *selective tolerance*. Tolerance to respiratory depression, nausea, vomiting, sedation, and euphoria all occur rapidly. Tolerance to cognitive effects, however, is not as quick to develop and tolerance to miosis and constipation rarely occurs. Dependence, or a state of adaptation that results in withdrawal symptoms upon abrupt cessation of opioids, often coexists with tolerance. Both tolerance and dependence differ from addiction, the discussion of which exceeds the limits of this chapter.

Patients receiving long-term opioid therapy often have increased opioid requirements to manage acute pain in the postoperative period as their baseline regimen will prove inadequate. Careful titration of opioid analgesics is important given the requirements are often higher than expected. In patients whose pain is expected to improve following surgery (e.g., tumor resection, joint replacement), it is imperative that the patient is closely monitored for oversedation as the stimulus:opioid ratio may shift quickly leaving them at risk. Similarly, if regional anesthesia is used for patients receiving long-term opioid therapy, the ensuing lack of pain may negate the stimulus requisite to counter the sedative effects of the patient's baseline opioid regimen. Therefore, careful monitoring and, possibly, adjustment to the baseline regimen may be required. Anesthesia providers should consider the addition of nonopioid analgesics to aid in the management of postoperative pain.

IMPLICATIONS OF BUPRENORPHINE IN THE PERIOPERATIVE ENVIRONMENT

While more commonly used to manage opioid addiction, buprenorphine can be used to manage pediatric chronic pain.[3,4] It may also be used in combination with naloxone. Buprenorphine is a partial mu-opioid receptor agonist that also acts as an agonist at the opioid-receptor-like 1 (ORL-1) receptors. It is also an antagonist at the kappa- and delta-opioid receptors.[3,5] Buprenorphine exhibits a higher affinity to the mu receptor, with slower association and dissociation when compared to other opioids or naloxone. Anesthesia providers should be aware that traditional opioids become less efficacious with concomitant buprenorphine therapy. Thus, the perioperative administration of buprenorphine can make perioperative pain control difficult.

There are multiple proposed guidelines regarding perioperative buprenorphine, but evidence is lacking resulting in a paucity of evidence-based guidelines to guide clinical practice. Proposed options for management of buprenorphine include discontinuation, reducing the dose, substitution with traditional opioids or methadone in advance, or continuing buprenorphine throughout the perioperative period. Administration of opioids with high mu-receptor affinity, such as hydromorphone or sufentanil, during the perioperative period is commonly recommended.[6-8] A multimodal approach is often recommended, with reliance on regional anesthesia and nonopioid analgesics prominent in the care of this population. Coordinating with the team managing the long-term opioid therapy is critical to lessen the risks associated with discontinuation and resumption of the patient's regimen.

NALTREXONE IN THE OPERATING ROOM

Naltrexone is similar to naloxone and acts as a potent competitive opioid antagonist at the mu-opioid receptors and as a partial agonist at kappa-opioid receptors. Preoperatively, naltrexone may be administered orally or via an intramuscular injection. Oral naltrexone is absorbed rapidly and has a 10-hour half-life, requiring repeated dosing. Intramuscular naltrexone (XR-NXT), however, yields opioid antagonism for 28 days.[9,10]

Naltrexone is used chronically in two scenarios: high dose for treatment of addiction and compulsive behaviors and low dose to manage chronic pain. Unfortunately, the impact of low-dose naltrexone on perioperative care remains unknown. For patients presenting on low-dose naltrexone therapy, anesthesia providers should adhere to the recommendations related to high-dose usage, which are largely based on opioid abuse treatment literature.

For elective surgery, it is recommended that oral naltrexone to be discontinued at least 72 hours prior to surgery and XR-NXT to be discontinued at least 4 weeks prior to surgery. Of note, chronic blockade of mu-opioid receptors may lead to upregulation of those receptors, increasing the potential for heightened sensitivity to opioids and risk for oversedation.[9,10] Thus, close monitoring is recommended. If opioid administration is required for management of acute pain during naltrexone therapy, opioids should be carefully titrated to effect under close observation. Perioperative pain management should be optimized using systemic nonopioid analgesics such as ketamine and techniques, as well as regional anesthesia.[10] Naltrexone should be reinitiated under the guidance of a specialist several days following the last dose of opioids.

GENERAL APPROACH TO THE CHRONIC PAIN PATIENT

Given the complexity of this patient population, a team approach including all stakeholders (the patient, family, anesthesia provider, pain physician or prescriber of long-term analgesics, and surgeon) is advised to ensure safe, effective care, especially for moderate to extensive surgical procedures (Figure 133.1).

While a variety of medications are used to manage chronic pain, it is important anesthesia providers are aware that some of the frequently used medications do not have IV formulations and may cause withdrawal syndromes if stopped abruptly. Procedures associated with brief NPO times usually will not require major

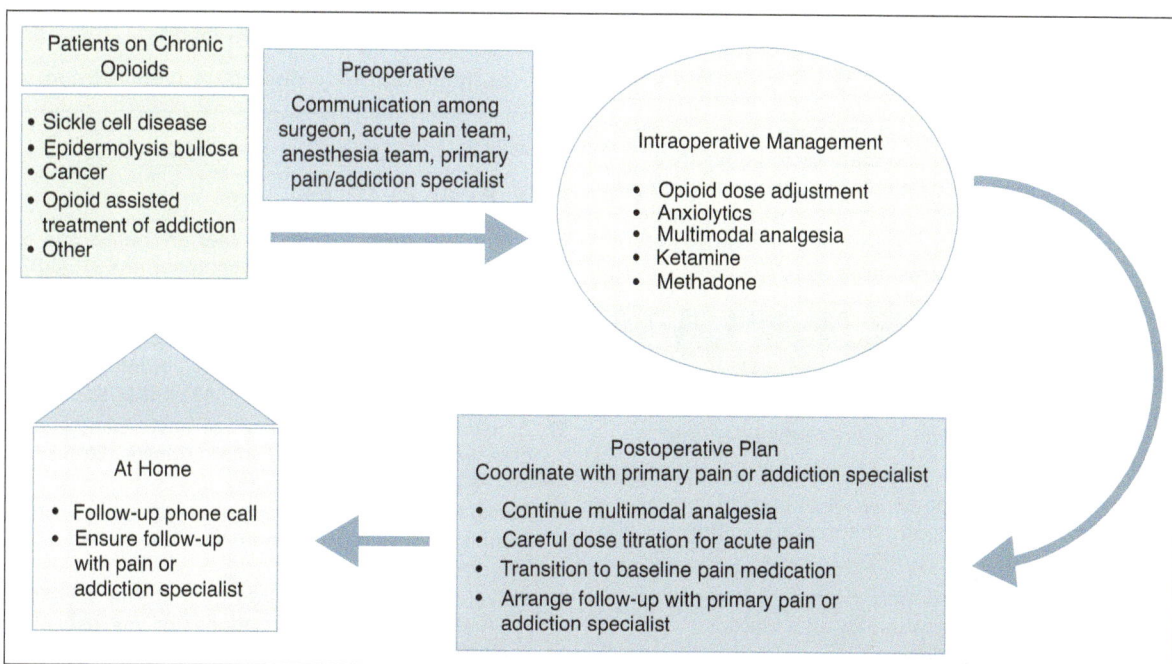

Figure 133.1: Workflow when caring for chronic pain patients presenting to the operating room.

Table 133.1 Approach to Analgesic Management With Chronic Pain

Medication Class	Preoperative Action	Postoperative Action
Anticonvulsants	Wean if prolonged NPO planned	Resume as soon as eating
Antidepressants (tricyclic, SSRI, and SNRI)	Wean if prolonged NPO planned, otherwise continue	Resume as soon as eating
Clonidine	Continue	IV while NPO if rebound phenomena seen, or oral when taking PO
Herbal agents (research each for specific risk profile)	Stop, with timing based on risk profile	Resume as risk of interactions and primary effects subside
Opioids	Continue	Plan to wean to baseline with guidance of chronic pain care provider
NSAIDs	Hold per surgical preference	Resume per surgical preference
Muscle relaxants	Continue	IV equivalent while NPO, then resume enteral form

NPO, nothing by mouth; NSAIDs, nonsteroidal anti-inflammatory drugs; SNRI, serotonin and norepinephrine reuptake inhibitors; SSRI, selective serotonin reuptake inhibitors.

interruptions of medications, but more prolonged NPO times can be problematic. It is optimal to coordinate with the chronic pain provider prior to elective surgeries regarding weaning and resuming all medications to reduce side effects, minimize risk of withdrawal, and reduce risk of misuse. Preoperative discussion to set realistic pain management goals and to address postoperative pain expectation is also very important tool in enhancing patient and family satisfaction.[9,11] Part of this discussion is the need for alterations in existing medications and plans for perioperative management and the rationale for changes made. Table 133.1 provides general guidance regarding approaches to each major class of chronic pain medication.

COMPLEX REGIONAL PAIN SYNDROME

Complex regional pain syndrome (CRPS) is a painful condition characterized by pain in extremities, which is disproportionate in time or degree to a previous trauma. CRPS pain is nondermatomal and is associated with disturbances in sensory, motor, sudomotor, vasomotor, and/or trophic findings. Two types are identified, with CRPS type II uniquely associated with a definable nerve lesion.[12]

Preventing CRPS is a difficult task, because the incidence is small after surgery, and there are no markers to know ahead of time who is at risk. However, principles of good perioperative pain care can reduce the incidence of chronic postoperative pain. For patients with active CRPS or a history of it, several aspects of care should be overserved as shown in the Box 133.1.[13,14]

KEY TAKEAWAYS

- The biopsychosocial model of pain care applies to both chronic and acute pain is crucial in caring for pediatric chronic pain patients who present to the operating room.
- Chronic opioid agonism and antagonism present special challenges in perioperative care that require planning and communication.
- Multimodal therapy for perioperative pain is the single most consistent recommendation for all scenarios involving chronic pain patients.

BOX 133.1 KEY POINTS WHEN CARING FOR PATIENTS WITH COMPLEX REGIONAL PAIN SYNDROME (CRPS)

- Coordination of pain care should take place with the patient's pain physician whenever possible.
- Surgeries should be postponed until CRPS I signs are minimal to absent when possible.
- Regional anesthesia techniques should be used whenever possible.
- Multimodal analgesia may offer protection and should be pursued.
- Low-dose ketamine should be considered for use during the procedure.
- Gabapentin should be continued or started preoperatively if possible.
- Vitamin C 500 mg daily for 6 weeks from date of injury may reduce risk for CRPS.
- Early mobilization postoperatively is important.

KEY REFERENCES

Complete references for this chapter are online and available at https://connect.springerpub.com/content/book/978-0-8261-3875-0/part/part03/toc-part/ch133.

1. Liossi C, Richard F, Howard RF. Pediatric chronic pain: biopsychosocial assessment and formulation. *Pediatrics.* 2016;138(5):e20160331. doi:10.1542/peds.2016-0331
11. Brooks MR, Golianu B. Perioperative management in children with chronic pain. *Pediatr Anesth.* 2016;26(8):794–806. doi:10.1111/pan.12948
14. Asaad B, Glass P. Perioperative management for patients with complex regional pain syndrome. *Pain Manag.* 2012;2(6):561–567. doi:10.2217/pmt.12.62
15. Cravero JP, Agarwal R, Berde C, et al. The Society for Pediatric Anesthesia recommendations for the use of opioids in children during the perioperative period. *Paediatr Anaesth.* 2019;29(6):547–571. doi:10.1111/pan.13639

CHAPTER 134

Palliative Care

Mark John Meyer and Lori Ann McKenna

> **LEARNING OBJECTIVES**
>
> - Understand the current trends in pediatric palliative care.
> - Understand that while childhood mortality has decreased, symptom burden remains high, and many pediatric palliative patients benefit from curative as well as palliative procedures in the operating room (OR).
> - Understand how to manage a pediatric palliative patient with advance directives in the OR with required reconsideration.
> - Understand perioperative management for full suspension of advance directives, limited resuscitation based on procedures, and limited resuscitation based on patient's goals.

INTRODUCTION

For many anesthesia providers, the interaction with palliative care patients begins near the time of diagnosis, often during a biopsy, line placement, or other diagnostic test such as MRI, CT, lumbar puncture (LP), or bone marrow aspirate (BMA). This is a time of high anxiety for patients and families, not only because of the procedure itself but also due to the added concern of a new serious diagnosis. Although the frequency with which pediatric palliative patients undergo surgery is not well studied, it has been reported to account for less than 1% of all pediatric surgeries performed annually.[1] While this patient population presents to the operating room infrequently, they present significant challenges for anesthesia providers, surgeons, and perioperative staff alike during the perioperative period. This chapter explores the interface of anesthesia and pediatric palliative populations, with a focus on perioperative management of advance directives. Included is a description of the reconsideration and suspension of advance directives, limits of resuscitation based on procedures, and limits of resuscitation based on goals.

BACKGROUND

Over the last decade, the criteria for defining a pediatric palliative patient have expanded from a diagnosis that will end in death in the near term to a broader list of diagnoses comprised of life-limiting conditions for which there may be no cure. The latter group includes those with an uncertain prognosis and disease trajectory, though many will live into adolescence and adulthood. Another significant change in the past decade relates to the timing of the introduction into palliative care, as this now often begins at the time of diagnosis as opposed to historical approaches that initiated entry into palliative care near the end of life. These changes in practice have greatly expanded the services and support offered to many pediatric palliative patients, with a variety of patient populations now receiving prolonged periods of palliative care. For example, patients diagnosed with leukodystrophy who are expected to have a limited lifespan may live to their third decade and often enter palliative care shortly after diagnosis. Similarly, many boys with Duchenne muscular dystrophy will now live well into adulthood despite remaining at risk for sudden death. Patient populations such as these frequently require elective, and sometimes urgent, surgical procedures such as appendectomy, adenotonsillectomy, dental rehabilitation, and endoscopy in the first two decades of life. They may also need condition-specific procedures such as gastrostomy, central line placement, or tracheostomy placement. It is important to understand that when presenting to the operating room, many pediatric palliative patients will have advance directives and/or do not resuscitate (DNR) orders. It is imperative that the anesthesia provider have a sound understanding of the application of such orders in the perioperative setting.

MANAGEMENT OF ADVANCE DIRECTIVES

All too often when anesthesia providers are made aware that a patient has advance directives, it is interpreted as simply meaning a DNR is in place. Unfortunately, this does not provide the anesthesia provider any information regarding the patient's or surrogate's wishes beyond excluding chest compressions, intubation, defibrillation, or resuscitative medications. In reality, however, most interventions by anesthesia providers can be considered resuscitative making adhering to a patient's advance directives challenging. Historically, it was common practice to suspend DNR orders during the perioperative period to avert the aforementioned confusion. This is no longer common practice as the automatic suspension is ethically problematic. Not only is it a denial of the patient's or surrogate's autonomy, but it also fails to respect their participation in the decision-making process. In doing so, it may result in unwanted aggressive supportive care or conversely foregoing care that is appropriate. As such, the American Society of Nurse Anesthetists, American Society of Anesthesiologists, and American College of Surgeons recommend reconsideration of advance care directives rather than automatic suspension of the orders during the perioperative and intraoperative period.[2–4]

The recommendation to require reconsideration of existing DNR orders mandates a discussion involving the patient and/or their surrogate and the involved healthcare providers prior to the start of a procedure. The conversation should include a thorough discussion of the perioperative risks, the patient's treatment goals, and acceptable approaches to care that adhere to patient's goals and wishes. This includes interventions managed by all of the care team, including anesthesia, surgery, nursing, the intensive care, the primary treatment teams, and palliative care. The outcome of the reconsideration can be revoking the existing DNR orders allowing for (a) full attempt at resuscitation *or* modifications and (b) limits placed on resuscitation by procedure *or* (c) limits defined by the patient's goals.[5]

NO LIMITS ON RESUSCITATION

After reconsideration of DNR orders, it may be appropriate to suspend the advance directives during the perioperative period for a variety of reasons; many surgical procedures require airway manipulation or support, anesthetic medications may result in hemodynamic compromise, or the surgical procedure itself may be associated with temporary pulmonary and/or hemodynamic compromise requiring escalations in supportive care. Quite often, interventions at odds with preexisting advance directives are expected and temporary and are required only for the duration of the surgical procedure. Additionally, when the patient presents in their baseline state of health and their individual risks for surgery and/or anesthesia are not inordinate, it can be appropriate to use all resuscitative efforts. A clear advantage of suspension of advance directives is the reduction of interpretation errors on the behalf of the anesthesia provider. A well-developed plan is easy to define, communicate, and easily understood by all.

LIMITED RESUSCITATION BY PROCEDURE

An alternative suspension of DNR orders is the procedure-oriented approach that limits the action of the perioperative team members by procedure. In this scenario, it is important that the anesthesia provider thoroughly explain to the patient and/or their surrogate the necessary interventions to ensure the patient's safety throughout the procedure. This should also include a discussion of interventions or procedures that may not be essential to care. As patients and their surrogates are not experienced clinicians, it is common for them to not fully comprehend the breadth of interventions commonly employed during a general anesthetic. Misunderstanding or a lack of information may lead to refusal of medication administration as well. For example, many patients and surrogates are familiar with the use of epinephrine during cardiac resuscitation. This medication has far more utility in the perioperative period, however, and can be used to treat bronchospasm and/or anesthesia-induced hypotension. Failure to appreciate the full utility of the medication may inadvertently lead to refusal of all vasoactive medications. An advantage of procedure-oriented suspension of DNR orders is that it allows for clarity regarding what is acceptable by the patient and/or their surrogate (Box 134.1).

LIMITED RESUSCITATION BY GOALS

Many palliative care patients have advance directives based on a goal-directed approach. In this scenario, the anesthesia provider should use their clinical judgement to determine which medical interventions, including resuscitative measures, can be used to support the patient while aligning with their goals. Many patients with a life-threatening condition benefit from life-sustaining care and opt to undergo procedures that may prolong and improve their quality of life. Their goals are to continue to receive life-sustaining treatments and/or treatments that reduce symptom burden. Therefore, the use of resuscitation efforts for correctable respiratory or hemodynamic compromise induced in the operating room is consistent with their goals.

Often these patients and/or surrogates will decide to allow for a natural death or to forego resuscitation efforts for irreversible causes related to the primary condition, thereby making the treatment of hypotension following the induction of anesthesia appropriate but negating the ability to correct hypotension secondary to massive blood loss. One advantage to this approach is that patients and their surrogates are not always able to judge which procedures are appropriate and many are not interested in the technical conduct of the anesthetic and surgical procedure. Additionally, the anesthesia and surgical providers are afforded freedom in judgement and flexibility in action to correct patient and procedural variations. The challenge of a goal-directed approach is that patient or surrogate must be able to articulate their goals, and the anesthesia provers must be able translate the goals into a practical plan for intraoperative management. Goals such as "focusing on quality of life" are vague and require unguided interpretation by the anesthesia provider. In this scenario, the palliative care team and primary care team can help clarify patient goals. It is also important to convey to the patient and/or their surrogate that goals and intraoperative risks change as life-threatening conditions progress and that a reconsideration of goals is recommended with each successive anesthetic.

PERIOPERATIVE MANAGEMENT

Prior to arrival in the operating room, a thorough preoperative evaluation should take place, allowing ample opportunity to optimize critically ill patients. During the preoperative evaluation, the discussion regarding how advance directives will be managed during the perioperative period should be initiated. How long any departures from standing advance directives should remain in place should also be considered as full recovery from anesthesia and surgery may require 24 to 48 hours depending on the surgical procedure planned. Once a plan has been agreed on, it should be documented in the medical record, and the patient's orders should reflect any alterations made to the advance directives. The plan must also be communicated to the entiqre team caring for the patient. Quite often this is done via a preoperative brief involving the entire perioperative team allows all questions to be answered and for contingency planning to be discussed. Utilizing this approach not only improves staff performance, but it can also reduce staff distress with caring for these challenging patients.

BOX 134.1 PROCEDURES TO CONSIDER FOREGOING WITH PROCEDURE-SPECIFIC SUSPENSION OF DO-NOT-RESUSCITATE ORDERS

- **Airway support:** Supplemental oxygen, oral airway, intubation, bilevel positive airway pressure (BiPAP), suctioning, and bag and mask ventilation
- **Vascular access:** Arterial, central, and peripheral IV access
- **Medication administration:** With emphasis on resuscitate medications, including vasoactive medications, and antibiotic administration
- **Invasive procedures:** Thoracentesis, chest tube placement, cardioversion, defibrillation, extracorporeal membrane oxygenation (ECMO), blood product transfusion, Foley catheter placement

KEY TAKEAWAYS

- Pediatric palliative support begins at diagnosis and while mortality is declining symptom burden is on the rise necessitating surgical intervention.
- Automatically forgoing a DNR order during the perioperative period is no longer the norm for pediatric palliative patients.
- The policy of reconsideration of advance directives needs to be followed when pediatric palliative patients present for surgical procedures.
- The policy of reconsideration offers three choices for the pediatric palliative patient: no limits on resuscitation, procedure-based limitations, or goal-based limitations.
- A multidisciplinary approach is of utmost importance when caring for the pediatric palliative patient in the perioperative environment.

REFERENCES

1. Goudreault M, Humbert N, Gauvin F, et al. Interventions in the operating room for children near end of life: a multidisciplinary approach. *J Pediatr Surg*. 2018;53(5):1065–1068. doi:10.1016/J.JPEDSURG.2018.02.038
2. AANA Board of Directors. Reconsiderations of advance directives: practice guidelines and policy considerations. 2015. https://www.aana.com/docs/default-source/practice-aana-com-web-documents-(all)/reconsideration-of-advance-directives.pdf?sfvrsn=550049b1_6
3. American College of Surgeons. Statement on advance directives by patients: "Do not resuscitate" in the operating room. 2014. https://www.facs.org/About-ACS/Statements/19-Advance-Directives
4. Bastron R. Ethical concerns in anesthetic care for patients with do-not-resuscitate orders. 1996. https://pubs.asahq.org/anesthesiology/article/85/5/1190/35862/Ethical-Concerns-in-Anesthetic-Care-for-Patients
5. Truog R, Waisel D, Burns J. DNR in the OR. *Anesthesiology*. 1999;90(1):289–295. doi:10.1097/00000542-199901000-00034

CHAPTER 135

Procedures in Radiology

Christopher A. Allphin and Ali I. Kandil

LEARNING OBJECTIVES

- Identify the different imaging modalities utilized for the pediatric patient.
- Understand the unique considerations of each imaging modality for the pediatric patient.
- Describe anesthetic plans appropriate for each commonly used imaging modality.
- Recognize the most commonly used anesthetic and sedative medications for radiology procedures and understand the appropriate use of those medications.

INTRODUCTION

Anesthesia is often utilized in the pediatric population for imaging and radiological procedures. While radiologists historically managed sedation for these procedures, many factors have led to the involvement of anesthesia and nonanesthesia providers.[1,2] Much of the challenge associated with radiological studies relates to the requirement of a motionless patient to optimize image quality, oftentimes with little to no stimulation from the imaging study or procedure. Furthermore, the need for anesthesia in the pediatric population increases as the number of imaging studies increases.[3] Depending on the patient's age, comorbidities, and number of imaging studies required, this may necessitate anesthetic interventions ranging from anxiolysis to general anesthesia. Off-site anesthesia varies dramatically from institution to institution, with the required expertise increasing as the acuity of the patient increases. This chapter reviews some of the common imaging modalities and the associated unique aspects of anesthetic care.

COMMONLY USED IMAGING MODALITIES

MAGNETIC RESONANCE IMAGING

MRI is a medical imaging technique used to diagnose and evaluate different abnormalities, including developmental anomalies, seizures, neoplasms, and cerebrovascular disease.[4] The MRI suite is an environment with unique elements, especially when considering the pediatric population. The noise, confined space, and ever-present sources of artifact, whether it be physiological or metal-related, create different challenges in the care of the patient and often require anesthesia to yield impactful studies.

One unique characteristic is the emphasis on proper positioning. Unlike other imaging modalities, MRI requires the patient to remain in the same position for long periods in order to capture adequate images. An infant undergoing an MRI of the brain may fall asleep after being swaddled, thereby requiring no medications to facilitate imaging, but a toddler undergoing a similar study may require medications to achieve adequate positioning. Patient factors other than age may also contribute to positioning difficulties. Chronic back pain, anxiety, or the inability to lie flat for prolonged periods of time are only a few of the examples of conditions that prevent the patient from being able to remain motionless in order to capture adequate images. Abnormal anatomy, such as contractures or protruding tumors, may also make it difficult or impossible to achieve appropriate positioning without the administration of sedation or anesthetic medications.

Additionally, the MRI suite itself adds logistic challenges. The magnetic pull of the scanner, coupled with anesthesia providers' reliance on certain equipment to ensure patient safety, poses challenges not witnessed in other venues. The noise created by an MRI scanner during imaging is loud, requiring the patient to wear ear protection. A 3-Tesla (T) MRI scanner can reach a noise level of up to 130.7 dBA, which is higher than the noise level experienced when working with a jackhammer.[5] Prolonged exposure can lead to hearing loss. Ear protection will reduce the noise level, but even with ear protection healthy individuals can have a temporary shift in the hearing threshold.[5,6] Some age groups may not tolerate or become frightened with the placement of earplugs. In addition, the MRI scanner is an enclosed cylinder that may cause claustrophobia, depending on the type of scan and positioning of the patient. These environmental factors may require the need for sedation or anesthetic medications.

In other instances, an MRI study may require the administration of contrast to improve the diagnostic accuracy of the scan. The radiologist may need to give the contrast via either an IV catheter or orally, depending on the goals. For IV catheter placement, a pediatric patient may require sedation or anesthesia. If oral contrast is necessary, one needs to consider the timing of administration or that the patient may not tolerate oral contrast administration, further necessitating the placement of an endotracheal tube (ETT).[7]

COMPUTED TOMOGRAPHY

CT is a medical imaging technique used to differentiate low-density and high-density structures. Indications range from cerebral vascular accidents, stroke, and acute trauma, to evaluation of middle ear ossicles, and evaluation of nodules, cancer, or metastatic disease, or obstructive pulmonary processes. Imaging via CT is rapid, with scans typically complete in 10 to 80 seconds. Therefore, the short imaging time makes CT ideal for use with medically unstable patients requiring an expeditious diagnosis. Ultimately, the need for sedation and/or the anesthetic plan for the patient depends on the goals of the imaging study.

While most adult patients can likely undergo CT scans with no medication or with oral anxiolytic medications, some individuals in the pediatric population may not tolerate a short imaging study. Indications for anesthesia in the pediatric population may include combative or uncooperative patients, nausea and vomiting, need for oral contrast, angiography, medical instability, neck instability, and the need for breathholds. Additionally, some CT scans require special positioning which may require adjuvant medications. While not always indicated in these instances, anesthetics may be helpful in obtaining adequate imaging.

NUCLEAR MEDICINE

Nuclear medicine is a specialized field of radiology that uses radioactive medications to examine organ function and structure to facilitate diagnosis and treatment. Single-photon emission CT (SPECT) and PET are nuclear medicine studies commonly used in children. Like with MRI and CT, the patient needs to remain still for image recording. Procedural sedation is an option, but some patients may require general anesthesia depending on their medical history, age, or anxiety. The stakes are quite high with many of these images, as malignancy, spread of malignancy, or remission from previous malignancy may be captured.

INTERVENTIONAL RADIOLOGY

Procedures performed in interventional radiology (IR) allow radiologists to use image guidance modalities to facilitate vascular and nonvascular interventions. The interventions often performed include, but are not limited to, angiography, embolization, sclerotherapy, and biopsies. The anesthetic needs depend heavily on the procedure and location of the targeted pathology, in addition to the age and comorbidities of the patient.

Procedures on cerebral lesions often involve physiological considerations and alterations. Angiographic procedures may require access to the femoral vessels, necessitating the patient to remain in supine position during the procedure and for a prolonged period on completion. In the pediatric population, especially in moribund infants, vascular access for interventional procedures is exceedingly difficult in a nonsedated/anesthetized patient, necessitating anesthesia services.

RADIATION ONCOLOGY

Radiation oncology is the use of radiation therapy to destroy certain tumors in children. The therapy is usually very quick and painless. One of the reasons radiation oncologists request anesthesia is that they require the patient to remain motionless to be able to precisely target the tumor cells. One of the biggest challenges of radiation therapy is the frequency of the treatments, with treatments often occurring daily or multiple times per day over a period of several weeks. Radiation oncology procedures commonly witnessed in the pediatric population include stereotactic radiosurgery and total body irradiation.

Stereotactic radiosurgery is used to treat intracranial tumors and arteriovenous malformations. This procedure involves the placement of a head frame to maintain a still patient and facilitate accurate radiation targeting during subsequent treatments. Total body radiation, used in preparation for bone marrow transplant, is normally a twice-a-day treatment administered over a period of 6 weeks. Innovative anesthetic plans have been employed for children receiving consecutive anesthetics whereby repeated airway manipulation would otherwise be required. Drugs such as dexmedetomidine, ketamine, and propofol have made successfully completing treatment regimens more achievable.

SELECTION OF ANESTHESIA DEPTH

When creating an anesthetic plan for a patient who is undergoing a radiological procedure, it is important to consider the patient's medical history and age, as well as the scheduled procedure. Coordination between the ordering provider, the radiologist, and the anesthesia provider is imperative to ensure optimal imaging and patient safety. While some patients require minimal to no sedation, others may require moderate sedation, deep sedation, or even general anesthesia.

The American Society of Anesthesiologists (ASA) has published the definition of general anesthesia and the levels of sedation as a guide for providers. The definitions take into account the patient's responsiveness, need for airway intervention, adequacy of spontaneous ventilation, and cardiovascular function. The levels of sedation include minimal sedation, moderate sedation, and deep sedation, followed by general anesthesia (see Box 135.1).[8] While these are clear definitions, it is possible for the patient to pass between the different levels of sedation or in and out of general anesthesia very quickly. Thus, it can be challenging to definitively identify the current state of sedation or anesthesia.

Many nonanesthesia providers administer sedative medications in radiology suites to pediatric patients. The ASA has released guidelines on the administration of sedation by nonanesthesia providers.[9] Individuals administering sedative medications should receive adequate training in order to provide safe and effective care. In 2018, an ASA task force, in conjunction with the governing bodies of several other specialties, released the most recent guidelines on the administration of moderate procedural sedation and analgesia. These guidelines include adequate preoperative evaluation and preparation, monitoring, supplemental oxygen, medications, ability to treat airway compromise, and recovery care.[10] The American Academy of Pediatrics and the American Academy of Pediatric Dentistry produced guidelines for the safe administration of sedation.[11] There is no difference between nonanesthesia providers when comparing the rates of major complications, although further training is necessary for nonanesthesia providers performing deep sedation.[12,13]

When considering a patient for monitored anesthesia care (MAC; Box 135.2) or general anesthesia, it is very important to adhere to strict NPO guidelines.[14] In 2019, a multidisciplinary

---

BOX 135.1 LEVELS OF SEDATION

- **Minimal sedation:** The patient responds normally to verbal stimulation, while their airway, spontaneous ventilation, and cardiovascular function are unaltered.
- **Moderate sedation:** The patient responds purposefully to verbal stimulation or light touch and can maintain adequate spontaneous ventilation and a patent airway. Cardiovascular function is usually unchanged.
- **Deep sedation:** The patient responds purposefully after repeated or painful stimulation. They may not be able to maintain a patent airway or adequate spontaneous ventilation, requiring intervention. Cardiovascular function is usually unchanged.
- **General anesthesia:** The patient does not respond to surgical stimulation. Airway patency and spontaneous ventilation are often inadequate, requiring intervention. Cardiovascular function may also be compromised.

> **BOX 135.2 MONITORED ANESTHESIA CARE**
>
> - **Monitored anesthesia care:** direct involvement by a qualified anesthesia provider, which includes the provider completing a preoperative evaluation, understanding the patient's coexisting medical conditions, and converting to general anesthesia when necessary
>
> *Source:* From Distinguishing Monitored Anesthesia Care ("MAC") from Moderate Sedation/Analgesia (Conscious Sedation), n.d.

international committee[15] established NPO guidelines specifically for procedural sedation, due to the low aspiration risk for patients receiving procedural sedation. The guidelines take into account the risk factors for aspiration of both the patient and the procedure and provide more timing flexibility for patients who fall into the negligible and mild risk factor groups.

When selecting the anesthetic type for a patient in each location within the radiology department, providers must take into consideration the unique characteristics of each patient within that specific location.

ANESTHESIA FOR MRI

Some patients in the MRI suite require no sedation. For each age group in the pediatric population, providers have had success with different distraction strategies. With neonates and small infants, feeding, swaddling, and reducing noise and patient movement often are successful techniques that minimize the need for adjunctive medications.[17] For older children or adolescents, distraction or entertainment in the form of movies or music has proved to be an effective approach to tempering MRI-related anxiety and movement.[17] Abbreviating MRI protocols to shorten the duration of the total scan time may also potentially decrease the need for adjunctive medications.[18] Likewise, some institutions have reported success with behavioral training in children to avoid the use of medications.[19,20]

While providers may be able to avoid adjunctive medications for patients undergoing MRI studies, many pediatric patients continue to require sedation and/or anesthesia to achieve adequate imaging studies to overcome the aforementioned challenges. Additionally, some MRI studies have special considerations that require the use of general anesthesia. For example, MRI enterography to evaluate inflammatory bowel disease requires general anesthesia with an ETT, followed by placement of a nasogastric tube to administer oral contrast.[7] For other MRI studies, radiologists may need the patient to hold their breath for prolonged periods, requiring general anesthesia and possibly muscle relaxation.

When providing anesthesia in the MRI suite, it is important to have monitoring devices that are MRI-compatible. Prior to induction of anesthesia, anesthesia providers must evaluate which equipment is MRI-safe and can enter the MRI room in the event of an emergency. This includes laryngoscopes, anesthesia machines, ventilators, infusion pumps, and emergency equipment. Many pieces of equipment are not MRI-safe and have the potential to cause great harm to the patient and/or providers if allowed to enter the MRI scanner. Providers should also have screening methods for patients and providers prior to entering the MRI suite. Screening should include the presence of foreign bodies or implanted devices, such as pacemakers or defibrillators.[21,22]

ANESTHESIA FOR CT

Similar to MRI, many of the patients arriving for CT imaging do not need any sedative medications for adequate imaging. The significantly shorter duration required for CT studies makes such strategies as swaddling, distraction, or behavioral training effective. In many instances, the goals of the CT imaging study dictate sedation and anesthetic requirements.

Sedative medications can assist in various aspects of the care of patients arriving to the CT scanner. When considering medications for sedation, providers must take into account the duration of the scan compared with the medication duration. A medication with a long duration may not be appropriate for a patient undergoing a scan that takes seconds or minutes to complete.

General anesthesia may be the ideal plan for some patients requiring CT imaging. For pediatric chest CT imaging, for instance, the radiologist may need motionless images taken at different phases of the respiratory cycle, requiring a general anesthetic with the placement of an ETT and adequate lung recruitment to combat atelectasis.[23] Another factor that may dictate the need for a general anesthetic with an ETT is when oral contrast is administered prior to imaging. Timing is important with contrast studies, and preimaging intake of the oral contrast may violate the NPO guidelines.[14]

ANESTHESIA FOR NUCLEAR MEDICINE

The goal of a nuclear medicine study is to achieve adequate imaging of a motionless patient. Similar to other radiological studies, the choice of an anesthetic in nuclear medicine depends on the patient's age and medical history. The use of sedation or general anesthesia is rare and occurs most commonly in young children or in scans that require patients to remain absolutely still, such as brain SPECT or SPECT studies in children with cancer.[24]

ANESTHESIA FOR IR PROCEDURES

Many pediatric patients undergoing interventional radiology (IR) procedures require deep sedation or general anesthesia, even though these procedures may be done with minimal to moderate sedation in adults. Unlike most other radiology studies, many IR procedures involve some type of intervention that many pediatric patients have difficulty tolerating even with supplemental medications.[25]

Therapeutic neurointerventional procedures for patients with cerebral arteriovenous malformations, such as Moyamoya disease or cerebral aneurysms, often require special considerations, especially in pediatric patients. Most commonly, providers use general anesthesia with muscle relaxation as movement can be dangerous to the patient. Muscle relaxation allows the anesthesia provider to manipulate the ventilation, for breathholds or end-tidal carbon dioxide adjustment. Interventional radiologists often request specific blood pressure parameters be maintained during the procedure, which may require placement of an arterial line for monitoring and multiple points of IV access for administration of vasoactive medications.[26]

ANESTHESIA FOR RADIATION ONCOLOGY PROCEDURES

Some of the procedure and patient considerations that make the selection of anesthesia type for radiation oncology procedures challenging are that the patient must be motionless and the anesthesia provider has limited access to the patient. Anesthesia providers use remote monitoring, including video monitoring of the patient, and although adverse events are rare in these procedures they should consider taking extra precautions to ensure patient safety.[27] Also, due to the repeated nature of the procedures, adequate NPO guideline adherence can be challenging.

With these considerations, general anesthesia is often necessary. While adults and some adolescents can undergo stereotactic radiosurgery with local anesthesia or sedation, pediatric patients usually require general anesthesia. General anesthesia may be chosen for patients undergoing total body irradiation, but procedural sedation is also acceptable, even with the risk of aspiration for these patients.[28,29]

NONRADIOLOGICAL PROCEDURES IN THE RADIOLOGY DEPARTMENT

While many patients come to the radiology department solely for imaging studies, some patients also undergo other studies in combination with the imaging study. One reason for this is to limit exposure to the deleterious effects of anesthesia, especially in young children and children with severe comorbidities. These studies include echocardiograms, lumbar punctures (LP), drug-induced sleep endoscopies (DISE), and auditory brainstem response (ABR) hearing tests.

ECHOCARDIOGRAM

An echocardiogram is a common imaging modality which uses ultrasound to assess cardiac function. A transthoracic echocardiogram requires using an ultrasound probe on the skin at various locations on the chest and side of the patient. Anesthesia is not always necessary in this study but may be necessary in order for the patient to remain relatively still. A transesophageal echocardiogram is more invasive, requiring the placement of an ultrasound probe through the mouth and into the esophagus and stomach. This type of echocardiogram usually requires the patient to be under deep sedation or general anesthesia. It is important for providers to consider the effects of chosen medications as they may have cardiodepressant effects or effects that could lead to exacerbation of underlying cardiac pathology. It is recommended that an anesthesia provider with training in cardiac anesthesia be present in cases of known or suspected complicated cardiac pathology or physiology.

LUMBAR PUNCTURE

Indications for LP include suspected meningitis, encephalitis, or seizures. LP is usually requested in addition to an MRI of the brain to help identify certain pathology. Providers should consider combining the studies, especially when patients require administration of anesthesia. Some patients may need only local anesthesia for successful completion of the LP, some may need mild to deep sedation, and others may require general anesthesia. Positioning for LP is generally lateral decubitus. For additional information regarding LP, please see Chapter 22, "Lumbar Puncture."

DRUG-INDUCED SLEEP ENDOSCOPY

Providers often use DISE to diagnose and direct treatment of upper airway obstruction in patients with known or suspected obstructive sleep apnea (OSA). Surgery after DISE has led to improvements in sleep study parameters.[30] While patients often undergo DISE in the operating room setting, providers may choose to combine it with another study, such as cine MRI of the upper airway. DISE is relatively quick and does not require a sterile environment. Providers performing DISE want to mimic the airway reflexes of normal sleep, which requires the patient to remain spontaneously ventilating while tolerating visualization with a fiberoptic endoscope. In children, the most likely anesthetic to achieve these objectives safely in an off-site location is a combination of IV dexmedetomidine and ketamine.[31,32] For additional information regarding DISE studies, please see Chapter 71, "Drug Induced Sleep Endoscopy (DISE)."

AUDITORY BRAINSTEM RESPONSE

ABR testing is common in the evaluation of hearing in children. In order for the study to be reliable, children must remain still during the test. Some children may not need any medication to achieve this goal, while others may require mild sedation up to general anesthesia. Providers have had success with using a combination of medications to achieve adequate sedation.[33]

SELECTION OF MEDICATIONS

While it is possible to achieve adequate sedation with a variety of medications, one must consider the profile of the medications in order to safely achieve the desired goals. This includes considering the side effects, duration of action, routes of administration, and the like (see **Table 135.1**). When developing a plan for sedation or anesthesia for a patient, it is also important to consider the training of the individuals providing the medications.

PROPOFOL

Propofol is a sedative-hypnotic medication commonly used in induction and maintenance of anesthesia.[35] It is a gamma-aminobutyric acid (GABA) receptor agonist and is the most commonly used IV anesthetic. It can be given safely as a bolus dose or as a continuous infusion in a pediatric patient. The side effects of propofol include decreased blood pressure, bradycardia, infection, pain upon injection, upper airway obstruction, and respiratory depression. It has been shown to lead to propofol infusion syndrome with prolonged continuous infusion times, which results in metabolic acidosis, hyperkalemia, rhabdomyolysis, and cardiovascular collapse.[36] Providers who use propofol should have training and experience in providing general anesthesia.

Propofol is a common agent that providers use in radiological suites. Patients who receive propofol repeatedly for radiation therapy have not been shown to develop tolerance to the medication.[37] When used as a continuous infusion for longer studies, such as in MRI, propofol may lead to increased parental satisfaction and improved recovery, when compared with dexmedetomidine.[38] A meta-analysis of randomized controlled trials with trial sequential analysis compared propofol and dexmedetomidine as sedatives for children undergoing MRI. Patients receiving propofol took less time to initially sedate and recovered faster than patients who received dexmedetomidine. They were also discharged from the hospital faster.[39] Another meta-analysis comparing propofol and dexmedetomidine use for MRI showed that the duration of sedation was similar, but those who received dexmedetomidine had increased recovery times and increased delirium.[38,40] If used in combination, propofol and dexmedetomidine may lead to fewer adverse events than using propofol as the sole anesthetic.[41]

Table 135.1 Common Medications Used in Radiology

Agent	Site of Action	Side Effects	Route of Administration	Dose
Propofol	GABA receptor agonist	Hypotension, burning at injection site, apnea	IV Induction Maintenance Sedation (bolus + infusion)	 2.5–3.5 mg/kg 125–300 mcg/kg/min 1–2 mg/kg followed by infusion of 150 mcg/kg/min, with titration as needed

Ketamine	NMDA antagonist	Prolonged emergence, hallucinations, delirium	PO
			  Premed
			IM
			  Premed
			IV
			  Sedation
			  Induction
			Intranasal
			Rectal
				
				6–8 mg/kg
				
				4–5 mg/kg
				
				1–2 mg/kg/dose
				1–2 mg/kg
				3–6 mg/kg
				8–10 mg/kg

Pentobarbital	GABA potentiation	Hypotension, apnea, bradycardia	IV
			  Sedation
			IM
			  Sedation
				
				1–3 mg/kg (repeat every 5–10 min PRN; max 100 mg/dose)
				
				2–6 mg/kg (max 100 mg/dose)

Midazolam	Indirect GABA potentiation	Bradypnea, paradoxical reaction, hypotension	PO
			  Premed
			Intranasal
			  Premed
			  Sedation
			IV
			  Premed
			  Sedation
			
			IM
			  Sedation
			Rectal
			  Sedation
				
				0.25–0.5 mg/kg (max 20 mg)
				
				0.2–0.3 mg/kg
				0.2–0.3 mg/kg (max 10 mg/dose)
				
				0.05 mg/kg
				0.05–0.1 mg/kg (max 6 mg; age 6 mo–5 yr)
				0.025–0.05 mg/kg (max 10 mg; age 6–12 yr)
				
				0.1–0.15 mg/kg
				
				0.25–0.5 mg/kg

Dexmedetomidine	Alpha-2 agonist	Bradycardia, hypotension, hypertension	Intranasal
			  Premed
			  Sedation
			IV
			  Sedation
				
				1–2 mcg/kg
				2–3 mcg/kg
				
				Loading dose 0.5–2 mcg/kg over 10 min
				Maintenance 0.5–1 mcg/kg/hr

Chloral hydrate	Enhances GABA receptor complex	Nausea, vomiting, arrhythmias, hypotension	Oral Sedation	 25–100 mg/kg (max 1,000 mg)

GABA, gamma-aminobutyric acid; NMDA, N-methyl-d-aspartate.

Source: Lexicomp. Drug Information Handbook: A Comprehensive Resource for All Clinicians and Healthcare Professionals. Lexi-Comp Incorporated. 2013. https://books.google.com/books/about/Drug_Information_Handbook.html?hl=&id=GBx9lAEACAAJ.[34]

CHLORAL HYDRATE

Chloral hydrate is a medication commonly used for sedation in noninvasive procedures. It works by enhancing the GABA receptor complex and can be given rectally or orally. Onset time for sedation is between 30 and 45 minutes. The side effects include airway obstruction, hypotension, bradycardia, and vomiting. It has also been shown to have carcinogenic potential. It has a much longer half-life in preterm infants than in toddlers and medication effects may last for many hours after initial administration.[42]

Many providers have safely used chloral hydrate for procedural sedation in the inpatient or outpatient setting,[42–44] but there are reports of death after administration.[45] When compared with other methods of sedation, there is variable evidence. Given orally, it has similar rates of failure when given for neurodiagnostic procedures as compared with oral midazolam, oral dexmedetomidine, and oral hydroxyzine hydrochloride.[42] With the advent of newer medications, the use of chloral hydrate is waning.

PENTOBARBITAL

Pentobarbital is a barbiturate medication that provides sedation by potentiating the GABA effects. It can be given orally or intravenously. The side effects include oxygen desaturation, nausea and vomiting, paradoxical hyperreactivity, respiratory depression, agitation, and prolonged sedation.[46] The duration of sedation after administration of IV pentobarbital is about 86 minutes.[6]

When compared with dexmedetomidine for use in MRI, pentobarbital results in longer recovery time and total sedation time.[47] When compared with propofol for use in MRI, pentobarbital is less efficient, with longer recovery time and higher rate of failure.[48] Patients receiving pentobarbital compared with chloral hydrate not only have a more rapid onset of sedation but also experience prolonged recovery times and increased rates of paradoxical reaction.[46] While pentobarbital is a useful sedative agent, appropriate patient selection is necessary for optimal results. Duration of imaging/procedure coupled with age are important criteria to consider prior to using it for sedation.[49]

MIDAZOLAM

Midazolam is a benzodiazepine commonly used for its anxiolytic, hypnotic, and amnestic effects, and works through the GABA receptor. It can be given via different routes, including IV, PO, IN, and IM. The most significant side effect is respiratory depression. The administration of midazolam has been shown to reduce postoperative nausea. The elimination half-life of midazolam is approximately 2.5 hours.

Providers commonly use midazolam to achieve moderate sedation during procedures.[50] In a Cochrane review of randomized controlled trials in which midazolam was compared with placebo or other agents, there was no difference in the effectiveness of sedation by the agents or the placebo, with some evidence of lower anxiety with midazolam as compared with the placebo.[51] While some use it as a sole agent, others combine it with other medications. A systematic review and meta-analysis comparing individual use of nitrous oxide and midazolam with their combined use showed that the combined use led to a reduction in the required midazolam dose.[52]

DEXMEDETOMIDINE

Dexmedetomidine is a selective alpha-2 agonist that possesses analgesic, sedative, and anxiolytic effects. It is an effective medication in infants and children that causes minimal respiratory depression while maintaining airway patency. Dexmedetomidine can cause bradycardia, hypertension, or hypotension. It can be via different routes, including PO, buccal, IN, IM, and IV, and has a half-life of 1.8 hours.[53–55]

Providers commonly use dexmedetomidine for procedural sedation in patients of all ages. It has been used as a sole agent for pediatric patients undergoing noninvasive radiological imaging studies.[56,57] A systematic review and meta-analysis comparing intranasal dexmedetomidine with oral chloral hydrate for sedation in infants and toddlers showed that patients receiving dexmedetomidine had a higher success rate of sedation, a shorter time of onset of sedation, and a lower incidence of nausea and vomiting.[58] When compared with patients receiving midazolam for procedural sedation, those receiving dexmedetomidine experienced more comfort.[59] The sedation from dexmedetomidine is similar to normal sleep as it mimics non-REM sleep at the level of the locus coeruleus.[60]

Researchers have also studied the safety profile of dexmedetomidine. A continuous infusion after repeated boluses may cause hypertension most commonly in children <1 year of age.[1] Studies have shown that providers have achieved adequate sedation with dexmedetomidine in patients with OSA with limited airway support required when compared with sedation provided via administration of propofol.[61] When used as a sedative medication in patients without OSA, dexmedetomidine does not seem to cause airway obstruction.[62]

KETAMINE

Ketamine is an N-methyl-d-aspartate (NMDA) antagonist that provides sedation, analgesia, or anesthesia. It exhibits sympathomimetic effects, leading to increased blood pressure, heart rate, cardiac output, and coronary perfusion. The side effects of ketamine include hallucinations, nightmares, and agitation.

Providers have successfully used ketamine as a sedative for radiological procedures.[63] When combined with propofol, the necessary dose of both medications decreases and the cardiovascular effects of each are attenuated as well.[64,65] Due to the analgesic properties of ketamine, providers may also use it as a medication for more invasive procedures.

> ### KEY TAKEAWAYS
>
> - Each radiological imaging modality has unique considerations for the pediatric patient.
> - Providers must create an appropriate anesthetic plan, taking into account the imaging modality as well as the patient's characteristics (e.g., age and anxiety level).
> - When creating an anesthetic plan, providers must choose appropriate medications and dosing.

KEY REFERENCES

Complete references for this chapter are online and available at https://connect.springerpub.com/content/book/978-0-8261-3875-0/part/part05/toc-part/ch135.

1. Mason KP. Sedation trends in the 21st century: the transition to dexmedetomidine for radiological imaging studies. *Paediatr Anaesth.* 2010;20(3):265–272. doi:10.1111/j.1460-9592.2009.03224.x
2. Mason KP. Challenges in paediatric procedural sedation: political, economic, and clinical aspects. *Br J Anaesth.* 2014;113(Suppl 2): ii48–ii62. doi:10.1093/bja/aeu387
9. American Society of Anesthesiologists Task Force on Sedation and Analgesia by Non-Anesthesiologists. Practice guidelines for sedation and analgesia by non-anesthesiologists. *Anesthesiology.* 2002;96(4):1004–1017. doi:10.1097/00000542-200204000-00031

10. Practice guidelines for moderate procedural sedation and analgesia 2018: a report by the American Society of Anesthesiologists Task Force on Moderate Procedural Sedation and Analgesia, the American Association of Oral and Maxillofacial Surgeons, American College of Radiology, American Dental Association, American Society of Dentist Anesthesiologists, and Society of Interventional Radiology. *Anesthesiology*. 2018;128(3):437–479. doi:10.1097/ALN.0000000000002043

22. Practice advisory on anesthetic care for magnetic resonance imaging: an updated report by the american society of anesthesiologists task force on anesthetic care for magnetic resonance imaging. *Anesthesiology*. 2015;122(3):495–520. doi:10.1097/ALN.0000000000000458

23. Mahmoud M, Towe C, Fleck RJ. CT chest under general anesthesia: pulmonary, anesthetic and radiologic dilemmas. *Pediatr Radiol*. 2015;45(7):977–981. doi:10.1007/s00247-014-3250-3

CHAPTER 136

Ultrasound-Guided Vascular Access

Nathan Fagan and Manish N. Patel

> **LEARNING OBJECTIVES**
> - Discuss the basics of ultrasound physics.
> - Learn how to maximize the ultrasound image to improve chances of successful access.
> - Compare the two most common types of ultrasound vascular access: longitudinal and transverse.
> - Discuss the technique of ultrasound-guided vascular access.
> - Briefly describe the types of vascular access.

INTRODUCTION

Vascular access, both peripheral and central, is one of the most basic and essential tools utilized in the delivery of anesthesia. Situations in which reliable vascular access cannot be obtained present a unique challenge given the critical nature parenteral medications have in the delivery of safe and effective anesthetic care. Traditionally, vascular access has been guided by anatomical landmarks, palpation, and use of devices such as "vein finders" to locate vessels for cannulation. There has been a growing emphasis, however, placed on the use of ultrasound guidance to assist with securement of vascular access since the 1990s.[1-5] The shift toward utilization of ultrasound when securing vascular access is driven by the improved success rates and decreased complication rates associated with ultrasound-guided techniques.[1-5] The clear benefit and wide availability of ultrasound have led to many safety advocacy organizations and society guidelines advocating for the "global" use of ultrasound during vascular access for central lines and with difficult peripheral access.[6] Despite the advantages offered by ultrasound, it is estimated that ultrasound guidance is still only used routinely 20% to 55% of the time when obtaining central access.[1,2,7-16]

ULTRASOUND PHYSICS

The use of ultrasound has become ubiquitous in anesthesia practice. Before attempting to perform ultrasound-guided vascular access, however, it is imperative anesthesia providers have a basic understanding of ultrasound physics. While a deep understanding of how ultrasound works is unnecessary, having a rudimentary grasp of how an ultrasound image is produced is crucial. Comprehension of a few key concepts will allow anesthesia providers to optimize the ultrasound image, thereby facilitating successful vessel cannulation.

Ultrasound is the imaging of mechanical sound energy. When an electrical current is applied, the piezoelectric crystals housed on the surface of an ultrasound transducer are disrupted, inducing vibration responsible for generating a sound wave. The sound wave, or ultrasound beam, is transferred from the probe into the patient's tissues when the probe is held against a patient's skin. In the body, tissues such as fat, muscle, fluid, and bone serve as conductive mediums, with each having a unique interaction with the sound wave. Depending on the acoustic impedance of the tissue encountered, sound waves are attenuated, reflected, or refracted. An ultrasound image is produced by interpretation of the echoes returned to the probe following reflection, with the image produced based on the amplitude of the returned signal and depth of reflection.

IMAGE MANIPULATION

A full, in-depth explanation of all parameters an anesthesia provider can adjust on an ultrasound machine is beyond the scope of this chapter. However, there are a few simple adjustments that anesthesia providers can make to optimize imaging and maximize the rate of successful cannulation attempts. It should be noted that the parameters available for adjustment may vary from machine to machine, especially with dedicated vascular access ultrasound machines often used by anesthesia and vascular access providers. Many newer machines auto-optimize the image for the operator. Nonetheless, the parameters that have the most influence on image optimization are readily available on most machines; these are probe selection, gain, focal zone, and color Doppler.

PROBE SELECTION

Probe selection is a pivotal, yet simple choice to make when utilizing ultrasound as most anesthesia providers are limited to choosing between two probes: a linear high-frequency probe or curved low-frequency probe. High-frequency linear probes are ideal for imaging superficial structures as the sound waves generated are readily attenuated, with a diminished portion of the beam returning to the probe for image generation.[6,17] Structures 2 to 3 cm below the surface of the skin are best visualized with a high-frequency linear probe. The sound waves generated by low-frequency curved probes can penetrate deeper structures and subsequently are ideal for imaging structures 4 cm or more below the surface of the skin.

In practice, when attempting to secure vascular access in either superficial vessels or smaller patients, a high-frequency linear probe should be used to produce the best ultrasound image. Deep structures are of little concern in this scenario. However, if the vessel is deeper or the patient is larger, such as the femoral vein in an obese patient, a low-frequency curved probe should be used to mitigate the effects of attenuation and better visualize the targeted vessel.

GAIN

Adjustment of gain alters the amplification of the ultrasound signal across the field of view, effectively making an image either brighter or more subdued based on the direction of change.[6,17] Adjusting the gain simply brightens or darkens the image. The location of the gain function varies from machine to machine, but is usually assigned to an easily accessible rotating knob. A common misconception is that increasing the gain increases the "power" or energy delivered to the patient by the ultrasound probe. When adjusting gain, the ultrasound machine is using mathematical calculations that impact imaging processing in order to brighten the image.[6,17]

FOCAL ZONE

The focal zone refers to the area of the ultrasound beam where it is narrowest, which equates to optimal image quality.[6,17] Typically, the generated ultrasound beam will converge in the near field until it hits the focal zone.[6,17] Beyond the focal zone, the ultrasound beam rapidly diverges or spreads out.[6,17] It is important to remember that the best image possible will be produced when the target is in the focal zone as image quality rapidly degrades beyond the focal zone.

The set focal zone is typically displayed as a "triangle" or "arrow" on the size scale along the side of the monitor and denotes the exact depth at which the ultrasound beam is focused. The focal zone should be adjusted so that the targeted vessel is within the focal zone. The location of this parameter adjustment varies widely from machine to machine. If it is not on its own button on the control panel, focal zone adjustment can usually be found in the advanced settings of the machine. If this option is not easily accessible, it is possible that your unit may be setting the focal zone automatically. While it is possible to set more than one focal zone on some machines, it is not recommended. Setting more than one focal zone drastically decreases the frame rate, which will negatively impact image processing as it becomes increasingly more challenging for the ultrasound machine to produce consistent, live images.

COLOR DOPPLER

Color Doppler can be a key problem-solving tool when using ultrasound for vascular access. Color Doppler uses the same basic principles of ultrasound imaging, but in a unique way. Rather than simply processing the returned echoes to make a static, grayscale image, color Doppler incorporates information regarding flow velocity and direction relative to the probe to semiquantitate blood flow in a region of interest.[6,17] It should be noted that the color of the flow does not indicate arterial or venous flow; rather, this is dependent on the Doppler angle. The color on the images produced is determined by probe placement, with flow away from the probe typically depicted in blue and flow toward the probe typically depicted in red. The ability to analyze flow is particularly helpful in the assessment of a thrombosis or when determining if a vessel is an artery or a vein.

Color Doppler imaging is also highly variable depending on probe angle. No color/flow information will be produced when the angle of the probe is 90 degrees or perpendicular to the direction of flow.[6,17] In clinical practice, 60 degrees is a good target angle to aim for.

The color Doppler function is usually bound to a button or knob with "C" label. This will both activate the function and adjust the color gain. When color Doppler is activated, a secondary box overlays the grayscale image defining which portion of the screen will display color information. This box is user-controllable to allow manipulation of the portion of the screen displaying color Doppler. To maximize the information, it is recommended to keep the color box as small as possible to optimize image quality. The smaller the color box, the more likely the computer is to display the information correctly.

Two additional settings for color Doppler anesthesia providers should be aware of are color gain and Doppler angle. As previously mentioned, the color gain is usual assigned to the same knob used to activate it. Increasing the color gain increases the sensitivity to flow, which is useful in identifying flow in low-flow vessels. Decreasing the color gain lowers the sensitivity to slow flow. When dealing with low-flow vessels, the goal is to adjust the color gain until only flow in the target vessel is seen without color "noise" overlying the adjacent tissues. Doppler angle is the angle the computer employs during methodical calculation and production of color images. If the ultrasound machine does not have the ability to adjust the Doppler angle or if the color Doppler does not seem to be working appropriately after adjusting the other parameters, changing the angle of the probe to the targeted vessel may improve quality.

OBTAINING VASCULAR ACCESS

VASCULAR ANATOMY

Because ultrasound guidance is most often used for establishing central or difficult peripheral access, the potential risks of failed vessel cannulation should be minimized. This can be achieved by having a basic understanding of vascular anatomy, as well the knowledge of what an appropriate vascular target looks like. Vessels on an ultrasound image are normally round in the transverse plane (**Figure 136.1**) and tubular with the longitudinal plane (**Figure 136.2**). In addition, they are usually anechoic (black) unless there is slow or turbulent flow, which may appear as echogenic (gray) debris within the vessel.

Veins tend to be thin-walled, oval, and compressible structures when compared with arteries, which are thick-walled, round, and not as easily compressible as veins. When compressed, normal veins will completely collapse, while an artery is not only difficult to compress but will often demonstrate hallmark pulsations. With color Doppler, veins will often produce a uniform color appearance, while arteries will produce color turbulence due to their pulsations (**Figure 136.3**). Additionally, veins will distend with the use of tourniquets and in dependent positions (i.e., internal jugular vein with reverse Trendelenburg position), while arterial size remains fixed. While simplistic, a sound understanding of the variations in appearance between veins and arteries will aid the anesthesia provider in choosing appropriate vessels to cannulate and minimize failed attempts.

STEPS FOR ULTRASOUND-GUIDED VASCULAR CANNULATION

The use of ultrasound guidance has become the accepted standard when central vascular access is required, when conventional techniques for obtaining peripheral access are not possible, if there are patient-related factors increasing the likelihood of bleeding, or if target vessel is small. Although the type of access required may vary from central to peripheral to arterial, the discussed techniques are universal and can be applied to all access procedures.

Prior to attempting to obtain central venous access, it is imperative the anesthesia provider obtain a brief, concise history of prior access.[12] While not always possible, attempting to incorporate this into the preoperative evaluation will help to minimize failed attempts due to issues related to prior access or complications of prior access. The history should include history of prior central access, laterality of access, known complications of prior access, such as a deep vein thrombosis or stenosis, and history of surgery that may have impact on vasculature. Any history of bleeding or current anticoagulation use should also be elicited.

CHAPTER 136: ULTRASOUND-GUIDED VASCULAR ACCESS | 677

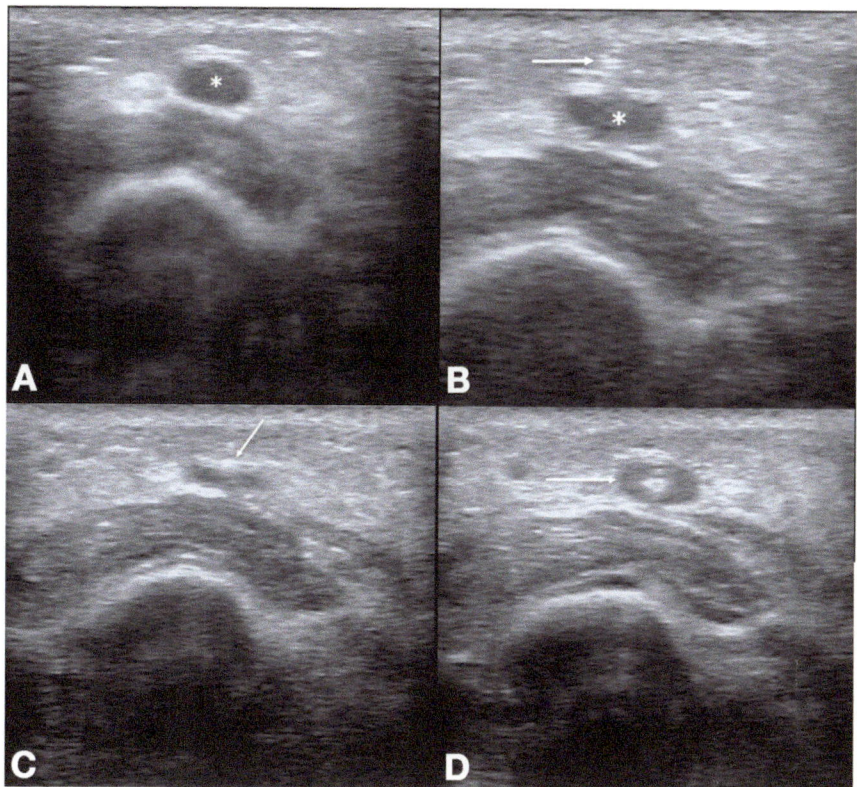

Figure 136.1: Venous cannulation under ultrasound using a transverse approach. Transverse ultrasound-guided vessel access images from an upper extremity peripheral IV placement. The initial image (A) demonstrates an oval compressible peripheral vein (*). The angiocatheter and target vessel are aligned on the ultrasound image followed by advancement of the angiocatheter into the SC tissues superficial to the vessel (arrow; B); note that the probe has been moved proximally along the arm to visualize the tip of the angiocatheter in relation to the target vessel during advancement; (C) further advancement of angiocatheter tip (arrow) is now "tenting" the target vessel, and the ultrasound probe has again been advanced proximally to ensure visualization of the venipuncture; (D) the angiocatheter tip is visualized in the target vessel during further advancement to ensure adequate purchase; note the centered tip appears as a "bull's-eye" (arrow).

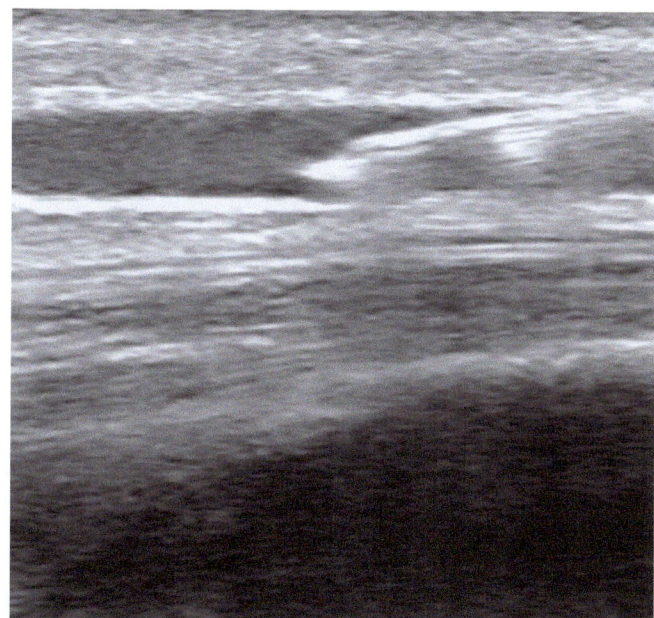

Figure 136.2: Venous cannulation under ultrasound using a longitudinal approach. Longitudinal ultrasound-guided vessel access image. Note that the access needle length as well as the target vessel are visualized in one plane during access.

After a brief history or chart review, the operator should then choose the optimal ultrasound probe for the task at hand. It is possible that the "optimal probe" may be the only one in your department. If multiple probes are available, things to keep in mind are probe size, probe shape, and probe frequency. Superficial access or access in smaller patients can almost always be performed with a high-frequency linear probe. For deeper access, such as the femoral vein in an obese patient, anesthesia providers should opt for a lower frequency curved probe. If possible, using a linear probe is always recommended as it translates the operator's hand motions more precisely. While curved probes distort the edges to give the operator a wider field of view, the operator's hand motions are not translated well, especially at the edges. This becomes most apparent when longitudinal techniques are used to obtain vascular access.

Once a probe has been selected, ultrasound interrogation of the intended vascular access site should be performed. This evaluation should identify the vessel of interest for the access desired, course of the vessel, including identification of abrupt changes in caliber or direction, and a survey of surrounding structures, including adjacent vessels and nerves. If access at the thoracic inlet is desired, such as when cannulating internal jugular or subclavian veins, attention should also be paid to the pleural reflection and the lung. Ultrasound does not travel well through air; thus, the pleural reflection will appear as a bright line, followed by shadows produced by sound-reflecting material.

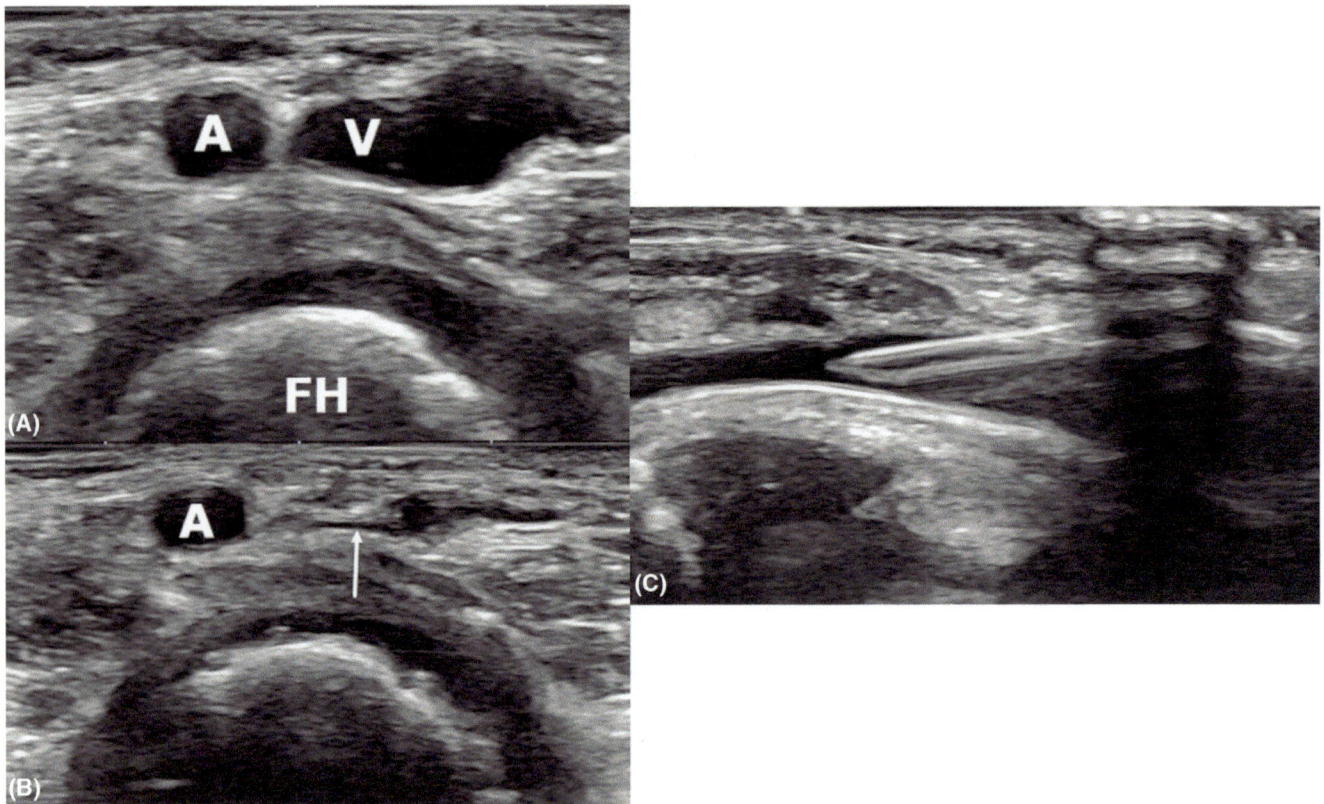

Figure 136.3: Comparison of veins and arteries under ultrasound. Ultrasound of the right groin to access the femoral vein for central line placement. The femoral artery (A) and vein (V) are identified on the transverse ultrasound of the groin (A and B). The artery is round and compressible. The vein is oval-shaped and nears the insertion of the greater saphenous vein and is compressible (arrow). Transverse venous access for central line placement is shown (C).

FH, femoral head..

Insertion Technique

There are two approaches to vascular access, the longitudinal and the transverse approach.[18,19] With the longitudinal approach, the entire length of the vessel is visualized as opposed to a cross-sectional view. The vascular access needle or IV cannula is inserted through the soft tissue toward the intended vessel and subsequently into the vessel (see Figure 136.1). Using this approach affords anesthesia providers the benefit of visualizing the entirety of the needle during insertion. While this approach offers an accurate depiction of the needle tip depth, longitudinal imaging with adjacent vessels in small patients may be difficult due to poor spatial resolution.[18,19] This may result in cannulation failures, with the needle being lateral to the targeted vessel. The key to success with longitudinal access is keeping the probe as flush with the patient skin as possible and finding the point of vessel in which the back wall appears the brightest (see Figure 136.2). The point at which the back wall of the vessel is the brightest denotes the center of the vessel. If the path of the needle is visualized in its entirety, the tip of the needle or IV cannula is more likely to be within the lumen of the vessel.

In the transverse approach, the ultrasound probe is placed perpendicular to the vessel such that it is seen as a round or oval structure within the soft tissues.[18,19] The access needle or IV cannula is inserted through the skin and directed under direct ultrasound guidance toward the top of the vessel and subsequently into the lumen. The needle or cannula is guided to the target vessel by localizing the needle tip, which appears as a bright, "echogenic" dot on the ultrasound image (see Figure 136.1). With the needle held at roughly a 45-degree angle, the needle is slowly advanced toward the target in a dynamic fashion. The anesthesia provider should advance the echogenic tip of the access needle toward the target vessel in small increments, moving the ultrasound probe so the tip is constantly visualized. Once near the target vessel, the needle or IV cannula may tent the vessel prior to actual puncture. The needle or IV cannula should be advanced into the intended vessel until a good portion of the needle or IV cannula is within the vessel (usually about 1–2 cm). This can be accomplished by repeating the steps used for initial access, except now the echogenic tip should be kept within the center of the vessel.

The goal of either approach is single wall puncture with minimal vessel wall injury and hematoma formation. Although higher success has been reported with transverse approach vascular access, each technique has its advantages and disadvantages.[18,19] The authors advocate learning both techniques as successfully obtaining access may require the use of a combination of the two techniques.

Various Types of Vascular Access

The most common form of vascular access used by anesthesia providers is peripheral venous and/or arterial access either within the upper or the lower extremity (Figure 136.4). The previously mentioned techniques can be used with any ordinary IV cannula for IVs or arterial access for monitoring. However, when access is desired in a deeper vessel, especially

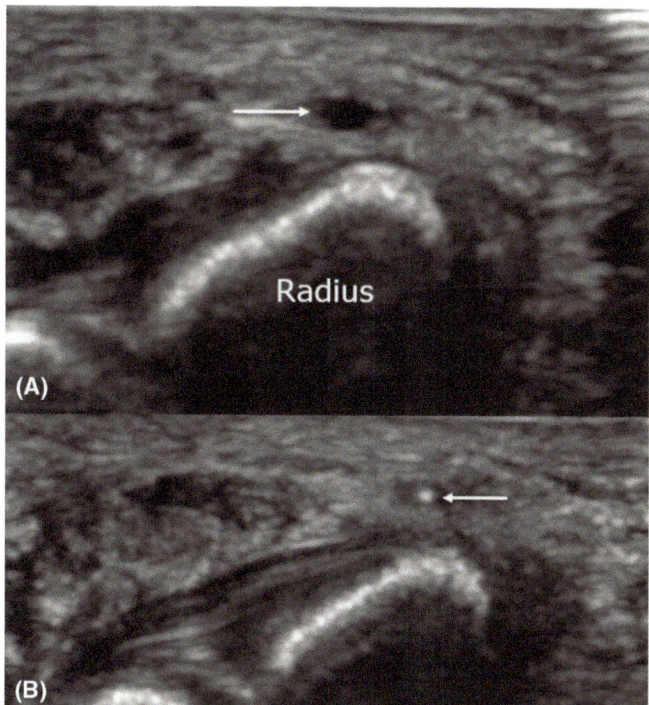

Figure 136.4: A 1-day-old premature infant requiring arterial access for monitoring. (A) The radial artery (arrow) measures approximately 8 mm. (B) A 24-gauge angiocatheter was placed into the right radial artery (arrow).

be able to be easily moved in and out of either the dilator or the line lumen. When possible, the placement of the line should be confirmed with fluoroscopy or x-ray.

KEY TAKEAWAYS

- An in-depth understanding of ultrasound physics and how the machine works is unnecessary to perform good ultrasound-guided vascular access. However, knowing a few techniques to optimize an ultrasound image can help to maximize the anesthesia provider's chance of successful vessel cannulation.
- Both arteries and veins can appear as black channels or as circles/ovals when viewed in the longitudinal or transverse plane.
- Veins are thin-walled and easily compressible, while arteries have a thicker wall and are less likely to compress. Small arteries may be compressed but will pulsate with the patient's heart rate.
- Ultrasound cannulation of a vessel can be performed in either the transverse or longitudinal plane. While transverse is typically the method of choice for beginners, each technique has advantages and disadvantages. Because ultrasound is dynamic, if one method is not working, do not hesitate to abandon it and try the other.
- Every attempt should be made to cannulate the vessel in one stick, thereby limiting the potential of vessel rupture, hematoma formation, or vessel spasm.
- Ultrasound can not only be used for initial cannulation in central line placement but also for troubleshooting such things as vessel spasm, hematoma, or location of the wire (intraluminal or not).

mid-arm, upper arm, or lower extremity, longer IV cannula should be utilized. We routinely use a 1.88-inch 20-gauge IV or 1.75-inch 22-gague IV for deeper vessels. Midline catheters are placed in a similar fashion to peripheral IVs. The midline catheter is inserted into the peripheral vein using either the longitudinal or the transverse approach, with subsequent advancement of the cannula once secure access into the desired vein is achieved with ultrasound guidance.

Frequently, anesthesia providers are required to place central lines prior to or during a surgical procedure. Either the jugular vein or the femoral vein may be utilized for these types of access depending on patient- and surgery-related factors. The central line kit should be appropriately selected for the number of lumens desired and the caliber and length of the central line. These kits typically contain all the supplies needed for access (an access needle, guide wire, dilator, the central line itself). Using the technique discussed previously, central access is obtained within the desired vessel (internal jugular or femoral vein) using ultrasound guidance and the access needle. The wire provided with the kit is then placed via the access needle into either the superior vena cava or the inferior vena cava. The wire should advance without resistance into the desired vessel. The intraluminal wire placement can be evaluated with ultrasound guidance when there is question. If the wire is appropriately within the vessel, it will appear as either an echogenic line or dot within the dark lumen on either longitudinal or transverse imaging, respectively. The needle is removed, and the vascular access site is dilated with the dilator followed by placement of the central line and removal of the wire. Both the dilator and the line should glide easily over the wire. While some resistance going through soft tissue is normal, the wire should always

KEY REFERENCES

Complete references for this chapter are online and available at https://connect.springerpub.com/content/book/978-0-8261-3875-0/part/part03/toc-part/ch022.

1. Practice guidelines for central venous access 2020: an updated report by the American Society of Anesthesiologists Task Force on central venous access. *Anesthesiology*. 2020;132(1):8–43. doi:10.1097/ALN.0000000000002864
10. AIUM practice parameter for the use of ultrasound to guide vascular access procedures. *J Ultrasound Med*. 2019;38(3):E4–E18. doi:10.1002/jum.14954
11. Lamperti M, Biasucci DG, Disma N, et al. European Society of Anaesthesiology guidelines on peri-operative use of ultrasound-guided for vascular access (PERSEUS vascular access). *Eur J Anaesthesiol*. 2020;37(5):344–376. doi:10.1097/EJA.0000000000001180
12. Spencer TR, Pittiruti M. Rapid Central Vein Assessment (RaCeVA): a systematic, standardized approach for ultrasound assessment before central venous catheterization. *J Vasc Access*. 2019;20(3):239–249. doi:10.1177/1129729818804718
13. Franco-Sadud R, Schnobrich D, Mathews BK, et al. Recommendations on the use of ultrasound guidance for central and peripheral vascular access in adults: a position statement of the society of hospital medicine. *J Hosp Med*. 2019;14:E1–E22. doi:10.12788/jhm.3287

CHAPTER 137

Ethical Considerations in Pediatric Anesthesia

Megha Karkera Kanjia and Julie Schackman

LEARNING OBJECTIVES

- Explain the differences between informed consent and assent in the pediatric patient.
- Discuss the role of an emancipated minor in a pediatric care setting.
- Distinguish among end-of-life care, futility, and potentially life-sustaining medical treatment.
- Analyze the differences between organ donation through brain death and donation after cardiac death.

INTRODUCTION

Primum non nocere. "First do no harm." This statement is the underlying principle and ideal behind the Hippocratic Oath, which, to this day, stands as the foundation of medicine.[1] The expression compels us to protect our patients from more than just physical harm but also any potential mental, emotional, and psychological harm while in our care.

As pediatric anesthesia providers, we are first and foremost patient advocates. Children and parents may have a myriad of concerns; for this reason, it is important to address both the child and their family as individuals as well as a unit. Based on the age and development of the patient, appropriate information should be given to best ensure that the patient feels comfortable in this setting.

INFORMED CONSENT

Informed consent is a formal agreement made between an anesthesia provider and a patient or surrogate to proceed with a treatment after a discussion about the "nature of the illness or condition [being treated]; proposed diagnostic steps and/or treatments and the probability of their success; the potential risks, benefits, and uncertainties of the proposed treatment; and alternative treatments, including the option of no treatment other than comfort measures."[2] Designed to ensure that a patient's autonomy is protected during medical decision-making, consent must be given by an appropriate person who displays competence and has autonomy.[3] Competence means that the patient or surrogate has the ability to comprehend the information as it relates to the treatment as well as understand the consequences of the decisions made.[3] A formal agreement should be made after a proper history and physical has been performed and a frank discussion of anesthetic risks and benefits has taken place.

Without consent, performing any type of treatment could be considered assault. The American Academy of Pediatrics also strongly recommends seeking assent from pediatric patients whenever possible.[2] Other topics that should be discussed with families as appropriate are alternative methods of delivering anesthesia; preoperative medications; common, uncommon, and major complications of anesthesia; and postoperative expectations, such as postoperative ventilation.

Potential liability may revolve around failure to discuss alternatives to the planned treatment or the risks and benefits as they apply to the patient. To be considered liable, the anesthesia provider must be considered negligent regarding the explanation of the procedure. Language should not be a barrier to obtaining consent from a patient; limitations in literacy should be addressed with appropriate interpretation, live or virtually, by the care team or institution.[3]

"WHAT IF THIS WERE YOUR CHILD?"

Parents may be looking for support in the decisions they are making regarding their children. Anesthesia providers should remember to offer guidance while remembering that the values of the providers should not be weighed as would be the values of the family. It may be prudent to offer help and support by involving other people, such as a chaplain, if the family agrees.

ASSENT

As pediatric anesthesia providers, we have both the fortune and responsibility of caring for a wide range of children, both in terms of age and development. For this reason, each individual patient must be considered as just that: an individual. While legally consent is obtained from an adult guardian, ethically the anesthesia provider must also receive assent from the patient as appropriate. One common way to initially assess a pediatric patient's ability to assent based on maturation is known as the Rule of Sevens. This rule suggests that in a typically developing child, the presumption holds that anyone younger than the age of 7 irrefutably has no capacity to assent, from 7 to 14 refutably has no capacity to assent, and older than the age of 14 refutably has capacity to assent.[4] To obtain proper assent, honest discussions about expectations should be geared toward their understanding. For example, honesty with a 3-year-old patient may include a conversation about "puppy dog nose stickers" to prepare for cold ECG leads and "blowing up a balloon" to explain the need for inflation of the reservoir bag. Conversely, more straightforward explanations may be given to a 15-year-old child who is undergoing an open reduction of a radial fracture.

Patients who are 14 years of age or older may be able to comprehend the risks and benefits of anesthesia because they are typically able to formulate abstract thoughts and ideas by this age. They may feel as though they are adults, so addressing them independently may help instill confidence in the anesthesia provider. Older patients may also realize the gravity of surgery and the consequences that may arise leading to increased anxiety. A prudent anesthesia provider should take extra time to discuss the specific concerns of the patient. Further explanation of certain procedures or gentle reassurance specifically related to any concerns may be helpful.

A survey performed by Lewis et al. explored the attitudes of anesthesia providers regarding pediatric patients' refusal of anesthesia.[5] Of the respondents, 45% reported that they had cancelled at least one case in their career due to patient refusal,[5] and 44% were willing to restrain patients <1 year of age, while only 2% were willing to restrain children >11 years of age.[5] Incorporating the family's preferences is key to pleasing both the patient and the family. A request for or against a premedication or specific medication is often valid.

RIGHTS OF MINORS AND EMANCIPATED MINORS

While minors generally require the consent of a legal guardian to receive medical care, certain scenarios allow minors to seek care without the presence of an adult. In most states, minors of a certain age, known as mature minors, do not require consent from a parent or guardian for treatment of substance abuse, sexually transmitted diseases, and reproductive health.[3] However, as there are important differences in the laws, providers must be up-to-date on local rules and regulations.[6] Without exception, physicians are given the authority to treat minors without parental consent in emergent or life-threatening situations, although attempts should be made to notify the adult legal guardians when feasible.

Along these lines, one should be careful when notifying a child of a positive pregnancy test. While pregnancy tests are routinely run preoperatively for female patients of childbearing age, anesthesia providers must consider the risks of informing the family of these results. By law in some states, under no circumstances should the parents of the child be informed of this result. The anesthesia provider should discuss the results with the patient in a private setting and encourage the patient to share this information with her family. In addition, if the surgical team opts to cancel the scheduled procedure, ambiguous comments may be necessary to protect the patient's privacy.

An emancipated minor is an individual who is a minor by age but an adult by law. Generally, they must meet certain criteria such as being married, economically independent, or military.[3,4] Emancipation may be granted for a variety of reasons but typically aims to protect children who are independent from their parents.[3] These patients should be treated as adults in all medical decision-making regardless of age.

JEHOVAH'S WITNESSES

As healthcare professionals, pediatric anesthesia providers must be sensitive to the diverse needs of all families while also providing the highest level of care for the minor patient. When caring for a family that identifies as Jehovah's Witnesses, the perioperative team must be prepared to discuss at length concerns regarding resuscitation, blood transfusion, and the potential ethical and legal limitations of adhering to the family's requests.

Many Jehovah's Witnesses refuse products derived from blood based on religious beliefs. However, as each member may have their own particular requests dependent on the situation, anesthesia providers must discuss specific options at length, including cell saver, autonomous blood donation, acute normovolemic hemodilution, and others. Providers should make their best attempt to formulate a plan based on the patient's personal belief system, surgical risk, and comorbidities. A frank discussion should be conducted with the family prior to surgery to set expectations, including a conversation about the provider's ethical and legal obligation to protect the child and transfuse blood products, if necessary, even without a court order.[7]

LIFE-SUSTAINING CARE AND CONSIDERATIONS

END-OF-LIFE CARE

Previously denoted as do not intubate/do not resuscitate (DNI/DNR), labels have more recently evolved into "life-sustaining medical therapy" (LSMT).[7] When patients identified as LSMT are preparing for surgery, the anesthesia provider must have a conversation with the patient and their family to ensure their preferences regarding specific therapies during the perioperative period are understood by the team providing care (Box 137.1). In addition, it is imperative appropriate supporting documentation be signed and placed in the patient record prior to the start of the procedure. Because surgery and anesthesia routinely require intubation and possibly even medications to alter hemodynamic status, specific situations must be discussed prior to entering the operating room. Appropriate procedures must be discussed in these specific cases for palliation, providing appropriate vascular access, and treating urgent problems.[7]

Once goals of care are defined, decisions regarding therapies and procedures will likely become clearer. The majority of patients and families may opt to focus on goal-directed approaches as many patients prefer to plan for treatments if the outcome is more likely to be beneficial or if the condition is reversible.

WITHHOLDING AND WITHDRAWING TREATMENT

Withholding treatment and *withdrawing treatment* are often used interchangeably and, while there are subtle differences between the two, they are the same legally, morally, and ethically.[8] When choosing to withhold or withdraw treatment, certain treatments may not be administered, yet patients should still be cared for and must not be abandoned. Discussing withdrawal and withholding of care is an unimaginable course for a family to go through. The family will likely require a significant amount of support from other family members, social workers, healthcare team members, clergyman, or other staff. The responsibility of these discussions falls principally on the primary staff member caring for the patient. Anticipated case scenarios need to be discussed with the family so that realistic expectations can be established.[8] Some families may not want treatments that may be considered to be "medically indicated"; it is also important to respect these wishes when possible.[9] As previously mentioned, involvement of the

---

BOX 137.1 KEY QUESTIONS FOR PERIOPERATIVE LIFE-SUSTAINING MEDICAL TREATMENT DISCUSSION

- Planned procedure and anticipated benefit to the child
- Likelihood of requirement of resuscitation
- The benefits of resuscitation and reversibility of causes
- Potential venues of postoperative care
- Postoperative expectations

Source: From Coté CJ, Lerman J, Anderson BJ. *A Practice of Anesthesia for Infants and Children.* Elsevier; 2019: Table 5.3.

institution's ethics committee is reasonable if there is confusion or misunderstanding regarding the plans being made for the care of the patient.

Many healthcare professionals regard withholding treatment and withdrawing treatment as separate entities, while legally these courses fall under the same heading. Anesthesia providers should be trained in understanding these two practices. Ideally, the same physician who has initiated treatment should also be withdrawing treatment; this ideal holds true also in dealing with donation after cardiac death (DCD).

FUTILITY

Futility is a term that describes a situation when the potential treatment fails to extend a reasonable chance of survival or will fail to result in a patient's end goal. Some may describe futility as a treatment or procedure with no value, while others may consider an intervention futile if the likelihood of benefit is extremely low, such as less than 1%.[10,11]

A prospective cross-sectional study was conducted in the United Kingdom that requested pediatric intensivists to complete a survey regarding care in cases that were seemingly futile. This survey noted that in 79% of cases, care was deemed appropriate, 8% of cases were deemed futile, and care was deemed inappropriate in 13%.[12] The majority of cases that were deemed futile in this study were those with respiratory failure and all of these had other comorbidities, developmental delay being predominant. This study recognized that there was a high number of futile and inappropriate cases in the pediatric ICU noted during the study. Several studies quoted in this chapter note that subjective prediction of the medical staff yields a better prediction of the outcome of these patients than the use of the Acute Physiology and Chronic Health Evaluation (APACHE II) score.[13]

ORGAN DONATION AND DONATION AFTER CARDIAC DEATH

Organ donation is most commonly performed after designation of brain death by the primary physician according to the brain death protocol. After brain death is declared and if the family consents, the patient is brought to the operating room under the care of the anesthesia provider for organ procurement.

DCD differs from the former process in that the child is declared dead after withdrawing care leading to cardiac arrest. The family along with the healthcare team make a joint decision to donate the patient's organs after the patient passes away. Due to the time constraints for organ survival, care is often withdrawn in the operating room instead of at bedside. As with brain death, there must be a protocol in place for withdrawal of therapy. The National Academy of Medicine, formerly called the Institute of Medicine, has deemed DCD to be an ethically appropriate option.[14] Withdrawal of therapy may take place in the operating room and protocols may vary by institution; if cardiac death takes longer than 1 hour, the patient is no longer a candidate for DCD and should be taken back to the ICU.

Between 2000 and 2007, the number of available organs via DCD had doubled. Approximately 74% of kidneys and 90% of livers that were obtained from DCD donors were able to be transplanted.[14] While pediatric patients may not directly benefit from other pediatric DCD donors, these additional organs will continue to add to the total number of available organs. The physician who would typically withdraw care of the child should also be responsible for withdrawing care in the operating room. The anesthesia provider should only do so if they are the person responsible for the patient otherwise. Otherwise, the anesthesia provider should function as a facilitator. Ethical issues have arisen around DCD due to concerns about whether the process is in the "best interest" of the child; however, the child should always undergo extensive observation and opportunity to regain function prior to this decision. This situation may be particularly difficult for families as the therapy is not typically withdrawn in their presence and they are not able to remain with the child as they are dying. To avoid conflict of interest, the primary team responsible for the care and healing of the patient should never be involved in discussing the possibility of organ donation with the family.

PATIENT SAFETY

Consideration of patient safety should be given even during times of emergency and production pressures that are common in the operating room setting. Anesthesia providers are obligated to provide safe care and work to minimize patient harm, decrease the flaws within our system, and continually work toward improving the quality of care delivered to our patients.

PERSONAL BELIEFS OF ANESTHESIA PROVIDERS

The personal beliefs of anesthesia providers should be regarded with respect, just as the anesthesia provider regards the values of the patient. If an anesthesia provider has beliefs that preclude them from providing care for certain procedures, these should be followed when possible. In the case of an emergency, the current culture leans toward the anesthesia provider subordinating their beliefs to those of the patient. Anesthesia providers who feel strongly about organ donation, pregnancy termination, or other ethical positions should make these clear to the anesthesia team with ample time to find an adequate replacement for the case.

KEY TAKEAWAYS

- Pediatric anesthesia providers should always strive to care for patients in a thoughtful and ethical manner.
- While minors and those with developmental delay may be unable to legally consent for themselves, the anesthesia provider should seek assent from the patient as appropriate.
- The rights of minors and emancipated minors should be understood and respected.
- Anesthesia providers should do everything possible to respect the beliefs of the patient and the patient's family while ensuring the safety of the patient at all times.
- End-of-life care should always be approached sensitively and involve a multidisciplinary approach.
- Organ donation is a revered practice with very specific protocols that should be followed rigorously to support the family and avoid any concern for conflict of interest.

REFERENCES

1. Smith CM. Origin and uses of primum non nocere-above all, do no harm!. *J Clin Pharmacol.* 2005;45(4):371–377. doi:10.1177/0091270004273680
2. Committee on bioethics. Informed consent in decision-making in pediatric practice. *Pediatrics.* 2016;138(2):e20161484. doi:10.1542/peds.2016-1484
3. Davis PJ, Cladis FP, Smith RM. *Smith's Anesthesia for Infants and Children.* Elsevier; 2017.
4. Arshagouni, P. But I'm an adult now ... Sort of-Adolescent consent in health care decision-making and the adolescent brain. *J Health Care L. & Pol'y.* 2006;9:315.
5. Lewis I, Burke C, Voepel-Lewis T, Tait AR. Children who refuse anesthesia or sedation: a survey of anesthesiologists. *Pediatr Anesth.* 2007;17(12):11341142. doi:10.1111/j.1460-9592.2007.02331.x
6. Kives SL. Adolescent consent in reproductive and sexual health decision-making: should there be an arbitary age of consent or should it be based on the 'evolving capacities of the child'? *J Pediatr Adolesc Gynecol.* 2008;21(1):47–51. doi:10.1016/j.jpag.2007.08.002
7. Coté CJ, Lerman J, Anderson BJ. *A Practice of Anesthesia for Infants and Children.* Elsevier; 2019.
8. Wellesley H, Jenkins IA. Withholding and withdrawing life-sustaining treatment in children. *Pediatr Anesth.* 2009;19(10):972–978. doi:10.1111/j.14609592.2009.03027.x
9. Consensus statement of the society of critical care medicine's ethics committee regarding futile and other possibly inadvisable treatments. *Crit Care Med.* 1997;25(5):887891. doi:10.1097/00003246-199705000-00028
10. Miles SH. Medical Futility. *Law Med Health Care.* 1992;20(4):310–315. doi:10.1111/j.1748-720x.1992.tb01209.x
11. Schneiderman LJ. Medical futility: its meaning and ethical implications. *Ann Intern Med.* 1990;112(12):949. doi:10.7326/0003-4819-112-12-949
12. Vemuri G, Playfor SD. Futility and inappropriate care in pediatric intensive care: a cross-sectional survey. *Pediatr Anesth.* 2006;16(3):309–313. doi:10.1111/j.14609592.2005.01761.x
13. Marks RJ, Simons RS, Blizzard RA, Browne DR. Predicting outcome in intensive therapy units — a comparison of Apache II with subjective assessments. *Intensive Care Med.* 1991;17(3):159–163. doi:10.1007/bf01704720
14. Durall AL, Laussen PC, Randolph AG. Potential for donation after cardiac death in a children's hospital. *Pediatrics.* 2007;119(1):e219–24. doi:10.1542/peds.2006-0375

CHAPTER 138

Quality Improvement and Safety in Pediatric Anesthesia

Megha Karkera Kanjia

> **LEARNING OBJECTIVES**
> - Define common terminology regarding safety events in the perioperative setting.
> - Define common terminology regarding quality improvement planning tools.
> - Explain the basic differences between the Model for Improvement and the Lean methodology.

INTRODUCTION

In today's world of pediatric anesthesia, many patients and families are equally, if not more, concerned about anesthesia than they are about the surgery itself. As a field, anesthesia has progressed in the safety world through increased understanding about anesthetic agents and various anesthetic techniques, as well as improved monitoring over time. These improvements have shown a decrease in mortality related to anesthesia from 2 in 10,000 to less than 5 in 1,000,000.[1]

As a member of the healthcare team, anesthesia providers are consistently focused on the safety of their patients and many routinely aim to improve the quality of care that is provided on a daily basis, regardless of whether that is recognized by each individual team member. Quality improvement (QI) in many fields, such as aviation, manufacturing, and healthcare, is a true science that must be understood to ensure that changes made reflect improvement and that the improvement reflects the desired direction of the providers, leaders, and institution. The importance of safety and QI is vital to establishing the high reliability that all organizations strive for: Those that are successful before actual failure may display their resilience during times of desperation.

Safety and QI have gained increasing interest over the past several years to improve the overall care provided to patients and have now been included in the required competencies for many graduate healthcare curriculums. Patient safety, QI, and professionalism are significant pillars of this pyramid and are deemed crucial to patient care. *Safety* may be defined as freedom from unacceptable risk, which is dependent on the controlled as well as the uncontrolled aspects of any system. The Occupational Safety and Health Administration (OSHA) as well as other regulatory boards determine the national benchmarking for particular events, such as for needlestick injuries, along with specifications of how to manage these risks and treat the consequences. Establishing a "culture of safety" will also allow a system to operate within the appropriate confines of the boundaries of safety while allowing the members of the team to feel secure and safe within systems with many moving parts.

REGULATORY BODIES

Regulatory bodies such as OSHA, The Joint Commission (JCO), the Surgical Care Improvement Project (SCIP), and the American College of Surgeons (ACS) are governing bodies that both create and uphold specific standards of practice and safety in the hospital and perioperative setting. Each of these groups plays a role in accreditation, compliance, and safety to help generate appropriate benchmarking metrics for hospitals to follow. Each group has a slightly different focus; however, there should be committees within the hospital, as well as appointed individuals, to uphold the standards set forth by each regulatory body. For example, OSHA examines reports of needlestick injuries, personal monitoring (radiation), exposure rate to tuberculosis, and personal protective equipment (PPE) availability and appropriateness. These injuries are required to be reported to the government regulatory board to appropriately monitor these potential public health issues. This is both an opportunity to contribute to establishing the national benchmark, as well as an opportunity for various hospitals to work toward QI within their given areas.

Within the field of pediatric anesthesia, the Wake Up Safe (WUS) program was created and works in parallel with the Society for Pediatric Anesthesia to continue monitoring and investigating events with the aim of continuously improving care provided to pediatric patients undergoing anesthesia. The WUS has formulated a database to which various pediatric anesthesia departments from the United States contribute data for the purpose of gathering data to further examine adverse events as it relates to this specialty.[2]

Patient safety events can be correlated with production pressure and systemic flaws that typically involve multiple moving parts. Other hazards in anesthesia include fatigue and sleep deprivation, which can cause a delay in reaction times as well as weakened judgment. Organizations such as the Accreditation Council for Graduate Medical Education (ACGME), the National Academy of Medicine (NAM), and the Federal Aviation Administration (FAA) have implemented work-hour restrictions in an attempt to minimize fatigue.[1] Other areas of improvement that have gained popularity in recent years is the emphasis on communication and patient care hand-offs.

KEY TERMINOLOGIES

Some important terminologies to understand safety discussions include *near-miss events*, *sentinel events*, and *root cause analysis (RCA)*.

NEAR-MISS EVENTS

Near-miss events include events in which there is a discrepancy in how a process should have been completed and how it was completed, leading to an event that could cause potential harm or death. OSHA defines this as an incident in which "no property was damaged and no personal injury was sustained, but where, given a slight shift in time or position, damage or injury easily could have occurred."[3]

SENTINEL EVENTS

According to the JCO, a *sentinel event* is defined as a patient safety event that results in death, permanent harm, or severe temporary harm.[4] These events are critical to address not only because of the potential patient harm but also to address system-wide issues that can continue to stress the system in which healthcare team members and patients coexist. Sentinel event alerts may be generated to alert team members of hazardous conditions and medication errors/interactions as evidenced by our ever-changing systems in healthcare. Working in the operating room both under emergent and a routine basis provides a fast-paced environment that can potentially lack double-checks in areas that typically require these throughout the rest of the healthcare system. This seemingly small concept provides a perfect agar for a petri dish of potential events, errors, and even disaster. The importance of addressing each near-miss is crucial for this reason as it should be viewed as an opportunity to minimize the potential for a future event.

ROOT CAUSE ANALYSIS

When a sentinel event or a near-miss occurs, it is important to examine all moving parts of the system to gain more than a cursory understanding of the events leading up to the event. These discussions may occur in the form of an RCA, or another analysis, including more Safety II concepts. RCA is a methodology of investigation that examines a problem by understanding the root causes of a problem. The most crucial components of any analysis selected should be that the process is examined with and without biases and that the conversations are nonpunitive to potentially move forward with positive changes. Often, utilizing an RCA for a more profound understanding of the event is done by use of the "5 whys."[6] This technique is performed by continuously asking the question "Why did this happen?" repeatedly until it is felt that the root cause is uncovered. The idea behind an RCA is to attempt to uncover a systemic-type cause rather than a more immediate cause.[4] For example, an RCA may be conducted to examine "betadine prep solution spilled on the operating room floor causing a workplace fall." An RCA does not always account for the moving parts of a system as well as other methodologies may do so. This type of framework can potentially fail to examine specific areas that may be considered "deficient" due to the cognitive bias that could be presented. Additionally, an RCA tends to examine one specific incident to find root causes, while it may not be very likely for this event to recur in the exact same scenario in the future.

Some institutions and other QI teams feel as though the RCA methodology tends to exhibit more finger-pointing than other methodologies of examining event. The Safety II concepts tend to examine how scenarios go "well" or why "things go right" rather than why things go wrong. Other opportunities for examining a process include a fault-tree analysis to examine potential causes of a problem *before* the failure occurs.

Opportunities for improvement may revolve around automating certain processes, utilizing information technology, and planning other processes to mitigate human factors, which are often nearly impossible to circumvent. The closer examination of human factors through failure mode and effect analysis (FMEA) and better understanding concepts such as efficiency–thoroughness trade-off may improve both the resiliency of both the team and from an organizational standpoint.

ROLE OF PATIENT HAND-OFFS

In recent times, communication has been highlighted as an opportunity to improve patient care through hand-offs during transfer of patients between units and shift changes; in the 1970s and 1980s, several articles cited these failures in communication as a cause of a safety event.[5] For this reason, emphasis on patient hand-offs has gained traction in many healthcare settings as fundamental parts of patient care and safety; they are also a common piece of QI projects in the patient care arena.[1] Today, many previous and ongoing QI projects aim to improve communication around patient care, often involving hand-offs. Additionally, medication errors are more common in pediatric anesthesia given the opportunities for failure in the operating room setting. Careful calculation of weight-based dosages must be completed by the anesthesia provider; as a group, we are the only providers who prescribe, dose, dispense, administer, and document a medication administered to a patient. We often go through all these mental steps alone while our "mental workload" is consumed in a fast-paced operating room setting. Most physicians and other providers outside of the operating room do not administer medication without the double-check of another provider or pharmacist, which can mitigate the opportunity for error.

WHAT IS QUALITY IMPROVEMENT?

QI is a *science* of methodical planning and multiple iterations and interventions to yield improvements in a process or area. QI combines ideas of how to associate effective processes along with clinical practice into practical methods to improve overall patient care. This may include clinical guidelines to develop pathways based on a national benchmarking, or even a more streamlined process meant for use for specific institutions. Aligning the goals of the organization and leadership priorities is crucial to project planning as well. For example, if a project is initiated to improve patient wait times in a radiology preoperative area, but the leadership's primary goal is to focus on increasing research grants, it may be difficult to get buy-in for this project at this time. Additionally, if there is minimal leadership buy-in for specific goals and projects, they are much less likely to be successful.[7] It is important to consider the importance of how pathways or protocols are best applicable to a particular area, as it may not be appropriate or helpful to apply certain pathways blindly without appropriate methodology, and one should consider the various environments in which the same process may be planned.

QUALITY IMPROVEMENT METHODOLOGY

There are several methodologies to follow in pursuit of QI; two popular methods include the Model for Improvement, initially theorized by Edward Deming, and Lean Six Sigma methodology, which is credited in part to the Toyota Production System. Lean Six Sigma looks to enhance effectiveness by mitigating defects and seeking errors less than $1/10^6$ (to the sixth power) in frequency.

All improvement requires change; however, change is not necessarily an improvement. This is a concept of paramount importance to QI work as it is crucial that team members and leaders have an understanding of QI methodology and project planning to best lead improvement. Common, yet incorrect, responses to ongoing systemic problems may include "the organization is running as best as possible," "Should we make our providers do better?" or even expecting significant improvement without making changes.

Model for Improvement Methodology

In order to fulfill the components of the QI project, one must first identify a problematic area that is also seen by leadership

> **BOX 138.1 THE MODEL FOR IMPROVEMENT QUESTIONS**
>
> 1. What are we trying to accomplish?
> 2. How will we know that a change is an improvement?
> 3. What changes can we make that will result in an improvement?[7]
>
> *Source:* From Langley GL, Moen R, Nolan KM, Nolan TW, Norman CL, Provost LP. *The Improvement Guide: A Practical Approach to Enhancing Organizational Performance.* 2nd ed. Jossey-Bass; 2009.

> **BOX 138.2 FIVE MAJOR PRINCIPLES OF THE LEAN APPROACH**
>
> 1. Defining *value* (what a customer is willing to pay for) based on the "customer's perspective"
> 2. Identifying *value streams* required to provide to the customer
> 3. Making the value-added steps move smoothly
> 4. The *customers "pull"* services as needed (as opposed to a "push" system)
> 5. Everyone is pursuing "*perfection*"
>
> *Source:* From Langley, Gerald J. *The Improvement Guide: A Practical Approach to Enhancing Organizational Performance.* Jossey-Bass; 2014:463–465.

as problematic at the organizational level to establish appropriate "buy-in." The problem should be identifiable and quantifiable by some metric or baseline data so that there is a solid understanding of where the problem started and what is the desired direction of improvement. The Model for Improvement methodology may accelerate QI projects by posing three crucial questions (Box 138.1). Baseline data are critical because initiating interventions without initial data makes the improvement data questionable.

SMART Aims

The next important goal in organization of a QI project is to develop a *SMART aim*; SMART is an acronym for "Specific, Measurable, Attainable, Relevant, and Timebound." The characteristics of a SMART aim will allow for a project to display both the goal of the project as well as the starting point. An example of a thoughtful SMART aim is "the aim of this project is to decrease late case starts in the Main Campus Texas Children's Hospital operating rooms from 12% to 5% by April 31, 2021." There should also be an *operational definition* to explain the significance of "late case starts" such that any individual who is looking at the project should understand what is considered late and not late; you may designate this by saying, "Late starts are considered if they enter the room more than 5 minutes after the scheduled time."

Failure Mode and Effect Analysis

The process to approach any QI project is typically more complex than initially projected in many cases. Many QI project leaders uncover several "mini-projects" in an attempt to tackle a larger initiative. To start a project, it is important to examine a process that has had some issues; a recommended tool for this would be to start by developing a process map of the steps of any process. After this step, an FMEA can be utilized to examine the failures and successes in a process and often can be high yield in examining potential interventions for a given QI project.

An important component of QI projects is that it should reflect a change over time; in other words, the results should be displayed in a graph that can show that a change has occurred as a result of an intervention. Without analyzing a metric over time, results can be misleading because it may not be possible to correlate the intervention with the measured results. Results over time should be displayed in a *run chart*; however, additional statistical charts can be used based on the type of results being displayed. Annotations on a run chart may also indicate chronological events and interventions that are reflected in the results over time on the x-axis.

Lean Methodology

Lean is similar to the Model for Improvement in that both methodologies seek to make a change that would lead to improvement; however, several differences exist (Box 138.2). The main premise of Lean includes "How do we reduce 'waste' in a system to make it seem more 'lean'?" Lean improvement strives to eliminate waste by utilizing a "systematic approach to identifying and eliminating waste (nonvalue added activities) through continuous improvement by following the product at the pull of the customer's pursuit of perfection."[7] This includes minimizing wasted energy and products in the system, removing anything that is not required and not felt to be of value to the customer, as well as making any process simpler for the team. The "customer" does not necessarily need to be one who walks into the storefront but may be the healthcare team members utilizing some part of the ongoing system.

Finally, if the solution is already known, a QI project may not be necessary. For example, if the operating room staff do not use gloves because the glove box is routinely on the floor rather than close to the providers, moving the box to an accessible location does not necessarily constitute a project but may be a solution to a known problem.

> **KEY TAKEAWAYS**
>
> - Sentinel events can be precursors to significant events and can reflect grave problems within a system and expose system flaws.
> - Quality improvement (QI) should follow a true science and methodology in an attempt to follow improvement.
> - Consider what you intend to change and how you will know that change is an improvement.
> - Understanding the tools of QI and how to utilize them will assist in structuring a more successful QI project.

KEY REFERENCES

Complete references for this chapter are online and available at https://connect.springerpub.com/content/book/978-0-8261-3875-0/part/part05/toc-part/ch003.

1. Davis, PJ, Cladis FP. *Smith's Anesthesia for Infants and Children.* 9th ed. Elsevier. 2016;1315.

2. Kurth CD, Tyler D, Heitmiller E, et al. National pediatric anesthesia safety quality improvement program in the united states. *Anesth Analg.* 2014;119(1):112–121 doi:10.1213/ANE.0000000000000040
3. "UNITED STATES DEPARTMENT OF LABOR." *Safety and Health Topics | Incident Investigation | Occupational Safety and Health Administration,* www.osha.gov/dcsp/products/topics/incident-investigation/index.html
4. Sentinel Event. *The Joint Commission.* www.jointcommission.org/resources/patient-safety-topics/sentinel-event
5. Cooper JB, Long CD, Newbower RS, Philip JH. Critical incidents associated with intraoperative exchanges of anesthesia personnel. *Anesthesiology* 1982;56:456–461. doi:10.1097/00000542-198206000-00010
6. 5 Whys: Finding the Root Cause: IHI. *Institute for Healthcare Improvement.* www.ihi.org/resources/Pages/Tools/5-Whys-Finding-the-Root-Cause.aspx
7. Langley GJ. *The Improvement Guide: A Practical Approach to Enhancing Organizational Performance.* Jossey-Bass; 2014:46-3465.

APPENDIX A

Common Adjunct Medication Dosing

Table A.1	Frequent Preoperative Sedative Medications		
Medication	**Oral Dose**	**Onset**	**Notes**
Chloral hydrate	25–100 mg/kg/dose, max: 1000 mg	15–30 min	May repeat after 30 min with 25–50 mg/kg/dose if necessary
Diazepam	Infants ≥6 mo: 0.2–0.3 mg/kg/dose, max: 10 mg	15–60 min	Onset not available in Lexi-Comp and Micromedex
	Children: 0.2–0.5 mg/kg/dose, max: 10 mg	15–60 min	
	Adolescent: 0.2–0.3 mg/kg/dose, max: 10 mg	15–60 min	
Melatonin	0.5 mg/kg/dose, max: 20 mg	20–30 min	
Midazolam	0.5–1 mg/kg/dose, max: 20 mg	10–20 min	Sedation: 0.25–0.5 mg/kg/dose (usual 0.5 mg/kg), max: 20 mg

Table A.2	Combination Antiemetic Therapy	
Risk Category	**Medication(s)**	**Breakthrough Options**
High	5-HT3 receptor antagonist + corticosteroid + neurokinin receptor antagonist	Lorazepam, diphenhydramine + promethazine, olanzapine, dronabinol
Moderate	5-HT3 receptor antagonist + neurokinin receptor antagonist (aprepitant) OR 5-HT3 receptor antagonist + corticosteroid (dexamethasone)	Lorazepam, diphenhydramine + promethazine, scopolamine, aprepitant, olanzapine
Low	5-HT3 receptor antagonist (ondansetron, granisetron, palonosetron)	Lorazepam, diphenhydramine + promethazine, scopolamine
Medications	**Dosing**	**Notes**
5-HT3 receptor antagonist		
Ondansetron	0.15 mg/kg/dose IV OR PO q8h (max dose: 8 mg)	
Granisetron	IV: 40 mcg/kg/dose (×1 dose prior to procedure) OR PO: 40 mcg/kg/dose q12h (max dose: 0.6 mg/dose)	
	IV: 1 mcg/kg (max dose: 75 mcg/dose)	Higher doses in chemotherapy-induced nausea and vomiting prevention, long duration of action
Corticosteroid		
Dexamethasone	Children: 5 mg/m²/d or 0.1 mg/kg/dose	
	Adult: 12 mg IV (Day 1), 8 mg IV (Day 2), 5 mg IV daily (as needed)	
Neurokinin receptor antagonist		
Aprepitant	<10 kg: 40, 20, and 20 mg	
	10–20 kg: 80, 40, and 40 mg	
	21–40 kg: 80, 80, and 80 mg	
	>40 kg (adult dosing): 125, 80, and 80 mg	

(continued)

Table A.2	Combination Antiemetic Therapy (*continued*)	
Medications	**Dosing**	**Notes**
Additional agents		
Olanzapine	0.1 mg/kg (rounded to 2.5, 5, and 10 mg) QHS	Patients receiving 10 mg/d (divide BID)
Scopolamine	Children <6 yr of age: 1/2 patch	Do NOT cut, 72-hr duration
	Children >6 yr of age: 1 patch	
Lorazepam	0.02 mg/kg/dose IV q6h (max dose: 2 mg)	
Diphenhydramine	0.5–1 mg/kg/dose IV q6h PRN	Side effects: sedation and dry mouth
Promethazine	0.25 mg/kg/dose IV q6h PRN	Do NOT use in children <2 yr of age; black box warning: severe tissue damage
Prochlorperazine	0.1–0.15 mg/kg/dose IV q3–4h (max dose: 10 mg, max daily dose: 40 mg)	
Dronabinol	5 mg/m^2 TID or QID (round to 5, 7.5, or 10 mg dosing) (max dose: 10 mg)	
Metoclopramide	0.1–0.25 mg/kg/dose IV (max dose: 10 mg)	Black box warning: tardive dyskinesia, max. rate: 5 mg/min

Table A.3	Recommended Prophylactic Antibiotics in Infective Endocarditis				
Risk Factors	**Medication**	**Dose**	**Scenario**	**Route**	**Timing**
Dental procedures involving manipulation of gingival tissue OR					
Mechanical or prosthetic valve **OR**	Amoxicillin	50 mg/kg/dose (max: 2 g)	Oral therapy in patients NOT allergic to penicillins	Oral	One-time antibiotic dose should be administered 30–60 min prior to procedure
Periapical region of the teeth OR					
Cyanotic lesions not fully repaired (including surgical shunts or conduits) **OR**	Ampicillin **OR**	50 mg/kg/dose (max: 2 g)	Unable to take oral antibiotics and NOT allergic to penicillins	IV or IM	
Perforation of the oral mucosa					
Heart defect completed repaired with prosthetic material or device within the first 6 mo after repair	Cefazolin **OR**	50 mg/kg/dose (max: 1 g)		IV or IM	
Endothelialization of prosthesis occurs within 6 mo after procedure **OR**	Ceftriaxone	50 mg/kg/dose (max: 1 g)		IV or IM	
Repaired heart defect that has residual defects	Cephalexin (or equivalent first or second gen) **OR**	50 mg/kg/dose (max: 2 g)	Oral therapy in patients allergic to penicillins	Oral	
For example persistent leaks or abnormal flow around a prosthetic patch or device	Clindamycin **OR**	20 mg/kg/dose (max: 600 mg)		Oral	
	Azithromycin/ clarithromycin	15 mg/kg/dose (max: 500 mg)		Oral	

(*continued*)

Table A.3 Recommended Prophylactic Antibiotics in Infective Endocarditis (continued)

Risk Factors	Medication	Dose	Scenario	Route	Timing
For example persistent leaks or abnormal flow around a prosthetic patch or device	Clindamycin OR	20 mg/kg/dose (max: 600 mg)		Oral	
	Cefazolin OR	50 mg/kg/dose (max 1 g)	Unable to take oral antibiotics and allergic to penicillins	IV or IM	
	Ceftriaxone OR	50 mg/kg/dose (max 1 g)		IV or IM	
	Clindamycin OR	20 mg/kg/dose (max 600 mg)		IV or IM	
	Clindamycin OR	20 mg/kg/dose (max 600 mg)	History of anaphylaxis, angioedema, or urticaria to penicillin	Oral or IV OR IM	
	Azithromycin/ clarithromycin	15 mg/kg/dose (max 500 mg)			

Table A.4 Preoperative Pharmacology

Drug	Route	Dose	Onset Time	Comments
Benzodiazepines				
Midazolam	PO	0.5–1 mg/kg/dose (max: 20 mg)	10–20 min	
	IN	0.2 mg/kg/dose (max: 10 mg)	<10 min	
	IV	0.05–0.1 mg/kg/dose (up to 2 mg/dose) OR 10 mg (adolescent)	1–5 min	Dose-dependent
Lorazepam	IV/PO	0.05–0.1 mg/kg/dose (max dose: 4 mg)	IV: 15–20 min, PO: 20–30 min	
Diazepam	IV	Infants/children: 0.05–0.1 mg/kg (max total dose: 0.25 mg/kg)	4–5 min	
		Adolescents: 0.2–0.3 mg/kg (max dose: 10 mg/dose)		
	PO	Infants ≥6 m: 0.2–0.3 mg/kg (max dose: 10 mg)		
		Children: 0.2–0.5 mg/kg (max dose: 10 mg)		
		Adolescents: 0.2–0.3 mg/kg (max dose: 10 mg/dose)		
Opioids				
Fentanyl	IV	1–2 mcg/kg/dose (max: 50 mcg)	Immediate	
Morphine	IV	0.05–0.1 mg/kg/dose	5–10 min	
Hydromorphone	IV	0.01–0.02 mg/kg/dose	5 min	
Barbiturate				
Pentobarbital	IV	1–2 mg/kg/dose (max: 100 mg), additional dose of 1–2 mg/kg q3–5 min to desired effect	3–5 min	

(continued)

Table A.4 Preoperative Pharmacology (*continued*)				
Drug	**Route**	**Dose**	**Onset Time**	**Comments**
Alpha agonists				
Clonidine				
Dexmedetomidine	IV	0.5–2 mcg/kg/dose	5–10 min	
	IN	2–3 mcg/kg/dose	45–60 min	Higher doses recommended for children ≥5 yr of age
NMDA antagonist				
Ketamine	IV	1–3 mg/kg/dose (no max dose)	30–60 sec	
	IM	5–10 mg/kg/dose		
	IN	≥6 mo: 3 mg/kg/dose		
		<2 yr: 3–5 mg/kg/dose		
		2–7 yr: 3–6 mg/kg/dose		
Other				
Ketorolac	IV	0.5 mg/kg/dose (max dose: 15 mg)	30 min	Should NOT exceed 5 total days of therapy, 15 mg sufficient in most cases
Etomidate	IV	0.2 mg/kg/dose (max: 10 mg)	30–60 sec	
Chloral hydrate	PO	25–100 mg/kg/dose (max: 1000 mg)	15–30 min	
Melatonin	PO	0.5–1 mg/kg/dose (max: 20 mg)	10–20 min	

NMDA, N-methyl-D-aspartate

APPENDIX B

Age-Based Parameters

Table B.1 Normal Pediatric Respiratory Rates

Age Category	Age Range	Normal Respiratory Rate
Infant	0–12 mo	30–60 per min
Toddler	1–3 yr	24–40 per min
Preschooler	4–5 yr	22–34 per min
School age	6–12 yr	18–30 per min
Adolescent	13–18 yr	12–16 per min

Table B.2 Normal Heart Rate and Blood Pressure Parameters for Children

Age	Heart Rate (Beats/Min)	Blood Pressure (mm Hg)	Respiratory Rate (Breaths/Min)
Premature	110–170	SBP 55–75 DBP 35–45	40–70
0–3 mo	110–160	SBP 65–85 DBP 45–55	35–55
3–6 mo	110–160	SBP 70–90 DBP 50–65	30–45
6–12 mo	90–160	SBP 80–100 DBP 55–65	22–38
1–3 yr	80–150	SBP 90–105 DBP 55–70	22–30
3–6 yr	70–120	SBP 95–110 DBP 60–75	20–24
6–12 yr	60–110	SBP 100–120 DBP 60–75	16–22
>12 yr	60–100	SBP 110–135 DBP 65–85	12–20

DBP, diastolic blood pressure; SBP, systolic blood pressure.
Source: From Zeno R, Kosla J, Melnyk BM. Evidence-based assessment of children and adolescents In KS Gawlik, BM Melnyk, AM Teall, eds. *Evidence-Based Physical Examination: Best Practices for Health and Well-Being Assessment.* Springer; 2020;57. Table 4.1.

Table B.3 Anticipated Glomerular Filtration Rate Based on Age

Age	Range GFR (mL/min/1.73m²)
*≤30 WGA	<10
*34 WGA	<15
1–3 d	20.8 ± 5.0
3–4 d	39.0 ± 15.1
4–14 d	36.8 ± 7.2
15–19 d	46.9 ± 12.5
1–3 mo	85.3 ± 35.1
4–6 mo	87.4 ± 22.3
7–12 mo	96.2 ± 12.2
1–2 yr	105.2 ± 17.3
2.7–11.6 yr	127.1 ± 13.5
16.2–34 yr	112 ± 13

GFR, glomerular filtration rate; WGA, weeks of gestational age.

Table B.4 Pediatric Anesthesia Quick Reference

Age	Wt(kg)	Bag	Blade	OA	ETT	LMA	Mask	BP	HR	SBP	RR
Prem	<3.3	.5	P1,M0	4.5	2.5–3	1	Red	White	120–180	40–60	55–60
0–6 mo	3.3–6	.5	P1,M1	5.5	3.5	1	Green	Orange	95–145	50–70	35–40
6–12 mo	7.5	.5	P1,M1	6	4	1.5	Green	Orange	110–180	60–110	25–30
1 yr	10	1	P1,M1	7	4–4.5	1.5–2	Green	Green	100–160	65–115	20–24
2 yr	10	1	P1,M1	7	4.5	1.5–2	Clear	Green	90–150	75–125	16–22
3 yr	12–14	1	P1,M2	7	4.5–5	2	Clear	Green	65–135	80–120	14–20
4 yr	14–19	1	P1,M2	7	5	2	Clear	Green	65–135	80–120	14–20
5 yr	14–19	1	P1,M2	7	5–5.5	2	Yellow	Light blue	70–115	90–120	12–20
6 yr	14–20	1	P1,M2	7	5.5	2	Yellow	Light blue	70–115	90–120	12–20
7 yr	20–25	1	P1,M2	8	5.5–6	2.5	Yellow	Light blue	70–115	90–120	12–20
8 yr	20–25	1	P2,M2	8	6	2.5	Yellow	Light blue	70–115	90–120	12–20
9 yr	20–28	1	P2,M2	8	6–6.5	2.5	Yellow	Light blue	55–110	90–130	12–20
10 yr	28–42	1	P2,M2	8	6–7	3–4	Yellow	Light blue	55–110	90–130	12–20
11 yr	28–42	2	P2,M2	8	6–7	3–4	Clear	Navy	55–110	90–130	12–20
12 yr	28–45	2	P2,M2	8	6–7	3–4	Clear	Navy	55–110	90–130	12–20
13 yr	45–56	2	P2,M2	8	6–7	4–5	Clear	Navy	55–105	100–140	12–20
14 yr	45–56	2	P2,M2	8	6–7	4–5	Clear	Navy	55–105	100–140	12–20
15 yr	45–56	2	P2,M2	8	6–7	4–5	Clear	Navy	55–105	100–140	12–20
16 yr	45–56	2	P2,M2	8	6–7	4–5	Clear	Navy	55–105	100–140	12–20

BP, blood pressure; ETT, endotracheal tube; HR, heart rate; LMA, laryngeal mask airway; OA, oral airway; RR, respiratory rate; SBP, systolic blood pressure; Wt, weight.

APPENDIX C

Antibiotic Prophylaxis

GENERAL PRINCIPLES

- All dosing recommendations are for patients with normal renal and/or hepatic function.
  - Prior to using **Table C.1**, a reliable estimation of glomerular filtration rate must be verified.
  - Other questions to ask/consider:
    - Is the patient receiving dialysis or renal replacement therapy?
    - Has the patient ever or recently experienced acute kidney injury (AKI)?
    - Does the patients have any chronic renal or urologic condition that may predispose them to renal injury?
    - Does the patient have low muscle mass?
- All dosing recommendations are based on prophylaxis in patients not on antibiotic therapy for existing infection.
- Preoperative and intraoperative doses may be different from doses used for treatment purposes.
- Recommend checking with your institution's pharmacy for the following circumstances:
  - patients with suspected or known hepatic or renal dysfunction, including those who have required prolonged infusion times or administration intervals of vancomycin or aminoglycosides and
  - patients receiving ongoing antibiotic therapy initiated before surgery, especially aminoglycosides or vancomycin (**Table C.1**).

Table C.1   Intraoperative Antibiotic Dosing and Suggested Redosing Interval

Antibiotic	Dose (mg/kg)	Maximum per Dose (mg)	Redosing Interval (Determined by GFR)			
			Normal GFR >60	GFR 30–60	GFR 10–29	GFR <10, dialysis
Ampicillin + sulbactam (dose in amp + sul)	75	3,000	q2h	q3h	q6h	q8h
Aztreonam	30	2,000	q4h	q4h	q8h	q12h
Cefazolin	40	2,000 (3,000 if >100 kg)	q3h	q6h	q8h	N/A
Cefepime	50	2,000	q4h	q6h	q8h	q12h
Cefotaxime	50	2,000	q3h	q6h	q8h	q12h
Cefoxitin	40	2,000	q3h	q6h	q8h	q12h
Ceftazidime	50	2,000	q3h	q6h	q8h	q12h
Ceftriaxone	50	2,000	q12h	q12h	q12h	q12h
Cefuroxime	50	2,000	q3h	q3h	q6h	q12h
Ciprofloxacin	10	400	q12h	q12h	q12h	N/A
Clindamycin	10	900	q6h	q6h	q6h	q6h
Gentamicin (single dose <40 kg)	4.5	160	q12h	N/A	N/A	N/A
Gentamicin (single dose ≥40 kg)	4.5	360	q24h	N/A	N/A	N/A
Gentamicin (>6-hr case, large blood loss or continued postoperative dosing)	2.5	160	q6h	N/A	N/A	N/A
Linezolid	10	600	q8h	q8h	q8h	q8h
Meropenem	20	1,000	q3h	q6h	q8h	q12h

(continued)

Table C.1	Intraoperative Antibiotic Dosing and Suggested Redosing Interval (continued)					
Antibiotic	Dose (mg/kg)	Maximum per Dose (mg)	Redosing Interval (Determined by GFR)			
			Normal GFR >60	GFR 30–60	GFR 10–29	GFR <10, dialysis
Metronidazole	15	1,000	q12h	q12h	q12h	q12h
Piperacillin–tazobactam	100	3,375	q2h	q3h	q6h	q8h
Vancomycin	15	No max	q8h	q8h	q12h	N/A

GFR, glomerular filltration rate; N/A, not applicable.

PRE- AND INTRAOPERATIVE ANTIBIOTICS

- Patients who screen positive for MRSA should be given a single preoperative dose of vancomycin in addition to routine prophylaxis.
- Preoperative antibiotics should be complete within 60 minutes of surgical incision.
- Patients receiving treatment antibiotics should generally receive routine preoperative prophylaxis in addition to their concurrent therapy.
  - If receiving vancomycin or aminoglycosides therapeutically, consult pharmacy.
- Redose prophylactic antibiotic according to times in the table or if the patient has experienced excessive blood loss.
  - After skin incision is closed, follow postoperative guidance (Table C.2).

GENERAL SURGERY PROCEDURES

- For patients who are MRSA positive on screening, a single dose of preoperative vancomycin is indicated in addition to the recommended agent in Table C.3.
- All antibiotics should be completed within 60 minutes of surgical incision.

CARDIOTHORACIC SURGERY PROCEDURES

- For patients who are MRSA positive on screening, a single dose of preoperative vancomycin is indicated in addition to the recommended agent in Table C.4.
- All antibiotics should be completed within 60 minutes of surgical incision.

Table C.2	Intraoperative Prophylactic Antibiotic Dosing		
Drug	Preincision Dose	Redose	Maximum Single Dose
Piperacillin–tazobactam	100mg/kg	In 2 hr	3,375 mg
Ampicillin	50 mg/kg	In 2 hr	2,000 mg
Ampicillin–sulbactam	75 mg/kg (a + s components)	In 2 hr	3,000 mg
Cefazolin	40 mg/kg	In 3 hr	2,000 mg (3,000 mg if >100 kg)
Cefuroxime	50 mg/kg	In 3 hr	2,000 mg
Cefoxitin	40 mg/kg	In 3 hr	2,000 mg
Cefotaxime	50 mg/kg	In 3 hr	2,000 mg
Aztreonam	30 mg/kg	In 4 hr	2,000mg
Clindamycin	10 mg/kg	In 6 hr	900 mg
Gentamicin <40 kg	4.5 mg/kg	In 12 hr	160 mg
Gentamicin ≥40 kg	4.5 mg/kg	In 24 hr	360 mg
Vancomycin	15 mg/kg	In 8 hr	No maximum
Ciprofloxacin	10 mg/kg	In 8 hr	400 mg
Ceftriaxone	50 mg/kg	In 12 hr	2,000 mg
Metronidazole	15 mg/kg	In 12 hr	1,000 mg

Table C.3 Antibiotic Dosing for General Surgery Procedures

Procedure		Recommended Prophylactic Agent	Alternate for β-Lactam Allergic
Appendectomy			
	Uncomplicated	Cefoxitin	Clindamycin + gentamicin
	Perforated	Piperacillin–tazobactam	Clindamycin + gentamicin
Biliary tract			
	Lap-low risk	None	
	Lap-high risk or open	Ampicillin–sulbactam or ceftriaxone	Clindamycin + gentamicin
Gastroduodenal—including bariatric, antireflux for high risk		Cefazolin	Clindamycin + gentamicin
Small bowel			
	Nonobstructed	Cefazolin	Clindamycin + gentamicin
	Obstructed	Cefoxitin	Clindamycin + gentamicin
Colorectal		Cefoxitin	Clindamycin + gentamicin
Hernia–hernioplasty, herniorrhaphy		Cefazolin	Clindamycin
Pectus/Nuss bar		Cefazolin	Clindamycin

Table C.4 Antibiotic Dosing for Cardiothoracic Procedures

Procedure		Recommended Prophylactic Agent	Alternate for β-Lactam Allergic
Median sternotomy			
	Uncomplicated	Cefuroxime	Clindamycin (+aztreonam if PD catheter)
	Heart transplant	Cefuroxime	Clindamycin
	Heart transplant, previous VAD	Cefuroxime + single-dose vancomycin	
Cardiac device			
	Pacemaker	Cefuroxime	Clindamycin
	VAD	Cefuroxime	Clindamycin
Video-assisted thoracoscopy		Ampicillin–sulbactam	Clindamycin
Thoracic, non-cardiac/vascular		Ampicillin–sulbactam	Clindamycin

PD, peritoneal dialysis; VAD, ventricular assist device.

Table C.5 Antibiotic Dosing for Neurosurgical Procedures

Procedure	Recommended Prophylactic Agent	Alternate for β-Lactam Allergic
Craniotomy	Cefazolin	Clindamycin or vancomycin
Craniectomy	Cefazolin	Clindamycin or vancomycin
CSF shunt placement	Cefazolin	Vancomycin
Baclofen pump insertion/revision	Cefazolin	Clindamycin or vancomycin
Meningomyelocele (neonate)	Ampicillin + gentamicin	
Meningomyelocele (nonneonate)	Cefazolin	Clindamycin + gentamicin
Spinal fusion	Cefazolin	Vancomycin or clindamycin

Table C.6 Antibiotic Dosing for Orthopedic Procedures

Procedure	Recommended Prophylactic Agent	Alternate for β-Lactam Allergic
Arthroscopy	Cefazolin	Clindamycin
Implantation of internal fixation devices	Cefazolin	Clindamycin
Osteotomy	Cefazolin	Clindamycin
Spinal fusion (idiopathic)	Cefazolin	Clindamycin or vancomycin
Spinal fusion (neuromuscular)	Cefazolin	Clindamycin or vancomycin + gentamicin
Laminectomy	Cefazolin	Clindamycin

ORTHOPEDIC PROCEDURES

- For patients who are MRSA positive on screening, a single dose of preoperative vancomycin is indicated in addition to the recommended agent in Table C.6.
- All antibiotics should be completed within 60 minutes of surgical incision.

OTOLARYNGOLOGY PROCEDURES

- For patients who are MRSA positive on screening, a single dose of preoperative vancomycin is indicated in addition to the recommended agent in Table C.7.
- All antibiotics should be completed within 60 minutes of surgical incision.

Otolaryngology Procedure-Specific Recommendations

- Recommended antibiotic: ampicillin–sulbactam.
- Alternate antibiotic for beta-lactam allergic: clindamycin.
- For patients who are MRSA positive on screening, a single dose of preoperative vancomycin is indicated in addition to the recommended agent in Table C.8.
- All antibiotics should be completed within 60 minutes of surgical incision (Table C.9).

Table C.7 Antibiotic Dosing for Otolaryngology Procedures

Procedure	Recommended Prophylactic Agent	Alternate for β-Lactam Allergic
Head and neck		
Clean	None	
Clean + prosthetic material	Ampicillin–sulbactam	Clindamycin
Clean-contaminated	Ampicillin–sulbactam	Clindamycin
Cancer surgery	Ampicillin–sulbactam	Clindamycin

Table C.8 Otolaryngology Procedures Requiring Antibiotic Prophylaxis

Procedures for Which Prophylaxis Is Recommended

Ear		Neck	
	Cochlear implant		Laryngotracheoplasty (LTP)
	Tympanomastoidectomy for chronic ear disease		Slide tracheoplasty
	Stapedectomy		Graft placement
	Ossicular chain reconstruction (OCR)		Open laryngeal cleft repair
Larynx/pharynx			Malignancy
	Endoscopic cleft repair		Lymph node dissection/incision (suspected malignancy)
	Vocal cord injection		Thyroglossal duct cyst excision
	Pharyngeal flap		Drool
	Pharyngeal injection—add cefuroxime (CSF coverage)		Brachial cleft cyst excision
Nasal/Sinus			Neck infection
	Septorhinoplasty (SRP): revision or grafting		
	FESS		

CSF, cerebrospinal fluid leak functional; FESS, functional endoscopic sinus surgery

Table C.9 Otolaryngology Procedures Not Requiring Antibiotic Prophylaxis

Procedures for Which Prophylaxis Is Not Recommended

Neck	Larynx/Pharynx	Nasal/sinus
Thyroidectomy	Microlaryngeal surgery	Septorhinoplasty
Parotidectomy	Adenotonsillectomy/uvulopalatopharyngoplasty (UPPP)	Septoplasty
Submandibular gland excision		

UPPP, uvulopalatopharyngoplasty

Table C.10 Antibiotic Dosing for Urologic/Gynecologic Procedures

Procedure		Recommended Prophylactic Agent	Alternate for β-Lactam Allergic
Urologic			
	Lower tract instrumentation with risk of infection	Trimethoprim-sulfamethoxazole (TMP-SMX) or a fluoroquinolone	Clindamycin
	Clean without entry into the urinary tract	Cefazolin ± gentamicin	Gentamicin ± clindamycin
	Clean with entry into the urinary tract	Cefazolin ± gentamicin	Gentamicin or fluoroquinolone +/- clindamycin
	Clean contaminated	Cefoxitin	Clindamycin + gentamicin
Hysterectomy (abdominal or vaginal)		Ampicillin–sulbactam or cefoxitin	Clindamycin + gentamicin

TMP-SMX, trimethoprim-sulfamethoxazole

UROLOGIC/GYNECOLOGIC PROCEDURES

- For patients who are MRSA positive on screening, a single dose of preoperative vancomycin is indicated in addition to the recommended agent in **Table C.10**.
- All antibiotics should be completed within 60 minutes of surgical incision.

POSTOPERATIVE ANTIBIOTICS

- For routine prophylaxis, antibiotics are not continued after the incision is closed.
- Redosing in the operating room should be considered if closure is close to the usual redosing time.
- For selected procedures, prophylaxis may continue up to 48 hours postincision closure.
- The first postoperative dose is timed off of last dose given prior to incision closure (may be a preoperative or intraoperative dose).
- Be sure to check your institution's formulary for institution-specific dosing and intervals.

BIBLIOGRAPHY

Bratzler DW, Dellinger EP, Olsen KM, et al. Clinical practice guidelines for antimicrobial prophylaxis in surgery. *Surg Infect (Larchmt)*. 2013;14(1):73–156. doi:10.1089/sur.2013.9999

Cincinnati Children's Hospital Medical Center. Institutional guidance e, 2021.

Lexicomp, 2021.

Munoz-Price LS, Bowdle A, Johnston BL, et al. Infection prevention in the operating room anesthesia work area. *Infect Control Hosp Epidemiol*. 2019;40(1):1–17. doi:10.1017/ice.2018.303

APPENDIX D

Case Plan Template

PEDIATRIC CASE PLAN   First Name _____   Nickname _____

Age ____ Weight (kg) _____ BMI _____ Allergies _____

| Fluids (4, 2, 1 rule): | Maintenance | _____ mL/hr | Deficit | _____ mL | 3rd Space | _____ mL/hr |

Est. Blood Volume (EBV): _____ mL   HCT _____ %   Allowable blood loss   EBV X (HCT - target HCT)/HCT _____ mL

ETT Size: _____   cuffed _____   Ø cuff _____   LMA size _____   Cultural needs y/n _____

Comorbidities: _____

Special considerations: _____
_____
_____

EMERGENCY MEDS

Epinephrine	Atropine	Glycopyrrolate	Succinylcholine: IV	IM
.01 mg/kg (10 mcg/kg)	.02 mg/kg	.005-.01 mg/kg	1.5-2 mg/kg	3-4 mg/kg
mg/ mcg	mg	mg	mg	mg

| Defibrillation | 2j/kgX1; 4j/kg | j | j | | |

BMI, body mass index; ETT, endotracheal tube; HCT, hematocrit; LMA, laryngeal mask airway

INDEX

abnormal automaticity, 459
absorption, pharmacologic agent, 43–44
acetaminophen, 65, 66, 650
achalasia, 526
achondroplasia
    airway assessment, 229
    anesthetic management, 229–231
    anesthetic technique, 230–231
    cardiopulmonary assessment, 229–230
    clinical features, 229, 230
    neurological assessment, 230
    pathophysiology, 229
    postoperative care, 231
    preoperative pharmacology, 230
acid–base management, cardiopulmonary bypass, 443
acidosis, 23
ACL reconstruction. *See* anterior cruciate ligament reconstruction
acquired cardiac disorders
    acute rheumatic fever (RF), 198
    Kawasaki disease (KD), 197–198
    multisystem inflammatory disease syndrome, 197
    myocarditis, 197
acquired esophageal strictures, 527
acromegaly, 176
active humidification, 83
acute appendicitis (AA), 477
acute compartment syndrome (ACS), 587–588
acute kidney injury determinants, 23
acute normovolemic hemodilution (ANH), 131
acute otitis media (AOM), 156, 333
acyanotic defects, noncardiac surgery, 466–467
Addison's disease, 177–178
adenotonsillar hypertrophy, 342
adenotonsillectomy
    anesthetic management, 342–346
    anesthetic technique, 343–344
    complications, 342, 345
    obstructive sleep apnea (OSA), 368
    postoperative care, 345–346
    preoperative evaluation, 343
    preoperative pharmacology, 343
    surgical techniques, 342
    tonsillar size evaluation, 343
adrenal disorders, 177–178
adrenal dysgenesis, 177

adrenal neuroblastoma, 545
adrenergic receptor, 71
adult congenital heart disease (ACHD), 450
advanced mask ventilation techniques, 103–104
afferent thermal sensing, 28-29
afterload, stroke volume, 8–9
age-based pediatric airway guide, 104
agenesis, incomplete lung development, 16
agent analyzers, 85
airway anatomy and physiology
    larynx, 12–14
    nasal cavity and nasopharynx, 11, 12
    oral cavity, 11–12
    oropharynx, 12
    trachea, 14–15
airway assessment
    Down syndrome, 251
    Hurler and Hunter syndromes, 266–267
airway considerations, preterm infant, 149
airway fire management, 348
airway management
    advanced mask ventilation techniques, 103–104
    difficult airway, 111–118
    endotracheal tubes (ETTs), 105–111
    mask management, 102–103
    nasopharyngeal airways, 103, 105
    preoperative assessment, 102
    sleeve gastrectomy, 498–499
    supraglottic airways, 105, 106
    tracheostomy patient, 111
    trauma, 618
airway obstruction, 99
airway resistance, ventilation, 19
albumin, 45
alpha-1-acid glycoprotein (AAG), 45
alpha-agonists, autism spectrum disorder (ASD), 237
alveolar cleft repair, 416–418
    anesthetic technique, 417
    complications/emergencies, 417
    indications/contraindications, 416
    postoperative care, 417–418
    preoperative evaluation, 416–417
    preoperative pharmacology, 417
amblyopia, 162
AMMs. *See* anterior mediastinal masses
amputation

anesthetic technique, 594–595
    indications/contraindications, 593
    postoperative care, 595
    preoperative evaluation, 593
    preoperative pharmacology, 593–594
anal fissures, 208
Anderson–Hynes pyeloplasty, 563
anemia, world health organization classifications, 130
anesthesia adjuncts, 65, 66
anesthesia induction
    asthma, 99–100
    bronchopulmonary dysplasia (BPD), 100
    complications, 98–99
    inhalation induction, 96–97
    intravenous induction, 97–98
    obesity, 100
    patient preparation, 95–96
    stages, 97
anesthesia machine
    capnography, 84–85
    carbon dioxide absorption, 82–83
    check, 83, 84
    electrical system, 82
    oxygen analyzers, 83–84
    pneumatic system, 82
    scavenging system, 82, 83
ANH. *See* acute normovolemic hemodilution
anophthalmia, 389
anorectal disease, 208–209
anorectal malformations, 512
anorectal renal malformations (ARMs), 294
anterior cruciate ligament (ACL) reconstruction
    anesthetic technique, 579–580
    complications/emergencies, 580
    indications/contraindications, 578
    postoperative care, 580–581
    preoperative evaluation, 579
    preoperative pharmacology, 579
    regional anesthesia, 578
anterior mediastinal masses (AMMs)
    anesthetic technique, 535–537
    case study, 539
    management, 536
    preoperative evaluation, 535
    risk stratification, 536
anticholinergic agents, 70
anticholinergics, 80
anticipated difficult airway management
    flexible bronchoscopy, 114–115

video laryngoscopy, 115
video laryngoscopy–assisted fiberoptic intubation, 115–116
antiemetic agents, 79
    anticholinergics, 80
    atypical antipsychotics, 70
    butyrophenone, 66, 70
    dopamine antagonist, 66
    glucocorticosteroid, 70
    H1 antagonist, 66
    5-hydroxytryptamine (5-HT3) antagonists, 66, 79
    neurokinin antagonist (NK-1 receptor), 70
    pharmacokinetic properties, 67–69
antiemetic medications, 142
antiepileptic drugs
    adverse effects, 315
    perioperative management, 314
antifibrinolytic agents
    hemophilia, 213
    perioperative blood loss minimization, 130
anxiety and anxiolysis
    assessment, 654–655
    nonpharmacological approaches, 80
    perioperative period, 654
    postoperative pain, 654, 656
    treatment, 655–656
AOM. *See* acute otitis media
Apert syndrome
    anesthetic management, 232–233
    anesthetic technique, 232–233
    clinical manifestations, 232
    incidence, 232
    pathophysiology, 232
    postoperative care, 233
    preoperative evaluation, 232
    preoperative pharmacotherapy, 232
aplasia, incomplete lung development, 16
aplastic anemia, 214–215
apnea, preterm infant, 149
apneic oxygenation, 113–114
appendectomy
    anesthetic technique, 478
    complications and emergencies, 479
    indications/contraindications, 477
    laparoscopic, 477, 511
    positioning concerns, 478
    postoperative care, 479
    preoperative evaluation, 477–478
    preoperative pharmacology, 478
aprepitant, 69, 70
arginine vasopressin, 72
Arnold-Chiari malformation, 151–152

arrhythmogenic right ventricular cardiomyopathy (ARVC), 196
arterial blood pressure monitoring, 87–89
arteriovenous malformations (AVMs), 153
arthrogryposis
  anesthetic management, 234–235
  anesthetic technique, 234–235
  clinical manifestations, 233
  pathophysiology, 233–234
  postoperative care, 235
  preoperative evaluation, 234
  preoperative pharmacotherapy, 234
asthma, 99–100
atlantoaxial instability, Down syndrome, 251
atracurium, 59
atrial flutter (AF), 459
atrial septal defect (ASD)
  cardiac surgery, 438
  noncardiac surgery, 468
  pathophysiology and clinical manifestations, 183–184
  postsurgical repair assessment, 184
  types, 183
atrioventricular septal defects (AVSDs), 185–186, 438–439
atropine, 59
atypical antipsychotics, 70
auditory brainstem response (ABR), 671
Augmentation cystoplasty, 565–586
authorized agent-controlled analgesia (AACA), 649
autism spectrum disorder (ASD)
  anesthetic management, 236–238
  anesthetic technique, 238–239
  clinical manifestations, 236
  pathophysiology, 236
  postoperative care, 239
  premedication, 239
  preoperative evaluation, 236
  preoperative pharmacotherapy, 236–238
autonomic nervous system (ANS), 3, 4
AVMs. See arteriovenous malformations
AV nodal reentrant tachycardia (AVNRT), 459
axillary temperature, 133–134

BA. See biliary atresia
balanitis xerotica obliterans (BXO), 547
balloon dacryoplasty, 379
barbiturates, 51
Beckwith–Wiedemann syndrome
  anesthetic management, 240–242
  anesthetic technique, 240
  clinical manifestations, 240
  pathophysiology, 240
  postoperative care, 240
  preoperative evaluation, 240

preoperative pharmacology, 240
special considerations/concerns, 242
behavioral and developmental milestones
  evaluation, 32
  factors influencing, 38
  guidelines, 33–38
Benjamin–Inglis classification, laryngotracheoesophageal clefts, 15
benzodiazepines, 51
  autism spectrum disorder (ASD), 236–237
  reversal, 58
bifid uvula, 171
bilateral sagittal split osteotomy, 404–405
bile synthesis, 26–27
biliary atresia (BA)
  anesthetic management, 614
  diagnosis, 613
  hepatic portoenterostomy (HPE), 614
  incidence, 613
  pathogenesis and etiology, 614
bilirubin metabolism, 26
biotransformation, liver, 27–28
bispectral index (BIS), 93
bladder temperature monitoring, 134–135
Blalock–Taussig shunt (BTS), 447–449
bleeding, hypospadia repair, 552
blepharoptosis, 163
blood–gas partition coefficient, 49
blood loss
  cranial vault reconstruction, 325–326
  spinal fusion, 574
blood therapy
  conservation strategies, 130–131
  cryoprecipitate, 129
  fresh frozen plasma, 129
  management, 128
  monitoring, 131
  packed red blood cells, 129
  perioperative blood loss minimization, 129–130
  platelets, 129
  transfusion, 128
blood transfusion, trauma, 616–617
blunt abdominal trauma, 622
bone-anchored hearing aid (BAHA), 287
  anesthetic management, 336
  anesthetic technique, 336
  contraindication, 335
  indication, 335
  postoperative care, 336
  preoperative evaluation, 336
  stump/implant and removable processor, 335
  surgical procedure, 335
botulinum toxin injection, 527
bowel resection
  anesthetic management, 492
  anesthetic technique, 492–493

indications/contraindications, 491
laparoscopic surgery, 491
postoperative care, 493
preoperative evaluation, 492
vomiting and abdominal distension, 492
BPD. See bronchopulmonary dysplasia
brachycephaly, 323
bradycardia, 99
brain-gut axis disorders, 209
brain tumors, 152–153
breast reduction
  anesthetic technique, 419–421
  bilateral, 421–422
  complications/emergencies, 420–421
  indications/contraindications, 418
  postoperative care, 421
  postoperative nausea and vomiting (PONV), 418
  preoperative evaluation, 419
  preoperative pharmacology, 419
bronchiolitis obliterans syndrome (BOS), 220–221
bronchopulmonary dysplasia (BPD), 100, 148
brown adipose tissue (BAT), 31
buccal mucosa, pathology, 171
bupivacaine, 73, 644
buprenorphine, chronic pain, 663
burn injuries
  classifications, 623
  fluid resuscitation, 623
  inhalation injury, 623
  management, 623–624
  pain management, 624
  pathophysiology, 622–623
  thermoregulation, 623
burns
  anesthetic technique, 429
  complications/emergencies, 429–430
  indications/contraindications, 426
  inhalational injury, 428
  pathophysiological changes, 426–428
  postoperative care, 430–431
  preoperative evaluation, 426, 429
  preoperative pharmacology, 429
  scald, 431
butyrophenone, 66, 70
BXO. See balanitis xerotica obliterans

caffeine halothane contracture test (CHCT), 601–602
calvarium, 323
capnograms, 84
capnography, 84–85
carbohydrate drinks, 78
carbon dioxide absorption, 82–83
cardiac arrhythmias, 459
cardiac catheterization
  indications/contraindications, 452–454
  left heart catheterization, 453

new onset pulmonary hypertension, 457
right heart catheterization, 452
therapeutic, 454
cardiac injuries, 621–622
cardiac output
  heart rate and rhythm, 9
  invasive and noninvasive monitoring, 90, 92
  oxygen-carrying capacity, 9
  stroke volume, 8–9
  variations in, 9
cardiac surgery
  off-pump, 446–452
  on-pump, 437–444
cardiac tamponade, 622
cardiac total anomalous pulmonary venous return (TAPVR), 441
cardiac transplantation
  anesthetic management, 625
  cardiopulmonary bypass (CPB), 626
  heart failure, 625
  indications, 625
  monitoring, 626
  organ allocation, 625
cardiomyopathies
  arrhythmogenic right ventricular cardiomyopathy, 196
  dilated cardiomyopathy, 195–196
  hypertrophic cardiomyopathy (HCM), 193–195
  left ventricular noncompaction, 196–197
  restrictive cardiomyopathy, 196
  types, 194
cardiomyopathy, noncardiac surgery, 470
cardiopulmonary assessment
  achondroplasia, 229–230
  Down syndrome, 251
  Hurler and Hunter syndromes, 267
cardiopulmonary bypass (CPB), 626
  cannulation, 442
  circuits and prime volume, 442, 443
  coagulation, 442
  complications/emergencies, 444
  flow while, 442
  initiation, 442
  physiological impact, 442–444
  postoperative care, 444–445
  weaning, 444
cardiopulmonary interactions, 9–10
cardiovascular considerations, preterm infant, 149
cardiovascular system
  anatomy, 6–8
  cardiopulmonary interactions, 9–10
  embryology, 6
  laparoscopic surgery, 509
  physiology, 8–9
cataract, 162
catheter ablation, 461
caudal epidural, 645

caudal epidural blockade, 552
celiac disease, 207
cell savage, 131
central chemoreceptors, 17
central nervous system, anatomy, 3
central venous catheters (CVCs)
    cardiac output (CO) monitoring, 90–91
    central venous pressure monitoring, 90
    complications, 91, 92
    femoral veins, 89
    internal jugular vein, 89
    mixed venous oxygenation monitoring, 91
    subclavian vein, 89
    venous access, 89
central venous pressure (CVP) monitoring, 90
cerebral blood volume (CBV), 307
cerebral palsy (CP), 154, 320
cerebral perfusion pressure (CPP), 307
cervical mediastinoscopy (CM), 535
CHARGE syndrome
    anesthetic management, 244–245
    anesthetic technique, 244–245
    cardiac malformations, 244
    clinical features, 244
    clinical manifestations, 243
    cranial nerve (CN) dysfunction, 244
    hypogonadotropic hypogonadism, 244
    incidence, 243
    pathophysiology, 243
    postoperative care, 245
    preoperative evaluation, 244
    preoperative pharmacotherapy, 244
CHD. *See* congenital heart disease
chest wall compliance, 19
chloral hydrate, radiology, 672–673
choanal atresia, 12, 232
cholecystectomy
    anesthetic technique, 521–522
    complications/emergencies, 522
    incidence, 520
    indications/contraindications, 520
    postoperative care, 522
    preoperative evaluation, 520–521
    preoperative pharmacology, 521
    signs and symptoms, 520
cholesteatoma, 337
chondrodysplasia punctata, 353–354
chondrolysis, 592
chordee, 550
choroid plexus tumors, 153
chronic diarrhea, 206
chronic ear disease, 157
chronic exertional compartment syndrome (CECS), 588
chronic kidney disease (CKD)
    blood pressure control, 24
    electrolytes and acidosis, 23
    fluid balance, 23-24
    glomerular filtration rate assessment, 24
    nephrotoxic medications, 24
chronic otitis media with effusion (COME), 156
chronic pain
    analgesic management, 664
    buprenorphin, 663
    complex regional pain syndrome (CRPS), 664
    dependence, 662
    general approach, 663–664
    long-term opioid therapy, 662
    naltrexone, 663
    tolerance, 662
circulation, trauma, 618
circumcision
    anesthetic technique, 548
    dorsal penile nerve block, 549
    dorsal slit technique, 547
    indications/contraindications, 547
    postoperative care, 548
    preoperative evaluation, 547
    preoperative pharmacology, 547–548
    prevalence, 547
cisatracurium, 60
classic bladder exstrophy (CBE), 224
cleft lip and palate (CLCP), 170
cleft lip and palate repair
    alveolar cleft repair, 416–418
    anesthetic technique, 408
    classification, 406
    indications/contraindications, 406
    postoperative care, 408
    preoperative evaluation, 407
    preoperative pharmacology, 407
    syndromes commonly associated, 417
clonidine, 650–651
coagulation, cardiopulmonary bypass, 442
coarctation of the aorta (CoA)
    anomalies associated, 187
    case study, 451–452
    end-to-end repair, 448–449
    magnetic resonance imaging, 186
    noncardiac surgery, 469
    off-pump cardiac surgery, 446–447
    pathophysiology and clinical manifestations, 186–187
    postsurgical repair assessment, 187
    symptoms, 186
cochlear implants
    anesthetic management, 340–341
    anesthetic technique, 340–341
    components, 339
    contraindications, 339
    postoperative care, 341
    preoperative evaluation, 340
    preoperative pharmacology, 340
codeine therapeutic recommendations, 65
Cohen cross-trigonal technique, 565
COLDS scoring system, 76–77
colloids, 127–128
colonic conditions
    colonic polyps, 209
    Hirschsprung's disease, 208
    inflammatory bowel disease (IBD), 207–208
    intractable functional constipation, 208
    noninflammatory bowel disease colitis, 208
colonic polyps, 209
colonoscopy, 523–525
COME. *See* chronic otitis media with effusion
commotio cordis, 621–622
compartment syndrome
    acute compartment syndrome (ACS), 587–588
    chronic exertional, 588
    management, 588
complete tracheal rings, 14–15
complex regional pain syndrome (CRPS), 664
compliance, lung, 18–19
computed tomography, 668–670
conduction, heat loss, 31
conduction system disturbances
    long QT syndrome (LQTS), 201–203
    supraventricular tachycardia (SVT), 200–201
congenital anomalies of the kidney and urinary tract (CAKUT), 21–22
    anesthesia considerations, 224
    antenatal diagnosis, 222
    congenital ureteral obstruction, 223
    electrolytes and acidosis, 23
    fluid balance, 23
    incidence, 222, 223
    long-term consequences, 222
    nonobstructive nephropathy, 223–224
    obstructive nephropathy, 222–223
congenital blepharoptosis (ptosis), 386–387
congenital diaphragmatic hernia (CDH)
    anesthetic management, 606–607
    bilateral lung hypoplasia, 605
    diagnosis, 604
    diaphragmatic closure, 604
    ECMO support, 606
    embryological basis, 604
    incidence, 604
    inhaled nitric oxide (iNO), 606
    invasive blood pressure monitoring, 605–606
    lung hypoplasia, 604–605
    lung-to-head ratio (LHR), 605
    mechanical ventilation, 605
    outcome predictors, 605
    pathophysiology, 604–605
    perinatal management, 605
    physical examination, 605
    pulmonary vasculature reduction, 605
    ventricular dysfunction, 605
congenital esophageal stenosis (CES), 526–527
congenital hearing loss (CHL)
    causes, 340
    cochlear implants, 339–341
    etiologies, 339
    prevalence, 339
congenital heart disease (CHD), 10, 100
    adult, 470
    cyanotic, 188–193
    incidence, 466
    issues related, 461–462
    left-to-right shunts, 181–188
    patient risk stratification, 181
congenital high airway syndrome (CHAOS), 638
congenital hypothyroidism (CH), 173
congenital limb deformities, 227, 228
congenital scoliosis, 570
congestive heart failure (CHF), noncardiac surgery, 470
continuous pulse oximetry, 86
contractility, stroke volume, 8
contractures, arthrogryposis, 234
controlled hypotension, 325
controlled ventilation, 120
convection, heat loss, 30
core body temperature, 133
corticosteroids, 79
Cotton–Myer subglottic stenosis grading scale, 13, 14
CPB. *See* cardiopulmonary bypass
cranial suture lines, 323
cranial vault reconstruction
    anesthetic technique, 324–326
    postoperative care, 326
    preoperative evaluation, 324
    preoperative pharmacology, 324
    total, 324
craniofacial microsomia, 263
craniosynostosis, 152, 153, 323. *See also* cranial vault reconstruction
craniotomy
    anesthetic management, 301–303
    anesthetic technique, 301–302
    cerebral blood flow (CBF), 300–301
    cerebrospinal fluid, 300
    contraindications, 300
    indications, 300
    postoperative care, 302
    preoperative evaluation, 301
    preoperative pharmacology, 301
Cri du chat syndrome
    anesthetic management, 246–247
    anesthetic technique, 246–247
    clinical manifestations, 246
    pathophysiology, 246
    postoperative care, 247
    preoperative evaluation, 246
    preoperative pharmacotherapy, 246

critical congenital heart defects (CCHD), 188
Crohn's disease (CD), 207–208
Crouzon syndrome (CS)
  anesthetic management, 248–250
  anesthetic technique, 249–250
  clinical manifestations, 247
  pathophysiology, 248
  postoperative care, 250
  preoperative evaluation, 248
  preoperative pharmacotherapy, 248
cryoablation, 461
cryoprecipitate, 129
cryptorchidism, 225, 555
  congenital anomalies, 556
  definition, 555
crystalloids
  glucose-containing fluids, 127
  Lactated Ringer's solution, 126–127
  normal saline, 127
  Plasma-Lyte, 127
Cushing's disease, 176
cyanosis, 437
cyanotic congenital heart disease (CCHD)188–193
  dextro-transposition of the great arteries (d-TGA), 191–192
  noncardiac surgery, 469
  single-ventricle congenital heart disease, 192–193
  tetralogy of fallot, 189–191
  truncus arteriosus, 192
cyanotic defects, noncardiac surgery, 469
cystatin C, 24
cystoscopy
  anesthetic technique, 559
  complications/emergencies, 559
  indications/contraindications, 558
  postoperative care, 559–560
  preoperative evaluation, 559
  preoperative pharmacology, 559
cytochrome P450 (CYP450) monooxygenases, 27

dantrolene sodium, malignant hyperthermia, 601
dead space, 120, 121
deliberate hypotension, 131
dental caries, 168, 169
dental rehabilitation
  anesthetic technique, 394–395
  case study, 395–396
  indications/contraindications, 393
  postoperative care, 395
  preoperative evaluation, 393–394
  preoperative pharmacology, 394
dental trauma, 170–171
depolarizing neuromuscular blocking (NMB) agents, 59
desflurane, 50
desmopressin
  hemophilia, 213

perioperative blood loss minimization, 129
dexamethasone, 70, 79, 651
dexmedetomidine, radiology, 673
dextromethorphan, 651
dextro-transposition of the great arteries (d-TGA), 191–192, 439
diabetes insipidus (DI), 153, 176–177
diabetes mellitus (DM), 172–173
diabetic ketoacidosis (DKA), 172
diazepam, 51
dietary thermogenesis, 32
difficult airway management
  algorithm, 117
  anesthesia induction, 112–113
  anticipated, 114–116
  congenital and acquired airway abnormalities, 112
  difficult bag-mask ventilation, 113
  extubation, 116–118
  oxygenation strategies, 113–114
  prevalence and predictors, 111–112
  unanticipated, 116
difficult bag-mask ventilation (DBMV), 113
diffuse esophageal spasm, 526
dilated cardiomyopathy (DCM)
  anesthetic considerations, 196
  pathophysiology and clinical manifestations, 195–196
direct laryngoscopy, 108–109
dismembered pyeloplasty, 562
disseminated intravascular coagulation (DIC), 210–211
distal hypospadias, 549–550
distribution, pharmacologic agent, 44–45
diverting gas analyzers, 84
dobutamine, 72
dolasetron, 66
dominant dystrophic epidermolysis bullosa (DDEB), 256
donation after cardiac death (DCD), 682
dopamine, 70–71
dopamine antagonist, 66
dorsal rhizotomy
  anesthetic management, 320–321
  anesthetic technique, 321
  contraindications, 320
  indications, 320
  poor oropharyngeal control, 321–322
  postoperative care, 321
  preoperative evaluation, 320
  preoperative pharmacology, 321
double aortic arch, 447
double-lumen endotracheal tube (DLT), 284
Down syndrome
  anesthetic management, 251–252
  anesthetic technique, 251–252
  clinical manifestations, 250
  common features, 251
  pathophysiology, 250

postoperative care, 252
  preoperative evaluation, 251
  preoperative pharmacotherapy, 251
droperidol, 66
drug elimination, 47–48
drug-induced sleep endoscopy (DISE), 671
  anesthetic management, 371–374
  anesthetic technique, 372
  complications/emergencies, 373–374
  indications/contraindications, 371
  postoperative care, 374
  preoperative evaluation, 371–372
ductal coarctation, 446–447
duodenal atresia
  anesthetic management, 615
  incidence, 614
  pathophysiology and clinical manifestations, 614–615
dystrophic epidermolysis bullosa (DEB), 256

ear conditions, 156–158
  chronic ear disease, 157
  otitis media, 156
  sensorineural hearing loss (SNHL), 157–158
early childhood caries (ECCs), 393
early-onset scoliosis (EOS)
  elongation–derotation–flexion (EDF) casting technique, 581
  serial casting technique, 581
EBV. See estimated blood volume
echocardiogram (ECHO), 671
  atrioventricular septal defects (AVSDs), 186
  dilated cardiomyopathy, 195
  hypertrophic cardiomyopathy, 195
  hypoplastic left heart syndrome (HLHS), 193
  left-to-right shunting lesions, 472
  patent ductus arteriosus (PDA), 185
  repaired truncus arteriosus, 193
  restrictive cardiomyopathy, 196
  single-ventricle defects, 473
  tetralogy of fallot (TOF), 190
  unrepaired coarctation of the aorta (CoA), 187
Eckardt Symptom Score (ESS), 527
ectopic atrial tachycardia (EAT) treatment, 458
EGD. See esophagogastroduodenoscopy
Ehlers–Danlos syndromes (EDS)
  anesthetic management, 254–255
  anesthetic technique, 254–255
  clinical manifestations, 254
  pathophysiology, 253–254
  postoperative care, 255
  preoperative evaluation, 254
  preoperative

pharmacotherapy, 254
electrocardiogram, 86-87
electroencephalography (EEG), 93
electrolyte abnormalities, 23
electrophysiology studies (EPS)
  anesthetic management, 462–464
  complications/emergencies, 464
  indications/contraindications, 458–459
  postoperative care, 466
  preoperative evaluation, 462
  preoperative pharmacology, 462
  Wolff-Parkinson-White (WPW) syndrome, 464–465
elongation–derotation–flexion (EDF) casting technique, 581
embryonic development, 2, 3
emergence delirium (ED), 50, 142, 379
encephalocele, 151, 152
endocarditis, cardiac conditions, 473
endocrine conditions
  diabetes mellitus (DM), 172–173
  hypothalamic–pituitary–adrenal (HPA) axis, 174–178
  parathyroid dysfunction, 174
  polycystic ovary syndrome (PCOS), 178
  sepsis, 179
  surgery-induced stress, 179
  thyroid disease, 173–174
  thyroidectomy/goiter, 179
endoluminal functional imaging probe (EndoFLIP), 526
endoscopy, gastrointestinal, 523–525
endotracheal tubes (ETTs)
  direct laryngoscopy, 108–109
  flexible bronchoscopy, 110
  Mehta cast application, 582
  nasal intubation, 110–111
  orchidopexy, 557
  rapid-sequence intubation (RSI), 111
  video laryngoscopy, 109–110
end-stage liver disease (ESLD), 626, 627
end-stage renal disease (ESRD), 24
end-tidal carbon dioxide, 120
enhanced recovery after surgery (ERAS)
  congenital cardiac surgery, 660
  gastrointestinal surgery, 658
  idiopathic posterior spinal fusion, 659–660
  lower urinary tract reconstructive surgery, 567, 568
  pectus excavatum repair, 658–659
  urological procedures, 660
enhanced recovery after surgery (ERAS) protocols, 78
entropy monitors, 93
enucleation
  anesthetic technique, 392

anophthalmia and microphthalmia, 389
considerations and concerns, 392
indications/contraindications, 389
postoperative care, 392
preoperative evaluation, 391
surgical procedure, 390
trauma, 389
ephedrine, 72
epicardial pacemaker systems, 470
epidermolysis bullosa (EB)
anesthetic management, 258–260
anesthetic technique, 259–260
clinical manifestations, 255
incidence, 256
pathophysiology, 255–256
postoperative care, 260
preoperative evaluation, 258–259
subtypes, 256-257
epilepsy, 154
stereotactic grid placement, 307–310
vagal nerve stimulator placement, 310–313
epilepsy surgery
anesthetic management, 315–318
anesthetic technique, 316–318
contraindications, 313–314
indications, 313–314
ketogenic diets and anesthesia, 315
perioperative management, 314
preoperative pharmacology, 316
types, 314
epinephrine, 71
equipment and monitoring
anesthesia machine, 82–83
arterial blood pressure monitoring, 87–89
central venous catheters (CVCs), 89–91
electroencephalography (EEG), 93
near-infrared spectroscopy (NIRS), 93
physiologic monitoring, 85–87
transesophageal echocardiography (TEE), 91-93
during transport, 93–94
ERAS. See enhanced recovery after surgery
Erector spinae plane block, 488, 489
eruption of teeth, 167–168
ESLD. See end-stage liver disease
esmolol, 651–652
esophageal atresia (EA), 294
esophageal conditions
achalasia, 205
atresia, 204
duplications, 204
esophagitis, 204–205
foreign body ingestions and food impactions, 205
stenosis and strictures, 204
trachea esophageal fistula (TEF), 204

webs and rings, 204
esophageal dilation, 526–527
Esophageal Injury Score, 527
esophageal manometry
indications/contraindications, 526
preoperative evaluation, 527–528
esophageal motility disorders, 526
esophageal temperature monitoring, 134
esophagitis, 204–205
esophagogastroduodenoscopy (EGD)
anesthetic technique, 524–525
complications/emergencies, 525
contraindications, 523
indications, 523
postoperative care, 525
preanesthetic evaluation, 523
preoperative pharmacology, 524
estimated blood volume (EBV), 128
ethical considerations
assent, 680–681
emancipated minor, 681
end-of-life care, 681
futility, 682
informed consent, 680
Jehovah's witnesses, 681
organ donation, 682
patient safety, 682
personal beliefs of anesthesia providers, 682
rights of minors, 681
withholding and withdrawing treatment, 681–682
etomidate, 58, 97
ETTs. See endotracheal tubes
euthyroid goiter, 174
evaporation, heat loss, 30
evisceration, 390
exenteration, 390
EXIT procedures. See ex utero intrapartum therapy procedures
extraocular eye conditions, 163
extubation, 116–118
exudative retinal detachment (RD), 382–383
ex utero intrapartum therapy (EXIT) procedures
anesthetic technique, 641–642
fetal anesthetic considerations, 639–641
indications/contraindications, 638–639
maternal anesthetic considerations, 639
multidisciplinary team involvement, 639
postoperative care, 642
potential risks associated, 642
preoperative evaluation, 641

Face, Legs, Activity, Cry, Consolability (FLACC) scale, 239
facial cellulitis/infection, dental caries, 168, 169

factor concentrates, perioperative blood loss minimization, 129
failure to thrive (FTT), 207
FAS. See fetal alcohol syndrome
fasciotomy
anesthetic technique, 588–589
incisions, 588
indications/contraindications, 587–588
postoperative care, 589
preoperative evaluation, 588
preoperative pharmacology, 588
fatty acid metabolism, 26
femoral nerve blockade, 570
fentanyl, 463
fetal alcohol syndrome (FAS)
anesthetic management, 261–262
anesthetic technique, 262
clinical manifestations, 261
facial abnormalities, 261
pathophysiology, 261
postoperative care, 262
preoperative evaluation, 262–262
preoperative pharmacotherapy, 262
fetal circulation, 7
fetal pulmonary circulation, 20
fetal surgery, minimally invasive fetal surgery, 636–638
fever
EXIT procedure, 638–642
hematopoietic stem cell transplant, 219
FFP. See fresh frozen plasma
first-order multiple-compartment kinetics, 49
first-order single-compartment kinetics, 48
flexible bronchoscope for intubation via supraglottic airway (FOI-SGA)
air-Q, 114
continuous ventilation, 115
procedural steps, 115
flexible bronchoscopy
airway management, 110
supraglottic airway, 114
fluid management
age-related heart rate, 125
daily caloric requirements, 124
intraoperative, 125–131
normal fluid requirements, 124
physiological considerations, 124
preoperative fasting guidelines, 124–125
total pancreatectomy and islet autotransplantation (TPIAT), 633
trauma, 616
fluid/metabolic status, preterm infant, 149
fluid resuscitation, burn injuries, 623
fluid warmers, 137, 138
flumazenil, 55, 58
FOI-SGA. See flexible bronchoscope for intubation via supraglottic airway
forced-air warming device, 137
fospropofol, 57, 58

Fowler–Stephens procedure, 556
fresh frozen plasma (FFP), 129
frictional resistance, lung, 19
functional gastrointestinal disorders (FGIDs), 209
futility, 682

gabapentinoids, 652
galvanic/fuel cell analyzers, 83
gas exchange, 20–21
gastric and gastrojejunal tube placement
anesthetic technique, 495
complications/emergencies, 495
indications/contraindications, 493
laparoscopic, 493–495
postoperative care, 495–496
preoperative evaluation, 494
preoperative pharmacology, 494
gastric conditions
gastritis, 205–206
gastroparesis, 206
gastropathy, 205–206
GI bleeding, 206, 207
gastritis, 205–206
gastroesophageal reflux disease (GERD)
incidence, 502
Nissen fundoplication, 502–504
gastrointestinal (GI) conditions
bleeding, 206, 207
brain–gut axis disorders, 209
colonic and anorectal conditions, 207–209
esophageal conditions, 204–205
gastric conditions, 205–206
small bowel conditions, 206–207
gastroparesis, 206
gastropathy, 205–206
gastroschisis
anesthetic management, 609–610
clinical manifestations, 607–609
diagnosis, 609
incidence, 608
pathophysiology, 607–609
general endotracheal anesthesia (GETA), 533
genioplasty, 404–405
genitourinary cancers, 224, 225
genitourinary conditions
congenital anomalies of the kidney and urinary tract (CAKUT), 222–224
renal injury, 224–225
gingiva, pathology, 171
gingivitis, 169
glanuloplasty, 550
glaucoma, 163
glenohumeral joint instability, 584
glomerular filtration rate (GFR), 22
chronic kidney disease (CKD), 24
creatinine-based measurements, 48
Schwartz equations, 47
glucocorticosteroid, 70
gluconeogenesis, 26

glucose-containing fluids, 127
glycogenolysis, 26
glycolysis, 26
goiter, 174
Goldenhar syndrome (GS)
  anesthetic management, 263, 265
  anesthetic technique, 265
  clinical features, 264
  clinical manifestation, 263
  pathophysiology, 263
  postoperative care, 265
  preoperative evaluation, 263, 265
  preoperative pharmacotherapy, 265
graft-versus-host disease (GVHD), 220
granisetron, 66
Graves' disease, 173
Gross Motor Function Classification Scale (GMFCS), 227
GS. See Goldenhar syndrome

Haller index (HI), 486
handoff checklist, 140, 141
H1 antagonist, 66
Hashimoto's thyroiditis (HT), 173
head and neck conditions
  hyperparathyroidism, 160
  neck masses, 160–161
  salivary gland disease, 160
  thyroidectomy, 159–160
HEAR MAPS Classification Method, 423
heart
  cardiopulmonary interactions, 9–10
  electrical system, 6–7
  embryology, 6
  fetal circulation, 7
  functional anatomy, 6
  physiology, 8–9
  transitional circulation, 7–8
heart failure, cardiac transplantation, 625
heart rate, 9
heat and moisture exchanger (HME), 30
heat generation, 31–32
heat loss
  conduction, 31
  convection, 30
  evaporation, 30
  mechanisms, 30–31
  radiation, 30
hematologic conditions
  aplastic anemia, 214–215
  disseminated intravascular coagulation (DIC), 210–211
  hemophilia, 211–214
  immune thrombocytopenia, 211
  sickle cell disease, 215–216
hematopoietic stem cell transplant (HSCT)
  bronchiolitis obliterans syndrome (BOS), 220–221
  conditioning, 219
  fever and infection, 219
  graft-versus-host disease (GVHD), 220
  normal hematopoietic stem cell infusion, 218–219
  sinusoidal obstructive syndrome (SOS), 219–220
  transplant-associated thrombotic microangiopathy (TA-TMA), 220
hemodilution, cardiopulmonary bypass, 444
hemophilia
  antifibrinolytic agents, 213
  desmopressin, 213
  factor correction, 212–214
  female carriers, 212
  fresh frozen plasma/cryoprecipitate, 213
  hemophilia A, 212
  hemophilia B, 212
  high-titer inhibitor, 212–213
  incidence, 211
  low-titer inhibitor, 213
  mild, 212
  moderate, 212
  postoperative management, 213–214
  severe, 211–212
  symptoms, 212
  vascular access, 214
  venous thromboembolism, 214
hemorrhage, bowel resection, 493
hemorrhoids, 208
hemostasis, TPIAT, 633
hepatic portoenterostomy (HPE), 614
hepatic system
  anatomy, 25, 26
  bilirubin metabolism and bile synthesis, 26–27
  biotransformation, 27–28
  glucose regulation, 26
  lipid/fatty acid metabolism, 26
  physiology, 25–28
  protein synthesis, 26
hepatocytes, 25
hepatopulmonary syndrome (HPS), 626
hernia, 484
hernia repair
  anesthetic technique, 485
  indications/contraindications, 484
  postoperative care, 485
  preoperative evaluation, 485
  strangulation, 484
high-flow nasal cannula (HFNC), 112
high-pressure system, 82
high-resolution esophageal manometry (HREM), 526
  anesthetic technique, 528
  complications/emergencies, 528
  preoperative pharmacology, 528
hip disorders, 227–228
Hirschsprung's disease, 208
Hoarseness, case study, 349–350
HPS. See hepatopulmonary syndrome; hypertrophic pyloric stenosis
humidification, 83
Hurler and Hunter syndromes
  anesthetic management, 266–268
  anesthetic technique, 267–268
  incidence, 266
  pathophysiology, 266
  postoperative care, 268
  preoperative evaluation, 266–267
  preoperative pharmacotherapy, 267
  signs and symptoms, 267
  symptom presentation, 266
hydrocephalus, 151, 305–306
  congenital causes, 330
  obstructive, 330
  third ventriculostomy, 330–331
  ventriculoperitoneal (VP) shunt, 330
hydrophilic pharmacologic agents, 45
5-hydroxytryptamine antagonists, 79
5-hydroxytryptamine (5-HT3) antagonists, 66
hyperaldosteronism, 177
hyperoxia, cardiopulmonary bypass, 444
hyperparathyroidism, 160, 432
hyperthermia, 136
hyperthyroidism, 173–174
hypertrophic cardiomyopathy (HCM)
  anesthetic considerations, 194–195
  diagnosis and treatment, 194
  pathophysiology and clinical manifestations, 193–194
hypertrophic pyloric stenosis (HPS)
  anesthetic management, 613
  clinical presentation, 612
  diagnosis, 612
  fluid resuscitation plan, 612
  pathophysiology and clinical manifestations, 612
  physical examination, 612
  pyloromyotomy, 612
hypocalcemia, thyroidectomy and parathyroidectomy, 436
hypogonadotropic hypogonadism, 244
hypoparathyroidism, 174
hypoplasia, incomplete lung development, 16
hypospadia repair
  anesthetic technique, 552
  buccal mucosal graft, 553–554
  complications, 550
  components, 550
  indications/contraindications, 549–550
  postoperative care, 552–553
  preoperative evaluation, 550–552
  preoperative pharmacology, 552
  surgical techniques, 551
hypospadias, 225, 549
hypotension, 616
hypothalamus disorders, 175
hypothermia, 136, 443
hypothyroidism, 173
hypovolemia, 616

ICU ventilators, 120
idiopathic scoliosis, 227
ileocolic intussusception, 505
imaging techniques
  computed tomography, 668–669
  interventional radiology, 669
  magnetic resonance imaging, 668
  nuclear medicine, 669
  radiation oncology, 669
  sedation levels, 669–670
immune thrombocytopenia, 211
infant ECG electrodes, 86
infection, hematopoietic stem cell transplant, 219
infective endocarditis
  antibiotic prophylaxis, 80
  prevention, 474
inflammation, cardiopulmonary bypass, 444
inflammatory bowel disease (IBD), 207–208
informed consent, 680
infracardiac cardiac total anomalous pulmonary venous return (TAPVR), 441
inguinal hernia, 484
inguinal hernia repairs (IHR), 484
inhalation induction
  desflurane, 96
  with parental presence, 96
  proper mask fitment, 96
  sevoflurane, 96
  single-breath inhalation induction, 96–97
  steal induction, 96
inhaled anesthetics
  cardiovascular effects, 50
  characteristics, 50
  desflurane, 50
  drug solubility, 49
  efficacy and potency, 49
  emergence delirium (ED), 50
  halothane and enflurane, 49
  isoflurane, 50
  malignant hyperthermia (MH), 51
  neurotoxicity, 51
  nitrous oxide, 50
  sevoflurane, 50
inotropic agents, 70–72
inspiratory-to-expiratory ratio, 117
insulinoma, 172–173
interdependence model, lung, 17–18
intermediate-pressure system, 82
International Neuroblastoma Risk Group Staging System (INRGSS), 543, 544
International Neuroblastoma Staging System (INSS), 543
interventional radiology, 669
intractable focal epilepsy, 318–319
intractable functional constipation, 208
intraocular eye conditions, 162–163
intraoperative fluid management
  blood, 128–131
  colloids, 127–128
  crystalloids, 126–127
  physiological processes, 125
  third spacing, 125, 126
  volumetric chambers, 126

ontraoperative neuromonitoring (IONM), scoliosis surgery, 574, 575
intravenous anesthesia induction
  etomidate, 97
  ketamine, 97
  propofol, 97
  rapid-sequence induction (RSI), 97–98
intravenous anesthetic agents
  barbiturates, 51
  benzodiazepines, 51, 58
  pharmacokinetic and pharmacodynamic properties, 52–57
  sedative-hypnotic agents, 58
intraventricular hemorrhage (IVH), 148
intussusception
  anesthetic technique, 507
  complications/emergencies, 507–508
  cuffed endotracheal tube (ETT), 507
  diagnosis, 505
  differential diagnoses, 505
  etiology, 504
  ileocolic, 505
  indications/contraindications, 504–506
  nonidiopathic cases, 504
  non-operative pneumatic reduction, 506
  perforation, 506
  preoperative evaluation, 506–507
  rapid sequence induction (RSI), 507
  symptoms, 505
irritant receptors, 17
isoflurane, 50
isoproterenol, 71–72

junctional epidermolysis bullosa (JEB), 256

Kawasaki disease (KD), 197–198
ketamine, 58, 97, 652
  autism spectrum disorder (ASD), 237–238
  radiology, 673
ketogenesis, 26
KFS. See Klippel–Feil syndrome
kidney transplantation, 629–631
  allograft kidney, 629
  anesthetic technique, 630–631
  complications and emergencies, 631
  indication/contraindications, 629
  postoperative care, 631
  preoperative evaluation, 629
  preoperative pharmacology, 629
  size-related considerations, 629
King–Moe classification, scoliosis, 570
Klippel–Feil syndrome (KFS)
  anesthetic management, 269–270
  anesthetic technique, 270
  clinical manifestation, 269
  clinical triad, 269

pathophysiology, 269
postoperative care, 270
preoperative evaluation, 269–270
preoperative pharmacotherapy, 270
knee ligament reconstruction, 578–581
kyphosis, 570

Lactated Ringer's solution, 126–127
laparoscopic hernia repair (LHR), 484
laparoscopic surgery
  anesthetic technique, 510
  appendectomy, 511
  carbon dioxide pneumoperitoneum, 509
  cardiovascular system, 509
  complications, 510–511
  neurological system, 508
  postoperative care, 510
  preoperative evaluation, 510
  preoperative pharmacology, 510
  renal system, 510
  respiratory system, 509
laryngeal edema, thyroidectomy and parathyroidectomy, 436
laryngeal mask airway (LMA), 105
  Mehta cast application, 582
  orchidopexy, 557
laryngomalacia, 13–14
laryngospasm, 98–99
  incidence, 141–142
  postanesthetic care, 142
laryngotracheoesophageal clefts, 15
larynx, 12–14
  airway obstruction, 13–14
  iatrogenic webs, 13
  motor and sensory innervation, 13
  normal, 12
  rigid framework, 12
  stenosis, 13, 14
  subsites, 12
lean methodology, 686
LeFort fractures, 401
LeFort osteotomy
  anesthetic technique, 402–403
  complications/emergencies, 404
  indications/contraindications, 401
  postoperative care, 404
  preoperative evaluation, 401–402
  preoperative pharmacology, 402
left-sided frontalis sling, 388
left-to-right shunts
  atrial septal defect (ASD), 183–184
  atrioventricular septal defects, 185–186
  coarctation of the aorta (CoA), 186–187
  patent ductus arteriosus (PDA), 184–185
  vascular rings and slings, 187–188

ventricular septal defect (VSD), 181–183
left ventricular noncompaction (LVNC), 196–197
Lenke's classification, scoliosis, 570
levobupivacaine, 73
lidocaine, 73, 652
life-sustaining medical therapy (LSMT), 681
light meal, 78
Lindholm laryngoscopes, 347
linear effect model, 43
lipid/fatty acid metabolism, 26
lipophilic pharmacologic agents, 45
lip, pathology, 171
liver
  cell types, 25
  development, 25
  physiology, 25–26
  segments, 26
liver transplantation
  anesthetic technique, 628
  indication/contraindications, 626
  postoperative care, 629
  preoperative anesthetic assessment, 627–628
  pulmonary concerns, 626–627
local anesthetics, 72, 73
long QT syndrome (LQTS)
  anesthetic considerations, 202–203
  pathophysiology and clinical manifestations, 201–202
lorazepam, 51, 55, 58, 65, 66
lower urinary tract reconstructive surgery
  anesthetic technique, 566–568
  augmentation cystoplasty, 565–566
  indications/contraindications, 564
  postoperative care, 568–569
  preoperative assessment, 566
  preoperative pharmacology, 566
  ureteral reimplantation, 564–565
low-pressure system, 82
LP. See lumbar puncture
LSMT. See life-sustaining medical therapy
lumbar and thoracic epidurals, 645–646
lumbar puncture (LP), 671
  acute lymphoblastic leukemia, 542
  anesthetic technique, 541
  complications, 540
  indications/contraindications, 539–540
  postoperative care, 541
  preoperative evaluation, 540
Lund–Browder diagram, 427
lung compliance, 18
lung development
  postnatal, 16
  prenatal, 15–16
  stages, 16
lung-to-head ratio (LHR), 605
lung volumes and capacities, 17

MABL. See maximum allowable blood loss
magnesium, 652–653
magnetic resonance imaging (MRI)
  anesthesia for, 668
  stereotactic grid placement, 308
mainstream gas analyzers, 84
major aortopulmonary collateral arteries (MAPCAs), 439
major vascular disease, 469–470
malignant hyperthermia (MH), 77
  Clinical Grading Scale, 599
  clinical presentation, 601
  diagnosis, 601–602
  epidemiology, 598
  incidence, 598
  inhalation anesthetics, 51
  malignant hyperthermia-susceptible children, 598–601
  pathophysiology, 598
  phenotypes associated, 600
  treatment, 601
Malignant Hyperthermia Association of the United States (MHAUS), 601
malignant hyperthermia-susceptible children, 598–603
Mallampati classification, 12
malnutrition, 207
malocclusion, 169
mandibular distraction osteogenesis (MDO)
  anesthetic technique, 397–398
  indications/contraindications, 396–397
  postoperative care, 398–399
  preoperative evaluation, 397
mask management, 102–103
Masseter muscle rigidity (MMR), 601
mast cell activation syndrome (MCAS), 254
maxillary osteotomies, 402
maximum allowable blood loss (MABL), 128
maximum effect model, 43
McGill Oximetry Scoring System, 366
MD. See muscular dystrophy
mechanical ventilation
  congenital diaphragmatic hernia (CDH), 605
  controlled ventilation, 122
  default mode, 121–122
  invasive positive pressure, 121
  pressure-controlled ventilation, 122
  pressure support ventilation (PSV), 122
  synchronized intermittent mandatory ventilation (SIMV), 122
  volume-controlled ventilation (VCV), 122
medial patellofemoral ligament (MPFL) reconstruction
  anesthetic technique, 579–580
  complications/emergencies, 580
  indications/contraindications, 578
  postoperative care, 580–581
  regional anesthetics, 578

mediastinoscopy
  anesthetic considerations, 536
  anesthetic technique, 535–537
  complications, 537–538
  indications/contraindications, 535
  postoperative care, 538
  preoperative evaluation, 535
Mehta cast application
  anesthetic technique, 582–583
  complications/emergencies, 583
  indications/contraindications, 581
  postoperative care, 583
  preoperative assessment, 582
melatonin, 79
mesonephros, 22
metabolic and bariatric surgery (MBS), 498
metanephros, 22
methohexital, 51
microlaryngoscopy
  anesthetic management, 347–349
  anesthetic technique, 347–349
  indication/contraindications, 346, 347
  laser applications and precautions, 348
  postoperative care, 349
  preoperative evaluation, 347
  preoperative pharmacology, 347
microphthalmia, 389
microtia, 423
microtia repair
  anesthetic technique, 425
  complications, 425
  indications/contraindications, 423
  postoperative care, 425
  preoperative evaluation, 423–424
  preoperative pharmacology, 424–425
midazolam, 51, 673
milrinone, 72
minimally invasive fetal surgery
  anesthetic management, 637
  anesthetic technique, 638
  complications, 638
  indications/contraindications, 636
  myelomeningocele (MMC) repair, 636–637
  preoperative evaluation, 638
  twin–twin transfusion syndrome (TTTS), 636, 637
minimally invasive Nuss procedure, 486
minimally invasive surgery, neuroblastoma, 545
minimum alveolar concentration (MAC), 49
mitochondrial myopathy
  anesthetic management, 271
  anesthetic technique, 272
  clinical manifestation, 271
  pathophysiology, 271
  postoperative care, 272
  preoperative evaluation, 271
  preoperative pharmacotherapy, 272

mixed cardiac total anomalous pulmonary venous return (TAPVR), 441
mixed venous oxygenation monitoring, 91
Model for Improvement methodology, 685–686
modified Cormack–Lehane grading system, 13
Modified Yale Pediatric Anxiety Scale (MY-PAS), 655
Monro–Kellie hypothesis, 307
mucopolysaccharidosis (MPS), 266
multiple wavelength pulse CO-oximetry, 86
multisystem inflammatory disease syndrome (MIS-C), 197
muscle involvement, ventilation, 18
muscular dystrophy (MD)
  anesthetic management, 273–274
  anesthetic technique, 273–274
  clinical manifestation, 273
  pathophysiology, 273
  postoperative care, 274
  preoperative evaluation, 273
  preoperative pharmacotherapy, 273
musculoskeletal conditions
  congenital limb deformities, 227, 228
  hip disorders, 227–228
  spinal disorders, 226–227
  sports-related injuries and fracture, 227
myelomeningocele repair
  anesthetic technique, 328–329
  antenatal correction, 327
  indications/contraindications, 327–328
  postoperative care, 329
  prenatal correction, 327
  preoperative evaluation, 328
  preoperative pharmacology, 328
  ventriculoperitoneal shunt placement, 328
myelomeningocele (MMC) repair, 636–637
myocarditis, 197
myringotomy, 333–334

naloxone, 65
naltrexone, chronic pain, 663
Narcotrend monitors, 93
nasal cavity, 11, 12
  choanal atresia, 12
  posterior, 11
  turbinates, 11
nasal conditions
  obstruction, 158
  sinusitis, 158–159
nasal intubation, 108–109
nasal septum deviation and obstruction, 364
nasolacrimal duct obstruction (NLDO), 163, 379–380
nasolacrimal duct probing, 379
nasopharyngeal airways, 103, 105
nasopharyngeal temperature monitoring, 134

nasopharyngeal tonsillar tissue, 12
nasopharynx, 11
near-infrared spectroscopy (NIRS), 93
NEC. See necrotizing enterocolitis
neck masses, 160–161
necrotizing enterocolitis (NEC)
  anesthetic management, 611–612
  medical management, 611
  mortality rates, 611
  pathophysiology and clinical manifestations, 610–611
  risk factors, 610
  symptoms, 611
neonatal emergencies
  biliary atresia (BA), 613–614
  congenital diaphragmatic hernia (CDH), 604–607
  duodenal atresia, 614–615
  hypertrophic pyloric stenosis (HPS), 612–613
  necrotizing enterocolitis (NEC), 610–612
  omphalocele and gastroschisis, 607–610
  sacrococcygeal teratomas (SCTs), 607
neonate
  pulmonary circulation, 20
  ventilation, 17
neostigmine, 60
nephrolithiasis, 224–225
nephrotoxic medications, 24
nervous system
  central nervous system (CNS), 3
  embryonic development, 2, 3
  newborn reflexes, 3–4
  peripheral nervous system (PNS), 3
neuraxial analgesia
  caudal epidural, 645
  lumbar and thoracic epidurals, 645–646
neuroblastoma, 543–546
neuroblastoma resection
  anesthetic technique, 545–546
  indications/contraindications, 543
  postoperative care, 546
  preoperative evaluation, 543–544
  preoperative pharmacology, 545
neurocognitive implications, 4, 6
neurogenic bladder, 224
neurokinin antagonist (NK-1 receptor), 70
neurological conditions
  Arnold–Chiari malformation, 151–152
  arteriovenous malformations, 153
  cerebral palsy, 154
  craniosynostosis, 152
  encephalocele, 151, 152
  epilepsy, 154
  hydrocephalus, 151
  spina bifida, 152, 153
  tethered cord, 152
  tumors, 152–153

neuromuscular blocking agents, 463
neuromuscular blocking (NMB) agents
  characteristics, 59
  depolarizing, 59
  neuromuscular junction, 59
  nondepolarizing, 59–61
neuromuscular scoliosis, 227
  nonoperative treatment, 570–571
  postoperative complications, 576
  types, 570
neuroskeletal assessment, Hurler and Hunter syndromes, 267
neurotoxicity, inhaled anesthetics, 51
newborn reflexes, 3–4
  postural, 5
  primitive, 5
Nissen fundoplication
  anesthetic management, 503
  comorbidities, 502
  complications/emergencies, 503–504
  indications, 502
  physiological changes, 503
  postoperative care, 504
nitrous oxide, 50
NLDO. See nasolacrimal duct obstruction
noncardiac surgery
  anesthetic technique, 474–475
  complications/emergencies, 475–476
  considerations, 470
  crisis resource management, 470
  indications/contraindications, 466–470
  postoperative care, 476
  preanesthetic evaluation, 471–473
  preoperative pharmacology, 473
  timing of, 471
  upper respiratory infection (URI), 471
nondepolarizing muscle relaxant (NDMR), 274, 321
nondepolarizing neuromuscular blocking (NMB) agents, 59–61
  reversal, 60, 61
noninflammatory bowel disease colitis, 208
noninvasive blood pressure (NIBP) measurement, 85, 87
non-MH-induced rhabdomyolysis, 601
nonobstructive nephropathy, 223–224
nonopioid analgesics, 79
nonshivering thermogenesis (NST), 31
nonsteroidal anti-inflammatory drugs (NSAIDs), 65, 589, 653
norepinephrine, 72
normal larynx, 12
normal saline, 127
normothermia

fluid warmers, 137
forced-air warming device, 137
humidification of inhaled gases, 137–138
radiant warming devices, 137
room temperature, 136–137
transport warming devices, 138
nuclear medicine, 669, 670
Numeric Rating Scale (NRS), 654

obesity, 100
obstruction, nasal conditions, 158
obstructive lesions, noncardiac surgery, 467
obstructive nephropathy
 congenital obstructions, 222
 congenital ureteral obstruction, 223
 posterior urethral valves (PUV), 222–223
 prune belly syndrome (PBS), 223
obstructive-noncommunicating hydrocephalus, 330
obstructive sleep apnea (OSA), 275
 adenotonsillectomy, 368
 anesthetic management, 366–368
 anesthetic technique, 367
 clinical manifestation, 365
 diagnosis, 365
 McGill Oximetry Scoring System, 366
 multiple organ systems, 370
 pathophysiology, 365
 polysomnography (PSG), 365, 366, 371
 postoperative care, 367–368
 preoperative assessment, 366–367
 prevalence, 365
 sleeve gastrectomy, 499
 upper airway resistance, 365
ocular trauma, 163
odontogenesis
 bell stage, 167
 bud and cup stage, 167
 eruption, 167–168
 histodifferentiation and morphodifferentiation, 167
 morphological development, 167
 neural crest cell migration, 166–167
off-pump cardiac surgery, 446–452
 anesthetic technique, 448–450
 coarctation of the aorta, 446–447
 indications/contraindications, 446
 pacemaker generator placement, 448
 PDA ligation, 448
 postoperative care, 450–451
 preoperative evaluation, 448
 preoperative pharmacology, 448
 pulmonary artery (PA) banding, 447
 vascular ring division, 447
oil–gas partition coefficient, 49

omphalocele
 anesthetic management, 609–610
 clinical manifestations, 607–609
 diagnosis, 609
 incidence, 608
 pathophysiology, 607–609
oncologic-bone marrow transplantation conditions
 anesthesia considerations, 217–218
 brain tumors, 217
 hematopoietic stem cell transplant (HSCT), 218–221
 leukemias and lymphomas, 217
 nausea and vomiting, 218
 pain management, 218
 steroid administration, 217–218
ondansetron, 66, 67, 79
on-pump cardiac surgery, 437–444
 anesthetic technique, 438–442
 cardiopulmonary bypass, 442–444
 indications/contraindications, 437
 postoperative care, 444
 preoperative evaluation, 437–438
 preoperative pharmacology, 438
 STAT score, 437
open hernia repair (OHR), 484
ophthalmic conditions
 anesthetic management, 165, 166
 examination under anesthesia, 164
 extraocular eye conditions, 163
 intraocular eye conditions, 162–163
 ocular trauma, 163
 surgical procedures, 163–164
 syndromes associated with, 164–165
 visual acuity, 162
ophthalmologic exam under anesthesia
 anesthetic management, 375
 indications/contraindications, 375
opioid analgesic agents
 metabolizers, 65
 opioid receptor agonists and antagonists, 61
 pharmacokinetic properties, 62–64
 reversal, 60–61
opioid-free anesthesia
 acetaminophen, 650
 adenotonsillectomy, 653
 anxiety and anxiolysis, 654–656
 clonidine, 650–651
 dexamethasone, 651
 dextromethorphan, 651
 esmolol, 651–652
 gabapentinoids, 652
 ketamine, 652
 magnesium, 652–653
 nonsteroidal anti-inflammatory drugs, 653
oral cavity, 11–12
oral clefts malformations, 406

oral cleft surgery, components, 406
oral pathology, 171
orchidopexy
 anesthetic technique, 556–557
 case study, 558
 complications/emergencies, 557
 indications/contraindications, 555–556
 postoperative care, 557
 preoperative evaluation, 556
 preoperative pharmacology, 556
organ donation, 682
oropharyngeal airway devices, 102–103
oropharynx, 12
orthodontics
 malocclusion, 169
 tooth impaction, 170
otitis media, 156
otitis media with effusion (OME), 156, 333
otolaryngologic conditions
 anesthetic management, 155–156
 anesthetic planning, 156
 ear conditions, 156–158
 head and neck conditions, 159–161
 nasal conditions, 158–159
 physical examination and assessment, 156
 preoperative evaluation, 155
 throat conditions, 159
overwhelming postsplenectomy infection (OPSI), 532
oxycephaly, 323
oxygen analyzers, 83–84
oxygenation strategies, 113–114

packed red blood cells (pRBCs), 129
PAD. See preoperative autologous donation
Pain Catastrophizing Scale (PCS), 655
pain management
 burn injuries, 624
 fasciotomy, 589
 opioid-free anesthesia, 650–653
 patient-controlled analgesia (PCA), 648–649
 pectus excavatum (PE), 489–490
 regional anesthesia, 643–645
 total pancreatectomy and islet autotransplantation (TPIAT), 633–634
palliative care
 advance directives, 665–666
 limited resuscitation, 666
 perioperative management, 666
palonosetron, 66
pancreatitis, 632
pancuronium, 60
PAP. See pulmonary alveolar proteinosis
paramagnetic oxygen analyzers, 83, 84
paraphimosis, 547

parathyroid, 433
parathyroid dysfunction, 174
parathyroidectomy, 160
 anesthetic technique, 434–436
 indications/contraindications, 432, 433
 postoperative care, 436
 preoperative evaluation, 433–434
 preoperative pharmacology, 434
Parkland formula, 623
parotidectomy
 anesthetic management, 359
 anesthetic technique, 359
 complications and emergencies, 359
 indications/contraindications, 358–359
 postoperative care, 360
 preoperative evaluation, 359
 preoperative pharmacology, 359
 sialendoscopy, 359
 surgical approaches, 358
parotid glands, 358
partial anomalous pulmonary venous return (PAPVR), 184
partition coefficient, 49
passive humidification, 83
patent ductus arteriosus (PDA), 20, 184
 ECHO image, 185
 ligation and division, 449–450
 pathophysiology and clinical manifestations, 185
 postsurgical repair assessment, 185
patent foramen ovale (PFO), 20
patient blood management (PBM) protocols, 128
patient-controlled analgesia (PCA)
 advantages, 649
 authorized agent-controlled analgesia (AACA), 649
 disadvantages, 649
 indications, 648–649
PBS. See prune belly syndrome
PE. See pectus excavatum (PE)
peak inspiratory pressure (PIP), 119–120
pectus excavatum (PE)
 anesthetic technique, 487–489
 complications/emergencies, 489
 Haller index (HI), 486
 indications/contraindications, 486
 postoperative care, 489–490
 preoperative evaluation, 487
 preoperative pharmacology, 487
pediatric and congenital cardiac catheterization laboratory (PCCCL), 452
 anesthesia technique, 455–457
 complications/emergencies, 456–457
 postoperative care, 457
 preoperative evaluation, 455
 preoperative pharmacology, 455
 radiation exposure, 454–455
 work environment challenges, 454

pediatric sedation handoff checklist, 141
PEEP. See positive end-expiratory pressure
penile anomalies, 225
pentobarbital, 51, 673
perfusion, 19–20
　postnatal ventilation, 20
　West's zones, 21
perfusion mismatch, ventilation, 20–21
perianal abscess, 209
periodontal conditions, 168–169
periodontitis, 169
peripheral airway resistance, 19
peripheral chemoreceptors, 17
peripheral nerve blockade (PNB)
　complications/emergencies, 647–648
　ultrasound-guided, 646
peripheral nervous system (PNS), 3
persistent pulmonary hypertension (PPHN), 20
phantom limb pain, 593, 594
　preoperative medications, 595
　treatment timeline, 594
pharmacodynamics, 42–43
pharmacokinetics
　absorption, 43–44
　distribution, 44–45
　elimination, 47–48
　metabolism, 45–47
　pediatric versus adult patients, 44
　principles, 48–49
pharmacologic considerations
　anesthesia adjuncts, 65, 66
　anticholinergic agents, 70
　antiemetic agents, 65–70
　growth and development, 41–42
　IV anesthetic agents, 51–58
　limitations, 41
　local anesthetics, 72, 73
　neuromuscular blocking agents, 58–61
　opioids, 61–65
　pharmacodynamics, 42–43
　pharmacokinetics, 43–49
　pharmacologic agents, 49–51
　potency, 43
　vasoactive and inotropic agents, 70–72
pharyngoplasty, 414–415
pharyngotonsillitis, 159
phenylephrine, 72
pheochromocytoma, 178
physiologic monitoring
　electrocardiogram, 86–87
　noninvasive blood pressure (NIBP) measurement, 85, 87
　precordial stethoscope, 85
　pulse oximetry, 86
　temperature monitoring, 87
　urine output, 87
Pierre–Robin sequence (PRS), 12, 399–400
　anesthetic management, 275
　anesthetic technique, 276–277
　clinical manifestation, 275
　pathophysiology, 275

postoperative care, 277
preoperative evaluation, 275–276
pilonidal cyst, 518–519
pilonidal sinus surgery
　anesthetic technique, 518
　complications, 518
　indications/contraindications, 518
　postoperative care, 519
　preoperative evaluation, 518
　preoperative pharmacology, 518
PIP. See peak inspiratory pressure
pituitary disorders, 175–177
pituitary gigantism, 176
plagiocephaly, 323
Plasma-Lyte, 127
plasmapheresis, 213
platelets, 129
pneumatic system, 82
pneumothorax, 621, 425
polarographic electrodes, 83
polycystic ovary syndrome (PCOS), 178
PONV. See postoperative nausea and vomiting
portal vein thrombosis (PVT), 628–629
portopulmonary hypertension (POPH), 626
positive end-expiratory pressure (PEEP), 118
postanesthetic care
　complications, 141–144
　discharge, 144–145
　patient transport, 140
　safe handoff, 140
postbreast surgery pain syndrome (PBSPS), 419
postductal coarctation, 447
postdural puncture headache (PDPH), 540
posterior fossa tumor, 302
posterior glottic stenosis (PGS), 13
posterior sagittal anorectoplasty (PSARP)
　cardiac involvement, 512–513
　complications/emergencies, 514–515
　indications/contraindications, 512
　limb anomalies, 513
　postoperative care, 515
　preoperative evaluation, 512
　preoperative pharmacology, 513–514
　renal dysfunction, 513
　revision, 516–517
　VACTERL association, 512
posterior urethral valves (PUV), 222–223
postnatal lung development, 16
postoperative bleeding, 143–144
postoperative hematoma, thyroidectomy and parathyroidectomy, 436
postoperative nausea and vomiting (PONV), 58, 142–143, 464
　adenotonsillectomy, 345
　breast reduction, 418

microtia repair, 425
orchidopexy, 557
sleeve gastrectomy, 499–500
splenectomy, 534
posttonsillectomy bleeding (PTB), 98, 345–346
postural newborn reflexes, 5
postural orthostatic tachycardia syndrome (POTS), 254
Prader–Willi syndrome
　anesthetic management, 278–279
　anesthetic techniques, 279
　clinical manifestation, 278
　facial features, 278
　pathophysiology, 278
　postoperative care, 279
　preoperative evaluation, 278–279
　preoperative pharmacotherapy, 279
precordial stethoscope, 85
preductal coarctation, 446
preload, stroke volume, 8
premedication and optimization
　melatonin, 79
　nonopioid analgesics, 79
　preoperative anesthesia clinics, 78–79
　sedatives, 79
prenatal lung development, 15–16
preoperative autologous donation (PAD), 131
preoperative evaluation
　medical history, 76
　preoperative fasting, 77–78
　respiratory infections, 76–77
preoperative fasting
　ASA guidelines, 77–78
　carbohydrate drinks, 78
　clear fluids, 78
　gastric ultrasound, 78
　noncompliance, 77
　patient compliance and clear communication, 78
pressure-controlled ventilation, 122
pressure equalization tube (PET), 333–334
pressure support ventilation (PSV), 122
preterm birth, 148
preterm infant
　airway considerations, 149
　cardiovascular considerations, 149
　fluid/metabolic status, 149
　neurodevelopmental consideration, 148
　postoperative care, 149–150
　preoperative evaluation and care, 149
　pulmonary considerations, 148–149
　thermoregulation, 149
primary hyperparathyroidism, 174
primitive newborn reflexes, 5
propofol, 58, 97, 463, 671
propofol-related infusion syndrome (PRIS), 58
protein binding, pharmacologic agents, 45

protein synthesis, liver, 26
PRS. See Pierre–Robin sequence
prune belly syndrome (PBS), 223
　anesthetic management, 280–281
　anesthetic techniques, 281
　clinical manifestation, 280
　incidence, 280
　pathophysiology, 280
　postoperative care, 281
　preoperative pharmacotherapy, 281
PSARP. See posterior sagittal anorectoplasty
pseudosyndactyly, 259
PSV. See pressure support ventilation
ptosis repair, 386–387
pulmonary alveolar proteinosis (PAP)
　anesthetic management, 283–285
　anesthetic techniques, 284–285
　congenital, 282
　diagnosis, 282
　pathophysiology, 282
　postoperative care, 285
　preoperative evaluation, 283–284
　preoperative pharmacotherapy, 284
　prevalence, 282
　primary, 282
　radiography and histology, 283
　secondary, 282
　therapeutic strategies, 282–283
pulmonary artery catheter waveform, 91
pulmonary artery monitoring, 134
pulmonary circulation, 19–20
pulmonary considerations, preterm infant, 148–149
pulmonary contusion, 620–621
pulmonary hypertension (PH)
　anesthetic considerations, 199–200
　noncardiac surgery, 470
　pathophysiology and clinical manifestations, 198–199
　WHO classification, 199
pulmonary hypoplasia, 16
pulmonary resistance, 19
pulse oximetry, 86
pyeloplasty
　anesthetic technique, 563
　dismembered, 562
　indications/contraindications, 562–563
　postoperative care, 563
　preoperative evaluation, 562
　preoperative pharmacology, 563
pyloric stenosis, 98
pyloromyotomy, 612

quadratus lumborum (QL) block, 563, 567
quality improvement and safety
　failure mode and effect analysis, 686
　hand-offs, 685
　lean methodology, 686

methodology, 685–686
near-miss events, 684
regulatory bodies, 684
root cause analysis, 685
sentinel event, 684–685
SMART aims, 686
radiant warming devices, 137
radiation oncology, anesthesia for, 670–671
radiofrequency catheter ablation (RFCA), 461
radiology
 imaging techniques, 668–671
 medication selection, 671–673
 nonradiological procedures, 671
rapid-sequence induction (RSI), 97–98, 302, 507
Ravitch procedure, 486
RB. See retinoblastoma
recessive dystrophic epidermolysis bullosa (RDEB), 256, 258
recombinant factor concentrates, perioperative blood loss minimization, 129
rectal temperature monitoring, 135
recurrent laryngeal nerve (RLN) damage, thyroidectomy and parathyroidectomy, 435, 436
Reentry tachycardia, 459
regional anesthesia
 anatomic considerations, 643
 and combined general anesthesia, 643–644
 indications/contraindications, 643
 local anesthetics, 644–645
 neuraxial analgesia, 645–646
 peripheral nerve blockade, 646–648
 postoperative care, 648
 preoperative evaluation, 644
regional blocks, bowel resection, 493
remifentanil infusions, 463
renal blood flow (RBF), 22
renal developmental anomalies, 223–224
renal function and metabolism, cardiopulmonary bypass, 444
renal system
 embryology and development, 22
 end-stage renal disease (ESRD), 24
 laparoscopic surgery, 510
 pathophysiology, 23
 physiology and homeostasis, 22–23
 transplantation, 24
residual limb pain, 593
respiratory infections, preoperative evaluation, 76–77
respiratory rate, 119, 120
respiratory system
 gas exchange, 20–21
 laparoscopic surgery, 509
 lung development, 15–16

lung volumes and capacities, 17
perfusion, 19–20
ventilation, 17–19
restrictive cardiomyopathy, 196
retina, 381
retinal detachment (RD), 163
 exudative, 382–383
 incidence, 381
 rhegmatogenous, 382
 tractional, 383
 trauma-related, 382
retinal surgery
 anesthetic management, 383–386
 considerations and concerns, 383
 indications/contraindications, 381–383
 postoperative care, 385–386
 preoperative evaluation, 383–384
retinoblastoma (RB), 163, 389–390
retinopathy of prematurity (ROP), 163, 382
rhabdomyolysis
 muscular dystrophy (MD), 274
 non-MH-induced, 601
rhegmatogenous retinal detachment (RRD), 382
rheumatic fever (RF), 198
rocuronium, 60
room temperature, 136–137
root cause analysis (RCA), 685
ropivacaine, 73, 644, 645
ryanodinopathies, 599

sacral spine, 551
sacrococcygeal teratomas (SCTs), 607
salivary gland, 171
salivary gland disease, 160
saturation kinetics, 49
scald burns, 431
scaphocephaly, 321
scavenging system, 82, 83
Scheuermann's kyphosis, 570
Schwartz equations, 47
sciatic nerve block, 580
scissors mouth-opening technique, 109
scoliosis, 570
 congenital, 227
 idiopathic, 227
 impaired lung function, 226
 neuromuscular, 227
 syndromic, 227
sedative-hypnotic agents, 58
sedatives, 79
selective dorsal rhizotomy (SDR), 320
sensorineural hearing loss (SNHL), 157–158
sepsis, 179
septal defects, 438, 467, 468
septic arthritis, 584
septorhinoplasty
 anesthetic technique, 362–363
 complications/emergencies, 363
 indications/contraindications, 362
 postoperative care, 363
 preoperative evaluation, 362

preoperative pharmacology, 362
sevoflurane, 50
SGA. See supraglottic airway
shivering thermogenesis, 31
shock assessment, trauma, 616
shoulder arthroscopy, 584–585
shoulder surgery
 anesthetic technique, 585–586
 indications/contraindications, 584
 physeal damage, 585
 postoperative care, 586
 preoperative evaluation, 585
 preoperative pharmacology, 585
sialendoscopy, 359
sickle cell disease (SCD), 215–216
sigmoidal maximum effect model, 43
single-breath inhalation induction, 96–97
single-incision laparoscopic surgery (SILS), 532–533
single-ventricle congenital heart disease, 192–193
single-ventricle palliation, cardiac surgery, 440–441
sinusitis, 158–159
sinusoidal obstructive syndrome (SOS), 219–220
skin temperature monitoring, 134
sleep-disordered breathing (SDB), 159
sleeve gastrectomy
 anesthetic technique, 499–500
 case study, 500–501
 complications/emergencies, 500
 indications/contraindications, 498
 postoperative care, 500
 preoperative evaluation, 498–499
 preoperative pharmacology, 499
slipped capital femoral epiphysis (SCFE), 227–228
 anesthetic technique, 591–592
 childhood obesity, 591
 classification, 590
 complications/emergencies, 592
 diagnosis, 590, 591
 endocrine abnormalities, 591
 incidence, 590
 indications/contraindications, 590–591
 postoperative care, 592
 preoperative evaluation, 591
 preoperative pharmacology, 591
 symptoms, 590
small bowel conditions, 206–207
SNHL. See sensorineural hearing loss
Society of Thoracic Surgeons-European Association for Cardio-Thoracic Surgery (STAT) score, 437
somatic nervous system, 3
somatosensory-evoked potentials (SSEP)
 scoliosis surgery, 574, 575

spina bifida, 152, 153, 569
spinal disorders, 226–227
spinal fusion
 anesthetic technique, 573–575
 complications/emergencies, 575
 idiopathic scoliosis, 576–577
 indications/contraindications, 570–572
 postoperative care, 575–576
 preoperative evaluation, 572–573
 preoperative pharmacology, 573
splenectomy
 anesthetic technique, 532–533
 complications/emergencies, 533
 emergency, 532
 indications/contraindications, 531–532
 overwhelming postsplenectomy infection (OPSI), 532
 partial, 532
 postoperative care, 534
 preoperative evaluation, 532
 preoperative pharmacology, 532
spontaneous ventilation, 120–121
spring-assisted cranioplasty, 324
Stagnara wake-up test, 574
STAI. See State-Trait Anxiety Inventory
State-Trait Anxiety Inventory (STAI), 654–655
stenosis, larynx, 13, 14
stereotactic grid placement
 anesthetic management, 308–310
 anesthetic technique, 308–309
 anticonvulsant medications, 307
 contraindications, 307
 head frame, 307
 indications, 307
 intracranial physiology, 307
 magnetic resonance imaging considerations, 308
 postoperative care, 310
 preoperative evaluation, 308
 preoperative pharmacology, 308
stereotactic radiosurgery, 669
strabismus, 163
strabismus surgery
 anesthetic management, 376
 anesthetic techniques, 377–378
 complications/emergencies, 377–378
 indications/contraindications, 376
 postoperative care, 378
 preoperative evaluation, 376
 preoperative pharmacology, 376–377
stress, cardiopulmonary bypass, 444
stretch receptors, 17
stroke volume
 afterload, 8–9
 contractility, 8
 preload, 8

subacute bacterial endocarditis prophylaxis, 80
subglottic stenosis (SGS), 14
    Cotton–Myer system, 13, 14
    current rates, 13
subglottis, 13
submandibular gland excision, 361–362
succinylcholine, 59
sugammadex, 60, 61
supracardiac total anomalous pulmonary venous return (TAPVR), 441
supraglottic airway (SGA), 105, 106
    flexible bronchoscopy, 114, 115
    obstruction, 232
supratentorial tumor symptoms, 153
supravalvular aortic stenosis (SVAS), 296
supraventricular tachycardia (SVT), 459–460
    anesthetic considerations, 200–201
    pathophysiology and clinical manifestations, 200
surface tension, 17–18
surfactant, 18
surgery-induced stress, 179
sympathetic and parasympathetic innervation, 4
synchronized intermittent mandatory ventilation (SIMV), 122
syndrome of inappropriate antidiuretic hormone secretion (SIADH), 176–177
syndromic scoliosis, 227

tachycardia
    differential diagnosis, 460
    mechanism, 459–461
tear system, 379
TEF repair. See tracheoesophageal fistula repair
temperature monitoring, 87
    core body temperature, 133
    hyperthermia, 136
    hypothermia, 136
    locations, 133–135
    normothermia, 136–138
    thermoregulation, 135–136
testicular torsion, 225
tethered cord, 152
tetralogy of fallot (TOF)
    cardiac surgery, 439
    clinical manifestations, 189
    postsurgical repair assessment, 190–191
    repair, 190, 445
therapeutic cardiac catheterization, 454
thermogenesis
    dietary, 32
    nonshivering, 31
    shivering, 31
thermoreceptors activation, 29
thermoregulation, 135–136
    afferent thermal sensing, 28–29
    burn injuries, 623
    central regulation, 29
    efferent response, 29

heat generation, 31–32
heat loss, 30–31
    inadequate, consequences, 32
    physiology, 28–29
    preterm infant, 149
    trauma, 618
thiopental, 51
third ventriculostomy
    anesthetic technique, 331
    complications, 331, 332
    considerations and concerns, 330
    postoperative care, 331–332
    preoperative evaluation, 331
    preoperative pharmacology, 331
thoracic neuroblastoma, 545
Thoracic paravertebral spinae plane block, 488
thoracic trauma
    cardiac injuries, 621–622
    pneumothorax, 621
    pulmonary contusion, 620–621
    tracheobronchial tree injuries, 621
throat conditions, 159
thymectomy, 537
thyroid, 433
thyroid disease
    hyperthyroidism, 173–174
    hypothyroidism, 173
thyroidectomy, 159–160
    anesthetic technique, 434–436
    indications/contraindications, 432
    postoperative care, 436
    preoperative evaluation, 433–434
    preoperative pharmacology, 434
thyroidectomy/goiter, 179
thyroid storm, 173–174
    thyroidectomy and parathyroidectomy, 435–436
tidal volume, 119, 120
tissue–blood partition coefficient, 49
tongue base reduction
    anesthetic management, 369–370
    anesthetic technique, 369–370
    complications and emergencies, 370
    indications/contraindications, 369
    postoperative care, 370
    preoperative examination, 369
    preoperative pharmacology, 369
tongue lip adhesion (TLA), 275
tongue, pathology, 171
tooth development and eruption
    dental caries, 168, 169
    odontogenesis, 166–168
    tooth impaction, 170
total anomalous pulmonary venous return (TAPVR), 441–442
total body radiation, 669
total knee arthroplasty (TKA), 580
total pancreatectomy and islet autotransplantation (TPIAT)

anesthetic concerns, 633–634
case preparation, 632–633
outcomes, 634–635
pancreatitis, 632
preoperative evaluation, 632
surgical approach, 632
TPIAT. See total pancreatectomy and islet autotransplantation
trachea, 13–15
trachea esophageal fistula (TEF), 204
tracheal resection
    anesthetic management, 355–357
    anesthetic technique, 356
    case study, 357
    complications/emergencies, 356
    indications/contraindications, 354–355
    postoperative care, 356–357
    preoperative evaluation, 355
    preoperative pharmacology, 356
tracheobronchial tree injuries, 621
tracheoesophageal displacement index (TEDI), 640
tracheoesophageal fistula (TEF) repair
    anesthetic technique, 481–482
    clinical presentation, 480
    complications, 482–483
    genetic syndromes, 481
    Gross classification, 480
    indications/contraindications, 480
    postoperative care, 483
    preoperative evaluation, 481
    preoperative pharmacology, 481
tracheoesophageal fistulas (TEF), 294
tracheomalacia, 15, 436
tracheostomy
    age-dependent trachea variations, 351
    airway management, 109
    anesthetic management, 351–352
    complications/emergencies, 353
    indication/contraindications, 351
    intraoperative management, 352–353
    postoperative care, 353
    preoperative evaluation, 351–352
tractional retinal detachment (RD), 383
transcutaneous monitoring of the partial pressure of carbon dioxide (TcCO$_2$), 89
transdermal scopolamine, 80
transesophageal echocardiography (TEE), 91, 93
    contraindications, 92
transitional circulation, 7–8
transplant-associated thrombotic microangiopathy (TA-TMA), 220
transplant surgery
    cardiac transplantation, 625–626

kidney transplantation, 629–631
liver transplantation, 626–629
transpulmonary gradient (TPG), 441
transversus abdominal plane (TAP) blocks, 563, 567
trauma
    abdominal and solid organ, 622
    anesthetic technique, 617–618
    blood transfusion, 616–617
    burn injuries, 622–624
    cognitive aids, 617
    definition, 616
    enucleation, 389
    fluid management, 616
    management, 616–617
    preoperative evaluation, 617
    shock assessment, 616
    thoracic trauma, 620–622
trauma-related retinal detachment (RD), 382
traumatic brain injury (TBI)
    assessment, 619–620
    Glasgow Coma Scale (GCS), 619–620
    treatment, 620
traumatic lumbar puncture (TLP), 540
Treacher Collins syndrome (TCS)
    anesthetic management, 287–288
    anesthetic technique, 288
    clinical features, 286
    clinical manifestation, 286–287
    pathophysiology, 286–287
    postoperative care, 288
    preoperative evaluation, 287
    preoperative pharmacotherapy, 287
Triggered automaticity, 459
truncus arteriosus, 192, 440
tuberous sclerosis complex (TSC)
    anesthetic management, 289–290
    anesthetic techniques, 290
    clinical manifestation, 289
    pathophysiology, 289
    postoperative care, 290
    preoperative evaluation, 289–290
    preoperative pharmacotherapy, 290
tubular secretion, 48
tumors, 152–153
Turner's syndrome
    anesthetic management, 291–293
    anesthetic techniques, 293
    clinical manifestations, 290
    pathophysiology, 290–291
    postoperative care, 293
    preoperative evaluation, 291–293
    preoperative pharmacotherapy, 293
turricephaly, 323
twin-twin transfusion syndrome (TTTS), 636
tympanoplasty
    anesthetic management, 337–338
    considerations and concerns, 337, 338
    contraindication, 337

indication, 337
intraoperative management, 337–338
postoperative care, 338
preoperative evaluation, 337

ulcerative colitis (UC), 207–208
ultrasound-guided vascular access
  cannulation, 676–679
  color Doppler, 676
  focal zone, 676
  gain adjustment, 675–676
  insertion technique, 678
  physics, 675
  probe selection, 675
  various types, 678–679
  vascular anatomy, 676
unanticipated difficult airway management, 116
undescended testicles, 555
UPJ obstruction. *See* ureteropelvic junction obstruction
upper respiratory infections (URIs), 76
ureteral reimplantation, 564–565
ureteropelvic junction (UPJ) obstruction
  CHARGE syndrome, 562
  enlarged renal pelvis/ hydronephrosis, 562
  pyeloplasty, 562–563
urinary stent, 553
urine output monitoring, 87
urolithiasis
  anesthetic technique, 561
  complications/emergencies, 561
  indications/contraindications, 560
  medical expulsion therapy, 560
  postoperative care, 561
  preoperative evaluation, 560–561
  preoperative pharmacology, 561
uterotonic medications, 642
uvula, pathology, 171

vagal nerve stimulator placement, 310–313
  anesthetic management, 311–313
  anesthetic techniques, 311–312
  indications/contraindications, 310–311
  postoperative care, 312
  preoperative evaluation, 311
valvular lesions, noncardiac surgery, 467, 469
vascular rings, 447
  cardiac surgery, 449
  noncardiac surgery, 469
  and slings, 187–188
vasoactive agents, 70–73, 464
VATER association
  anesthetic management, 295
  anesthetic techniques, 295
  clinical manifestation, 294–295
  pathophysiology, 294–295
  postoperative care, 295
  preoperative evaluation, 295
  preoperative pharmacotherapy, 295
VCUG. *See* voiding cystourethrogram
VCV. *See* volume-controlled ventilation
vecuronium, 60
velopharyngeal dysfunction (VPD), 414–415
velopharyngeal insufficiency (VPI), 414
venous air embolism, cranial vault reconstruction, 326
venous malformations (VMs)
  anesthetic technique, 412–413
  complications/emergencies, 413
  head and neck, 410
  indications/contraindications, 410
  laser treatment, 410–411
  postoperative care, 413
  preoperative evaluation, 411
  preoperative pharmacology, 411
  treatment, 410
venous thromboembolism, hemophilia, 214
ventilation

airway resistance, 19
compliance, 18–19
elasticity and recoil, 17–18
mechanics, 17–19
muscle involvement, 18
neonatal, 17
neurochemical control, 17
and perfusion mismatch, 20, 21
and perfusion ratio, 21
postnatal, 20
trauma, 618
ventilation management
  dead space, 120, 121
  end-tidal carbon dioxide, 120
  ICU ventilators, 122
  inspiratory-to-expiratory ratio, 119
  mechanical ventilation, 121–122
  modes, 120–122
  peak inspiratory pressure (PIP), 120
  positive end-expiratory pressure (PEEP), 120
  respiratory rate, 119, 120
  spontaneous ventilation, 120–121
  tidal volume, 119
ventricular septal defect (VSD)
  cardiac surgery, 438
  names and locations, 182
  noncardiac surgery, 467, 468
  pathophysiology and clinical manifestations, 181–183
  postsurgical repair assessment, 183
  types, 181
ventriculoperitoneal shunt placement
  anesthetic management, 304–305
  anesthetic techniques, 304–305
  contraindications, 303
  indications, 303
  postoperative care, 305–306
  preoperative evaluation, 304
  preoperative pharmacology, 304
vertical expandable prosthetic titanium ribs (VEPTR), 571
vesicoureteral reflux (VUR), 223

classification, 564
Cohen cross-trigonal technique, 565
cystoscopy, 564
extravesical approach, 565
indications/contraindications, 564
minimally invasive procedure, 564
Pfannenstiel skin incision, 564–565
primary, 564
secondary, 564
video laryngoscopy, 109–110, 116
visual acuity, 162
Visual Analog Scale (VAS), 654
vocal cords, 13
voiding cystourethrogram (VCUG), 564
volatile anesthetic agents, 463
volume capnogram, 85
volume-controlled ventilation (VCV), 122
volume of distribution, pharmacologic agent, 45
VUR. *See* vesicoureteral reflux

Wake Up Safe (WUS) program, 684
warming infant transport mattress, 138
water-soluble pharmacologic agents, 45
Williams syndrome
  anesthetic management, 296–297
  anesthetic technique, 297–298
  clinical manifestation, 296
  pathophysiology, 296
  postoperative care, 298
  preoperative evaluation, 296–297
  preoperative pharmacology, 297
withholding and withdrawing treatment, 681–682
Wolff-Parkinson-White (WPW) syndrome, 459, 461

X-linked retinoschisis (XLRS), 382

zero-order kinetics, 49